PHARMACOLOGY
AND DRUG THERAPY
IN NURSING

PHARMACOLOGY AND DRUG THERAPY IN NURSING

MORTON J. RODMAN, B.S., Ph.D.

Professor of Pharmacology and Chairman, Department
of Biological Sciences, College of Pharmacy, Rutgers,
The State University of New Jersey

and

DOROTHY W. SMITH, R.N., M.A., Ed.D.

Professor and Chairman, Department of Medical-Surgical
Nursing, Rutgers, The State University of New Jersey

J. B. LIPPINCOTT COMPANY
Philadelphia and Toronto

Distributed in Great Britain by
Blackwell Scientific Publications, Oxford and Edinburgh

Copyright © 1968 by J. B. Lippincott Company

Library of Congress Catalogue Card Number 68-17437

Printed in the United States of America

Sixth Printing

ISBN-0-397-54075-2

Preface

In planning this book, the authors—one a pharmacologist, the other a teacher of medical and surgical nursing—shared similar aims: to show how knowledge of the nature of our respective areas of specialization could contribute to more effective patient care. We were both well aware that pharmacology is, under the best of circumstances, not an easy subject to teach. Students are often asked to assimilate masses of detailed data concerning countless drugs. All too often, such factual knowledge is learned and then forgotten without the student ever having gained any real understanding of the basic principles of drug therapy. Thus, we knew that we wanted to stress not only factual data but fundamental principles. However, certain complications became evident.

Teaching pharmacology to nursing students in this way poses special problems. Some students come to the study of this subject well grounded in such essential prerequisites as physiology, biochemistry, and other basic biological-medical sciences; others study pharmacology before having had any real exposure to the sciences essential for an understanding of how drugs really act and what they are intended to accomplish.

A related difficulty is seen in the differing views among nursing educators concerning the way in which pharmacology should best be fitted into the curriculum. Some schools teach pharmacology as a separate course; in others information concerning drugs is conveyed as only one part of an integrated course dealing with all the varied aspects of the care and treatment of a particular type of patient.

Nursing education is currently faced with the dilemma of differentiating the levels of practice to be undertaken by nurses prepared in different types of programs. Yet, in most clinical settings, it is extremely difficult to separate the technical and professional functions which nurses perform in relation to drug therapy. Thus, this book has been written with the thought that it should be useful in any program preparing registered nurses, and that it should also serve as a useful reference sourcebook for the practicing graduate.

Any nurse who is responsible for administering medicines has responsibilities far exceeding mere administration. She must understand the actions of the drugs that she gives and know the correct doses required for producing desirable effects and avoiding adverse reactions. She should also be capable of making intelligent observations of the effects that administered drugs have upon her patients; and she should be aware that patients and their families must often be taught how to use drugs most effectively and safely. In short, she must employ professional nursing knowledge and make judgments that are based upon a professional person's insights. For if knowledge of the technical aspects of giving a drug is not accompanied by true understanding of the principles underlying the drug's administration, patient care tends to become routinized, and the patient fails to gain all the benefits that he might from drug therapy. Worse yet, he may be subjected to unnecessary hazards.

In practice, this view led to our decision to present information about drugs in a manner calculated to foster insights into fundamental pharmacological principles as they relate to the nurse's functions. Such insights cannot be acquired by mere memorization of lists of drug actions and uses, offered without any attempt to explain their true significance. The student should, instead, be shown the reasoning behind the ways in which drugs are used in treating patients ill with various disorders.

In order to offer adequate explanations of drug action in a manner most meaningful to the student, we have attempted to discuss the various classes of drugs in their most practical contexts: first, in relation to the basic sciences, particularly physiology; and secondly, in terms of the patient, his illness, and of the nurse's responsibility to see that he gains the greatest good from his medication. The latter context does not apply only to the final section which deals with the management of various common clinical conditions. This section differs from the others only in the sense that the disorders discussed therein require treatment with several different types of drugs. However, even in the other sections, which are organized in terms of single specific drug categories, the treatment of the patient rather than the mere response of a particular organ or system receives the main emphasis.

In order to emphasize the principles of drug action in relation to the nurse's responsibilities in patient care, it was necessary to make certain compromises. It quickly became clear that we could not include detailed specific data about a great many individual drugs in the body of the text. To do so would tend to obscure the truly significant points we wished to make concerning drug actions and their application to treatment. Therefore, we have attempted to point up basic principles and maintain the students' interest by taking up primarily the *prototype drugs* of each class. Other drugs of the same general category are discussed mainly in terms of their similarity to and differences from the prototypes. In almost every case, the detailed discussions of the actions of prototype drugs are preceded by a review of the physiological functions that they affect and of the pathophysiology of the conditions that they are used to treat.

Although we have avoided the inclusion of comprehensive discussions of large numbers of drugs within the various chapters, detailed factual data about numerous individual agents may be found in the *Drug Digest* section. These monographs contain the basic facts about such matters as actions, uses, side effects and dosage of many drugs which are mentioned briefly in the main text but not discussed in detail there, in order not to interfere with the free-flowing narrative of the chapters or obscure the more general points which we wished to make. We hope that these Drug Digests will also serve practicing nurses as a succinct source of practical information, when they wish to check the main facts about various drugs that they are called upon to administer.

Other material in this text is also intended to facilitate rapid reference and review. Most chapters, for example, contain *tabular summaries* of such aspects of each drug class as the actions, clinical indications, side effects, cautions and contraindications, and dosage and administration of the prototype drugs. In addition, the material considered of greatest significance to practicing nurses is also summarized separately in tabular form.

Each chapter also contains a list of *Review Questions* and many contain *Nursing Study Situations*. The review questions are keyed to the contents of the text in a sequential manner, so that the student may determine how well she is succeeding in finding and understanding the most important points as she reads each chapter. The study situations are intended to help the student check, not only her grasp of the factual material presented in each chapter, but also her ability to *apply* this knowledge about the drug in various situations commonly encountered in actual nursing practice.

Each chapter also offers a list of references for further reading. These have been selected primarily for the aptness with which they illustrate more fully some of the principal points made in the chapter. They are drawn largely from medical and nursing journals that are readily accessible and clinically oriented, with the intention of offering a guide to sources of more detailed information for those who require it.

Acknowledgments

We wish to acknowledge here the help of several individuals who played significant roles in the production of this book.

Mr. Barton Lippincott originally conceived this project in company with the senior author. Mr. David Miller, Nursing Education Editor, brought both authors together. His was the task of exhorting the reluctant writers to turn out manuscript at a pace a good deal less glacial than they would have held to if left to their own devices. His combination of friendly encouragement and humorously couched cries of outrage eventually overcame an almost equally stubborn combination of sloth and unrealistic perfectionism on the writers' part.

The book was finally brought to fruition by two other members of the Lippincott staff whose efforts went far beyond the routine of their jobs. Miss Naomi Coplin brought to bear on the manuscript a knowledge of pharmacologic writing and the taste and competence of a skillful medical editor. Mr. J. Stuart Freeman, Jr., Production Editor of the Medical Division, skillfully coordinated all the other complex tasks involved in converting a manuscript into a printed text.

Others, less immediately involved than the publisher's staff, also offered support to this project. Mrs. Barbara Finneson created the line drawings. Dr. Roy A. Bowers, Dean of the College of Pharmacy of Rutgers University, not only gave encouragement to what he viewed as a significant scholarly contribution, but also aided materially by allowing the senior author to set himself a more convenient schedule for research and writing than his teaching duties would ordinarily have permitted. Thanks are also due to L. Bernice Chapman, Dean of the College of Nursing of Rutgers.

Miss Doris Sholk, Secretarial Assistant at the College of Pharmacy, dealt efficiently with a voluminous correspondence and aided in many other ways that eliminated complications that could have consumed the authors' time and energy. Mrs. Gilda Waldron typed some 2,500 pages of manuscript cleanly, efficiently, and with a personal concern and involvement that helped keep matters moving forward.

Finally, Beatrice Rodman, R.N., a best friend and severest critic, contributed endless hours to reading and commenting on the manuscript. In addition, she gave sustenance to morale when, as often happened, it became shaky; and she took on burdens that were not rightfully hers in order to spare the senior author and allow him time for completion of his part of this collaborative task.

Contents

Section Three

DRUGS ACTING ON AUTONOMIC NEUROEFFECTORS

Section Four

DRUGS ACTING ON THE HEART AND
CIRCULATION

Contents

General Principles of Pharmacology

In this introductory section, we shall set the scene for the later study of the many different classes of drugs used in treating patients. Although the other sections of this text may be studied without prior exposure to the orientation offered in these first four chapters, the student who begins by gaining some understanding of the general principles of the subject is more likely to be able, later, to put detailed factual data concerning individual drugs in proper perspective. Therefore, it should prove profitable for the student to devote some time to the preliminary study of the topics taken up here.

We shall begin (Chapter 1) by indicating how drugs were discovered in the past and by describing the processes by which drug products are developed and tested today. Our purpose in doing so is not to present a detailed historical and technical discussion of these topics. Rather, we wish to introduce certain *terms* and *concepts* that the student should learn early in her study of this subject in order to facilitate later learning. In addition, advice is offered here in regard to methods of studying about drugs and of developing those attitudes that will help to widen and deepen one's knowledge of drug actions and their application to the treatment of patients.

After this initial, general orientation to the subject of drugs, we shall (Chapter 2) examine in some depth certain of the fundamentals of drug action that have been derived from modern scientific studies of the interactions between body chemicals and the molecules of drugs entering the living system. Although looking at drug and tissue interactions in this way may, at first, seem far removed from using drugs in actual clinical situations, the deeper understanding of drug action that can be developed by considering such basic concepts should serve the student well when such knowledge is later applied to actual patient care.

Because drugs are a two-edged sword, the nurse must always be aware of their potential toxicity as well as their utility. Thus, the several major classes of adverse drug effects are described (Chapter 3). The student will see, here, in broad outline, the scope of the hazards that may be encountered in practice when drugs are misused. The importance of administering drugs properly and the nurse's responsibilities in this regard are then taken up (Chapter 4), in order to indicate the kinds of precautions that must be habitually practiced if the patient is to gain maximum benefit from drug therapy with minimal danger.

· 1 ·

An Orientation to Drugs

DEFINITION AND SCOPE OF PHARMACOLOGY

You are about to embark upon the study of drugs, a subject of considerable importance in the present-day practice of nursing. In this chapter we shall discuss what the nurse ought to know about the drugs that she administers to patients and how she should go about acquiring pharmacological knowledge both as a student and as a practicing nurse. However, let us begin by defining our subject and indicating what aspects of it will be important to us.

Pharmacology is, in the broadest sense, the branch of knowledge that has to do with those chemicals that have biological effects. We, however, are concerned only with the biological and medical aspects of the subject. For our purposes, then, pharmacology is the study of the *actions of chemicals on living organisms.*

Actually, of course, nurses are concerned mainly with what chemicals can do, for better or worse, when they come in contact with the tissues of human beings. Thus, they are concerned primarily with *pharmacotherapeutics,* the branch of pharmacology that deals with drugs—chemicals that are used in medicine for the treatment, prevention and diagnosis of disease. This area is sometimes called *clinical pharmacology,* because it deals with the effects of the drugs that the doctor orders for treating *human patients.*

In addition, the nurse must study some aspects of still another offshoot of pharmacology. This is *toxicology, the study of poisons—chemical substances that are harmful to health or injurious to life.* Since overdoses of drugs often are toxic, we shall be concerned with learning the signs and symptoms of adverse drug actions and the measures to be taken to counteract the poisonous effects of drugs.

This book, then, deals mainly with the actions of drugs on human beings and with the application of such knowledge to problems that arise in treating patients. However, we think that the nurse should also

know something about the experimental science upon which drug treatment is based. This science is called *pharmacodynamics* and deals with the interactions between the chemical components of living systems and the foreign chemicals, including drugs, that enter living organisms.

Pharmacologists (scientists who specialize in the study of pharmacodynamics) employ all kinds of biochemical, physiological and other techniques. Although the technical details of their studies are beyond the scope of this book, we think it important that the professional nurse know something about the ways in which drugs are discovered and developed.

HISTORICAL DEVELOPMENT OF PHARMACOLOGY

Although experimental pharmacodynamics is one of the youngest of the medical sciences, pharmacotherapeutics is one of the most ancient branches of man's knowledge. We know this not only from the discovery of Sumerian clay tablets dating back beyond 2000 B.C., and Egyptian papyri from about 1500 B.C., but also from the activities of present-day primitive peoples living in Stone Age type cultures—Australian aborigines, for example, and New Guinea natives.

Men everywhere came upon potent natural chemicals as they foraged for food among the plants of the field. Gradually, they learned which fruits, roots, berries and barks were safe to eat and which had discomforting effects on body function. Through this slow system of trial and error and by observing which growing things animals ate and which they avoided, a great deal of knowledge was acquired and passed along as part of the peoples' folklore.

Primitive Pharmacology. The type of natural product first used internally for medical purposes was probably a cathartic, since laxative chemicals are very frequently found in nature in the form of purgative plants and mineral salts. Such substances were very likely used for religious purposes, because it seemed reasonable that something which cleansed the bowel might also drive out the evil spirits that were thought to be defiling a sick person.

Thus, drugs were first used for their mystical or magic powers rather than for their physiological effects; and, indeed, it is true today that a drug's effects are not limited to what it does to body function directly. People still respond not only physiologically but psychologically to the taking of a drug—a point that the nurse can sometimes use to advantage in administering medicines. The nature of this psychological response is not fully understood, but it is related to the patient's hopes and expectations and to his anxieties and fears concerning the effects of the drug he is getting.

Ancient, Medieval and Modern Medicines. Through experience, and by trial and error—the method we call *empiricism*—a number of natural substances of plant, animal and mineral origin that seemed to have been proved useful for relief of symptoms came into use and were handed down, first, through oral tradition and, later, in the form of pharmacopeias, or books of drug preparations.

Many of the medicines discovered empirically by the ancient Egyptians, Hebrews and Greeks are still in use today, as are substances employed as medicines by the Arabs of the Middle Ages and by the Indians whom the white men met in their voyages of exploration which ushered in the Modern Era.

The famous Ebers Papyrus, an Egyptian compilation of drug lore dating from around 1500 B.C., refers to the use of opium, castor oil and squill among many other medicines. The ancient Greek physician Dioscorides makes mention of colchicum in his encyclopedic work on materia medica. The herbals of the medieval monasteries included belladonna; and the Swiss physician, Paracelsus, introduced mercury for treating syphilis in the 16th century. The North American Indians made use of the cathartic properties of Cascara bark; and cinchona, the quinine-containing Fever Bark, was a standard remedy for malaria and other ills among the Indians of South America.

Although a few of the remedies handed down in this way were effective, the vast majority of them were actually quite worthless. Most illnesses, of course, clear up spontaneously as a result of the body's own ability to heal itself; yet, as often happens even today during poorly controlled clinical trials, medicines that happened to be administered simultaneously were credited with the cure. Uncritical acceptance of such seeming successes led to the retention of countless worthless substances in the medicinal compendia. Even though a few enlightened skeptics tried to rid the pharmacopeias of the relics and rubbish which accumulated over the centuries, Dr. Oliver Wendell Holmes could still say, as late as 1860, that "if the whole materia medica . . . were sunk to the bottom of the sea, it would be all the better for mankind and all the worse for the fishes."

Pharmacology Becomes a Science. This sort of therapeutic nihilism—the view that all drug treatment was worthless—was never shared by the patients, whose need for help bred a simple faith in the efficacy of medicines. In addition, some doctors trained in the basic medical sciences which began to develop during the 19th century came to feel that *rational* therapy was, indeed, possible if it could be based upon knowledge of normal physiology and the pathological processes underlying the disease to be treated.

At about this time, chemical science began to make the first of its remarkable advances. Early in the 19th century, chemists became skilled in the extraction and isolation of the active pure principles from crude drugs of vegetable and animal origin. The isolation, in about 1805, of morphine, the active alkaloid of opium, by a young German pharmacist, Friedrich Sertürner, was followed in the next few years by the extraction of strychnine, quinine, emetine and other potent plant principles in pure form.

The availability of these potent biologically active chemicals with constant physical properties that could be relied on stimulated the development of studies using the methods of experimental physiology. As a result, the first pharmacodynamic studies conceived and carried out in the *quantitative* manner characteristic of modern medical science were reported at this time. Thus, the French physiologist and pioneer pharmacologist François Magendie, in his work with strychnine, was able to determine exactly how much drug was needed to cause a particular effect in most of his experimental animals. Today, the first thing the pharmacologist tries to do in studying a biologically active chemical is to establish its *dose-response relationships*—that is, exactly how much of the pure drug it takes to bring about its various effects.

Further advances in pharmacology were related to the rise of organic synthetic chemistry. One of the first drugs to be produced synthetically was the anesthetic ether. Later, in the 19th century, the search for quinine substitutes led to the synthesis of the salicylates; and a chemist trying to find a safer form of these drugs discovered that he could improve the original molecule by treating it with acetic acid to get aspirin.

This procedure—preparing whole families of drugs related in chemical structure to a natural or synthetic chemical known to possess biological activity—opened up a new field of pharmacological study called *biochemorphology,* the study of the relationships between chemical structure and biological activity. Such *SAR (structure-activity relationships)* studies have resulted in the development of many classes of modern drugs, as we shall see in the following section.

Besides physiology and organic chemistry, other areas of biology and chemistry—notably biochemistry—are today making important technical contributions to the pharmacodynamic study of drugs. For example, one branch of biochemical pharmacology is concerned with attempts to trace the pathways that drugs take after they enter the body. Through the use of isotopically labeled drugs and other techniques such as paper chromatography, pharmacologists can now learn the final fate of a drug molecule by following it from the time it is absorbed until its biochemically altered molecular fragments leave the body.

Most recently, pharmacologists have employed the methods of enzyme chemistry and molecular biology to learn *where* a drug is acting and exactly *how* its molecules interact with the macromolecules of living cells. The study of the exact mechanisms by which drugs act to affect the functioning of body cells and systems is still in its infancy. However, it is hoped that this still largely theoretical area of study will lead some day to the development of drugs that will selectively kill viruses and cancer cells without harming normal human cells at all; and intimate knowledge of the cellular actions of drugs is useful even now for increasing our understanding of fundamental life processes.

THE DEVELOPMENT AND EVALUATION OF DRUGS

In the preceding section, we have seen in a general way how pharmacologists work to establish the pharmacodynamic properties of drugs. Once a substance has been shown to be biologically active, the pharmacologists perform studies mainly of four kinds:

1. To determine the *dose-response relationships* of the drug—that is, *how much* of the agent it takes to produce various effects;

2. To investigate its *structure-activity relationships* (SAR)—that is, the extent to which the drug's actions resemble and differ from those of compounds of closely related chemical structure;

3. To determine the drug's *metabolic fate* in the body—that is, how the body handles the foreign chemical from the time it enters the body and is absorbed into the system, until it, or the metabolites into which it has been transformed, are excreted;

4. To investigate the drug's *site* and *mechanism of action*—that is, just *where* in the body the drug acts to exert its various effects and just *how* it affects the metabolism of the reactive cells through the interaction of its molecules with those of the responsive tissues.

In this section, we shall discuss in somewhat more detail certain aspects of studies of the first two types listed above, with emphasis upon the terms and concepts that are most pertinent to the needs of nurses.

The studies of the third and fourth types will be discussed in Chapter 2—again in terms of what nurses need to know about drug action.

Few of us realize how many years of scientific study are required before a newly discovered chemical may be marketed for medical use. The processes by which new drugs are discovered, developed and tested for efficacy and toxicity are long and difficult.

We shall say something next about these procedures, because, by becoming aware of what is necessary to determine a drug's safety and true value, the nurse will begin to appreciate the need for all the precautions that are required in administering drugs to patients.

Sources of New Drugs. As we have already seen, drugs were once found by a random search for active substances among the plants, minerals and animals of the countryside. Today, scientists are still searching for new drugs in plant and animal tissues and in the soil. The main difference from the earlier approach lies in their use of systematic methods for uncovering specific kinds of actions caused by chemicals coming in contact with living tissues.

The biological methods called *screening tests* are relatively simple, inexpensive procedures for quickly determining whether or not substances of natural or synthetic origin have any activity of the particular kind that is being sought. Such screening procedures are sometimes applied to thousands of chemicals in programs designed to find drugs for various diseases. During World War II, for example, when the Japanese cut off the sources of quinine, scientists set up a "crash" program to find substitutes for quinine: they screened thousands of new and old chemicals and discovered a few valuable new antimalarial drugs. Later, the thousands of soil samples from all over the world that were screened for antibiotic activity produced a handful of useful antimicrobial agents including chloramphenicol, chlortetracycline and streptomycin. Today, vast numbers of chemicals are being screened for antineoplastic activity.

Once the presence of a particular action has been recognized in a crude extract, the relative amount of such activity can be determined in a roughly quantitative way by procedures called *biological assays* because they utilize animals or microorganisms rather than chemical or physical tests. As increasingly pure and potent plant or animal tissue extracts are obtained, their activity is compared with that of a preparation of known strength. This so-called reference standard is used as a measure of the amount of activity present only until the hormone, antibiotic, vitamin or plant principle becomes available in pure form and can be standardized by chemical assay.

Such screening and bioassay techniques, which were the basis for the early discovery of some of the potent drugs of natural origin, are being again applied to crude drugs used by the natives of various lands. Among the alkaloids extracted from anciently employed plants and made available in pure form in relatively recent years are: reserpine, the tranquilizing and blood-pressure-reducing drug obtained from *Rauwolfia serpentina*, a plant used in India for thousands of years; vinblastine, an antileukemic chemical extracted from a species of the decorative, flowering periwinkle plant; d-tubocurarine, the pure active principle of one of the crude curare extracts ("tube curare") that South American Indians have used as arrow poisons since prehistoric times.

The same methods have been used as a guide to the extraction and purification of vitamins from foods and hormones from animal glands. However, these substances are sometimes present in quantities so minute that scientists must seek other sources in order to bring down the cost. This was the case with *cortisone*, an adrenal cortex hormone which is present in amounts so small that it was impossible to extract enough to determine what uses it might have in human patients. Therefore, once its chemical structure was worked out, efforts were made to synthesize this steroid hormone. Finally, by starting with simpler steroids and laboriously building the complicated cortisone molecule from them, enough was prepared to permit clinical testing on patients with severe arthritis.

Structure-Activity Relationship Studies. The discovery of the remarkable antiarthritic power of cortisone and recognition of its useful anti-inflammatory activity in many other illnesses set off a search for even better corticosteroid compounds. The procedures employed in the discovery of the newer synthetic corticosteriods serve as an example of another experimental approach to the development of new drugs. This involves attempts to modify the chemical structure of a compound of known activity in ways that produce a closely related chemical with improved properties.

It may seem strange that chemists should be able to make chemicals that never existed before and yet are capable of acting more powerfully than hormones and other body chemicals produced by millions of years of evolution. Yet, this proved to be true with various of the synthetic corticosteroids, such as prednisolone, triamcinolone and betamethasone. These substances are as effective as the natural adrenal cortex hormones, cortisone and hydrocortisone, even when administered in such smaller doses. The synthetically tailored molecules are also free of certain undesirable actions of the natural hormone molecules.

Many other classes of drugs have come into being as a result of attempts to produce new compounds that would be better in some respect than a *prototype*—a chemical of a particular chemical configuration that produces a therapeutically desirable effect.

The very many "chemical cousins" built by making slight changes in the molecular structure of the prototype are called its *congeners* or *analogues*. Among the classes of drugs derived in this way were the local anesthetics, the antihistaminics, the anticholinergics, and, more recently, the phenothiazine-type tranquilizers and the benzothiazide-type diuretics.

Starting with a "lead" compound of known activity, the organic chemist often can produce dozens or even hundreds of derivatives by tinkering with the structure of the basic molecule in various ways. These are then screened for activity by pharmacologists in the hope that some relatively small change in chemical structure has resulted in the synthesis of a new compound that is an improvement over those that were previously available.

Sometimes, a small change in structure—the addition of a chlorine atom at a particular point in the molecule, for example—may give the new congener significant advantages over the parent compound. For example, the new drug may be effective when taken by mouth, whereas the prototype had to be given by painful injections (the synthetic progestins have this advantage over the natural female hormone, progesterone).

Sometimes, a new analogue may bring about the clinically desired effect when administered in much smaller doses than the prototype drug—perhaps because the new molecule fits more specifically into sites in the reactive cells. Altering the architecture of a prototype molecule to obtain compounds of increased potency is not, in itself, necessarily desirable, and the fact that the new drug can be administered in a smaller dose does not in itself make it superior to the parent compound. Thus, it is doubtful that the prototype benzothiazide diuretic *chlorothiazide* is less useful than various newer congener compounds, even though its milligram dosage may be about a hundred times as large as that of the more potent "improved" compounds produced by the molecule-manipulating chemists. This is because the *ratios* between the amounts of all these drugs required to produce *the desired effect* (i.e., removal of excess sodium from the body by way of the kidneys) and the amounts that cause an *undesired effect* (i.e., loss of excessive quantities of potassium) are essentially similar in all these chemically related substances.

Sometimes, however, a slight change made in the molecule of a prototype drug does more than merely lower the dose needed to produce the desired action. It may, for example, lead to a reduction in some undesired or toxic effect. This occurs when the tailoring of the molecule allows it somehow to seek out the target cells for therapeutic activity while avoiding other tissues. Such *selectivity* or *specificity* of action is one of the properties most sought for in modifying the molecular structure of natural and synthetic prototype drugs. Yet, there are few clear-cut rules for rationally predicting which modifications will produce new compounds of greater selectivity. So the search for better drugs by these methods is still mainly a matter of trial and error.

Preclinical Pharmacological Evaluation. Only a tiny minority of chemicals that display biological activity in a screening program are ever marketed as drugs. According to one recent survey, less than 2,000 of over 100,000 compounds screened by the pharmaceutical industry in one year were cleared for trial in human patients. Less than fifty of these chemicals eventually became medicines. Most of the active compounds that failed to become drugs were discarded because the doses required to produce a therapeutically desirable effect were too close to those that produced toxicity in preliminary laboratory tests in animals.

Once screening has revealed that a chemical is capable of producing a particular effect, it is often subjected to a battery of other tests in animals to determine its entire *spectrum* of activity. *No drug has only a single action;* it is essential to learn, at an early stage, *all* of a drug's varied actions and how much of the drug is required to produce each of its different effects. For example, a drug discovered in a search for antihistaminic activity may also have anticholinergic-antispasmodic effects on smooth muscle; it may possess a local anesthetic action that blocks nerve impulse conduction in peripheral nerves; and, often, it may cause drowsiness by depressing the central nervous system.

A drug that produces its desirable primary action only at dose levels very close to those that cause various secondary effects (side-effects) of a kind likely to be uncomfortable probably would be judged not likely to prove clinically useful. Thus, a drug may show ability to protect laboratory animals from the ill effects of inhaled histamine; but if it did so only at dose levels that made the animals drowsy, it would probably be discarded, since it would be less useful than some of the already available antihistaminic drugs that are relatively free of this adverse side effect.

On the other hand, if the new drug's *pharmacological profile* appears interesting and its *dose-response relationships* seem favorable in comparison to certain standard drugs already in clinical use, it may be put through several series of *toxicity tests*. These tests, which are designed to predict whether the drug can be safely administered to human subjects, are carried out in groups of small animals such as mice, rats and rabbits.

Groups of animals are used in order to reduce the chance of error resulting from differences in the way individual animals respond to drugs. This is necessary because no two animals (or people) react to

drugs in the same way. Even when the animals are litter-mates of the same sex and weight, they may differ from one another physiologically and biochemically in ways which are not readily apparent. Such biochemical or physiological individuality may profoundly influence the way in which the bodies of related animals handle a drug or the ways in which their tissues respond to the same dose of the drug. Thus, drugs are tested in *groups* of animals, in order to minimize mistakes in evaluation of a drug that stem from *individual variations* among animals of the same species.

Acute Toxicity Tests. Several species of animals receive a range of doses of the test drug and are observed for pharmacological effects and symptoms of toxicity. The data obtained by the laboratory pharmacologist in such tests serve as a guide to the clinical pharmacologist who wants to know what the drug is likely to do in human patients. The ratio between the dose of a drug that produces a desirable effect and that which causes toxic effects gives the doctor an idea of the drug's *safety margin.*

The test drug's *relative safety* in comparison to already available standard drugs—that is, its *therapeutic index*—is a factor used in considering whether it should be discarded or studied further. Most chemicals that are found to have a particular effect in pharmacodynamic screening tests fail to pass the acute toxicity studies. That is, the drug produces potentially desirable effects only when given in doses that are too close to those that cause acute toxic reactions, or the test chemical proves less effective or more toxic than other drugs of the same class that are already marketed.

Chronic Toxicity. If a drug seems to have a relatively wide safety margin, long-term studies are initiated, in which several species of animals receive large daily doses. The animals are closely observed for long periods and are tested frequently to determine the state of vital organ systems, including the liver, kidneys, blood and bone marrow. Adverse laboratory reports in such chronic toxicity studies usually keep a drug from going on to further trials in humans unless it seems potentially useful for treating a previously incurable disease.

Information is also obtained by gross and microscopic pathological studies of the tissues of dead animals. The drug's effects on the fertility of female animals and on the fetuses of pregnant females is also carefully observed. At the same time, studies of the drug's metabolism are conducted to determine how rapidly and completely it is absorbed by various routes of administration, and how it is distributed in the body and finally broken down and excreted. (Such studies furnish information concerning how frequently the drug should be administered and by which routes it should be given to get the most rapid or long-lasting effects).

If the results of all these preclinical trials indicate that the compound is reasonably safe, potentially useful in the treatment of one or more clinical conditions, and possibly superior to presently available drugs, it may be cleared for clinical trial in human beings. The doctors who are to act as clinical investigators are then supplied with a brochure containing detailed data of all aspects of the preclinical studies, as a guide for planning their clinical trials.

Clinical Evaluation of Drugs. Drugs are tested in humans only after the preclinical toxicity tests in animals have shown them to be reasonably safe. Yet, the occurrence of unforeseen toxicity in man always exists, as was demonstrated by the thalidomide disaster of 1962. Hundreds of mothers who took this seemingly harmless sedative drug gave birth to dreadfully deformed babies. This tragedy, which occurred largely outside of the United States, served to spur passage of new legislation regulating investigational drugs—the Kefauver-Harris amendments to the Federal Food, Drug and Cosmetic Act, which became effective in 1963.

Under these regulations, drugs are evaluated in humans under very carefully controlled conditions. The legal details need not concern us here; however, nurses should be aware of the basic philosophic principles underlying the evaluation of so-called investigational drugs in humans. Therefore, we shall review some of the terms, concepts and premises employed in such clinical research.

Evaluations of the effects of drugs on humans are generally conducted in three stages, which differ mainly in the number of patients and doctors involved and in the kinds of data collected. The purposes of all three phases of clinical investigation are essentially the same: first, to prove that the drug is reasonably *safe* for most patients under conditions of clinical use; and second, to demonstrate that the drug is in fact *useful* in one way or another to treat patients suffering from an actual illness. The Food and Drug Administration now demands proof of *efficacy* as well as safety before a new drug may be marketed.

The *first phase,* or *pilot study,* which is conducted in a very limited number of people, usually by a single very well qualified clinical investigator, is intended to determine whether the drug is active and safe in humans. These tests are designed to eliminate errors that may have gone undetected in the tests carried out in animals.

Species variation in response to drugs is a common occurrence. It is often the result of differences in the way animals of other species may metabolize a drug. Thus, a drug that may have caused no ill-effects in animals of a particular species may still prove toxic to humans, because the livers of the animals contained enzymes (lacking in human liver) that were capable of rapidly destroying the drug before it reached toxic levels in the tissues.

In addition, species differences may have obscured the presence of a *desirable* action. This is due, in part, to the difficulty of duplicating human disease states in laboratory animals. It is, for example, especially difficult to tell from animal studies how a drug is likely to affect the mental state of human beings. Thus, the phenothiazine-type tranquilizers were not shown to affect psychotic symptoms favorably until they were actually tried in mental patients rather than experimental animals.

Safety in Human Studies. Most investigational drugs are first tried out in healthy human volunteers in order to select a safe starting dose. In other situations, the doctor begins by giving the drug to sick patients in a dose much smaller than had caused toxic effects in animals. The dose is raised gradually in first one subject and then others, until either a toxic effect is detected or a therapeutic response is seen.

In almost all such cases, the patient *knows* that he is participating in an experiment and has given his *consent* to the procedure. The clinical investigator usually gives the subject a full explanation of the purpose of the experiment and makes it clear to him that there is an element of uncertainty involved concerning the drug's potential usefulness and toxicity—unless in his professional judgment, the patient's best interests are not served by informing him or his family of such matters. This ethical and moral obligation has recently been codified in guidelines for clinical investigation set by the Food and Drug Administration. However, controversy continues in regard to just how fully the experimenter must inform the patient about what drug effects may be expected.

The second phase of the clinical drug study is an expanded version of the first cautious tests. It is conducted by several doctors who are specialists both in drug investigations and in the illness that the drug is designed to treat. These physicians watch their patients for signs of both improvement and possible toxicity. They are especially alert for signs of toxicity of the same type seen in animals during the preclinical trials, but they also sometimes spot unusual reactions that require halting of the test.

Even before they begin administering the drug, these doctors have a whole battery of laboratory tests performed on the patients. Most important are tests of *liver* and *kidney* function and the status of the *blood forming organs.* Such studies are repeated at regular intervals over the months of second stage testing. If abnormalities appear, the clinical investigators have to decide whether the drug's value to the patient is worth the risk of continuing the drug treatment.

Drugs that cause reactions involving the bone marrow and skin or affecting hepatic or renal function often have to be withdrawn. There are, however, some circumstances in which drugs may continue to be employed clinically despite the occasional development of such reactions in some patients during long-term therapy. For example, few of the drugs introduced in recent years for preventing epileptic seizures are free of potentially dangerous long-term effects on vital organ systems. Yet clinical investigators have recommended their acceptance and the F.D.A. has cleared them for marketing (and only rarely called for their withdrawal) because they feel that the risk of therapy with these drugs in such chronic neurological diseases is worth taking, since these drugs often help people who otherwise might become invalids, or even have to be institutionalized, to lead normal useful lives.

Similarly, in fatal or life-threatening diseases, the investigators often decide that the benefits to be gained by continued administration of a potentially dangerous drug outweigh its hazards. Most of the compounds used in cancer chemotherapy, for instance, have very narrow safety margins. Yet they are cleared for use in leukemia and other neoplastic diseases despite clinical tests that reveal the risk of bone marrow damage and hematopoietic and digestive toxicity.

On the other hand, drugs that are intended for use in relatively minor ailments are withdrawn if this phase of clinical testing turns up evidence of toxicity. This is especially true when safe and effective drugs of the same class are already available. Thus, if an analgesic-antipyretic being tested showed even the smallest incidence of blood dyscrasias, it would very likely be promptly discarded, because the risk of causing dangerous depression of bone marrow function in even one patient would not be warranted by the drug's ability to relieve a headache or reduce a fever. This is especially true when a comparatively safe drug such as aspirin is available for the same purposes. (That is why in this country aminopyrine is prescribed infrequently.)

By the time that the *third stage* of clinical testing is reached definite dosage schedules have been determined and the doctors have acquired enough information on necessary precautions to permit the drug to be put into the hands of dozens of practicing physicians, who are treating hundreds or even thousands of patients. These doctors have been advised of all the known possibilities of drug-induced toxicity and are aware of all the precautions required for safe use of the investigational drug.

The nurse who works with physicians in such studies should also be fully informed about the drugs that are being employed. In dealing with investigational drugs, she should learn, for example, what changes to watch for in the patient's condition and what actions she is expected to take in case signs of adverse effects appear. Such information may often be obtained from the brochure prepared by the pharmaceutical company for the physician. In addition, the nurse should not hesitate to ask questions of the physician about any aspect of the procedure that puzzles her. She should not be so awed by the mystique of participating in a scientific experiment that she fails to act with the knowledge and prudence which are always required when she is charged with the responsibility of administering *any* drug.

During this phase of the study, the doctors watch the patients carefully for side effects. If the patient's safety or comfort seem to be compromised, the drug may have to be withdrawn and the experiment brought to an abrupt end. The nurse should be aware of her duty to the individual's safety as well as to the success of the study. Thus, she can encourage the patient to talk to his doctor about his discomfort. The physician can then determine whether the patient's complaints are actually caused by the test drug or by the disease. If the symptoms are, indeed, drug-induced, the doctor may order the drug discontinued; if, on the other hand, the symptoms are part of the patient's illness, the doctor explains this to him. And the clinical investigator, in reporting the patient's reactions, will not attribute them unfairly to the drug that is on trial.

Many useful drugs can cause side effects so severe as to seem prohibitive. Yet, if the drug is a very useful one, its administration may be continued despite the discomfort that it causes. Thus, although colchicine often causes diarrhea when given in the doses required to abort an acute gout attack, this agent is so specific and so superior to other available treatments that it is used in spite of its drawbacks. For similar reasons the trial of a new drug may be continued in the face of obvious side reactions.

Drugs are sometimes given even when the therapeutically effective doses are very close to those that are capable of causing severe toxicity. Thus, digitalis is the drug of choice for treating congestive heart failure, despite the frequency with which it causes gastrointestinal upset and its potential cardiac toxicity. The curare-type alkaloids and related muscle relaxant drugs can paralyze respiratory muscles when injected in doses intended only to relax the abdominal musculature. In all such cases, the real criterion is whether the seriousness of the patient's condition warrants the continued administration of a new and apparently useful drug despite its evident dangers. Of course, the people on the medical team are obligated to use every means of detecting toxicity at an early stage, so as to counteract it promptly. In the case of a new curare-type compound, for example, supplies and equipment for resuscitating the patient must be immediately available, should his respiration fail.

The nurse can best serve the patient who is forced to bear a test drug's discomforts in order to gain its benefits by helping him to recognize the drug's usefulness for him. Although the patient has the right to ask his doctor to discontinue the trial at any time, he should also be helped to see the positive as well as the negative aspects of the situation. Often, after the nurse has said something to remind the patient of the relief the drug may have given him during the acute phase of his illness, he is better able to think his problem through and decides to continue therapy.

Efficacy Evaluation. We have up to now emphasized the need for seeing that the patient is protected from the possible *adverse effects* of drugs undergoing clinical trial. However, we should also consider the ways of avoiding actions that increase the difficult task of determining whether a new drug is truly *beneficial* or not.

Determining the therapeutic usefulness of a new drug in human patients is often a formidable task. Many of the difficulties that arise in attempting to evaluate a drug's efficacy stem from the very humanity of the people involved—the patient, his doctor and the nurses. Indeed, the concern of physicians and nurses with the patient's welfare is one of the main complications that sometimes prevents scientific evaluation of a drug.

In some studies, the effects of the drug can be measured objectively. Thus, the efficacy of a diuretic drug may be determined by collecting and measuring the patient's urine output and noting the loss of body weight as edema fluid leaves his tissues. The effects of other drugs can be judged by recording changes in body temperature, blood sugar levels, or electrocardiographic readings. On the other hand, difficulties arise when the patient's *subjective response* is the sole basis for deciding if a drug has been effective for relieving pain, itching, nausea, nervousness or mental depression and other symptoms.

In such cases, conscious and unconscious psychic forces often operate in ways that make it difficult to determine a drug's true pharmacological activity and therapeutic value. All of us are subject to suggestion to some extent. However, some patients (known as *positive placebo reactors*) are unusually susceptible to the positive symbolic implications of receiving medications. These patients tend to report that they feel better even when they have received only a *placebo*—a "blank" or "dummy" medication. Or, if they are *negative placebo reactors*, they may complain of adverse side effects even when they have actually received no active drug.

One technique often used by clinical investigators for reducing unconscious bias is the *double-blind study*. This is a procedure in which neither the patient nor the doctor and nurse who check his responses to medication know what the patient is actually receiving. That is, both are kept in the dark as to whether the capsule or other dosage form being administered is the drug being tested, a standard drug of known activity, or a placebo. The identity of the coded contents of each dose is known only to another member of the research team, who is often the pharmacist or another doctor or nurse. This technique is intended to keep the doctor and nurse from unconsciously communicating their attitudes about the new drug to the patient, who is often so responsive to positive or negative suggestion about his therapy.

Ordinarily, in administering medications to patients, the nurse tries to take advantage of placebo responses by offering patients subtle positive suggestions, which are often as potent as the drug's own pharmacodynamic effects in helping relieve symptoms and for making patients feel better. However, when assisting in the clinical evaluation of an *investigational drug*, she should make every effort to avoid influencing the patient's attitude toward the test drug.

This is especially important during the final phase of broad clinical trials, when it is often not feasible to employ the double-blind method of evaluation. Since even the inflection of her voice may influence the patient's response to the test drug, the nurse should avoid conveying her enthusiasm for the treatment or her distrust of a new drug. She should never discuss the nature of the drug and its actions or the anticipated benefits and possible side effects with the patient or his family.

This does not mean that the patient taking an "on-trial" drug does not have his usual right to discuss the treatment he is getting. However, to avoid the possibility of conveying her conscious or unconscious approval or disapproval of the drug and the testing procedure, the nurse should tell the patient that she is referring his question to the doctor, and then, of course, actually do so.

Thus, instead of brusquely brushing off the patient with, "you'll have to ask the doctor," or answering a query about what a drug is supposed to do with a vague "Oh, it's to help you get well," the helpful nurse explains in a concrete way that the patient's question will be dealt with, "when Dr. Jones comes here between two and three P.M. today." The patient's visitors, if they are concerned about his treatment and need information or reassurance, should also be brought into touch with the doctor.

Post-release Studies. Even after a drug has been permitted to be marketed, much may still be learned about its potential toxicity and usefulness. Occasionally, some toxicity has been encountered only when the drug was being used on hundreds of thousands of patients. The manufacturer and the F.D.A. are then faced with deciding whether to withdraw the approved drug from the market, or whether the risk to a small minority of patients is warranted by the benefits gained by the majority of patients. Several drugs for treating mental depression were withdrawn in recent years when evidence of toxicity appeared belatedly in some patients; yet, one drug—tranylcypromine—was reinstated, with certain restrictions, because doctors claimed that they found it very valuable for some of their suicidal patients.

Just as the nurse should always keep her eyes and ears open for signs of adverse effects in patients taking newly marketed drugs, she should also look for signs that might contribute useful information about the drug's potential for doing good. Alert observation of the way patients respond to new drugs has sometimes led to the discovery of new uses for such agents. The ability to recognize and exploit an accidental observation is called *serendipity* and is a phenomenon that has led to the discovery of new and useful drugs as well as to other scientific advances.

The antidepressant action of iproniazid—the first of the powerful modern drugs for treating depression—was first recognized in patients receiving the drug as a treatment for tuberculosis. The tranquilizing effect of chlorpromazine, the first phenothiazine tranquilizer, was first noted in patients receiving the drug as an adjunct administered before and after anesthesia. The antihistaminic drug dimenhydrinate was found useful against motion sickness by allergists who were giving it to patients with hay fever. And certain observed side effects of the early sulfonamide anti-infective drugs—an increased urine flow and a drop in blood sugar in a few patients being treated for infections—provided the leads that resulted eventually in the development of two entirely new classes of drugs: the sulfonamide-type diuretics, such as acetazolamide and its successors, and the oral hypoglycemic drugs used against diabetes, such as tolbutamide and its sulfonylurea relatives.

LEGAL REGULATION AND DRUG STANDARDS

Federal Government Regulations. In the preceding discussion of how modern drugs are developed and how their safety and efficacy are evaluated, our main concern has been to convey the meanings of certain terms and concepts that the nurse who handles and administers drugs should understand. Now let us look at some of the legislation through which the federal government is empowered to regulate and control the manner in which drugs are manufactured and marketed.

The Food and Drug Administration (F.D.A.). This agency of the Department of Health, Education and Welfare is charged with the enforcement of a body of law that has gradually grown up during this century in recognition of the fact that the manufacture and sale of drugs requires close regulation, in order to protect the public's health. The legislation under which this regulatory agency operates is primarily the *Federal Food, Drug, and Cosmetic Act of 1938* and its various amendments. We shall not discuss the many detailed provisions of this law; however, a brief history of how such legislation developed may illustrate the need for ensuring that all drugs meet high standards of strength and safety.

The earliest federal legislation regulating the quality of medicines was the *Pure Food and Drug Act of 1906.* Its passage followed a quarter of a century fight to give the government some control over the then totally unrestricted sale of drugs, many of them worthless or dangerous. The law was intended primarily to prevent the marketing of adulterated drugs; and a later amendment in regard to the labeling of medications was designed to eliminate false and misleading claims concerning therapeutic usefulness.

Although this Act corrected various flagrant abuses, the law of 1906 really did little to assure the *safety* of drug products, and bills that were intended to do so made little headway during the next generation. It required a tragic accident in 1937 to arouse public pressure on Congress for the passage of new legislation to guarantee greater safety of prescription drug products. The Elixir of Sulfanilamide incident, which took over 100 lives, occurred when a drug manufacturer seeking a solvent for the then new anti-infective chemical, sulfanilamide, selected diethylene glycol. This substance proved to be an excellent vehicle for the drug, but, because its pharmacological effects had not been tested in animals, its toxicity was unknown until the reports of illness and death in patients taking the product began to pour in.

The Federal Food, Drug and Cosmetic Act of 1938, which was then passed, made it mandatory for manufacturers to perform toxicity tests in laboratory animals before seeking from the F.D.A. approval to market any drug. The law provided procedures by which that agency could keep a drug from being marketed, or order its recall, if its scientists decided that the drug's safety had not been adequately tested, or if they felt that the drug was too dangerous for use in the clinical situations for which it was intended.

The F.D.A. was further empowered by the Durham-Humphrey amendment of 1952 to determine which medications could be dispensed only on a doctor's order. This modification of the law, which also deals with rules for the refilling of prescriptions, was intended to limit unsupervised self-medication. It was aimed most particularly against abuse of the barbiturates, a problem which had recently begun to be recognized and one which could not be controlled under the provisions of the Harrison Narcotics Act (see p. 13).

Although this amendment made it somewhat more difficult for people to harm themselves with drugs bought "over-the-counter" and taken without medical advice or supervision, the problem of drug abuse continued to grow greater. The most recent legislative attempt to restrict the availability of potentially dangerous drugs was the passage of the *Drug Abuse Control Amendments of 1965.* These regulations attempt to exert more stringent control than ever before over the manufacture, distribution and sale of barbiturates, amphetamines, and a long list of products containing combinations of various other central nervous system depressants and stimulants.

Prior to this latest legislation, the Food, Drug and Cosmetic Act had been markedly modified in 1962. The *Kefauver-Harris Drug Amendments* of that year were again the result of a wave of public alarm and revulsion which rose as the result of another near disaster involving an inadequately tested drug. Thalidomide, a seemingly safe sleep-producing drug marketed in Europe, was shown to have been the cause of dreadful deformities in newborn babies whose mothers had taken the drug during pregnancy. The drug was then undergoing mass clinical trials in this country, and the public's realization of how readily it might have been released here helped to marshal support for new restrictive legislation.

These legal changes gave the F.D.A. broad new powers for regulating all aspects of drug research and development. Among these powers was one long sought by the government agency—the right to pass judgment not only on the safety of every new drug but also upon its *effectiveness.* The F.D.A. took the view that safety and efficacy are closely linked, for the patient who takes a worthless drug for a serious condition is wasting not only money but time, during which his ailment may be advancing. In addition, since the thalidomide incident had once again shown that *no* drug is really ever entirely safe, including seemingly harmless ones, the patient who takes an ineffective drug may also be exposed to unnecessary danger.

We need not attempt to review here the regulations for government monitoring of new drugs, except to note that many of the points made in the earlier discussion of the preclinical testing procedures and the clinical investigations of new drugs are part of the new requirements of the F.D.A. for the regulation of so-called investigational drugs.

Such controls did not, however, originate with this legislation. Reputable drug manufacturers have, of course, always made every effort to ensure the safety and quality of their products. Unfortunately, because such self-regulation was not adopted throughout the pharmaceutical industry, restrictive measures have had to be enforced and have become increasingly stringent after each much publicized mishap. The present somewhat stultifying federal control over almost every aspect of drug research and development and marketing probably reflects the public's desire for drug safety above all other considerations. Most

people, it seems, now recognize that a drug is no ordinary commodity but one which, they feel, must meet the most demanding standards that industry can devise.

Drug Standards. Many of the standards which the F.D.A. now maintains were orginally set by scientists employed by the drug industry and by others outside of government. The need for standards for quality of drugs has long been recognized, and physicians, pharmacists and others have long made up compendia of the most useful drugs and formulations, which were intended to ensure uniformity and purity of these products. The very first federal regulation passed in 1906 recognized two of these compendia—the *United States Pharmacopeia* (the *U.S.P.*) and the *National Formulary* (the *N.F.*)—as official standards (the term "official," indicating the pharmacopeial status of a drug, means that the standards set for that drug have the force of federal law).

The United States Pharmacopeia was first published in 1820 as a guide for apothecaries, who then sometimes still collected the plants from which vegetable medicinal products were prepared, and for physicians, who at that time often did their own compounding. Later, as pharmacists came to rely on chemical and pharmaceutical manufacturers for supplying the new synthetic drugs and purified plant principles, the scientists employed by these companies developed the analytical tests and biological assays that served as the basic objective standards of drug quality.

Today, representatives from medical and pharmacy schools and state associations, and from various professional and scientific groups, including the American Medical Association, the American Pharmaceutical Association, and the American Chemical Society serve on a Committee of Revision of the U.S.P., which works to develop and publish specifications for modern potent drugs.

Under the supervision of this Committee, the U.S.P. is now revised and published at five-year intervals. The present pharmacopeia is the seventeenth revision. U.S.P. XVII, like earlier editions, contains monographs dealing with drugs chosen because of their demonstrated usefulness in the diagnosis and treatment of disease or because they are considered so-called pharmaceutic necessities (substances that aid in the manufacture of the therapeutically valuable medications).

Although the U.S.P. is a "bible" mainly for pharmaceutical chemists and pharmacists, nurses should acquaint themselves with this standard book, which is available in most medical libraries and contains much valuable reference material. For one thing, the U.S.P. is the most authoritative source of information in regard to safe dosage ranges for the important drugs discussed in its pages. Most of the dosage details listed in the tables of this book comes from the

U.S.P. and from the other official compendium, the National Formulary (N.F.).

The N.F. is similar to the U.S.P. in its subject matter and aims and serves to supplement it. Drugs are now admitted solely on the basis of their therapeutic value—reflecting the current concern that drugs be proved effective as well as safe and pure. The N.F. XII continues to follow the objectives of its founders and present publishers, the American Pharmaceutical Association, by setting high standards of quality for the drugs deemed worthy of admission. The latest edition includes tests and assays which make use of the most modern methods of instrumental analysis and assay for seeing that such standards are met. This is a book that the nurse will sometimes have occasion to use when she needs certain kinds of information not included in drug package inserts or other sources.

Nomenclature of Drugs. The Drug Amendments of 1962 made it mandatory that the monographs of the U.S.P. and the N.F. provide only one *official name* for each drug. This attempt to reduce the proliferation of confusing names that have all too often been applied to a particular drug in the past is a step in the right direction. For the same drug often has a chemical name, a code name while in an investigational status, and a variety of synonyms or "trivial" common names and proprietary, or trade, names.

The F.D.A. has now been given the authority to designate a single, simple official name for any drug that does not have one; however, it has, in practice, permitted this task to be taken over in almost every case by a special committee on nomenclature called the *USAN Council*. (USAN stands for United States Adopted Name.) This group, which is made up of representatives from the U.S.P. Convention, the American Pharmaceutical Association, and the American Medical Association, selects suitable *nonproprietary names* for new drugs. These will later be adopted automatically as the U.S.P. or N.F. titles of any compound that becomes officially recognized.

The use of the *non*proprietary name is desirable for teaching purposes, because it aids communication and reduces confusion. Thus, this name is used to designate the drugs discussed in this book wherever possible. However, respect for the realities of the presently existing state of affairs makes it necessary to refer in many cases to the *proprietary, or trade,* name of certain drugs. Thus, when a drug is far better known by its manufacturer's trade-mark designation than by its *non*proprietary, official, generic or USAN name, we shall of necessity use that name. (The manufacturer's name is always capitalized, whereas nonproprietary names begin with a lower case letter.)

Sometimes, an older name which has been discarded in favor of a newly coined official designation refuses to die, and we shall there list it parenthetically as a synonym. However, in the labeling of prescription drug packages, only the established *non*proprietary name may appear in addition to the manufacturer's *trademark,* or *brand name,* and the drug's chemical designation.

Other Regulations and Agencies. The *Harrison Narcotic Act* of 1914 and related laws and amendments are administered by the U.S. Treasury Department and enforced by the Bureau of Narcotics of that agency. Although this law takes the form of a tax measure under the government's Internal Revenue Code, it is actually devised to control the traffic in narcotic drugs. Under its provisions, federal control is exerted over the manufacture, importation, transportation and distribution of opium and coca and their derivatives, and certain synthetic drugs that are judged capable of causing and sustaining addiction.

The nurse must, of course, familiarize herself with those provisions of this law that apply to her professional practice. In addition, she should learn the local regulations concerning her role in the administration of narcotic drugs. Not only do the states—and sometimes even municipalities—have legislation that differs in some respect from the federal act, but various hospitals have set up their own rules and procedures for handling and accounting for narcotics. (We cannot cover the complex legal aspects of narcotic control here. We shall say a great deal more about the nature of addiction in the next chapter and at various other places in this book.)

Federal regulations control not only narcotics, but also antibiotics, biological products, and the advertising of drugs. All antibiotics must meet standards of purity and potency set by the F.D.A. However, biologicals are regulated by a division of the Public Health Service—the *Division of Biological Standards* of the *National Institutes of Health.* This agency sets the control requirements that must be met by each lot of such biological products as vaccines, antitoxins, immune serums, immunologic diagnostic aids and blood derivatives. These immunologic agents, though used in the diagnosis and treatment of disease, are not truly drugs. Thus, in this book, their use in the prophylaxis and therapy of certain infections is discussed only briefly in the final section. However, the nurse who has occasion to make frequent use of any of these drugs should obtain detailed information concerning their storage and administration from other available sources.

The *Federal Trade Commission* (F.T.C.) has jurisdiction over the advertising of nonprescription drugs, among other commodities. Under the Wheeler-Lea Act of 1938 the F.T.C. is charged with protecting the public from false advertising and deceptive practices. The agency has also in the past exerted some control over advertisements directed at the medical profession, but such jurisdiction is now largely in the hands of the F.D.A. as a result of the Kefauver-Harris amendments of 1962. Some authorities on the subject of drug advertising feel that the interests of the general public would be better served if the promotion of products advertised for purchase without a prescription were subject to the greater power of the F.D.A. Many who are disturbed by the tastelessness of much radio and television advertising of drugs and the tendency to sacrifice full disclosure of factual information for less than completely honest statements feel that further controls would be desirable.

Although the F.T.C. frequently has been criticized for its failure to put a stop to advertising claims for home remedies which are, at the very least, misleading, the agency has in fact at times conducted vigorous, though largely futile, campaigns against such abuses. In one attempt to keep a company from claiming that its cathartic promoted the flow of "golden" liver bile, the Commission fought a fifteen year battle against a battery of company lawyers who always managed to find legal loopholes for nullifying the agency's "cease and desist" orders.

The nurse, in her daily contacts with people, can do a good deal to counteract the more odious kinds of drug advertising by quietly and repeatedly pointing out the facts of the matter in the simplest possible terms. Of course, she may often feel frustrated by the odds against the probable success of her efforts to counteract the psychological impact on the public mind of a multimillion-dollar advertising campaign. Yet, because she is truly concerned with the public's health and welfare, she will persevere in this aspect of her role in health education. For, as we have indicated, drugs and medicines are different in character from the countless other commodities that are constantly being hawked to the public.

A consumer who is bilked when he buys some other gadget or service can always say, "Oh well, it was only money!" However, when he buys a worthless or potentially harmful medicine, his health and even his life may be at stake. Thus, the very least that the nurse can do is encourage people to seek medical diagnosis and treatment instead of trying to treat their own symptoms with a proprietary remedy that may be misleadingly advertised.

Advertisements for arthritis remedies, for example, often suggest that a more expensive product is superior to aspirin, when actually salicylates would be preferable for most people. More odious and potentially dangerous, however, are those that reinforce the hesitancy that some people have in seeing a doctor about rectal or genitourinary tract symptoms. Some advertisements for nonprescription medications play skillfully on ignorance, fear, prudery and personal embarrassment in this regard.

Thus, a patient who is beguiled by claims that a product will eliminate the spectre of surgery by shrinking hemorrhoids medically may too long put off seeing a doctor for proper diagnosis and treatment. He may get temporary relief of minor symptoms through the use of such a palliative (symptom-relieving) product, but his underlying condition may deteriorate until his hemorrhoids require surgical correction in any case. More serious still is the possibility that the patient's self diagnosis that led him to listen to the advertisement and buy the product may have been mistaken. The masses which he took for hemorrhoids may actually be rectal cancer—a condition for which treatment should, of course, never be delayed by the application of palliative remedies.

INTRODUCTION TO THE STUDY OF PHARMACOLOGY

We will close this chapter with some suggestions as to how the student may best approach the study of pharmacology. The subject is a difficult one, because it requires attending to a great deal of detailed information. The number of potent new drugs introduced into clinical practice continues to be greater than the number of older drugs being discarded. Thus, the subject seems to grow ever greater in scope and complexity.

Nonetheless, the nurse who approaches the study of drugs *systematically,* and with the feeling that pharmacology is an exciting and rewarding aspect of the world of patient care, can readily learn all she needs to know in order to carry out her professional responsibilities relative to drug therapy with confidence and zest. The nurse is fortunate in one important respect: she gets ample opportunity to translate theoretical considerations into very practical applications as she functions in a clinical setting, and can actually see sick patients respond to the drugs about which she is studying.

Thus, the study of a drug such as digitalis becomes more meaningful when one sees how its cardiac actions make the difference between a dyspneic, edematous exhausted woman and one who can return home able to care for her family once more. The factual details concerning the pharmacology of morphine also become easier to retain when one has seen this drug assuage the agony of a severely injured accident victim in a seemingly miraculous fashion. The term "miracle drug" is often reserved for certain recently discovered agents which open up ways of controlling conditions not previously treatable; but some of the tried and true drugs handed down through the generations are often just as dramatic in their effects.

Despite the intrinsic interest of observing how the actions of drugs help to improve the condition of sick patients, it would be wrong to imply that the task of learning the details of drug action is ever an easy one. Some aspects of any discipline are tedious, and learning the details calls for concentration and perseverance. Thus, in using this book the student will soon find that there is no substitute for seeking out the answers to the *review questions* at the end of each chapter and then writing out the correct answers in a notebook. The points which the review questions seek to bring out all appear somewhere in the chapter—in the narrative body, the tabular summaries, or elsewhere; and your learning will be reinforced if you *write out* the answers in your own words, rather than simply checking off the various points in your head, as you come across them in the text.

One way of *systematizing* your study is to concentrate first on the most important and well-established drugs in each class. For example, once one has learned the main facts, about the *prototype* agents digitalis, morphine, atropine, and epinephrine, it becomes easier to understand most of the other drugs that are classed as cardiovascular drugs, analgesics, and autonomic nervous system stimulants and depressants. The nurse will find it relatively easy to learn the main facts about totally new drugs if she understands the pharmacology of the older agents.

If the nurse thinks of each new drug that she encounters in terms of its significant *similarities to* and *differences from* the *prototypes* of each major drug category, she will be on her way to mastery of this important but difficult subject. If, instead, she looks upon every agent that she deals with as an isolated entity, the nurse may soon find herself swamped in a mass of unrelated details which will keep her in a constant state of bewildered frustration.

What kinds of information should the nurse try to retain about the prototype drugs of each major class? A good point at which to begin is with each drug's *primary* and *secondary pharmacological actions.* When one knows what a drug does to alter normal physiological function, it is often easy to guess how it may have a favorable effect on a pathologically functioning organ. Thus, it becomes easier to remember rationally that the drug is indicated in the treatment of a particular clinical disorder.

Similarly, knowledge of some of the secondary actions of a drug helps us to understand why side effects of certain types are likely to occur even when ordinary doses are administered. In addition, this kind of information makes us aware of the factors that are most likely to cause a patient to react poorly to the drug— that is, those conditions in which the use of a given drug may be *contraindicated* or require special precautions. Knowledge of a drug's actions also helps us predict the likely signs and symptoms of a toxic reaction to massive overdosage and the antidotal drugs and other measures that may need to be employed.

The above listing of the kinds of data that the nurse should try to learn about each prototype drug is not meant to imply that she should really ever rely solely on reason or memory. A rational approach to the study of drugs and a willingness to employ brute memory in retaining as much detail as possible are requisites for the most profitable *study* of drugs, but one should never depend upon these mental tools alone when *administering* drugs to patients.

Look it up when in doubt is an essential rule for any nurse, no matter how experienced she is in drug therapy. The vast number and variety of medications makes it impossible for anyone to carry around in her head all the details of drug dosage and action that may apply to any particular case. Thus, it is essential to have available up-to-date reference materials on the ward and to seek the assistance of the physician and the advice of the pharmacist to resolve any doubts about a drug which is to be administered.

Although the nurse should have learned the essential facts about the drugs that she uses, from her organized study of pharmacology through textbook, lectures, and practical experience, she may require more specific information when dealing with a new and relatively unfamiliar drug or with a patient who has special problems. Thus, it is always desirable to discuss with the doctor what special observations he wants made in regard to the therapeutically desirable effects and the side effects for which he wishes you to watch.

In the last analysis, however, no matter how much the nurse knows about drugs or how helpful it may be to talk to the doctor or pharmacist concerning the details of particular drugs, there is no substitute for having available the necessary reference books concerning the drugs that one is called upon to employ. While one's own personal library dealing with drugs may be limited to a single definitive textbook on pharmacology and drug therapy such as this one, the nurse working in a hospital setting should demand that she be given easy access to all the material on drugs that she is expected to employ on patients in her care on the ward.

Reference Sources

The following is a list of books and journals which will serve as excellent supplements to the kind of data concerning drugs that is found in this book. Although this list is by no means all-inclusive, nor, on the other hand, is it necessary to have all of them available, the nurse should familiarize herself with all these sources of drug information and learn how to use them.

New Drugs (Council on Drugs, American Medical Association, Chicago). This book, published annually, is organized into chapters and sections summarizing the most significant points about most of the major groups of drugs. Within each chapter, there are authoritative summaries of the current status of individual drugs of that class which have been introduced relatively recently. Many statements similar to these monographs appear each year in the pages of the

Journal of the American Medical Association, evaluating the most recently marketed drugs. The nurse who subscribes to this journal can clip and file these Council Reports, but they can also be obtained by simply requesting that they be sent regularly.

Physicians' Desk Reference (P.D.R.) (Medical Economics, Inc., Oradell, N. J.). This annual publication is a very well cross-indexed compendium of factual information about currently available drug products. Although the information about these products is furnished by their manufacturers rather than coming from disinterested authorities, the important data on available dosage forms, methods of administration, therapeutic indications, precautions and contraindications, side effects and toxicity are usually quite fully stated, especially for the most widely used products of the major pharmaceutical companies.

Similar information about drug products may be obtained by requesting product brochures from the pharmaceutical companies or by examining copies on file in pharmacies. Such information can also be found in the package inserts which come with each unit of the drugs. Since the data therein concerning the drug's uses, dosage, possible adverse effects, contraindications and required precautions is considered a part of the product's labeling, it has been approved by the Food and Drug Administration and thus does not constitute mere advertising puffery for the product.

The Medical Letter (published by Drug and Therapeutic Information Corporation, Inc., 305 East 45th St., New York, N. Y.). This is an independent, nonprofit publication that provides evaluations of new drugs and periodic summaries of the drug therapy of various clinical conditions. Its appraisals express the consensus of the authorities who serve as consultants to the publication. The reports, which are released twice a month, offer critical and unbiased opinions about relatively new drugs which are often being promoted in the advertising pages of the journals with a fanfare that may tend to obscure their true value. Although the consultants' comments on such drugs must by their nature be tentative, they often serve to put heavily promoted drug products into a more proper pharmacological perspective than can be gained from the occasional reading of one or two publications on the new drug in medical or nursing journals.

Journals. Journals are, in fact, an excellent source of information on drug therapy. The nurse who writes to the author for reprints of published papers reviewing drugs in which she is interested can painlessly and inexpensively build up a file of current drug data to supplement her books on pharmacology and drug therapy. Among the journals which offer papers dealing with drugs on a practical, clinical level are those whose publicatons make up the bulk of the bibliographical references cited at the end of each chapter

of this book. These include: (1) The Journal of the American Medical Association, (2) The New England Journal of Medicine, (3) Medical Clinics of North America, (4) Modern Treatment, (5) Clinical Pharmacology and Therapeutics, and the nursing publications, (6) American Journal of Nursing, and (7) R.N.

Encyclopedic Sources. Nurses who occasionally may have to study the details of a drug's sources, chemistry, toxicology, mechanisms of action and so forth in depth can often gain a great deal of information by consulting the following massive compendia of factual information about various aspects of individual drugs.

The United States Dispensatory and Physicians Pharmacology, Osol, Pratt and Altschule (eds.), 26th Ed. (Philadelphia, Lippincott, 1967) The present edition is a collection of articles dealing with individual drugs and with pharmacologic classes of drugs. Although smaller in size than earlier editions because of elimination of much technical and historical material related to manufacture, its close to 1300 pages now contain a greater proportion of the kinds of information that are most useful for those engaged in prescribing, dispensing and administering drugs.

The Pharmacological Basis of Therapeutics, Goodman and Gilman (eds.), 3rd Ed. (New York, Macmillan, 1965) This classic text is directed mainly at medical students, interns, residents and practicing physicians. However, many nurses also will often profit from perusal of this excellent encyclopedic treatment of drug actions as related to therapeutics and related medical sciences when they require detailed factual information about the basic scientific aspects of pharmacodynamics.

Drill's Pharmacology in Medicine, DiPalma, J. R. (ed.), 3rd Ed. (New York, McGraw-Hill, 1965) This book offers ninety chapters prepared by numerous contributors, and as its editor says, it is "not for the lazy or weakhearted."

The Pharmacologic Principles of Medical Practice, Krantz and Carr, 6th Ed. (Baltimore, Williams & Wilkins, 1965) A less massive text than the others, but one which is ample enough in the detail that it offers and easier to read than the others because of its co-authors' continued concern with the art of communication.

Drugs of Choice 1966–1967, Modell, W. (ed.) (St. Louis, Mosby) This biennially issued book is intended as a practical guide to the physician who is trying to select the best available drug for dealing with a particular therapeutic problem. The contributions of close to fifty authors are edited by the distinguished clinical pharmacologist, Walter Modell.

CONCLUSION

Although the greater part of this book will be devoted to practical considerations in regard to what happens when drugs are administered to sick people, we hope that the nurse will recognize that the drugs and chemicals in our environment have much broader significance both in our society and in science.

The following two chapters of this section will offer some indication of this to the discerning reader. Thus, although in the next chapter's discussion of what happens to drug molecules in the body we shall emphasize the practical clinical significance, it will also be apparent that such knowledge is of fundamental importance in many other areas of biological and physical sciences. Similarly, subjects such as drug addiction and accidental poisoning—discussed in Chapter 3—are obviously social as well as medical problems. That is, the misuse of drugs and chemicals raises serious ethical and moral issues concerning the right of man to injure his own health and that of other human beings and other species through the careless use of chemical substances with biological activity.

REVIEW QUESTIONS

1. (a) What does the term *pharmacology* mean in its broadest sense? in the context of its use by nurses and other medically oriented people?

(b) What is meant by a *drug?* a *poison?*

2. What is meant by (a) *pharmacodynamics?* How does this aspect of pharmacology differ from (b) *pharmacotherapeutics* and (c) *toxicology?*

3. (a) List several drugs still in use today which were discovered empirically by ancient and primitive peoples.

(b) List several pure plant principles, the availability of which first permitted drugs to be studied scientifically on a quantitative basis.

(c) List several substances, the synthesis of which led to further pharmacological advances.

3. List four types of studies that pharmacologists commonly carry out in appraising the biological activity of a chemical or drug.

4. What is meant by (a) screening tests? (b) biological assays?

5. (a) List several alkaloids recently extracted from anciently employed plants with bioassay as a guide to the purity of the extracts.

(b) List several synthetic corticosteroids prepared by modification of the molecule of the natural adrenal cortex hormones.

6. What is meant by (a) the prototype or "lead" of a class of drugs, and (b) its congener compounds or analogues?

7. (a) What types of improvement may chemists make in the therapeutic usefulness of a compound by altering its basic molecular structure?

(b) List several classes of drugs that have been largely derived by starting with a particular chemical structure and altering the basic architecture of the molecule in various ways.

8. (a) What is meant by a drug's *spectrum of activity* or its *pharmacological profile?*

(b) What is meant by a drug's *primary* and its *secondary* effects?

9. (a) What is the main purpose of preclinical acute toxicity tests in several species of animals?

(b) What is meant by a drug's *therapeutic index*, as determined in acute toxicity testing?

10. (a) What types of observation are made during chronic toxicity studies on several species of animals?

(b) What kind of information is gained from studies of a drug's metabolism in several species of animals during long-term studies?

11. (a) What is the practical significance of individual (biologic) variation in response to drugs?

(b) What is the significance of species variation?

12. (a) What are the two main objectives of all three phases of clinical testing procedures in humans?

(b) What information does the clinical investigator ordinarily give to volunteer subjects and patients taking an investigational drug?

13. (a) What *types of toxicity* are especially watched for in clinical studies of drug safety?

(b) Under what circumstances may clinical studies of a drug be continued despite the detection of signs of such toxicity in some patients?

14. (a) What responsibility does the nurse have to the patient and to the investigator of a drug on clinical trial and what should she do to best meet her obligations in terms of both the patient's welfare and the success of the investigation?

(b) What are some examples of drugs that are clinically useful despite their relatively high toxicity?

15. What is meant by (a) the *subjective response?* (b) the *double-blind* technique? (c) the *placebo reactor?*

16. (a) How should the nurse use her knowledge of patients' suggestibility: (1) in administering drugs ordinarily? (2) in administering a new drug during a clinical investigation of its efficacy?

(b) How should the nurse deal with questions about drugs that are under investigation?

17. (a) Why should the nurse be especially observant of the responses of patients to a drug that has been only recently approved by the F.D.A. for marketing?

(b) What is meant by *serendipity*, and what are some examples of useful uses for new drugs discovered in this way?

18. (a) What was the first federal law regulating the qualities of medicines, and what aspects of drug marketing was it intended to control?

(b) What incident led to passage of the Federal Food Drug and Cosmetic Act of 1938, and in what way did this law try to provide for greater safety of drug products?

19. (a) What amendment to the FDC Act makes it

mandatory that certain drugs may be obtained only by prescription and that such medications require the physician's permission for refilling of prescriptions?

(b) What types of drugs are subjected to further restrictions relative to their distribution and sale in accordance with the provisions of the Drug Abuse Control Amendments of 1965?

20. (a) What was the nature of the so-called "thalidomide incident" of the early 1960's?

(b) What powers did the Kefauver-Harris Drug Amendments of 1962 confer upon the Food and Drug Administration?

21. (a) What is the main function of the monographs in the United States Pharmacopeia, and on what basis are drugs chosen for inclusion in this official compendium?

(b) Which organization publishes the National Formulary and what are the objectives of its publishers?

22. (a) What are some of the kinds of names by which drugs are sometimes designated?

(b) How can the manufacturer's proprietary, or brand, name ordinarily be distinguished from the same drug's *non*proprietary name?

23. (a) What are some types of drugs which are regulated under the provisions of the Harrison Narcotic Act?

(b) What government agency administers and enforces this law?

24. (a) What educational function can the informed nurse perform relative to the effect of the advertising of drugs for self-medication?

(b) What kind of harm can come to a patient who heeds certain types of advertising for nonprescription drug products?

25. (a) What is meant by a prototype drug and how can acquiring knowledge of such a drug be utilized in systematizing one's study of pharmacology?

(b) What kinds of information should one look for in studying the prototype drug of a pharmacological category or any new drug that we may need to know about?

BIBLIOGRAPHY

Beckman, H.: In defense of tinkers. New Eng. J. Med., *267*:72, 1962.

Beecher, H. K.: The powerful placebo. J.A.M.A., *159:* 1602, 1955.

Burger, A.: Approaches to drug discovery. New Eng. J. Med., *270*:1098, 1964.

Dowling, H. F.: What's in a name? J.A.M.A., *173*:1580, 1960.

Irwin, S.: Drug screening and evaluative procedures. Science, *136*:123, 1962.

Kautz, H. D.: The development of new drugs. Am. J. Nurs., *53*:145, 1953.

Greiner, T.: Subjective bias of the clinical pharmacologist. J.A.M.A., *181*:92, 1962.

Jerome, J. B.: Current status of nonproprietary nomenclature for drugs. J.A.M.A., *185*:256, 1963.

Kohlstaedt, K. G.: Introduction to clinical investigation. J.A.M.A., *187*:344, 1964.

Leake, C. D.: The scientific study of pharmacology. Science, *134*:2069, 1961.

Miller, L. C.: Doctors, drugs, and names. J.A.M.A., *177:* 14, 1961.

Modell, W., and Houde, R. W.: Factors influencing clinical evaluation of drugs. J.A.M.A., *167*:2190, 1958.

Modell, W.: Safety in new drugs. J.A.M.A., *190*:141, 1964.

Peck, H. M.: Adequacy of the preclinical safety evaluation. J.A.M.A., *187*:341, 1964.

Rodman, M. J.: What's behind the new drug drought? R.N., *28*:78, 1965 (March).

Starr, I.: The testing of new drugs and other therapeutic agents. J.A.M.A., *177*:14, 1961.

The Interactions of Drugs and Body Tissues

FACTORS INFLUENCING THE EFFECTS OF DRUGS

Drug Dosage. We indicated in the previous chapter that the pharmacologist tries to determine first, the *dose-response relationships* of a new drug and, then, the drug's relative safety—the difference between the amounts that produce, respectively, desired and undesirable effects, expressed in terms of a figure called the *therapeutic index* (T.I.). Ordinarily, test drugs with too low a T.I. in animal studies are discarded; those with a higher T.I. are often evaluated clinically in humans.

This concern with drug dosage that produces a therapeutically desired effect without causing adverse effects is part of the doctor's everyday practice as he writes his orders for medication. He is, in addition, concerned with *maintaining* the desired effects of the drug over a period ranging from days to months or more. To do so he must know both the *dose* that will produce the desired effect and the *frequency* with which that amount must be administered.

The doctor is ordinarily guided in his choice of dose and dosage scheduling by the data compiled during the drug's pharmacological evaluation. Dosage information based upon such studies appears in the insert that is found in each drug package; in a product brochure approved by the Food and Drug Administration; and in advertisements for the drug, which under F.D.A. regulations must now meet many of the same standards that apply to the product's actual labeling. In addition, dosage information appears in the official compendia (U.S.P. and N.F.) and in all other compilations of drug data, including a book of this kind, with its many dosage tables.

Usually, when the doctor prescribes the drug in accordance with such directions and the nurse ad-

ministers it as ordered, the patient responds as expected. Yet, the young nurse, in administering drugs to patients and in observing how they react, soon becomes aware of a disquieting fact—the dose that ordinarily produces the desired effect sometimes causes quite unexpected reactions. That is, some patients react atypically to the usual dose of a drug; and indeed, the same patient may react in quite different ways when he receives the identical dose of a drug at different times.

The nurse, who has been urged to familiarize herself with the dosages of the drugs that she administers, now learns that the so-called "usual dose" given by such authoritative compendia as the U.S.P. and N.F. is not a "universal" dose. And it should not surprise us that the same factors of *individual variation* that make test animals respond differently to drugs affect human reactions to drug dosage. That is—biochemically and physiologically at least—all men are *not* created equal. Thus, the recommended usual dose which is safe and effective for the so-called average patient may prove to be too much or too little for other people whose body metabolism and physiological functions differ from the norm.

In this chapter and the next one, which deals in more detail with the adverse effects of drugs, we shall offer some practical examples of how individual differences influence the ways in which people respond to drugs. Insight into such matters is most important for the physician, whose responsibility it is to order drugs; and nurses also should understand the nature of the underlying differences that account for the variability with which people respond to the usual therapeutic doses of drugs. The nurse who gains such understanding can make more meaningful observations of the patient's responses to drugs. Signs that might otherwise have escaped her attention, or

19

seemed unimportant, become significant. When these are reported to the physician, he can make the kinds of dosage adjustments that improve the patient's response to treatment.

In recent years, a great deal of knowledge has been acquired about the real reasons for differences in the way patients respond to drugs. Let us examine in some detail the physiological, biochemical, psychological and even immunologic and genetic factors that alter the responses of patients to drug dosage.

Weight, Age, and Sex. Many of the factors that make one person very sensitive to a dose of a drug to which others may be very resistant are relatively obscure. All that the doctor can do is to start with the usual dose for the "average" patient and alter the amount administered if this dosage proves to be too little or too much for the particular patient being treated. Ideally, it is desirable for the doctor to adjust the dosage to fit the individual patient at the time that he writes the original drug order, and, to the extent that his knowledge of the patient permits, the doctor does do so routinely.

Most commonly, he takes the *patient's weight* into consideration in determining whether to reduce or raise the usual dose of a potent drug, since there is a definite relationship between the mass of administered chemical and the mass of body tissues and fluids through which it is distributed and diluted. Generally speaking, the greater a person's body weight, the smaller the amount of the administered dose likely to arrive at the reactive target tissues; the less the person weighs, the greater the portion of the dose reaching the reactive cells, and, of course, the more powerful the effect.

This relationship of body size to dosage has been recognized most clearly in the case of *women* and *children,* for whom it has been customary to make downward adjustments of dosage. Children's dosage has been adjusted traditionally in accordance with formulas based on body weight and age. However, doctors have become aware in recent years that many factors less obvious than body weight play a part in determining the reactions of children, the elderly, and women to administered drugs. The dosage for infants is now often calculated from formulas that are based upon body surface, and the pediatrician gives consideration to factors related to the baby's maturity also.

Other Factors. Even when the doctor gives careful consideration to basic aspects of drug dosage such as the patient's weight and age, the person may react in an unusual or "un-average" way. Sometimes the initial dose of a drug produces the desired effect, but with continued administration of the same dose at the recommended intervals, the patient may suffer toxic effects. This can occur when the drug is administered in amounts greater than the patient can metabo-lize and eliminate before the next dose is added to the residue remaining in his body. Such *cumulative toxicity* shows only one of the ways in which differences in the interactions between a drug and the body tissues of different patients may result in reactions other than those expected.

Drugs and Living Systems

In order to understand the operation of these influential factors, it is best that we think for a while in terms of molecular pharmacology rather than clinical pharmacology and to look at drug and tissue interactions at the molecular level rather than in terms of the pharmacological effects useful in therapy.

The living body and each of its cells can be considered as the site of countless chemical reactions that go on continuously and endlessly (as long as life lasts) at split-second speed. A dose of an administered drug may be thought of in terms of its millions and millions of reactive molecules. Thus, when a drug enters a living system, we can think of its molecules immediately beginning to react with those of the cells and tissues with which they come in contact. Most such chemical reactions result in the inactivation and removal of the molecules of foreign chemical from the body; but some of the body's chemical constituents react with the drug molecules in a manner that alters cellular function.

The factors that influence the effects that a dose of a drug will have may be divided into: (1) Those factors that determine *how much* of the drug actually arrives at the reactive tissues, and (2) those factors that influence the *responsiveness* of these target tissues to the amount of the administered dose that reaches them.

FACTORS INFLUENCING DRUG METABOLISM

In its broadest sense, the study of a drug's metabolism deals with everything that happens to the drug, from the time the foreign chemical enters the biological system until it and all of its products have been eliminated from the body. The manner in which the body deals with every different kind of drug molecule is unique. The biochemical pharmacologist who studies the metabolic fate of drugs has to determine how the body handles each new drug; he cannot infer what will happen to it from what he may know about the metabolism of related drugs with similar, but not identical, molecular structures.

The analytical chemical techniques that the biochemical pharmacologist employs in studying the metabolism of drugs are beyond the scope of this text, as are the physicochemical principles that form the theoretical basis of his scientific studies. However, the results of drug metabolism studies have important practical applications in determining the directions that the doctor writes on a drug order and that the nurse follows in administering the drug to a patient.

As we have seen in the previous chapter, the biochemical pharmacologist determines first, in several species of animals and, later, in humans, exactly how the body handles a new drug. He works out the ways in which the drug is *absorbed, distributed, inactivated* and *excreted.* The data obtained by such studies tell the clinical investigator when to expect the *onset* of a drug's activity, when its *intensity* is likely to reach a peak; and how long its effects will last—that is, the probable *duration* of the drug's action. Such information, in turn, helps to determine the *dose* of the drug to be administered; the *dosage form* and *route of administration;* and the *frequency* with which the drug must be repeated in order to maintain its desired effects.

In Chapter 4, we shall discuss the various dosage forms that are available and the specific points that the nurse must keep in mind in administering them. Here, we shall discuss the scientific basis for administering medications. Our purpose is to show, by examples of specific drugs and clinical situations, how various factors operate to determine the concentration of the drug that reaches the tissues capable of reacting to it to produce the desired (or the undesired) pharmacological effects.

Critical Concentration. Before a drug can act to produce its effects on physiological functions, it must reach a certain concentration in the fluids bathing the tissues that are capable of responding to the drug. That is, the molecules of the chemical must make their way from the point at which they enter the body to the vicinity of those tissues with which they react. When the systemically active drug has reached a certain minimal level in the reactive tissues, the functioning of these tissues is changed—usually in the direction of greater activity (stimulation) or reduced activity (depression).

Dynamic Equilibrium. The concentration attained by the drug at any time after its administration depends upon a constantly shifting balance between the rate and extent to which the drug is (1) absorbed into the body fluids from the site of its entry into the body; (2) is transported or distributed to distant points in the body; (3) is detoxified, inactivated, or transformed into breakdown products, and (4) is excreted or eliminated from the body, via various routes.

Let us look more closely at some examples of how a drug's concentration in the tissues, and, consequently, its pharmacological effects, can be altered by the presence of factors that influence the absorption, distribution and disposal of drugs.

DRUG ABSORPTION

Before a drug can begin to exert its actions, it must reach the tissues with which it reacts. In order to do so, the drug molecules must be able to move from the point at which they enter the body to the sometimes distant reactive tissues. In the process of making its way from the site of entry to the site of action, the drug must pass many barriers. It is also subjected to mechanisms that tend to destroy drugs and eliminate these foreign substances from the body.

The term *absorption* refers to the processes involved in transferring the drug molecules from the place in which they are deposited in the body to the *circulating fluids.* A drug that is taken by mouth must pass through the gastrointestinal mucous membranes in order to enter the venous and lymphatic circulation; a drug that is injected into a muscle mass or into the layer of fat and connective tissue just beneath the skin must diffuse from these sites into the blood stream.

Oral Absorption. The oral route of administration is the one most commonly employed, because it is the most convenient, the safest and the cheapest way to get a drug into the patient's system. Most drug molecules are readily absorbed from the mucosal surface of the gastrointestinal tract. Drugs that cannot pass into the blood stream intact and in adequate amounts must be given by parenteral injection. Injection of such substances assures their more rapid and complete absorption, but it also increases the danger of accidental overdosage and possible infection (Chap. 4).

Orally administered drugs are most readily absorbed from small intestine, the inner lining of which is covered with millions of villi which, with their network of capillaries, offer a vast mucosal surface area through which the drug molecules can pass into the systemic circulation. Thus, although some substances such as the salicylates and alcohol begin to be absorbed almost immediately from the mucosa of the stomach, most drugs are more rapidly and completely absorbed when the stomach quickly empties its contents into the duodenum.

Drugs and Food. Because the stomach empties more slowly when filled with food, orally administered drugs are more rapidly absorbed when taken between meals. Besides delaying gastric emptying into the intestine, food often binds the drug molecules to its protein components. This tends to reduce irritation of the G.I. mucosa by drugs such as the iron salts used in the treatment of anemia. However, it also often ties up drug molecules in complexes that cannot readily pass through the mucosal lining of the intestine. Also the increased acidity and peptic activity of the gastric contents during the digestion of a meal may destroy more of the drug and thus reduce the amount that is finally absorbed.

For example, most oral penicillin products are best given between meals to prevent their destruction and increase the chances of the antibiotic's reaching effective antibacterial levels in the infected tissues. Other drugs are wrapped in special enteric coatings (See Chap. 4) to help them escape digestion in the upper G.I. tract or to keep them from causing irritation and vomiting. Some substances must be administered parenterally because they are inactivated by digestive secretions before they can be absorbed. The hormones insulin and corticotropin, for example, are protein molecules that are digested when taken orally; and the anticoagulant drug heparin, a natural polysaccharide, also must be given by injection rather than orally.

Lipid Solubility and Ionization. Still other substances are stable enough in the G.I. tract, but they are inadequately absorbed because of physicochemical properties that make it difficult for their molecules to penetrate the mucosa of the intestinal tract. This mucous membrane is made up of epithelial cells that let some substances pass through readily and prevent others from penetrating. The membranes of these cells, like those of all cells, are made up of a sort of "sandwich" of lipids, or fatty substances, bounded by protein on both sides. Small water-soluble drug molecules may pass through tiny pores in the cell membrane. Larger molecules must, however, diffuse through the nonporous portion which makes up the largest part of the membrane surface.

Substances that are *soluble in lipids* (alcohol, for example) pass readily through the mucosal surface of the stomach and intestine. Substances that are low in lipid solubility, such as certain sulfonamides, are not likely to be absorbed when taken by mouth. Thus, when succinylsulfathiazole and phthalylsulfathiazole are taken in tablet form, their molecules do not penetrate the intestinal mucosa in amounts that permit them to reach effective anti-infective concentrations in the blood and tissues. Instead, they accumulate in the lumen of the lower bowel, and the high concentration that these sulfonamide drugs attain there makes them useful for "sterilizing" the gut.

Similarly, certain antibiotics, such as streptomycin and neomycin, must be given by injection for treating tuberculosis or other systemic infections, because the poor solubility of their ions in lipids make their passage through the intestinal mucosa difficult. (Drugs that are *highly ionized*—that is, present mostly in the form of electrically charged particles—tend to be repelled by the cell membranes of the intestinal mucosa and by other cell walls also.) Yet, the poor solubility and strong ionization are the physicochemical factors that account for the usefulness of these antibiotics in treating bacterial diarrhea. Because of

their poor absorption from the intestinal tract these antibiotics, like the sulfonamides, tend to pile up there and reach the levels required for control of gastrointestinal pathogenic bacteria.

Other highly ionized drugs that pass poorly through the intestinal mucosa include the so-called quaternary ammonium compounds, some of which are used in treating peptic ulcers and high blood pressure. When ganglionic blocking agents (Chap. 17) of this kind are given by mouth, they are irregularly and incompletely absorbed. In most patients with hypertension the oral route is used because of its convenience, although the uncertain rate and degree of absorption of these drugs from the G.I. tract often makes it difficult to keep the patient's blood pressure properly stabilized.

On the other hand, substances such as the salicylates (including aspirin), which are *not* ionized to any great extent in gastric secretions, begin to be rapidly absorbed from the stomach soon after they are swallowed. In fact, aspirin is so readily absorbed from both the stomach and the small intestine—whether given by itself or combined with buffers or in carbonated form—that all the television commercial "controversy" as to which pain-relieving product acts fastest is essentially pointless.

Parenteral Absorption. The speed of a drug's absorption after injection of a watery solution in which it is dissolved depends, in part, upon the blood supply of the injection site. Thus, drugs are absorbed from muscles, which are abundantly supplied with blood vessels, more rapidly than from subcutaneous tissues, with their relatively poor blood supply. In general, therefore, the intramuscular route would be preferred in an emergency when more rapid onset of action is desired. On the other hand, when the doctor wants the drug to act more slowly but with a steadily sustained effect—e.g., when epinephrine is used in treating bronchial asthma—he may prefer to place the drug in a subcutaneous depot site.

Of course, the absorption of drugs from injection sites can be retarded or accelerated by other means. For example, massaging the area into which epinephrine was injected can force more of the drug into the asthmatic patient's blood stream if his breathing becomes difficult. On the other hand, a drug may be administered in a pharmaceutical dosage form that delays its absorption. Since a drug is eliminated from the body only after it has entered the blood stream and has been carried to the detoxifying and excretory organs, the length of the drug's activity can sometimes be considerably prolonged by measures that slow its passage into the circulation.

Repository Dosage Forms. One way to slow a parenterally administered drug's absorption and increase the duration of its action is to suspend it in a colloidal or a fatty substance from which it is only slowly released. The antidiabetic hormone insulin, for example, requires much less frequent injection when it is suspended in protamine. Patients who require anticoagulant drug therapy can be kept heparinized around the clock with relatively few injections of a gelatin suspension of heparin into an intramuscular depot. The duration of action of corticotropin (ACTH) can be similarly extended.

Drugs that are so rapidly absorbed and eliminated that they require inconveniently frequent and possibly painful injections are sometimes converted into relatively insoluble salts and esters. Penicillin G, for example, is available in the form of the benzathine and the procaine salts. When watery suspensions of these substances are deposited deep in a muscular site, the antibiotic dissolves only gradually in tissue fluids, and so it is absorbed slowly into the circulation. Thus, this dosage form serves as a muscular depot that keeps penicillin in the blood and tissues for long periods by slowly and steadily replacing the portion of the circulating antibiotic that is being excreted by the patient's kidneys.

The hormones testosterone and estradiol are now available as relatively insoluble esters such as the cypionate or the enanthate. Dissolved in a suitable vegetable oil, these substances provide long-lasting hormonal activity. The patient is spared the pain and expense of the frequent injections that were required when the rapidly absorbed and quickly metabolized hormone was employed. (It is imperative to take every precaution with oily solutions or suspensions of particulate material to avoid intravascular injection, which might cause formation of a fat embolism.)

Intravenous Administration. When a drug solution is injected directly into a vein, its absorption is instantaneous. Sometimes (though not always) its onset of action also is all but immediate. This has both advantages and dangers. Thus, when a patient is in a state of shock, morphine I.V. is much more effective than the same drug injected subcutaneously, which would have to make its way to the brain through an inadequately functioning peripheral circulatory system.

On the other hand, dumping an entire dose of morphine directly into the patient's blood stream might result in further depression of his circulation and respiration, and adverse drug reactions could not be counteracted by applying a tourniquet or ice packs to slow absorption, as is possible in the case of most other parenteral injections. Therefore, intravenous injections usually are made slowly to avoid having the drug reach the brain, heart or other vital organ in so high a concentration that it exerts too powerful an effect. The patient is observed closely before the plunger is pressed to inject each new increment of the drug, in order to detect any signs of adverse effects that might make it necessary to discontinue the injection.

DRUG DISTRIBUTION

The fact that a drug gains immediate access to the blood stream does not necessarily mean that it produces a rapid and powerful pharmacological effect. For, once the drug has been absorbed into the circulation, it must still make its way from the blood into the fluids bathing the tissues of the organ on which it acts. Many factors may keep the molecules of the drug from penetrating into particular tissues and exerting its effects on their cells.

The term *distribution* refers to the manner in which a drug is *transported* by the blood stream to various areas of the body and to those factors which are involved in its ability to accumulate in some tissues or in its failure to enter other regions in significant amounts. The pattern of a drug's distribution often determines how rapidly it acts and how long its effects last, or even whether it will act at all. Recent studies of the complex physicochemical factors responsible for the pathways taken by individual drugs have revealed what happens to the molecules of various drugs as they move about the body. Thus, we can now offer some relatively simple explanations for the specific actions observed when certain drugs are used clinically.

Plasma Binding. When some drug molecules enter the blood stream, they immediately become attached to the plasma proteins. As long as the drug stays tied to these macromolecules, it cannot exert any effect on other tissues, because the drug-protein complex cannot diffuse out of the blood stream through the pores of the capillary walls. However, such protein binding is not irreversible, and some of the drug molecules are constantly being released from their loose complex with the albumin of the blood. The freed molecules may then diffuse into the tissue fluids and make the kinds of connections with cellular receptors that result in drug actions. Of course, such freedom also exposes the drug to forces that can destroy it or remove it from the body.

Drugs that are tightly bound to plasma proteins and are only gradually freed tend to have a long half-life. (The term *half-life* refers to the time it takes for the body to eliminate half of the peak quantity that a drug has reached in the circulation; it serves as an index of a drug's duration of action.) A drug that does not leave the blood stream cannot be destroyed by enzymes in such tissues as the liver, nor can it be excreted by the kidneys. Thus, a long-acting sulfonamide drug such as sulfamethoxypyridazine, owes its long-lasting anti-infective action to the fact that it is released only slowly from this circulating storage depot.

Other Storage Sites. The fact that a drug tends to concentrate in certain tissues from which it is only slowly released does not necessarily mean that these tissues are the site of its pharmacological actions. Thus, the fact that the antimalarial drugs quinacrine and chloroquine tend to accumulate in the skin and liver does not mean that this is where they act. Nor does the fact that most of any administered dose of the barbiturate thiopental winds up eventually in the body's fat depots indicate that these inactive tissues are where it has its significant pharmacological effects. Likewise, although digitalis accumulates in kidneys, liver and skeletal muscles, its main action is exerted on the myocardium.

The Blood-Brain Barrier. The affinity of thiopental for fatty tisue, or lipids, plays an important part in its ability to enter the brain and produce sleep. When this fat-soluble substance is injected intravenously, it is carried swiftly to the brain and immediately penetrates the so-called blood-brain barrier. This is *not* an actual membrane like the meninges, but the cells of which it is made up behave like other biological membranes in their ability to let in lipid-soluble, non-ionized substances and to bar the entrance of molecules that are strongly ionized and poorly soluble in fat.

Thus, thiopental, a drug of very high lipid solubility, passes promptly from the blood into the brain, and the relatively high concentration that it immediately attains there produces sleep within seconds. On the other hand, other less lipid-soluble barbiturates, such as phenobarbital or barbital, may take half an hour to forty-five minutes to bring about the same degree of central nervous system depression, even when they are injected directly into the blood stream.

Redistribution. Drugs ordinarily do not remain in the tissues to which they are first transported. Thus, a drug such as thiopental, which first piles up in the brain because of that organ's rich blood supply, does not ordinarily stay there very long but is redistributed to the much larger mass of body tissues for which it has an equal (or even greater) physicochemical affinity. After a very short time, during which the blood circulating through the brain carries the drug molecules to the rest of the body, the level of thiopental in the nervous system falls below that needed to keep the patient asleep, and he quickly awakens.

Where does the drug go, as it drains out of the brain? It is carried to the fat depots, skeletal muscles, connective tissues, skin and bones. These regions do not have as rapid a rate of blood flow as the brain and, thus, did not get as much of the lipid-soluble drug immediately after its injection as did the nervous system. Eventually, however, most of the drug

makes its way to this greater mass of tissue and accumulates there.

Because the drug is still present in the body in an active form, some of its molecules continue to move from fat and muscles back into the blood stream which then carries them to the brain. Ordinarily, the drug's concentration in the nervous system stays well below the level needed to put the patient back to sleep. In some circumstances, however, the so-called "ultra-short-acting" barbiturate may keep the patient asleep for an unexpectedly long time—for example, when a patient has received large amounts of thiopental by continuous intravenous infusion, in order to keep him unconscious during a lengthy surgical procedure. Eventually, the depots of fat and muscle become completely saturated with the barbiturate which they receive directly and by redistribution from the brain. The excess spills over into the blood and is carried back to the brain to accumulate there once more, and the brain levels can then be reduced only by the body's metabolizing the drug or excreting it.

DRUG METABOLISM AND EXCRETION

Although the action of thiopental is usually terminated by its rapid redistribution from the brain to other tissues, its actual removal from the body is a much slower process. As is the case with most other drugs, this barbiturate is first broken down to pharmacologically inactive fragments by liver enzyme systems. These metabolites are then removed from the body by the kidneys. If the body did not possess such mechanisms for converting drugs to more easily excreted compounds, a drug such as thiopental could, theoretically, never leave the system once it had entered it.

Cumulation of Drugs. The ability of the body to transform drugs into inactive metabolites or to eliminate drugs intact is a very important factor. If a person's mechanisms for detoxifying and excreting drugs are not functioning normally, even ordinarily safe doses of a drug may accumulate sufficiently to produce undesired toxic effects. In fact, overdosage can occur even in healthy people when they ingest a chemical in amounts greater than the body's metabolic and excretory mechanisms can handle it. For example, in *alcoholic intoxication*, the drinker absorbs more of an alcoholic beverage than his tissues can destroy and eliminate in the time between drinks. The cumulative action, as each new increment of alcohol is added to the residues remaining in the body, causes effects much more severe than those produced by any one drink.

On the other hand, some drugs are so swiftly transformed into inactive metabolites and excreted that it is difficult to keep them at tissue levels that allow their actions to be maintained for any length of time. In such cases, an extra-large priming dose may be administered, followed by some special dosage form that delays the drug's release and thus prolongs the duration of its presence at active levels.

Priming dosage is often used with sulfonamides and with digitalis glycosides to assure that active levels of these drugs are reached rapidly in the tissues by giving amounts that temporarily exceed the body's capacity for eliminating these agents. Once an active level of drug is established by such rapid cumulation, the doctor orders smaller doses—just enough of the drug to replace that which has been eliminated by the body since the previous dose. Thus, in administering digitalis, we must note the difference between the first, large priming or digitalizing doses and the later, much smaller maintenance doses of this drug.

Biotransformation. The bodies of human beings and those of other animals possess mechanisms for converting foreign molecules to harmless substances. These chemical alterations are brought about by enzyme systems in the blood and in all body cells but particularly those of the liver. The enzyme systems capable of catalyzing these chemical reactions have, of course, been developed over the ages by evolutionary processes.

It may seem strange that the body should have the means for dealing with newly synthesized drugs in the same manner in which it protected itself against foreign compounds taken in with foods in ages past. Actually, however, almost all of the biochemical reactions in which drugs and chemicals are transformed to harmless substances are based upon a relatively few broad, general processes. These biochemical reactions, which occur with all kinds of chemical compounds, may be classified into four main types: *oxidation, reduction, hydrolysis,* and *conjugation,* or *synthesis.*

We shall not take up the nature of these reactions in detail; however, we should note that all these metabolic transformations usually result in the formation of new chemicals which are *less active* pharmacologically than the parent compound and *more readily eliminated.* Occasionally, the metabolite formed by chemical alteration of a drug may prove to be *more* toxic than the agent originally administered. Certain of the early sulfonamide drugs, for example, were changed to substances more poorly soluble in the urine. These acetylated sulfonamides then tended to precipitate out of the urine as sharp crystals capable of cutting and damaging delicate kidney tubes (Chap. 35).

The liver is the single most important site of drug detoxification. Hepatic cells contain tiny particles called microsomes, which are packed with enzymes capable of catalyzing the oxidation, reduction and hydrolysis-type reactions responsible for the breakdown of most drug molecules to inactive metabolites. The duration and intensity of the actions of drugs that are metabolized in the liver can be profoundly influenced by many conditions that affect the functioning of these hepatic microsomal enzyme systems.

Excretion. The body eliminates drugs and their metabolites by many routes. Drugs may be excreted through the sweat glands onto the skin surface; they may appear in saliva, bile, or even mother's milk. The volatile general anesthetics and other drugs are eliminated largely by the lungs. The gases cyclopropane and nitrous oxide, for example, are exhaled after returning intact to the alveoli from the central nervous system; and alcohol excreted in the breath can be measured chemically in the so-called drunkometer tests employed to determine blood-alcohol concentrations.

The kidneys are the organs that play the most important part in the elimination of drugs. The molecules of the unchanged drug or of its metabolites are first filtered through the glomeruli. Sometimes, more of the drug's molecules are added to the glomerular filtrate by the process of tubular secretion—the transport of substances from the blood into the renal tubular fluid. Penicillin, for example, is excreted rapidly by glomerular filtration and tubular secretion.

With most drugs, another process—tubular reabsorption—plays a part in returning most of the filtered molecules to the blood stream before they can leave the body in the urine. The drug molecules filtered by the glomeruli into the tubular fluid diffuse back into the plasma through the membranes of the epithelial cells that line the tubules. Interestingly, the metabolites of most drugs are less readily reabsorbed and more rapidly excreted than their parent compounds. The biotransformations of these drugs convert them into compounds which are more highly ionized and less lipid-soluble—physicochemical properties that reduce a drug's ability to penetrate cell membranes. Thus, the metabolite molecules that appear in the glomerular filtrate do not readily make their way through the tubular cell membranes and back into the blood but are largely carried off in the urine and excreted.

Reabsorption of drug molecules by the renal tubules may be reduced artificially, in order to speed their elimination. In poisoning by aspirin or barbiturates, for example, the patient's urine is alkalinized by injecting sodium bicarbonate intravenously, in order to raise the number of ionized drug particles in the glomerular filtrate. This, in turn, reduces the amount of the drug that returns to the blood and increases the amounts excreted by the kidneys. As a result, the patient recovers more readily from poisoning by these drugs.

METABOLIC AND EXCRETORY FACTORS INFLUENCING DRUG ACTION

Many factors may influence the body's ability to inactivate and excrete drugs. If a drug enters the body and is absorbed at a rate greater than it can be eliminated, it can accumulate until it reaches toxic levels in the reactive tissues. When, on the other hand, conditions occur that speed a drug's breakdown and elimination, the effects of an average dose may be much less than one would have predicted. Thus, individual variation in the response to drugs can often be traced to differences in the rates at which different people metabolize and excrete administered drugs.

Age and Drug Elimination. The patient's age often makes a difference in the way he reacts to drugs. Recent evidence indicates that newborn infants require much smaller doses than would be expected on the basis of size and body weight because they have not yet developed adequate mechanisms for metabolizing and excreting foreign chemicals. For example, penicillin is poorly secreted by the renal tubules of such infants, and therefore therapeutic antibacterial blood levels of this antibiotic can be maintained by administering only small doses at relatively infrequent intervals.

Unfortunately some premature infants have died because their incomplete metabolic and excretory mechanisms permitted the accumulation of toxic amounts of other anti-infective agents. The antibiotic chloramphenicol, for example, has caused fatalities in infants who had not developed the capacity to metabolize and excrete the drug in the amounts that were administered. Similarly, the sulfonamide drug sulfisoxazole has caused jaundice and kernicterus in premature infants. This has also been traced to their metabolic immaturity—resulting, in this case, in a piling up of bile pigments in the blood and brain.

Genetic Abnormalities and Drug Elimination. The sensitivity of newborn infants to some drugs has a counterpart in adults who lack certain enzymes required for drug detoxification. Such enzyme deficiencies have been traced to a hereditary defect. For example, some members of a few families are born with an abnormal plasma cholinesterase, an enzyme that catalyzes the hydrolytic breakdown of various esters, including the drugs procaine and succinylcholine.

Ordinarily, the latter drug, which is injected by vein in order to produce relaxation of skeletal muscles during anesthesia, is rapidly detoxified. However, patients with a genetically induced lack of the plasma enzyme *pseudocholinesterase* have suffered prolonged paralysis of the respiratory muscles after administration of relatively small amounts of succinylcholine. The abnormally slow metabolic activity of the altered,

or atypical, plasma pseudocholinesterase enzyme permits the undestroyed drug to exert its effects on the muscles of respiration for long periods. The patient then requires mechanical oxygenation during the period of prolonged apnea that results.

Pathology and Drug Elimination. In the same way, drugs administered in doses that cause no difficulties for most patients may prove dangerous for those with diseases of the liver or kidneys. This is why so many drugs that require detoxification or excretion by these organs are considered contraindicated in patients with *hepatic* or *renal* disease.

Unexpectedly severe drug reactions sometimes develop in patients with undetected pathology of these drug-metabolizing and excreting organs. The administration of only a small dose of morphine, for example, may precipitate hepatic coma in a patient with cirrhosis of the liver. This occurs, in part, because the liver cells which ordinarily dispose of the narcotic have been destroyed by disease and replaced by scar tissue. Because the liver lacks detoxifying enzymes, the patient cannot adequately metabolize the morphine, which stays in the brain in unusually high levels for long periods.

Similarly, a patient with a severely damaged liver is not a good candidate for basal anesthesia with a barbiturate such as thiopental. Lack of the liver enzymes that ordinarily destroy this drug may lead to long persisting and abnormally large blood and brain levels of this depressant drug. Thus, in patients with unsuspected partial hepatic insufficiency, the use of this usually ultra-short-acting barbiturate may cause unexpectedly deep and prolonged unconsciousness or death from respiratory failure.

Drugs that are ordinarily excreted by the kidneys can cause unusual reactions when administered in seemingly safe doses to patients with renal insufficiency. The drug, which the kidneys cannot transfer to the urine, stays in the blood and tissues at unexpectedly high levels. If further doses are administered, the drug can accumulate to toxic levels in various tissues.

The antibiotics streptomycin and kanamycin, for example, which are administered parenterally for tuberculosis or other infections, are readily excreted by the kidneys. In patients with impaired renal function, however, these drugs may pile up, first in the kidney tissues and later in other organs, including both branches of the eighth cranial nerve. This may lead to further kidney damage from the nephrotoxic effects of these drugs. In addition, continued accumulation of unexcreted drug in the auditory and vestibular nerves may cause deafness and loss of equilibrium, even though only seemingly safe doses had been injected at what was thought to be proper intervals.

The presence of kidney disease may convert a quite harmless drug into a dangerous one. Magnesium sulfate (Epsom salts) is an example: solutions of this drug are sometimes given by mouth to produce a local cathartic action in the intestine. The small amounts of magnesium ions that manage to make their way into the blood stream by passing through the intestinal mucosa are promptly passed out in the urine by the excretory action of healthy kidneys. Occasionally, however, in children or elderly patients with impaired renal function, failure to excrete magnesium ions results in coma, because the abnormally high levels of this substance depress brain function. The hypersusceptibility of elderly patients to some drugs can often be traced to failing kidney or liver function.

Tolerance. As we have seen, some patients may be hypersusceptible to drugs because they lack adequate amounts of drug-detoxifying enzymes. Others may, on the other hand, be *hypo*susceptible to the actions of certain drugs—that is, these patients do not respond as strongly as expected when they receive an ordinary dose of the drug. One reason for such unusual resistance or ability to tolerate drugs is the presence in the patient's body of enzymatic biotransformation mechanisms of increased efficiency. Thus, the patient's body is able to dispose of the drug so rapidly that it does not readily attain and maintain the concentration in the reactive tissue that is needed to produce pharmacological effects.

Some people and some strains of animals (see *species differences*, Chap. 1) are born with such an increased capacity to metabolize certain kinds of drugs. Such congenital tolerance is thought to account for the fact that people from some families react quite differently to doses of the antituberculosis drug isoniazid (INH), for example, than do patients from other families. Some patients metabolize isoniazid so rapidly that they require unusually large daily doses to maintain the blood and tissue levels effective for controlling the bacteria. These "rapid inactivators" show congenital tolerance to isoniazid because they possess a gene that produces an active enzyme system. On the other hand, patients who lack this gene inactivate isoniazid so slowly that it often tends to accumulate to toxic levels in certain of the peripheral nerves.

Tolerance to the actions of some drugs may be *acquired* when patients continue to take the drug over a period of time, so that a patient may soon require doses much larger than he did at first in order to obtain the drug's desired pharmacological effects. One reason for such resistance may be the fact that, in the presence of the drug, the body develops the ability to remove the chemical in larger amounts and more rapidly. For example, it has been found recently that the administration of barbiturates and other drugs somehow induces the synthesis of additional drug-oxidizing enzymes in liver cell microsomes. Thus,

such *enzyme induction* may account in part for the patient's increased ability to tolerate doses of the depressant drugs which had at first made him drowsy and produced sleep. (Other aspects of the phenomenon of tolerance are discussed on pp. 33–34.)

Combined Effects of Drugs. One of the most important factors influencing the effect that a dose of a drug may produce is the presence in the body of some other drug at the same time. The fact that the effect produced by a dose of one drug may be modified by other drugs that the patient is taking has considerable practical importance. Thus, two or more drugs often may be given in combination deliberately to produce a better therapeutic result than could be obtained if each one were given singly. On the other hand, drugs may sometimes interact in ways that were not foreseeable and that may result in serious adverse effects in some circumstances.

When one drug is administered while another is exerting its effects at the same time, the action of the primary agent may be either increased or decreased. Drugs that work together or cooperate to bring about a particular effect are said to be *synergistic* * (Gr. *syn* = together + *erg* = work); drugs that act simultaneously in ways that produce opposing effects are called *antagonistic*.

Some drugs, when given in combination, work together to bring about effects that are simply the sum of the effects which each produces separately (e.g., effect x + effect x = 2x). Such *simple summation,* or *addition,* is often sought by the doctor when he orders that certain drugs be given in combination.

Sometimes, combining drugs causes a more dramatic intensification or prolongation of the actions of one or both agents than that observed in simple summation. One form of such synergism—positive summation—is sometimes called (some say, incorrectly) potentiative. The term *potentiation,* when used in this way, means that the two drugs given together cause an effect that is more than merely additive. That is, their effects are *greater* than the expected sum of their separate actions. (E.g., effect x + effect x = effect 3x or effect 5x, etc.)

Potentiation is most impressive when the effect of one of the drugs in a combination is markedly increased by the addition of a drug that does not even

---

* The various terms used to describe the combined actions of drugs currently are used in different ways by different writers. Thus, some authorities reserve the term *synergism* to describe only what we have defined as *potentiation*. Others, on the other hand, speak of "synergism" when the total effect of combining two drugs is merely *additive*. In fact, some writers—usually those who prepare advertising copy for drug product manufacturers—refer to the "synergistic effects" of combinations of drugs which may even have quite *different* effects, but which are claimed to be better for accomplishing a particular therapeutic aim than competing products containing only a single ingredient.

share the same kind of activity. Such intensification of the effect of the active drug often occurs because: the second drug (1) does something to raise the concentration of the active drug in the vicinity of the reactive tissues or (2) keeps the first drug at active concentrations for an unusually long period.

For example, the action of an active drug ordinarily may be rapidly terminated through the detoxifying effect of a specific enzyme system. If a drug of another class *interferes* with the enzymes responsible for the destruction of the active drug, the effects of the active drug are likely to be *intensified* and *prolonged*. The powerful neurohormone acetylcholine, for example, is ordinarily destroyed by a hydrolytic reaction catalyzed by the enzyme acetylcholinesterase. When an enzyme-inhibiting drug such as neostigmine (Prostigmin) is administered, the enzyme's substrate, acetylcholine, is not inactivated as rapidly as usual. Instead, this neurohormone accumulates in the vicinity of the reactive cells to produce effects much more powerful than the usual ones.

Similarly, certain other drugs tend to suppress the activity of the enzyme monoamineoxidase (MAO), which participates in the inactivation of another neurohormone, norepinephrine. If norepinephrine or certain related sympathomimetic drugs are then administered, their effects are markedly increased. Such potentiation of sympathetic nervous system effects has led to serious reactions when patients receiving monoamineoxidase inhibitor drugs happen to take sympathomimetic drugs in cold remedies or in weight-reducing products. The potential hazards in store for patients who medicate themselves with nonprescription drugs while taking various prescribed drugs are only now beginning to be understood. However, enough is known so that the nurse should warn patients *not* to purchase remedies for self-medication while taking prescribed drugs, without first consulting their physician.

Potentiation of an active drug can also be brought about by combining it with a drug that *interferes with its renal excretion*. For example, when the drug probenecid (Benemid) is administered together with penicillin, it tends to prevent the secretion of penicillin by the renal tubules. As a result of the reduced rate of renal excretion, the antibiotic remains in the blood and tissues at relatively high levels for longer periods. Thus, the addition of the potentiating agent probenecid intensifies and prolongs the antibacterial effect of penicillin.

Finally, another way in which one drug may raise the concentration of another at the reactive tissue may be illustrated by the commonly used injectable which is a combination of local anesthetic agents with vasoconstrictor drugs such as epinephrine. By reducing the local flow of blood, the latter drug prevents the local anesthetic from being absorbed too swiftly into the systemic circulation. Instead of being swept away into the blood stream, the anesthetic stays at the injection site in effective concentration. This lengthens its desired local anesthetic action. (See p. 34 for further examples of synergism and potentiation.)

THE RESPONSES OF REACTIVE CELLS TO DRUGS

We have examined some of the complex physico-chemical and biochemical factors that determine how great a concentration of an active drug accumulates in the tissues that are capable of responding to it. Now we shall discuss the ways in which the reactive cells respond to drugs that reach them in amounts adequate for bringing about changes in function—that is, to drugs that attain critical concentration in the tissues.

In broadest terms, we may think of therapeutic agents as acting in two ways: (1) By producing *pharmacodynamic* changes in the functioning of various of the patient's cells, organs and systems, and (2) by acting as *chemotherapeutic agents* to interfere with the functioning of cell populations foreign to the body, such as invading microorganisms. The term *chemotherapy* which was originally employed to describe the use of chemicals, in the treatment of infectious diseases, is now often used to indicate also the action of drugs employed for selectively destroying cancer cells.

The specific pharmacodynamic effects of drugs on cells can be broadly divided into (1) *stimulation* and (2) *depression*. In addition, some substances act in a nonspecific manner to elicit tissue reactions of a more fundamental nature such as inflammation (e.g., the so-called "irritant" effects of chemicals).

Drugs that are derived from animal tissues are also often used in physiological amounts as replacement therapy. For example, the powdered thyroid glands of cows or pigs may be used to substitute for the thyroid hormone that a human patient lacks; and insulin obtained from animal pancreas often takes the place of the hormone absent in the patient with diabetes.

Stimulation refers to a drug-induced *increase* in the activity of certain reactive cells, with the result that some functions over which they exert control may be intensified. This is perhaps best illustrated by the action of drugs that imitate the effects of neurohormones or otherwise add to their activity. Thus, the so-called sympathomimetic drugs stimulate those functions of the heart that are under the control of the sympathetic nervous system and its neurohormone norepinephrine.

Depression refers to the *reduction* in cellular activity brought about by the actions of some drugs.

This drug-induced decrease in activity is best seen in the effects of drugs that block the normal effects of neurohormones. Thus, the cholinergic blocking agent atropine reduces the responsiveness of the smooth muscle and exocrine gland cells which are ordinarily activated by the neurohormone acetylcholine. Other depressant drugs, such as the barbiturates, specifically reduce the functional activity of groups of nerve cells in the brain stem and elsewhere in the central nervous system.

Actually, the effects of interactions between drugs and living tissues are much more complicated than our casual use of the terms stimulation and depression suggests. For example, although a drug depresses some cellular biochemical reaction, the end result of this may be an *increase* in the activity of some interrelated physiologic system. Thus, the depressant effect of atropine on certain inhibitory cardiac cells actually results in an acceleration of the heart rate. Within the central nervous system, too, drug-induced depression of cells that ordinarily exert an inhibitory function releases other neurons, whose activities are then intensified.

Sites and Mechanisms of Drug Action. Pharmacologists frequently conduct studies to determine exactly *where* in the body a drug acts to bring about the observed pharmacological effects. Then, when the group of cells that serves as the *locus* or *site* of a particular drug action has been identified, these scientists often try to find the locus of action on the cellular level and to determine the *mechanism* by which the effect is brought about—that is, they attempt to learn just *how* the drug influences some crucial biochemical or physicochemical step in cellular function.

Some studies of the manner in which drug molecules interact with living molecules—that is, *molecular pharmacology*—are technically difficult to do. They are also somewhat frustrating in the sense that the more the scientist learns about drug-cell interactions, the more he realizes how much still remains to be learned. He is not, however, concerned if his findings seem to have no immediate practical application. For the investigator of drug and tissue interactions is advancing the search for new knowledge, and he knows that, through the use of drugs as research tools, he is contributing to a deeper understanding of the nature of cellular chemistry and function.

Nurses also often find it intellectually stimulating and professionally fruitful to study some of the more intimate reactions by which drugs and poisons bring about their effects. For this reason we shall try to indicate throughout this text *where* and *how* certain important drugs act to produce their therapeutically useful and their toxic effects. Instead of merely saying that a drug does something—causes a fall in blood pressure, for example, or relieves pain—we shall explore its actions at somewhat deeper levels. For we think that when the nurse has a deeper understanding of precisely where and how a drug is acting, she is able to offer the patient more intelligent care, as well as gain greater satisfaction from her practice. Thus, we offer the following generalizations about the locus and mechanism of drug action as background for the more specific discussions of these aspects of the action of individual drugs that will be discussed later.

Locus of Drug Action. The site of a drug's action may sometimes be far distant from the organ which it stimulates into increased activity or which reacts with reduced function. Conversely, as indicated earlier in this chapter, the fact that a drug accumulates in a particular tissue does not mean that this is where it exerts its important pharmacological effects. This may seem strange in view of the emphasis we have previously laid on the importance of factors that influence a drug's ability to concentrate in reactive tissues.

The term *reactive tissues* is the key to the seeming contradiction. Thus, in the case of skeletal muscles, the drug-reactive tissues responsible for muscle relaxation or contraction may often be not the muscles themselves but the central nervous system cells which send out the impulses that control muscular activity. On the other hand, a drug may accumulate in skeletal muscles without producing any effects in these structures because, although tissues are capable of binding the drug, the resulting drug-tissue complexes do not have any intrinsic ability to alter the physiological functioning of the muscles. Thus, to produce an effect a drug must have more than a mere chemical affinity for any tissue in which it accumulates. Not only does the presence of a drug not assure changes in physiological function of that tissue, but such binding to "silent" receptors may actually keep the drug from acting elsewhere in the body.

A physiological state may be altered by drugs that act at any of several different sites. For example, drugs can reduce high blood pressure by acting either at central nervous system sites or peripherally in the heart or blood vessels. Thus, one drug may act at the vasomotor center, another at the sympathetic ganglia, a third at the sympathetic nerve endings and still another in the smooth muscles of the blood vessels or in the myocardium. The end result of the actions of all these drugs is the same—a drop in blood pressure.

Similarly, pain may be relieved by any of several different classes of drugs, each of which acts at a different site. The pain caused by spasm of a muscle may be made to vanish by administering an antispasmodic drug that causes the muscle to relax. Pain also disappears when the peripheral nerve fibers that carry sensory impulses toward the central nervous system are blocked by injecting a local anesthetic drug. Other agents—analgesics and general anesthetics—can reduce awareness of muscle pain through their actions upon groups of nerve cells in the brain.

Knowledge of a drug's exact sites of action has practical value in various ways. Drugs with different sites of action are sometimes combined, in order to gain their additive effects in producing a particular therapeutically desirable action. Thus, in treating a patient with hypertension, the doctor commonly orders combinations of two or more drugs that lower blood pressure by actions at different sites. The sum of the actions of relatively small doses of several drugs is often greater than the action that could be produced by a large dose of one drug acting at a single site, and the side effects of each may be diminished.

Mechanisms of Drug Action. Once the action of a drug has been localized, attempts are sometimes made to determine the nature of the affinity between drug molecules and cellular constituents that accounts for the functional changes in cellular activity. Scientists try to learn whether the drug acts on the surface of the cell to alter the characteristics of the cell membrane, or whether it penetrates into the cell to react with some intracellular structure, such as the nucleus, mitochondria or microsomes. They may even try to pinpoint the drug's action at a particular enzyme system or seek to understand the nature of the physical and chemical forces that drive an active group of atoms in the drug molecule toward a complementary chemical grouping on the surface of an enzyme molecule or other cell constituent.

THEORIES OF DRUG ACTION

It is generally agreed that most potent drugs produce their effects by interacting with cellular components that are chemically specialized to combine and react with the foreign molecules. However, there is no one theory capable of explaining all of the different ways in which drugs act. Broadly speaking, we may say that drugs act: (1) by combining with cellular constituents called *receptors;* (2) by interacting with cellular *enzyme systems,* and (3) by affecting the *physicochemical properties* of the outer cell membrane and of intracellular structures in ways still not well understood. Let us now look briefly at each of these modes of action.

Receptor Theory. Many potent drugs are believed to act by combining with chemical groups, on the cell surface or within the cell, for which they possess a *specific affinity.* Such a specific cellular reagent is called a *receptor* or the *receptive substance.* In no case do we know the exact chemical nature of a cellular receptor. However, it is believed that receptors contain chemical groups that attract drug molecules that have a shape that permits them to approach

the receptor surface and fit into it. When the foreign chemical key fits this cellular lock in the same way as natural body chemicals do, the drug may be able to set off the same chain of biochemical reactions as the natural chemical, thus resulting in increased cellular activity.

Thus, the natural body chemical acetylcholine combines with receptors in the membranes of muscle and nerve cells that are chemically specialized to receive it. This binding of acetylcholine with the cholinoceptive substance then sets off changes that may, for example, make muscle cells contract or trigger nerve cell signals. Certain synthetic drugs that resemble acetylcholine chemically can fit the same cellular receptors. As a result, these foreign chemicals interact with the receptors in ways that bring about functional changes similar to the ones that occur naturally. Drugs that have a chemical affinity for a receptor and form a complex with it of a kind that produces a functional change are called *agonists.*

Not all drugs with chemical structures that fit cellular receptors are capable of acting as agonists. A foreign chemical may be bound to tissue components for which its molecules have a chemical affinity, without initiating any pharmacological action. The drug-receptor complex formed in such cases is *not* capable of setting off the sequence of biochemical events that result in a pharmacological effect. Such a drug may, in fact, act as an *antagonist* to a natural agonist.

If, for example, a chemical such as atropine or curare, which is capable of attaching itself to a cholinergic receptor, forms a complex that *lacks intrinsic activity,* the natural agonist, acetylcholine may not be able to initiate the series of steps responsible for normal cellular activity. That is, the atropine or curare molecules *compete* with acetylcholine for the cellular receptor sites. If these bulky molecules occupy the receptors, they block acetylcholine's access to these cellular sites and, thus, interfere with the normal activity of the muscle, gland or nerve cells. Although such *competitive antagonists* of acetylcholine as atropine and curare do not produce the kind of activity that results when the natural chemical combines with cellular receptors, these drugs are, of course, anything but "inactive." On the contrary, by interfering with the normal agonist-receptor reactions, these blocking drugs produce powerful pharmacological effects—that is, changes from normal physiological functions.

Drug-Enzyme Interactions. Many drugs are believed to act by affecting the functioning of cellular enzyme systems. Enzymes are the molecules that control all the chemical reactions constantly going on within living cells. Each cellular enzyme controls only one chemical reaction; that is, an enzyme is capable of reacting with only one specific molecule—its *substrate.* Thus, a drug that affects the functioning of an enzyme does so because its molecular configuration resembles that of the enzyme's substrate in some respect.

Many of the principles of drug-receptor reactions apply also to drug-enzyme interactions. Just as the receptor surface possesses chemical groups specialized to receive the molecules of agonist—molecules with a complementary shape or configuration—the surface of each enzyme has special *active sites* or *"centers"* that are designed to receive certain atomic groupings of the substrate molecule. The enzyme-substrate complex formed by the binding of these complementary chemical groups is broken in a tiny fraction of a second, but not before the substrate has been converted into new chemical products. These new products in turn form the substrates for still other enzymes in the series of continuing chemical reactions by which the cell produces its energy and synthesizes its own substance. The freed enzyme molecule is ready to react with still another molecule of its substrate within thousandths of a second.

A foreign chemical may have a structure similar in some respects to that of the natural substrate of an enzyme. Thus, the drug molecule may be able to approach the enzyme surface and form a complex with the active centers. However, the enzyme cannot work on the foreign chemical in exactly the way it acts on its natural substrate. As a result, the products needed for normal cellular activity fail to be formed.

Competitive inhibition of an enzyme in this way is the manner in which many drugs produce their effects. A natural chemical needed by the cell (i.e., a metabolite) may often be kept from combining with its specific enzyme because of the presence of a foreign chemical that closely resembles the essential substance. The cell then is unable to produce other substances that it and the whole organism require. Such *antimetabolite* drugs are used to kill neoplastic cells in the treatment of cancer (Chap. 44). Similarly, bacterial cells can sometimes be deprived of natural nutritive substances by the use of drugs that possess chemical structures similar to those of the essential metabolites. The antibacterial sulfonamide drugs, for example, are believed to act by competing for bacterial enzyme systems that normally take up the vitamin para-aminobenzoic acid (PABA). Although the sulfonamide molecule closely resembles PABA, the bacterial cells cannot use it in the series of enzymatic steps by which the bacteria make certain other substances that are essential for their growth and reproduction (Chap. 35).

The competitive nature of such mechanisms of drug action is evidenced by the fact that the drugs' actions can be overcome by the administration of large enough amounts of the natural metabolite. Thus, bacteria whose growth had been suppressed by sulfonamides can be made to grow again by adding PABA to the growth medium. The natural metabolite molecules apparently compete successfully with the drug for the active sites of the enzyme system in which they are the normal substrate. Similarly, poisoning by drugs that act by competitively inhibiting human cellular enzyme systems that require vitamin K or folic acid can sometimes be reversed by administering the natural metabolites or closely related substances which can then participate in the essential enzymatic steps.

Noncompetitive inhibition occurs when the drug that has suppressed the activity of an enzyme *cannot* be displaced from the active sites of the enzyme surface by any amount of the natural substrate. Various poisons become so firmly bound to the active sites of cellular enzymes that the natural substrate can never make the necessary attachments required for carrying on normal cellular activity.

This does not mean, however, that such poisoning is irreversible. Often, specific chemical antidotes are capable of breaking the bond between the active groups on the enzyme surface and the poison molecule. For example, arsenic molecules can be removed from poisoned tissue systems by the antidotal drug dimercaprol (Chap. 3). Similarly, poisoning by certain organic phosphates that combine irreversibly with the enzyme acetylcholinesterase can be counteracted by the antidotal chemical pralidoxime, which pries the poisonous organic phosphate molecules loose from their tight attachment to the active sites of the enzyme. The enzyme is then once more able to take up and destroy its natural substrate, acetylcholine, which had been piling up to toxic levels in the patient's tissues.

Metal-binding is still another mechanism by which some drugs, poisons and antidotes act. Certain enzymes require tiny traces of metal ions in order to function properly. Substances that tie up these metals can knock out the enzymes and, with them, certain chemical reactions essential to the life of the cell and of the organism itself.

The highly active poison cyanide, for example, inactivates the enzyme cytochrome oxidase, which plays a key part in the series of reactions by which all cells use oxygen to burn foodstuffs for the production of energy. Cyanide ions do their deadly work by combining with iron atoms dispersed at the active points on the surface of this enzyme. When cyanide binds these bits of metal that control the activity of this important enzyme, the cells cannot utilize the oxygen brought to them by the blood, and death swiftly follows.

On the other hand, certain other metal binding drugs can counteract poisoning when carefully employed to remove an excess of an offending metal. A drug called edetate sodium, for example, has the capacity to pick up calcium ions and remove them from the body. This may be desirable in treating poisoning by digitalis, because calcium ions tend to intensify the adverse effects of digitalis on the heart. A related drug, calcium disodium edetate, ties up not calcium but lead ions. This makes it useful for treating lead poisoning (Chap. 3). Other metal-binding agents grasp and remove iron and copper and, thus, are of value in cases of poisoning by those metals.

Physicochemical Mechanisms. Apparently, the activity of many drugs depends on their molecules possessing groups of atoms that fit into specific sites on the surfaces of cellular receptors or enzymes. However, not all drug molecules act by combining with cellular molecules for which they have a special chemical affinity. Some drugs alter cellular function by what seem to be physical rather than chemical reactions.

The general anesthetics, for example, are thought to act on the cells of the central nervous system by affecting the physical properties of their membranes. These volatile substances are inhaled and carried from the lungs to the brain, where they dissolve in the lipids of the nerve cell membranes.

This physical effect could affect neuronal function in any of several ways. For one thing, solution of the drug molecules in the membrane might change the permeability characteristics of the membrane. This, in turn, would affect the flow of ions in and out of the cell and thus alter the polarity upon which nerve impulse generation and conduction depend (Chap. 5). The physically stabilized nerve cell membranes could not then carry on their normal cycles of depolarization and repolarization.

A more recent view of volatile anesthetic action mechanisms is that these anesthetics combine physically with water molecules to form hydrated microcrystals called clathrates. The presence of these tiny "icebergs" may alter the physical properties of nerve cell membranes by interfering with the flow of ions through the pores in the membranes or by affecting the functioning of energy-producing enzymes. In any case, the depressed nerve cell function stems from a nonspecific physical change and not a specific chemical interaction.

Selective Activity. Most drugs produce their particular effects because of their ability to seek out cellular components for which they have a chemical affinity. In order to be useful for altering physiological functions, this selective action upon living molecules in the patient's tissues must be a reversible one. That is, inhibition of an enzyme or blockade of a receptor by a drug molecule must be only temporary when the drug is given to bring about a functional change in a person's tissues. On the other hand, when a drug is administered, not to produce a pharmacodynamic effect, but to destroy parasitic cells which have invaded the patient's tissues, it is desirable that the reaction between the molecules of the drug and those of the infectious microorganisms or the cancer cells be an irreversible and permanent one that will destroy the invasive cells. Ideally, such chemotherapeutic agents should have a selectively toxic effect upon an enzymatic reaction that is essential to the life of the parasitic cells but not important for the functioning of the cells and tissues of the patient.

Selective toxicity of such a degree is relatively rare. A rare example is penicillin—a drug that affects a life process unique to bacteria. More commonly, as in the case of anticancer drugs, the tissues of the patient also may be poisoned because they employ enzymatic reactions essentially similar to those of the neoplastic tissues. However, cancer cells, which grow more rapidly, require more of the essential metabolites for survival, growth and reproduction than do normal, healthy cells. Consequently, leukemic and other neoplastic cells are selectively poisoned, and the patient's disease can be kept under control, for a while at least, with only minimal toxicity to his own tissues. Scientists continue to seek biochemical differences between cancerous cells and normal tissues, in order better to exploit this principle of selective toxicity.

FACTORS INFLUENCING THE REACTIVITY OF CELLS TO DRUGS

We have previously noted that many factors influence the effects that the same dose of a drug may have on different individuals or even on the same person at different times. We have seen that many of these factors are important because they influence the concentration of the drug attained at the reactive tissues—by affecting the rate of the drug's detoxification, or in other ways. Now, let us look at a few examples of factors that account for differences in response by their influence upon the capacity of the target cells to respond.

The physiological state of the cells and systems of the patient plays an important part in determining how he will react to the dose of a drug at different times. Thus, a hypnotic, or sleep-producing, drug is much less effective in the morning than at night, presumably because the body's diurnal rhythms make the nervous system more resistant to drugs early in the day. Of course, as with drug tolerance of all types, increased resistance to hypnotics is limited, and a patient can be put to sleep by increasing the dose of the drug.

Changes in acid-base balance and in the degree of tissue hydration are other physiological factors that sometimes influence the response of patients to drugs. For example, patients who are alkalotic or hypochloremic, respond only sluggishly to treatment with mercurial diuretics. If excess hydrogen and chloride ions are supplied by pretreatment with an acidifying agent such as ammonium chloride, the mercurial diuretic produces copious diuresis.

The tissues of the uterus vary in their responsiveness to certain drugs, depending upon the physiological state of the smooth muscle cells. During the early months of pregnancy, oxytocic drugs such as the ergot alkaloids and posterior pituitary hormones (Chap. 39) exert little or no effect on the uterus. However, as pregnancy advances, this organ undergoes changes that make it increasingly sensitive to drugs that stimulate uterine contractions. Finally, at term, quite small doses of these drugs can elicit powerful contractions.

The sex of the patient makes a difference in the way a person responds to drugs. Women may require smaller doses of certain drugs, not only on account of their generally lower weight but because drugs may affect them differently—for example, during pregnancy, lactation or menstruation. Also, they may show subtle differences in responsiveness to certain drugs. For example, women are said to be more susceptible than men to the excitatory effects of morphine.

The age of a child influences his reaction to drugs that affect the central nervous system. For example, children seem more prone to suffer drug-induced convulsions than do adults. High overdoses of certain antihistaminic drugs, which would only make adults drowsy, sometimes set off seizures in youngsters. Drugs such as the salicylates also have unexpectedly strong effects on the nervous systems of children. Those who are feverish and dehydrated are especially prone to suffer from salicylate poisoning.

Pathological State. The patient's *pathological state* often alters his responsiveness to drugs. A person suffering from hyperthyroidism, for example, is especially sensitive to epinephrine and other adrenergic drugs. On the other hand, he is relatively resistant to depressant drugs, including opiate analgesics. Similarly, a person with fever will often respond to aspirin with a drop of a degree or two, whereas one with normal temperature will show no change in that respect when this analgesic-antipyretic is given only for its pain-relieving effect.

The presence of severe pain tends to increase a patient's resistance to opiates, and an extremely anxious patient can prove resistant to very large doses of sedative drugs. Therefore, if the doctor has ordered analgesics or sedatives on a p.r.n. basis, it is best to administer these drugs soon after the symptoms arise rather than wait until the pain has grown more severe or the patient's anxiety has progressed to the point of agitation, when very much larger doses will be required. (On the other hand, the nurse may wisely decide that the symptoms can be relieved and the need for drugs postponed by talking to the patient to find out what is troubling him and by helping reduce his emotional reactions to his pain or his feelings of fear and helplessness.)

Patients who are in severe pain are able to resist the respiratory depression produced by morphine more readily than when their pain is only moderately severe. Thus, if the source of a patient's pain is suddenly removed—as when a biliary or kidney stone is passed—a morphinized patient's respiration may become slower or shallower than it was while the pain persisted. Similarly, in the patient with cardiac decompensation and congestive heart failure, digitalis increases the cardiac output, whereas this heart stimulant fails to increase the strength and efficiency of a more normally dynamic heart and may, indeed, cause a reduction in its output.

Tolerance of reactive cells to the presence of various drugs, alters the patient's response to ordinary doses. The cause of such tissue tolerance, or cellular resistance, is not very well understood. Unlike the *disposal type* of tolerance discussed earlier, it does *not* depend upon an increased capacity of the body to handle the drug and thus to keep its concentration at the reacting tissues abnormally low. In tolerance of this type, the reactive cells seem to have acquired the capacity to function more or less normally even in the presence of high blood and tissue concentrations of the drug.

A dramatic example of increased *adaptability* of reacting cells to the presence of a drug is the remarkable degree of resistance to opiates often acquired by nervous system cells. Addicts often become capable of taking heroin in doses many times the amount that would kill a nontolerant person. Unfortunately, this phenomenon also occurs in patients who require morphine and other potent pain-relieving drugs for long periods. As a result, the doctor must keep raising the dose and the frequency of administration, in order to keep the patient's pain under control.

Attempts are made to delay the development of tissue tolerance in such patients by giving them only small doses of narcotic analgesics in combination with nonaddicting agents. Dosage of these tolerance-producing drugs is raised only gradually, and they are given on an irregular dosage schedule. The drugs are discontinued temporarily whenever the patient's condition improves and his pain eases. Tolerance diminishes in such circumstances and can even be lost if the period of drug abstinence is long enough. Addicts sometimes deliberately have themselves committed for detoxification treatment only because they want to reduce their tolerance and thus regain the desired effects of the drug when it is taken in smaller, less costly amounts.

Cross tolerance is a phenomenon that develops with different drugs that act at the same cellular sites to produce similar pharmacological effects. Thus, a person who acquires tolerance to the vasodilator effects of glyceryl trinitrate is also relatively resistant to other nitrate and nitrite vasodilators. Addicts tolerant to heroin also withstand the effects of morphine and other opiate and opioid drugs. Alcoholic patients often prove resistant to ether and other general anesthetics that depress the central nervous system in much the same way as alcohol does.

Physical dependence is a phenomenon that often—but not always—accompanies the development of tolerance. In such cases, not only are the cells of the central nervous system adapted to the presence of the drug—they cannot, indeed, function normally when the level of the drug in their vicinity is lowered. Thus, the presence of the drug—opiates, or barbiturates, or alcohol, for example—is required to preserve normal equilibrium; and when the drug is withdrawn, the abnormal activities of the neuronal cells result in a characteristic abstinence syndrome (Chap. 3).

Psychological and **emotional factors** play an important part in the way people respond to drugs. We see this most clearly in the ways in which people respond to placebos. Thus, a person may respond positively or negatively, according to his personal makeup, even though the blank dosage forms that are administered have no pharmacological action at all.

The influence of a person's temperament upon his response to drugs is not, however, limited to placebos. A person's underlying personality structure and the circumstances or setting in which he takes a drug may make his reaction to active drugs quite different from what may be excepted. Such *subjective responses* occur most often when people take drugs that affect their mood or their thought processes—whether alcoholic beverages, marihuana, psychotropic drugs for the treatment of mental and emotional illnesses. Thus, the nurse should be especially observant of the responses of depressed or agitated patients to mood-elevating and tranquilizing drugs (Chap. 7), and she should note whether these drugs are having the desired mental effects or are merely making the patient restless or drowsy. Similarly, a patient's temperament helps to determine the dosage of potent analgesic drugs that he may require for relief of pain.

Combined Drug Actions. The effects of a drug will be different from those expected for the dose given if drugs of the same type or of some different types are already present in the vicinity of the reactive cells. That is, the effect of one drug is altered by the *additive* or *antagonistic* actions of the others. Such synergism and antagonism have many practical applications in situations in which drugs are being taken or administered.

Sometimes, two drugs that have similar pharmacological effects can cause an unexpectedly severe reaction when both are taken. People who drink an alcoholic beverage after taking a barbiturate may suffer a dangerous degree of central depression, because the combined actions of the two drugs on the nervous system reduce the activity of the same groups of brain cells and to a much greater extent than either substance alone would have done.

On the other hand, the combined effects of two depressant drugs on the nervous system need not be harmful and may even be used to advantage. For example, the pain-relieving properties of potent analgesic drugs are often synergized by the administration of a depressant drug of the phenothiazine-tranquilizer type. Chlorpromazine (Thorazine), for example, increases the sedative and analgesic power of morphine.

This reduces the amount of narcotic needed to keep patients comfortable and tends to slow the development of tolerance and physical dependence in patients suffering from chronically painful conditions. Similarly, the addition of promethazine (Phenergan) to meperidine (Demerol) permits reduction of the dosage of the latter analgesic during labor.

Drugs with similar primary effects may be combined most advantageously when the drugs differ in their secondary actions. In such circumstances, combination of fractions of the full therapeutic dose of each drug permits the doctor to attain the desired effect without proportional increase in undesired side effects. Thus, in the management of grand mal epilepsy, the full dose of phenobarbital required to keep their seizures under control may make some patients uncomfortably drowsy. On the other hand, a fully effective dose of diphenylhydantoin (Dilantin) may cause gastrointestinal upset, nervousness, and a feeling of unsteadiness when moving about. However, when the two anticonvulsant drugs are combined in only fractions of the fully effective dose of each, the patient's seizures may be kept under complete control and the side effects of both drugs reduced.

An ideal drug combination is one in which the therapeutically desirable effects of two drugs are additive and their secondary side effects are actually antagonistic and cancel each other out. For example, a product for treating colds and allergies may contain two antihistaminic drugs. The primary actions of each drug in counteracting allergic symptoms may be simply additive—i.e., both drugs protect the reactive tissue cells from the effects of histamine. However, one drug may cause excessive sedation as a result of a secondary depressant effect on the nervous system, and the other a jittery feeling because of its central stimulating effect; then, combining the two tends to reduce both of the antagonistic adverse effects.

Antagonism between the actions of different drugs on the reactive cells is often used in formulating prescriptions and drug products. Obviously, it is not the primary actions of both drugs that antagonize one another, since this would reduce or nullify the therapeutically desired action. Actually, the doctor takes pains to avoid such therapeutic incompatibilities in his drug orders; however, he often adds some antagonistic agent to a prescription to counteract a secondary, undesired side effect of the chief effective ingredient.

Thus, when phenobarbital and diphenylhydantoin in combination continue to produce drowsiness in an epileptic patient, the doctor may order the addition of an amphetamine derivative such as desoxyephedrine. Such a central stimulant counteracts the patient's tendency to become sleepy, without in any way antagonizing the anticonvulsant effects of the two antiseizure drugs. Similarly, mild psychomotor stimulants such as caffeine, dextroamphetamine or methylphenidate (Ritalin) are commonly combined with antihistaminic drugs in products designed to achieve antiallergic effects and, at the same time, keep the patient alert and able to carry on his normal activities.

Antagonism of one drug's action by another drug with opposite pharmacological or chemical effect is often very useful in counteracting toxic effects from overdoses of drugs or from poisons. As we shall see in the next chapter, overdosage of a depressant drug may be treated by administering stimulants, and of a stimulant, by depressants. Poisoning by certain metals is counteracted by administering their chemical antagonists to neutralize them. Overdosage of certain anticoagulants that cause bleeding by competing with the essential metabolite vitamin K can be counteracted by administering drugs that act like the vitamin, to displace the anticoagulant molecules.

SUMMARY

We have tried in this chapter to illustrate by practical examples some of the current concepts of how drugs and other foreign chemicals interact with the chemical constituents of the cells of the patient's body. These aspects of biochemical and molecular pharmacology may seem extremely complex and not directly related to what the nurse—or the physician, for that matter—needs to know in caring for the patient who is receiving drug therapy.

It is true that the material presented in this chapter is not as immediately practical as that offered in the chapters that follow. Yet it is knowledge that will help to broaden and deepen the nurse's growing understanding of how drugs achieve their therapeutic effect. The nurse who develops a more sophisticated understanding of what is happening within the body when a drug is administered can very often take pride in being able to provide her patients with better care when pharmacotherapeutic agents have been ordered.

REVIEW QUESTIONS

1. (a) What are some sources of drug dosages that are approximations of the proper amounts to be administered to most patients?

(b) What is meant by the "usual dose" of a drug, and why may this amount be too little or too much for some patients?

2. (a) Why is the patient's body weight a factor to be considered in individualizing drug dosage?

(b) What factor other than body weight is often the basis for formulas used by pediatricians in calculating dosage for infants?

3. (a) Broadly speaking, what happens to the molecules of a drug that is administered to a living animal or person?

(b) In terms of the way a drug is dealt with by the body, what are the two general classes of factors that influence the effects that an administered drug is likely to produce?

4. (a) What happens to a drug when it is administered to a patient? By what four general processes is the drug handled by the body?

(b) What aspects of a drug's actions are determined by the ways in which the body handles it?

5. (a) What is meant by the *critical concentration* of an active drug that has been administered?

(b) What is meant by *dynamic equilibrium*, in reference to the processes by which a drug is handled in the body after its administration?

6. (a) What is meant by *absorption* of an administered drug?

(b) What effects do the presence or absence of food in the stomach have upon the extent to which orally administered drugs are likely to be absorbed?

7. (a) What, in general, is the effect of a drug's lipid solubility upon its absorption from the intestinal tract?

(b) What, in general, is the effect of the degree of a drug's ionization upon its ability to be absorbed from the G.I. tract?

(c) Give examples of some drugs that are readily absorbable or poorly absorbable on the basis of their lipid solubility or ionization constants.

8. (a) Why is a watery solution of a drug absorbed more rapidly when injected intramuscularly than when administered by the subcutaneous route?

(b) What are some means by which a drug's absorption from the site of its injection may be delayed? Give examples.

9. (a) What is meant by the *distribution* of a drug after it has been administered and absorbed into the blood stream?

(b) What is meant by *plasma binding*, in regard to drugs?

10. (a) What is meant by the *half life* of a drug?

(b) What is meant by the term *blood-brain barrier*, and what physicochemical properties tend to make it relatively easy for a drug to pass this "barrier"?

11. (a) What are the four main kinds of enzymatically catalyzed biochemical reactions by which the body breaks down active drugs to form inactive metabolites?

(b) What organ plays the most important role in the biotransformation of drugs to more readily excreted chemicals, and which organs play the most important part in eliminating such metabolites?

12. (a) Give an example of how the immaturity of the excretory mechanisms of premature infants may affect the concentration in the tissues of an administered drug.

(b) Give an example of how immaturity of metabolizing mechanisms has caused drug toxicity in infants.

13. (a) Give an example of how a drug's action may be lengthened and intensified in patients with a hereditary lack of the enzyme which ordinarily detoxifies that drug.

(b) Give an example of how a pathological condition that prevents enzymatic destruction of a drug may intensify the effects of the drug to the point of toxicity.

(c) Give an example of how a pathological state that interferes with a drug's excretion can cause the drug to accumulate to toxic levels.

14. What is meant by each of the following terms:

Congenital tolerance; acquired tolerance; cross tolerance

Enzyme induction; disposal-type tolerance; tissue tolerance

15. (a) Give an example of how one drug may potentiate the effects of another by interfering with the enzymatically catalyzed biotransformation reactions by which the second drug is ordinarily inactivated.

(b) Give an example of potentiation resulting from one drug's ability to interfere with the renal excretion of another.

16. (a) How do drugs that produce pharmacodynamic effects differ from those that act as chemotherapeutic agents?

(b) How do stimulating drugs differ from depressants?

17. (a) Give examples of several sites at which different drugs may act to produce a fall in the blood pressure of a hypertensive patient.

(b) Do the same for pain-relieving drugs.

18. (a) What is meant by the terms *receptor* and *agonist*?

(b) What is meant by the terms *competitive antagonist* (at a receptor) and *competitive inhibition* (of an enzyme-substrate reaction)?

19. (a) Give an example of how a drug may produce poisoning by its ability to bind trace metals in the body.

(b) Give an example of how a drug with metal-binding properties may serve as a chemical antidote against some kinds of poisons.

20. (a) Give an example of how the physiological state of a person's organs or systems may alter the responses of his tissues to the same drug at different times.

(b) Give examples of how the patient's pathological condition may alter the manner in which he reacts to various drugs.

21. (a) How can the nurse make practical use of the relationship between the severity of a patient's pain and his capacity to resist or tolerate the effects of opiate analgesics, sedative-hypnotics, and tranquilizers?

(b) What attempts are made to delay the development of tolerance to opiates in patients with chronically painful conditions who are likely to require long-term administration of opiates or other potent analgesics?

22. (a) What phenomenon offers the clearest proof of the fact that psychological factors very often influence a patient's response to drugs?

(b) What are some examples of types of drugs to which the patient's response is often influenced by factors related to his personality, temperament, emotional state, and the circumstances in which the drugs are taken?

23. (a) Give an example of how the administration together of two drugs that act at similar reactive cells may provide a more effective therapeutic response.

(b) Give an example of how taking two similarly acting drugs simultaneously may have an unexpectedly severe additive effect.

24. (a) Indicate how a combination of two drugs with comparable primary effects and antagonistic secondary effects may prove therapeutically more desirable than giving either drug separately.

(b) Indicate, by examples, how knowledge of the antagonistic effects of drugs can be employed to counteract adverse side effects and toxicity.

BIBLIOGRAPHY

Albert, A.: Selective Toxicity, 3rd ed. New York, Wiley, 1965.

Berblinger, K. W.: The influence of personalities on drug therapy. Am. J. Nurs., 59:1130, 1959.

Burns, J. J.: Implications of enzyme induction in drug therapy. Am. J. Med., 37:327, 1964.

Conney, A. H., and Burns, J. J.: Factors influencing drug metabolism. Advances Pharmacol., 1:31, 1962.

Di Palma, J. R.: Drug doses: the scheduling is what counts. R.N., 28:51, 1965 (April).

Evans, D. A. P.: Pharmacogenetics. Am. J. Med., 34:639, 1963.

Friend, D. G.: Some useful principles and practices for modern drug therapy. Clin. Pharmacol. Ther., *1*:135, 1960.

Furchgott, R. F.: Receptor mechanisms. Ann. Rev. Pharmacol., *4*:21, 1964.

Kalow, W.: Genetic factors in relation to drugs. Ann. Rev. Pharmacol., *5*:9, 1965.

Loewe, S.: Antagonism and antagonists. Pharmacol. Rev., *9*:237, 1957.

Mark, L. C.: Metabolism of barbiturates in man. Clin. Pharmacol. Ther., *4*:504, 1963.

Rodman, M. J.: What happens to drugs in the body. 1. Absorption, distribution, and termination of action. R.N., *28*:73, 1965 (July).

———: What happens to drugs in the body. 3. Receptor action, drug-enzyme interaction. R.N., *29*:73, 1966 (Jan.).

———: What happens to drugs in the body. 4. Synergism and antagonism. R.N., *29*:72, 1966 (May).

Williams, R. T.: Detoxication mechanisms in man. Clin. Pharmacol. Ther., *4*:234, 1963.

Wolf, S.: The pharmacology of placebos. Pharmacol. Rev., *8*:339, 1956.

The Toxic Effects of Drugs and Chemicals

The chemicals employed in treating disease are capable of producing not only the therapeutically desired effects but also many that are undesirable. In Chapter 1, it was pointed out that, even after drugs had been carefully screened and tested for toxicity in animals, they often cause unexpectedly severe reactions in patients, under clinical conditions. In Chapter 2 we studied some of the factors that may make an ordinarily safe dose of a drug dangerous for some patients. In this chapter we shall examine in more detail the main types of drug toxicity.

The undesirable effects of drugs may be broadly classed as follows:

1. Effects that are *predictable* from what we already know of a drug's pharmacodynamic properties. These side effects of therapy can often be traced to a particular patient's *hypersusceptibility* to the primary or secondary pharmacological actions of the therapeutic agent.

2. Effects that are *not* readily predictable, because they are the result of a patient's *unusual reactivity* or *hypersensitivity* to the drug in ways which usually have little to do with the drug's main pharmacological actions. *Allergic drug reactions* come in this category.

3. Effects that occur when drugs are chronically abused by people who take them without medical advice, because they crave the drug's psychological effects or because drug taking serves some symbolic personal purpose. *Drug addiction* is an important aspect of this type of adverse drug effect.

4. *Drug poisoning,* which occurs when chemicals are taken in massive overdoses either accidentally or in the act of suicide. The detection and treatment of acute and chronic toxic reactions of this kind require special measures, based upon the principles of *toxicology.*

The nurse can do a great deal to keep all these adverse drug effects to a minimum. Thus, throughout this book we shall emphasize the kinds of observations that the alert nurse should make in relation to drug therapy. We shall also point out the things that nurses must teach patients to look for when they are taking various kinds of drugs at home. In addition, nurses are often in a position to play a part in the prevention of poisoning by household chemicals other than drugs; also, they often assist the physician in the treatment of poisoning.

ADVERSE REACTIONS TO DRUGS

There has, of course, always been evidence that drugs are capable of doing harm as well as helping patients. However, the problem of coping with the adverse effects of drugs has never been as serious as it is today. The many newly synthesized chemicals that are now being introduced as therapeutic and diagnostic agents are capable of causing a much greater variety of reactions than those that resulted with medicines from natural sources. Such reactions are also often much more severe than those caused by the relatively weak medicines with which the doctor once had to treat his patients' ills. Thus, the same actively potent drugs that have brought such benefits to so many people in this golden age of drug therapy are often the very ones that are also responsible for the rising tide of adverse reactions.

The exact extent of drug-induced illness is uncertain. Reports range from as few as one half of one per cent in some hospitals to as many as five per cent of all admissions in others. It seems certain that many drug reactions are never reported. In any case, it is safe to say that *every drug* is capable of causing adverse reactions in some patients and that the nurse must therefore be constantly alert to detect the signs of such reactions.

Pharmacological, or Predictable, Toxicity

Primary Actions. One of the most common occurrences when drugs are being administered is the development of adverse effects from simple overdosage. In such cases, the patient suffers from effects that are merely an extension of the desired action of the compound. Thus, a patient taking a dose of phenobarbital that was intended only to reduce his nervous tension may become excessively drowsy and find that he cannot carry on his ordinary activities. More serious, but still similar in principle, is the case of the patient receiving an anticoagulant drug in a dose that produces the intended effect to a greater degree than was expected. Instead of lowering the clotting factors in his blood only to the point at which the chances of clot formation are reduced, the drug's action may lead to development of spontaneous bleeding.

Such excessive reactions to a drug's main action can usually be avoided by adjusting the dosage carefully to the needs of the individual patient instead of having him take the "usual" or "average" dose. Thus, when the nurse reports that the patient is reacting in the expected way but more strongly than was intended, the doctor will order a reduction in dosage or an increase in the intervals between doses. If, for example, the nurse notes that a hypertensive patient taking a blood-pressure-reducing drug gets weak, dizzy and faint upon arising, the physician will usually adjust the drug's dosage in a manner intended to limit the drug-induced fall in pressure. Similarly, when the nurse reports certain abnormalities in the pulse of a heart failure patient receiving digitalis, the doctor will waste no time in lowering the dosage of the drug to a level that will produce the desired cardiac effects and not the toxic ones.

The presence of pathological conditions other than the one being treated may make some patients unusually susceptible to the main action of a drug which is being given in a dose that would ordinarily be quite safe. For example, patients with liver and kidney disease are hypersusceptible to the actions of drugs that depend upon healthy hepatic and renal functions for their elimination from the body. Thus, as we have noted, many drugs are administered only with great caution, and others are contraindicated, because of the dangerous reactions that can occur when an unmetabolized or unexcreted drug accumulates to toxic levels in elderly patients or others with disorders of these vital organs.

Other illnesses may make it unsafe to administer certain drugs because their ordinary actions may produce adverse effects in those patients, who are particularly susceptible to them. Thus, a hyperthyroid patient may react excessively to the stimulating effects of an adrenergic drug such as epinephrine or ephedrine; and an ordinary dose of morphine may produce excessive depression in a hypothyroid patient. Similarly, the use of many other potent drugs may be contraindicated in the presence of pre-existing disease, because the effect desired in most patients cannot be safely attained in those with illnesses of certain types.

Secondary Actions. We have already noted that drugs rarely possess a single specific action but can usually produce a wide variety of effects in addition to the primary one. Many of these multiple actions are uncovered during the initial screening tests, on the basis of which the pharmacologist draws the drug's profile of pharmacological activity. Fortunately for most patients, it is usually possible to find a dose that brings about the desired effect without producing undesired secondary reactions. Sometimes, however, this is not possible and the occurrence of a side effect is almost inevitable when a patient receives an ordinary therapeutic dose of the drug.

For example, a patient being treated for allergy with an antihistaminic drug may become drowsy because the dose of the drug required for controlling his allergic symptoms may also depress parts of the patient's brain. If the patient or nurse reports this, the doctor may discontinue the drug and try another antihistaminic agent; or he may prescribe a small dose of a central stimulant in an attempt to counteract the depressant effects of these drugs. Interestingly, some antihistaminic drugs are actually employed for treating insomnia. Thus, the very action which is considered undesirable in one patient may be the one for which a drug is employed in another patient.

Some patients may be more susceptible to one of a drug's secondary actions than they are to its therapeutic action. Thus, atropine and similar natural and synthetic anticholinergic drugs used for treating peptic ulcer are contraindicated in certain patients, who may suffer severely from one or another of several secondary effects when these agents are administered in doses intended only to reduce gastric acid secretion and relax gastrointestinal smooth muscle spasm. These drugs may, for instance, precipitate an attack of glaucoma when administered to patients especially susceptible to this condition, even though the ocular effects of such atropinelike drugs cause only some annoying but bearable blurring of vision in most people. Similarly, atropine and other drugs of this class are contraindicated in elderly men with an enlarged prostate gland, because a secondary action that most people are hardly aware of may lead to bladder paralysis and urinary retention, requiring catheterization in this especially susceptible group of patients.

The important point about side effects that stem

from a drug's primary and secondary pharmacological actions is that they are largely predictable and are therefore able to be prevented or, at least, kept to a minimum. Thus, if the doctor and nurse are aware of a drug's fundamental actions and apply their knowledge of the drug's basic pharmacodynamic data to the case of the particular patient being treated, severe side effects of this type need never develop.

In the weighing of potential benefit against potential risk, the primary responsibility is, of course, the physician's. For example, in a patient with a history of asthma, the doctor may avoid treating postoperative abdominal distention or urinary retention with a smooth muscle stimulant such as bethanechol, because he knows that muscle-contracting drugs of that class may constrict the patient's bronchial tubes and interfere excessively with his respiratory exchanges. If the doctor, having weighed all the risks, decides to employ a drug despite its potentially adverse pharmacological effects, he keeps a close watch on his patient to detect early laboratory and clinical signs of the onset of toxicity. The nurse also must be aware of what toxic effects to watch for, and she promptly reports any such signs to the physician.

Hypersensitivity and Idiosyncracy

Drugs sometimes cause adverse effects that have little or nothing to do with the ordinary pharmacological effects of the drugs. Sometimes a drug that had been well tolerated previously produces toxic effects when administered in what had before been a safe dose. Once such a reaction has occurred, it may recur every time the person is exposed to even tiny amounts of the drug. These ill effects, which do not develop in experimental animals or in most patients to whom the drug is administered, are most often allergic in origin. On the other hand, the extreme sensitivity of certain people to some chemicals sometimes cannot be proved to have such an immunologic basis and in these cases the cause often evades identification.

Drug Allergy. The nature of allergic reactions (see Chap. 40), briefly, is as follows: Substances foreign to the body act as antigens to stimulate the production of antibodies. Later, when such a previously *sensitized* individual is again exposed, the antigen reacts with the antibodies in ways that are damaging to many body tissues. A few drugs that are protein in nature can act as complete antigens. Most drugs are not themselves proteins, but apparently combine with body proteins to form a foreign protein which then stimulates the production of antibodies. Drug-protein combinations that serve as incomplete antigens of this kind are called *haptenes.*

The reactions that occur when sensitized individuals are exposed to even minute amounts of the chemical to which they are allergic are classified as (1)

Immediate (urticarial reactions; anaphylactoid reactions) and (2) *Delayed* (tuberculin type reactions; serum sickness type reactions).

Immediate-type reactions to drugs develop within minutes of exposure to a chemical to which the person has previously been sensitized. The antigen-antibody reaction is believed to result in the release of active chemical substances, such as *histamine,* from the tissues themselves. These chemical mediators that are suddenly set free from a bound form exert their pharmacological actions on the smooth muscles of small blood vessels and other organs.

Allergic reactions of this kind may be relatively mild, or they may be severe enough to be rapidly fatal. The less severe reactions may be manifested by the appearance of raised, itchy wheals, or swellings in the skin (urticaria—"hives"). The anaphylactoid-type reactions can lead to swift circulatory collapse or to asphyxia from swelling of the larynx and blockage of bronchial passages. Small doses of otherwise safe drugs such as aspirin and penicillin have caused fatally severe immediate reactions.

Delayed-type reactions to drugs differ from the immediate type in both the pathological and the clinical picture, as well as the response to treatment. Reactions of this type develop only several hours after exposure to the drug to which the person is sensitized. The skin lesions that appear are inflammatory in nature rather than urticarial and may be of many different kinds. Drug fever, swelling of the joints, and reactions involving the blood-forming organs, liver, and kidneys may also occur.

Idiosyncracy is a term sometimes used to describe abnormal sensitivity to drugs in some people. The basis for the inability of such individuals to tolerate small doses of drugs that are safe for most others is not well understood. Such reactions are thought to be the result, not of allergic hypersensitivity and subsequent antigen-antibody reactions, but of an inherited inability to handle chemicals of certain types. The genetic flaws that predispose some people to idiosyncratic reactions to certain drugs have begun to be elucidated in recent years.

It is often difficult to differentiate between delayed-type immunologic reactions to drugs and nonimmunologic idiosyncratic reactions, because, in the delayed, or tuberculin-type reactions, it has not often been possible to demonstrate the presence of antibodies in the blood. Therefore, in the following discussions of the adverse reactions to drugs in specific organs such as the skin, bone marrow and blood, and liver, we shall discuss both types of reactions together. The important point with both kinds of reactions is that they occur only in a minority of predisposed individuals and that their development is not readily predictable, except, occasionally, from a knowledge of the patient's prior history.

Dermatological Reactions (Drug Eruptions). Drugs that are taken internally and carried to the skin by way of the blood can cause eruptions similar to those seen in dermatoses of almost every type. Most common are the urticarial reactions observed with salicylates, penicillin, etc. However, drugs may cause rashes resembling those of measles (morbilliform eruptions), acne, psoriasis, pemphigus, eczema and other dermatological disorders.

People who already have skin difficulties sometimes seem predisposed to react to certain drugs in specific ways. Thus, youngsters with acne tend to be most susceptible to the acneiform eruptions induced by bromides, iodides and the male sex hormone. People with atopic dermatitis are prone to respond to procaine or to penicillin with eczematous reactions marked by redness, blistering, weeping and crusting of the skin. Actually, however, generalizations are difficult, because almost all drugs are capable of causing any of various kinds of reactions under certain circumstances.

Skin reactions that have elicited special interest in recent years are: (1) photosensitivity and (2) the erythema-multiforme-type reaction. Both have occurred following the use of sulfonamide-type drugs, and have also appeared in patients treated with other agents. Drug-induced photosensitivity usually takes the form of sunburnlike lesions. Such reactions are sometimes a manifestation of the delayed type of allergy. Sunlight, in such cases, reacts with the drug in the skin to create a new molecule that then acts as a haptene to sensitize the skin. Other cases of photosensitivity are *non*immunologic in origin, with severe reactions occurring the very first time the patient takes a drug and exposes himself to light.

The *erythema-multiforme-type* reaction (as seen in the Stevens-Johnson syndrome, Chap. 43), may be very serious. Here the skin lesions may take the form of blisters as in pemphigus. Often, bleeding into the center of the lesion causes a red circle—the so-called bull's-eye lesion. Patients with this severe skin reaction and accompanying systemic illness require very careful nursing care, since the incidence of fatalities is relatively high.

Exfoliative dermatitis, another skin eruption that may be life-threatening, also is often associated with the administration of certain drugs to sensitive individuals.

Blood Dyscrasias. Among the most serious side effects of drugs are agranulocytosis, thrombocytopenia, aplastic anemia, hemolytic anemia, and others that affect the blood. Because of the dangerous nature of such reactions, the Council on Drugs of the A.M.A. has established a Registry on Blood Dyscrasias to which doctors are encouraged to report any cases of drug-induced hematotoxicosis. A Study Group on Blood Dyscrasias then investigates the possible relationship between the patient's hematological illness and the drugs that he may have been taking. Reports are tabulated and summaries are published or sent out periodically. Because nurses must often teach patients who are taking certain drugs to watch for early signs and symptoms of blood disorders, we shall summarize here some pertinent points about the types of blood dyscrasias most commonly encountered.

APLASTIC ANEMIA is one of the most serious of the blood disorders that may be induced by drugs. More than half the patients who develop this condition die in spite of all treatment efforts. The condition is characterized by damage to the patient's bone marrow, with the result that the blood-cell-forming tissue is largely replaced by fatty tissue. As a result of this there is a reduction in *all* the formed elements of the circulating blood (pancytopenia). The patient becomes pale and weak and is subject to hemorrhages and infections.

Among the drugs reported to have produced this condition are chloramphenicol, phenylbutazone, trimethadione and certain sulfonamides and their derivatives. The manner in which these and other chemicals damage the bone marrow is not known. The fact that the vast majority of patients who receive these drugs do not develop this blood dyscrasia indicates that the reaction is idiosyncratic. However, the specific nature of the sensitivity of some people to these drugs is still a mystery. There is, unfortunately, no test to help determine which patients are susceptible to drug-induced aplastic anemia.

Doctors now try to order these drugs only when they feel that their usefulness for treating certain serious illnesses far outweighs the chance—however slight, statistically—that the particular patient may be one of the very small minority to develop aplastic anemia. When such drugs are being employed over prolonged periods, the doctor orders frequent blood tests in order to detect the earliest signs of hematological abnormalities. He and the nurse warn patients to report signs of illness such as sore throat, weakness, pallor and bleeding. Early detection through such signs and by the blood tests permits the immediate discontinuation of therapy with the potentially dangerous drug before irreversible bone marrow aplasia sets in.

AGRANULOCYTOSIS, a very marked reduction in the number of circulating white blood cells, is the most common of the drug-induced hematological adverse reactions. The condition in its acute form is characterized by a sharp drop in the total leukocyte count and an almost complete absence of granulocytes. As a result, patients are deprived of one of the body's main defense mechanisms against infection. Thus, the condition is often first detected when the patient comes down with a severe prostrating infection—usually a sore throat.

Aminopyrine is the drug most commonly associated with blood dyscrasia of this type. Most American doctors prefer to employ analgesics with less potential for doing harm than this one. However, the related drug phenylbutazone is relatively widely used for treating rheumatic disorders that have proved resistant to salicylate therapy. When he has to employ this drug or other agents often associated with agranulocytosis—chlorpromazine or propylthiouracil, for example—the physician takes frequent white blood cell and differential counts. Here, too, the doctor and nurse warn the patient to report immediately the development of signs of infection, such as fever and sore throat or the occurrence of a skin rash or jaundice. Since it is sometimes, but not always, possible to demonstrate leukocyte-agglutinating antibodies in the patient's serum, agranulocytosis apparently may be sometimes an allergic response to certain drugs.

Once the condition is detected, the offending drug is immediately withdrawn, and any infection that may be present is vigorously treated with antibiotics. Patients are told to inform future physicians whom they consult of their sensitivity to the drug in question, since taking even a single small dose years later may set off a similar reaction.

THROMBOCYTOPENIA, a deficiency of blood platelets, develops occasionally during treatment with various types of drugs. Unless the condition is quickly detected and the drug promptly discontinued, serious bleeding, and even death from brain hemorrhage, may result. Some drugs, such as the antibiotic ristocetin, damage the circulating platelets by a direct action; others—meprobamate, and chlorothiazide, for example—may do so by an allergic mechanism. Thrombocytopenia that results from damage to the bone marrow elements that produce the platelets is most dangerous. Certain drugs used in treating epilepsy and diabetes have caused irreversible damage of this kind. Patients are watched for possible development of purpura, and most cases respond rapidly when the condition is detected and the drug discontinued.

HEMOLYTIC ANEMIA. A number of drugs are now known to cause the destruction of circulating red blood cells. This results not only in the symptoms of anemia (pallor, weakness and heart palpitations) but also, sometimes, in renal complications that may lead to anuria. The condition is occasionally the result of an allergic sensitization reaction in which the patient produces antibodies that cause his red cells to clump together when he later takes another dose of the sensitizing drug—phenacetin, for example.

More commonly, drug-induced hemolytic anemia is caused by an idiosyncrasy which makes the red cells of some people particularly sensitive to certain kinds of chemicals. This type of toxicity is one of the few manifestations of drug intolerance that scientists have been able to trace back to its source. It is now known that some people produce red blood cells in which the protective enzyme called glucose-6-phosphate dehydrogenase (G-6-PD) is abnormal and deficient in activity. Persons with this defect, which is hereditary, are sensitive to the action of certain "oxidant" drugs, including primaquine, acetanilid and some sulfonamides.

This sensitivity was noted in Negro soldiers returning from the Korean conflict, who were given the antimalarial drug primaquine. They showed a much higher susceptibility to drug-induced hemolytic anemia than their white comrades. The condition was then shown to be genetic in origin. Since that time, the gene controlling the deficiency of this dehydrogenase enzyme has been found in other racial and ethnic groups. The erythrocytes of such people are now known to be susceptible to destruction by many drugs that are more commonly prescribed than primaquine, including aspirin and phenacetin and anti-infective drugs such as the sulfonamides, nitrofurantoin and sulfoxone.

Several simple tests for detecting this genetically transmitted enzyme deficiency have been devised. Thus it is now possible for the doctor to recognize hypersusceptible patients in advance and avoid treating them with drugs capable of precipitating hemolytic anemia. In actual practice, since physicians rarely employ such tests before prescribing drugs, the nurse may be the first to note signs and symptoms of a hemolytic reaction—complaints of weakness, back pain, and the passage of dark urine. She should promptly report these to the doctor, who will have the laboratory check the patient's hemoglobin levels and order the drug withdrawn if necessary.

Scientists are studying *pharmacogenetics*—the relationship between hereditary influences and the response to drugs—in the hope of discoveries that will lead to a reduction in other kinds of idiosyncratic reactions.

Hepatic Drug Reactions. Substances that directly damage the liver are ordinarily detected in routine laboratory screening tests and are rarely used as drugs. Yet drug-induced liver injury is not uncommon. Such adverse hepatic reactions are believed to be the result of individual hypersensitivity in most cases, but the cause is unknown in others.

Liver toxicity of one type seems to be the result of a reaction affecting the lining of the bile channels. Patients taking chlorpromazine, for example, have suffered jaundice resembling that caused by biliary obstruction. It is believed to be the result of an allergic reaction in which the narrow biliary canals are blocked and the bile backs up into the blood. Other drugs that have caused intrahepatic cholestasis include certain male hormone derivatives and the antibiotics erythromycin estolate and triacetyloleandomycin.

Another kind of acute liver damage induced by drugs is more serious, because it involves the functioning liver cells rather than merely the bile drainage channels. Under the microscope, the damaged liver tissue resembles the histological picture seen in viral hepatitis. Thus it has sometimes been argued that the patient's liver ailment was viral in origin and not drug-induced at all. Other authorities have suggested that the hepatic necrosis is the result of some action of the drug which makes the patient's liver more susceptible to the lurking hepatitis virus.

The occurrence of serious hepatotoxicity of this type has resulted in removal from the market of many drugs that had passed all the usual safety tests. This indicates that the safety of any drug is always uncertain and that its status may change in the light of continued clinical experience. Thus, even though a drug causes liver damage in only a small minority of hypersusceptible patients, injury to this vital organ is so serious that withdrawal of the drug is considered warranted.

On the other hand, when a particular agent is considered especially valuable, it may be retained despite some occasional reports of hepatotoxicity. This has been true of the antibiotic tetracycline, for example. In such cases, however, doctors are cautioned against the use of high doses of the drug with liver-damaging potential; and nurses must be especially alert for possible signs of liver involvement such as nausea, vomiting, and abdominal pain—signals that usually appear before actual jaundice is evident.

Other Types of Drug-induced Toxicity. Drugs may act directly or indirectly to cause many other kinds of adverse effects. Kidney damage induced by drugs, for example, may be especially serious, since it can interfere with further excretion of the drug. A number of antibiotics, including polymyxin, colistin, bacitracin, streptomycin, neomycin, and kanamycin are potentially nephrotoxic. In the case of many of these antibiotics, failure to excrete the drug can also cause permanent damage to inner ear structures when the drugs accumulate and reach neurotoxic levels. (Ability to damage specifically the auditory and vestibular branches of the eighth cranial nerve is called ototoxicity.) Patients who drive a car while taking drugs of certain types must be warned that their driving skill may be impaired by the effects of these agents on brain function. Among the drugs most likely to affect a patient's judgment and motor coordination are the barbiturates and other hypnotics, sedatives, and minor tranquilizers. The adverse effects of these drugs and of certain antihistaminic agents may be intensified if the patient drinks even a relatively small amount of an alcoholic beverage.

Recently, considerable attention has been given to the possibility that drugs may adversely affect not only the person taking them, but also, in the case of pregnant women, the developing fetus. It is, at present, very difficult to evaluate an experimental drug's capacity to cause fetal malformations. Thus, to avoid the danger of possible teratogenic (literally, "monster-producing") effects of drugs, doctors are now administering very few drugs to women during pregnancy. In fact, many physicians now keep their prescribing of drugs to a minimum for *all* women of childbearing age, because of the possibility that pregnancy may have occurred without yet having been detected. A teratogenic drug administered to a woman during this period might be injurious to the rapidly developing embryo.

THE NATURE OF ADDICTION AND DRUG ABUSE

Among the adverse effects of drugs, some of those most commonly encountered occur as a result of drug abuse and the development of addiction. The nurse is often required to care for patients hospitalized as the result of deliberate misuse of certain medications. In her role of administering narcotic analgesics, such as morphine and meperidine (Demerol), and sedative-hypnotic drugs, such as the barbiturates, she learns to avoid any action that might tend to foster addiction in her patients. In addition, preventing addiction becomes a more personal matter for the student when she learns that the abuse of drugs is a common occupational hazard of nurses as well as of pharmacists and physicians.

The dangers inherent in the abuse of drugs of various types are discussed in several places in this book, as is the manner in which patients are managed who have been harmed by chronic overindulgence in drugs. We shall also later discuss the adverse effects of addiction to opiates and related drugs (Chap. 9), and of the abuse of barbiturates (Chap. 6) and stimulants such as the amphetamines (Chap. 16). Alcoholism is taken up in Chapter 12, which is devoted to the pharmacology of ethyl alcohol. These are not, however, the only agents that people misuse; therefore references are made also to the abuse of nonprescription headache remedies, and laxatives, and also to the corticosteroid drugs often used for treating arthritis, asthma, and very many other disorders.

In this chapter, we shall deal only in general terms with certain phenomena which seem to underlie the abuse of many different drugs and chemicals. That is, we shall discuss some of the *psychological* and *physiological* factors which are usually involved in one way or another in the development of drug abuse and addiction. We must warn, however, that these phenomena are quite complex and that there still remains a good deal to be learned about both the psychic factors which make some people turn to drugs and the biochemical factors that tend to perpetuate their enslavement to certain agents.

Definition of Terms. The terms that are employed in discussing the misuse of drugs are themselves in need of definition. The words *addiction* and *habituation,* for example, have been used in so many different ways by different people that their use now seems to cause confusion and controversy. The World Health Organization's Expert Committee on Addiction-Producing Drugs has recently suggested that these terms be abandoned in favor of the more general one, *drug dependence.* Yet, both this term and the even broader one *drug abuse* also require considerable explanation of what is meant when they are used in specific situations.

Dependence is a general term intended to indicate the high degree of involvement with drugs that develops when people take them repeatedly, whether continually or periodically. The nature and degree of dependence that different drugs produce varies considerably. Some agents, such as the stimulants, cocaine and amphetamine, cause only a *psychological dependence,* whereas others, such as the opiates and barbiturates, produce a *physical dependence* as well.

Drug abuse is a somewhat broader term because it can encompass both psychological and physical dependence, but it may also be used to describe behavior in which these phenomena need not be present. This term refers to the use of any chemical in a way that is not sanctioned medically, culturally, or socially. The drug abuser takes drugs without medical advice, and he takes them in amounts that produce changes in his behavior of which most other people disapprove. The abuser's behavior is not condoned by the majority because they fear that his conduct is detrimental not only to himself but to others. Thus, they may be concerned that the drug may lead to violence or to a general downgrading of the moral tone of the community.

Psychological dependence upon drugs may be only mild or, on the other hand, so strong that satisfying the psychic need for the drug's effects becomes the most important matter in the person's life. The lesser degree of psychic dependence is what is often meant when we say that a person is "habituated" to the use of a drug. People can become habituated to almost anything that gives them an improved sense of well-being. A habit need not necessarily be harmful; indeed, it may help a person to keep small tensions from building up into big ones by releasing his minor nervous tensions in a relatively harmless way.

The habit-forming drugs most commonly used in our society are the nicotine that people inhale in smoking and the caffeine that they take in with coffee, tea and other beverages. Typically, people indulge in these habit-forming substances because, weighing one thing against another, they feel better when under the benign influence of tobacco or coffee than when they are without them. People do not readily give up things to which they are habituated and they tend to feel uneasy when deprived of them.

Yet mild psychic dependence is not ordinarily considered very serious, because many people when adequately motivated do have enough will power to break their habit permanently; others who have come to rely more strongly on a chemical substance may require professional help in overcoming habituation to nicotine, but they do nevertheless accomplish the task without suffering intolerable personal travail. Besides, any harm that may result from overindulgence in drugs that are merely mildly habituating is largely limited to the individual himself. Society as a whole does not ordinarily concern itself with such manifestations of the human tendency to seek sources of personal pleasure as a tension-relieving device.

A *craving* for a drug which is so powerful that it outweighs all of the drug-dependent person's ordinary drives and concerns is an indication of a much more intense degree of psychological dependence. The need for the feeling that a particular drug gives the person and the compulsive efforts to regain that feeling are primary characteristics of *addiction* rather than mere habituation. The behavior of the drug-obsessed person usually becomes harmful to himself and to others. He devotes so much of himself to the business of getting, taking and staying under the influence of the drug that he has little time or energy left for activities that are constructive personally and socially. The abuse of drugs to this degree usually calls down the wrath of society on the individual, because his behavior makes the general community feel threatened.

Psychiatrists generally believe that people who are capable of becoming so compulsively concerned with drug taking were emotionally disturbed to begin with. Without involving ourselves in the various psychodynamic theories of the causes of drug dependency, we can certainly suggest that it is usually *not* the drug but the personality of the individual who is exposed to it that determines whether the drug is going to be compulsively abused in ways that are harmful to the individual and to society.

Thus, many people can take barbiturates on a doctor's prescription for long periods without ever developing a strong craving for these depressant drugs; yet others quickly require larger and larger doses to give them the peculiar feeling of release which they find that these drugs offer them. Before long their drug-seeking and -using behavior becomes socially unacceptable, because they and those with whom they come into contact are endangered by their abusive use of the barbiturates.

Similarly, most people who must receive morphine or meperidine (Demerol) for the relief of pain do not find the feeling that the drug gives them so over-whelmingly pleasant that they develop a strong crav-ing for opiates. On the contrary, many patients find the sensations so disagreeable that they would rather try to bear their pain than receive these narcotic analgesics. In addition to suffering this *dys*phoria rather than the expected *eu*phoria, or state of well-being, such people may also worry about the pos-sibility of becoming dependent upon these drugs.

The nurse can help in such cases by reminding patients who need narcotics to provide temporary relief of pain—following a fracture, for example, or after surgery—that the pain will subside spontaneously in a few days, after which they will no longer re-quire analgesic medication. She can make it clear that the brief use of these drugs for relief of pain is not ordinarily hazardous, as the vast majority of patients quickly discontinue them once their painful condition is relieved.

On the other hand, there are occasional patients who quickly become psychologically dependent upon drugs once they have been exposed to them. Ap-parently, the opiates offer some people a release from inner tensions that they find extremely gratifying. Thus, the nurse may note that a particular patient continues to ask for a narcotic pain-reliever long after most patients with the same condition no longer need it. Such reactions are much more rare than one would believe from the stories often told by sympathy-seeking addicts about how they became "hooked" by taking drugs prescribed for pain. None-theless, the nurse should promptly discuss such occa-sional situations with the patient's physician, and, in general, she should follow procedures that will mini-mize drug dependence in susceptible individuals.

Psychological dependence upon drugs, it seems, stems mainly from some sort of personality dis-turbance. Once a person with this type of psychologi-cal difficulty experiences the kind of drug-induced gratification that is especially meaningful to him, he will compulsively seek to maintain himself in such a state at all costs. Unless such a person's psychological difficulties are successfully treated, he is likely to resume the abuse of drugs even after his dependence seems broken—by a long jail term or by detoxification in an institution. That is, although his dependence seems broken, he still remembers the pleasant feeling and seeks out the drug once he is free again to do so. This, and *not* physical dependence, accounts for the high relapse rate among drug-dependent individuals.

Tolerance and Physical Dependence. The taking of larger and larger doses of certain drugs in order to gain and maintain their desired effects is a com-mon characteristic of drug abuse. This need to in-crease the dose to keep getting gratification is coupled with varying degrees of ability to withstand the drug's adverse effects. Such *tolerance* is partly the

result of an increased capacity for metabolizing and eliminating the drug; it is also the result of the ability of a person's cells and tissues to adapt somehow to the presence of the drug, so that, up to a point at least, they function more or less normally.

Actually, tolerance has its limits, and doses are finally reached with any drug that can result in in-toxication and death. The true importance of toler-ance is that its occurrence so often leads to the de-velopment of *physical dependence*, a phenomenon that tends to reinforce the drug-seeking behavior of people whose personalities make them susceptible to drug abuse. This type of dependence is the result of drug-induced changes in tissue function that make the presence of the drug necessary in order to main-tain a normal state of activity.

The biochemical basis for physical dependence upon drugs is still obscure, as is its relationship to tol-erance. In the case of the opiates, it is thought that the same cellular changes in the central nervous system that lead to ability to withstand the drugs' actions may also play a part in the development of physical dependence upon these agents. With other drugs, the amphetamines for example, the chronic abuser may become quite tolerant and require larger and larger doses without ever becoming physically dependent.

Withdrawal Syndromes. The fact that a person has become physically dependent upon a drug is dem-onstrated, not by any detectable biochemical changes but by what happens when the drug is abruptly withdrawn. When this happens in a person who has been taking large amounts of certain drugs, a char-acteristic pattern of signs and symptoms develops. Apparently, as the level of drugs in the tissues of a physically dependent person drops after he stops taking the drugs, the drug-adapted cells fail to func-tion normally.

In the case of depressant drugs, the systems that are released from the state of reduced activity seem to become hyperactive. Two main patterns of hyper-excitability are now recognized upon withdrawal of depressant drugs: (1) The withdrawal of opiates and other potent narcotic analgesics is marked by many signs and symptoms of autonomic nervous system hyperactivity as well as by increased central nervous system excitability. (2) *The barbiturates* and other hypnotics and sedatives and the minor tranquilizers, on the other hand, produce a different picture when they are abruptly withdrawn after long abuse. As happens when the alcoholic is deprived of liquor, the abstinence syndrome with barbiturates and pharmacologically related drugs is marked by excita-bility of the portions of the nervous system controlling motor and mental functions. Patients become tremu-lous and may suffer seizures of the grand mal type;

they also tend to become confused and disoriented and may suffer severe psychotic reactions.

The physical discomfort that develops when a person is deprived of a drug that he has been taking to excess for a prolonged period tends, of course, to make it more difficult for him to stop abusing the drug, even if he makes an effort to do so. That is, the withdrawal syndrome is a negative factor which reinforces such positive factors as the euphoria that the psychologically susceptible person feels when he begins to take the drug. Actually, however, the pangs of withdrawal are less important in perpetuating addictive behavior than many people think.

Some people tend to assume that the addict's main reason for continuing to take drugs is his desire to avoid the physical suffering brought on by abstinence. Yet, authorities on addiction to opiates say that the withdrawal sickness with these drugs is usually no worse than we experience when we have a case of the "flu." They argue that the difficulties of so-called "cold turkey" withdrawal are overrated and that the heroin addict's abstinence agonies are part of a purposeful bid for sympathy. In any case, we can agree that the person who goes back on narcotics soon after his release from long incarceration does so for psychological rather than physical reasons, since he is, of course, no longer suffering a withdrawal sickness. We must note, however, that while the opiate syndrome may be relatively mild in individuals withdrawing from the highly diluted heroin to which they are addicted, barbiturates, alcohol, and other general depressants of the central nervous system can cause a much more dangerous withdrawal illness in individuals who have become physically dependent upon these substances.

Treatment of Addiction. The management of drug-dependent patients is discussed in some detail in the chapters dealing with commonly abused substances such as the barbiturates, opiates, amphetamines and alcohol. Here, we shall consider generally the goals of therapy and the kind of attitudes that health personnel should develop in order to help people who are prone to misuse medications and to deal with their difficulties.

WITHDRAWAL of the abused drug under controlled conditions is the first step in treating any person who has been hospitalized as a result of difficulties caused by drug dependency. Most withdrawal programs make use of some temporary substitute for the drug that the patient has been abusing. In the case of heroin, for example, the longer-acting narcotic, methadone, is administered to reduce the severity of withdrawal. When barbiturates and other abused sedatives, hypnotics or tranquilizers are being withdrawn, pentobarbital is commonly employed to stabilize the patient. Both substitutes are themselves dependency-producers—they would not work otherwise to mini-

mize the abstinence syndrome—and must themselves be gradually withdrawn.

Most patients are weaned away from opiates in a week or two or from barbiturates over a period of several weeks. Some drug abusers may complain during this period of all sorts of symptoms in an effort to get more medication. Although some of the patient's discomfort is the direct physical result of withdrawal, his complaints may also stem from a desire to persuade doctors and nurses to give him more medication to satisfy his psychic dependency on drugs. The nurse must then use good judgment in determining how much medication to administer in response to the patient's complaints. She should not, on the one hand, assume a punitive attitude and withhold drugs when she has a choice in the matter; on the other hand, giving in too readily to the patient's demands for a chemical crutch tends only to delay his recovery.

In general, it is desirable to make the patient as comfortable as possible by means other than drugs. Physical measures such as back rubs, soothing tubs, and warm blankets are often better than medications. Similarly, staying with the anxious patient as much as possible offers him much needed psychological support. Nevertheless, if the doctor has left a p.r.n. order for salicylates, these should be administered without hesitation for relief of muscular aches and pains; and insomnia may well be controlled by sleep-producing substances such as chloral hydrate or phenobarbital without fear of fostering further addiction, when the physician has left their use to the nurse's discretion.

Detoxifying the patient does not, of course, do anything to alter the underlying emotional difficulties that led him to take drugs to excess in the first place. Then, to quiet the uneasiness that he may feel when deprived of drugs, the abuser may try every sort of subterfuge in an effort to get depressant drugs. The nurse must be alert to the patient's attempts to acquire drugs, without at the same time assuming the attitude of policeman. The patient and his visitors should be watched to see that he receives no forbidden drugs, and they should be told courteously but firmly that no tricks will be tolerated.

REHABILITATION of drug addicts and abusers is by far the most difficult part of the whole treatment procedure. The rate of recidivism is very high—over 90 per cent in opiate addiction, for example. Thus, one who deals with addicts may readily feel frustrated and discouraged. It then becomes easy to blame the patient and scorn him as a weak-willed antisocial parasite. Such attitudes, to which the patient is extremely sensitive, serve only to interfere with the nurse's effectiveness in caring for him.

Quick cures should not be expected in drug-dependency. It is best to look upon the condition as a chronic illness marked by periods of relapse. The defects of character and inadequacies in the addict's personality are the result of long development; so treatment can be expected to be a long-term matter too. Thus, the nurse does what she can to help the patient cope with his problems until he becomes better able to deal with his difficulties effectively.

The nurse sometimes has an opportunity to work closely with such a patient and his family during the long period of rehabilitation. The public health nurse may, for example, offer emotional support and guidance and help them to profit from the services offered by local community mental health centers.

Various private voluntary organizations seem to be having some success in salvaging people with addictive personalities. The most successful of such rehabilitative programs, including Narcotics Anonymous and Synanon, try to get the drug abuser to take a realistic look at himself and his life situation. The leaders of these groups are usually themselves former addicts who have suffered the same kind of experiences as the patient. Thus, knowing all the tricks that the addict uses to fool himself and others, these counselors do not err in the direction of excessive permissiveness. This is apparent both during the detoxification process, which is carried out "cold turkey" in such facilities, and later in the rehabilitation process when immature attitudes are greeting with disdain. The patient, however, takes such verbal dressings-down and, often, profits from them because he can identify with former addicts who have succeeded in rehabilitating themselves.

Prevention of Drug Abuse and Addiction. The nurse's role in minimizing the likelihood of dependence developing in patients receiving potent narcotic analgesics is discussed in detail in Chapter 9. In addition, the nurse's knowledge of the actions of other commonly abused drugs gives her an opportunity to help combat the misuse of drugs in her community. She can do this, both as a public health and school nurse and as a citizen, by taking part in activities intended to disseminate accurate information concerning the hazards of taking drugs without supervision.

The nurse should be aware that the abuse of drugs is not necessarily limited to economically disadvantaged individuals or to people who are emotionally disturbed in any very obvious way. Drug-taking occurs in people of every class, including not only dwellers in our urban slums but also suburban housewives, high school and college students, and members of the medical, dental, and nursing professions.

Self-Experimentation With Drugs. At the present time, there are even those who advocate the use of certain drugs as a means of gaining more meaningful experiences than the everyday realities of our culture offer. The so-called psychedelic, or mind-expanding,

drugs such as lysergic acid diethylamide (LSD), psilocybin, and mescaline are touted to college students as agents that offer them opportunities to gain new insights and set free blocked creative powers. This kind of appeal to people seeking "kicks" is pernicious. For although it is true that marihuana smoking, glue sniffing, and LSD "trips" do not produce addiction in the classic sense, these practices can be extremely hazardous.

The dangers of LSD, for example, have not yet been fully elucidated. Most people who have experimented with this and other hallucinogens have had only transient reactions, which some find rapturous and others fearful. Yet a small but significant number of others have been precipitated into prolonged psychotic episodes. Some recent reports indicate that LSD may do damage to chromosomes. This raises the possibility that a young person beguiled into "exploring inner space" by taking a drug that temporarily disorganizes his mental processes may actually suffer genetic changes affecting future generations.

Just why young people who have no knowledge of a drug's real potential for doing harm would want to run the risk of taking such a chemical is puzzling to people of older age groups—and particularly to pharmacologists whose work makes them aware of the hazards inherent in almost all drugs. Perhaps there is a certain satisfaction in defying the hypocrisies of the "square" world of one's elders, especially when the glories of certain drugs are glamorized by some academic people with intellectual pretensions. Actually the "acid" (LSD) cultists are no smarter than the junior high schooler who inhales the vapors of model airplane glue, all the while blissfully unaware that some of these volatile solvents are capable of causing blood dyscrasias and liver damage.

In addition, of course, the effects of such substances upon a person's perceptions, thinking, and motor coordination often expose him to physical injury. This is, of course, also true of the abuse of alcoholic beverages, as the professional "potheads" who argue for the legalization of marihuana are quick to proclaim. However, the fact that our society accepts the moderate use of one substance that is capable of being abused by some individuals does not necessarily make the use of other potentially dangerous drugs more acceptable.

Some so-called intellectuals argue that laws aimed at preventing the abuse of these drugs tend to curtail their personal freedom—yet society has increasingly accepted the responsibility of protecting immature or emotionally disturbed people from the consequences of their own rash acts and impulsive behavior. Thus, although marihuana and LSD have not been shown to produce dangerous withdrawal reactions, the unrestricted availability and widespread use of these substances cannot be sanctioned. For substances with psychic effects that can lead people to injure themselves or others do require legal control, and their use, except in legitimate scientific experimentation, is correctly categorized as drug abuse.

Drug-Taking Among Medical Personnel. The fact that drug abuse is not limited to people who lack adequate knowledge of the physical and mental damage that drugs can do is apparent from the high incidence of addiction among medical personnel. One reason for the higher proportion of addiction among doctors, nurses, dentists and pharmacists is that drugs are so readily available to these professional people. In addition, of course, these people, being human, may share the human weakness for seeking relief of tension with drugs. It is often hard to know who of us—despite no lack of money, opportunity, or education—may be susceptible to drug abuse as a solution for inner tensions created by our life situations.

Thus, the nurse must be alert to the possibility that a colleague may occasionally be stealing narcotics or other drugs from the stores of the ward. Someone may, for example, be substituting falsely labeled solutions or tablets for drugs that have been taken for personal use. Sometimes one may begin to suspect this when several patients fail to get relief of pain after routine administration of morphine, meperidine (Demerol) or other potent analgesics. This could be because sterile saline has been used to replace the actual narcotic drug in the labeled vial or because an inert tablet (resembling codeine or Dilaudid, for example) has been substituted for the actual analgesic. In all such situations, one should avoid being the source of rumors that might arouse unnecessary suspicion and distrust. The possibility of illegal diversion of drugs should, however, be suggested to the nursing supervisor who will be in a better position to take constructive measures in such cases.

The nurse herself should, of course, never yield to the temptation to take a dose of a narcotic that has not been specifically prescribed for her by a physician. Nurses are subject to pain and anxiety just as is anyone else, and these symptoms may well require treatment with potent and potentially addicting medications. The nurse should never fear to take such medication under medical supervision. She should *not*, however, administer such drugs to herself for symptomatic relief without medical advice and supervision. Even occasional self-treatment of this kind might lead to the habitual use of a dangerous drug and to eventually disastrous dependency upon it.

POISONING BY DRUGS AND CHEMICALS

Toxicology is the science that deals with poisons—chemical substances that cause harm when they come into contact with living tissues, even in very small amounts. Actually, the term *poison* is more difficult than that to define. Most of the drugs that are used to treat disease may prove to be poisonous under some circumstances. Although most people think of poisons as chemicals so dangerous that their effects on living tissues can never be anything but injurious and life-endangering, many medically useful substances can also act as poisons when taken in doses above those administered in pharmacotherapy.

Throughout this text, we shall discuss the toxicological aspects of those drugs that experience has proved most likely to cause poisoning in overdosage. In this chapter, we shall make some generalizations about the nature of poisoning and the measures which are taken to treat and prevent poisoning. We shall emphasize accidental poisoning, caused not only by drugs but also by other chemicals commonly found in the home and on the farm.

Our concern with these aspects of toxicology stems from the frequency with which nurses are called upon to play a part in the detection, prevention and treatment of poisoning. The nurse's observations of the patient's signs and symptoms often help the physician to make his diagnosis of poisoning. She also aids in the management of poisoned patients, not only by applying first aid measures and by assisting the physician with more complicated treatment regimens, but also by keeping in readiness the antidotal drugs and equipment required for treatment. Finally, the nurse often helps to prevent poisoning both by avoiding accidents when she herself handles and administers medicines and by helping to educate the public.

Scope and Seriousness of Poisoning. The seriousness and extent of poisoning as a public health problem has become apparent during recent years as a result of more efficient collection of epidemiologic data by municipal, state and national health agencies. Most cases of chemical toxicity are the result of either suicide attempts or the accidental ingestion of drugs or of chemical substances which were never intended for human consumption.

The incidence of accidental poisoning is highest in children under five years of age, but elderly patients and other adults often mistakenly take drugs or other chemicals in toxic quantities. In one recent year close to 500 children died from accidental poisoning as did over 1,000 individuals in the older age groups. These statistics refer only to fatalities resulting from substances taken internally through mischance in the home; they do not include deaths from industrial chemicals or from the inhalation of gases such as carbon monoxide, nor fatal suicidal poisonings.

Such mortality statistics do not truly reflect the actual dimensions of the accidental poisoning problem. There are, apparently, about 600 cases of accidental chemical ingestion for each reported fatality. Thus, in one recent one-year period, the National

Health Survey estimated that there occurred close to a million poison emergency cases. Many of these cases required little treatment beyond gastric lavage, and the individual suffered few ill effects other than possible psychological trauma. On the other hand, many victims of poisoning that did not prove fatal suffered serious injuries, which required prolonged medical and surgical treatment. (A child who swallows a lye solution, for example, may be hospitalized for many months for dilation of an esophagus constricted by scar tissue and finally for surgical correction of the damage.)

Chemical Causes. DRUGS AND MEDICINES are the cause of more cases of poisoning than are all other chemicals combined. Aspirin alone accounts for about half of all drug deaths in children; barbiturates and other hypnotics are the agents most frequently involved in adult fatalities. Other medications commonly reported as the cause of poisoning include antihistaminic drugs in products for treating the common cold; laxatives (especially those containing strychnine); opiate-containing analgesic and cough preparations, and, most recently, various tranquilizer drugs.

CHEMICAL SPECIALTY PRODUCTS constitute the other main cause of poisoning. These include not only pesticides (insecticides, rat poisons and weed destroyers) but also substances employed for cleaning and painting tasks about the home. Among the substances of this sort most frequently ingested are: bleaches, soaps and detergents; furniture polishes and waxes containing kerosene and other petroleum distillates; paint and varnish solvents and thinners; disinfectants such as cresol and lye; and an endless array of other chemicals in close to a quarter million such products. Despite the passage of the Federal Hazardous Substances Labeling Act in 1960, the labeling on many of these products is still far from fully informative.

Poison Control Centers. The inadequacy of labeling was one of the factors that led physicians and others in the public health professions to pool their resources to gain the information required for coping with poison emergencies. The first formal program for the collecting and disseminating of data concerning accidental poisoning was set up in Chicago in 1953. This pilot project proved so successful that other cities, states and regions soon initiated similar centers for fact gathering and for the interchange of information. Today, about 500 such groups are represented in the American Association of Poison Control Centers.

The manner of operation of such centers is varied to fit different local needs. In general, however, poison control centers provide services of two types. Some, located in hospitals, offer facilities for the treatment of victims of accidental poisoning. They are organized to offer not only immediate first aid measures but also medical and surgical specialty services, which require advanced technical equipment and extensive laboratory facilities.

Other centers—usually located in the health departments of large cities or states or in medical and pharmacy schools—function as sources of information rather than treatment. Often they can be reached 24 hours a day for answers to the questions most commonly asked by doctors faced with a poison emergency: "What is in it?" "How toxic is it?" "What's the best treatment?" Treatment centers and hospital emergency rooms also are often called upon to furnish such information. Thus, the nurse, who, with the physician and pharmacist, is often a key member of a team for handling emergencies of this kind, should be aware of available reference materials and other sources from which the answers to such questions may be found.

Sources of Information. Very many books are available dealing with toxicology, pharmacology, the chemical contents of various kinds of household products, etc. (See Bibliography.) However, two comprehensive compendia have proved especially useful as sources of information in poison emergencies. These are (1) The massive card file prepared by the National Clearinghouse for Poison Control Centers, and (2) the book *Clinical Pharmacology of Commercial Products* by Gleason, Gosselin and Hodge.

Both are sources of the kinds of information that the physician is most frequently seeking—the chemical contents of a specific trade-named product; how hazardous its ingestion is likely to prove; the signs and symptoms to look for; and first aid and more comprehensive treatment measures that should be employed. The Clearinghouse File consists of a constantly expanding set of alphabetized cards of two types—*white ones* which deal with the management of cases in which any one of thousands of *specific products* may have been ingested; and *orange cards* which outline in greater detail the procedures for treating poisoning by the most toxic *chemical ingredients* of some of these products. The manual published in book form furnishes similar information in its seven sections, together with an illustrative chart on how to use the text in the most efficient manner for acquiring the data that may be needed in a poisoning emergency.

OTHER RESOURCES. Occasional cases cannot be readily dealt with by consulting such sources. Calls of this kind are relayed to regional information centers which have the facilities for tracing down specialized data. Sometimes, they make long-distance calls to the manufacturers of the ingested products or to expert consultants who may possess vital specialized information, and can often furnish the information needed in managing poisoning by plants, venomous animals, foods, and pharmaceuticals.

Pharmacists close to home can almost always furnish factual information that will help in the identification of drug products that have been accidentally ingested. The pharmacist may do so by referring to the *Identification Guide for Solid Dosage Forms* made available by the American Medical Association or by consulting the section in the Physician's Desk Reference in which pictures of many common capsules and tablets are shown. Other useful compendia of drug data include the *American Drug Index;* the *United States Dispensatory,* and the *Modern Drug Encyclopedia.*

Conveying of Information. The handling of poisoning emergencies requires considerable teamwork and a willingness to be flexible in carrying out functions of various kinds, including some that do not ordinarily fall within one's professional duties. Poisoning often constitutes such a grave emergency that each person simply tries to contribute whatever knowledge and skill he has in the best way he can. Thus, the more the nurse knows about poisons and antidotes, reference materials, and other resources, the more effectively can she function in caring for the patient and in furnishing information to physicians and laymen who may call the emergency ward.

Such information relative to the management of cases of poisoning is so varied that no physician could possibly keep it all in his head. Thus, if a doctor telephones for advice and no fellow physician is available to give it, the nurse can certainly try to find the necessary information and transmit it to the inquiring doctor in a tactful manner. Lay people who telephone for information about handling a pediatric emergency are best advised to hurry the child to the family physician or, in his absence, to the nearest hospital.

Laymen may, however, be given first aid information in such an emergency. If the nature of the ingested substance is known, the person may be told whether or not to induce vomiting and how best to do so; or if the question concerns contamination of the skin and eyes with chemicals, the person should be urged to wash these areas immediately with copious quantities of tap water. Of course, the patient should be brought in for further medical attention after first aid has been administered. The caller should be advised to save the container of the product and to bring it, or the suspected poison itself, to the hospital or to the physician's office.

Prevention of Poisoning

There may be little beyond the advice indicated above that the nurse may be able to tell the lay person once a poison accident has occurred. However, the nurse *can* tell people a great deal that may help to *prevent* poisoning. Public health and school nurses have an especially important part to play in advising people concerning the safe handling and storage of drugs in the home. However, the nurse serving in a hospital setting can teach patients who are about to return home how to avoid overdosage and other poison accidents.

This is especially true of elderly patients who are often forgetful and tend to become confused. The nurse sometimes has to help the aged person who lives alone to devise systems for remembering what drugs he has taken, so that he does not inadvertently take an overdose. Thus, the nurse may make a chart for the patient taking digitalis and show him how to place a check mark on it after he takes each day's medication. She can also teach him to read the labels and to follow instructions carefully before taking any drug. Such a patient should not, in any case, be given responsibilities beyond those that he is capable of handling. If at all possible, another family member should keep the patient's medication and see to it that it is administered only exactly as ordered.

The Public Health Nurse is usually called upon to make follow-up visits to homes in which poison accidents have occurred. Often, even casual observation of the home environment indicates various hazardous conditions which could result in future accidents. She then makes suggestions concerning safer storage and use of drugs and household chemicals. School nurses are sometimes called upon to participate in campaigns in regard to poison control aimed at educating parents through their school age children. The nurse often gives such children simple safety instructions and distributes any of the many poison prevention pamphlets—and even comic books—which are made available by the U. S. Public Health Service, the National Safety Council, the American Medical Association and other groups concerned with poison prevention. Such instruction is especially valuable when the school child has preschool siblings—the group most prone to poison accidents.

The measures most commonly emphasized in educational programs aimed at the general public can best be summarized as follows:

1. *Read the label before using any drug or chemical product.* Many individuals and consumer organizations have led long, hard fights for informative labeling of chemical products. Many accidents could be prevented if people would read the labeling carefully. This applies not only to obviously hazardous substances such as pesticides and caustic chemicals, but to cosmetics such as hair dyes and to nonprescription drugs, including laxatives and corn removers.

2. *Never take any medicine in the dark.* This applies especially to elderly patients who read uncertainly at best and often totter to the bathroom during the night, remove the wrong bottle from the medicine cabinet and pour themselves a dose. Aged patients—and others—have, for example, taken medicines intended only for external use in this way. They may take a tablespoonful of camphorated oil or a liniment

containing methyl salicylate—both dangerous substances—instead of the intended cough medication. Others have reached for a box containing sodium bicarbonate powder and have instead picked up a similarly shaped container and taken a teaspoonful of boric acid—dangerous when taken internally.

3. *Keep all chemicals in their original containers.* Most accidents with caustic liquids such as lye solutions, furniture polishes containing kerosene and other petroleum distillates, turpentine, and insecticides occur when these liquids are poured into pitchers, drinking glasses, measuring cups and soda pop bottles. Then a thirsty child comes along and takes a drink of the dangerous liquid that has been left where he can reach it. Adults, too, can become confused, if a thick yellow furniture or floor polish is transferred to a mayonnaise jar that is then left unlabeled.

4. *Never store nonedible products on shelves used for food.* Insect powders containing toxic fluorides have been placed next to flour in an unlabeled container. The poison has then been employed in cooking with fatal results. Similarly, poisonous chemicals such as carbon tetrachloride should never be stored in the medicine cabinet next to cough medications and other household remedies.

5. *Destroy all old medicines instead of just discarding them.* A nurse once gave such a good talk about the dangers of keeping old prescriptions that the P.T.A. members promptly went home and cleaned out their medicine cabinets. However, the mothers threw the drugs into trash cans from which they were promptly salvaged by scavenging children. Pets also have sometimes been poisoned by carelessly discarded medications, which should have been poured into the sink or flushed in the toilet.

6. *Keep all drugs, household chemicals, and other potentially poisonous substances out of the reach of children.* This is, of course, the most basic rule of all in homes where youngsters live or are likely to visit. In such households, even the medicine cabinet is an undesirable place to keep drugs, unless it can be locked. Yet medications are constantly left about on bedside tables, living room chairs, and handbags where exploring tots can readily find and swallow them. Similarly, floor-level kitchen cabinets containing bleaches and other cleaners are convenient for the crawling child as well as for his mother. Thus, the cardinal rule in households with very young children should be to keep all products containing chemicals stored up high and preferably under lock and key in order to thwart climbers whose motor abilities have outdistanced their experience and understanding of danger.

Diagnosis and Treatment of Poisoning

Diagnosis of poisoning is, of course, the doctor's task, and it may, indeed, pose many problems for the physician. The signs and symptoms of poisoning are essentially the same as those seen in other disorders, and the combinations of toxic effects produced by many drugs resemble syndromes seen in various diseases. Thus, drug-induced convulsions may not differ from status epilepticus, and coma caused by a depressant drug may not be easily differentiated from the same state developing as a result of disease.

The nurse may note various signs and symptoms in the course of making her observations of the patient, which may prove useful for the physician in making his diagnosis.

A comatose patient may, for example, have fresh needle marks on parts of the skin overlying veins that addicts use in "mainlining" opiates. These and the presence of characteristic "tracks" may be an indication that the patient is a heroin addict who has suffered an "O.D.," or overdose. Similarly, suspicion may be aroused by an unusual odor on the breath, which may serve to differentiate diabetic coma from alcoholic stupor or cyanide poisoning. Burns about the mouth and adjacent skin may indicate the recent ingestion of a caustic chemical solution. Marked darkening of a urine sample may signify that phenols have been swallowed and absorbed systemically.

All such specific observations are reported to the doctor along with those relating to the patient's pulse, blood pressure, respiration characteristics, and the state of central nervous system function. The events observed and reported by the nurse before the physician arrives on the scene serve to supplement his own later observation in ways which often permit earlier detection of the fact that the patient is a victim of poisoning.

Treatment. The management of poisoning emergencies requires the use of measures of several types: (1) Emergency measures for *removing the substance from the skin*, eyes and gastrointestinal tract before significant local damage or systemic absorption occur. (2) Administration of locally and systemically acting *antidotes* to counteract the poison chemically or to antagonize its effects by an opposing chemical or pharmacological action. (3) Application of *supportive treatment* measures to maintain the patient's vital functions and to minimize his discomfort, pain and suffering. Some pertinent aspects of each of these types of treatment will now be discussed in the above order. However, the actual management of the poisoned patient may not necessarily follow this sequence. Thus, although emptying the stomach is commonly an initial measure, it is often first necessary to administer a specific antidote parenterally or to support the patient's respiration artificially before proceeding to remove the poison.

Removing toxic chemicals from the skin and eyes requires quick and prolonged rinsing with large amounts of running water, after first removing contaminated clothing; the patient's eyelids are held open. Later, a paste of sodium bicarbonate can be applied to skin burned by acid, or a dressing soaked in dilute vinegar may be placed over any area contaminated by caustic alkali. The pain of eye burns may be relieved by topical anesthetics, and a corticosteroid ophthalmic solution or ointment is instilled into an injured eye. Special solvents may be preferred for removing certain chemicals—for example, fixed oils such as olive oil and castor oil remove phenol more readily than water does. However, speed is so essential in such cases that valuable time should not be wasted in locating or preparing special solutions.

Vomiting may be induced by physical or chemical measures at the scene of the accident, prior to arrival of medical help; gastric lavage, which is more certain but also requires more technical competence, may be carried out later in the emergency room or doctor's office. Often the patient can most rapidly be made to vomit by having him drink several glasses of tepid water containing about one tablespoonful of salt in each. Emesis may then be hastened by touching the back of the patient's throat with a finger or the handle of a spoon.

In addition to this procedure and the use of such other household emetic substances as mustard powder, emesis may be induced by drugs. Laymen are now often advised to keep a 1-ounce bottle of ipecac syrup at home for emergency use in case of suspected poison ingestion. The F.D.A. now permits the sale of this quantity of ipecac syrup without the prescription that was formerly required. This change is based on recent evidence indicating that administration of half an ounce of this preparation induces vomiting in the vast majority of patients in 15 to 30 minutes. It had been previously feared that this drug's onset of action was too slow to be useful in a poisoning emergency and that it might itself prove toxic if vomiting failed to occur and its alkaloids (including emetine) were systemically absorbed. Fluidextract of ipecac, a more concentrated preparation containing fourteen times as much of the alkaloids, has indeed proved poisonous when administered by mistake in place of the syrup.

Although it may be desirable to administer ipecac syrup as a first aid measure prior to arrival of the doctor, the physician himself is more likely to employ apomorphine to induce vomiting. This opium alkaloid usually acts quickly after 5 mg. are injected subcutaneously. If it fails to act, no more than one more injection is ordinarily made, because this drug can cause excessive central depression. Ipecac syrup, on the other hand, may be repeated when a first dose fails to induce vomiting.

The label on bottles of ipecac syrup states that the patient should call the physician, or the Poison Control Center, or hospital emergency room for advice before using this emetic. If the emergency room nurse answers the telephone, she should try to learn what the patient has taken and what condition he is in, for such facts have a bearing on whether or not emetics may be administered.

The nurse relays such information about what the patient took, and how much, to the emergency room physician, along with what she was able to learn about the condition of the poison accident victim. The doctor may telephone the family, whose number the nurse had taken, and tell them what emergency measures to employ, including emesis if desirable. Of course, if prompt medical assistance is not available, the nurse herself may give immediate advice to the family to the best of her ability; she then uses every possible means to obtain the treatment of a physician for the patient.

Emetics are contraindicated in the following circumstances: (1) *If the patient is comatose or only semiconscious.* In such cases, emetics may fail to act and may themselves prove toxic. (2) *If the patient has taken a convulsant poison* such as strychnine and is already showing some signs of central excitement. Retching and vomiting may precipitate seizures in such circumstances. (3) *After ingestion of strong acids, corrosive alkali or other caustic substances.* The stress of vomiting may lead to rupture of the walls of the stomach or esophagus, which have been weakened by chemical corrosion. (4) *Following ingestion of petroleum distillates* such as kerosene, gasoline, coal or fuel oil, or paint thinners and cleaning fluids. Aspiration of such substances into the lungs during retching and vomiting may lead to development of pneumonitis.

Gastric lavage possesses similar contraindications, except that the likelihood of aspiration pneumonia may be less when a stomach tube is skillfully employed in comatose patients and in those who have swallowed kerosene or products containing petroleum distillates. The nurse is often called upon to restrain children while the doctor inserts the lavage tube orally or intranasally. (Full discussion of the various aspects of this technical procedure should be sought from appropriate texts.)

The stomach tube may be left in place after the lavage fluid—usually tap water—has been introduced and syringed out repeatedly, and may then be used for administration of any of a variety of other substances. These include demulcent fluids, for soothing local irritation; concentrated solutions of saline cathartics, for speeding the removal from the intestinal tract of any toxic material that may already have passed the pyloric sphincter; and specific chemical antidotes designed to neutralize, precipitate, oxidize or otherwise alter the poison to a relatively harmless form.

Chemical antidotes include the so-called *Universal Antidote*, a mixture of activated charcoal, tannic acid, and magnesium oxide. A half dozen or so teaspoonfuls of the light, fluffy powder are mixed with water to make a thin paste which is then further diluted to make a glassful of liquid. When instilled into the stomach, the charcoal in this antidote *ad*sorbs large amounts of alkaloidal poisons such as strychnine, and other substances; the tannic acid precipitates alkaloids and also some metallic poisons; the magnesium oxide acts as a mild antacid to neutralize strong mineral acids without the danger of gas formation such as accompany the use of carbonate-type alkalinizers. The mixture is finally siphoned out of the stomach to avoid the possibility that the temporarily inactivated poison may once more be released in toxic form.

Other chemical antidotes include potassium permanganate, which in dilutions of 1:10,000 to 1:5,000 oxidizes various alkaloids and other organic poisons; sodium chloride, which precipitates soluble silver salts as insoluble silver chloride; and copper sulfate, which coats phosphorus particles with inactive copper phosphide. In addition, certain foods make excellent poison precipitants. Milk and raw egg whites contain proteins that combine with mercury, arsenic and other heavy metals to form insoluble and inactive albuminates. Starch is an especially effective precipitant of iodine when tincture of iodine has been swallowed. These substances also have a soothing demulcent action on the irritated gastrointestinal mucosa. Vinegar and citrus fruit juices contain weak acids—acetic and citric—which may help to neutralize stronger alkali.

Support of the patient's vital functions is especially important in poisoning, because the poison not only may adversely affect the patient's respiratory and circulatory systems but also may interfere with its own elimination by way of the liver and kidneys. Some supportive measures must be applied immediately—artificial respiration and treatment for shock, for example—but others are often carried out long after the poison has been removed from the body and emergency antidotal drugs have been administered. Supportive care is sometimes required for days and weeks, and its success often depends upon the quality of the nursing that the patient receives.

The medical and nursing measures employed in support of the poisoned patient are essentially similar to those employed in treating any seriously ill patient. We shall review only briefly some examples of the supportive measures most pertinent to the care of patients poisoned by various of the drugs and chemicals most commonly involved in such cases. More detailed discussions of the management of poisoning by individual agents such as the barbiturates, opiates, strychnine, and the anticholinesterase-type insecticides

will be found at appropriate points in the text (*see Index*).

RESPIRATION is often interfered with by drugs that depress or overstimulate the central nervous system. In such cases, the nurse looks for signs and symptoms of hypoxia such as early restlessness and confusion, which, along with lethargy, often appear well before the onset of cyanosis. The nurse's functions include the reporting to the physician of the presence of signs of obstruction such as wheezing. However, the nurse herself must often take immediate action to keep the patient's airway open. She also assists the physician with intubation and suctioning procedures and preparation for tracheotomy.

Artificial respiration and oxygen inhalation are commonly employed when the patient's own breathing is inefficient and hypoxia is developing. In an extreme emergency, mouth-to-mouth and manual techniques applied by the nurse may be lifesaving. More commonly, the nurse is responsible for the observation and care of a patient whose lungs are being rhythmically inflated by a mechanical resuscitator. She also works with patients receiving oxygen by means of nasal catheters, face masks, and tents.

Patients with prolonged drug-induced respiratory depression run the risk of contracting hypostatic pneumonia and other infections. The nurse may help to minimize these dangers by application of careful nursing measures. Patients deeply depressed by barbiturates, for example, should have their position in bed changed frequently to counteract the adverse effects of stasis upon pulmonary function. Those whose cough reflex is sluggish should be assisted to cough in order to expel mucus from the lungs. Nurses caring for such patients must wear masks and gowns to keep the patient's exposure to infection at a minimum. If atalectasis occurs, the nurse may assist with bronchoscopy and other measures for aiding drainage. Among the drugs employed in pneumonia and pulmonary edema are antibiotics and detergents or other agents for reducing surface tension in the tracheobronchial tree.

CIRCULATORY FUNCTION must be maintained in poisoned patients not only to keep vital organs functioning as effectively as possible, but because inadequate circulation delays the elimination of the poison and reduces the effectiveness of parenterally administered antidotal drugs. Administration of intravenous fluids to counteract shock is a very important aspect of circulatory system support. The nurse checks the patient's blood pressure frequently, sees that the materials required for intravenous infusion are available, and takes the necessary measures to assure that fluid is flowing into the vessel at the proper rate.

In addition to replacement fluids such as whole blood, plasma, isotonic saline and the synthetic plasma expanders, vasopressor drugs are often employed to raise the poisoned patient's blood pressure. A very useful but potentially dangerous drug often used for this purpose is levarterenol. In such cases, the nurse does not leave the patient during infusion of the drug, and she takes his pressure as often as every five minutes. She is especially attentive in seeing that the needle is taped properly to the patient's skin or the catheter securely held in place, and that the patient's limb is well restrained. This is not only to assure continued intravenous flow of the pressure-raising drug, but also to prevent the ischemia and subsequent tissue necrosis that may occur if this drug leaks into the surrounding tissues. If any swelling appears at the site of the needle, indicating that fluid is extravasating, the nurse stops the flow and reports the situation to the doctor immediately, so that the intravenous infusion can be promptly restarted.

The nurse is often part of the hospital cardiac arrest team. One of her important responsibilities relative to cardiac resuscitation involves seeing that emergency supplies and equipment are available and in good condition. Thus, the supply of drugs such as digitalis, quinidine, atropine and epinephrine, which are often employed in counteracting the adverse effects of poisons upon the heart, must be kept constantly replenished. Equipment for meeting critical cardiac emergencies also includes such apparatus as defibrillators, artificial pacemakers, and the electrocardiograph.

LIVER FUNCTION may be interfered with or even fail as a result of direct damage by hepatotoxic agents such as the halogenated hydrocarbons carbon tetrachloride and chloroform and other organic solvents, or as a result of poisoning by phosphorus, or the toxin of the poisonous mushroom *Amanita phalloides*. Once the poison is removed from the body and the more immediately dangerous drug effects are counteracted, the main treatment may consist of measures to keep the patient alive while liver tissue is being regenerated.

The nurse must often encourage the patient to eat the diet prescribed for him despite his persistent anorexia. Diets high in calories, carbohydrates and protein are considered more important than any drugs in the management of patients with acute liver damage. High doses of many vitamins are often administered, and an antiemetic phenothiazine tranquilizer-type drug may occasionally be administered to control nausea, vomiting and restlessness. More potent central depressants such as barbiturates and opiates are ordinarily avoided, since these drugs may precipitate hepatic coma in patients with severe liver damage.

KIDNEY FUNCTION may fail after a person has been poisoned, either as a result of prolonged circulatory collapse and renal ischemia or because of direct damage to the tubular epithelium by nephrotoxic chemi-cals such as mercury bichloride. In addition to the early use of drugs such as dimercaprol and osmotic diuretics to protect the kidneys during the renal excretion of the poison, many measures are employed to support the patient's body water and electrolyte balance during the period of several weeks that may be required for renal tubular regeneration.

The nurse has many responsibilities in the medical management of the patient with drug-induced acute renal failure. She makes observations of the oliguric patient's daily urinary output and the changes in his body weight during this time of limited intake of fluids, electrolytes and food. She encourages the patient to sip the small amounts of carbohydrate solutions that he is allowed or supervises the slow intravenous infusions of glucose solution that may be required if nausea keeps the patient from taking such substances by mouth.

The nurse also now often cares for poisoned patients who have to undergo hemodialysis. This is a procedure in which poisons and other substances present in excess in the blood plasma are removed by diffusion through a membrane and into a dialysis solution. These so-called artificial kidneys are used both for patients with acute renal failure and for speeding the elimination of poisons in patients whose kidneys are not damaged but merely unable to excrete the high levels of poison in the plasma as rapidly as is necessary. Rapid removal of salicylates, barbiturates and other drugs by dialysis has hastened the recovery of patients who might not have survived if the physician had depended upon the patient's own relatively slow renal excretory mechanisms for removing these poisons.

Other supportive measures are concerned with maintaining the patient's comfort and well being. Here too, nursing care is of major significance in hastening the patient's recovery from poisoning. For example, patients suffering from drug-induced delirium or from one of the withdrawal syndromes following chronic depressant drug toxicity must be kept from hurting themselves during delirium. They are assisted in orienting themselves, in regard to where they are and what is being done to help them. Other poisoned patients may require more than the usual amount of mouth and skin care following contact with irritant chemicals. Patients in pain require not only analgesic drugs but measures such as massage, changes of position, and physical support when they must be moved. The poisoned patient with chills and fever profits from the same nursing measures that afford symptomatic relief to those with infections.

Systemically Acting Antidotes

Systemically acting antidotes are drugs that are used to counteract the actions of poisons that have already been absorbed into the systemic circulation and have begun to exert their toxic effects on various tissues. Some of these drugs are referred to as *physiological antidotes* because they alter tissue function in a manner directly opposed to the action of the poison. Thus, if a person is suffering from strychnine poisoning, which is marked by excessive stimulation of the central nervous system, his symptoms of nervous hyperexcitability may often be best counteracted by administering a barbiturate to produce depression of the overstimulated nerve cells. Similarly, groups of nerve cells that have been too deeply depressed by barbiturates to function efficiently—the medullary respiratory center, for example—may be returned to more normal function in some circumstances by administration of central stimulants such as the analeptics pentylenetetrazol, picrotoxin, or bemegride. The use of antidotes of this type is taken up in the discussions of the treatment of overdosage by specific drugs at the appropriate points in the text.

Other systemic antidotes also act only after absorption but differ from the physiological antidotes in the manner of their actions. These are the *chemical antidotes*—drugs that act by combining with and, thus, inactivating toxic chemicals that have entered the tissues, rather than by counteracting their effects. They are like the chemical antidotes discussed earlier, except that the chemical reactions take place in tissues other than the gastrointestinal tract. Specific antidotes of either the chemical or physiological type are relatively few. Some specific chemical antidotes not taken up elsewhere will be discussed here, together with the treatment of poisons not dealt with at other places in the text.

Antidotes for Heavy Metal Poisoning

The so-called heavy metals, including lead, arsenic, mercury, copper and gold, are all toxic to living tissues. They are thought to exert their various adverse biological effects through their ability to tie up in living tissue chemicals that must be free in order for cells to function normally. When these substances (sulfhydryl (SH) or thiol groups, carboxyls, phosphoryls, and others) are bound by the metals, certain cellular enzyme systems are inactivated, cellular functions fail, and, finally, the cells die.

In the past quarter century, a number of new drugs have been developed for counteracting heavy metal toxicity. These drugs act by breaking the bond between the metal and the vital cellular constituents. Administered early enough, these antidotal chemicals can prevent the development of the very many severe signs and symptoms of heavy metal toxicity. The poisonous metallic ions are clasped by the antidote molecules and carried out of the body before they can harm the tissues. (These metal-binding antidotal chemicals are called *chelating agents*—a name derived from the Greek word *chele,* which means claw.)

Lead poisoning is the most commonly encountered heavy metal toxicosis. Lead encephalopathy—an especially severe form of poisoning—affects mainly children. The metal-induced brain damage causes convulsions, coma and, in about one quarter or more of the victims, death. The condition often develops in children who eat flakes of paint containing white lead. When toxic levels of the poorly excreted metal accumulate in the tissues, symptoms are seen that range from gastrointestinal upset, through muscle weakness ("lead palsy"), to the fatal convulsions mentioned earlier.

Modern treatment of lead poisoning is based upon the use of the chelating agent calcium disodium edetate. Administered by vein, this antidote gives up its calcium and takes on the free lead ions in the tissues, for which it has a higher affinity. The metal mobilized in this manner is then removed from the body by way of the kidneys without doing damage to these or other organs. Unfortunately, this antidotal treatment often fails to halt the explosive course of acute lead encephalopathy in children. Thus, early detection of the presence of lead in the tissues, followed by removal of the child from the dangerous environment, is the most important preventive measure against lead poisoning.

Poisoning by salts of mercury and arsenic, as well as the effects of overdosage with the gold salts used for treating rheumatoid arthritis can be counteracted by the early administration of the chemical antagonist dimercaprol. Dimercaprol, also known as British Anti-Lewisite, or BAL, was developed by British scientists during World War II for use against the arsenical chemical warfare gas, lewisite, which it was feared the Germans might employ. It was synthesized and studied because of the belief that arsenic toxicity was the result of reactions of the metalloid with cellular sulfhydryl (SH) groups. Dimercaprol, a dithiol, furnishes sulfhydryl groups which grasp arsenical compounds and thus keep them from inactivating essential sulfhydryl enzyme systems in the tissues.

Arsenic, especially in the form of the nearly tasteless arsenic trioxide, was a poison traditionally employed in criminal homicides in the Middle Ages and even into this century. The development of chemical methods for detecting its presence in body tissues has discouraged the use of arsenic compounds as a means of committing murder. However, arsenic compounds are commonly employed as weedkillers and for other pesticidal purposes. Thus, arsenic still causes often fatal poisoning of children who gain access to and ingest such dangerous products.

Accidental ingestion of even small amounts of sodium arsenite or other inorganic arsenic compounds causes severe gastroenteritis after a brief latent period. This leads to severe loss of fluids and electrolytes, circulatory collapse, and death in about 24 hours.

Occasionally, absorption of the drug into the central nervous system results in a more rapidly fatal outcome after a period of convulsions and coma.

In addition to the prompt injection of dimercaprol, supportive measures such as correction of dehydration and treatment of shock may also be required. First aid immediately after ingestion requires the use of gastric lavage, followed by a freshly prepared solution of ferric hydroxide or sodium thiosulfate and, finally, a saline cathartic such as sodium sulfate. In the absence of these chemical antidotes, induction of emesis and administration of milk is indicated, until the patient can receive more active medical treatment.

Mercury in the form of mercuric chloride (corrosive sublimate) was once a common cause of acute poisoning. This salt, which is used to prepare solutions used for the disinfecting of inanimate objects, is available in the form of the official (N.F.) Mercury Bichloride Large Poison Tablets. These are required to be distinctive in color and shape to minimize the possibility of their being mistakenly taken internally. (The tablets are often stained blue and come in the angular shape of a stylized coffin.)

Acute poisoning by ingestion of soluble mercury salts is marked by immediate burning pain in the mouth, throat, esophagus and stomach. The patient may die of circulatory collapse after a few hours of continuous vomiting and severe, bloody diarrhea. Gastric lavage with a solution of egg white or of the reducing agent sodium formaldehyde sulfoxylate may help to inactivate and remove the corrosive mercuric salts. In the absence of these substances, a mixture of egg whites and milk may be drunk to help to precipitate the mercury in the upper G.I. tract; the patient may then be made to drink a dilute solution of sodium bicarbonate.

If the patient survives the first phase of mercury poisoning, signs of systemic poisoning often appear in a day or two. Unless dimercaprol administration is vigorously maintained, renal tubular necrosis de-

velops in two or three days. This results in oliguria, azotemia, and death, unless the patient's renal insufficiency can be successfully managed by supportive measures until tubular regeneration and recovery occur in about two weeks. (The organic mercurial compounds employed as diuretics rarely cause severe toxicity. Metallic mercury, or quicksilver, is not hazardous; the main danger from a broken oral or rectal mercury thermometer lies in the broken glass.)

Antagonists of other heavy metals occasionally employed to chelate poisonous metals include the recently introduced compounds penicillamine (Cuprimine) and desferrioxamine (Desferal). The use of the latter drug in the treatment of acute iron poisoning is briefly discussed in Chapter 25. The former agent, penicillamine, has been used experimentally in the treatment of mercury and lead poisonings. It is also employed in the treatment of Wilson's disease, or hepatolenticular degeneration, a condition caused by a metabolic defect which permits the accumulation of copper in certain tissues. The degenerative changes of this disorder may be delayed by a dietary regimen low in copper and by the administration of penicillamine capsules for chelating this metal.

Poisons affecting oxygen transport and utilization include carbon monoxide (CO) and cyanide (CN). Poisoning from inhalation of gas containing CO is said to occur more frequently than all other kinds of poisoning combined. Its treatment by the inhalation of pure oxygen is intended to displace CO from the hemoglobin molecule, so that oxygen can again be carried by the blood to all the body tissues including those of the brain. Cyanide ion does not keep the blood from carrying oxygen to the tissues, but it prevents the tisues from using the oxygen in the series of cellular oxidation-reduction reactions essential to life. Treatment of cyanide poisoning depends upon the rapid administration of systemically acting chemical antidotes (See Table 3-2). These are intended to bind the cyanide ion before it can fatally interfere with cellular respiration.

TABLE 3-1

SOME DRUGS FOR USE IN POISON EMERGENCIES

AGENT	QUANTITY	ACTION
Drugs for Chemically Antidoting and Removing Poisons from the Gastrointestinal Tract		
Acetic acid 5% (or vinegar)	1 pt.	Neutralizer
Aluminum hydroxide gel	8 oz.	Antacid-demulcent
Apomorphine HCl hypo-tabs	5 mg.	Emetic
Calcium hydroxide (lime water)	sat. sol.	Precipitant
Charcoal, activated	1 Gm.	Adsorbent

TABLE 3-1 (Continued)

AGENT	QUANTITY	ACTION
Drugs for Chemically Antidoting and Removing Poisons from the Gastrointestinal Tract (Continued)		
Ipecac syrup	30 ml.	Emetic
Liquid petrolatum (mineral oil)	8 oz.	Solvent-demulcent
Magnesium oxide	30 Gm.	Antacid
Magnesium sulfate (Epsom salt)	8 oz. (50% sol.)	Cathartic
Milk, evaporated	1 can	Demulcent-precipitant
Milk of magnesia	1 pt.	Antacid-laxative
Oil (olive, cottonseed, salad)	8 oz.	Demulcent-laxative
Potassium permanganate tabs, to make	1:5,000 to 1:10,000 sol.	Oxidizing agent
Sodium bicarbonate powder, to make	5% sol.	Precipitant
Sodium sulfate (Glauber's salt)	8 oz. (40% sol.)	Cathartic
Sodium thiosulfate crystals to make	1% sol.	Neutralizer
Starch, powder	3 oz.	Precipitant
Tannic acid, powder	1 oz.	Precipitant
Tincture of iodine	(dil. 1 ml. to 4 oz. with water)	Precipitant and oxidizer
Universal Antidote	1 lb.	Adsorbent, antacid, precipitant
Drugs for Neutralizing Absorbed Poisons Chemically or for Antagonizing Their Effects by Systemic Pharmacologic Action		
Amobarbital (Amytal) sodium, ampules		Anticonvulsant
Amyl nitrite, perles		Cyanide antidote
Atropine sulfate, ampules or hypo tabs		Anticholinergic
Caffeine sodium benzoate, ampules		Analeptic
Calcium chloride (or gluconate), ampules		Fluoride antagonist
Calcium disodium edetate, ampules		Lead antagonist
Dimercaprol (BAL) in oil, ampules		Heavy metal antagonist
Ethyl alcohol, sol. for injection		Methyl alcohol antagonist
Methylene blue sol., ampules		Cyanide antidote; methemoglobinemia antagonist in poisoning by nitrites
Nallorphine (Nalline), ampules		Narcotic antagonist
Nikethamide (Coramine), ampules		Analeptic
Pentobarbital (Nembutal) sod., ampules		Sedative-anticonvulsant
Phenobarbital (Luminal) sodium, tab. and ampules		Sedative-anticonvulsant
Picrotoxin, ampules		Analeptic
Pralidoxime (Protopam), ampules		Organic phosphate antagonist
Secobarbital (Seconal), caps. and ampules		Sedative-hypnotic
Sodium nitrite sol., ampules		Cyanide antidote
Sodium thiosulfate sol., ampules		Cyanide antidote
Thiopental (Pentothal) sod., ampules		Anticonvulsant

TABLE 3-1 (Continued)

AGENT	QUANTITY	ACTION
Drugs for Supportive Therapy		
Aminophylline sol., ampules		Cardiac stimulant
Ammonia, aromatic spirits		Reflex respiratory stimulant
Codeine sulfate or phosphate, hypo tabs.		Analgesic
Corticotropin (ACTH), ampules		Anti-stress
Dextrose 5% and 50% sol., ampules		Nutrient-diuretic
Digitoxin or digoxin, tabs.		Cardiac stimulant
Diphenhydramine (Benadryl), ampules		Antihistamine
Epinephrine, 1:1000 sol., ampules		Cardiac stimulant-broncho-dilator
Glyceryl trinitrate, sublingual tabs.		Coronary vasodilator
Meperidine (Demerol) HCl, tabs. or ampules		Analgesic
Morphine sulfate, hypo tabs. or ampules		Analgesic
Norepinephrine (Levophed) bitartrate, ampules		Circulatory stimulant
Paregoric (Camphorated tr. of opium)		Antidiarrheal
Procainamide (Pronestyl) HCl sol., ampules		Antiarrhythmic agent
Quinidine HCl or gluconate, ampules		Antiarrhythmic agent
Ringer's solution, bottle		Fluid-electrolyte therapy
Sodium bicarbonate sol., ampules		Systemic alkalinizer
Sodium lactate sol., ampules		Systemic alkalinizer
Tetracaine, sterile ophthalmic sol.		Topical anesthetic
Miscellaneous		
Vitamins C, K, B complex, etc.; Antibiotics; Oxygen; Ether; Nitrous oxide		

TABLE 3-2

POISONING BY COMMON CHEMICALS *

POISON AND SOURCES	SIGNS AND SYMPTOMS	EMERGENCY TREATMENT
Acids (corrosive)		
Hydrochloric, sulfuric, nitric, phosphoric, and other concentrated corrosive acids. *Toilet bowl cleaners* sometimes contain hydrochloric and phosphoric acids, and, more frequently, the less corrosive substance *sodium bisulfate*.	1. Burns about the mouth and throat. 2. Stomach pain, nausea, and vomiting of shreds of mucoid tissue. 3. Circulatory collapse, indicated by weak, rapid pulse, cold clammy pale skin, etc. 4. Death may result rapidly from shock or from asphyxia as a result of respiratory tract edema. 5. Surviving patients may suffer obstructive strictures or stenoses requiring surgical repair.	1. DO NOT USE EMETICS OR GAVAGE. 2. Give milk of magnesia, aluminum hydroxide gel, or dilute soap solution. 3. Large quantities of water. 4. Demulcents such as milk, egg whites, olive oil. 5. External skin burns should be flooded with large amounts of water, followed by application of sodium bicarbonate paste. 6. Eye burns should also be flushed with water, possibly after use of a topical anesthetic.

* Based in part upon a lengthier list of chemical poison monographs published in Physicians' Desk Reference, 15th ed., 1961, by M. J. Rodman. See index for references to discussions of poisoning by drugs and chemicals not taken up here.

TABLE 3-2 (Continued)

POISON AND SOURCES	SIGNS AND SYMPTOMS	EMERGENCY TREATMENT
	Alkali (corrosive)	
"LYE" includes sodium and potassium hydroxides, caustic soda, alkaline carbonates. (Drain pipe cleaners, paint removers, Clini-test urine testing tablets, and stove grease removers contain caustic alkali.)	1. Burns about the mouth and throat edematous, white then turning brown. 2. Burning pain in esophagus and stomach; mucoid, then bloody vomitus. 3. Circulatory collapse indicated by cold, clammy skin and rapid, weak pulse. 4. Death may result rapidly from shock or occur later from this cause as a result of perforation of viscera; early asphyxia, or more slowly developing respiratory tract infections may also prove fatal.	1. DO NOT INDUCE EMESIS OR EMPLOY GASTRIC LAVAGE. 2. Give weak acids such as vinegar or lemon juice after having patient drink large quantities of water or milk to dilute the alkali. 3. Demulcents, including olive oil, and egg white, may be given. 4. External burns are washed with large amounts of water or with dilute vinegar. 5. Doctor may order potent analgesics, I.V. fluids and electrolytes, antibiotics, and corticosteroids.
	Arsenic Compounds	
Arsenic trioxide and pentoxide; sodium arsenite and arsenate, etc.; inorganic and organic forms are found in weed killers, rat killers, insecticides, paints, etc.	1. Burning, cramping pains in G.I. tract; throat constricted; swallowing difficult; severe watery or bloody diarrhea. 2. Dehydration, thirst with sweetish, metallic taste; garlicky odor on breath. 3. Death may result from circulatory collapse following fluid and electrolyte losses and gastrointestinal bleeding. 4. Nervous system toxicity may appear in advanced chronic cases. This is manifested by headache, dizziness, delirium, coma and convulsions.	1. Emetics, gastric lavage, and saline cathartics. 2. Milk, sodium thiosulfate solution, or freshly prepared ferric hydroxide solution may follow the lavage or emesis. 3. *Dimercaprol* (BAL) is administered intramuscularly. 4. I.V. fluids and electrolytes to correct dehydration and deficiencies and to counteract shock.
	Bleaches	
Household laundry bleaches contain the *hypochlorite* salts of sodium, potassium, and calcium; e.g. *Clorox*, etc.	1. Burning pain in mouth, throat, esophagus and stomach. 2. Vomiting is common, but the vomitus rarely contains the shreds of mucous membranes and blood seen after ingestion of caustic alkali or acid. 3. Cold, clammy cyanotic skin may indicate impending cardiovascular collapse. 4. Confusion, delirium, and coma may occur. 5. Swelling, blocking and perforation of the G.I. tract are infrequent but signs and symptoms should be watched for.	1. AVOID USE OF ACIDS, but administer mild *antacids* such as milk of magnesia, aluminum hydroxide gel, etc. 2. Gastric lavage may be carefully employed, using tap water, or sodium thiosulfate solution. 3. Demulcents such as egg white or milk may be left in the stomach. 4. Measures to counteract shock (e.g., I.V. fluids) may be used. 5. Skin should be washed with large amounts of water and a paste of sodium bicarbonate applied.

TABLE 3-2 (Continued)

POISON AND SOURCES	SIGNS AND SYMPTOMS	EMERGENCY TREATMENT

Camphor

An ingredient of the liniment, *camphorated oil,* which is sometimes mistakenly taken internally instead of castor oil, or otherwise accidentally ingested; camphor moth repellents, balls and flakes, may also be ingested.

1. Nausea, and vomiting following a feeling of warmth in the stomach; vomitus smells of camphor.
2. Headache, dizziness, confusion, restlessness, delirium, and possible hallucinations.
3. Grand mal type seizures followed by postconvulsive depression, and possible coma or respiratory failure.

1. Gastric lavage or induction of emesis may be employed immediately after ingestion, but not if signs of central excitement have developed (gavage may be done carefully following sedation).
2. Sedation or light sleep may be induced by administration of barbiturates by slow intravenous infusion.

Carbon Monoxide

This gas from automobile exhausts, stoves and heaters causes more cases of poisoning than any other chemical. It acts by combining with hemoglobin in the blood to form carboxyhemoglobin which keeps the blood from picking up oxygen in the lungs and transporting it to the tissues, including the brain.

1. Inhalation of low concentration of CO may cause only mild headache; higher concentrations cause severe throbbing headache.
2. Exposure to very high concentrations can cause loss of consciousness with few symptoms; occasionally, coma may be preceded by confusion and ataxia.
3. The skin often shows a characteristic, cherry-red discoloration.

1. Remove patient to fresh air immediately and apply artificial respiration if breathing has stopped.
2. Inhalation of pure oxygen displaces CO from hemoglobin and restores the oxygen-carrying capacity of the blood; oxygen is then transported more readily to the brain and other body tissues.
(Hyperbaric treatment increases the efficiency of this process.)

Carbon Tetrachloride

This chlorinated hydrocarbon volatile solvent is used in dry cleaning as a stain remover; as an industrial degreaser; and occasionally in home fire extinguishers.

1. Nausea, vomiting, abdominal pain.
2. Headache, confusion, dizziness, drowsiness, visual disturbances, coma and possible death from respiratory failure, especially during *inhalation* of high concentrations of the volatile vapors.
3. Late liver and kidney damage may cause death from acute hepatic necrosis or acute kidney failure. Look for anorexia, nausea, vomiting, jaundice; or oliguria, anuria, albuminuria, edema and weight gain.

1. If inhaled, remove patient to fresh air; if ingested, perform gastric lavage with water or induce emesis; if spilled on skin, remove contaminated clothing and wash skin with water and soap.
2. Oxygen inhalation is desirable after both inhalation and ingestion to protect liver from effects of hypoxia.
3. Prophylactic and supportive measures vs. liver and kidney complications.

TABLE 3-2 (Continued)

POISON AND SOURCES	SIGNS AND SYMPTOMS	EMERGENCY TREATMENT

Cyanides

The gas hydrogen cyanide is used as a fumigant by exterminators of rodents and other vermin in ships' holds, warehouses, greenhouses, etc.; the salts such as sodium or potassium cyanide are used in silver and other metal polishes, in photography, metallurgy and electroplating.	1. Rapid death as a result of respiratory failure can occur from exposure to even small amounts. 2. Less immediately lethal quantities of cyanide cause signs and symptoms of hypoxia which are the result of inability of brain cells and other tissues to *utilize* oxygen due to inhibition of cellular enzymes, including cytochrome oxidase. 3. Signs and symptoms include headache, dizziness, rapid, difficult breathing; coma followed by generalized muscle tremors and convulsions.	1. Immediate artificial respiration and inhalation of oxygen supplied under positive pressure. 2. Inhalation of amyl nitrite vapors from ampules, followed by intravenous injection of sodium nitrite solution. (This converts part of the blood's hemoglobin to methemoglobin which combines with cyanide.) 3. Injection of sodium thiosulfate solution to convert cyanide to the safer thiocyanate. 4. Whole blood infusion may be necessary.

Fluorides

Sodium fluoride and sodium fluosilicate are ingredients of certain insecticides such as roach powders; the minute amounts of sodium fluoride in fluoridated water supplies are *not* toxic, neither in the acute sense described here nor chronically.	1. Nausea, salivation, vomiting, abdominal pain and cramps, diarrhea. 2. Dehydration, pallor, cardiac irregularities, cardiovascular collapse. 3. Muscle weakness, tremors, partial paralysis, spasms and, occasionally, convulsions of the tetanic type. 4. Death may occur in a few hours from cardiac or respiratory failure, or circulatory collapse.	1. Neutralize chemically by having the patient drink milk or other fluids containing soluble calcium salts; then do a careful gavage. 2. I.V. injections of calcium salts are used to control muscle spasms. 3. Parenteral fluids are used to control shock.

Kerosene, etc.
Petroleum Distillates, including gasoline, mineral spirits, etc.

These volatile liquids are used not only as fuels for heat, light, and motor vehicles, but also as the solvents for furniture polish waxes, in paint thinners, and in cleaning fluids. They are especially dangerous when aspirated into the lungs; acute bronchopneumonia is a frequently fatal complication.	1. Ingestion may cause a burning sensation in the upper G.I. tract, nausea and vomiting. Coughing or choking may occur if some of the liquid was inhaled into the lungs while being swallowed. 2. Drowsiness, stupor and coma may develop. 3. Lung involvement may be indicated by the presence of rales, pulmonary edema with dyspnea, cyanosis, and fever. Death may result from pulmonary edema and cardiac dilatation with irregularities, and finally failure.	1. DO <u>NOT</u> INDUCE EMESIS. 2. Very carefully carried out gastric lavage with large amounts of water or sodium bicarbonate solution (3%) may be desirable in some circumstances. 3. This may be followed by olive oil or mineral oil and by a saline cathartic to prevent further absorption. 4. Supportive treatment to overcome or minimize the respiratory tract inflammation may include the use of corticosteroids, antibiotics, and oxygen. Epinephrine is contraindicated.

TABLE 3-2 (Continued)

POISON AND SOURCES	SIGNS AND SYMPTOMS	EMERGENCY TREATMENT

Nicotine

This tobacco plant alkaloid is available as Black Leaf 40, a 40% solution of the sulfate salt, which can be rapidly fatal if ingested. Although the nicotine content of tobacco is high, the ingestion of cigarettes or other tobacco products has not proved dangerous, apparently because vomiting occurs and absorption is poor.

1. Small amounts cause salivation, nausea, vomiting, abdominal pain and diarrhea.

2. Larger amounts at first cause central and cardiovascular effects including headache, dizziness, weakness, visual disturbances and confusion, cardiac irregularities and high blood pressure.

3. Later, in severe poisoning, the blood pressure drops, breathing becomes labored, convulsions are followed by loss of reflex activity; and death may result from respiratory muscle paralysis.

1. Gastric lavage with a solution of potassium permanganate 1:5000 may be followed by administration of the universal antidote in water to oxidize or precipitate the ingested alkaloid and remove it.

2. If spilled on the skin wash off immediately with water to prevent systemic absorption.

3. Measures for controlling convulsions and supporting the patient's respiration and circulation may be ordered.

Phenol (Carbolic Acid)

This substance and the related cresols are locally irritating and destructive and cause severe systemic toxicity when absorbed. Disinfectant solutions containing phenols have sometimes been ingested with suicidal intent; the small amounts (1–2%) in skin lotions is generally safe, but should not be applied frequently to large areas of damaged skin.

1. White burns of the skin and mucous membranes.

2. Burning pain of the mouth, esophagus and stomach; nausea, vomiting, diarrhea.

3. Pulse weak and irregular, skin pale or cyanotic, breathing shallow indicate shock.

4. Transient stimulation of the nervous system may cause excitement followed by depression.

5. Death may result rapidly from respiratory failure; if patient does not die early, he may suffer late kidney damage. Urine is scanty and turns dark on standing.

1. Delay absorption of ingested phenols by administering olive oil or other vegetable oils, which act as solvents. This is followed by gastric lavage, and milk, eggs or other demulcents.

2. If spilled on skin, remove contaminated clothing immediately and wash with large amounts of running water. Special solvents such as alcohol solutions and fixed oils are unnecessary, although olive oil or castor oil may serve as emollients.

Turpentine

This oil from pine wood is a solvent for paints and varnishes commonly found in the home; its toxicity is similar to that of other volatile oils, including *pine oil*, which is a common constituent of disinfectant and cleansing solutions.

1. Ingestion is followed by a burning pain in the mouth and throat, pain in the stomach, and nausea, vomiting and diarrhea.

2. Inhalation into lungs may cause coughing and choking and other respiratory difficulties.

3. Systemic absorption can cause central nervous system stimulation (excitement, delirium, occasional convulsions) followed by depression (stupor, coma and respiratory failure).

4. Kidney irritation may cause albuminuria and hematuria. The urine has an odor like that of violets.

1. The stomach is lavaged with water or weak sodium bicarbonate solution.

2. Demulcents, including milk or mineral oil, are left in the stomach to allay irritation.

3. Fluids may be forced to produce a copious dilute urine and thus prevent renal irritation.

4. Measures to support respiration may be employed.

5. Relieve pain with codeine rather than with morphine, which may further depress respiration.

TABLE 3-2 *(Continued)*

POISON AND SOURCES	SIGNS AND SYMPTOMS	EMERGENCY TREATMENT

Xylene and related aromatic hydrocarbons, including *Benzene* and *Toluene*

POISON AND SOURCES	SIGNS AND SYMPTOMS	EMERGENCY TREATMENT
These substances are used as *solvents* for removing paints and lacquers, and as degreasers; they also sometimes serve as the base or vehicle for insecticidal solutions and are often ingredients of *glues* used by hobbyists and others. Glue sniffers sometimes seek the central effects of such volatile solvents.	1. Local irritation of skin, eyes, and mucous membranes; when swallowed, a burning sensation is felt in the upper G.I. tract, followed by nausea, salivation, and vomiting. 2. Systemic absorption of the inhaled vapors causes effects similar to those of alcoholic intoxication. Continued absorption can result in coma with hyperactive reflexes, and finally respiratory failure. 3. Chronic exposure to benzene can cause bone marrow damage and blood dyscrasias.	1. Skin and eyes should be thoroughly washed; if ingested, the material should be removed by gastric lavage, and mineral oil or a saline cathartic left in the stomach. 2. Supportive measures include artificial respiration, administration of fluids parenterally, and measures for treating pulmonary complications. 3. Epinephrine must *not* be administered, nor should vegetable fats or alcohol be given.

SUMMARY OF POINTS FOR THE NURSE TO REMEMBER CONCERNING POISONING

- The nurse has an important role in educating the public about ways to store and handle chemicals safely in the home, in order to avoid poison accidents. She also advises people about the kinds of first aid measures that they should know in order to cope with chemical emergencies.

- The nurse should observe patients in the emergency room or at the time of their admission to medical services for signs that may arouse suspicion of poisoning as a possible cause of illness.

- The nurse whose duties may involve caring for poison accident victims should request that adequate reference materials be available in the emergency room and other departments. She should learn how to use these and other sources to quickly find required information concerning the chemical contents of various products, their potentially toxic effects, and the recommended antidotes and other treatment measures.

- The nurse's role in poison emergencies is a flexible one, in which she cooperates with the physician, the pharmacist, and the family to make the most effective use of community resources, such as poison control centers, in order to treat the patient as quickly and effectively as possible.

- In the actual treatment of the poisoned patient the two most important aspects of the nurse's role involve: (1) participating in measures designed to remove the poison from the patient's body as rapidly as possible (e.g., gastric lavage and emesis) in order to minimize absorption of the poison into the systemic circulation, and (2) aiding in the support of the patient's vital functions (e.g., maintaining a patent airway; administering intravenous fluids, etc.) and offering longer term nursing care aimed at hastening the patient's recovery and reducing his pain and discomfort.

REVIEW QUESTIONS

Drug Reactions of the Hypersusceptibility, Hypersensitivity, and Idiosyncratic Types

1. What are two general ways by which nurses can help to minimize the potentially adverse effects of drugs?

2. (a) What is the most common cause of adverse side effects from an administered drug?

(b) What measure does the doctor take to lessen such side effects?

3. (a) What pathological conditions may cause a drug to accumulate to toxic levels upon continued administration?

(b) What other kinds of pre-existing pathology may make a particular patient react adversely to a dose of a drug that is safe for most people?

(c) How can the nurse best prepare herself to help prevent adverse effects stemming from a drug's primary and secondary pharmacological actions?

4. (a) How do *non*protein drugs sometimes become antigens capable of sensitizing a person so that he suffers an allergic reaction upon later exposure to the drug?

(b) What are the two main allergic reactions that may be set off by drugs that act as haptenes; and how are the pathological effects of each of these types likely to be manifested clinically?

5. (a) What is meant by the term *drug idiosyncracy?*

(b) How does an idiosyncratic drug reaction differ from the delayed-type reactions that occur in some drug-sensitive individuals?

6. Describe briefly the nature of drug eruptions of each of the following types: (a) urticarial; (b) morbilliform; (c) photosensitivity; (d) erythema multiforme.

7. (a) What is the hematological result of a drug reaction that causes aplastic anemia?

(b) What are some drugs which have sometimes caused this very serious kind of blood dyscrasia?

8. (a) What signs and symptoms might the nurse note in a patient who suffers agranulocytosis as the result of exposure to a drug to which he is sensitive?

(b) What is the hematological picture which the laboratory would report for a patient with this blood dyscrasia?

9. (a) What enzymatic defect is present in people whose erythrocytes are unusually susceptible to destruction by certain drugs?

(b) What are some drugs that sometimes set off hemolytic reactions in such susceptible individuals?

10. (a) Liver disorders of what two types are sometimes induced by certain drugs in some susceptible patients?

(b) What are some signs of possible liver damage for which the nurse should be alert when patients are receiving drugs that are known to cause occasional liver damage?

11. (a) What is meant by the terms *nephrotoxicity* and *ototoxicity* and what are some examples of drugs that sometimes cause these adverse effects?

(b) What is meant by the term *teratogenic,* and what prescribing policy is being employed to minimize the possible occurrence of teratogenic effects?

Addiction and Drug Abuse

1. (a) What are two common chemicals upon which very many people are psychologically dependent?

(b) What are some ways in which the relatively mild habituation to these substances differs from the more severe degree of psychic dependence induced by drugs in addicted individuals?

2. (a) Why are most people who receive narcotic analgesic drugs for a brief period *un*likely to become psychologically dependent upon them, whereas a few soon show signs of such dependence?

(b) What kinds of reactions to the administration of narcotics might lead the nurse to suspect that the patient may be becoming psychologically dependent upon these drugs?

(c) What should the nurse do in such a situation?

3. (a) What sort of factors may account for the development of tolerance to certain drugs?

(b) What part do tolerance and the often related phenomenon, physical dependence, play in the perpetuation of drug abuse behavior with regard to some drugs and individuals?

4. (a) What are the two main patterns of withdrawal syndromes seen when patients are abruptly deprived of drugs that they have been taking in large amounts for long periods?

(b) What measures may the nurse take to make the patient more comfortable during the withdrawal period?

5. (a) What are some arguments for making marihuana, LSD and similar drugs legally available for self-experimentation?

(b) What are some arguments for keeping such substances under sanctions that restrict their ready availability to all who might wish to experiment with them?

6. (a) What are some reasons for the high incidence of drug addiction among medical personnel?

(b) What might make a nurse suspect that drugs are being diverted for improper use in a hospital setting?

(c) What measures might the nurse take to protect herself from the hazard of drug addiction?

Poisoning

1. In what general ways can the nurse participate in the detection, treatment and prevention of poisoning?

2. (a) What age groups appear to be most susceptible to accidental poisoning?

(b) List some statistics that indicate the scope and seriousness of accidental poisoning in this country.

3. (a) List some types of drug products commonly involved in cases of accidental poisoning.

(b) List some classes of chemical specialty products that are often accidentally ingested.

4. (a) List two comprehensive compendia of information concerning all aspects of poisoning.

(b) List several sources of information useful for identifying the contents of pharmaceutical products.

5. (a) Give some examples of how hospital and office nurses, public health nurses, and school nurses can offer people advice and guidance that can help to prevent poisoning.

(b) List the kinds of measures that all nurses can offer to patients as part of general programs for preventing poisoning through public education.

6. (a) List some observations that may arouse suspicion of poisoning and aid the doctor in making his diagnosis.

(b) What general observations that the nurse makes may be helpful to the physician for diagnosing a case of poisoning?

7. Of what three general types are the measures employed in the management of cases of acute poisoning?

8. (a) What household substances are used for first aid induction of vomiting, and what emetic may now be obtained without a prescription for use by the layman in a poison emergency?

(b) What injectable emetic may the physician employ for emptying the patient's stomach in a poison emergency?

9. List four circumstances in which the use of emetics may be contraindicated.

10. (a) List several kinds of antidotal substances that may be administered by means of the gavage tube after the patient's stomach has been repeatedly syringed with tap water.

(b) What are the ingredients of the Universal Antidote?

(c) List several kinds of foodstuffs which may be effective for precipitating or neutralizing certain poisons of specific types.

11. (a) What measures may the nurse take to help prevent hypostatic pneumonia from developing in patients who have taken an overdose of barbiturates?

(b) What are some of the nurse's duties in efforts to support the circulation of the poisoned patient?

12. (a) How can the nurse help support hepatic function in patients with liver damage from drugs and chemicals?

(b) What are some of the nurse's responsibilities in the medical management of patient's with drug-induced renal damage?

13. (a) What chemical can serve as a specific antidote for treating lead poisoning?

(b) What is the manner of action of this chemical antidote and what term is used to describe chemicals that act in this way?

14. (a) What is the specific chemical antidote for poisoning by heavy metals such as arsenic and mercury?

(b) Which organ system is most readily damaged by the ingestion of arsenic salts used in weed killers and other products?

(c) Which organ suffers the most severe damage from systemically absorbed mercury salts?

15. (a) In what way does carbon monoxide act as a poison, and how is poisoning by inhalation of this gas treated?

(b) What is the manner in which cyanide causes poisoning, and what chemical antidotes are employed in its treatment?

BIBLIOGRAPHY

Adverse Drug Reactions

Baer, R. L., and Harber, L. C.: Photosensitivity induced by drugs. J.A.M.A., *192*:989, 1965.

Cahen, R. L.: Evaluation of the teratogenicity of drugs. Clin. Pharmacol. Ther., *5*:480, 1964.

Di Palma, J. R.: What to do about adverse drug reactions. R.N., *28*:57, 1965 (Oct.).

Done, A. K.: Developmental pharmacology. Clin. Pharmacol. Ther., *5*:432, 1964.

Erslev, A. J.: Drug-induced blood dyscrasias—aplastic anemia. J.A.M.A., *188*:531, 1964.

Feinberg, S. M.: Allergy from therapeutic products. J.A.M.A., *178*:815, 1961.

Friend, D. G.: Adverse reactions to drugs. Clin. Pharmacol. Ther., *5*:257, 1964.

Huguley, C. M., Jr.: Drug-related blood dyscrasias. J.A.M.A., *177*:23, 1961.

Kautz, H. D., Gwinn, R. P., and Berryman, G. H.: Suspected adverse effects of drugs. J.A.M.A., *189*:269, 1964.

Kirshbaum, B. A., Beerman, H., and Stahl, E. B.: Drug eruptions, a review of some of the recent literature. Am. J. Med. Sci., *240*:512, 1960.

Modell, W.: Hazards of new drugs. Science, *139*:1180, 1963.

Perry, C. J. G., and Morgenstern, A. L.: Drugs and driving. J.A.M.A., *195*:376, 1966.

Rodman, M. J.: The rising tide of dangerous drug reactions. Nursing Forum, *1*:105, 1962.

——: Intolerance, allergy and idiosyncracy. R.N., *28*:51, 1965 (Oct.).

Rostenberg, A., Jr., and Fagelson, H. J.: Life-threatening drug eruptions. J.A.M.A., *194*:660, 1965.

Schreiner, G. E.: Toxic nephropathy. J.A.M.A., *191*:849, 1965.

Tumen, H. J. *et al.*: Hepatic reactions to drugs. J.A.M.A., *191*:405, 1965.

Drug Addiction and Abuse

Blomquist, E. R.: The doctor, the nurse, and drug addiction. G.P., *18*:124, 1958.

Eddy, N. B.: Addiction producing versus habit forming. J.A.M.A., *163*:1622, 1957.

Essig, C. F.: Addiction to nonbarbiturate sedatives and tranquilizing drugs. Clin. Pharmacol. Ther., *5*:334, 1964.

Fraser, H. F., and Grider, J. A.: Treatment of drug addiction. Am. J. Med., *14*:571, 1953.

Glaser, H. H., and Massengale, O. N.: Glue sniffing in children. J.A.M.A., *181*:300, 1962.

Isbell, H., and White, W. M.: Clinical characteristics of addictions. Am. J. Med., *14*:558, 1953.

Isbell, H., and Fraser, H. F.: Addiction to analgesics and barbiturates. Pharmacol. Rev., *2*:355, 1950.

Ludwig, A. M., and Levine, J.: Patterns of hallucinogenic drug abuse. J.A.M.A., *191*:92, 1965.

Prescor, M. J., and Walker, P. K.: The treatment of drug addiction. Am. J. Nurs., *51*:611, 1951.

Rodman, M. J.: Management in drug abuse and addiction. R.N., *27*:59, 1964 (Dec.).

————: Drug abuse and its medical management. R.N., *30*:47, 1967 (Aug.).

Seevers, M. H.: Medical perspectives on habituation and addiction. J.A.M.A., *181*:93, 1962.

Seevers, M. H., and Woods, L. A.: The phenomena of tolerance. Am. J. Med., *14*:546, 1953.

Wikler, A., and Rasor, R. W.: Psychiatric aspects of drug addiction. Am. J. Med., *14*:566, 1953.

Poisoning by Drugs and Chemicals

Adams, W. C.: Poison control centers: Their purpose and operation. Clin. Pharmacol. Ther., *4*:293, 1963.

Cann, H. M., Neyman, D. S., and Verhulst, H. L.: Control of accidental poisoning—a progress report. J.A.M.A., *168*:717, 1958.

Done, A. K.: Clinical pharmacology of systemic antidotes. Clin. Pharmacol. Ther., *2*:750, 1961.

Jacobziner, H.: Causation, prevention, and control of accidental poisoning. J.A.M.A., *171*:1769, 1959.

Pfeiffer, C. C.: Emergency treatment of common poisons. Am. J. Nurs., *55*:1382, 1955.

Press, E.: Poison control centers. Nursing Outlook, *5*:29, 1957.

Rodman, M. J.: A survey of potentially harmful household products. J. Pediat., *46*:171, 1955.

————: Drug poisoning. R.N., *25*:68, 1962 (May).

Smith, H. D., and Houston, S.: Lead poisoning in children. Am. J. Nurs., *54*:736, 1954.

Stern, G.: The emergency treatment of poisoning. G.P., *21*:139, 1960.

Stewart, R. D.: Poisoning from chlorinated hydrocarbon solvents. Am. J. Nurs., *67*:85, 1967.

Thoman, M. E., and Verhulst, H. L.: Ipecac syrup in antiemetic ingestion. J.A.M.A., *196*:433, 1966.

Tonyan, A., and Jensen, J. S.: The nurse's part in poison control. Am. J. Nurs., *58*:96, 1958.

Williams, F. J.: Nurses have much to do about poison control. Nursing Outlook, *6*:93, 1958.

Woody, N. C., and Kometani, J. T.: BAL in the treatment of arsenic poisoning of children. Pediatrics, *1*:372, 1948.

Information Related to Poisoning and Its Management

Arena, J. M.: Poisoning. Springfield, Ill., Charles C Thomas, 1963.

Browning, E.: Toxicology of Industrial Organic Solvents. New York, Chemical Publishing Co., 1953.

Buckley, E. E., and Porges, N. (eds.): Venoms. Washington, D. C., Am. Assoc. Adv. Science, 1956.

Clinical Handbook on *Economic Poisons*. Toxicology Section. Atlanta, Communicable Disease Center, Public Health Service, 1963.

Dack, G. M.: Food Poisoning. 3rd ed. Chicago, Chicago Univ. Press, 1956.

Deichmann, W. B., and Gerarde, H. W.: Symptomatology and Therapy of Toxicological Emergencies. New York, Academic Press, 1964.

Dreisbach, R. H.: Handbook of Poisoning. 5th ed. Los Altos, Calif., Lange Medical Publications, 1966.

Dubois, K. P., and Geiling, E. M. K.: Textbook of Toxicology. New York, Oxford University Press, 1959.

Gleason, M. N., Gosselin, R. E., and Hodge, H. C.: Clinical Toxicology of Commercial Products. 2nd ed. Baltimore, Williams and Wilkins, 1963.

Goodhart, R. S.: Modern Drug Encyclopedia and Therapeutic Index. 10th ed. New York, The Reuben H. Donnelley Corp., 1965.

Identification Guide for Solid Dosage Forms. J.A.M.A., *182* (No. 12), Dec. 22, 1962.

Kaye, S.: Handbook of Emergency Toxicology. 2nd ed. Springfield, Ill., Charles C Thomas, 1961.

Muenscher, W. C.: Poisonous Plants of the United States. 2nd ed. New York, Macmillan, 1951.

New Drugs. Council on Drugs. Chicago, Ill., American Medical Association, 1967.

Physicians' Desk Reference. Oradell, N. J., Medical Economics, 1967.

Polson, C. J., and Tattersall, O. B. E.: Clinical Toxicology. Philadelphia, J. B. Lippincott, 1959.

Press, E.: Accidental Poisoning in Childhood. Am. Academy of Pediatrics. Springfield, Ill., Charles C Thomas, 1956.

Thienes, C. H., and Haley, T. J.: Clinical Toxicology. 3rd ed. Philadelphia, Lea & Febiger, 1955.

U. S. Dispensatory and Physicians' Pharmacology. 26th ed. (Osol, A., Pratt, R., and Altschule, M. (eds.). Philadelphia, J. B. Lippincott, 1967.

Von Oettingen, W. F.: Poisoning, A Guide to Clinical Diagnosis and Treatment. 2nd ed. Philadelphia, W. B. Saunders, 1958.

Wilson, C. O., and Jones, T. E.: American Drug Index, 1968. Philadelphia, J. B. Lippincott, 1968.

4

The Administration of Drugs

THE NURSE'S RESPONSIBILITY IN DRUG THERAPY

The professional nurse carries important responsibilities relative to drug treatment. Her duties include more than the actual administering of the medication. She must also observe how the patient responds to drug therapy. Further, with the growing tendency to permit some patients to take some of their own medicines, it is more important than ever that the nurse instruct patients in proper self-administration of drugs and watch for the effects of such treatment.

The nurse's responsibilities in these respects are growing rapidly. Thus, to carry out these important functions properly, she must continually keep broadening and deepening her understanding of drug therapy in relation to the particular illness that is being treated. She needs, first, to know the actions of both the well-established drugs and those most recently introduced and, then, how to apply this pharmacological knowledge in the context of what she has learned about all other aspects of nursing care. The nurse who has some understanding of the nature of the patient's underlying illness and understands how the patient's pathophysiological functioning can be favorably altered by the drugs that are being used to treat his disorder, is better able to integrate drug administration into her total plan of care. Thus, the nurse's knowledge of what actions to expect from an administered drug are used along with those nursing measures that will most enhance the desired effect of the medication or minimize its adverse effects.

LEGAL AND ETHICAL RESPONSIBILITIES. The nurse is legally and ethically obligated, in giving drugs, to be in possession of all the knowledge that is essential for their safe administration. Therefore, before giving an ordered drug, she should acquaint herself with the pertinent facts in regard to the drug's expected effects, untoward actions, dosage, and manner of administration. To do so she must have available the books and other sources of essential information, and she has to have the time to consult such resource materials.

All too often, nurses tend to jeopardize the patient's safety and their own professional reputation and welfare by their reluctance to tell persons in charge that adequate drug data and time to check them are basic necessities of safe practice. If something goes wrong, it is no excuse that the ward was very busy, and the doctor or head nurse had said, "I'll take the responsibility." Whenever you administer a drug, you do in fact accept the responsibility for giving it safely. Many court decisions make it abundantly clear that the nurse is held legally responsible for her own actions when administering drugs. Thus, if a doctor orders a dangerously large dose of a drug and the nurse fails to question it and administers the drug as ordered, she may be held responsible for whatever harm the patient sustains.

On the other hand, the nurse should not let herself be overwhelmed by the responsibility of administering medications and become so tense and fearful of making a mistake that her judgment is impaired—a state of mind that would predispose any person toward making more, rather than fewer, errors. Rather, she should gain the knowledge necessary for safe practice and then proceed with confidence.

The best insurance against making errors in medication is to have a thorough understanding of the nature of the drugs that are being given and to practice habitually certain time-tested measures for assuring maximum safety. In the following discussion we shall try to familiarize the student first with the nature and sources of drugs and then with the principal methods by which they are administered. With some knowledge of where drugs come from, the dosage forms into which they are formulated, and the routes by which they enter the body, the subject of drug administration may seem less awesome. Finally, lest the student think that administration of medication can ever be carried out properly in a casual, mechanical way, we shall discuss some of the many factors that the nurse must keep in mind as she carries out this task. This, we hope, will make it clear that this aspect of patient care requires the application of knowledge and judgment in ways that go far beyond the mechanical skill of pouring and measuring a solution or even the skill required to give an injection.

SOURCES OF DRUGS

In Chapter 1 we traced the development of drug therapy, in a general way, from its prehistoric origins to the present day. We saw that both primitive witch doctors and modern medical men make use of certain *natural substances* in treating disease. *Plant* and *animal* parts and *minerals* dug from the ground are still sources of drugs today as they were in the earliest days of pharmacotherapeutics. In addition, for only the past century or so doctors have been able to draw on a fourth source of drugs—the laboratories of the organic chemists who *synthesize* substances that never before existed. Let us now look a bit more closely at each of these sources of drugs. For knowing something about where our drugs originate will add to our understanding of the dosage forms of drugs—the pharmaceutical formulations which the nurse finally administers to the patient.

Botanicals and Their Constituents

Until this century, the plant world was the chief source of substances for treating disease. At first, physicians used the crude drugs themselves—the bark of trees (e.g., cinchona); the leaves of flowering ornamental plants (e.g., digitalis); or the roots of shrubs (e.g., belladonna)—after such plant parts had been gathered, dried, and ground to a fine powder. Later, liquid pharmaceutical preparations were made by treating the crude drug with water or alcohol which extracted the active constituents and left behind the inert plant residues.

Tinctures are made usually by extracting the useful principles of plants with solvents containing alcohol. (Alcoholic solutions of some nonvegetable chemicals also are called tinctures, e.g., tincture of iodine.) Tinctures of therapeutically potent drugs such as opium and belladonna have a drug strength of 10 per cent. That is, 10 ml. of a tincture contains the active constituents extracted from 1 Gm. of drug. Thus, for example, if 1 Gm. of opium contains 100 mg. of morphine, that amount of the active constituent would be contained in 10 ml. of tincture of opium. Similarly, belladonna tincture contains about 30 mg. of active constituents such as atropine and hyoscine in 100 ml. —the same amount of these alkaloids contained in 10 Gm. of the coarsely powdered leaf from which the tincture is prepared. Less potent drugs are made into tinctures that contain the active principles of 20 Gm.

of drug in every 100 ml. Compound tinctures such as paregoric (camphorated tr. of opium) and compound tincture of benzoin contain amounts of the various active constituents which vary in accordance with traditionally established formulations.

Fluidextracts are much more concentrated liquid preparations of vegetable drugs. The strength of the alcoholic solution is such that each milliliter contains the active constituents of 1 Gm. of the drug from which it is made. Thus, fluidextract of belladonna contains in 10 milliliters the 30 mg. of extractives that are found in 10 Gm. of powdered belladonna leaf (or in 100 ml. of the tincture).

Extracts are concentrated preparations made by evaporating the hydroalcoholic extractive solvents until a syrupy liquid, plastic mass, or dry powder is left. The strength of extracts is adjusted so that they are usually several times stronger than the crude drug itself. Thus, for example, belladonna extracts contain between three and four times the active constituents of the leaf itself.

Plant Constituents

In recent years, the prescribing trend has been away from such so-called *galenicals* (after the Greek physician, *Galen*, who practiced in Rome in the second century). Instead, doctors tend to prefer the purified crystalline chemicals isolated from the most potent extracts of plants or, in many cases, prepared synthetically in the laboratory. Among the most important classes of vegetable drug constituents are the *alkaloids* and the *glycosides*.

Alkaloids are nitrogenous chemicals that can be extracted from various parts of many plants. They are usually quite active pharmacologically. The doctor can depend upon getting a rapid, powerful action when he gives his patient a pure medicinal alkaloid; however, the danger from overdosage is also greater from these constituents than from the galenical preparations or crude drugs that contain them.

The nurse will often know that she is handling an alkaloid, because its name ends in "ine"—for example, morph*ine*, atro*pine*, pilocar*pine*, strychn*ine*. These are not, however, the only drugs with names that end in this suffix. The names of certain other nitrogenous substances of natural origin, such as the hormone epinephrine from animal adrenal glands, bear this ending. Similarly, certain synthetic substances with chemical structures and pharmacological actions that resemble alkaloids of natural origin are sometimes so named. The local anesthetic, procaine, for example, is not correctly classed as an alkaloid, despite its relationships to cocaine, an alkaloid extracted from the leaves of the coca plant.

Glycosides are active plant principles containing a sugar such as glucose in the molecule. Actually, it is the noncarbohydrate portion of the molecule, or aglycone (genin), that accounts for its pharmacological activity. However, in the case of the digitalis glycosides (medically, the most important of the drugs of this class), the sugar portion of the molecule is very important because it permits the aglycone to penetrate into cardiac muscle cells and exert its stimulating effect on myocardial function. The glycoside digitoxin is a thousand times more potent in this respect than the powdered digitalis leaf. Interestingly, it is now cheaper for a heart patient to be maintained on this purified crystalline glycoside than on the crude drug itself. The names of the official glycosides usually end in "in," as in digox*in*, digitox*in*, strophanth*in*.

Other Plant Constituents

Plants also yield oils, gums, resins and tannins, which are still used in medicine. Among the *fixed oils* are olive, cottonseed and castor oils; the *volatile* oils include aromatic flavoring essences such as peppermint, spearmint and clove. *Gums* are exudative plant secretions that form thick mucilaginous masses when mixed with water. Some, such as psyllium seed and agar, are used internally as laxatives; others, e.g., tragacanth and acacia, are often used externally in soothing lotions or as pharmaceutical suspending agents. *Resins* include substances such as the rosin found in pine tree sap. Some are pharmacologically active local irritants with minor uses in medicine as laxatives and caustics. *Tannins* are phenol derivatives found widely in the vegetable kingdom. They are used mainly in industry to tan hides; in medicine, this capacity to precipitate protein has led to their employment as astringents and for forming protective coverings over burn surfaces.

Drugs Derived from Animal Sources

The organs of animals—and, indeed, those of men—were once used in medicine on a mystical basis. Today, some of our most potent drugs are obtained by extraction from animal tissues, for use as substitutes for human glandular secretions that may be lacking. The hormone insulin, which is used in treating diabetes, is an active principle from animal pancreas; corticotropin (ACTH) is isolated from the pituitary glands of animals that are slaughtered for food. The thyroid glands of animals are dried, defatted and powdered for use in replacement, or substitution, therapy of hypothyroid patients. Recently, the pituitary glands of human corpses have been employed for extracting the human growth hormone (HGH), which is more effective than animal-derived somatotrophin for treatment of certain types of dwarfism.

Inorganic Chemicals

Metallic salts, such as those of iron, and some elements such as sulfur and iodine have long been used in medicine. The salts of silver and mercury are still employed as antiseptics and disinfectants. Clays such as kaolin and attapulgite are ingredients of certain products for treating diarrhea; and aluminum hydroxide and the phosphate salt of that metal are used for counteracting excessive amounts of hydrochloric acid in the upper gastrointestinal tract. The hydroxide of magnesium also is used for digestive disorders, as both an antacid and laxative, and salts of the same mineral—the sulfate and the citrate—are employed as saline cathartics. Most recently, the radioactive isotopes of inorganic substances such as gold, phosphorus and iodine have come into use in the diagnosis and treatment of disease.

Synthetic Organic Chemicals

More than half a million carbon-containing chemicals that do not exist in nature at all have come from the laboratories of synthetic organic chemists, since Wohler's discovery early in the last century that man might make what it was previously believed could be formed only by living organisms (animals and plants). Only a small fraction of all these synthetic chemicals possess biological activity, and an even smaller proportion are both safe and effective enough to be used in the treatment of disease. Yet, synthesis is the single most important source of modern medicinal chemicals.

As we have previously indicated (Chap. 1), it is often preferable to produce certain natural substances synthetically, even when they occur in natural animal or plant products. Of the line of alkaloids, hormones and other plant and animal principles that have been prepared synthetically, one of the most recent is oxytocin. This principle of the posterior pituitary gland thus synthesized is free of vasopressin—a persistent impurity that was characteristic of the natural extract of the neurohypophysis.

Other reasons for preparing natural products synthetically are mainly economic. Thus, it is less costly to prepare the adrenal corticosteroids synthetically from cheap, readily available intermediates than to extract and purify the minute quantities obtainable from animal adrenal glands by laborious extraction processes. In addition, the organic chemist can often come up with entirely new chemicals that are much more potent and, in many instances, less toxic than their natural counterparts.

ROUTES OF ADMINISTRATION OF DRUGS

The manner in which a drug is administered is one of the most important factors influencing its action. Depending upon how a dose of a drug is given, it may produce a profound effect or none at all. Thus, when a solution of magnesium sulfate (Epsom Salts) is taken by mouth, it acts only within the intestine to exert a cathartic effect; when the same magnesium salt is injected intramuscularly, its molecules reach the central nervous system and produce deep depression.

As we saw in Chapter 2, the path by which a drug is introduced into the body influences primarily the rate and completeness of its absorption into the blood stream. This, in turn, plays a primary part in determining how quickly the drug begins to act and the intensity with which it acts. In addition to influencing the speed of *onset* and the degree of *intensity* of a drug's action, the dosage form and manner of administration also often influence the *duration*, or length of action.

We shall review briefly the main routes by which drugs are administered so that they can enter the systemic circulation and exert their effects on the distant tissues that have the capacity to react to them. At the same time, we shall offer some information about the *dosage forms* in which drugs are available. However, we will not attempt to take up in detail the techniques for administering medications by various routes, since these are presented in texts on the fundamentals of nursing; nor shall we discuss the ways in which the various solid and liquid dosage forms are put together, since such aspects of pharmaceutical preparations come within the province of the pharmacist rather than the nurse.

Oral Administration

As we have already indicated, the most desirable way to give drugs is by mouth. Wherever it is possible to do so, pharmaceutical companies try to make drugs available in dosage forms suitable for oral administration. Swallowing such a preparation is the simplest way to get a drug into the body and on its way into the blood stream and the other tissues. Given by mouth, the drug produces effects that are more readily controllable than when it is administered by injection. In addition to their convenience and relative safety, oral dosage forms are less costly than injectable forms that have to be prepared as sterile solutions which must then usually be administered by a professionally trained person.

Solid oral dosage forms include *tablets, capsules, powders* and *pills.* Pills are now largely passé, even though people still persist in calling tablets "pills." (Pharmacists are still sometimes referred to as "pill rollers," despite the fact that a modern druggist almost never prepares a pill after leaving pharmacy school; and, of course, the term which the popular press commonly employs in discussing oral contraceptives—"The Pill"—is also a misnomer.)

Powders also are relatively rare today and are limited mainly to products for relief of gastrointestinal distress. Perhaps people are impressed by the ritual of pouring a measured amount of a fine powder or rough granules into a quantity of water, stirring as the powder dissolves with effervescence, and then drinking the solution. Such bulky effervescent antacids and laxatives are today being made available more frequently as big tablets that form a bubbling solution, which is apparently just as effective and psychologically satisfying as the older form.

Tablets are made by compressing powdered or granulated drugs into a compact form that is readily swallowed and that then breaks up into a finely divided powder in the stomach. In regard to disintegration and absorption, tablets are much more reliable than pills, which often dried out during storage and were then likely to pass through the entire G.I. tract without ever dissolving. Tablets frequently are coated, to improve their palatability, with substances that promptly dissolve in the stomach.

Enteric coatings on tablets and capsules have another purpose. They are intended to delay the release of stomach-irritating drugs that might cause nausea and vomiting. Once the tablet has passed the pylorus, the acid-insoluble coating dissolves in the alkaline intestinal secretions, and the drug is absorbed from that site without having caused stomach upset. Irritating drugs are often given with food which coats the gastric mucosa and thus reduces epigastric distress.

Prolonged-action tablets and capsules also have a delayed action. However, the purpose here is not to protect the stomach from irritation but to produce a long-sustained drug action. Some of the contents of the capsule or tablet are released almost immediately and absorbed to bring about quick action. The remainder of the material is released gradually as the capsule gives up its contents for absorption over a period of several hours. For example, a Spansule capsule is so prepared that one therapeutic dose of dextroamphetamine or any other drug put up in this form is promptly set free in the stomach, and the rest is released further down in the G.I. tract to exert a steady action for 10 to 12 hours.

These so-called sustained-action or timed-disintegration products are available in a variety of physical forms based on different biopharmaceutical principles of release and absorption. These forms include capsule products that release pellets with soluble coatings of varying thickness, and controlled-release tablets (e.g., Gradumets) made up of an inert, porous plastic impregnated with drugs that dissolve and leach out slowly as the tablet passes down through the G.I. tract.

The principles and the intricacies of product design do not concern us here. The important point for the nurse to know is that *these oral dosage forms must never be tampered with in any way.* Altering the dosage form may easily result in overdosage. The pellets of a Spansule, for example, must *not* be poured out of the capsule or crushed, nor should the Gradumet tablet ever be broken up and mixed with anything else. (Single dose tablets, on the other hand, are sometimes crushed to help a person who is convinced that he cannot swallow the intact dosage form or to make the medication more palatable to a child by mixing it with jam, jelly, honey, etc.)

The main purpose in making drugs available in timed-release form is to reduce the number of doses that the patient has to remember to take. A patient is much more likely to get the benefits of prescribed drug therapy when he needs to take only two rather than four to six doses a day.

Liquid dosage forms for oral use are popular, especially in widely advertised nonprescription cough medications. The purpose of such products differs from that of the liquid extracts of vegetable drugs mentioned earlier. Here, the intent is to offer medication in a form that not only is readily absorbable but also is palatable and easy to take. This, of course, reflects the current view that the patient benefits more by being kept comfortable than by being distracted and overawed. (In the past, we suspect, it was thought that a patient would be duly impressed by a disagreeable tasting medicine, on the theory that "it tastes so terrible that it must be good for me.") Thus, the *vehicles*, or solvents for medications, are usually pleasantly flavored liquids, which may be watery, alcoholic, or hydroalcoholic.

Syrups are solutions of sugar in water, to which flavors of various types are usually added. Children like to take syrupy liquids and are less likely to balk when bitter, salty, or insipid substances are disguised in one of the official syrups—the fruit flavors cherry, orange and raspberry, or in chocolate (Cocoa Syrup) or licorice (Glycyrrhiza) syrup. Although it is true that it is better for the child to enjoy the taste of medicine that he must take instead of gagging on it and struggling against efforts to give it to him, too much emphasis must not be placed on flavor.

It is never desirable to fool a child into taking medication by calling it "candy." For it should not be surprising if the child then eats the entire contents of the bottle—and becomes ill. Similarly, television commercials for cough syrups, which put excessive emphasis on palatability, do a disservice ("Gee, Mom, it tastes just like the syrup you put on ice cream"). It is hardly an accident if a child so conditioned downs the entire contents of a cold product containing salicylates and antihistamine drugs and is poisoned by a product promoted in this way.

Nonetheless, when used with discretion, syrups are a desirable form of liquid medication. Often, they add a demulcent, or soothing, action of their own that is transiently helpful to the raw mucous membranes of a cough-inflamed pharynx. Their use is often preferable to the practice of putting drugs in milk or fruit juice to disguise their disagreeable taste.

This is, of course, often done with salty drugs such as potassium iodide, ammonium chloride, or sodium bromide, and usually works with adults, but children may later refuse to eat or drink foods that they have come to associate with an "off" taste or odor.

Watery solutions and suspensions of various kinds are often ordered. *Aromatic waters* are aqueous solutions saturated with various volatile substances, such as cinnamon oil, spearmint oil and peppermint. The amount of the oil that dissolves in water is relatively low compared to the quantities contained in alcoholic solutions. However, the flavoring is often adequate as an aid in disguising certain salty substances dissolved in the watery vehicle. Other substances such as iodine and potassium iodide dissolve so readily in water that they are sometimes made available in highly concentrated aqueous solutions containing large amounts of the drug in doses of only a few drops (e.g., strong iodine solution, and saturated solution of potassium iodide).

SUSPENSIONS of insoluble or immiscible drugs include emulsions and gels, among others. *Emulsions* are mixtures of oil and water made possible by the artful introduction of certain pharmaceutical agents that keep the oil particles dispersed in tiny droplets throughout the aqueous phase of the emulsion. Like homogenized milk, which is also an emulsion, these pharmaceutical forms can be readily diluted with water if so desired, just prior to administration. The advantage of these products lies in the increased palatability that they give to oily liquids such as mineral oil and cod liver oil—substances that are therefore commonly made available as emulsions.

Gels and *magmas* are more or less viscous suspensions of mineral precipitates in water. The antacid, aluminum hydroxide, is available as a gel made palatable with sweetening and flavoring substances. Magnesium hydroxide is made available as a magma (Milk of Magnesia). Preparations, of both types like other mixtures of suspended solids, should be well shaken before use, because the finely divided particles tend to settle out on standing, leaving a layer of clear watery liquid on top. The use of disposable medicine cups is especially desirable in administering such suspensions. Esthetic considerations alone dictate that the peptic ulcer patient should not be surrounded by glasses coated with the residues of the thick, milky antacid suspensions that he is taking. It is also more sanitary and more efficient to administer such oral medications in this way.

Hydroalcoholic liquids include *elixirs*, which contain about 25 per cent of alcohol, flavored with volatile oils and slightly sweetened. These clear liquids are often preferred by adults who may detest downing a heavy viscous syrup. Elixirs used as vehicles include the official Aromatic Elixir, which tastes like an orange cordial and can be colored red by the addition of amaranth; *Glycyrrhiza Elixir,* with an anise flavor that helps to hide the presence of salty or bitter drugs; and *Compound Benzaldehyde Elixir,* with a bitter almond odor and vanilla flavor and a low alcohol content. Among the substances often administered in this way are codeine (e.g., in the well-known Elixir of Terpin Hydrate and Codeine) and bromides, phenobarbital, and the antihistamine, diphenhydramine. The pharmacist uses a combination of low strength and high strength hydroalcoholic solutions—Iso-Alcoholic Elixir—to adjust the amount of alcohol needed to keep different drugs in solution. Such liquids should be administered undiluted in order to avoid upsetting the delicately adjusted hydroalcoholic balance and inadvertently precipitating one or more of the drugs from solution.

Alcohol in still higher concentrations—often 50 per cent and more—is sometimes required for keeping certain substances in solution. *Spirits,* for example, contain volatile oils such as peppermint or orange in much larger amounts than can be dissolved in water. Some spirits are used to flavor elixirs, others for exerting a medicinal effect of their own (in carminative products for treating gastric distress, for example). Aromatic spirit of ammonia, an alcoholic solution of an ammonium salt, has a pungent odor that does as much psychologically as the irritant solution does medically. Certain *tinctures,* in addition to those made by extracting potent vegetable drugs, are highly alcoholic solutions of the flavoring principles obtained from such substances as lemon or orange peel.

Timing of oral medications in relation to meals is often an important consideration. The doctor usually determines whether a particular medication is best given before or after meals (a.c. or p.c.; see Table 4-1), but he often leaves this to the nurse's judgment. Irritating drugs are ordinarily taken with food to avoid causing nausea and perhaps precipitating vomiting which may result in loss of the medication. Patients with acute rheumatic fever, for example, often require some milk and crackers or other snack to lessen salicylate-induced gastrointestinal irritation, when such aspirin-type drugs are being pushed to maintain high salicylate blood levels around the clock.

On the other hand, other drugs are best given between meals if the presence of food in the stomach may delay their absorption unduly, or if the digestive secretions can destroy too great a proportion of the dose. Most oral penicillin products, for example, are given before, rather than after meals, for this reason. However, if there is any doubt about the best timing for oral administration of a particular drug, the nurse should consult the physician about it.

The doctor's advice should also be sought as to whether an ordered oral medication should be omitted when a patient is vomiting or so nauseated that giving anything by mouth might precipitate vomiting. If the drug has been prescribed for relief of nausea, and the patient seems able to retain the antiemetic medication, it should be given. However, when vomiting is persistent, the physician should be consulted concerning the possibility of giving the drug rectally, or by some parenteral route in order to avoid irritating the upper G.I. tract.

Non-Oral Routes

Other factors besides a drug's irritating properties may make it necessary for the doctor to bypass the upper G.I. tract in order to get the medication into the patient's blood stream. Some drugs simply do not attain adequately high plasma concentrations when given by mouth. This, as we have seen (see Chap. 2) may be because the drug is destroyed by digestive secretions or fails to pass through the epithelial barrier lining the intestinal tract. In addition, some drugs, such as glyceryl trinitrate, are largely destroyed in the liver when carried to that organ from the intestine by way of the portal circulation. In such cases, the drugs are sometimes given via the sublingual, buccal, or rectal routes.

Parenteral administration is preferred when it is important that all of the drug be absorbed rapidly and as close to completely as possible. The term, parenteral, means literally by any route other than the gastrointestinal, or enteral, tract. This, of course, includes the inhalation of volatile vapors of a drug through the lungs. However, although this is indeed a way of attaining high drug blood levels quickly in a controllable manner, the inhalation route is limited to a relatively few drugs. Thus, parenteral routes refer ordinarily to all the various ways by which solutions or suspensions of drugs are injected beneath the skin and deposited within the body.

Injection of drugs requires skill and special care, because parenteral administration is more hazardous than the oral dosage form. This is mainly the result of the rapidity and efficiency with which drugs are absorbed from most injection sites. The effects of overdosage resulting from an error in calculating and measuring the dose or in administering it is much more likely to prove disastrous when the drug is given parenterally. Once the drug is injected, it is usually difficult—and, in some situations, impossible—to keep it from being fully absorbed and from producing all of its effects, including adverse ones.

Injections may be painful, cause local tissue damage, or permit the entrance of infectious microorganisms. However, all of these difficulties can be kept to a minimum by the use of proper equipment and procedures. For example, an injection need not hurt if the needle is sharp and is inserted and withdrawn quickly, except, of course, when the injected solution is itself irritating to the tissues. Similarly, infection is unlikely when the medication is furnished in sterile form, the patient's skin is properly cleansed, and the sterility of needles and syringes is assured. (The nurse, as she learns the technical details of injection procedures, learns also all the practices and rules that ensure maximum safety.)

We have left to the textbooks of fundamental nursing the full discussion of all the technical procedures involved in preparing for safe and effective parenteral administration. We may note, however, that most injectable medications come in sterile ampules, disposable cartridges, rubber stoppered vials, or in bottles, and that there are now available—in addition to the traditional needles and glass syringes—other means of delivering the medication such as jet spray devices (e.g., Hypospray) and throw-away plastic syringes that come with a needle which is used only once (e.g., Tubex sterile needle units).

Parenteral administration employs various routes. Some—such as the subcutaneous, intramuscular, intraperitoneal, and intravenous routes—are used when a drug's systemic actions are desired; others—for example, intracutaneous and intrasynovial injections—are employed for achieving local effects with minimal generalized activity. Some significant aspects of the more commonly employed parenteral methods of administering drugs will now be briefly discussed.

Subcutaneous, or hypodermic, injections are made into the loose connective tissue underneath the skin (both the above Latin and the Greek-derived terms mean exactly that). Soluble drugs deposited at sites such as the outer surface of the arm or the front of the thigh are rapidly absorbed into the blood ordinarily, and the drug's effects come on promptly. However, if the patient is in shock, this route is undesirable because the sluggish circulation slows the drug's absorption. The drug solution is best delivered directly into the blood stream by intravenous injection ("I.V.") in such situations.

Not all drugs are suited to subcutaneous injection. Since no more than 2 ml. can ordinarily be deposited at such sites, the drugs given in this way must be highly soluble and potent enough to be effective in small volume. (Epinephrine, morphine, and insulin are commonly administered in this manner.) The subcutaneous tissues contain nerve endings that transmit pain impulses when the injected solutions are irritating. Sometimes sterile abscesses develop as a result of chemical irritation, and the tissues may become necrotic and slough off. Thus, the I.V. route is preferred for irritating drug solutions, although some are now also administered by deep intramuscular injection.

HYPODERMOCLYSIS is a form of subcutaneous injection that permits the slow administration of large amounts of fluids such as isotonic saline and glucose solutions. A larger bore needle is inserted into the loose tissues to the outer sides of the upper body or into the anterior aspect of the thigh, or elsewhere, and the fluid is slowly infused. This procedure helps to counteract thirst in a dehydrated patient unable to take fluids by mouth; however, the amount of fluid that can be administered is self-limited by the pressure of the infused fluid upon the vessels which must absorb it.

Occasionally, the spread of such locally injected fluid is facilitated by adding the enzyme *hyaluronidase* to the hypodermoclysis solution. This enzyme helps to break down one of the main components of the intracellular connective tissues and thus open up more space for fluid diffusion. These temporary enzyme-induced changes in the intracellular subcutaneous ground substances aid the dispersal of the fluid from the injection site and thus lessen painful tissue tension. This is particularly useful for infants and young children, but care is required to avoid too rapid absorption with resulting overload of the circulatory system.

The rate of absorption from subcutaneous injection sites can sometimes be slowed when a more prolonged action is desired. Addition of the vasoconstrictor epinephrine to local anesthetic solutions, for example, keeps the desired action localized and reduces the likelihood of systemic toxicity from too rapid absorption. Substances such as insulin may be suspended in a protein colloid solution, and heparin and corticotropin may be administered in gelatin solutions, to reduce the rate of absorption and thus prolong their action. Application of an icebag above the site of subcutaneous injection slows absorption still further, as does application of a tourniquet in cases in which a reaction occurs.

Intramuscular injections are made with a longer, heavier needle that penetrates past the subcutaneous tissues and permits the drug solution or suspension to be deposited deep between the layers of muscle masses. Watery drug solutions spread over a larger area than when injected subcutaneously, and absorption is even more rapid than by the latter route. On the other hand, finely divided suspensions of insoluble substances are only very slowly absorbed when deposited in an intramuscular depot. Thus, this route is employed for administering the long-acting esters of sex hormones and corticosteroid drugs or poorly soluble salts, such as benzathine penicillin G and procaine penicillin G, which are absorbed over periods of days or even exert their antibacterial effects for weeks.

The intramuscular injection site contains fewer sensory nerve endings than the subcutaneous sites, so that I.M. injections tend to be less painful. However, with irritating substances, a small amount of the local anesthetics procaine or xylocaine is often added to the injection solution. Irritation is less likely to lead to tissue necrosis deep in the muscle than when irritants are placed under the skin. However, the danger of inadvertent intravenous injection is greater when the needle is placed deep down into these more vascular muscular tissues. Thus, it is essential—especially with oily suspensions of insoluble particles—to ascertain that the needle has not entered a blood vessel by pulling up the plunger after inserting the needle. If blood is aspirated and appears in the syringe, the needle is withdrawn and reinserted at another site. Care is also taken to avoid injury to the sciatic nerve in making injections into the gluteal muscles.

Intravenous injection bypasses all barriers to drug absorption. As a result, this is the most rapidly effective and, at the same time, the most dangerous route of administration. For, once a drug is placed directly into the blood stream it cannot be recalled, nor can its action be slowed by tourniquets or other means. Thus, every effort must be made to avoid errors and to detect early signs of adverse reactions. This route is usually reserved for the emergency administration of potent drugs when very rapid action is required, as in the use of epinephrine for anaphylactic shock or norepinephrine for circulatory collapse.

Sometimes substances that would be very irritating to subcutaneous and intramuscular tissues (highly alkaline sulfonamide sodium salt solutions, for example) are given by slow I.V. injection, since they do not harm the inner lining of the veins. Care is taken to avoid leakage of such solutions into the surrounding tissues, because pain, sterile abscesses, and necrotic sloughing can develop if highly irritating substances or potent local vasoconstrictors such as norepinephrine extravasate.

INFUSIONS of large amounts of fluid are often made by venoclysis, to overcome dehydration and supply nutritive substances when patients are unable to take fluids or foods orally. The technique of inserting the needle into the vein under sterile conditions is similar to that used when small quantities of drug solutions are injected. In this case, however, the nurse must adjust the rate of flow and see that it is kept at the speed that the doctor ordered, in order to avoid overloading the patient's circulation and, at the same time, to assure an adequately rapid flow of fluids and electrolytes. Occasionally, solutions may be infused into the bone marrow of the sternum or the extremities when the patient's veins are very small or have collapsed.

Intrathecal or intraspinal injections are made by doctors trained in the special techniques. Spinal anesthesia is accomplished by careful placement of a local anesthetic solution in the subarachnoid space. Similarly, anti-infective drugs are sometimes injected intrathecally in the treatment of meningitis, to attain a high local concentration of an antibiotic or sulfona-

mide which does not readily penetrate the subdural and other membranes by way of the blood stream.

Intradermal or intracutaneous injections are made for local rather than systemic effects. Injection of a small amount of solution just below the surface of the skin promptly produces a wheal, which delays further absorption into the lymphatics. Local anesthetics are sometimes injected in this way and further deeper injections are then made through the superficially deadened tissues. Tuberculin testing and allergic sensitization tests are also carried out by this method of pricking the skin or by scratching the material into the upper skin surfaces.

INTRASYNOVIAL OR INTRA-ARTICULAR injections are used mainly to attain high local concentrations of corticosteroid drugs to reduce acute inflammation in a joint without much danger of systemic steroid toxicity. Even when the doctor uses great care, local discomfort is ordinarily increased for a few hours before the drug's palliative effects develop. Steroids of the same kind are now often injected into bursae, tendons and nerve sheaths for their local effects, and intralesional injections of steroids are often employed in dermatology. (These are essentially intradermal or sometimes subcutaneous injections made through a small bore needle for locally limited actions.)

Application to Skin and Mucous Membranes. Drugs are often applied to the skin and to the mucous membranes of the mouth and throat, the nose and other parts of the respiratory tract, the eyes, and the genito-urinary and gastrointestinal tracts. In the case of the skin, such applications are almost always intended to have only a local effect and any systemic absorption that occurs is only incidental and unintended. On the other hand, drugs are sometimes brought into contact with the mucosa of the mouth and rectum as a means of getting them into the blood stream when swallowing the agents is undesirable or impossible. The dosage forms that are administered for both systemic mucosal absorption and local dermatomucosal drug effects will be briefly discussed here.

Sublingual tablets are placed under the tongue and *buccal* tablets between the gums and the cheek, in order to attain therapeutic concentrations of certain drugs in distant tissues. The drugs administered in these ways are agents that either tend to be destroyed by the digestive juices (for example, the polypeptide hormone oxytocin) or, even if absorbed, are so rapidly detoxified by liver enzymes that high plasma levels are difficult to attain rapidly by the oral route. Glyceryl trinitrate (nitroglycerin) is a drug of the latter type: when a nitroglycerin tablet is placed under the tongue, it is so rapidly dissolved and absorbed by way of the venous capillaries beneath the tongue that its therapeutic effects on the heart of a person suffering anginal pains are usually felt in one to five minutes.

Patients taking sublingual tablets must be instructed in their proper use. They are told not to chew or swallow the tablet and not to take water with it, but simply to place it under the tongue and let it dissolve. Buccal tablets are best placed next to the upper molar teeth, and the patient is instructed to avoid disturbing the dosage form after it is placed in the parabuccal space. As with sublingual tablets, the patient avoids eating, chewing, drinking or smoking, lest the tablet be swallowed and destroyed instead of being absorbed by way of the mucosa of the buccal pouch between gums and cheek.

The mucous membranes of the mouth and throat are often treated with local applications of antiseptic, anesthetic and astringent drugs. The public is subjected to a good deal that is obviously nonsense, in advertisements for nonprescription mouth washes, gargles, throat lozenges or troches, and medicated chewing gums and much of the folklore of mouth and throat therapy must be discounted. However, oral hygiene is an important part of patient care. Thus, the nurse should be familiar with the principles of mouth cleanliness.

The throat is sometimes sprayed with local anesthetics during surgical or diagnostic procedures. In this way, sensory receptors are deadened to avoid gagging and thus permit passage of instruments such as endotracheal tubes, laryngoscopes and bronchoscopes. Topically applied anesthetics may be absorbed systemically in amounts that can prove toxic; thus, the doctor may ask the nurse to record the amounts of solution being employed in this way, in order to be sure that, in the administration of the drug, safe amounts are not exceeded.

The nasal mucosa is commonly treated with drug solutions applied as sprays, nose drops and tampons. Among the drugs applied in this way are decongestants for opening blocked nasal passages and hemostatics to stop nosebleeds. Here, too, the public is often led to expect too much from such topical application, with the result that nonprescription preparations are misused in ways that can prove harmful. The nurse should be familiar with the correct procedure for instilling drops into the nose, so that they do not pass wastefully down into the throat. Systemic absorption of the drugs contained in nasal medications can have adverse effects on the cardiovascular and the central nervous systems.

Occasionally, drugs are deliberately applied to the nasal mucosa for absorption into the systemic circulation. Patients with diabetes insipidus, for example, often take vasopressin in the form of a snuff. "Snowbirds" sniff cocaine and opiate addicts often "snort" heroin to attain the central stimulating and depressant effects of these addicting drugs.

Inhalation of drugs into the deeper respiratory tract passages is used for both local and systemic effects.

Volatile drugs that are drawn in as vapors with inhaled air reach the blood stream very rapidly by passing through the thin mucosal covering that lines the lung surfaces. General anesthetics are given in this way, as are the gases oxygen and carbon dioxide. A number of other drugs that require rapid absorption are also administered by inhalation.

Among the drugs that are inhaled for systemic activity are amyl nitrite, the vapors of which reach the heart very rapidly to relieve an anginal attack when the patient breaks the vial in a handkerchief and inhales the volatile contents; ergotamine, which is now sometimes given in this way to abort a migraine headache; and isoproterenol and other bronchodilators, which are commonly inhaled for relief of emphysema and bronchial asthma. In addition, drugs are often inhaled for their local effects on the respiratory mucosa. These include detergents and enzymes, for liquefying thick obstructive secretions, and antibiotics which reach distant local areas in the lungs when inhaled in the form of very fine particles nebulized by a stream of air or oxygen.

Rectal administration of drugs in the form of enema solutions and glycerinated gelatin or cocoa-butter-based suppositories is commonly employed for local effects as well as a means of getting drugs into the systemic circulation when the oral route cannot or should not be used. The nurse is often responsible for administering medications rectally in a manner that facilitates their absorption from the mucosa of the lower G.I. tract.

The best time for administering drugs rectally is immediately after the patient has moved his bowels. The lower tract may be emptied by administering an evacuant enema or by the use of suppositories that act locally to set off the defecation reflex. After the lower bowel has been cleansed, the suppository or the retention enema containing the dose of the drug for systemic absorption and action is inserted, and the patient is kept lying down for at least 20 minutes in the case of a suppository and about half an hour for an enema. If the patient gets up too soon, the unmelted suppository may be evacuated or the unabsorbed enema fluid may be expelled. The patient should lie still and breathe deeply, to help to prevent loss of the medication.

One of the drugs commonly administered rectally is aminophylline, a substance that often causes gastric distress when given by mouth. It must be noted, however, that this drug—like the organic mercurial suppositories, which are also given in this way—may cause rectal irritation in some patients. Solutions are less likely to cause local irritation and proctitis, because they are absorbed more rapidly and completely than is the material erratically released from suppository bases. On the other hand, the amount of fluid that can be retained is relatively small, and the more rapidly absorbed drug may have too fleeting an action.

Rectal administration of depressant drugs is sometimes employed to put children to sleep prior to general anesthesia with other agents. Thiopental sodium, for example, is available as a rectal suspension for producing preanesthetic hypnosis or basal narcosis and is administered by use of a disposable plastic syringe and applicator. Antiemetic drugs such as prochlorperazine (Compazine) are commonly administered as rectal suppositories, since the vomiting patient may not be able to retain these drugs when they are given by mouth.

In the genitourinary tract, medication is usually intended for local effect, but drugs can reach the systemic circulation by being absorbed from the urethral or vaginal mucosa. Dangerously high plasma concentrations of local anesthetics, for example, have been reached when solutions were instilled into a traumatized urethra prior to passage of a sound or a cystoscope. Urethral suppositories containing soothing substances are sometimes employed after dilatation or other painful procedures. Vaginal suppositories containing estrogens combined with anti-infective drugs are applied in vaginitis, and irrigating solutions, or douches, are sometimes instilled to cleanse and acidify the vaginal mucosa.

The skin is treated mainly with liquid lotions and liniments and with semisolid ointments and pastes containing oily bases such as petrolatum or lanolin, or water-miscible bases such as surface-active, or wetting, agents. The dermatologist chooses the dosage form and bases that are best-suited for application to the particular area and skin condition which require treatment. The nature of the most common dermatological disorders and the drugs and dosage forms used for relief of skin symptoms are more fully discussed in Chapter 43.

Ordinarily, the skin acts as a barrier to most drugs that are applied to it. This is an advantage in minimizing the absorption of potentially toxic drugs. The corticosteroids, for example, relieve itching and other skin symptoms when applied topically, without causing the systemic side effects that can occur upon oral administration.

The usefulness of the skin as a route by which drugs may enter the body is limited; however, some substances applied by inunction (dermal application with friction) attain therapeutic blood levels. Mercury ointment, for example, was once applied this way for treating syphilis in the pre-penicillin era; and enough methyl salicylate (oil of wintergreen) is sometimes absorbed by way of the sebaceous glands to produce a central analgesic effect. (Actually, most of the action of liniments containing this potentially toxic substance is local in nature, and pain is relieved by a combination of rubefacient (skin-reddening) and

counterirritant effects rather than by depression of the pain-perception centers of the brain.)

Drugs are sometimes driven into the skin by means of an electric current, in a rarely employed procedure called iontophoresis. A solution of an ionizable drug such as methacholine is applied to the skin. A galvanic current from an electrode then moves the small ions into the upper layers of the patient's skin, where the drug then exerts a local action.

Lotions and ointments are best applied in small amounts, to avoid both waste and messiness. Applications are made gently, by patting rather than rubbing, in order to avoid damaging irritated, inflamed areas. A firm stroke is desirable, since too lightly dabbing the pruritic skin tends to increase itchiness. If the preparation is one that stains clothing, the patient should be warned about it and advised to avoid having the medication come in contact with his clothing or, if this is not possible, to wear old clothes during the treatment period. Ointments should be removed from jars with a tongue blade and never with the fingers, in order to avoid contaminating the remainder of the contents.

Moist dressings are often applied as a means of keeping heat on inflamed areas or for producing a cooling vasoconstrictive effect on the skin. *Compresses* may be made by soaking sterile towels in solutions of aluminum acetate, potassium permanganate, or plain water. These are then wrung out and applied to the painful areas. *Poultices* are home remedies sometimes used for local inflammation. They are made by mixing substances such as linseed meal or bread crumbs with boiling water, spreading the moist mass on fabric and placing it over the affected part. The pharmacist may occasionally make a kaolin poultice for hot application by making a paste of kaolin and glycerin and scenting it for psychological effect.

Actually, only the use of moist compresses has any reputable professional status in modern dermatological therapy.

THE TASK OF ADMINISTERING MEDICINES

Many systems are being developed for relieving nurses of some of the tasks connected with the administration of medicines. Various kinds of cabinets and dispensers are being devised (e.g., the Brewer System) to facilitate the dispensing of medications. In some hospitals, the Pharmacy Department has taken over the entire mechanical task. Elsewhere, it is even thought desirable for selected patients to take their own medicines.

Such approaches may facilitate drug administration, but the nurse's major responsibilities are not diminished by such devices. The nurse must still see that the patient actually gets the drug as it was prescribed, and she must note and report how the patient reacts to drug therapy. When the patient has permission to take his own medication, the nurse has the task of instructing him as to the amount he is to take, the time intervals at which it is to be taken, and so forth. She must also teach the patient's family important aspects of the patient's medication regimen that they need to know when his treatment is to be continued at home.

No system can be a substitute for the nurse's own good judgment in dealing with the countless situations that arise in translating a doctor's order that medication be given into the administration of the drug in a way that is most beneficial and safe for the patient. Thus, we shall, in the following discussion, offer various rules for proceeding with the task of administering medicines safely and efficiently, but the policies and procedures established on the experience of others must be supplemented by each individual nurse's application of her own thought and experience to best advantage in every case.

Receiving the Drug Order. No medication should ever be administered without a doctor's order. Ideally, this should always be in writing, since a written record best protects the patient, physician and nurse from the traumatic experience of medication errors. In emergencies, the physician may have to give a verbal order by telephone or in person. In that case, the nurse should write down the order immediately and have the physician sign or initial it as soon afterward as possible.

In any relationship with a colleague, it is sometimes necessary for one person to remind another of the framework of rules and regulations under which they must both function. Thus, it is entirely proper for the nurse to ask the physician to please write down the order, when, while he is hurriedly departing, he throws over his shoulder a brisk, "Oh, and give her 15 mg. of phenobarbital three times daily!"

Often the physician's order for drugs is not adequately communicated. This can result in confusion, misunderstanding, and interruption of the patient's course of treatment. Sometimes, for example, the doctor tells the patient that he is going to have him get a laxative or a sleeping pill and then forgets to write the order on the patient's chart. Later, the patient is puzzled when he fails to receive the promised medication at bedtime. When he asks the nurse for it, and she has to reply that the doctor left no order for it, all concerned suffer as a result of the breakdown of communication. To avoid such situations, every effort should be made to set up and adhere to a clearly established system for handling medicine orders.

Prescriptions are special orders for medication which the doctor writes for the pharmacist to fill. Such prescribed instructions tell the pharmacist the drugs and the dosage form he is to dispense. In addition, the pharmacist is directed to write certain directions to the patient on the label of the medication container. These directions ordinarily tell the patient how much of the medication he is to take and at what intervals.

It was once the practice to use various devices for keeping the patient in the dark about what medication he was receiving. Today, this practice of hiding a drug's identity from the patient is being abandoned in many instances when it is to the patient's benefit to know what drug he is taking. Thus, doctors often now ask the pharmacist to put the exact names and strengths of the drugs on the label. Whether the container lists the contents or not, the nurse should find out exactly what she is administering when she is called in to care for a patient who is receiving prescribed drugs.

When, for instance, the public health nurse gives the patient a medicine which has come from the pharmacy with a label indicating only directions for taking it, she should telephone the pharmacist for more information. She should give him the number of the prescription and ask him to tell her what drug or drugs it contains and what amounts are being ingested each time the patient takes the medication as directed.

Doctors are also supposed to indicate on the prescription the number of times that they want the patient to have it refilled without visiting them again. If the doctor does not indicate the number of permissible refills, the pharmacist may refuse to issue the medication until he receives further authorization. Under the Drug Abuse Control Amendments of 1965, no prescription for depressant or stimulant drugs may be refilled more than five times, or more than six months after the original date of issue, unless the doctor authorizes renewal by issuing a new prescription. In the case of prescriptions for narcotics, the Harrison Narcotic Act forbids any refilling at all, and, since oral orders for narcotics are illegal, the doctor must *write* a new prescription each time that he wants the patient to receive more of the drug.

Measuring Systems. Prescriptions are written in either the metric or the apothecary system, and there is not much that the nurse can do to influence the physician to use the much preferred metric system. In hospitals, however, the nurse who is charged with the chief responsibility relative to the administration of medicines should be vocal in encouraging adoption of a single system—the simpler metric one—on drug orders. The use of both systems offers unnecessary opportunities for error, and the need to convert dosage from one system to the other is a flagrant waste of nursing time.

Dosage Accuracy. The nurse may be called upon to calculate dosage and prepare solutions in various dilutions, and she should, of course, learn to do so with the aid of a book on dosage and solutions. Although the required arithmetical calculations are simple enough, it is easy for a nurse to misplace an elusive decimal point or make some other mistake when harassed by work pressures. Thus, to avoid error, every calculation should be checked by another person. Without abrogating her responsibility for making correct calculations, the nurse is justified here, too, in using her influence to minimize the need to make calculations on the ward.

For example, if the ward has only 15 mg. morphine tablets, and the doctors are ordering 10-mg. doses, the nurse should ask the pharmacy to provide the 10 mg. size. This saves nursing time spent in making unnecessary calculations of a kind that could lead to error. Similarly, in the case of solutions used for soak, irrigations, etc., the pharmacy should be requested to prepare dilutions in the strengths that the doctors are ordering.

CHILDREN'S DOSAGE must often be determined in terms of preparations that are intended for adults. Particular care must be taken in making the necessary dilutions, since sick children are especially sensitive to drugs. As ordinary a drug as aspirin can have profoundly adverse effects when administered to a dehydrated, feverish child in even relatively small overdoses. Children often tend to react with unexpected severity to drugs that affect the functioning of the central nervous system, including sedatives and antihistaminics. Overdoses of the latter that only make adults sleepy can cause convulsions in youngsters.

Although calculation of the dose that a child is to receive is, of course, the doctor's responsibility, the nurse should be aware that most of the dosage rules developed for converting adult dosage to children's dosage are not very reliable and may thus serve as a built-in source of error. The child's age is often a dangerous basis for determining how much of a potent drug he should receive. Body weight is also not a reliable basis for determining dosage, for children of the same weight may still be different in size. Pediatricians now feel that a child's body surface area is the best basis for calculating drug dosage, and more and more of these doctors are employing tables for determining the dose for a child in this way.

CHECKING THE DOSE that has been ordered whenever there is any doubt about its accuracy is an essential habit to acquire. If the doctor seems to have ordered a dose that is outside the usual range, the nurse should check this with him before proceeding to administer the drug. Alertness and frankness between nurses and doctors is necessary in this regard, if errors are to be avoided. Thus, a doctor in one instance was writing an order on the patient's chart and gave it verbally at the same time, saying, "Give Mrs. Jones 2 mg. of digitoxin." The nurse, who realized that the usual

dose of digitoxin is 0.2 mg., said, "Do you mean 0.2 mg., doctor?" The doctor then found that he had also written 2 mg. on the order sheet.

Later that evening, the nurse was assisting the same physician in the care of a patient in status asthmaticus. Under the stress of what was her third emergency in three hours, she went to the medicine closet to prepare the 0.5 cc. of epinephrine prescribed by the doctor. Under the pressure of the moment, she drew up 1 cc. instead. Fortunately, the physician was still with the patient when she returned with the medication. This time it was he who noticed that the syringe contained an excessive dose and called the error to her attention. In both cases, of course, it was the patient who profited from the fact that the doctor and nurse both recognized that they shared a responsibility to help each other avoid errors.

Less dramatic measures for assuring accuracy of dosage involve maintaining the legibility of labels. Care should be taken in pouring liquids, so that the labels do not become soiled. If they do become worn or dirty, the bottles should be returned to the pharmacy for relabeling. Take special care, too, to write dosage information legibly on medicine cards, Kardex, and patient's charts. Do not yourself give medication when the order or the label of the container is not legible.

Proper storage of patient's drugs helps to promote safety by preventing the kinds of errors that tend to occur when medications are misplaced. Ward managers and, in some instances, pharmacists may now often be responsible for the storing of drugs on the ward; still, the nurse continues to carry this responsibility in many situations. In some hospitals, drugs are arranged alphabetically (from aspirin to zinc oxide, for example); in others, patient's medications are arranged according to their room numbers, in which case the nurse knows that medicines for the patient in room 405, for example, will be found in one place on the shelf and no other.

Preparation of medicines should be carried out in a quiet room, away from the nurse's station, where one is unlikely to be interrupted while working. The rooms where drugs are stored and prepared are not open to patients or the public. Narcotic drug cabinets are kept double-locked, but all drugs—whether narcotics or not—should be stored in locked cabinets for which the nurse carries the keys. Drugs that are commonly employed in emergency situations are checked daily to make certain that they, and the equipment required for their administration, are available for immediate use at all times. New nurses must always be informed about where emergency medications are kept, so that they need lose no time in searching for them.

Distribution of medications is facilitated and chances for error are reduced if the drugs are arranged in advance on the cart or tray in the order in which patients will be visited. The common practice in an adult medical-surgical or obstetrical unit of pushing a cart of medicine down the corridor is best avoided when distributing drugs to psychiatric patients or to children who might impulsively snatch medication from the cart. In general, medications should not be left unguarded, and it is important to take the medication tray with you when called from any patient's room. Some patients may steal drugs for suicidal purposes; others may hoard medication instead of taking it, for the same reason. Thus, it is important to stay with the patient and see that he actually swallows all oral medications.

Identifying the patient properly before administering his medication is, of course, crucial. It may seem unnecessary to go through the ritual of checking a patient's identification band against the name on the medication card when you are caring for only three patients and are well acquainted with each of them. Yet this habit can stand the nurse in good stead later when she may be working under more stressful situations. When the nurse works during the night and may have to give medicines to many sleepy patients, this habit can help to prevent mistakes. Patients often respond affirmatively when addressed by the wrong name; if a patient's identity is at all in doubt, do not give the drug without double checking in various ways, including asking the patient himself to state his name.

Patient's questions about the medication that they are receiving should always be given attention, although the matter of how much the patient should be told about this or any aspect of his treatment must be determined on an individual basis through consultation with his physician. Certainly, if a patient comments that he "can't take a particular medicine," the nurse should check with the doctor before giving the drug. Generally, the patient's questions about the nature of his drug therapy should be carefully considered, because they sometimes serve as an important safeguard against error.

In general, there is no pat answer to the question of how much the patient should be told about the nature and the purpose of the drug that is being administered. As we indicated earlier, it was once assumed that the patient should know little or nothing about the medicine that he was receiving. However, just as many physicians now have the pharmacist put the name of the medication on the prescription label, they also often explain the drug's expected therapeutic action to the patient and warn him of what side effects to expect.

This attitude is based on the idea that many patients profit in various ways from having an opportunity to participate in their own treatment rather than just passively following instructions. Thus, when a diabetic patient whose doctor has deliberately educated him about his condition asks his nurse how much insulin she is administering, it is silly for her to say, "I can't tell you that. You'll have to ask your doctor." Such a patient is likely to become angered—and with reason—by a secretive attitude, after he has been conditioned to inquire about the nature of his illness and encouraged to cooperate in his own treatment.

On the other hand, it is not always necessary or desirable to tell the patient the exact name of the drug that he is receiving. It may not be wise to say, "Here is your injection of morphine" to a patient being prepared for an operation or to one who is in temporary pain from trauma. The patient may be so disturbed by the thought of narcotic addiction that he will derive little benefit from the medication. Thus, it is probably better simply to say, "The doctor has ordered this medicine to help you rest and relax before you go to the operating room," or something similar.

Psychological factors must constantly be considered in approaching the patient and in the actual administration of his medication. In this regard, the nurse should look into her own attitudes toward the medications that she is administering, as it is quite easy to communicate wordlessly feelings that will have a negative influence on the patient's response to drug therapy.

It is all too easy to convey the thought that the patient does not really need a drug and that it is being given to him only because he does not have the courage to withstand a little pain or because he is an overemotional type who needs chemical calming as a substitute for the strength of character that he lacks. Medication given grudgingly may do more harm than good, just as can drugs administered with an air of distrustfulness that clearly states, "you never know how harmful medicine like this can be."

POSITIVE SUGGESTION, on the other hand, can be conveyed in the attitude of the nurse, in a quiet, subtle way. The act of giving medication is in itself one which conveys the idea that you are concerned with the patient's welfare and want him to get well. Thus, the nurse should offer medication to the patient as a tangible sign that the people charged with his care wish to help him. Most patients want to feel better and are emotionally prepared to expect relief from pain and discomfort when they receive medication. The nurse takes advantage of this belief in the efficacy of drugs and reinforces such expectations by her words and actions. If, for instance, the nurse takes the time to explain that a drug is going to bring about desired rest and relaxation, it is much more likely to do so than if she rushes in and administers an injection with no word of explanation.

LISTENING to the patient and letting him ventilate feelings of fear, anxiety and even anger or frustration concerning his treatment will often add to the effectiveness of the administered medication and to the patient's total response to therapy. While she may not agree with him, the nurse usually gives the patient a chance to voice his doubts about the efficacy of his treatment or to complain that his drug-induced discomfort is worse than what he can hope to gain from treatment.

REDUCING the patient's discomfort by physical and psychological measures should be attempted during and after the administration of medicines. As desirable as the use of a fresh, sharp needle and scrupulous injection technique is a brief, reassuring explanation of what the patient may expect, since this helps to lessen his apprehension and, in this way, to minimize the pain which he experiences.

After an injection has been completed, it is desirable to stay with the patient until his pain has subsided. The nurse can, for example, hold a child and rock or soothe him for a few minutes while he cries until he settles down. Adult patients can be helped to assume a more comfortable position, or to resume reading or be prepared for sleep. Nursing measures such as a soothing back rub following the administration of a pain-reliever such as morphine or a sedative-hypnotic barbiturate will aid in bringing about the desired effects of these drugs.

Nursing measures of this kind may minimize the need for drugs or even make them unnecessary in some cases. A restless patient can often be helped to drift off to sleep by bringing him a glass of warm milk, putting out a bright light, by talking with him or letting him tell you about things that may be troubling him.

Even in administering medications that produce only a bad taste or a dry mouth, the nurse can do things to lessen the patient's discomfort. Chilling certain medications in the refrigerator for a while helps to lessen their disagreeable taste and odor. Offering the patient a candy mint or chewing gum following such a dose may also be desirable. It sometimes helps, too, to mention in advance that a drug such as atropine will likely make the patient's mouth dry and that this will wear off before long. Similarly, if a child asks whether a medicine tastes bad, he should be told the truth, and efforts should be made to disguise the taste if this is at all possible.

ESTHETIC CONSIDERATIONS also have a place when medicines are being administered. Medicine should be offered with as much concern for cleanliness as when food is served. If medicine glasses are used, they should be well washed, scalded and dried. However, nurses should suggest the use of individual disposable containers in the interest of cleanliness and efficiency. Such paper cups should not, of course, be permitted to pile up when a patient is taking frequent doses of a medication such as sticky antacid

suspensions for treating peptic ulcer. Water for washing down medication should be fresh, cold and offered in adequate quantity.

Wasting of medication through carelessness can add greatly to the cost of the patient's treatment. It is easy to forget, when dispensing medications on a busy ward, that many modern drugs are quite expensive. Thus, medications should be carefully handled to avoid spilling them or rendering them unfit for use. However, one should not return an unused dose of a drug to a bottle from which medicines are dispensed. When the patient is discharged, any unused medicine should be returned to the pharmacy, so that he will receive credit for it and not have to pay for medication never received.

Recording the administration of all medications is, of course, essential. Methods of putting information down on the patient's chart vary from place to place. In general, it is considered necessary to see that each dose and the time of its administration is recorded along with an indication of who gave it. How the patient responded to medication is an important point of information for charting. Various measures are now in use for reducing the amount of time spent in recording medications. If, for example, the same medicine is administered four times daily, only the time of each dose need be charted in some institutions, and the name of the drug need not be entered each time.

SUMMARY

We have tried to take up some of the things that the nurse must consider in carrying out one of her most important patient-care functions—the administration of medicines. The reason for offering so much detailed, step-by-step advice is this: Once the nurse has developed habit patterns based upon safe and efficient ways of administering medicines, she will be able to concentrate on the broader aspects of the patient's total care. Freed of the need to keep myriad details in mind, she can observe the patient's reactions to drugs and integrate her observations into what she knows of the patient's condition and the purpose of treatment with the drug that is being given. This does *not*, of course, mean that she ever acts *mechanically*, for habit can never be relied upon to that degree. Nurses are, for example, often instructed to read the label three times—once, when removing the medicine from the cabinet; once, when taking the dose of the drug from the bottle, and once, when returning the medication to its storage place. It is certainly true that reading the label more than once can help to prevent mistakes—but it is entirely possible to read a label wrong three times when you are really not attending to the task!

Actually, attentiveness is the most significant aspect of safety—attentiveness to the label, attentive to the identification band that you are checking. No one is optimally alert at all times. It helps, however, to develop insight into one's own mental processes in this regard. Thus, the nurse who learns to recognize signs of her own inattentiveness and knows that this happens when she is harrassed and anxious, can make an extra effort to interrupt such reactions and to concentrate on the task confronting her.

The dispensing of pills and capsules of various colors day after day can become boring. So, for that matter, can the administration of injections, once one's skill has been perfected and even that once challenging procedure becomes a matter of routine. Nevertheless, these tasks can remain interesting to the nurse who looks at them in the total context of how the nurse contributes to effective patient care.

Certainly, it is thrilling to the nurse to see a pneumonia patient with a 104° temperature and severe dyspnea respond to penicillin therapy by becoming afebrile and comfortable and begin to breathe normally. A nurse can treasure the experience of seeing a patient in shock, whose pulse and blood pressure were unobtainable, recover in response to an infusion of norepinephrine which she prepared for intravenous administration. Such rewards of nursing are in store for those who acquire the necessary skill and judgment and who make a constant effort to understand the relationships between the actions of drugs and the manner in which the patient's malfunctioning organ systems respond to the presence of pharmacotherapeutic agents.

TABLE 4-1

SOME COMMONLY EMPLOYED ABBREVIATIONS EMPLOYED IN PRESCRIPTION ORDERS

ABBREVIATION	LATIN DERIVATION	MEANING
aa	ana	of each
a.c.	ante cibos	before meals
ad lib.	ad libitum	as freely, or as often, as is desired
Aq. (dest)	aqua (destillata)	water (distilled)
b.i.d.	bis in die	twice a day
c̄	cum	with
Caps.	capsula	capsule
Chart.	chartula	a medicated powder in a paper wrapping
Comp.	compositus	compound
dil.	dilutus	dilute
d.t.d.	dentur tales doses (no.)	give as many doses as indicated by the number
dis.	dispensa	dispense
elix.	elixir	elixir
ext.	extractum	extract
et	et	and
F, or ft.	Fac. or fiat	make; let be made
Flext.	fluidextractum	fluidextract
Gm.	gramma	gram
gr.	granum	grain
gtt.	gutta	a drop
h.	hora	hour
h.s.	hora somni	at bedtime
M.	misce	mix
non rep.	non repetatur	do not repeat
no.	numerus	number
noct.	nox, noctis	night
o	omnis	every
o.d.	omni die	every day
o.h.	omni hora	every hour

TABLE 4-1 (Continued)

Abbreviation	Latin Derivation	Meaning
o.d.	oculus dexter	right eye
o.s.	oculus sinister	left eye
os	os	mouth
pil.	pilula	pill
p.c.	post cibos	after meals
p.r.n.	pro re nata	literally, as the occasion arises; occasionally; when it seems to be desirable or necessary
q. or qq	quaque	every
q.h. or qqh	quaque hora	every hour
q. or qqd.	quaque die	every day
q.i.d.	quater in die	four times a day
q.s.	quantum sufficit	a sufficient amount
℞	recipe	take
s̄	sine	without
s.o.s.	si opus sit	if needed
S. or Sig.	signa	write (on the label)
Sp.	spiritus	spirit
sol.	solutio	solution
ss	semis	half
stat.	statim	immediately
Syr.	syrypus	syrup
tab.	tabella	tablet
t.i.d.	ter in die	three times a day
Tr.	tinctura	tincture
Ung.	unguentum	ointment
ut dict.	ut dictum	as directed
Vin.	vinum	wine

SUMMARY OF POINTS FOR THE NURSE TO REMEMBER

• Timing the administration of drugs is often left to the nurse's judgment. She should consider whether to give the drug with food or between meals, as well as the relationship of administration of the drug to the patient's hours of sleep. When in doubt about when would be preferable to administer a drug, the nurse should confer with the physician.

• The nurse must be alert to the possibility that the route of administration ordered by the physician may not be feasible in a particular situation and be ready to discuss this with the doctor. For example, if the patient is vomiting, administering a previously pre-scribed oral medication may be unwise. It is then desirable to get permission to substitute another dosage form to be administered by a different route.

• Be especially alert to avoid any error in administering parenteral dosage forms, since their more rapid and complete absorption makes mistakes particularly hazardous.

• Teaching the patient and his family how to take or to administer drugs with the greatest efficiency and safety is often the nurse's responsibility, as is observing and reporting the patient's response to drug therapy.

- The individual nurse must assume the responsibility for her own safe practice in administering medication. Such responsibility involves (1) the habitual employment of measures which lessen the chances of error (e.g., properly identifying the patient before administering any medication); (2) the acquiring of fundamental knowledge about the medication, such as its therapeutic use, side effects and potential toxicity, and usual dosage range; (3) working toward the establishment of institutional policies and procedures that foster safety and efficiency in the administration of medications.

- The nurse's actions and attitudes can increase or impede the effectiveness of drug therapy. Thus, her attitude should be one that conveys positive suggestions that foster realistic expectations of the benefits to be derived from treatment with the drug that is being administered. Her actions (for example, promoting the patient's physical comfort) should also contribute to the total objectives of patient care and treatment.

REVIEW QUESTIONS

1. (a) What characteristic do tinctures and fluidextracts have in common? How do they differ in strength?

(b) What do alkaloids and glycosides have in common and how do they differ chemically?

2. (a) What are some advantages of oral dosage forms over parenterally administered medications?

(b) List some examples of oral dosage forms.

3. (a) What is the main purpose of enteric-coated tablets?

(b) What is the main purpose of timed-release type medications?

4. (a) What is the main advantage of syrups as a dosage form of drugs?

(b) What aspect of the promotion of proprietary products of a syrupy nature is not a desirable one?

5. (a) What are emulsions and what is their main advantage?

(b) What is a common drug preparation which is available as a magma, and what procedure should always be followed before using such a preparation?

6. (a) Give an example of a situation in which drugs are administered with food.

(b) Give an example of a situation in which the administration of a drug is timed for between meals.

7. (a) List some advantages and disadvantages of parenteral administration.

(b) What are some ways by which some of the disadvantages of parenteral therapy can be kept to a minimum?

8. (a) List some advantages and disadvantages of subcutaneous administration.

(b) How may the rate of absorption from subcutaneous sites be speeded up or delayed?

9. (a) List some advantages of intramuscular over subcutaneous injections.

(b) What are some precautions that are routinely taken in administering drugs by the intramuscular route?

10. (a) What is the main advantage of intravenous administration of drugs?

(b) What precautions are required in making an intravenous injection or infusion?

11. (a) List three types of injections that are made for local rather than systemic effects.

(b) Indicate some clinical situations in which injections of each of these types are employed.

12. (a) Give examples of drugs administered by sublingual or buccal route, and explain the advantage of giving them by these routes.

(b) What should the patient be told about the proper way to take tablets by the sublingual and buccal routes?

13. (a) When is the rectal route of administration preferred to the oral route? What are some drugs commonly administered in suppository form?

(b) What are some measures taken to assure retention and systemic absorption of rectally administered medication?

14. (a) List some dosage forms which are applied to the skin for local actions in dermatological disorders.

(b) List some measures that make for more efficient use of locally acting dermatological products.

15. (a) What are some suggestions that the nurse can make relative to the writing of orders for drugs which can help promote greater safety for the patient and a saving of the nurse's time in institutions and elsewhere?

(b) List several measures that the nurse should employ habitually to avoid making medication errors.

16. (a) Discuss briefly why it may or may not be desirable to answer a patient's questions about what drugs he is receiving.

(b) Give an example of a situation in which the patient's best interests may be served, and one in which they would not be well served, by his knowing what he is receiving.

17. (a) Give an example of how the nurse's attitude toward the medication that she is administering conveys the positive suggestion that the drug is going to prove beneficial.

(b) Give an example of nursing actions that can be used to enhance the effectiveness of drugs administered to relieve pain or produce sleep.

18. (a) What fundamental knowledge must the nurse have about each drug that she administers in order to fulfill her legal and ethical responsibility relative to administration of medications?

(b) What information concerning drugs that are being administered should be recorded on the patient's chart?

BIBLIOGRAPHY

Apple, W. S., and Abrams, R. E.: Problems in prescription order communication. J.A.M.A., *185:*291, 1963.

Byrne, A. K.: Errors in making medication. Am. J. Nurs., *53:*829, 1953.

Campbell, J. A., and Morrison, A. B.: Oral prolonged-action medication. J.A.M.A., *181:*102, 1962.

Friend, D.: Principles and practices of prescription writing. Clin. Pharmacol. Ther., *6:*411, 1965.

Hanson, D. J.: Intramuscular injection injuries and complications. G.P., *27:*109, 1963.

Labeling of Prescription Drugs. Editorial. J.A.M.A., *185:* 316, 1963.

Lesnik, M. J., and Anderson, B. E.: Nursing Practices and the Law. 2nd ed. Philadelphia, J. B. Lippincott, 1962.

Nelson, E.: Pharmaceuticals for prolonged action. Clin. Pharmacol. Ther., *4:*283, 1963.

Schwartz, D.: Medication errors made by aged patients. Am. J. Nurs., *62:*51, 1962.

Shirkey, H. C.: Drug dosage for infants and children. J.A.M.A., *193:*443, 1965.

Skipper, J. K., Tagliacozzo, D. L., and Mauksch, H. O.: What communication means to patients. Am. J. Nurs., *64:*101, 1964.

To Label or Not to Label. Editorial. J.A.M.A., *194:*1311, 1965.

Drugs Acting on the Central Nervous System

The drugs that we shall discuss in this section are those that act primarily by affecting the functioning of nervous tissue. The most important agents of this type are the ones that are able to penetrate the blood-brain barrier and exert their effects upon the *brain* and the *spinal cord*—the central nervous system.

Drugs that interfere with the functioning of the C.N.S. may affect only a single activity, such as the perception of pain. They are more likely, however, to have multiple effects, because the various parts of the C.N.S. are functionally interrelated, so that stimuli that affect one area also alter the functioning of others. In addition, since the C.N.S. acts to coordinate the activity of all the other systems of the body—including the other great integrating system, the endocrine glands—drugs that act upon the cells of the C.N.S. can profoundly influence the functioning of organs and structures far removed from the nervous control centers.

Most of the chapters of this section deal with drugs that act centrally to affect sensory, motor, mental and emotional functions in ways that are therapeutically useful in the management of many illnesses. However, before discussing the various types of centrally acting drugs, it is desirable first to review those aspects of the anatomy and physiology of the C.N.S. that are most pertinent to an understanding of the actions of drugs on this complex system. Such a review is presented in the next chapter, and at the same time some general concepts concerning the actions of centrally acting drugs are introduced.

5

Introduction to the Pharmacology of the Central Nervous System

NERVOUS SYSTEM STRUCTURE AND FUNCTION

The Neuron. The structural unit of the nervous system is the neuron, or nerve cell, of which there are about 14 billion in the body—about 10 billion being concentrated in the brain alone. Neurons come in many different sizes and shapes, but all are essentially similar in basic structure.

Each neuron is made up of a cell body containing cytoplasm, a nucleus, and other particles or granules. Thin threads of protoplasm project from the surface of the nerve cell body. Most of the cell's surface is covered by short processes that subdivide and send off branches and smaller twigs to form a treelike crown—the *dendrites*. These receive signals from many other interconnecting neurons.

One point on the nerve cell body sends out a more elongated process which does not branch until it comes close to other neurons. This is the *axon*, which transmits messages to the dendrites, or directly to the cell body or soma of other neurons. Such junctions between the axon of one cell and the dendrites of other neurons are called *synapses*.

The axons of the nerve cells packed closely together in the brain may extend only a few thousandths of an inch before synapsing with other neurons. However, some axonal fibers run for several feet before synapsing. The corticospinal nerve tracts—bundles of axons that run between nerve cell bodies in the brain and the spinal cord and make up much of the white matter of the C.N.S.—are one example of the latter. Another example may be seen in the bundles of fibers that pass from the C.N.S. to the skeletal muscles and other peripheral organs.

These axonal cables make up the peripheral nervous system. The nerve fibers that transmit *sensory* signals to the C.N.S. from peripheral receptors are called *afferent* fibers. Those that conduct impulses from the C.N.S. that elicit responses from muscles and glands are called *efferent*, and include *motor* and *secretory* fibers.

The C.N.S. also contains sensory and motor neurons. However, most of the nerve cells in the brain are neither sensory nor motor but are connecting links between these two types of neurons. The human cerebral cortex is especially rich in such interneurons, or internuncials. It is the presence of vast numbers of cerebral cortex interneurons with their almost infinite synaptic connections that accounts for the endless variety of ways in which human beings can respond to incoming sensory signals, in comparison with the more stereotyped responses of lower animals with fewer interneurons and synaptic connections.

The Nerve Impulse. Nerve cells are specialized for sending out electrical signals. Actually, all living cells possess electrical properties that stem from the nature of their membranes. However, the thin threads of neuronal tissue are capable of conducting electrical signals at a speed much greater than that of other kinds of tissue. The drugs that we shall be discussing act by altering the excitability of neurons and their ability to conduct and transmit nerve impulses.

The porous membranes of neurons, like those of other cells, let some substances into the interior of the cells and keep others out. The cell ordinarily pumps sodium ions * out of its interior and into the fluids that surround it, whereas potassium ions tend to become concentrated within the interior of the cell. The differential in the distribution of ions on either side of the cell membrane is maintained by an expenditure

---

* Ions are electrically charged particles formed when the atoms of various elements gain or lose electrons.

of cellular energy. This leads to the build-up of an electrical *potential* between the two sides of the membrane—the interior of the nerve cell being negative compared to the more positively charged outside of the cell.

In the resting, or unstimulated, nerve cell the membrane that has concentrated the positive ions on the outside and negative ions on the inside is said to be *polarized.* Stimulation of the neuron by an incoming signal briefly changes the permeability of the stimulated portion of the membrane. The resulting inrush of sodium ions reduces the resting potential still further. The loss of polarity when the ionic concentrations on the inside and outside of the membrane at the point of stimulation are suddenly equalized is called *depolarization.* Such local depolarization some-

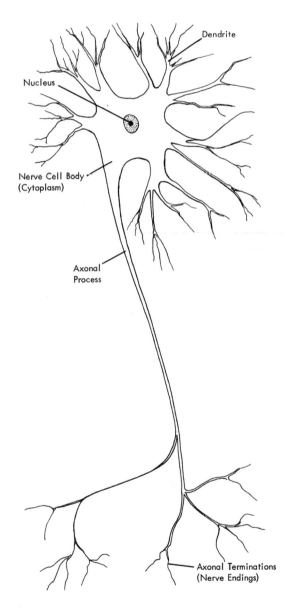

FIG. 5-1. A neuron—the structural unit of the nervous system.

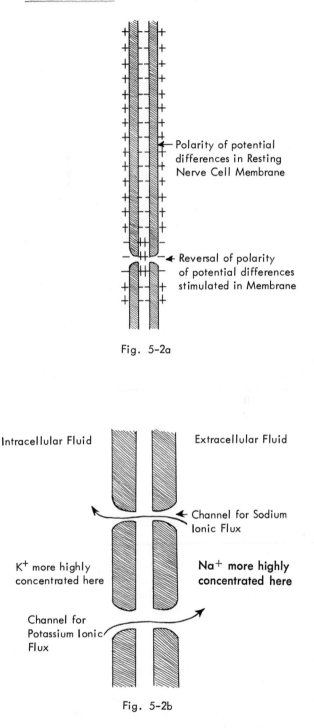

FIG. 5-2. Events during development and propagation of an action potential. (*Top*) Diagram of section of myelinated nerve cell membrane, showing ion concentrations in resting cell and at site of stimulation during depolarization and start of action potential propagation. (*Bottom*) Changes in ion concentration gradient as membrane is stimulated.

how acts as a stimulus to the adjacent portion of nerve cell membrane.

Apparently, the difference in potential between the stimulated section of nerve membrane and the unstimulated part directly adjacent to it serves as an electrical stimulus to the inactive portion. This depolarizes the next segment of membrane and sets off the wave of similar depolarizations down the entire length of the axon, which constitutes *conduction* of the nerve impulse. As this change of electrical potential races along, the membrane behind it is rapidly restored to its normal polarity. This happens because the cell's sodium pump expels the excess sodium ions from its interior, thus resulting in repolarization.

Until its membrane has been repolarized in this way, the nerve fiber cannot respond to new stimuli. This *refractory period* ordinarily lasts only one to three thousandths of a second. Thus, the nerve cell fiber can conduct several hundred signals per second, if it is itself stimulated by impulses strong enough to depolarize its membrane at such a rapid rate. These trains of tiny electrical pulsations are all the same whether they are signaling the input of sensory information, or sending out commands to the muscles, or storing data away in the brain's memory bank.

Drugs, as we shall see, affect nerve cell function by altering neuronal responsiveness to such signals and by changing the rate of nerve impulse conduction and transmission. For example, depressants such as phenobarbital may reduce the responsiveness of nerve cells by affecting the permeability of their membranes directly. By partially blocking the ionic exchanges in this way, these drugs are thought to alter the electrical activity of the neurons in ways that are useful for preventing convulsive seizures.

Synaptic Transmission. When the waves of depolarization, or *nerve action potentials* (NAP), arrive at the branching ends of the axon, they activate other nearby neurons. However, there is a delay of a few thousandths of a second in the spread of the electrical signals to the secondary nerve cells. One reason for this is that the neurons in a chain do not actually make contact with one another. Electron microscope studies of such synapses have demonstrated that a narrow space separates the membrane of the axonal ending from the membranes of the dendrites or the cell bodies of the next neurons.

How then do the weak electrical currents get across this synaptic gap? Synaptic transmission is now known to be chemical in nature. That is, the nerve impulse arriving at the ending of the first nerve cell (the *presynaptic fiber*) causes certain blisterlike granules (the *synaptic vesicles*) concentrated there to release molecules of a transmitter substance. This chemical is believed to bridge the gap between the presynaptic nerve endings and the membrane of the *postsynaptic cell*. That is, the molecules float across the microscopic gap, make contact with the postsynaptic membrane, and change its permeability in a way that triggers a new wave of electrical activity in the postsynaptic nerve cell.

The details of chemical transmission of nerve impulses in the autonomic nervous system by the neurohormones acetylcholine and norepinephrine are taken up in Chapter 14. The nature of neurohormonal transmission in the C.N.S. is thought to be essentially similar, but because of the difficulty of studying brain synapses, the details of what takes place there are still uncertain. However, evidence indicates that the autonomic neurotransmitters acetylcholine and norepinephrine (and perhaps other substances such as serotonin and gamma-amino butyric acid) transmit nerve impulses at central synapses also. As scientists learn more about the nature of central synaptic transmission, many drugs will probably be shown to produce their effects on the functioning of the C.N.S. by affecting the chemical reactions that take place at the junctions between adjacent nerve cells.

Central Excitatory and Inhibitory Systems. Many neurons of the C.N.S. send forth streams of messages that influence the functioning of other groups of nerve cells elsewhere in the C.N.S. Some of these neuronal control systems are *excitatory*, others exert *inhibitory* effects. The integrated activity of regulating impulses of both types determines the rates at which the affected nerve cell fibers fire. Many centrally acting drugs produce their effects by altering the functioning of such systems.

Individual nerve cell fibers fire impulses in an *all or none* fashion. That is, weak signals call forth no response at all, while impulses that exceed a certain

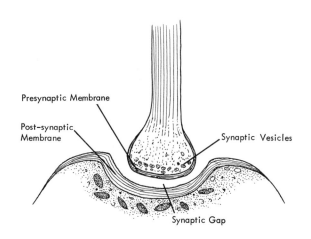

Fig. 5-3. A synapse. Here neurotransmitter from synaptic vesicles makes contact with post-synaptic membrane.

critical level, or *threshold,* make the nerve cell fiber send along a signal of maximum strength. However, the response of *postsynaptic* nerve cell bodies is *not* all-or-none in nature, but varies instead with the strength of the signals reaching it. The reason for this is that each nerve cell receives signals from the endings of not one but *many* other axons. Thus, the receiver neuron responds not to one signal but to the sum of many impulses reaching it within the same brief period. Once such summation exceeds a critical threshold level, the second cell sends out its own signals. The frequency with which such signals are conducted down the axon depends on the strength of the excitatory stimuli.

The impulses arriving at the postsynaptic nerve cell can change its membrane potential in either of two opposite directions. The *excitatory* presynaptic fibers are thought to release neurochemicals that tend to depolarize the second neuron of the synapse; at the same time, signals reaching this same nerve cell from still other fibers may tend to reduce its responsiveness. It may be that these *inhibitory* fibers release a type of chemical transmitter that tends to stabilize, or *hyperpolarize,* the postsynaptic membrane. The second cell in the synaptic chain will fire an impulse only when the sum of the excitatory, or depolarizing, stimuli impinging upon it in a brief period exceeds the sum of the inhibitory, or hyperpolarizing, stimuli that are simultaneously tending to reduce its responsiveness.

Many centrally acting drugs exert their effects by altering the balance between the excitatory and the inhibitory impulses impinging upon postsynaptic nerve cell membranes. They may do so by *increasing* either excitatory or inhibitory activity, or *by blocking* nerve impulses of one or the other of the two types.

Most depressant drugs, for example, produce their primary effects by keeping excitatory stimuli from depolarizing nerve cell membranes. On the other hand, these same depressants can increase the over-all excitability of some nerve cells by blocking out inhibitory impulses. Obviously, nerve nuclei that are released from the influence of inhibitory control in this way will respond with increased activity, at least until their excitatory stimuli are also blocked out.

Similarly, most C.N.S.-stimulant drugs act mainly by facilitating impulse transmission at excitatory synapses. However, some of those drugs may sometimes increase the activity of inhibitory presynaptic neurons. In this way, such stimulants may actually reduce the over-all excitability of the second nerve cell in such synaptic links.

THE FUNCTIONAL ORGANIZATION OF THE CENTRAL NERVOUS SYSTEM

The central nervous system is extremely complex. Indeed, the human brain has been called "the most complex organ in all creation." Yet, despite its anatomic and functional complexity, neurological scientists are continually filling in gaps in our knowledge of the neuroanatomy of the C.N.S., the functional relations between the various structures, and the manner in which the activity of one part affects that of others.

Central Nervous System Anatomy (See Figs. 5-4 and 5-5)

The brains of all vertebrate animals show certain basic similarities, despite their many differences and modifications, and are built along the same general lines. All contain an older, underlying portion that is connected by many nerve tracts to the more recently developed parts of the brain above and the even more primitive spinal cord below.

The brain has three major divisions—the *hindbrain,* the *midbrain,* and the *forebrain*—and each of these may be subdivided into other related groups of nerve cell bodies (nerve *nuclei*) and fiber *tracts.* We shall review only those parts that will be referred to later as sites at which various drugs act to bring about important changes in C.N.S. functions.

The hindbrain runs from the top of the spinal cord into the *midbrain.* It includes the *medulla oblongata* and the *pons,* the most primitive parts of the brain; these form the *brain stem,* a slender three-inch stalk upon which the cerebrum seems to be balanced. Above and behind the brain stem and connected to it by thick bundles of nerve fibers is the *cerebellum.* This organ, which lies in the lower, back part of the skull, works together with brain stem and certain cerebral structures to coordinate the activity of the muscles that are concerned with maintaining resting posture and in the control of the body's balance during complex voluntary movements.

The forebrain is composed of (1) the centrally located *diencephalon,* or 'tween brain, which is flanked by the two cerebral hemispheres that make up (2) the *telencephalon,* or end brain.

The diencephalon includes the *thalamus* and the *hypothalamus,* groups of nerve cells that connect with the cerebral cortex above and with various subcortical structures, including the brain stem. The thalamic nerve nuclei serve as a receiving and relay station for sensations such as heat and cold, pain, touch and muscle position sense. Some of these are sent directly to the appropriate receiving stations in the cerebral cortex; other sensory impulses are shunted to nerve cells in the core of the brain stem for further processing before being passed on to cortical areas.

The hypothalamic nuclei that lie below the thalamus help to make continuous adjustments in the control of body temperature, water balance, blood sugar levels, appetite and sleep. They also seem to play a central part in the expression of emotions.

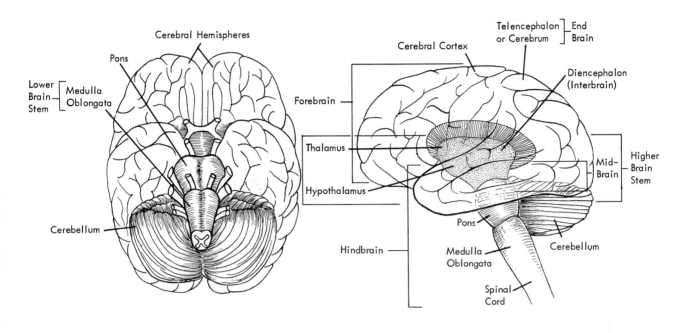

FIG. 5-4. View of underside of the brain.

FIG. 5-5. Median view of the brain.

The cerebral hemispheres of the telencephalon—and especially their frontal lobes—have grown to relatively tremendous size in humans. Their outer layer, the *cerebral cortex,* is made up of masses of nerve cell bodies, the gray matter. This, the most recently evolved part of the brain, has buried beneath it the more primitive parts of the cerebral cortex—the *rhinencephalon,* or "nose brain"—that in lower animals is concerned with the sense of smell. The cerebral cortical cells also cover over the subcortical structures of the diencephalon and the brain stem.

This folded cloak of cortical nerve cells contains not only the sensory neurons by means of which we receive information about our environment, and the motor neurons through which we act upon such information, but also the interneurons which make up the machinery that plays so important a part in the mental processes that are thought to account for the intellectual superiority of human beings.

Embedded in the strands of subcortical whitish nerve fibers, or white matter, are still other masses of gray matter, the *basal ganglia.* These groups of nerve cells include the caudate, amygdaloid, and lentiform nuclei. These cells send out fibers that connect with other subcortical motor centers and are, in turn, connected with the motor area of the cerebral cortex. Together with the cerebellum, the basal ganglia make up an *extrapyramidal* motor system, which

influences the functioning of the upper motor neurons of the motor cortex, and which—by way of its connections with the reticular core of the brain stem (see below)—affects the activity of the lower motor neurons of the spinal cord.

The reticular formation is a network of neurons located in the core of the brain stem. It is made up of several different kinds of nerve cells scattered diffusely among a tangled mass of fibers running from the top of the spinal cord up through the medulla, pons and midbrain into the thalamus and hypothalamus. Located at a crucial crossroad for nerve fibers passing into and out of the brain, the reticular formation plays a very important part in the integration of both sensory and motor activity.

Such coordination by the reticular formation seems to involve first a sifting of sensory data, and then the picking out of the appropriate motor response to fit the pattern of incoming information. All of the main sensory pathways passing toward the cerebral cortex send collateral branches to the reticular formation, where most of the 100 million sensory signals generated every second are filtered out.

Only the most significant messages are then relayed to the cerebral cortex. Such ascending impulses pass to all parts of the cerebral cortex by way of diffusely spreading polysynaptic nerve chains. Other reticular formation nerve cells send their signals downstream to modify the rate at which the spinal motor neurons fire their impulses out to the muscles. Thus, this neurological "middleman" can help to cope with environmental changes by influencing muscular (and glandular) reactions to the incoming messages which it also helps to monitor.

Central Nervous System Functions

The C.N.S. has several different kinds of functions, which it carries out through the interactions of nerve cells located at all levels. In general, however, all of these varied activities serve the same broad purpose—coordinating the reactions of the individual to a constantly changing external and internal environment. In this respect, humans are not essentially different from lower animals, except that their cerebral cortex with its innumerable interneuronal connections is capable of an enormously increased number and variety of responses to environmental stimuli.

In reviewing some of the main activities of the brain in terms of the operation of certain of its functional systems we shall consider the systems involved in *sensory, motor, mental,* and *emotional* activities separately. However, these systems actually work together in many ways. That is, the various parts of the C.N.S. do not operate independently but as a unit. Thus, although we tend to speak of various drugs as acting at particular central sites, we should be aware that the same drug may cause changes in many different functions through its indirect effects on other parts of the brain. In addition, a drug may act at one dose level to affect only one area of the brain and one main function, while larger doses of the drugs may affect several functions besides the most sensitive one.

Sensory Circuits and Consciousness. Millions of sensory impulses—perhaps 100 million a second—are constantly streaming into the central nervous system from peripheral receptor outposts. Many of these messages reach specialized areas of the cerebral cortex by way of special sense organs in the eyes, ears, nose, and tongue. Other sensations stem from receptors and nerve endings in the skin and internal organs. Some receptors are specialized for reporting touch, pressure, heat and cold, and pain; others—the proprioceptors—inform the brain of changes in the position of the body's parts.

Much of this stream of sensory data makes its way directly to terminals in the sensory, visual and auditory areas of the cerebral cortex. From there, signals are flashed to nearby associative cortical areas where the data is analyzed to determine what messages should be sent to the motor cortex which controls voluntary movements.

However, more primitive parts of the brain also have a role in the handling of sensory messages. These include the thalamus, hypothalamus, and the several parts of the brain stem. Recent neurophysiological research has helped to clarify the role of the brain stem's reticular formation in the sorting and efficient processing of incoming sensations.

Certain studies that have concentrated on the nature of what we call "consciousness" and on the wake-sleep cycles have recently revealed the role of the *reticular activating system* (RAS), the *ascending* portion of the reticular formation, which receives sensory stimuli by way of collateral fibers and then relays selected nerve impulses up to the cerebral cortex from the inner core of the brain stem. It is these signals, rather than those that pass to the sensory cortex by way of more direct pathways from the periphery, that help to keep the cortex awake.

Arousal of the cortex apparently depends upon the spraying of a particular pattern of nerve impulses from the RAS to various cerebral cortical areas. However, the cortex itself also seems to have something to say about its own state of excitability. It feeds a continuous stream of impulses back down to the reticular formation in the brain stem and hypothalamus. These messages can both reduce and increase the activity of the reticular activating system.

The control mechanisms involved in sleep are complex; however, it has been suggested that sleep is controlled neurologically in two ways: (1) A lessened input of external stimuli may deactivate the RAS and thus result in fewer facilitatory impulses passing upstream to stimulate the cerebral cortex. (2) Inhibitory impulses descending from the cerebral cortex can dampen down reticular activity and thus induce sleep.

In any case, it is now known that damage to the brain stem can cause coma of indefinite length. In addition, the central depressant drugs that produce sleep and anesthesia are now believed to affect cerebral cortical functioning not by a direct action on the cortex but by their ability to cut the connections between the tangled axons and dendrites of nerve cells located in the reticular activating system. The RAS then fails to send up to the higher cortical areas the specific patterned spray of signals that is required for maintaining consciousness. As a result, the anesthetized patient feels nothing, even though electroencephalographic evidence indicates that sensory impulses are continuously reaching his cerebral cortex by way of the direct sensory pathways.

Motor Circuits for Muscular Activity. The sensory stimuli that enter the C.N.S. set off responses that are mediated by motor and glandular cells. Muscular movements may be involuntary or purposeful. The simplest reflex contractions can be carried out in response to motor messages sent by the spinal cord alone, but voluntary acts require the planning and command functions of the cerebral cortex. In addition, muscular coordination calls for constant modification of the motor commands from above by the nerve cells of the cerebellum, basal ganglia and reticular motor system.

Two main bundles of motor nerves in the brain influence the activity of the spinal motoneurons that finally send out the messages that make muscles move. One of these fiber tracts—the *pyramidal system*—has its origin in the cells of the motor cortex. Most of its fibers cross over to the opposite side of the spinal cord at a point in the base of the brain stem. The other nerve fiber bundles, which make up the *extrapyramidal system*, help in carrying out the complex automatic adjustments needed for maintaining balance and posture in response to constantly changing environmental situations. The extrapyramidal system also interacts with the upper and lower motoneurons to assure the smooth performance of all voluntary movements.

Damage to the different parts of these motor systems can result in permanent muscular malfunction. Some drugs may temporarily interfere with the nervous control mechanisms for smoothly coordinated movements; other drugs may sometimes help to relieve neuromuscular disability. For example, certain tranquilizer drugs sometimes induce reversible disorders of the extrapyramidal motor system as an undesired side effect; alcohol and other depressants may, of course, cause incoordinated motor activity or ataxia; still other chemicals are capable of controlling disordered motor function. Certain centrally-acting drugs can, for example, relieve the rigidity and tremors of the basal ganglia disorder, Parkinson's disease. Others can reduce the writhing movements of athetosis and other manifestations of cerebral palsy; and the explosive neuronal activity responsible for epileptic seizures can be dampened by drugs that reduce the responsiveness of the cells that lie in the motor circuits.

Nervous Circuits for Intellectual and Emotional Functions. The cerebral cortex is considered the seat of the higher intelligence of humans. Actually, however, no single site for intellectual activity has ever been localized in the cortex. Apparently, the kind of behavior which is considered to be uniquely human depends upon the neural connections between all of the different areas of the cortex and between the cortex and certain subcortical sites. The latter include the hypothalamus and several groups of nerve cell bodies, or nuclei, which make up the subcortical part of the so-called limbic system. These structures, the amygdala, the hippocampus and the fornix, form a closed nerve cell circuit together with the limbic lobe of the primitive "nose brain" cortex.

The more recently developed parts of the cerebral cortex—the neopallium—are connected with these lower centers by fiber tracts that run between the frontal lobes and the underlying subcortical areas. The cortex plays a major role in intellectual function

such as learning, memory, judgment and creative thinking. That is, it receives sensory data, stores it in coded form, and then recombines all these bits of information in countless ways. The hypothalamic and limbic system nuclei seem to play a part in automatically selecting the program of behavior best suited to the particular situation. The two systems act together in translating thought into behavioral responses that are appropriate to the situations which must be dealt with.

These two interconnecting systems sometimes seem to influence one another in ways that are harmful to the individual. For example, under the influence of the frontal lobes of the cortex, which control the experiencing and the expression of emotion, the subcortical areas sometimes seem to shower the visceral organs with messages that call forth psychosomatic symptoms. Conversely, excessive impulses ascending from the areas that control *responses* to emotion seem to play a part in disrupting cortically controlled mental or intellectual function.

Cutting the fiber bundles between the frontal lobes and subcortical areas—as in the psychosurgical operation known as a prefrontal lobotomy—brings about strange changes in the patient's personality and emotional reactions. For example, he does not seem to be disturbed by pain or other previously upsetting stimuli. However, his general lack of emotional reactivity tends to leave him dull and apathetic.

Nonetheless, there are clinical situations in which it seems desirable to break the circuits between cortical and subcortical areas and thus partially disconnect the patient's thought processes from his emotional responses. Various drugs seem capable of affecting the relationship between intellectual and emotional activity temporarily. As with lobotomy, people under the influence of these drugs may be benefited in some ways and hurt in others.

Morphine, for example, may keep a patient from minding pain even though he continues to feel it, perhaps because the drug performs a partial and reversible chemical lobotomy. People who become addicted to opiates often show the same lack of emotional drives that blunts the personality of the lobotomized patient. Similarly, the major phenothiazine tranquilizers which often offer symptomatic relief of mental illness symptoms—perhaps by their effects on the subcortical areas involved in emotional responses—may prove harmful if used only as a substitute for dealing constructively with emotional problems.

GENERAL PHARMACOLOGY OF THE CENTRAL NERVOUS SYSTEM

How and Where Drugs Act

Ideally, it should be possible to demonstrate how drugs act upon the nerve cells of various C.N.S. structures to alter central nervous system functions. However, there is at present no single acceptable basis for adequately explaining precisely how and where drugs generally act to affect the functioning of the C.N.S.

Actually, this is not surprising, since the complicated nerve pathways involved in the control of many functions are still not completely mapped. In fact, the intimate details of the functioning of individual nerve cells are still obscure, as is the neurochemistry of synapses. Thus, we can hardly hope to explain exactly how drugs affect synaptic transmission and such fundamental properties of nerve cells as their excitability and conductivity when these aspects of nervous function are not yet fully understood.

Nonetheless, we do know enough to make some useful generalizations about the nature of drug action on the C.N.S.: First, nervous tissue is characterized by excitability, and drugs may act by altering such neuronal irritability. Further, and somewhat more specifically, the state of excitability of various nerve nuclei at any moment in time is the result of the sum of excitatory and inhibitory stimuli impinging simultaneously upon the nerve cell membranes. Drug molecules can be considered a form of foreign intervention that alters the precarious balance between these facilitatory and inhibitory influences which ordinarily determines the degree of central neuronal excitability.

How do drugs exert the cellular actions that result in changes in central function? Individual drugs no doubt act in many different ways to modify the various functions of individual nerve cells and of the nervous system as a whole. Here, however, we need only say that drugs may affect: (1) the metabolism; (2) the cell membrane potentials of individual neurons, or (3) the manner in which nerve impulses are transmitted at the synapses between two or more neighboring nerve cells.

Metabolic Action. Some drugs may act by affecting the cellular respiratory *enzyme systems* responsible for the chemical reactions from which the nerve cell derives its energy. Since some of that energy is used to run the cell's "sodium pump," the drug could then affect the excitability of the nerve cell membrane in ways that increase or decrease the cell's activity as a receiver or sender of nervous signals. The antiepileptic drug, diphenylhydantoin (Dilantin), for example, is thought by some to reduce the excitability of normal neurons in this way, so that the explosive discharges from groups of disordered nerve cells, or epileptic foci, fail to fire off abnormal activity in the cells of the rest of the brain.

Action on Membrane Potential. Drugs may act directly on the nerve cell membrane itself. The general anesthetics are thought to act, according to one theory, by preventing the changes in brain cell membrane permeability which normally occur at the point at which they are stimulated. The resulting alteration in the normal flow of ions into and out of the nerve cell is then thought to keep the membrane from depolarizing and sending its signal down the axonal fiber. Local anesthetics are believed to act upon peripheral nerve fibers in the same manner.

Action at Synapses. Another way in which centrally acting drugs may produce their effects is through interference with the chemical processes that are involved in the transmission of nerve impulses at synaptic junctions. The exact nature of the chemicals involved in central synaptic transmission is still uncertain. However, it is believed that the drugs that affect excitatory and inhibitory postsynaptic potentials do so in ways that are essentially similar to those of the drugs that act at peripheral junctional sites (Chap. 14). They may, for instance, act by imitating, blocking or otherwise affecting the metabolism of certain chemicals localized in parts of the brain—acetylcholine, norepinephrine, serotonin and gamma-aminobutyric acid, for example. By altering the normal relationships of these and other neurochemicals at presynaptic (axonal) fibers and postsynaptic (dendritic fiber and nerve cell body) sites antipsychotic drugs (Chap. 7) such as reserpine, the phenothiazine tranquilizers and the antidepressant drugs may alter the rate of transmission of nerve impulses through various functional pathways in the C.N.S.

The sensitivity of central synapses to interference by foreign chemicals (i.e., drugs and poisons) is thought to account for the fact that those areas in the brain that contain the most synaptic connections are the ones most susceptible to drug action. Thus, the ascending reticular formation, which is very rich in the number of interconnected nerve cells that it contains, is one of the first areas affected by many central depressant drugs. Very small doses of barbiturates or of general anesthetics such as ether are thus able to block the transmission of impulses from the reticular activating system to the cortex. As a result of their actions on this multisynaptic site, these drugs quickly cause a loss of consciousness and produce sleep and stupor, or narcosis.

On the other hand, drugs that act selectively at central nerve pathways with relatively few synaptic connections do not as readily induce loss of consciousness or general depression. They tend, instead, to interfere with specific functions, such as the emotional reaction to pain or other disturbing stimuli.

For example, the major tranquilizers that are used for treating mental illness symptoms such as restlessness and agitation may act mainly on the closed nerve circuits between the frontal lobes of the cortex and the subcortical nuclei of the nervous system. These contain relatively few linked neurons compared to the more sensitive polysynaptic circuits of the reticular activating system. This may account for the ability of these drugs to reduce excitement without causing excessive sleepiness or loss of consciousness.

CLASSIFICATION OF CENTRALLY ACTING DRUGS

Despite such speculations, we really do not know enough about the intimate actions of drugs on the C.N.S. to categorize them on the basis of the ways in which they act. Even if we could speak with more confidence concerning the exact sites and manner of action of drugs, such a classification would still have relatively little meaning. One reason for this is that drugs rarely act on only one group of central cells, or affect only a single functional nerve circuit system. Certainly, when a drug's dosage is raised, its effects usually tend to spread from the most sensitive central cells to involve many more resistant pathways and often the entire C.N.S.

Nevertheless, it is usually possible to administer drugs in amounts that allow their actions to be kept more or less localized at particular neuronal nuclei. This permits their use in the treatment of conditions marked by specific functional disorders. Thus, centrally acting drugs are commonly classified in terms of the main pharmacological effect that the doctor desires to elicit in the treatment of patients with various nervous disorders or emotional symptoms—for example, sedative, hypnotic, analgesic, anticonvulsant, etc.

More broadly, of course, drugs may first be classified as central *stimulants* and *depressants,* and each of these groups may, in turn, be subdivided on the basis of whether their actions affect the entire C.N.S. in the same way or whether they act differently at various sites. Some drugs seem capable of stimulating specific central neuronal sites and of depressing others, but most of the centrally acting drugs tend either to depress or to excite the entire central nervous system.

General Depressants. In actual practice, the drugs that are capable of depressing all nervous tissue are never deliberately used in doses that would knock out nerve centers at every level of the C.N.S.—the result of which would, of course, be catastrophic. They are, instead, administered in amounts calculated to induce just the degree of functional loss required in the treatment of clinical conditions of specific type. Fortunately, this is relatively easy to do, since drug-induced depression of the C.N.S. follows a general pattern which is more or less predictable.

Generally speaking, these drugs first depress the most recently developed functions of the cerebral cortex, and the most primitive functions of the medullary centers are the last to fail. Thus, the first effects of drugs such as alcohol, ether and the barbiturates are upon the psychosensory and psycho-motor functions of the cerebral cortex. Later, the subcortical and spinal centers that control muscle tone are depressed; finally, the brain stem centers responsible for respiration and other automatically controlled vital functions stop sending out their signals.

Sometimes, certain centrally acting drugs of the general depressant type may seem to be causing stimulation of the C.N.S. Alcohol may, for example, appear to be producing excitement. Actually, however, such seeming stimulation always results from the drug's depressant action on the functioning of nerve cells somewhere in the brain. The depressed nerve cells are located in the inhibitory areas of the brain. As a result, the areas that are released from inhibitory control may send out their excitatory impulses at a more rapid rate. Such "pseudostimulation" accounts for the uninhibited behavior of alcoholic intoxication and for the so-called excitement stage of general anesthesia. Increased activity of the C.N.S. also occurs when depressant drugs are withdrawn abruptly from people who have been abusing these drugs by taking large doses for long periods to the point of becoming physically dependent upon them.

Depending upon the dose employed, the general depressant drugs can bring about every degree of depression from light sedation, through sleep, stupor or narcosis, and, finally, deep coma with loss of all reflex activity. Thus, depending on how they are used clinically, the general depressants are commonly classified as *sedatives, hypnotics,* and *general anesthetics* (see Chaps. 6 and 11). Although many of these drugs can also prevent convulsive seizures, relax skeletal muscles, and relieve pain, they are not classified on the basis of these secondary pharmacological actions. That is, these drugs are not ordinarily referred to as anticonvulsants, muscle relaxants, and analgesics; these terms are reserved for those depressants that produce these effects primarily and in a more selective manner when used in safe clinical doses.

Selective Depressants. Some drugs are capable of altering certain central functions when given in doses that do not affect the functioning of the C.N.S. in general. For example, those that are classified as *anticonvulsants* are capable of reducing epileptic seizure activity when administered in amounts that do not interfere with normal psychomotor or psychosensory function. That is, they are less likely to make the patient excessively drowsy or interfere with his judgment, muscle tone, or finely coordinated movements.

Similarly, the selectively acting *potent analgesics* such as morphine can reduce the patient's reaction to severe pain without rendering him unconscious, and the *major tranquilizers* can calm the emotionally disturbed patient without putting him to sleep. Other more or less specific C.N.S. depressants include the lissive, or skeletal muscle *antispasmodic,* drugs, the *antiparkinsonism* agents, the *antitussives* and *antiemetics* as well as the *analgesic-antipyretic* agents.

Some of the selective depressant drugs seem to stimulate certain central sites even as they depress others. Thus, an opiate pain reliever such as morphine may stimulate the vomiting center and the spinal cord, and some phenothiazine-type tranquilizers cause increased activity in extrapyramidal motor systems. Similarly, some of these drugs—the salicylate analgesic-antipyretics, for instance—may act peripherally as well as through a combination of central depressant and stimulating actions. The antiparkinsonism drugs often exert potent peripheral effects upon various organs innervated by cholinergic nerves.

Central Nervous System Stimulants. Certain drugs act to increase the general excitability of the central nervous system. Although they are sometimes classified on the basis of the central sites that seem most susceptible to their stimulating action, the effects of most of these drugs tend to spread to all levels of the C.N.S. when the dose is increased. For example, a so-called brain stem stimulant, such as pentylenetetrazol, may stimulate not only brain stem respiratory control mechanisms but also motor control areas throughout the C.N.S., including spinal motor centers.

Some central stimulants are somewhat more specific than others. Caffeine and the amphetamines affect mainly certain subcortical areas to produce increased cortical activity of the psychomotor type. Their effects do not spread to the spinal cord in humans, and thus typically spinal convulsive seizures do not occur even with massive overdoses. On the other hand, because the pharmacological actions of caffeine and the amphetamines are not limited to the C.N.S., these drugs are capable of causing frequent peripheral side effects.

Most stimulants generally act in any of several ways to increase central excitability through their effects at excitatory synapses; however, some convulsant drugs are now known to act by lessening the effectiveness of central *inhibitory* influences. Strychnine, for example, stimulates increased activity of spinal centers by blocking the effects of the inhibitory neurohormones which ordinarily tend to counteract many of the excitatory stimuli that are simultaneously reaching certain central nerve cells.

Central nervous system stimulants do not ordinarily produce direct depression of the C.N.S., although, theoretically, they could do so by stimulating inhibitory areas without at the same time affecting excitatory sites equally. In addition, excessive drug-induced activity is often followed by a period of relative inexcitability of the C.N.S. This is particularly apparent after the occurrence of drug-induced convulsions, which are often followed by a period of postictal depression.

As we have seen, the central nervous system is of awesome complexity, and the student who is aware of this will develop a healthy respect for the drugs that are capable of interfering with neuronal function. Fortunately, despite their manifold and seemingly mystifying mechanisms of action, these drugs can be used with safety and with great benefit to suffering patients.

In the following chapters of this section, we shall learn how these drugs are used in order to gain their desirable effects and what precautions are employed to avoid accidental overdosage leading to acute toxicity. The need to prevent the abuse of many of these centrally acting drugs by addiction-prone people will also be emphasized.

REVIEW QUESTIONS

1. (a) What is meant by the terms: axon; dendrite; synapse?

(b) What is meant by the terms: nerve; afferent fiber; efferent fiber; interneuron?

2. (a) What is meant by the terms: depolarization; repolarization; refractory period; nerve action potential?

(b) By what means may impulses be transmitted from one nerve cell to another at synapses?

3. (a) What is meant by the terms: excitatory fiber; inhibitory fiber; summation of excitatory and inhibitory impulses?

(b) How may a so-called depressant drug cause increased activity of some central nerve cells; how may a stimulant drug reduce the over-all activity of other C.N.S. nerve cells?

4. (a) What function is carried out by the cerebellum through its connections with certain brain stem and cerebral structures?

(b) What are the general functions of the diencephalic structures, the thalamus and hypothalamus?

5. (a) What are some functions of the cerebral cortex?

(b) What parts of the brain comprise an extrapyramidal motor system?

6. (a) How, in general, do cells located in the core of the reticular formation affect the transmission of sensory stimuli?

(b) How may the reticular formation affect motor response to incoming sensory data?

7. (a) What areas of the cerebral cortex receive stimuli by way of direct pathways from the periphery?

(b) What is the role of the reticular activating system in maintaining consciousness and in sleep?

8. (a) Of what three general types are the motor nerve cells involved in the control of coordinated muscular movements?

(b) What are some examples of drugs that affect the function of motor neuron circuits?

9. (a) How may certain cortical areas (frontal lobes, etc.) and subcortical areas (limbic system and hypothalamus) influence one another and thus affect intellectual and emotional activity?

(b) What are some examples of drugs that may affect these neuronal circuits?

10. (a) How, in general, may drugs act to affect the excitability of nerve cell nuclei within the C.N.S.?

(b) In what three ways may drugs act more specifically to affect the functioning of C.N.S. neurons?

(c) List some examples of centrally acting drugs that may act in each of these ways.

11. (a) Which central site is thought to be most sensitive to drugs that cause rapid loss of consciousness?

(b) How may various drugs that depress certain specific central functions without as readily causing unconsciousness differ in the type of neuronal pathways that they primarily affect?

12. (a) Broadly, of what two types are the effects drugs may have on the functioning of the central nervous system?

(b) What are some clinically important pharmacological effects by which certain centrally acting drugs are classified?

13. (a) What pattern of depressant action is characteristic of the general depressants of the C.N.S.? (I.e., What is the general order of neurological depression of the various central sites of action of these drugs?)

(b) What are the successive pharmacological effects of the several states of increasingly deep depression of the C.N.S. induced by raising the dosage of general depressant drugs?

(c) Under what circumstances may central depressant drugs appear to be causing increased stimulation of the C.N.S.?

14. (a) List several classes of central depressant drugs that act selectively to bring about particular effects without producing the pattern typical of general depression.

(b) Give an example of a C.N.S. stimulant capable of affecting functions of all levels of the C.N.S. and of a stimulant with more specific and limited activity.

(c) Give an example of a convulsant drug which may increase C.N.S. activity by reducing the activity of neurons that have an inhibitory function.

The Barbiturates and Other Sedative-Hypnotic Drugs

DRUG-INDUCED SEDATION AND HYPNOSIS

Sedatives are drugs that produce mild drowsiness while reducing restlessness. Given during the day, small doses of sedative drugs tend to calm the tense, excitable patient without—ideally, at least—interfering with his ability to function normally. In fact, the lightly sedated patient may think more clearly and perform his normal activities more efficiently, when relieved of bothersome bodily symptoms.

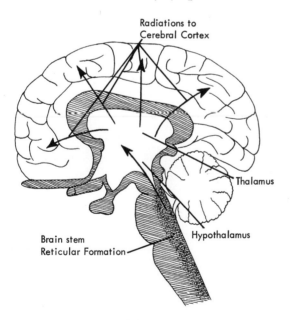

FIG. 6-1. The reticular activating system. Diffuse impulses from this area excite cerebral cortical activity. Depression of impulse transmission in this polysynaptic system reduces alertness and wakefulness.

Hypnotics or *somnifacients* are drugs that make it easier for the patient to fall asleep and stay asleep. Given at bedtime, in somewhat larger doses, the same drugs that serve as daytime sedatives induce a state similar to natural sleep. In still larger doses, these central depressants may make the patient stuporous, and massive amounts may cause coma and death due to respiratory and circulatory failure.

The drugs classified as sedative-hypnotics have a relatively selective action on the reticular formation in the brain stem (Chap. 5). Small doses deactivate this area which is so important in maintaining consciousness and wakefulness. By blocking some of the nerve impulses that normally ascend to the cerebral cortex by way of the reticular activating system, these drugs reduce excessive psychic activity and promote sleep. The effects of larger doses can, of course, spread to depress other parts of the nervous system including the spinal cord and the vital centers of the medulla oblongata.

THE BARBITURATES

Many chemically unrelated substances share the ability to produce the relatively mild degree of central depression needed for sedation and hypnosis. Some drugs still in use today—chloral hydrate and the bromides, for example—were introduced in the latter half of the last century; others such as glutethimide (Doriden) and methyprylon (Noludar) have come into use relatively recently. However, by far the most important sedative-hypnotics are the barbiturates, a class of compounds that first became available shortly before World War I.

Hundreds of these substances have been synthesized since barbital (Veronal) and phenobarbital (Luminal), the first of the series, were shown to be clinically useful. However, only a couple of dozen derivatives are in common use today, and the doctor can get good results in most cases by knowing how to use only three or four of these versatile drugs judiciously.

The doctor who has learned to pick the best barbiturate for a particular purpose and to employ it properly can produce any desired degree of depression from mild sedation to deep anesthesia. For although all the barbiturates possess essentially similar pharmacological effects, some are better suited than others for achieving different clinical goals. By selecting the best drug for producing a desired effect and by giving it in the right dose and by the best route of administration, doctors can use these drugs in the management of a wide variety of clinical conditions besides those requiring sedation and sleep.

Some of the barbiturates are, for example, better than others as anticonvulsants. Thus, phenobarbital is the preferred barbiturate for preventing grand mal epileptic seizures and thiopental (Pentothal) is considered best when a drug is needed to combat convulsions once they have begun. Similarly, in psychiatry, phenobarbital is an effective sedative for the long-term treatment of tension states and chronic psychosomatic conditions, and thiopental is a useful adjunctive agent for facilitating psychiatric interviews.

The various barbiturates differ mainly in the speed with which the effects come on and in the duration of action. How fast and how long a particular barbiturate acts depends, in turn, on how the body handles it after it has been administered and absorbed into the systemic circulation. For, although all are absorbed into the blood stream at about the same rate, the various barbiturates differ in their rates of entry into the nervous system and in the speed with which they leave the brain and the body.

Drugs of rapid onset, such as thiopental and secobarbital (Seconal), pass the blood-brain barrier more readily than do the relatively slow-acting agents, barbital and phenobarbital, which, for reasons previously discussed (Chap. 2), penetrate biological membranes more slowly.

The slow-onset agents have a longer duration of action, because they are excreted quite slowly, and largely unchanged, by way of the kidneys. On the other hand, the effects of the quick-acting barbiturates tend to wear off rather rapidly, because these compounds soon leave the brain and are redistributed to other body tissues including the liver, where they are detoxified. (Obviously, then, barbital and phenobarbital may be undesirable for patients with renal disease, and the thiopental and secobarbital types may be dangerous for people with severe hepatic disorders.)

Pharmacological Actions and Clinical Indications (See Table 6-3)

Anxiety and Insomnia

Few of us are always entirely free of emotional tension, nor would it be desirable if we were. Psychiatrists tell us that it is natural to get disturbed when we feel threatened. Such fears serve a useful purpose when they force us to take constructive action to correct a situation that is upsetting us. Sometimes, however, people become anxious about things that need no correcting and, in fact, without really knowing what it is that is bothering them.

In either case, whether triggered by actual events and situations or set off by internal emotional conflicts, anxiety produces essentially the same changes in physiological function. These changes may take the form of signs and symptoms such as cardiac palpitations, a rise in blood pressure, difficulty in breathing, or epigastric distress and diarrhea. People in a state of anxiety may feel dull, fatigued, and sleepy, or they may suffer from a feeling of inner tremulousness and tension, restlessness, and insomnia.

Such symptoms may range from mild to severe, and the person may be partially aware of the underlying emotional basis or entirely unconscious of it. Often, the doctor may try to determine the sources of the patient's emotional tension. However, before the doctor can begin to uncover the causes of underlying anxiety and help the patient to overcome his difficulties, he must first do what he can to make the patient more comfortable. That is, before the patient can be expected to think clearly about the nature of his emotional problems and begin to deal with them effectively, the physical manifestations of his anxiety, including sleeplessness, which is often an especially disturbing symptom, must be alleviated. The barbiturates are among the most effective agents for calming the patient and for counteracting symptoms such as insomnia.

The sedative action of the barbiturates can usually be brought about by relatively small doses of phenobarbital,* pentobarbital * (Nembutal), amobarbital * (Amytal), or butabarbital (Butisol). These and certain other barbiturates may thus be used to provide symptomatic relief in three kinds of clinical situations:

1. For patients experiencing anxiety symptoms as a reaction to temporary situational stress. Despite a recent trend toward the prescribing of the minor tranquilizers discussed in Chapter 7, which are more expensive, many doctors still feel that the barbiturates are unsurpassed for this purpose.

2. As an adjunct to psychotherapy in neuroses. Patients often find it easier to communicate their thoughts to the therapist when physical and mental

---

* See also Drug Digests.

discomforts arising from nervous tension are allayed by barbiturate sedation.

3. To reduce anxiety when it is thought to play an important part in causing symptoms of a physical disorder, or to reduce the patient's psychological distress over various symptoms of such organic or functional difficulties.

Among these so-called psychosomatic and somatopsychic conditions in which anxiety plays a role, either as cause or as effect, are the following:

Gastrointestinal disturbances marked by nausea, vomiting, painful smooth muscle spasm and diarrhea. Small sedative doses of barbiturates have little direct relaxing effects on visceral smooth muscles, nor do they significantly reduce the excitability of the central vomiting mechanism. However, the calmative action of the barbiturates has proved very desirable in many patients with peptic ulcer, pylorospasm, colitis or motion sickness, especially when the barbiturates are combined with drugs which act directly to reduce gastrointestinal hypermotility and hypersecretion.

Cardiovascular and other conditions marked by tachycardia, hypertension, or precordial pain and palpitations. For example, small doses of barbiturates are commonly prescribed as adjuncts to treatment with other drugs which act more specifically to reduce the heart rate and blood pressure or to dilate coronary and other blood vessels in patients with angina pectoris, hypertension, or hyperthyroidism.

Allergic disorders such as dermatoses and bronchial asthma. Here, barbiturate-induced sedation may reduce the patient's reaction to the stressful life situations that often set off attacks of dyspnea or neurodermatitis, and the drugs may also lessen the distress produced by such breathing difficulties or by persistent pruritus.

Menstrual and Menopausal Disturbances. Dysmenorrhea spasm and pain, for example, may prove less distressing when barbiturates are added to a regimen of analgesics and smooth muscle relaxants. The nervous and cardiovascular symptoms of premenstrual tension and of the menopause may also be benefited by combining barbiturate sedation with hormone therapy and other agents.

The hypnotic action of the barbiturates is widely employed in the management of insomnia. For this purpose the drugs are prescribed in doses three or four times those used for sedation. By reducing the apprehension of hospitalized patients or by lessening the unresolved emotional tensions of the patient who suffers from chronic insomnia, these drugs often produce restful sleep.

It should be noted, however, that these and other hypnotics are often misused by both patients and medical personnel. Since patients may become habituated to barbiturates quite readily, these drugs are best prescribed for brief periods only, and sleeping pills should not be passed out as part of the evening routine to suit the convenience of the hospital staff. Instead, a little time spent in talking to the patient reassuringly may minimize the need for soporific drugs.

Although hypnotic drugs are often required for hospitalized patients unable to sleep because of strange surroundings, worry over anticipated surgery, or pain and discomfort, attention should also be paid to reducing undesirable environmental factors. Thus, the nurse should see to it that the patient's room is well ventilated and at optimal temperature. His bedclothing should be adjusted so that it is neither too tight nor too loose, and not too light or too heavy. Often a warm drink or a bedtime snack adds to the patient's comfort in ways that help the hypnotic effect of the barbiturates to come on more readily.

Factors Affecting Choice of Hypnotic. The nurse, by noting and reporting the patient's sleep pattern, may be able to help the doctor decide which barbiturate is the best choice for him. Thus, if a patient has trouble in falling asleep but rests well afterwards, a single dose of a rapid-acting barbiturate of short to moderate duration such as secobarbital or pentobarbital may be best for him. When the patient is one who wakes too early, a drug from one of the intermediate (e.g., amobarbital) or long-acting (e.g., phenobarbital) groups may be most desirable.

Patients who have difficulty both in falling asleep and in staying asleep may be managed in various ways. The doctor may, for example, prescribe Tuinal, which is a combination of short-acting secobarbital with the intermediate-duration drug, amobarbital, or he may make use of any of several other preparations containing combinations of two or more barbiturates. On the other hand, he may give the patient a double dose of pentobarbital to produce deeper and more prolonged sleep, or he may prescribe a "repeat action" product containing butabarbital, for example, in order to give the patient the benefit of a second, delayed-action, dose when the effects of the first portion are wearing off.

Sometimes, for a hospitalized patient, the doctor leaves a "p.r.n." order permitting the hypnotic drug to be repeated if the patient seems to need further medication. Deciding whether to administer a second dose or to withhold additional somnifacient therapy requires mature nursing judgment.

It is important to ask yourself *why* the patient is unable to sleep in spite of the earlier administration of a hypnotic dose of the barbiturate. If pain is preventing him from falling asleep, the physician should be notified. Barbiturates, by themselves, are not very effective pain-relievers and may even make the patient more restless in the presence of pain. The doctor may order a barbiturate-analgesic combination, because these sedatives often add to the effectiveness of aspirin, codeine, and similar drugs. Of course, if the doctor has permitted the choice of either type of drug for a postoperative patient during the night, it is preferable to administer the analgesic rather than repeat the hypnotic barbiturate in such circumstances.

Administration of Hypnotics. There are times when the nurse must decide whether a dose ordered for administration at a particular time should actually be administered at all. Patients sometimes show symptoms of overdosage at the time their next dose is due. In such cases, the nurse should consult the doctor rather than follow his written order. Of course, if the patient is asleep when it is time for his next dose of the hypnotic, the ordered dose need not be administered. (The patient recalls with something less than affection and respect the nurse who—as in the classic story—wakes him to administer a sleeping pill!)

It is also important to remember that patients who have received sedation are especially vulnerable to injury. Special efforts must be made to protect these patients, especially when they are elderly, debilitated, or unused to the effects of barbiturates. Patients who tend to be unsteady on their feet are particularly so after administration of barbiturates. Thus, they should be reminded to put on their call light, if they want to get up to go to the bathroom during the night, so that they can be assisted.

Some patients are groggy in the morning, from the "hangover" effects of long-acting barbiturates administered the night before. The same is often true of those who required a second short- or intermediate-acting barbiturate during the night. Such second doses may be avoided and subsequent side effects reduced, if the nurse finds out *why* the patient is wakeful and uses measures other than drugs to help him get back to sleep.

Barbiturates are often ordered preoperatively, both the night before the operation and in the morning an hour or so before anesthesia and surgery are scheduled. Such sedation is intended to bring the patient to surgery well rested and with reflex nervous excitability reduced, so that anesthesia will be induced more smoothly. The nurse should be sure that such barbiturates are given on time. It is important, however, to remember that preoperative barbiturates are only one way to help calm the patient prior to surgery. Sedative drugs should not be relied upon to the exclusion of other measures (Chap. 11).

Other Actions and Uses. The anticonvulsant actions of the barbiturates are discussed in Chapter 8. The use of the ultra-short-acting agents of this class for basal anesthesia is taken up in Chapter 11, together with a description of how barbiturates of this and other types have been employed for facilitating psychiatric interviewing.

Side Effects and Contraindications

Contrary to popular belief, the barbiturates are relatively safe drugs. When administered in therapeutic doses on a doctor's order, compounds of this class do not cause many side effects in most patients. Most patients are not likely to acquire tolerance, become habituated or addicted, or suffer severe toxic effects in such circumstances.

It is true, however, that patients of some types may be prone to react poorly to barbiturates. The nurse should try to learn whether her patient has ever had a hypersensitivity reaction to these drugs. She should also be aware of factors in the personality or physical condition of a patient that might make him respond adversely to administration of barbiturates.

Some patients, especially elderly people, tend to become excited, instead of calmed, when they are given sleep-producing doses of certain barbiturates at night. This paradoxical excitement seems most likely to occur with the short-acting compounds, such as secobarbital. Patients with arteriosclerotic brain damage, who often become confused and disoriented in the dark, are the most likely victims of this idiosyncratic reaction. However, other patients may also become restless and even delirious, especially if they are in pain or feverish.

The nurse should always keep a close watch on the patient who has become confused by barbiturates. Side rails may be put up to keep him from being injured, but cuffs or other restraints should not be applied at the first sign of excitement because this may make the patient even more restless. Instead, the nurse often can calm the patient and help him orient himself by putting on the bedside light and talking to him. Such talk should, of course, consist only of simple, concrete statements that are made repeatedly and quietly, until the confused patient is calm and relaxed.

Sometimes, patients treated with a long-acting barbiturate such as phenobarbital may waken feeling dazed, dizzy and lethargic. Shorter-acting drugs may also leave the patient drowsy and with a headache, when they have to be given repeatedly during a night of interrupted sleep. Such a "hangover" effect may make it dangerous for a patient to drive or carry out any complex task requiring judgment and motor coordination. However, hospitalized patients are not usually harmed by some residual sedation from a long-acting barbiturate.

The barbiturates are relatively free of true toxic reactions involving injury to various of the vital organs. But, although these drugs do not themselves damage the liver, kidneys, or bone marrow, their use may be contraindicated in patients already suffering from diseases which impair the function of these organs. Thus, people with renal disease may not be able to take phenobarbital or barbital, drugs that are eliminated by the kidneys. Other barbiturates, which depend upon liver enzyme systems for their detoxication, may be contraindicated in patients with severe hepatic disease.

Allergic skin reactions are relatively rare, and a few patients may complain of persistent muscle or joint pains after treatment with barbiturates. Patients who prove truly sensitive to barbiturates may have to be treated with one of the older or new non-barbiturate sedative-hypnotics discussed on pages 103–106.

Chronic Toxicity or Addiction

The main problem with the barbiturates is that some of the people most in need of their calming effects are also the very ones who are most likely to abuse the drugs and become habituated and addicted to them. Many patients—epileptics, for example—often take small doses of barbiturates for years without running into difficulty of any kind; but some emotionally unstable individuals may get into trouble if these drugs are carelessly prescribed or administered. Also, mentally depressed patients with chronic insomnia may sometimes hoard sleeping pills and take a massive overdose for suicidal purposes.

The barbiturates are classed as habit-forming drugs. However, this in itself need not make them harmful, since—as we have seen (Chap. 3)—mere habituation need not be dangerous and people can become habituated to many substances without suffering any severe psychic or physical effects or feeling any compulsion to keep raising the dose to dangerous levels.

On the other hand, some individuals habitually take drugs in excessive amounts as a means of escaping from personal problems. These are the people who tend to develop a true barbiturate addiction. According to some authorities, physical dependence upon barbiturates is even more dangerous than addiction to the opiate derivatives. Daily ingestion of large doses of barbiturates does not cause the same sort of dependence pattern found with the narcotic analgesics, but it may lead to a greater degree of mental and physical deterioration.

The drugs most commonly abused are the short-acting barbiturates secobarbital and pentobarbital. These agents, and sometimes amobarbital, are taken in amounts several times the usual hypnotic dose. This does not usually put the barbiturate abuser to sleep but tends to produce a state of euphoria, or pseudostimulation, similar to the early effects of alcohol. Barbiturates and alcohol are commonly taken together to enhance these effects; other users alternate barbiturates with amphetamines or other stimulants that counteract the drug-induced depression.

Like the alcoholic, the barbiturate addict who loses control may hurt himself and others by causing an automobile accident or by setting a fire while smoking in bed. Although the barbiturate abuser may burn himself or get injured in an accident or a brawl, he usually eats better than the alcoholic, and, therefore, he is less likely to suffer nervous system damage of nutritional origin. However, the effects of drug-induced nervous damage may show up as coarse tremors and abnormal reflex responses. The presence of nystagmus may also mimic the neurological picture in alcoholism, or suggest the presence of cerebellar and other nervous diseases.

When the barbiturate abuser who has been taking large daily doses for several months is suddenly deprived of the drug, he may suffer a severe abstinence syndrome. This differs from the autonomic imbalance typical of the opiate withdrawal pattern; it is characterized instead by motor and psychic excitement. Without the drug, the addict becomes very nervous and increasingly restless. When he tries to sleep, he may have bad dreams or hallucinations. Prolonged sleeplessness often leads to delirium and sometimes to a fully developed psychotic episode. Muscle tremors and contractions may occur and may be the prelude to severe, sometimes fatal, grand mal convulsions.

Obviously, the barbiturates should be withdrawn very slowly in such patients. They should be prescribed only with great caution for patients diagnosed as severely psychoneurotic and others with a history of drug abuse. Narcotic addicts sometimes take barbiturates when opiates are unavailable or even simultaneously with opiates. Alcoholics, given barbiturates for insomnia and nervousness, tend to become dependent on them.

Acute Poisoning

Barbiturate overdosage ranks as the leading cause of drug-induced deaths. It is the publicity given to "sleeping pill" suicides of people prominent in the entertainment world, political life, and business that has aroused public distrust and fear of these drugs.

Sleep-producing doses taken on a doctor's order are ordinarily harmless, but only five to ten times this hypnotic dose can cause deep depression. Between ten and twenty times the therapeutic amount may produce stupor, coma, and death. Thus, a mentally depressed patient who deliberately ingests a dozen or more sleeping capsules is going to need prompt and vigorous treatment if his life is to be saved. This is why doctors use great caution in prescribing barbiturates for patients who seem depressed and possibly suicidal.

Accidental overdosage occurs often in children attracted to brightly colored capsules kept in a bedside table or other readily accessible place. Also, adults may take too many capsules unintentionally, especially if they have been drinking.

It is said that sometimes an insomniac becomes confused from the effects of the first couple of capsules and, in his dazed and disoriented condition, downs the contents of an entire bottle without realizing what he is doing. Whether such "twilight zone automatism" is a common factor in barbiturate poisoning has been disputed. However, the nurse should advise the patient never to keep a sleeping capsule container by his bedside; nor should a person take barbiturates while under the influence of alcohol.

Signs and symptoms of overdosage may be quite varied. Some patients may seem excited, instead of depressed, when first seen. Then, as in alcohol intoxication, they may lapse into stupor and coma. The chief danger, especially with large amounts of the quick-acting barbiturates, is that circulatory collapse or respiratory failure may occur. The slower-acting barbiturates cause deep, prolonged depression, during which the patient may develop hypostatic pneumonia.

Treatment in either case usually requires supportive medical and nursing care to prevent early death or the occurrence of late complications. Most important is the maintenance of an unobstructed airway. To achieve this, the patient is turned on his side and his tongue is kept from slipping back into his throat. Only then is it certain that oxygen is actually getting into the patient's lungs when it is given by mask or nasal catheter. Suctioning of mucus and foreign materials from the respiratory tract is necessary in order to prevent aspiration pneumonia in the comatose patient. (See pp. 108 to 109 for further details of nursing care.)

Analeptic drugs (Chap. 13) are sometimes used to help rouse the patient and to stimulate the depressed medullary centers. These drugs—pentylenetetrazol (Metrazol), picrotoxin, nikethamide (Coramine), bemegride (Megimide) etc.—have recently been condemned as dangerous, but they may sometimes make the difference between life and death when used judiciously.

Pentylenetetrazol (Metrazol) is sometimes given by vein to help determine the depth of depression. If a single injection brings about even a temporary arousal or return of reflexes, the patient's prognosis is good. No further stimulants need be administered, and the patient may be managed by supportive measures alone.

On the other hand, should the patient fail to respond to this "orientation dose" of pentylenetetrazol, more intensive analeptic treatment may be desirable. Sometimes patients begin to breathe spontaneously only after several successive doses of these drugs. Administration of these dangerous convulsant poisons should never, in any case, be a substitute for artificial respiration and other measures for supporting vital functions and preventing infection or other late complications.

Inasmuch as severe barbiturate poisoning resembles anesthesia in many ways, the drugs and techniques employed by nurse anesthetists and recovery room nurses are also used in the management of overdosage by these and other depressant drugs (see Summary, p. 108). In addition, the nurse may need to apply psychotherapeutic measures to support the patient who has swallowed these drugs in a suicide attempt.

The nurse should develop a plan of nursing care that takes into account the fact that the patient may remain emotionally disturbed after the failure of his suicide attempt. The patient requires emotional support as he faces the need to attack constructively the problems that had led him to take an overdose of barbiturates. The nurse should note the patient's attitudes and behavior, in order to be able to help give his physician or psychiatrist a clearer picture of his true emotional states so that further suicide attempts may be prevented.

Administration

Barbituric acid, the parent compound of this class, does not itself cause C.N.S. depression. However, the barbiturates prepared by chemically substituting various groups of atoms at certain positions in the basic molecule all possess the pharmacological actions previously described.

The barbiturates prepared this way are weakly acidic and poorly soluble, until combined with alkalies to form soluble salts. Remember that only the sodium salts made in this manner may be used for injection. For instance, only phenobarbital *sodium* is suitable for parenteral use: never try to dissolve and inject phenobarbital. Both types of products may be given by mouth, however.

The oral route of administration is preferred for producing sedation and hypnosis. Parenteral routes are employed usually only when the patient cannot take the drug by mouth or when rapid, dependable action is required—for example, in combating successive convulsive seizures.

The dangerous intravenous route is usually reserved for the ultra-short-acting agents when they are employed as basal anesthetics. Such injections should be performed preferably by an anesthesiologist or other physician with special experience. Equipment for maintaining respiration and for resuscitating the patient in case of accidental overdosage should be readily available.

The most important barbiturates in current use are classified in Table 6-1 (on p. 104), in accordance with the duration of sleep usually produced by oral administration of hypnotic doses.

NONBARBITURATE SEDATIVE-HYPNOTICS

Many drugs besides the barbiturates have the ability to produce sedation and sleep. Some, such as chloral hydrate, paraldehyde and the bromides, are very old drugs which have been largely replaced by the easier-

TABLE 6-1

BARBITURATES

Nonproprietary Chemical Name	Trade Name	Duration of Action *	Usual Dosage Range and Administration
Allylbarbituric acid		Short	200–800 mg. orally
Amobarbital U.S.P.	Amytal	Intermediate	100–300 mg. orally
Aprobarbital N.F.	Alurate	Intermediate	60–130 mg. orally
Barbital		Long	300 mg. orally
Sodium Butabarbital N.F.	Butisol	Intermediate	30–200 mg. orally
Butethal	Neonal	Intermediate	100–300 mg. orally
Butallylonal		Intermediate	200 mg. orally
Calcium Cyclobarbital N.F.	Phanodorn	Short	100–300 mg. orally
Diallylbarbituric acid	Dial	Intermediate	100–300 mg. orally
Heptabarbital	Medomin	Short	200–400 mg. orally
Hexethal	Ortal	Short	200–400 mg. orally
Sodium Hexobarbital N.F.	Evipal	Ultra-short	2–4 ml. of a 10% solution intravenously for anesthesia
Hexobarbital	Sombulex	Short	250–500 mg. orally
Mephobarbital N.F.	Mebaral	Long	30–100 mg. orally
Metharbital N.F.	Gemonil	Long	50–100 mg. orally
Methitural Sodium	Neraval	Ultra-short	Intravenously as a 5–10% solution for anesthesia
Sodium Methohexital N.F.	Brevital	Ultra-short	7–10 ml. of a 1% solution intravenously
Sodium Pentobarbital U.S.P.	Nembutal	Short	50–300 mg. orally
Phenobarbital U.S.P.	Luminal	Long	30–100 mg. orally
Probarbital Sodium	Ipral	Intermediate	50–500 mg. orally
Propallylonal		Intermediate	100–300 mg. orally
Sodium Secobarbital U.S.P.	Seconal	Short	50–200 mg. orally
Talbutal	Lotusate	Intermediate	30–120 mg. orally
Thialbarbitone Sodium		Ultra-short	Intravenously as required for anesthesia
Sodium Thiamylal N.F.	Surital	Ultra-short	3–6 ml. of a 2.5% solution intravenously
Sodium Thiopental U.S.P.	Pentothal	Ultra-short	2–3 ml. of a 2.5% solution intravenously
Vinbarbital Sodium	Delvinal	Intermediate	30–200 mg. orally

* *Duration:* Ultra-short—minutes
     Short—about 4 hours
     Intermediate—about 4 to 8 hours
     Long—about 6 to 10 hours

to-administer barbiturates. Others (See Table 6-2) are agents introduced rather recently with the hope that they would in turn replace the barbiturates.

Certain advantages are usually claimed for the newer non-barbiturate depressants. Actually, however, there is little proof that they are safer or otherwise superior to the barbiturates. In fact, most of them seem weaker and generally less dependable than the short-acting barbiturates, which they were designed to supersede.

Toxicity. These drugs were claimed, for example, to be safer than the barbiturates; yet all are capable of causing coma and death when taken in excess. Glutethimide * (Doriden) overdosage—accidental or deliberate—has become a rather frequent cause of fatal respiratory depression, as have difficulties following abuse of methyprylon (Noludar) and ethchlorvynol (Placidyl).

* See Drug Digest.

Addiction Liability. It was suggested at first that the new sedatives were not habit forming or addicting. However, drug abusers have used ethinamate * (Valmid), glutethimide, and other agents of this type to attain euphoria. Large daily doses of ethchlorvynol and other of these drugs have led to dependence similar to that which occurs with barbiturates. Sudden withdrawal has resulted in psychoses and grand mal convulsions of the same kinds seen when barbiturates are withdrawn too quickly from individuals who have been taking large amounts for months.

Other Claimed Advantages. It is also sometimes said that, because these drugs are detoxified relatively rapidly, residual sedation is rare. However, their short duration of action sometimes makes several doses necessary if the patient wakes repeatedly during the night. In such cases, "hangover" is as common as when the short-acting barbiturates are given in the same way.

The new drugs are no less likely than the barbiturates to cause excitement in elderly patients, those in pain, or emotionally upset people who react abnormally to light sedation. These drugs are relatively safe for patients with liver and kidney disease—and the same may also be said for the short-acting barbiturates when only small oral doses are administered for sedation and hypnosis.

* See Drug Digests.

In general, the newer sedative-hypnotics are preferred only for people who are allergic to barbiturates or have some idiosyncrasy that makes their administration dangerous.

The concern caused by reports of addiction to barbiturates and of fatal poisonings caused by them has led to a revival of interest in the older drugs. Chloral hydrate * and paraldehyde,* for example, are relatively safe, effective, and cheap sedative-hypnotics. The disagreeable taste and odor of these liquids can be disguised in various ways, and their pungency may even be an advantage, since it tends to discourage habituation.

Recently, chloral has become available in the form of several chemical complexes which are more convenient to take than the parent compound. Chloral betaine (Beta-Chlor), chlorhexadol (Lora) and petrichloral (Periclor) are examples of derivatives that are devoid of odor and aftertaste and less likely than chloral itself to cause stomach upset.

Proprietaries, Non-prescription. Bromides, scopolamine (hyoscine), and some antihistaminic compounds with sedative properties, are employed mainly in proprietary drug products. Combinations of scopolamine and centrally depressant antihistamines are promoted for "safe sleep." Actually, these products touted on radio and television commercials as containing "no barbiturates" are no safer than therapeutic doses of

TABLE 6-2
NON-BARBITURATE SEDATIVE-HYPNOTICS

NONPROPRIETARY OR CHEMICAL NAME	TRADE NAME OR SYNONYM	USUAL DOSAGE BY ORAL ADMINISTRATION
Acetylcarbromal	Abasin; Carbased; Sedamyl	260–600 mg.
Bromide Salts	In numerous products	300–1000 mg.
Bromisovalum	Bromural	300–900 mg.
Carbromal	Adalin; Uradal, etc.	300–900 mg.
Chloral betaine	Beta-Chlor	250–1000 mg.
Chloral hydrate U.S.P.	Noctec; Somnos, etc.	500–1000 mg.
Chlorhexadol	Lora	800–1600 mg.
Chlorobutanol U.S.P.	Chloretone	300–1000 mg.
Dichloralantipyrine	Sominat	600–1200 mg.
Ethchlorvynol N.F.	Placidyl	200–500 mg.
Ethinamate N.F.	Valmid	500–1000 mg.
Glutethimide N.F.	Doriden	250–500 mg.
Methapyrilene HCl	Lullamin, etc.	25–100 mg.
Methyprylon N.F.	Noludar	50–400 mg.
Methylparafynol	Dormison	250–500 mg.
Paraldehyde U.S.P.	Paral, etc.	8–15 ml.
Petrichloral	Periclor	300–600 mg.
Scopolamine HBr U.S.P.	Hyoscine	0.5–0.6 mg.

the latter and may in fact be more dangerous. Certainly, a patient who is taking a therapeutic dose of a barbiturate on a doctor's order is better off than someone who buys and uses a medicine without a prescription, merely on a radio announcer's recommendation. It is certainly preferable for the patient to bring his symptoms to the attention of a physician for evaluation and to follow the physician's recommendations rather than those of an advertising "pitchman."

The non-prescription products are weaker than the standard sedative-hypnotics, and it would require overdosage with a larger number of tablets to depress a person deeply. Otherwise, these mild depressants share the capacity of the other hypnotics for causing occasional untoward reactions. In addition, overdoses of scopolamine may produce atropinelike side effects of a kind especially undesirable in some patients (see Chap. 17).

The bromides do not work well when given as a single dose to produce sleep or sedation. They do dull the mind and dampen emotional reactions when continued administration during long-term therapy allows these cumulative drugs to build up gradually to therapeutic levels. The bromides, which were introduced around 1850 for treating epilepsy, will be discussed with other anticonvulsants in Chapter 8.

TABLE 6-3
PHARMACOLOGICAL ACTIONS AND CLINICAL INDICATIONS
OF BARBITURATES

PHARMACOLOGICAL ACTIONS	CLINICAL INDICATIONS	PREFERRED COMPOUNDS
Sedative	Anxiety state; excitement and restlessness; organic conditions involving gastrointestinal tract, cardiovascular system, endocrine system, and allergic reactions	amobarbital; butabarbital; pentobarbital; phenobarbital
Hypnotic	Insomnia; preanesthetic medication. (Intermediate-acting drugs at bedtime; short-acting drugs 1 hour prior to surgery in larger dose)	amobarbital; butabarbital; pentobarbital; secobarbital
Anticonvulsant	Epilepsy (long-acting drugs); control of acute convulsions in eclampsia, tetanus, and overdoses of convulsant poisons (short-acting drugs)	phenobarbital; mephobarbital; metharbital; thiopental; pentobarbital; amobarbital
Analgesia	Combined with salicylates and other analgesics, small doses are employed vs. headache, joint and muscle pain, etc.	amobarbital; butabarbital; pentobarbital
Amnesia	In obstetrics to reduce memory of delivery pain, without necessarily relieving the pain itself or producing anesthesia	pentobarbital
Anesthesia (general and basal)	Rapid, pleasant induction of anesthesia, prior to administration of other agents, or as sole anesthetic in short surgical operations and manipulative procedures	thiopental; thiamylal; methitural; methohexital; hexobarbital
Miscellaneous	In neuropsychiatry, for narcoanalysis, narcosuggestion, narcosynthesis, and narcotherapy	thiopental; secobarbital; pentobarbital; amobarbital

---

SUMMARY OF SIDE EFFECTS, TOXICITY, AND CONTRAINDICATIONS OF BARBITURATES

- *Side Effects from Moderate Doses*
  Paradoxical excitement and delirium
  Residual sedation ("hangover"): drowsiness, dizziness, lethargy, headache
  Hypersensitivity reactions: skin eruptions, angioneurotic edema, muscle and joint pains

- *Contraindications (Relative and Absolute)*
  Barbiturates should be employed very cautiously, if at all in:
  (1) Patients with a history of alcoholism or abuse of other drugs
  (2) Mentally depressed patients deemed potentially suicidal
  (3) Elderly patients, especially with senile psychosis
  (4) Extremely excitable persons and those in severe pain
  (5) Persons with hyperthyroidism, porphyria, fever, anemia, diabetes, and severe liver and kidney disease

- *Acute Toxicity from Large Doses*
  Mental confusion and excitement with possible delirium and hallucinations
  Deep sleep, stupor, coma, depressed reflexes
  Slow, shallow breathing
  Pulse weak and rapid when blood pressure falls to shock levels

Body temperature raised at first, falls later, and skin becomes cold and cyanotic
Pupils constricted and unresponsive to light in coma but may dilate with late, severe anoxia

- *Chronic Toxicity*
  Difficulty in thinking
  Poor judgment
  Sluggish responses
  Slurred speech
  Untidiness
  Emotional instability
  Nystagmus
  Strabismus
  Difficulty in accommodation
  Ataxia
  Tremors
  Withdrawal symptoms:
    Nervousness
    Anxiety
    Insomnia
    Hallucinations
    Delusions
    Tremulousness
    Muscle tremors
    Twitching
    Grand mal convulsions

SUMMARY OF POINTS THAT NURSES SHOULD REMEMBER IN ADMINISTERING SEDATIVE-HYPNOTIC DRUGS

- Remember that drug-induced sedation is only one of the ways to calm a nervous patient. Sedatives are no substitute for nursing care and should never be given to "save time" to listen to a patient who is anxious or worried.

- Remember that you can control the patient's environment in many ways that increase the effectiveness of hypnotic drugs. Among the measures that make for a climate conducive to sleep by reducing the stream of nerve impulses passing between the cerebral cortex and the reticular activating system are:
  1. Shutting out noise and reducing confusion
  2. Relaxing tense muscles with a back rub
  3. Listening sympathetically to the patient's fears and anxieties
  4. Regulating his daytime interests and activities in ways that reduce nighttime wakefulness

- Remember that people react differently to sleeplessness. Some are content just to rest, others are upset by broken sleep pattern, and those who are worried or fearful may find insomnia devastating. Thus, discretion in administering "p.r.n." sedative orders is necessary in avoiding the extremes of withholding medication when it is needed or, on the other hand, administering it too readily.

- Remember that although sedatives and sleeping pills may be habit forming and even addictive, they may be used rather freely with justification in some situations, especially in the hospital, because:
    1. The patient may be going through a period of crisis and tension, and his worries may be greatly magnified in the unfamiliar surroundings.
    2. He may have little to distract him mentally, or tire him physically, and he may take long naps during the day. (Despite this, he may have convinced himself that he is being hurt by lack of sleep during the night.)

- Remember to find out why the patient is restless or sleepless. If he is suffering pain, he may require analgesic medication; hypnotic medication may be worse than useless. Similarly, severe anxiety may require tranquilizers rather than hypnotics.

- Remember that any form of sedation increases the patient's vulnerability to accidents, such as falls, cigarette burns, etc., and take appropriate measures to protect the patient.

- Be aware of depressant drugs the patient may have had during the day, because some of these may cause an unexpected potentiation of hypnotics that may be given during the night.

- Be alert to the possibility that these drugs may cause mental confusion and other idiosyncratic responses, especially in elderly patients. Be sure to take immediate measures to prevent injury if the patient becomes restless and hyperactive.

- Be aware of the onset and duration of each drug's action and give it at the proper time for attaining desired effects with minimal untoward reactions. (For example, preoperative sedatives should be given *on time*, and hypnotics should be withheld when they are likely to cause sleepiness during the hours when the patient should be awake.)

- See that the patient actually takes the hypnotic drug. Never leave the drugs with the patient, as he may hoard them for a later suicide attempt.

- Advise patients against taking hypnotic drugs without medical supervision, and do not take them yourself unless prescribed by a physician for a specific purpose. Be alert to the signs of beginning drug dependence and discuss your observations with the physician.

- Advise that these drugs should be stored in a place inaccessible to children. They should, in any case, not be kept by the bedside because of the danger of possible accidental overdosage.

SUMMARY OF NURSE'S RESPONSIBILITY IN ACUTE POISONING BY BARBITURATES AND OTHER SEDATIVE-HYPNOTICS

- *Assisting the Physician with Diagnosis and Treatment*
    1. *With diagnosis* (e.g.): Save vomitus, gastric washings, and urine samples which may be useful for determining whether barbiturate or non-barbiturate depressants were taken.
    2. *With observations* of the patient's condition (e.g.): Keep careful check on the patient's respiration, pulse rate, blood pressure, and reflex responsiveness (i.e., loss or return of corneal, lid, and swallowing reflexes). Report any significant changes to the doctor.
    3. *With antidotal drug treatment* (e.g.): Be aware of the usual dosage range, uses, limitations, and possible toxic symptoms of the analeptic and pressor drugs

which the doctor may order for stimulating respiration, raising blood pressure, and reducing the level of central depression.
    4. *With supportive measures* (e.g.): Be prepared to administer intravenous fluids which may be ordered for feeding purposes, prevention of dehydration, and maintenance of kidney function. Help in the removal of certain barbiturates from the blood by hemodialysis with the artificial kidney and other means.

- *Protecting the Patient from Complications*
    1. Facilitate respiration by making certain that the patient's airway is not obstructed. Turn him on his

side and insert a tongue gag or assist the doctor in performing endotracheal intubation.

2. Move the patient frequently from side to side to prevent pulmonary atelectasis and hypostatic pneumonia. Suction the nose, oropharynx, and trachea as necessary.

3. Protect the patient's skin to prevent the development of decubital ulcers. Instill eye drops when these are ordered for lubrication of conjunctival membranes.

4. Observe the patient carefully but tactfully for indications of his mental and emotional state. Evaluate the likelihood of his attempting suicide again but avoid, as much as possible, giving him the impression that you are trying to police his every action.

5. Be aware of environmental hazards that might lend themselves to a successful suicide attempt (e.g., any window that the patient could open readily for a leap from the 15th floor should be fitted with a protective device to prevent its being opened. Razor blades and belts are examples of other hazards).

- *Supporting the Patient and His Family Emotionally*
1. Be sensitive to the patient's reaction to the failure of his attempt to end his life. Allow him to discuss some of his thoughts and feelings with you, if he wishes.

2. Avoid a punitive or judging manner. Try to understand your own reactions to persons who attempt suicide. In so doing you will be better able to avoid reactions to the patient which are likely to impede his recovery (blame, for example).

3. Allow the family opportunity to discuss their response to this event. Often they welcome an opportunity to talk of the effect of the patient's illness on them. Attempted suicide often makes family members reproach themselves, as they consider whether they may have contributed to the patient's illness. They may also wish to discuss ways by which they can help the patient to recover more readily.

- Discuss with the physician the patient's emotional responses that you observe, and work with him in developing a coordinated plan of care to help the patient with his emotional problems. The physician may recommend psychiatric treatment. If this is the case, the patient is sometimes helped by talking further with the nurse about psychotherapy. You may be able to help the patient to recognize that this is a desirable form of treatment and to accept it as such.

CLINICAL PROBLEM

Mrs. Caruso is being treated as an outpatient at the hospital's psychiatric clinic for a depression which she experienced after her only son was killed in an auto accident. In addition to psychotherapy, she is receiving 0.1 Gm. Nembutal at bedtime when necessary, in order to relieve her insomnia, and a glass of wine before lunch and dinner to encourage appetite. You are the public health nurse who visits Mrs. Caruso weekly.

- Mrs. Caruso comments: "I'm afraid to take the sleeping pills because I don't want to be addicted to them. But I can't sleep without them, and I'm so tired." How would you reply?

- What measures, in addition to taking the Nembutal, could you suggest which might help Mrs. Caruso to sleep?

- Contrast the potential hazards and benefits of Mrs. Caruso's taking Nembutal at home.

- Describe the ways in which alcoholic beverages are believed to stimulate appetite.

- During one of your visits, Mrs. Caruso mentions that she is constipated, and that she has never experienced this problem before. How would you reply to her question, "Shall I take some milk of magnesia?"

REVIEW QUESTIONS

1. (a) Define the terms *sedative* and *hypnotic*.
(b) Indicate the central nervous system sites most sensitive to the actions of sedative and hypnotic drugs.
2. (a) What are the most significant differences in the actions of the several types of barbiturates?

(b) Upon what factors do such differences in their actions depend?
3. (a) Give several examples of general clinical situations in which barbiturates are employed for sedative purposes.

(b) Give several examples of specific psychosomatic and somatopsychic conditions in which sedation with barbiturates is considered desirable.

4. (a) How may the nurse's observations help the doctor decide upon the best barbiturate for producing hypnotic effects in a particular patient?

(b) What are some points that the nurse must consider in deciding whether to administer a "p.r.n." barbiturate hypnotic?

5. (a) List some undesirable responses to barbiturates and indicate some measures that the nurse may take to minimize these difficulties by protecting the patient.

(b) In what patients may specific kinds of barbiturates be contraindicated?

6. (a) Describe briefly the mental and physical state of a patient who has been abusing barbiturates chronically and indicate the dangers to which he is exposed during such states of chronic intoxication.

(b) Describe briefly the nature of the syndrome which may be precipitated by the withdrawal of barbiturates from an addicted patient.

7. (a) List several types of measures which the nurse may be called upon to employ in assisting the doctor in treating a patient acutely poisoned by barbiturates and in regard to giving protection and support to the patient.

(b) List several analeptic agents and indicate briefly how these drugs may be used in determining the depth of barbiturate depression and in treating such overdosage states.

8. (a) In what clinical situations is phenobarbital often preferred over other barbiturates?

(b) What properties of phenobarbital account for its relative desirability in these conditions?

(c) Indicate some special purposes for which amobarbital and pentobarbital have been employed.

9. (a) List several claims that have been made for the superiority of certain non-barbiturate sedative-hypnotics, and evaluate the validity of such claims.

(b) Indicate the chief advantages and disadvantages of older sedative-hypnotics such as chloral hydrate and paraldehyde and list several special clinical uses of the latter.

10. (a) List some measures that the nurse may take to control the environment and thus increase the effectiveness of barbiturates and other hypnotic drugs.

(b) What advice can the nurse offer patients to help reduce the chance of acute and chronic intoxication occurring among members of their families?

BIBLIOGRAPHY

Blumenthal, M. D., and Reinhart, M. J.: Psychosis and convulsions following withdrawal from ethchlorvynol. J.A.M.A., *190*:154, 1964.

Clemessen, C., and Nillson, E.: Therapeutic trends in the treatment of barbiturate poisoning. Clin. Pharmacol. Ther., *2*:220, 1961.

Dobos, J. K., *et al.*: Acute barbiturate intoxication. J.A.M.A., *176*:268, 1961.

Fraser, H. F.: Tolerance to and physical dependence on opiates, barbiturates, and alcohol. Ann. Rev. Med., *8*: 427, 1957.

Friend, D. G.: Sedative hypnotics. Clin. Pharmacol. Ther., *1*:454, 1960.

Frohman, I. P.: The barbiturates. Am. J. Nursing, *54*: 432, 1954.

Horgan, P. D.: Caring for the drug-poisoned patient. R.N., *25*:62, 1962 (June).

Lasagna, L.: The newer hypnotics. Med. Clin. North Amer., *41*:359, 1957.

Newberry, W. B., Jr.: Sedatives have their place, but. Am. J. Nursing, *57*:1285, 1957.

Rodman, M. J.: Barbiturates, boon or bane? R.N., *20*:60, 1957 (June).

———: Drugs for safer sedation. R.N., *25*:61, 1962 (April).

Schreiner, G. E., *et al.*: Glutethimide intoxication. Arch. Intern. Med., *101*:899, 1958.

Shideman, F. E.: Clinical pharmacology of hypnotics and sedatives. Clin. Pharmacol. Ther., *2*:313, 1961.

Psychotherapeutic Agents

THE IMPACT OF MODERN DRUGS ON PSYCHIATRY

Drug treatment of mental and emotional disorders took a tremendous stride forward in 1952 with the introduction of two new agents for treating psychiatric patients. These drugs—*reserpine*, a derivative of the Indian snakeroot plant Rauwolfia serpentina, and *chlorpromazine,* a synthetic chemical of the phenothiazine class—were the forerunners of many new psychopharmacological agents that help to control psychiatric symptoms better than the drugs previously available.

Very many patients—some doctors in general practice set the figure at two out of every three patients they treat—show signs and symptoms that stem from emotional unrest. Most of these patients suffer mainly from physical complaints of psychosomatic origin. Others need help in coping with psychiatric difficulties ranging from mildly incapacitating psychoneuroses to major mental illnesses or psychoses.

About one million people in this country are patients in hospitals that specialize in psychiatric care. Those who respond well to intensive treatment of acute episodes are usually released within a short time. However, such patients still need outpatient medical attention, home care, and maintenance drug therapy to reduce the chance of relapses. The psychotherapeutic drugs developed in recent years have had their greatest success in reducing the severity of such acute reactions and the frequency of such relapses.

Drug Therapy. Drugs that affect the functioning of the mind are called *psychotropic* agents. Such substances, which include alcohol and the opiates, are of course not new, nor are they necessarily useful for treating mental illness. However, some new psychopharmacological agents have proved therapeutically effective in mental derangements and emotional upsets. Of the new classes of psychotherapeutic compounds the most important are (1) the *tranquilizers* and (2)

the *antidepressants;* these principally will be the kinds of psychotherapeutic drugs discussed in this chapter.

THE TRANQUILIZER DRUGS

Most important among the drugs used in mental, emotional, and behavioral disorders are those that relieve symptoms caused by anxiety. These so-called *psycholeptic* or *ataractic* agents (*ataraxia* is a Greek word meaning peace of mind) are commonly classified as *minor* and *major tranquilizers.* These terms reflect the relative effectiveness of the two broad subclasses of psycholeptics in calming the manifestations of anxiety of lesser and more severe degree.

The minor tranquilizers are used mainly as adjuncts in the management of psychosomatic conditions and in patients temporarily upset by some stressful life situation. The major tranquilizers are best reserved for treating psychotic patients, but smaller doses are often employed in many medical and psychiatric conditions including some psychoneuroses marked by mild to moderate degrees of anxiety.

Both types of tranquilizers differ from the barbiturates and other ordinary psychosedatives in not producing sleep, stupor, and coma as readily as do the older drugs. That is, there is a wider margin of safety between the doses of the tranquilizers that produce desirable calmness and the amounts that cause undesirable degrees of depression of consciousness, psychomotor performance and vital functions.

The Major Tranquilizers (Antipsychotic Agents)

The first drugs to produce an important impact upon the care of psychiatric patients were the *rauwolfia* alkaloids, of which reserpine was the most important. However, when administered in the large doses required in psychiatric cases, reserpine and the other rauwolfia plant products cause many disabling side effects. Because the same desirable tranquilizing effects can be achieved more conveniently with synthetic chemicals of the phenothiazine class, the rauwolfia alkaloids have been largely replaced recently by the latter drugs. Small doses of the rauwolfia alkaloids reduce blood pressure safely and are used today mainly in the treatment of hypertension. They are discussed more fully in Chapter 23 (Antihypertensive Agents) and the Drug Digests.

Neither the rauwolfia alkaloids nor the phenothiazine derivatives and other major tranquilizers are capable of *curing* psychiatric patients. The drugs are, however, often effective in alleviating the symptoms of severe anxiety and agitation. In doing so, these psychotherapeutic agents help the patient to profit from other forms of treatment such as psychotherapy. It is this that has led to a shortening of the time that most mental patients stay in psychiatric hospitals and to an increase in the number of patients who can be discharged from hospitals to home care.

The availability of effective drugs for calming excessively hyperactive patients has brought about a marked change in the atmosphere of mental hospitals. Agitated patients who once tore off their clothes and required physical restraint in packs, baths and jackets now walk about fully dressed both indoors and on the grounds. Many withdrawn patients who had to be given tube feedings are able now to eat with the other patients and attend to their own hygienic needs.

These changes in the behavior of patients under psychotropic drug therapy have had important effects upon the attitudes of the patients themselves and upon those of their families, and members of the hospital staff. The patient finds the present-day hospital quieter and more conducive to recovery. He can more readily re-establish relationships with other people, including the psychotherapist, and he is also better able to take advantage of occupational and recreational activities. His family may also be more understanding and cooperative when the patient returns home, since they are more hopeful of his eventual recovery. Nurses, too, have been freed of much of the need to restrain patients and keep them in custody merely; thus, they can spend more time in counseling them.

The Phenothiazine Derivatives (See also Drug Digests)

The phenothiazine drugs are capable of causing many pharmacological effects besides the special type of sedation for which they are noted. Some of these actions are clinically useful (e.g., the antiemetic effect which prevents vomiting from various causes) but others may sometimes be the cause of undesirable reactions. Therefore, once the usefulness and drawbacks of chlorpromazine (Thorazine), the first tranquilizer of this class, became apparent, chemists began to synthesize closely related chemical analogues of it.

The purpose of such molecular manipulations was to discover congener compounds with greater potency and fewer side effects than chlorpromazine.

At present, three main chemical subclasses of phenothiazines—the aliphatic or dimethylamine subgroup; the piperazine series; and the piperidyl derivatives—have been prepared (see Table 7-1). Each of these subgroups differs from the others in the nature of certain chemical side chains, and these differences are, in turn, thought to be responsible for differences in the tranquilizing potency and other C.N.S. and peripheral effects of the various compounds. In studying these drugs, it is desirable to note how the phenothiazine compounds of each of the chemical subclasses differ in their pharmacological effects, clinical utility, and adverse reactions.

The phenothiazines in use as tranquilizers are prepared by substituting radicals (atoms or side chains) in the number 2 (R_2) or the number 10 (R_{10}) position, or in both.

On the basis of chemical structure, phenothiazine derivatives are divided into:

The dimethylaminopropane group (also referred to as (1) *dimethylaminopropyl* and as (2) *dimethylaminoalkyl derivatives*), characterized by a *3 carbon* straight side chain at the number 10 position (e.g., promazine, chlorpromazine, methoxypromazine, and others).

The piperazine group (also referred to as *propyl piperidine subgroup*), characterized by a piperazine ring in the side chain at the number 10 position (e.g., prochlorperazine, perphenazine, thiopropazate, trifluoperazine, and fluphenazine).

The piperidine group (also referred to as (1) *piperidyl derivatives*, or as (2) *alkyl piperidyl derivatives*), characterized by a piperidine ring in the number 10 position side chain (e.g., mepazine; thioridazine).

A further factor of importance is whether or not there is a halogen substituent for the hydrogen in the number 2 position, and the nature of the halogen, i.e., whether chlorine or fluorine.

The relationships and the modifications are easily understood by study and comparison of the basic phenothiazine structure and the various formulas given in Table 7-1. It may be noted that the difference in the R_{10} substituent accounts for the different names of the chemical *sub*-classes to which reference will be made in the discussion of the differences in pharmacological actions and clinical uses.

Group 1: dimethylaminopropane side chain. Promazine (Table 7-1) and methoxypromazine are in the *"weak potency"* class (see dosage data, Table 7-2).

Group 1a. When this structure is *halogenated* at the number 2 position, there is significant change in activity of the resulting compounds of this subgroup. *Chlorpromazine* is about 2 to 4 times as potent as

TABLE 7-1

PHENOTHIAZINE DERIVATIVES (AMINO-PROPYL SIDE CHAIN) *

Basic structural formula of phenothiazine

Generic name Proprietary name	R_{10}	R_2
Propyl Dialkylamino Side Chain		
Promazine hydrochloride N.F. Sparine	$-(CH_2)_3N(CH_3)_2 \cdot HCl$	H
Chlorpromazine hydrochloride U.S.P. Thorazine	$-(CH_2)_3N(CH_3)_2 \cdot HCl$	Cl
Triflupromazine hydrochloride Vesprin	$-(CH_2)_3N(CH_3)_2 \cdot HCl$	CF_3
Alkyl Piperidyl and Pyrrolidinyl Side Chain		
Mepazine hydrochloride Pacatal		H
Thioridazine hydrochloride Mellaril		SCH_3
Propyl Piperazine Side Chain		
Prochlorperazine maleate U.S.P. Compazine		Cl
Trifluoperazine hydrochloride Stelazine		CF_3
Perphenazine Trilafon		Cl
Fluphenazine dihydrochloride Permitil, Prolixin		CF_3
Thiopropazate hydrochloride Dartal		Cl
Carphenazine Maleate Proketazine		

* Adapted from Wilson, C. O., and Gisvold, O.: Textbook of Organic Medicinal and Pharmaceutical Chemistry, ed. 5. Philadelphia, J. B. Lippincott, 1966.

TABLE 7-2

EFFECTIVE INITIAL DAILY DOSAGE RANGE *

	PERMITIL	STELAZINE	TRILAFON	DARTAL	COMPAZINE
Schizophrenic psychoses	2–10 mg.	10–60 mg.	32–64 mg.	50–100 mg.	75–100 mg.
Manic-depressive psychoses	10–20 mg.	20–80 mg.	32–96 mg.	60–150 mg.	75–150 mg.
Senile psychoses	1–5 mg.	2–8 mg.	4–12 mg.	10–40 mg.	10–40 mg.
Psychoneurotic disorders	1–5 mg.	4–20 mg.	8–24 mg.	15–60 mg.	15–60 mg.

	VESPRIN	THORAZINE	SPARINE	TENTONE	PACATAL
Schizophrenic psychoses	100–300 mg.	300–800 mg.	500–1,000 mg.	500–1,000 mg.	500–1,000 mg.
Manic-depressive psychoses	200–400 mg.	300–1,200 mg.	500–1,500 mg.	500–1,500 mg.	500–1,500 mg.
Senile psychoses	30–75 mg.	30–100 mg.	50–150 mg.	50–150 mg.	50–150 mg.
Psychoneurotic disorders	30–150 mg.	100–300 mg.	150–400 mg.	150–400 mg.	150–400 mg.

* Initial dosage is individualized according to the severity of symptoms such as anxiety, tension and psychomotor excitement. Maintenance dosages are determined by individual requirements.

promazine and methoxypromazine, and *trifluoromazine* is about 2 or 3 times as potent as chlorpromazine. These drugs are classified as "moderately potent."

Group 2: Piperazine ring substitutions in number 10 position. Prochlorperazine (Compazine) is formed by substitution of a *piperazine* ring for the simple amino group in chlorpromazine, which makes it at least five times as potent as the latter drug. *Perphenazine* and *thiopropazate* are essentially similar to prochlorperazine in potency, despite the further lengthening of the side chain.

Group 3: Trifluoromethyl substitutions, combined with a piperazine ring. Trifluoperazine (Stelazine) is identical with Compazine, except for the substitution of the latter's R$_2$ chlorine by a *trifluoromethyl* group (cf. Vesprin, which had *this* group but *not* the piperazine ring).

The incorporation of *both* the *piperazine ring* and the *trifluoromethyl* group still further increases the potency—to about *double* that of Compazine. *Fluphenazine* (Permitil; Prolixin) is identical with *Trilafon,* except for the substitution of the latter's R$_2$ chlorine by a *trifluoromethyl* group.

The incorporation of both the *piperazine ring* and the *trifluoromethyl group* still further increases the potency—to about double that of Trilafon.

The lengthening of the side chain probably doesn't make this compound very different from Stelazine.

Group 4: Piperidine ring substituents (one nitrogen atom instead of two). Mepazine (Pacatal), containing neither a halogen nor a 3 carbon side chain, is one of the least potent of the phenothiazines. *Thioridazine* (Mellaril) has a slightly longer chain on the number 10 position, with the *piperidine* ring. It also has a sulfur-containing (*thiomethyl*) radical in position number 2 of the phenothiazine ring.

These substitutions make for a *weaker* but *less toxic* compound (in terms of extrapyramidal effects).

Pharmacological Effects. The most useful action shared by all of the phenothiazines is their effect on certain *subcortical sites* that are involved in the emotional reactivity of the individual. Depression of these areas is believed to be responsible for the reduction in emotional excitability of anxious, agitated patients when they are treated with these agents. Drugs of the piperazine subgroup such as trifluoperazine (Stelazine) and fluphenazine (Permitil; Prolixin) are thought to have the greatest selective affinity for these subcortical sites. This may account for their ability to reduce emotional unrest when administered in relatively small doses that cause little or no drowsiness or motor incoordination—a true tranquilizing, or ataractic, action.

Drugs of the piperazine subgroup also possess the greatest *antiemetic* potency. This action is the result of their direct depressant effect on the chemoreceptor trigger zone (CTZ), the group of nerve cells that relays impulses to the medullary vomiting center. Prochlorperazine (Compazine) and perphenazine (Trilafon) are, for example, commonly used to prevent or overcome vomiting in various clinical conditions (see Chap. 38). All of the phenothiazines, with the possible exception of thioridazine * (Mellaril), are effective antiemetics.

----

* See also Drug Digest.

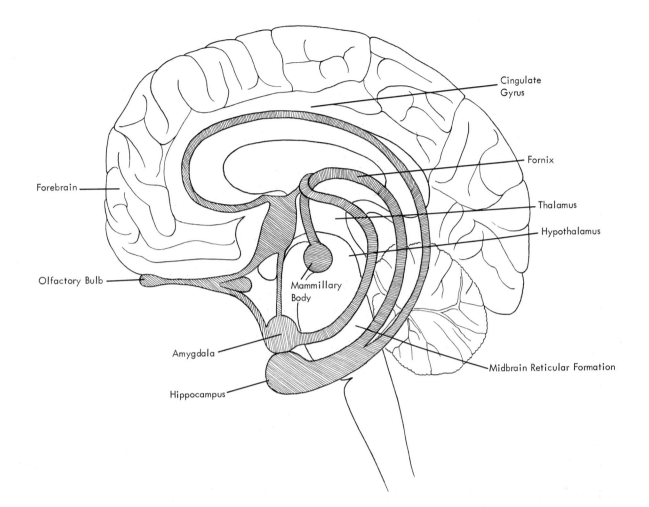

Fig. 7-1. The limbic system (the rhinencephalon (*nose brain*) and related structures) is thought to constitute a neuroanatomical emotional circuit. The phenothiazines and other antipsychotic drugs are believed to act primarily by affecting the excitability of subcortical centers in this "anatomical substrate of the emotions."

An important C.N.S. effect of the phenothiazines is their ability to intensify and prolong the action of other depressant drugs. The pain-relieving properties of the narcotic analgesics, for example, are potentiated by combining them with phenothiazines, especially those of the dimethylamine subgroup, such as chlorpromazine * (Thorazine). This action is due in part to their ability to reduce the patient's emotional reaction to pain and partly to their action in somehow increasing the effect of the narcotic analgesic drugs on pain perception. This is often useful for patients in severe pain; however, the potentiating action of the phenothiazines on barbiturates, alcohol, and narcotics may sometimes cause deep sleep, stupor, and even coma.

* See also Drug Digest.

(The pharmacological effects of the phenothiazines upon autonomic nervous system and endocrine gland functions also are undesirable; these are discussed in the section dealing with adverse reactions.)

Clinical Indications. The most dramatic effects of the phenothiazines are observed when they are used in the treatment of severely disturbed patients. All of these drugs are capable of quickly quieting patients who are hyperactive and highly agitated. This calming of psychomotor excitement is seen in patients diagnosed as suffering from many different psychiatric disorders. Thus the phenothiazines are commonly used for controlling extreme restlessness in: (1) acute schizophrenic reactions of the paranoid and catatonic (excitement swing) types; (2) the manic phase of manic depressive psychosis, (3) toxic confusional states including acute alcoholic intoxication, delirium tremens, and drug withdrawal syndromes, and (4) arteriosclerotic brain damage resulting in confusion and disorientation.

In acute excitement states such as those listed above, when the relieving of severe agitation is the first objective, the drugs of the dimethylamine series of phenothiazines are often preferred. Chlorpromazine (Thorazine) and promazine (Sparine), drugs that cause a relatively greater degree of sedation than those of the piperazine subgroup, may be most desirable, especially for patients who are exhausted for lack of sleep. Barbiturates were formerly used for this purpose, but the large doses, which were often needed, sometimes made patients comatose and depressed respiration dangerously. Even when smaller doses of barbiturates are employed, patients are often left deeply lethargic. With the phenothiazines, on the other hand, there is little likelihood of causing dangerously deep depression, and the patient can be readily aroused to take part in his own care and treatment.

Acute Agitation. Patients in states of acute excitement may have to be given the phenothiazine tranquilizers by injection. However, the oral form of these drugs is safer and more convenient to administer, and patients are transferred to oral medication regimens as soon as seems feasible. This is especially true if falls in blood pressure become a problem when promazine or chlorpromazine are administered by injection.

Maintenance Therapy. The doctor may decide to switch the patient to one of the less sedating piperazine-type phenothiazines during long-term maintenance therapy in order to minimize drowsiness and various side effects stemming from autonomic blockade. The potent piperazine class phenothiazines fluphenazine (Prolixin; Permitil) and trifluoperazine (Stelazine), for example, effectively control anxiety when administered in small daily doses that cause little, if any, drowsiness or hypotensive effects.

When these potent drugs or other phenothiazines, including prochlorperazine (Compazine), are employed regularly, symptoms of psychoses such as hallucinations and delusions tend gradually to disappear. This may be, as has been suggested, a unique effect of these psychotropic drugs—the result of an action that has been called "antipsychotic." On the other hand, the patient's greater ability to control his behavior may really be an indirect result of the reduction of his anxiety.

When his state of anxiety is lessened, the patient is better able to profit from psychotherapy. Because he is no longer reacting violently to his frightening hallucinations, he can often be helped to gain some insight into the causes of these disturbed sensory perceptions. Similarly, although his delusions may still persist, these twisted thought processes are less likely to disturb

him in ways that evoke abnormal behavior. Thus, a patient may, for example, admit that he still hears voices, or his talk may indicate that he is still subject to delusions. Yet, because he is less hostile and more readily reached by the psychotherapist and the nurses and other staff members, he may soon be judged sufficiently improved to return home and resume his usual occupation. These patients must, however, continue taking daily maintenance doses of the phenothiazine drugs, and they should of course receive continuing psychotherapy.

Chronic Conditions. Some of the potent phenothiazines of the piperazine class are claimed to be effective not only for controlling hyperactive patients but also for bringing about remissions in psychotic patients who are not at all overactive. That is, these drugs are said to improve the condition of certain chronic schizophrenics of the hypodynamic type—patients who are deeply withdrawn, mute, and seclusive.

Somehow, the phenothiazines of the "activating" type tend to stimulate such sluggish, lethargic patients out of their apathy. Under the influence of psychotropic drug therapy, a number of these "back-ward" or "hard-core" patients have become increasingly alert, recovered their drive and initiative, and regained their ability to think and talk logically.

Carphenazine * (Proketazine), a relatively new drug of this class, is claimed to have brought about recovery in up to 30 per cent of such cases. Others of this subgroup, including trifluoperazine (Stelazine) and fluphenazine * (Permitil; Prolixin) are said to have helped 10 to 20 per cent of regressed patients to recover. This may not seem remarkable, until we remember that many of the chronically ill patients who have now returned home had once been called "hopeless" and "incurable." Confirmation of the effectiveness of these phenothiazines for patients of such poor prognosis would be encouraging, indeed. Chronic schizophrenics would, of course, require maintenance drug therapy indefinitely to prevent relapse, and such patients should be seen regularly by a psychiatrist.

Non-Psychiatric Uses. The phenothiazines are sometimes prescribed for non-psychotic patients in relatively small doses. These cases include both general medical and surgical patients—in whom these drugs are used mainly to control nausea and vomiting and to help narcotic-analgesic drugs reduce severe pain—and psychiatric cases with relatively minor symptoms of anxiety. Chlorpromazine, for example, is useful in the management of cancer patients, in whom it relieves anxiety, potentiates the action of narcotics, and reduces nausea and vomiting caused by drugs or irradiation. Thioridazine (Mellaril), a phenothiazine of another type, has little antiemetic activity. It is equal to chlorpromazine in controlling anxiety and is less toxic than the latter; therefore, it is often prescribed in

* See also Drug Digests.

small doses for the relief of mild anxiety symptoms in patients reacting to stress. Somewhat larger doses are used for the control of moderate to severe symptoms in patients diagnosed as psychoneurotic.

Even drugs of the potent piperazine type are available in low dosage tablet form for treating nervousness in non-psychotic patients. Fluphenazine (Permitil) is prescribed for this purpose, and acetophenazine (Tindal) has been promoted as an adjunctive drug in the management of various physical illnesses, including cardiovascular disease. Larger doses of this drug have been recommended recently as especially effective for treating the paranoid form of schizophrenia.

Adverse Reactions. Unfortunately, the phenothiazines are capable of causing many kinds of side effects and toxic reactions. Therefore, doctors usually prefer to manage less severe anxiety states with one of the safer, "minor" tranquilizers. The phenothiazines are best reserved for use in more severe mental emotional illnesses which warrant the considerable risk that is involved in their long-term employment.

The side effects and toxic reactions of the phenothiazines may be grouped as follows: (1) *Central nervous system,* (2) *Autonomic,* (3) *Endocrine,* and (4) *Allergic.*

Central nervous system side effects may be the result of either excessive depression or excessive stimulation. Depression, manifested by drowsiness, dizziness, lethargy, and feelings of fatigue, is more common with drugs of the dimethylamine subgroup (e.g., promazine and chlorpromazine) and the piperidyl subtype (e.g., thioridazine) than with the piperazines (e.g., fluphenazine and trifluoperazine). On the other hand, drugs of the latter type seem more likely to overstimulate the extrapyramidal motor system.

Symptoms of *extrapyramidal stimulation* can be grouped in three categories: (a) *parkinsonism*—muscular tremors, rigidity and other signs resembling those seen in Parkinson's disease; (b) *dyskinesias*—sudden contractions of muscle groups in spasms resembling convulsive seizures, and (c) *akathisia*—extreme restlessness marked by increasing mental turbulence and motor activity. (Patients often complain of having "the jitters" or "restless legs.")

These reactions can usually be controlled by reducing the dose of the drug or withdrawing it entirely and administering drugs of the kind used in managing parkinsonism (Chap. 8), including benztropine (Cogentin) and diphenhydramine (Benadryl). Once these symptoms subside, the administration of a phenothiazine tranquilizer may be begun again at a lower dose level. The piperidyl derivative thioridazine (Mellaril) is said to cause fewer side effects of the extrapyramidal type than do other phenothiazines.

Autonomic blockade (Chap. 17) is a source of side effects seen most frequently with the dimethylamine and piperidyl type of phenothiazines. Injection of promazine (Sparine) to quiet an alcoholic may, for example, send his blood pressure plummeting. This hypotension occurs because the drug reduces vasomotor tone by cutting off some of the tonic vasoconstrictor nerve impulses passing to the arterioles by way of sympathetic nerve fibers. Promazine may also potentiate the depressant effects of alcohol and barbiturates in intoxicated patients and thus cause coma as well as falls in both blood pressure and in the rate and depth of respiration.

In addition to the adrenergic blockade described above, the phenothiazines may block cholinergic nerve impulses. This results in atropinelike symptoms, including mouth dryness, blurring of vision, and constipation. Such effects are most common with the piperidyl derivative mepazine (Pacatal) and occur to some extent with its relative, thioridazine. Both types of blockade are least likely with the potent piperazine-type phenothiazines, such as fluphenazine and trifluoperazine.

Endocrine Effects. The last mentioned drugs cause fewer endocrine effects than occurred with the earlier agents such as chlorpromazine. Glandular derangements include delayed menstruation and ovulation, false positive pregnancy tests, and abnormal lactation. Patients taking chlorpromazine for long periods put on excess weight, presumably because of the drug's effects on the pituitary gland and related hypothalamic mechanisms controlling various metabolic functions.

Skin discolorations and visual difficulties may be caused by melanin pigment deposited in the skin, eyes and other organs of patients taking high doses of phenothiazines. This excess pigment deposition may be the result of a drug-induced hormonal and neural imbalance, according to some medical scientists. Others suggest that such phenothiazine-induced *melanosic* may be the result of the action of certain wave lengths of light upon the drugs (and their metabolites) that have accumulated in the skin. In any case, whatever the mechanism by which it is brought about, the slate-blue to deep blue-black or purplish skin discolorations constitute a serious cosmetic problem. The nurse may be asked to help prevent such phototoxic reactions by keeping patients out of direct sunlight in the spring and summer months. The nature and significance of the ocular opacities are not well understood at present, but ophthalmologists suggest that all patients receiving prolonged treatment with high doses of phenothiazines be subjected to serial slit-lamp studies periodically.

Allergic Reactions. Many of the reactions reported in patients taking phenothiazines are the result of individual hypersensitivity. These reactions, which occur most commonly with chlorpromazine, include: (a) *Agranulocytosis* and other kinds of blood dyscrasias; (b) allergic skin reactions, such as *photosensitiv-*

ity (the development of dermatitis in patients who are exposed to the sun) and (c) *cholestatic hepatitis,* an obstructive type of liver disorder. Chlorpromazine jaundice is caused by swelling of the walls of the canaliculi, the tiny bile channels within the liver. When these become blocked, the bile backs up into the blood. The condition usually clears up when the drug is discontinued. However, because the symptoms resemble those of more serious obstructive biliary disorders, such as bile duct stones or cancer of the pancreas, exploratory abdominal surgery may be required to rule out the possibility that the patient's symptoms stem from such conditions.

Sudden Death. Recent reports of psychiatric patients who died suddenly and unexpectedly while receiving large doses of phenothiazine derivatives have created concern. It is still uncertain whether such fatalities can be dismissed as due to chance or, instead, constitute the most serious of all phenothiazine-induced complications.

Collapse and death have occurred without any clearcut post-mortem findings except an abundance of a brown glandular pigment in the heart and other viscera of these patients. Although the significance of this is not fully understood, some have suggested that these drugs may cause ventricular fibrillation or sudden cardiac arrest as a result of a quinidine-like effect (Chap. 21) of certain phenothiazine derivatives. Others think that these patients may be made subject to sudden seizures and that death may be due to asphyxia from food aspirated into the air passages.

The occurrence of side effects and severe toxicity of so many different types means that a close watch should be kept on patients taking phenothiazine-type tranquilizers. By reporting early signs of toxicity, the nurse can alert the doctor. To counteract the side effects he may order adjunctive drugs (e.g., antiparkinsonism drugs), or adjust the dose downward or discontinue the drug entirely.

Dosage and Administration. The dosage of any phenothiazine drug must be adjusted to meet the needs of the individual patient. Usually, patients suffering from acute psychotic reactions require much larger doses than those with milder symptoms. Once acute excitement has been controlled, dosage may be gradually reduced to lower levels for long-term maintenance therapy.

The phenothiazines are effective whether administered orally or parenterally. The latter route is usually reserved for treatment of the more severely agitated patient who needs large doses. The intramuscular route is preferred to intravenous administration because the danger of sudden severe falls in blood pressure is decreased when phenothiazines are more slowly absorbed. Hypotensive reactions may occur even with large *oral* dosage; therefore, all patients should be watched for signs such as dizziness

and faintness, and they should be warned to lie down with head lower than legs, if these signs of postural hypotension appear.

Instructions for diluting solutions with saline should be followed carefully, and the solutions should be injected into a muscle, not into subcutaneous tissues, because such tissues are more subject to irritation than are muscular sites. Injections are best made slowly, deep into the muscle, and the usual precautions taken to see that a vein has not been entered accidentally. The doctor may sometimes order the addition of procaine 2 per cent to reduce pain.

Rauwolfia Derivatives (See also Drug Digests)

The powdered root of the shrub *Rauwolfia serpentina* has been used for centuries in India to treat many medical conditions. Introduced here in the early 1950's for treating high blood pressure, rauwolfia also proved to have desirable effects on the behavior of psychiatric patients. Doctors noted that emotionally upset patients often became relaxed and less tense while under treatment with rauwolfia and its most important alkaloid, reserpine. Patients seemed less inclined to drowsiness than when they were treated with the barbiturates and other sedatives.

Reserpine soon replaced barbiturates in many products in which the latter had been employed for controlling anxiety and tension in patients with psychoneuroses and psychosomatic disorders. Psychiatrists, using much larger doses of reserpine, found that they were able to halt hostile aggressive behavior in agitated psychotic patients without the dangers and inconvenience of the older depressant drugs. Reports that reserpine reduced noise and violence in mental hospital wards and made patients more amenable to psychotherapy fired renewed interest in the drug therapy of mental illness.

However, the use of reserpine and other rauwolfia alkaloids in psychiatry has declined considerably. Most doctors now prefer to begin treatment with one of the phenothiazine derivatives, which have been found more dependable than the rauwolfia alkaloids in the management of psychotic patients. For psychoneurotic patients and those whose physical disorders are complicated by emotional tension doctors now usually prefer to try one of the minor tranquilizers rather than reserpine. The rauwolfia drugs are now used mainly in the management of hypertension and are discussed with the drugs used for reducing high blood pressure (Chap. 23).

Miscellaneous Antipsychotic Agents

Several relatively new tranquilizers may be tentatively classed as "major" on the basis of their ability to control severe symptoms in psychotic patients. One of these drugs, chlorprothixine (Taractan), is closely related chemically to chlorpromazine and other phenothiazines. It resembles these drugs in its pharmacological actions and clinical uses also. Like promazine and chlorpromazine, this non-phenothiazine is effective for producing rapid sedation in acute delirium states, including delirium tremens. Side effects include excessive sedation and postural hypotension, especially when the drug is used to quiet acutely intoxicated alcoholics.

Thiothixene (Navane) is another recently introduced antipsychotic agent that resembles chlorprothixene chemically but is claimed to cause less drowsiness than the latter when it is administered to acutely and chronically ill psychotic patients. Although its slight difference in chemical structure from the phenothiazines has also been linked to differences in pharmacological actions claimed to be clinically desirable, this compound shares many properties of the phenothiazine compound trifluoperazine—a fact that may be

related to the presence of the same sort of piperazine "tail" on both compounds (Table 7-1). Thus, it is not surprising that this drug has "activating" properties that are both useful in treating withdrawn chronic schizophrenics and also capable of causing undesirable extrapyramidal motor system stimulation. (Patients should be watched—as with the piperazine-type phenothiazines (p. 117)—for signs of parkinsonlike disorders and drug-induced restlessness, in order to prevent possible massive muscular contractions from continued administration of thiothixene.)

Haloperidol (Haldol), an antipsychotic agent recently made available in the United States after several years of wide use in Europe and South America, is said to be an alternative useful in treating patients who do not tolerate phenothiazines or who have proved resistant to treatment with the latter agents. This drug, a compound of the butyrophenone class, is

TABLE 7-3
MAJOR TRANQUILIZERS (ANTIPSYCHOTIC AGENTS)

Nonproprietary Name	Trade Name	Usual Daily Dosage Range *
Phenothiazine Derivatives		
Dimethylamine Subgroup		
Chlorpromazine HCl U.S.P.	Thorazine	30–1200 mg.
Methoxypromazine	Tentone	50–1500 mg.
Promazine HCl N.F.	Sparine	50–1500 mg.
Triflupromazine	Vesprin	20–200 mg.
Piperazine Subgroup		
Acetophenazine	Tindal	40–80 mg.
Carphenazine	Proketazine	25–400 mg.
Fluphenazine	Permitil; Prolixin	1–20 mg.
Perphenazine	Trilafon	6–64 mg.
Prochlorperazine N.F.	Compazine	15–150 mg.
Thiopropazate	Dartal	15–100 mg.
Trifluoperazine	Stelazine	2–30 mg.
Piperidyl Subgroup		
Mepazine	Pacatal	50–400 mg.
Thioridazine	Mellaril	30–800 mg.
Others		
Benzquinamide	Quantril	50–800 mg.
Chlorprothixene	Taractan	30–200 mg.
Haloperidol	Haldol	2–15 mg.
Prothipendyl	Timovan	100–400 mg.
Reserpine U.S.P.	Rau-Sed, Sandril Serpasil, Serpate, etc.	0.5–10 mg.
Thiothixene	Navane	6–30 mg.

* Dosage varies widely depending on the severity of the patient's symptoms and his response to the drug.

said to be especially effective in the manic phase of manic-depressive psychosis and for the paranoid type of schizophrenic patient. It tends to reduce paranoid delusions, hallucinations and psychomotor excitement when administered in doses that do not cause postural hypotension. (This may be an advantage in elderly patients.) However, haloperidol often causes extra-pyramidal motor system reactions, and severe—even suicidal—mental depression reactions of the kind seen in some patients taking reserpine (Chap. 23) have also sometimes been observed with this antipsychotic agent.

The Minor Tranquilizers (Antianxiety Agents)

Few people are entirely free of emotional tension. In fact, doctors sometimes say that most of their patients seem to be suffering from the effects of unresolved nervous tension. Most of these people do not require hospitalization or treatment with major tranquilizers such as the phenothiazines, with all of their potential side effects and toxicity (p. 117).

The barbiturates and other sedatives traditionally used for controlling mild or moderate anxiety symptoms have various drawbacks (Chap. 6). When the major tranquilizers were first introduced, it was hoped that they would provide safer sedation for the many people who have difficulty in coping with emotional

stress. Small doses of the phenothiazine and rauwolfia derivatives have been employed for this purpose, but the trend seems to be away from these drugs. Another group of tranquilizers, comprised of drugs that are much less likely to cause severe side effects, has come into use for managing the manifestations of anxiety in non-psychotic patients. These so-called minor tranquilizers (Table 7-4) are used for treating people of the same type that respond to the actions of the barbiturates. They are claimed, however, to have various advantages which make them preferable to the classic kind of sedatives.

Advantages. The minor tranquilizers do not cause the kinds of autonomic nervous system imbalances often seen with major tranquilizers such as chlorpromazine and reserpine. Also, extrapyramidal motor system stimulation does not occur with these drugs. The absence of side effects such as postural hypotension and pseudoparkinsonism together with the lower incidence of sensitization reactions give these drugs an advantage in the management of the many patients whose degree of emotional upset is not severe enough to require the more potent, potentially toxic phenothiazines.

The question of whether minor tranquilizers such as meprobamate * (Miltown, Equanil) and chlordi-

* See also Drug Digest.

TABLE 7-4
SOME MINOR TRANQUILIZERS (ANTIANXIETY AGENTS)

Nonproprietary Name	Trade Name	Usual Single Dose
Azacyclonol N.F.	Frenquel	20–100 mg.
Benactyzine	Suavitil	1–3 mg.
Buclizine	Softran; Vibazine	25–50 mg.
Chlordiazepoxide N.F.	Librium	5–10 mg.
Chlormezanone	Trancopal	300–800 mg.
Diazepam	Valium	2–5 mg.
Ectylurea	Nostyn; Levanil	150–300 mg.
Emylcamate	Striatran	200 mg.
Hydroxyphenamate	Listica	600–800 mg.
Hydroxyzine HCl N.F.	Atarax	25–100 mg.
Hydroxyzine Pamoate	Vistaril	25–100 mg.
Mephenoxalone	Trepidone	400 mg.
Meprobamate N.F.	Equanil; Miltown	400 mg.
Oxanamide	Quiactin	400 mg.
Oxazepam	Serax	10–30 mg.
Phenaglycodol	Ultran	300 mg.
Phenyltoloxamine	Bristamin	25–50 mg.
Pipethanate HCl	Sycotrol	3–6 mg.
Tybamate	Solacen	125–250 mg.

azepoxide * (Librium) offer any real advantage over the barbiturate-type sedatives is more complicated and controversial. Among the advantages claimed for the newer drugs are the following: (1) They relieve anxiety and tension without causing the drowsiness and confusion sometimes seen when barbiturates are employed. (2) They are less likely to lead to habituation in patients who tend to take excessive amounts of sedative drugs. (3) They are less likely to cause coma and other signs of severe toxicity, in the event of accidental or deliberate overdosage. (4) They have, in addition to their tranquilizing action, a wide variety of peripheral and C.N.S. effects, which may make them doubly useful in treating patients whose illnesses have both physical and emotional components.

Clinical Indications. Like the barbiturates, these drugs are used in a wide variety of clinical conditions ranging from the mild emotional upsets of people faced with stressful life situations to moderately severe psychiatric reactions in which the patient's behavior is for a time severely disturbed (e.g., acute alcoholic delirium). In addition, the combined mental and physical actions of these drugs are said to make them especially useful because they not only relieve anxiety but also allay other symptoms that occur secondary to tension. Conversely, the drugs may help to overcome emotional distress that is caused by disabling, painful, or annoying conditions.

For example, meprobamate and several more or less related compounds possess the ability to relax skeletal muscle spasm and tension. This, of course, makes these drugs doubly useful for patients who are emotionally upset because of painful musculoskeletal conditions, including arthritis. Neurotic and alcoholic patients in whom muscle tension and tremors are a source of discomfort may get relief by the use of these muscle-relaxing tranquilizers.

These drugs are useful for relieving the nervous tension that often accompanies other conditions also. Given alone, or combined with more specifically acting drugs, they are used to counteract the emotional component of various illnesses that are either caused or made worse by anxiety and tension.

Hydroxyzine * (Atarax, Vistaril), for example, has several actions which may be beneficial in such conditions. Its antihistaminic action may help counteract itching in allergic skin conditions; the antiemetic effect may overcome nausea and vomiting, and the antispasmodic action relieves painful gastrointestinal smooth muscle spasm. It should be noted, however, that hydroxyzine is commonly combined with a more potent antispasmodic drug in such cases. This may indicate that the drug's calming effects are considered more effective than its smooth muscle relaxing properties.

* See also Drug Digests.

Generally, in such psychosomatic and somatopsychic conditions, the minor tranquilizers are combined with other drugs. Thus, meprobamate (Equanil, Miltown) is available (1) in combination with estrogens, for treating menopausal symptoms, (2) in combination with corticosteroids, for arthritis, (3) in combination with nitrites, for angina pectoris and coronary artery insufficiency, (4) in combination with synthetic atropinelike drugs, for peptic ulcer, pylorospasm, and other gastrointestinal conditions. In all of these conditions, the tranquilizer plays the same part as do the barbiturates found in older drug products—it reduces the anxiety which may be either the underlying *cause* of the patient's condition or the *result* of the patient's response to pain and other discomforting symptoms.

Occasionally, the minor tranquilizers may be given by injection to control delirium and severe states of agitation. Chlordiazepoxide (Librium), for example, and its close relative, the somewhat more potent agent diazepam (Valium), have been employed during alcoholic withdrawal, in states of panic and hysteria, and even for quieting acute psychotic reactions in schizophrenia and agitated depression. However, these antianxiety agents of the benzodiazepine subclass, like the glyceryl derivatives, meprobamate, tybamate, and the other chemical classes of minor tranquilizers, are not ordinarily used in the long-term management of the psychoses but are reserved mainly for managing less severe degrees of anxiety related to stress and to somatic complaints.

Side Effects and Precautions. The minor tranquilizers cause fewer side effects than the phenothiazine or rauwolfia derivatives. They are now usually preferred for those patients whose degree of anxiety and tension is relatively mild. Nonetheless, these drugs do cause a fairly high incidence of minor side effects. Most commonly, patients who are taking these drugs for the first time may tend to become drowsy. This in itself is not very serious, but these patients should be warned that their mental alertness, reflex responsiveness, and motor coordination may be diminished and should be cautioned not to drive an automobile or operate dangerous machinery.

It is often claimed that these drugs do not lend themselves to the sort of abuse sometimes seen with barbiturates; nevertheless, they must be used with caution when patients have a history of alcoholism, drug addiction, or personality disturbances. Meprobamate, for example, has been taken in highly excessive doses by the patient who typically tends to use depressant drugs to the point of intoxication. When a patient is found to have been doing this daily for long periods, the drug should not be withdrawn abruptly, because he may suffer a severe abstinence syndrome similar to that seen with barbiturates. The physically dependent meprobamate abuser may become increasingly nervous and tremorous, or have hallucinations, delirium, or epileptiform convulsions when the drug is withdrawn.

Acute toxicity has not occurred as commonly with these tranquilizers as with barbiturates. People have taken as much as 200 times the therapeutic dose of chlordiazepoxide and survived. However, a few fatalities have been reported in patients ingesting massive overdoses of meprobamate. Death is the result of prolonged coma, circulatory collapse, and respiratory failure. Management of toxic reactions is essentially similar to the measures described in acute barbiturate poisoning (Chap. 6).

The relative difficulty of succeeding in a suicide attempt with the minor tranquilizers may make them preferable for managing anxiety in agitated-depressed patients who are considered suicide risks; however, the claimed superiority for these drugs over the barbiturate-type sedatives in other respects is debatable. Some doctors believe that properly selected doses of the less expensive barbiturate drugs will bring about all the desirable calming effects of the minor tranquilizers with no more drowsiness or other side effects than are caused by these supposedly safer agents.

ANTIDEPRESSANT DRUGS

The Nature of Depression

Mental depression is a very common psychiatric syndrome and a source of much anguish for many patients and their families. One authority has called depression "the most widespread, the most persistent, and the most frequently unrecognized emotional disorder that afflicts mankind." * He adds that "more human suffering has resulted from depression than from any other single disease." †

The term *depression* is used to describe a group of symptoms which vary widely in nature and severity. Such symptoms do not necessarily always require treatment. Thus, for example, depressed patients are often characterized as suffering from "feelings of sadness." However, all of us feel sad at times without necessarily being depressed in the sense of suffering from a symptom of mental illness. Indeed, it would be most remarkable if we did *not* feel sad after the loss of loved ones and other shocking events that are inevitable in the course of our lives.

Depression requires treatment only when its symptoms are severe and prolonged, that is, when the patient's reaction is entirely out of proportion to the event that triggered it or is caused by no readily

* Kline, N. S.: Depression: diagnosis and treatment, Med. Clin. North Amer., *45*:1041, 1961.

† Kline, N. S.: The practical management of depression. J.A.M.A., *190*:732, 1964.

discernible environmental difficulty at all. Among the depressive symptoms that most commonly indicate a condition needing treatment are feelings of fatigue, lack of interest in personal appearance, loss of appetite, and sleeplessness.

The patient may suffer a loss of self-esteem and say such things as "I am nothing" or "I am worthless." Typically, he may become apathetic and lose interest in people or affairs that had formerly engaged his attention. The patient may, for example, withdraw from participation in activities and decisions both at work and at home, perhaps saying "nothing seems worthwhile; nothing seems worth doing." Behavior cannot, however, be neatly categorized. Some patients may show mainly psychomotor retardation, a marked slowing down of all their activities; others may be in a state of psychomotor agitation, during which they move about constantly, complaining and voicing fears of impending disaster.

Treatments of various types are employed in the management of depression. Some kinds of neurotic depressive reactions respond only to psychotherapy. However, though support and reassurance are always desirable, deep or intensive psychotherapy is usually contraindicated in the more severe depressive reactions. Such patients often respond to a course of electroconvulsive therapy (ECT). Electroshock is employed less frequently for this purpose than it once was; however, many psychiatrists still depend upon it as a first line of attack in acutely suicidal patients.

In this section, we shall be concerned mainly with certain antidepressant drugs that have been introduced recently. Despite their dangers and drawbacks, these drugs are now considered the treatment of choice in most cases of depression.

Classes of Antidepressant Drugs

Until a few years ago the only drugs used in the management of depression were the psychomotor stimulants, such as the amphetamines and methylphenidate (Chap. 13), and sedatives such as the barbiturates, administered simultaneously or separately. At best, however, these drugs are useful only for patients with mild mood disturbances. For example, they may help to counteract fatigue and anxiety in someone suffering from grief after a family loss— a so-called *normal reactive depression*. Given alone or combined with barbiturates for a few days, the mood-lifting amphetamines may aid the saddened individual in making a quicker adjustment to his situation. However, these drugs are useless for more deeply depressed patients and may, in fact, make them worse by interfering further with their already disturbed sleep and appetite patterns.

Two important classes of antidepressant drugs have been developed in recent years. One group is referred to mainly as the monoamine oxidase (MAO) inhibitors; the other class is called by various names—central suppressants, psychostimulants, or tricyclic compounds—but it may be best to think of them as *non*-MAO inhibitors. In any case, despite suggestions that one type may be better than the other for certain categories of psychiatric depression, such specificity does not actually seem to exist. At present, there is no way for the doctor to decide in advance which of the two is better for a particular patient. In general, most doctors begin treatment with one of the *non*-MAO inhibitors, because these drugs cause fewer and less severe side effects, and patients do not have to be quite so closely supervised as do those who are taking one of the MAO inhibitors.

Clinical Indications. Antidepressant drugs of both types have brought about symptomatic relief in depression of varied clinical categories, including especially the following:

(1) The depressive phase of the manic-depressive psychosis, a condition characterized by alternating episodes of depression and elation. (2) Involutional melancholia, a condition occurring more commonly in women, especially those of menopausal age. (3) Certain so-called psychotic depressive reactions, in which patients misinterpret reality in ways that lead to suicidal ideas.

In all of these conditions, antidepressant drugs of each type may be used either alone or in conjunction with electroconvulsive therapy. If the patient fails to respond to one kind of drug, the doctor may gradually withdraw it and try an agent of the other class of antidepressants. Electroshock is reserved largely for patients unresponsive to drug therapy,

and even in such cases the drugs are often administered during the course of ECT as well as for a long time afterward. Used in this way, the drugs are said to reduce the number of shock treatments needed and the frequency of relapses.

Regardless of the treatment employed—drugs, ECT, psychotherapy, or a combination of all three—the nurse plays a most important role in helping the patient recover from his depressive episode. In consultation with the doctor, she may help the patient to understand the nature of his illness and what to expect from treatment, so that he can begin to cope more effectively with the stresses that he is experiencing. She helps the patient and his family to understand the need to follow his prescribed treatment very carefully. The nurse also aids the patient in performing his personal hygiene when he is still uninterested in his appearance, and she sees to it that he gets enough to eat despite his lack of interest in food. She should act at all times in a way that lets the patient and his family assume that his depression will eventually lift.

The MAO-Inhibitor Antidepressants (*Table 7-5*)

The prototype drug of this class, iproniazid (Marsilid), was introduced actually for treating tuberculosis. Psychiatrists who noted its tendency to make many tubercular patients euphoric decided to try it in mentally depressed patients. The drug proved dramatically effective for reducing symptoms of psychomotor regression and for providing relief of other aspects of depression. When iproniazid had to be withdrawn from the market because it caused liver damage, it was replaced by several antidepressant

TABLE 7-5
ANTIDEPRESSANT DRUGS

Nonproprietary Name	Trade Name	Usual Daily Dosage
Monoamine Oxidase Inhibitor Type (Psychic Energizers)		
Isocarboxazid	Marplan	10–30 mg.
Nialamide	Niamid	75–200 mg.
Phenelzine Sulfate	Nardil	45–75 mg.
Tranylcypromine Sulfate	Parnate	20–30 mg.
Non-MAO Inhibitor Type (Psychostimulants; Psychoanaleptics; Tricyclics)		
Amitriptyline HCl	Elavil	75–150 mg.
Desipramine	DMI; Norpramin; Pertofrane	75–150 mg.
Imipramine HCl N.F.	Tofranil	75–150 mg.
Nortriptyline	Aventyl	20–100 mg.

drugs that had a similar biochemical property—the ability to inhibit the brain enzyme, monoamine oxidase (MAO).

The Concept of MAO Inhibition. The exact role of the enzyme MAO, which is present in the liver and other body tissues as well as the brain, is not entirely understood. As indicated in Chapter 14, the enzyme plays a part in the inactivation of various biological amines. Among the amines detoxified by MAO are some substances ingested in foods (e.g., tyramine, a catecholamine present in large amounts in certain cheeses) and certain substances biosynthesized by the body itself such as serotonin and the adrenergic neurohormone, norepinephrine.

Since MAO is the enzyme mainly responsible for the inactivation of norepinephrine, drugs that interfere with MAO activity may lead to an increased level of that neurohormone in the brain, heart, and other organs. According to one view, this accumulation of norepinephrine and other amines in certain brain areas may account for the antidepressant effects of the MAO-inhibitor drugs. That is, the gradual increase in so-called psychic energy observed in depressed patients taking these drugs may be related to an increase, in the brain, in the amount of chemical transmitters of nerve impulses that lead to psychomotor activity.

Several MAO inhibitor antidepressants are presently in use. One chemical class, the hydrazines, includes nialamide * (Niamid), isocarboxazid (Marplan) and phenelzine (Nardil)—the most potent of this group. Another subclass, the *non*-hydrazines, includes pargyline (Chap. 23), which is used mainly for treating high blood pressure rather than depression, and tranylcypromine * (Parnate). Tranylcypromine differs from the others in possessing a more rapid onset of action. This early stimulation, which may be seen soon after treatment is started, may be the result of a direct amphetaminelike effect of tranylcypromine. However, its full antidepressant effects may not be manifested for two or three weeks or more, as is the case with the other MAO inhibitors, which act indirectly to increase brain amine stores.

The slow onset of antidepressant action is a drawback of these drugs that makes their use undesirable in acutely suicidal patients. In addition, the biochemical imbalance which the MAO inhibitors induce may persist long after the drugs have been withdrawn. This cumulative effect sometimes makes it difficult to deal with the various toxic actions caused by these drugs.

Side Effects and Toxicity. The MAO inhibitors cause serious reactions of several types, some of which have led doctors to question whether their therapeutic usefulness was high enough to warrant the risk of employing them. These ill effects include a variety

* See also Drug Digests.

of relatively minor side effects involving the central and autonomic nervous systems and very dangerous reactions such as drug-induced strokes and liver damage.

Hepatic damage resembling viral hepatitis has resulted from the use of iproniazid and pheniprazine, two hydrazine-type MAO inhibitors which had to be withdrawn from the market after a number of fatalities were reported. Hepatitis has not been a problem with newer antidepressants such as phenelzine and tranylcypromine. However, even with the safer enzyme inhibitors, the doctor orders liver function tests periodically as a precaution and avoids administering them to patients with a history of liver disease.

Central nervous system side effects of the MAO inhibitors seem to be the result of overstimulation. Some patients tend to become restless and hyperactive and may, in fact, show symptoms of agitation to the point of mania. To avoid such increased anxiety, antidepressants such as tranylcypromine are sometimes administered together with a phenothiazine tranquilizer (e.g., trifluoperazine). Another C.N.S. effect that sometimes occurs is the development of muscle spasm and tremors. Thus, special caution is required with these drugs in treating epileptic patients who are depressed.

The autonomic blocking effects of the MAO-inhibitor antidepressants include mouth dryness, constipation, blurring of vision, and cardiac palpitation. Much more serious, however, are the effects of these drugs on blood pressure. Most common and most difficult to deal with is postural hypotension, a sharp fall in blood pressure that occurs when the patient stands up. Signs of this drug-induced condition include dizziness or lightheadedness and, occasionally, fainting.

Less frequent but more serious is the rapid rise in blood pressure sometimes found with the MAO inhibitors. Tranylcypromine, for example, has caused hypertensive crises some of which have led to intracranial bleeding and death. This dangerous reaction, which is heralded by a sudden severe headache, is believed to be the result of the ability of the MAO inhibitors to potentiate the effects of circulating catecholamine vasoconstrictor chemicals. Such vasopressor substances may be produced by the patient's own adrenal glands and sympathetic nerves. Small amounts of pressor amines may also be contained in various cheeses and wines that the patient may ingest. Thus, patients must be warned not to indulge in these foods and beverages while under treatment with tranylcypromine and related MAO-inhibitor agents that may tend to convert ordinarily harmless amines into dangerous pressure raisers.

The effects of adrenergic drugs may be intensified by these antidepressant drugs. Thus, the use of amphetamine-type preparations or medications for the common cold or hay fever which contain vasoconstrictors (e.g., nasal decongestants) may lead to headaches and hypertensive reactions in patients on these antidepressant drugs. Therefore, such patients should be warned not to treat themselves with any medication not prescribed by the doctor.

The MAO inhibitors tend to delay the detoxification of many kinds of drugs, including central nervous system stimulants such as caffeine and depressants such as alcohol, barbiturates, antihistamines, and narcotics. Thus, the patient has to limit his intake of coffee, tea, and cola drinks, and the doctor has to prescribe the depressant drugs in low doses lest their effects be excessively potentiated.

Antidepressants of the MAO inhibitor type are never prescribed in combination with those of the psychostimulant or tricyclic type discussed below. Patients who have taken drugs of both types together have sometimes suffered very severe reactions, apparently because the MAO inhibitors potentiate certain atropinelike C.N.S. and peripheral effects of the agents of the second class. People taking overdoses of the two kinds of drugs have had bouts of extremely high fever (up to 109° F.) followed by muscular rigidity, collapse, coma, and death.

Thus, if a doctor wants to discontinue the use of MAO-inhibitor drugs because they have not helped his patient, he must wait at least a week after the drug is discontinued—and sometimes, in the case of the more cumulative drugs, as long as three weeks—before starting the patient on one of the *non*-MAO inhibitor antidepressants. On the other hand, patients may usually be switched from the latter drugs to one of the MAO inhibitors after a delay of only a few days.

The Non-MAO Inhibitor Antidepressants (Table 7-5)

Mechanism. A class of compounds that are similar in chemical structure to the phenothiazine tranquilizers has proved useful in the treatment of depressed patients. These drugs do not act by raising brain amine levels through the inhibition of MAO. It is thought that they may somehow make certain brain cells more sensitive to the stimulating action of the central neurohormones already present. In any case, the drugs that have been called central suppressants, psychostimulants, and—because of their chemical structure (Table 7-6)—tricyclic compounds, are considered the safest drugs with which to begin the treatment of depression.

Clinical Uses. One drug of this class, imipramine (Tofranil), has helped about two thirds of the severely depressed patients receiving it. Its effects come on more rapidly than those of the MAO inhibitors, but it takes several weeks for the action of this drug also to reach optimal effectiveness; there-

TABLE 7-6
NON-PHENOTHIAZINE ANTIPSYCHOTIC AND ANTIDEPRESSANT DRUGS

Antipsychotic Agents
Chloroprothixene (Taractan)

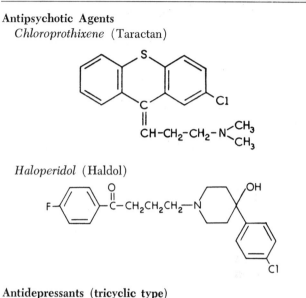

Haloperidol (Haldol)

Antidepressants (tricyclic type)
Imipramine (Tofranil)
Desipramine (DMI, and others) is identical except that
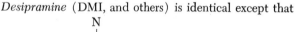
the side chain is CH—CH—CH—NHCH (one of the methyl groups has been dropped and replaced by a hydrogen attached to N)

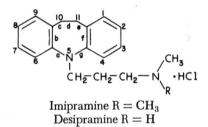

Imipramine R = CH₃
Desipramine R = H

Amitriptyline (Elavil)
Nortriptyline (Aventyl) is identical except that the side chain is —CHCH—CH—NHCH (one of the methyl groups has been replaced by a hydrogen)

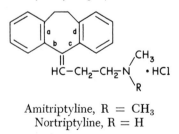

Amitriptyline, R = CH₃
Nortriptyline, R = H

Note the structural resemblance of these useful psychotropic drugs to the phenothiazine structure (Table 7-1).

fore, the doctor usually continues the drug for about four to six weeks even when few benefits are apparent.

Imipramine must first be converted in the liver to an active metabolite, desipramine, which is believed to be responsible for the desirable effects brought about in the brain. Recently, desipramine has been prepared synthetically and has been introduced commercially as Norpramin and Pertofrane. It is said to act more rapidly than imipramine. Its beneficial effects are often seen in two to four days and reach their peak in about ten days to two weeks. If no benefits have been obtained by then, the doctor may discontinue the drug and try treating the patient with one of the MAO inhibitors. Both imipramine and its derivative desipramine seem to work best in the depressed patients who show psychomotor retardation rather than agitation.

Amitriptyline * (Elavil), a drug closely related to imipramine, seems best for depressed patients who are also anxious and tense. That is, it seems to have some early tranquilizing effect as well as a slowly developing antidepressant effect. However, some patients tend to become very agitated during treatment with any antidepressant drug, and the addition of one of the major or minor tranquilizers to the regimen of these patients is required in order to keep them calm, even while they are taking amitriptyline.

Recently, a derivative of this drug, nortriptyline (Aventyl), has been introduced. This new non-MAO inhibitor antidepressant is said to have a more rapid onset of action than the parent compound, amitriptyline. It is claimed to be capable of producing both stimulating and quieting effects on behavior. Thus, its use is suggested for its early sedative and late antidepressant effects in cases of agitated depression and for its activating action on depressed patients with psychomotor retardation symptoms.

None of these drugs are given in combination with MAO-inhibitor antidepressants, but doctors may sometimes order the administration of both imipramine and amitriptyline for the same patient. For example, imipramine may be given early in the day at a time when psychomotor retardation is most marked in depressed patients. Later, amitriptyline or nortriptyline may be administered to provide sedation in the late afternoon and evening, along with the antidepressant action.

Side Effects and Toxicity. The tricyclic psychostimulant antidepressants have not caused the kind of liver damage or the severe hypertensive crises sometimes found with the MAO inhibitors. They are also much less likely to cause postural hypotensive episodes or potentiation of the effects of other medicines that are administered concurrently. These drugs do, however, produce side effects of one sort or another in about

* See also Drug Digest.

one out of four patients taking them. These discomforting effects are mainly the result of autonomic blockade and C.N.S. stimulation.

The autonomic side effects are mainly of the anticholinergic or atropinelike type and include mouth dryness, blurring of vision, constipation, and delayed urination. This means that imipramine, amitriptyline and their derivatives must be administered cautiously if at all to patients with a history of glaucoma and to elderly male patients with prostatic enlargement. These drugs can also cause excessive sweating and tachycardia, perhaps because of an adrenergic component in their action. Hypotension, jaundice, and blood dyscrasias are rare. However, the doctor may order laboratory tests of the patient's liver function and blood picture periodically.

The C.N.S. side effects may take the form of either drowsiness or restlessness along with confusion, dizziness and headaches. Depressed schizophrenic patients especially are likely to become unduly agitated when being treated with these psychostimulants and may require phenothiazine tranquilizers or sedation with other agents. The imipramine-type agents are most likely to cause insomnia and nervousness, or mild muscle tremors and twitching. Caution is required in epileptic patients because of hyperreflexia induced by these drugs.

The Status of Antidepressant Drugs

Most psychiatrists agree that, although drugs are not any more effective than electroconvulsive therapy against severe depressions, they have various advantages in many cases. For example, patients can continue to work while taking drugs, because they do not suffer the memory impairment that sometimes follows ECT. Patients are also much more willing to take drugs than to receive electroshock therapy. Finally, despite their side effects and occasional severe and even fatal reactions, drugs are considered safer than ECT when they are properly prescribed and the patient is closely supervised.

Once the depressed patient recovers from his depressive episode, an attempt is made to reduce the daily dosage gradually and, finally, to discontinue drug treatment entirely after a few months. However, patients who suffer from recurrent depressions may continue to receive the drug indefinitely to prevent relapses. If a depressive reaction does occur, the drugs seem to help reduce its severity and increase the patient's responsiveness to electroshock or chemoshock therapy.

OTHER PSYCHOTROPIC AGENTS

Two other types of psychotropic drugs deserve brief consideration here, although their use as psychotherapeutic agents is relatively limited. These are (1) the *pharmacoconvulsants* (drugs used occasionally as substitutes for electroshock therapy), and (2) the *psychotomimetics*—agents that produce hallucinations and other mental aberrations but, nonetheless, may have a place in the treatment of mental and emotional illness.

Pharmacoconvulsants. The first deliberately induced therapeutic convulsions were brought about by the administration of pentylenetetrazol (Metrazol) (Chap. 13). For reasons that are no better understood than is the theoretical basis for the other somatic psychiatric treatments, including insulin shock and electroconvulsive shock therapy, many schizophrenic and depressed patients seemed to improve after a series of chemoshock treatments with this central nervous system stimulant. However, pentylenetetrazol fell out of favor in comparison with ECT, which is easier to administer and does not precipitate the feeling of fear that patients complained about after the drug therapy. (When pentylenetetrazol is injected by vein, patients often experience a feeling of dread, or "impending doom" in the moments before the convulsions occur.)

Recently, however, interest has been aroused in a new pharmacoconvulsant, flurothyl (Indoklon). The drug was discovered accidentally during a search for fluorinated ether anesthetics (Chap. 13). Instead of producing unconsciousness, inhalation of this chemical caused strong tonic and clonic convulsions. Consequently, the drug has been studied for several years for its possible utility as a somatic treatment in psychiatry. The chemical was recently introduced commercially as a substitute for ECT in the treatment of schizophrenia and depressive psychoses. Despite various claims made for the advantages of flurothyl inhalation over ECT, the place of this pharmacoconvulsant in psychiatric therapy remains to be established.

Psychotomimetic Drugs. A group of psychotropic chemicals that tend to produce bizarre mental effects has had little psychotherapeutic utility. However, reports of these drugs—called, among other names, psychotomimetics, hallucinogenics, psychodysleptics, and psychedelics—have created so much public interest and medical concern that they deserve brief mention here.

The most intensively studied drugs of this class, lysergic acid diethylamide (LSD-25), mescaline, and psilocybin (Table 7-7), are similar in their ability to produce frequent visual hallucinations and illusions, and occasional paranoid delusions. For this reason, they have been called "psychotomimetics"—drugs whose effects mimic or imitate those of psychoses. Reports that such symptoms are sometimes elicited by extremely minute amounts of LSD have stimulated research concerning the concept that schizophrenia and other natural mental illnesses may stem from

TABLE 7-7

PSYCHOTOMIMETIC (HALLUCINOGENIC) AGENTS

Adrenochrome	Mescaline
Adrenolutin	Morning glory seeds
Bufotenine	Nutmeg (Myristica)
Dimethyltryptamine (DMT)	Peyote
Ibogaine	Phenycyclidine (Sernylan)
Lysergic Acid Diethylamide (LSD-25, Delysid)	Psilocybin
	STP (Dom)

biochemical imbalances in which metabolites produced in the body in small amounts may similarly affect brain function adversely.

However, despite their relative potency, the mental state produced by these drugs does not really differ significantly from toxic psychoses caused by overdosage with certain other drugs, and any resemblance to schizophrenia and other naturally occurring mental illness seems merely coincidental.

These drugs are not presently available for prescription use. They have, however, been widely employed on a research basis for psychotherapeutic purposes. LSD, for example, has been employed as an adjunct to psychotherapy in the treatment of chronic psychoneuroses, alcoholism, and other personality disorders that are difficult to treat. Despite occasional enthusiastic reports (some of which have been widely publicized) that remarkable changes in the basic attitudes and personality of these patients have been brought about by combined pharmacotherapy and psychotherapy, none of these drugs can be considered to be safe or effective treatment for any psychiatric condition at this time.

The use of these psychotropic drugs has reportedly precipitated prolonged psychotic reactions and suicide attempts, even in patients being treated by qualified psychiatrists. Thus, the dangers of self-administration are obvious. Yet there are indications that these agents are being widely abused, both by individuals of the type that commonly seeks "kicks" from chemical substances, and by others who claim that these drugs produce experiences that should be classed as religious or artistic.

The latter prefer to refer to the effects of these drugs as "psychedelic," a term that means "mind manifesting" and implies that these drugs have the ability to expand human consciousness into areas normally closed to us. It seems evident that some people do respond to these drugs with intense, highly personal emotional reactions; however, the validity of the implication that this is desirable has not been proved, whereas the undesirability of unsupervised and indiscriminate self-administration of these drugs seems clear.

Complications of self-experimentation with LSD include development of a sense of uncontrollable terror. Such panic reactions, or "bad trips," can usually be quickly controlled by the parenteral administration of a phenothiazine-type tranquilizer. Some patients—possibly prepsychotic or schizophrenic to begin with—have, on the other hand, had to be hospitalized for extensive periods after ingesting a single dose of LSD. Others have suffered from the sudden reappearance of hallucinations as long as a year or more after taking their last dose of LSD.

Although this drug has not yet been proved to cause permanent organic damage, recent studies indicate that LSD may be both neoplastic and teratogenic. Leukocytes of users have, for example, been shown to have a chromosome breakage rate considerably above normal. The offspring of rats injected with LSD early in pregnancy have been stillborn and stunted; and mice treated in the same way have given birth to litters with malformations and brain defects. At least one seriously deformed child has reportedly been born to a woman known to have taken a dose of LSD.

In addition to violent homicidal and suicidal deaths, several accidental fatalities have been reported in LSD users. Some have fallen from heights during attempts to fly; others have been hit while walking on busy roads in the belief that they were invulnerable to injury by speeding vehicles.

Thus, although this drug and such other psychotomimetics as the related agent dimethyltryptamine (DMT) do not cause physical dependence, and although tolerance to their actions disappears rather rapidly between periodic sprees, their potential hazards are considered very great. Unfortunately, the number of newly synthesized drugs of this class is likely to increase in the near future, and there will be no dearth of maladjusted young people willing to take such substances in the misguided belief that these drugs offer them an opportunity to gain insights into the nature of their "souls," their relationships to others and indeed, to the "cosmos."

Marihuana, a preparation of the leaves and flowering tops of the cannabis plant, may also be classed with these abused drugs. While technically not a psychotomimetic agent, it has the capacity to cause hallucinations in some circumstances. These reportedly appear with very large doses which may also set off acute panic reactions. Even occasional exposure to small doses may have adverse effects upon the personality and behavior of an individual already predisposed to mental imbalance. Inasmuch as users of marihuana probably include a disproportionately high number of young people with psychiatric problems, authorities generally agree that it would be undesirable to legalize the uncontrolled use of marihuana.

On the other hand, most of these same authorities also believe that the legal penalties presently imposed for possession and use of marihuana are disproportionately severe in comparison to the actual dangers of this substance, which has not yet been proved to produce any lasting mental or physical damage, nor physical dependence and tolerance. Despite the view of certain law enforcement groups that the smoking of marihuana leads almost inevitably to the use of heroin and other dangerous drugs, most people who experiment with marihuana do *not* go on to become addicted to narcotics. However, the attitudes of rebellion against authority and thrill seeking which foster much marihuana smoking may lead some youngsters into more seriously delinquent acts than the violation of the laws prohibiting possession of this substance.

Despite all the emotional controversy evoked by conflicting social attitudes toward this drug, surprisingly little scientific evidence has been available concerning the psychopharmacological effects of marihuana. This has been due in part to the difficulties of subjecting a crude plant product of variable content to quantitative pharmacological study. Recently, however, a substance believed to be the active constituent of cannabis has been isolated and synthesized. Pharmacologists hope that through the study of the effects of this intoxicant, called tetrahydrocannabinol (THC), on the brain it will soon become possible to gain factual data that will aid in determining what place, if any, marihuana should have in our society.

SUMMARY OF CLINICAL INDICATIONS FOR PHENOTHIAZINE DERIVATIVES

- *Psychiatric Indications*
  A. For control of extreme excitement and agitation in acute and chronic psychotic conditions, including: the schizophrenias; the manic phase of the manic depressive psychosis; acute alcoholic intoxication and delirium tremens; involutional and senile psychoses.
  B. For "activating" withdrawn, regressed types of previously refractory chronic schizophrenics. (Piperazine subgroup drugs such as fluphenazine, trifluoperazine, and carphenazine are preferred for this particular purpose.)
  C. For relief of anxiety, tension, and confusion in neurotic and psychosomatic patients. ("Minor" tranquilizers may be preferred for this purpose because of lower toxicity.)

- *Non-Psychiatric Indications* (general medicine and surgery)
  A. *Antiemetic* for control of nausea and vomiting in many medical conditions (see Chap. 38) and postoperatively during recovery from anesthesia. (Hiccups and retching may also be controlled.)
  B. *Potentiator* of narcotic-analgesic agents in the relief of intractable pain (e.g., in terminal cancer) and postoperatively. (The use of phenothiazines both permits and requires reduced dosage of narcotics, sedative-hypnotics, and anesthetics.)
  C. *Premedication* prior to anesthesia for surgery and obstetrics for desirable sedative, antiemetic, and analgesia-potentiating actions.

SUMMARY OF ADVERSE REACTIONS TO PHENOTHIAZINES AND WAYS TO PREVENT OR COUNTERACT THEM

- *Central Nervous System Side Effects*
  A. *Depression*
    a. Drowsiness, lethargy, feelings of fatigue, which can usually be controlled by reducing the dose or by administering psychomotor stimulants (e.g., dextroamphetamine) in small amounts.
    b. Patients under influence of alcohol, barbiturates, or narcotics may be made comatose by administration of phenothiazines. These drugs should never be given to patients already comatose.
  B. *Stimulation:* extrapyramidal or neuromuscular reactions.
    a. *Pseudoparkinsonism:* tremors, rigidity, drooling, characteristic masklike facies and shuffling gait. Discontinue drug, or lower the dose and administer an antiparkinsonism agent concomitantly.
    b. *Dyskinesias* or *dystonias:* sudden muscular spasms resembling convulsive seizures. Control by discontinuing drug and, if necessary, administering an antiparkinsonism agent. Both barbiturates and caffeine sodium benzoate, as well as diphenhydra-

mine, have been reported to be successful for terminating dystonic seizures.
    c. *Akathisia* or *motor restlessness:* feelings of inner tension or jitteriness, restlessness, and insomnia. Dosage should be reduced, *not* increased; barbiturates may be desirable during this temporary turbulent phase.

- *Autonomic-Blockade-Type Side Effects*
  A. *Adrenergic blockade:* Reduced vasoconstrictor tone may cause fall in blood pressure, especially upon standing (postural hypotension). To prevent dizziness or fainting, patient should be kept lying down. If shocklike state develops, vasopressor drugs (e.g., norepinephrine, but *not* epinephrine) may be administered.
  B. *Cholinergic blockade:* atropine-type side effects, including mouth dryness, constipation, and blurring of vision. Fever may occur in hot weather because of failure to perspire.

- *Endocrine Imbalance Effects*
  A. Breast engorgement and lactation may occur in females receiving large doses.
  B. Amenorrhea and false pregnancy tests.
  C. Increased appetite and weight gain.

- *Hypersensitivity-Type Reactions*
  A. *Cholestatic jaundice* has occurred with chlorpromazine. Condition usually clears up rapidly when the drug is withdrawn, but, because the symptoms resemble those of extrahepatic obstruction, laparotomy may be performed if symptoms fail to clear up after some time.
  B. *Blood dyscrasias,* including leukopenia and agranulocytosis, require discontinuance of drug and administration of antibiotics for prophylaxis and treatment of infections.
  C. *Dermatological reactions* include urticaria, rashes, and, rarely, exfoliative dermatitis. Possible photosensitivity reactions make it advisable that patients not be exposed to the sun for long periods.

SUMMARY OF CAUTIONS AND CONTRAINDICATIONS IN THE USE OF ANTIDEPRESSANT DRUGS

- Indirect stimulating drugs of the MAO-inhibitor type must not be given in combination with C.N.S. suppressants such as imipramine and amitriptyline. At least two weeks must be allowed to elapse after discontinuance of MAO-inhibitor therapy before the other kind of antidepressant medication is initiated.

- Patients receiving MAO-inhibitor antidepressants should be watched carefully for reactions when receiving other drugs, the effects of which may be intensified. Among the drugs which may be dangerously potentiated are sympathomimetics (e.g., in nose drops and weight-reducing medications); C.N.S. depressants such as alcohol, barbiturates, tranquilizers, narcotics, and antiparkinsonism drugs; antihypertensive agents. The patient's diet should also be considered, because ingestion of cheeses has reportedly caused hypertensive reactions in patients taking MAO-inhibitor drugs.

- These enzyme-inhibiting drugs must not be administered to patients with cerebrovascular defects and cardiovascular disorders, because of the danger to these patients of possible *hyper*tensive and *hypo*tensive reactions.

- Because of their atropinelike actions, the C.N.S. suppressants imipramine and amitriptyline are contraindicated in patients with prostatic hypertrophy and glaucoma. These drugs should be used with caution when patients are epileptic.

- Antidepressant drugs of either type should be used cautiously in patients who seem anxious or agitated. Concurrent administration of phenothiazine tranquilizers is desirable to prevent aggravation of excitement by the antidepressants.

- Patients taking the MAO inhibitors for a prolonged time should have liver function tests performed periodically. The drugs are contraindicated in patients with a history of hepatic disease or with impaired renal function.

- Patients with suicidal tendencies should be watched carefully, especially when their energy levels begin to rise in response to the actions of the antidepressant drugs. Electroconvulsive therapy may be desirable in such cases.

SUMMARY OF POINTS THAT THE NURSE SHOULD REMEMBER IN ADMINISTERING PSYCHO-THERAPEUTIC DRUGS

• Remember that suicide is an ever-present hazard, particularly with depressed patients. Because drugs may be hoarded and used later in a suicidal attempt, it is important to be observant when administering medication. For example, stay with the patient until he has taken his medicine, and be especially careful to keep the medicine cabinet locked. However, avoid assuming a manner that conveys distrust of the patient. Make your observations, and carry out safety practices in a matter-of-fact, not a punitive, way.

• Note the patient's physiological and emotional responses to drug therapy. For instance, observe whether he seems less anxious, and whether side effects such as weakness, drowsiness or nervousness occur. Does the patient take the drug willingly, or does he seem to fear it? Discuss with the physician any unusual reactions to the drug or to its administration. Help the patient to understand the purpose of the treatment, and the way in which it is expected to help him.

• Care should be taken when giving injections of phenothiazine tranquilizers intramuscularly to avoid accidental injection into a vein or leakage into subcutaneous tissues.

Patients should be kept lying down for at least one half hour after such injections, because of the danger of postural hypotensive reactions. Elderly patients are especially susceptible to such reactions; their period of rest in the horizontal position after such in-jections may need to be somewhat longer. Regardless of the route of administration of the drug, remember that side effects such as dizziness and fainting can result in falls. Observe carefully for these symptoms, and, if they occur, instruct the patient to sit down or, preferably, to lie down.

• Patients taking phenothiazines should not be exposed to excessive sunlight because of the possible occurrence of photosensitivity-type skin reactions. Patients should be kept cool in hot weather because of possible atropinelike fever reactions to both phenothiazines and antidepressants.

• Advise against taking psychotherapeutic drugs without prescription; encourage inquirers to consult physicians about symptoms such as nervousness and insomnia, so that appropriate therapy can be instituted.

• Avoid conveying to the psychiatric patient any implication that his illness is willful or that psychotherapeutic drugs are being administered as a somehow shameful necessity rather than as a legitimate aspect of therapy. Thus, your attitude should not say, in effect, "If you'd just get hold of yourself, you wouldn't need this medication." This is no more justified than it would be to tell the patient with pneumonia that he wouldn't need to be taking antibiotics if he would only cooperate and pull himself together.

REVIEW QUESTIONS

Major and Minor Tranquilizers

1. Differentiate between the following terms:
   (a) Psychotropic agents
   (b) Psycholeptic or ataractic agents
   (c) Psychotomimetic agents

2. (a) Differentiate between the so-called *major* and *minor* tranquilizers.
   (b) How do tranquilizers of both types differ from the barbiturates and other psychosedatives?

3. (a) List the three pharmacological actions of the phenothiazine derivatives upon the central nervous system that make them useful in several clinical situations, including non-psychiatric conditions.
   (b) List several psychiatric conditions in which the phenothiazine tranquilizers are used for controlling extreme restlessness and agitation.

4. List several drugs of each of the three chemical subgroups of phenothiazines and state the specific psychotherapeutic indications for which drugs of each subgroup may be preferred.

5. Indicate how the effects of the phenothiazines and other major tranquilizers may alter the behavior of a psy-

chiatric patient in ways that favorably influence his recovery both within the hospital and at home.

6. (a) How do the central nervous system side effects of drugs of the dimethylamine subgroup of phenothiazines tend to differ in general from those of the piperazine subgroup?

(b) What are the three categories of extrapyramidal system reactions commonly observed with large doses of phenothiazine drugs of the piperazine subgroup?

7. (a) List side effects caused by blockade of sympathetic and parasympathetic nerve impulses by the phenothiazine tranquilizers.

(b) List three types of hypersensitivity reactions reported to occur with phenothiazine tranquilizers.

8. (a) What precautions should be taken when injecting phenothiazine tranquilizers intramuscularly in order to avoid systemic and local side effects?

(b) What adjunctive drugs may the doctor order to counteract the various central nervous system side effects of the phenothiazines?

9. (a) What advantages of the minor tranquilizers often lead the doctor to order them rather than major tranquilizers for managing anxiety in non-psychotic patients?

(b) What advantages may the minor tranquilizers possess over the barbiturates and similar psychosedatives in the management of the kinds of anxiety in which drugs of both types are indicated?

10. (a) List some secondary (non-tranquilizing) actions of meprobamate and hydroxyzine and indicate some clinical conditions which may be especially benefited by the combination of these effects and sedation.

(b) List several conditions with psychosomatic or somatopsychic components which are treated by combining meprobamate with various drugs that specifically affect the physical component.

11. (a) What warning should be given to patients beginning treatment with minor tranquilizers such as meprobamate, chlordiazepoxide, and hydroxyzine?

(b) Why may the doctor be cautious in ordering minor tranquilizers for patients with a history of alcoholism, drug addiction, and personality disturbance?

12. (a) Why may the doctor order one of the minor tranquilizers rather than a barbiturate, for treating anxiety in a potentially suicidal patient?

(b) Why are both barbiturates and minor tranquilizers withdrawn slowly from patients who are found to have been taking large overdoses for long periods?

Antidepressant and Other Psychotropic Drugs

1. (a) List three categories of mental depression that are treated with antidepressant drugs.

(b) List some ways in which the nurse can help the depressed patient who is taking antidepressant drugs.

2. (a) Discuss briefly the theory of the manner in which the drugs of the monoamine-oxidase-inhibitor (MAOI) class produce their antidepressant effects.

(b) Discuss briefly one suggested way in which the non-MAOI antidepressant drugs may act to produce their desirable mental effects.

3. (a) List two drawbacks of the earlier MAOI drugs which have not been a problem when the newer antidepressant drug, tranylcypromine (Parnate) is employed.

(b) State a serious toxic reaction which has been encountered more commonly in patients treated with tranylcypromine than with other MAOI antidepressants and indicate in what type of patient this drug is contraindicated for this reason.

4. (a) What precaution does the doctor take in treating patients for long periods with drugs of the MAOI class?

(b) What other drugs must be especially avoided by patients taking MAOI antidepressants?

(c) What precaution does the doctor take in discontinuing therapy with MAOI drugs and in shifting to a non-MAOI antidepressant?

(d) What are some common C.N.S. and autonomic side effects seen with antidepressants of the MAOI type?

5. (a) For depressed patients of what type do the drugs of the non-MAOI or tricyclic class seem superior?

(b) What drugs are commonly added to the regimen of patients taking these antidepressants?

6. (a) List some side effects commonly seen in patients taking non-MAOI-inhibitor antidepressant drugs such as imipramine (Tofranil).

(b) In what patients must this drug and the related tricyclic compound, amitriptyline (Elavil), be administered with caution?

7. (a) What forms of treatment besides antidepressant drugs are employed in the management of mental depression?

(b) What is the relative status of the several types of antidepressant therapy at present?

8. (a) List two pharmacoconvulsant drugs and indicate their current status in psychiatric treatment.

(b) List several psychotomimetic drugs and indicate the possible dangers in their indiscriminate use.

BIBLIOGRAPHY

Tranquilizers

Ayd, F. J., Jr.: A survey of drug-induced extrapyramidal reactions. J.A.M.A., *175*:102, 1961.

Berger, F. M.: The similarities and differences between meprobamate and barbiturates. Clin. Pharmacol. Ther., *4*:209, 1963 (March–April).

Bross, R. B.: The modern mood-changing drugs. Am. J. Nursing, *57*:1142, 1957.

Boyd, L. J., *et al.;* Meprobamate addiction. J.A.M.A., *168:* 1389, 1958.

Domino, E. F.: Human pharmacology of tranquilizing drugs. Clin. Pharmacol. Ther., *3*:599, 1962.

Hollister, L. E.: Complications from psychotherapeutic drugs. New Eng. J. Med., *264*:291–293, 343–347, 1961 (Feb. 9 and 16).

———: Adverse reactions to phenothiazines. J.A.M.A., *189*:311, 1964.

———: Overdoses of psychotherapeutic drugs. Clin. Pharmacol. Ther., *7*:142, 1966.

Hollister, L., and Kosek, J. C.: Sudden death and phenothiazine derivatives. J.A.M.A., *192*:1035, 1965.

Hordern, A.: Psychiatry and the tranquilizers. New Eng. J. Med., *265*:584–588, 634–638, 1961 (Sept. 21 and 26).

Kinross-Wright, J.: Newer phenothiazine drugs in treatment of nervous disorders. J.A.M.A., *170*:1283, 1959.

Kurland, A. A., *et al.:* Pilot study of Navane (thiothixene) in chronic schizophrenics and acute psychotic patients. Curr. Ther. Res., *9*:298, 1967.

Lynn, F. H., and Friedhoff, A. J.: The patient on a tranquilizing regimen. Am. J. Nursing, *60*:234, 1960.

Margolis, L., and Goble, J. L.: Lenticular opacities with prolonged phenothiazine therapy. J.A.M.A., *193*:7, 1965.

Mohr, R. C., and Mead, B. T.: Meprobamate addictions. New Eng. J. Med., *259*:965, 1958.

Rodman, M. J.: Where we stand today with the tranquilizers. R.N., *23*:45, 1960 (Feb.).

———: Drugs for safer sedation. R.N., *25*:61, 1962 (April).

Satanove, A.: Pigmentation due to phenothiazines in high and prolonged dosage. J.A.M.A., *191*:263, 1965.

Schiele, B. C.: Newer drugs for mental illness. J.A.M.A., *181*:126, 1962.

Schiele, B. C.: Haloperidol. Dis. Nerv. System, *28*:181, 1967.

Antidepressants, etc.

Cole, J. O.: The therapeutic efficacy of antidepressant drugs—a review. J.A.M.A., *190:448*, 1964.

Council on Drugs: Paradoxical hypertension from tranylcypromine sulfate. J.A.M.A., *186*:854, 1963.

Goldberg, L. I.: Monoamine oxidase inhibitors. J.A.M.A., *190*:456, 1964.

Horwitz, D., *et al.:* Monoamine oxidase inhibitors, tyramine, and cheese. J.A.M.A., *188*:1108, 1964.

Kline, N.: The practical management of depression. J.A.M.A., *190*:732, 1964.

———: Depression: diagnosis and treatment. Med. Clin. North Amer., *45*:1041, 1961 (July).

Luby, E. D., and Domino, E. F.: Toxicity from large doses of imipramine and an MAO inhibitor in suicidal intent. J.A.M.A., *177*:68, 1961.

Rodman, M. J.: Drugs that help the depressed. R.N., *23:* 37, 1960 (April).

———: Drugs for treating emotional-mental illness. R.N., *26*:67, 1963 (June).

Symposium on Indoklon. J. Neuropsychiatry, *4*:152, 1963.

Psychotomimetic Drugs

Cohen, S., and Eisner, B.: Use of lysergic acid diethylamide in a psychotherapeutic setting. Arch. Neurol., *81:* 615, 1959.

Cohen, S.: Lysergic acid diethylamide—side effects and complications. J. Nerv. Ment. Dis., *130*:39, 1960.

Cole, J. O., and Katz, M. M.: The psychotomimetic drugs. J.A.M.A., *187*:758, 1964.

Frederking, W.: Intoxicant drugs (mescaline and LSD) in psychotherapy. J. Nerv. Ment. Dis., *121*:262, 1955.

Irwin, S., and Egozcue, J.: Chromosomal abnormalities in leukocytes from LSD-25 users. Science, *157*:313, 1967.

Ludwig, A. M., and Levine, J.: Patterns of hallucinogenic drug abuse. J.A.M.A., *191*:92, 1965.

Report of the Committee on Alcoholism and Drug Dependence: Dependence on cannabis (marihuana). J.A.M.A., *201*:368, 1967.

Report of the Council on Mental Health and the Committee on Alcoholism and Drug Dependence: Dependence on LSD and other hallucinogenic drugs. J.A.M.A., *202*:47, 1967.

Sherwood, J. N., *et al.:* Psychedelic experience, a new concept in psychotherapy. J. Neuropsychiat., *4*:69, 1962.

· 8 ·

Anticonvulsant and Antispasmodic Drugs

Skeletal muscles respond to commands that come from the central nervous system. Even the simplest movements require a closely coordinated sequence of contractions and relaxations. These are brought about by volleys of nerve impulses that originate in groups of nerve nuclei and pass to the muscles with split-second timing by way of a complicated network of fiber tracts (Chap. 5).

Diseases or injuries that disrupt the rate at which nerve cells fire or which alter the number of nerve impulses arriving at the muscles may result in disabilities marked by muscular paralysis or spasticity. Among the neuromuscular disorders caused by excessive and poorly controlled nerve impulse transmission to skeletal muscles are the *epilepsies, Parkinson's disease, cerebral palsy* and many other disabling conditions.

In this chapter, we shall discuss several classes of drugs that are used to reduce the hyperactivity of motor nerves. Although no drug can repair disease-damaged motor neurons, agents are now available that lessen the number and severity of epileptic seizures, reduce the rigidity and tremors of parkinsonism, and relax the spasms and spasticity of other musculoskeletal and neurological disorders.

ANTIEPILEPTIC AGENTS

The Nature of Epilepsy

Epilepsy is a general term employed to describe several different types of seizure syndromes. All are the result of a sudden discharge of excessive numbers of nerve impulses from a relatively few abnormal neurons among the billions in the brain. Spreading from these focal areas, the explosions of electrical energy disrupt the functioning of otherwise normal nerve cells.

The different patterns of signs and symptoms that occur during a seizure depend mainly on the location of the focus and on the pathways that the volleys of nerve impulses take in traveling to near or distant parts of the nervous system. Seizures are classified in accordance with their predominant symptoms, the site of the abnormal neuronal focus, and the nature of the electroencephalogram, or EEG—the tracing of spikes, waves, and domes that records the electrical activity of the brain.

Epileptic attacks are divided into four major classes: grand mal, petit mal, psychomotor, and focal, or jacksonian, seizures. An accurate diagnosis is considered the first step toward proper treatment, because the available antiepileptic drugs usually tend to vary in their ability to control the several types of seizures. Sometimes, treatment is further complicated by the occurrence of mixed seizures in some patients.

General Considerations in Antiepileptic Drug Therapy

Drugs have been developed that are capable of reducing the number and severity of epileptic attacks. These agents are often called *anticonvulsants,* although convulsions do not necessarily occur in all types of seizures. Anticonvulsant drugs are believed to act mainly by reducing the responsiveness of normal neurons to the sudden storms of nervous impulses arising at the focal disturbance sites. Some drugs may depress the hyperirritable focus itself.

The goal of drug treatment in epilepsy is the complete control of seizures with doses that cause no adverse effects. No drug is capable of doing this in all cases. To achieve maximal control of seizures with minimal side effects and toxicity, the doctor must first select the best drug or combination of drugs for the

134

individual patient and then gradually adjust the dose to fit his needs.

The doctor usually begins treatment with a drug that is well established as being effective for the patient's particular seizure type and known to be of relatively low toxicity. *Phenobarbital* is an example of such a safe and often effective drug. Its dose is gradually raised until maximal control of seizures is obtained, or drug-induced drowsiness becomes too severe. When this happens, the dose of phenobarbital is gradually reduced and a second drug such as *diphenylhydantoin* or *trimethadione* (see Drug Digests) is added to the patient's regimen.

Sometimes, when such combinations of safe drugs still fail to control the patient's seizures, the doctor may have to turn to more toxic drugs. Some antiepileptic drugs are capable of causing serious toxicity, including skin reactions, liver or kidney damage and blood dyscrasias. Since the patient may be taking these drugs for long periods when he is not being seen by a doctor, the nurse must tell him and his relatives to be alert for skin rashes and discolorations, sore throat, and fever. These may be the first signs of toxic drug reactions requiring the withdrawal of the antiepileptic agent.

It is important, however, that drugs be discontinued gradually, as too sudden cessation of medication may increase the number and severity of seizures. Usually, control can quickly be re-established by re-instituting the medication. Sometimes, however, abrupt discontinuance of anticonvulsant drugs may precipitate status epilepticus, a succession of severe seizures which may end fatally.

Thus, in shifting a patient from one drug to another in the trial-and-error period, the doctor usually decreases the first drug gradually, while slowly raising the dose of the new drug up to its optimal level. The nurse can help in this situation by teaching the patient and his family the importance of taking his medication exactly as directed by the doctor. Co-operation between patient, doctor, and nurse is necessary for complete success in seizure control.

To play her proper part in the management of the epileptic patient, the nurse must be aware of the kinds of personal problems that beset people with these conditions. Patients with epilepsy have always been the victims of prejudice. Because of misconceptions still prevalent in the public mind, they are often subjected to ridicule and ostracism.

The ancient superstition that these people had been seized by demons has its modern counterpart in the irrational notion that epileptics are mentally incompetent and personally unreliable. This often makes it difficult for the person who admits to having epilepsy to obtain and hold a job. Personal discouragement and poverty often are factors in failure to take prescribed medications.

Thus, the nurse must consider these matters in her approach to both the epileptic patient and the public. She should always take time to ask the patient how he is getting along on his medication in order to find out whether he is actually taking it. Because lack of work and of the funds to buy drugs may be responsible for a deterioration of his condition, the nurse should try to detect the presence of such problems and report them to the doctor or the social worker.

Three out of four epilepsy patients can be kept seizure-free with modern drugs. If the patient is to receive the full benefits of the new drugs, the great gains that have been made in medical treatment must be matched by similar strides socially. Nurses who strive to dispel fear concerning the disease and ignorance of the true nature of epilepsy in their communities can help all patients with epilepsy to live happier and more productive lives.

Use of Drugs in Managing Specific Kinds of Seizures

Grand mal epilepsy is characterized by the periodic occurrence of sudden severe convulsive episodes. The seizure may be preceded by a brief aura—a warning that may take the form of flashes of light, special sounds, or other visual, auditory, or sensorimotor phenomena. In the next moment, the patient falls unconscious with an involuntary cry. This is followed by a series of tonic convulsions, in which the limbs are rigidly extended or flexed, and the muscles of respiration fail to function usefully. Because breathing stops for a time, the person may become cyanotic. These symmetrical spasms give way to a series of muscular tremors or jerks—the clonic convulsive phase—and then the patient begins to breathe again. Finally, he recovers consciousness and may then fall into an exhausted sleep.

The drug most commonly employed for preventing such seizures is *diphenylhydantoin* (Dilantin), which may be administered alone or combined with phenobarbital. Unlike the barbiturate or the bromides (the first antiepileptic drugs), diphenylhydantoin depresses the motor areas of the brain without causing excessive drowsiness. The drug does, however, often cause other side effects involving the nervous system, the gastrointestinal tract, and the skin. (See Drug Digest, and Summary of Side Effects, p. 138.)

A parenteral form of diphenylhydantoin is often useful for bringing status epilepticus episodes to a halt. Administered by vein, this drug seems to be safer than intravenous barbiturates for this purpose. This injectable solution may also be given intramuscularly for preventing convulsions during neurosurgical procedures and in the postoperative phase. After the danger is past in these conditions, the patient may still have to be maintained on oral dosage of diphenylhydantoin for many months or years.

Diphenylhydantoin seems able to depress abnormal electrical processes in nervous and other tissues without interfering with normal functional activity. In patients who are susceptible to seizures, for example, this drug protects normal neuronal tissue against the periodic sudden spread of high frequency nerve impulses from an epileptogenic focus. This is thought to stem from the drug's ability to depress *post-tetanic potentiation* (PTP), a property of synaptic transmission observed mainly in sustained states of seizure activity rather than during ordinary neuronal excitation.

Diphenylhydantoin does so, it is believed, by counteracting excessive leakage of sodium ions into the interior of the cell through its permeable membrane. This action against the abnormal ionic transport processes observed in states of neuronal hyperexcitability may be the result of the drug's capacity to stimulate the intracellular metabolic mechanisms by means of which such cells extrude sodium ions from the interior —that is, the so-called "sodium pump."

This stabilizing action of diphenylhydantoin upon cell membranes is apparently not limited to central motor neuronal systems. Thus, the drug is being tried at present in various clinical conditions that are thought to result from excessive cellular electrical activity. These disorders include cardiac arrythmias, trigeminal neuralgia, and even states of mental, emotional, and behavioral abnormality as well as the epilepsies.

Some cases of grand mal epilepsy not readily controlled by diphenylhydantoin may respond to certain chemically related agents. One of these, *mephenytoin* (Mesantoin), tends to cause fewer minor side effects than the parent drug; unfortunately, its use has reportedly resulted in severe toxicity, including fatal blood dyscrasias. Another hydantoin derivative, *ethotoin* (Peganone), seems relatively free of such toxicity. The fairly large oral doses required for full control of grand mal epilepsy tend to cause gastrointestinal disturbances. Such stomach upsets may be minimized by having the patient take this drug with food; however, ethotoin is best employed in smaller doses, combined with reduced amounts of diphenylhydantoin or phenobarbital, rather than alone.

Petit mal epilepsy occurs mainly in children and tends to disappear as they grow up. Attacks are characterized, not by convulsions, but by brief lapses in consciousness. The child may suddenly stop what he is doing and stare blankly for a few seconds. Such trancelike states may happen dozens of times a day. Sometimes, the patient also has a tendency toward grand mal seizures, which may predominate in adult life. Other patients suffer from certain variations of the simple or pure petit mal; such so called

"myoclonic" and "akinetic" seizures do not respond readily to drug therapy.

The most effective drug for treating most petit mal seizures is *trimethadione* (Tridione). It is usually ineffective against grand mal seizures and may even increase the number of major attacks. Thus, patients with mixed seizure patterns require an increase in phenobarbital-diphenylhydantoin dosage, when trimethadione is being given for control of the petit mal component. (See also Drug Digest on trimethadione.)

The usefulness of this drug is limited sometimes by its tendency to cause adverse effects. Often these are relatively minor (nausea, vomiting, and photophobia), but rare dangerous reactions, including bone marrow damage which may lead to agranulocytosis and aplastic anemia, and kidney damage resulting in nephrosis, have also been reported. The threat of such severe toxicity means that the nurse must emphasize to the patient and his family the importance of returning for the frequent blood and urine examinations which the doctors will advise. If these routine studies reveal signs of drug-induced illness, the doctor will order trimethadione to be gradually withdrawn and replaced by some other agent.

One such substitute, *paramethadione* (Paradione), a close chemical relative, is said to cause a lower incidence of side effects. For example, the photophobia that occurs in about one quarter of the patients taking trimethadione seems to be found less frequently with this drug. More important is the relative rarity of blood dyscrasias with paramethadione. Thus, the drug is best reserved for patients who develop toxic reactions to trimethadione. Some patients are best controlled by a combination of these two oxazalidinedione derivatives.

Another class of chemical compounds, the succinimides, have also proved useful in a certain percentage of petit mal cases. These drugs are said to be safer than trimethadione; however, when employed for a long time, periodic blood, kidney, and liver studies are desirable, because toxic effects have been reported for all drugs of this class, including the newest of these agents, *ethosuximide* (Zarontin) (see Drug Digest). This derivative is also said to differ from the others in that its long-term use has not been marked by development of tolerance.

Psychomotor seizures are characterized by changes in behavior. These usually take the form of automatic repetitions of some pattern of movements. (The patient may, for example, go through the motions of lighting a cigarette, starting a car, or completing some other series of acts in a stereotyped manner.) On the other hand, the patient's acts may sometimes become bizarre and, by attracting public attention and comment, bring him into difficulty with the law, which may look upon him as a psychiatric case. These seizures are often the most difficult both to diagnose and to treat with drugs.

Phenacemide (Phenurone), a drug sometimes effective in grand mal and in petit mal epilepsy, has also benefited patients suffering from psychomotor epilepsy. Because of its potentially toxic effects, however, this drug is generally reserved for patients with severe seizures that are unresponsive to safer drugs. When such patients are transferred to phenacemide therapy, the doctor takes many measures for detecting toxicity in its earliest stages.

The patient usually has to be hospitalized during the first weeks of treatment while the drug's dosage is being adjusted to a safe and effective level. At this time, the nurse must watch for the appearance of signs indicating possible drug-induced toxicity on the liver, brain, or bone marrow and report these to the doctor.

Jaundice is, of course, an indication of possible hepatic damage by the drug; it may be preceded by anorexia, nausea and vomiting or followed by fever and general malaise. Early mental side effects may include headaches, insomnia, and restlessness, in some cases, and apathy, in others. The latter is more serious, since a loss of interest may signal the start of mental depression. The doctor will probably order the drug withdrawn in such cases, because some psychomotor epilepsy patients have committed suicide while taking phenacemide.

Laboratory reports of differential blood counts and liver function tests also aid the doctor in monitoring the patient's responses to this dangerous drug. However, complaints of a sore mouth or throat, relayed to the doctor by the patient's nurse, help to alert him to the presence of possible agranulocytosis in the period between blood studies.

A less toxic drug sometimes successful in treating psychomotor epilepsy is *primidone* (Mysoline). This agent, which is also effective in grand mal but not in petit mal epilepsy, is often preferred to phenacemide because of its greater safety margin. It does, however, cause various side effects, some of which are uncomfortable enough to make the patient want to discontinue the drug. Sometimes, for example, the very first dose causes an acute illness marked by nausea, vomiting, dizziness, drowsiness, and headache. (See Drug Digest for further information.)

Miscellaneous Minor Drugs Used in Epilepsy

The many and varied side effects that tend to appear during the long-term administration of drugs for controlling epilepsy have led to a search for safe and effective substitutes. A number of agents have been introduced that are sometimes employed as adjuncts to the more potent anticonvulsants. These drugs are best used, not alone, but in combination

TABLE 8-1
DRUGS USED IN EPILEPSY SEIZURE MANAGEMENT

Nonproprietary Name and Trade Name	Main Indications *	Usual Daily Dosage Range (in Gm.)
Acetazolamide U.S.P. (Diamox)	PM, GM	0.375–1
Bromides (sodium, potassium, calcium, ammonium, lithium)	GM	1–3
Diphenylhydantoin U.S.P. (Dilantin)	GM, Psych. M.	0.3–0.9
Ethosuximide (Zarontin)	PM	0.25–1.5
Ethotoin (Peganone)	GM, Psych. M.	2–3
Ethoxzolamide (Cardrase)	PM, GM	0.125–0.750
Mephenytoin (Mesantoin)	GM	0.3–1
Mephobarbital N.F. (Mebaral)	GM	0.2–0.8
Meprobamate N.F. (Equanil; Miltown)	PM	0.4–1.6
Metharbital (Gemonil)	GM	0.3–0.8
Methazolamide U.S.P. (Neptazane)	PM, GM	0.1–0.3
Methsuximide N.F. (Celontin)	PM	0.3–1.2
Paramethadione U.S.P. (Paradione)	PM	0.3–2.1
Phenacemide (Phenurone)	Psych. M., GM	1.5–3.0
Phenobarbital U.S.P. (Luminal)	GM, PM, Psych. M.	0.1–0.4
Phensuximide N.F. (Milontin)	PM	1.5–3.0
Primidone U.S.P. (Mysoline)	GM, Psych. M.	0.050–2.0
Trimethadione U.S.P. (Tridione)	PM	0.9–2.1

* GM = Grand Mal; PM = Petit Mal; Psych. M. = Psychomotor Seizures.

with the first line drugs. By making possible a reduction of the dosage of the main drug, the adjunctive agents tend to lessen the dangers of toxicity. Sometimes the addition of such a new drug to the patient's regimen brings about better control of his seizures than it had been possible to achieve previously.

Various minor tranquilizers, including *meprobamate* and *chlordiazepoxide* (Chap. 7), have helped some children with petit mal and minor motor seizures that had proved refractory to complete control by trimethadione, paradione, and the succinimides alone. Psychomotor stimulants such as the *amphetamines* and *methylphenidate* (Chap. 13) sometimes benefit a small minority of petit mal patients and others whose seizures seem to be activated by sleep. These drugs are sometimes added to the regimen of patients taking

large doses of phenobarbital and other depressants. Given this way, small doses of amphetamines or other drug of that class, tend to counteract excessive drug-induced drowsiness.

Certain diuretics of the carbonic-anhydrase-inhibitor type (Chap. 20) are sometimes effective additives in the management of petit mal and grand mal epilepsy. Drugs such as *acetazolamide* (Diamox) and *ethoxzolamide* (Cardrase) may act by altering the internal environment of the brain or the whole body. For example, they may have a dehydrating and acidifying effect on the body—actions that have long been recognized to reduce the frequency of epileptic attacks. On the other hand, the effects of these drugs may be the result of a build-up in the brain of carbon dioxide, a metabolic waste product which tends to depress nerve cell sensitivity.

SUMMARY OF SIDE EFFECTS AND TOXICITY OF ANTIEPILEPTIC DRUGS

- *The Hydantoins: Diphenylhydantoin, etc.*
  Neurological: unsteady gait, staggering, tremors
  Gastrointestinal: epigastric distress, nausea, vomiting
  Cutaneous: morbilliform and acnelike skin eruptions, and occasionally, hirsutism of face in girls
  Gingival: hyperplasia, or overgrowth of gum tissue

- *The Oxazolidinediones: Trimethadione, etc.*
  Ocular: photophobia of a distinctive type, the "glare phenomenon," hemeralopia
  Miscellaneous minor reactions: nausea, drowsiness, skin rash
  Blood dyscrasias: agranulocytosis, aplastic anemia (watch for fatigue, sore throat, bruising of skin and bleeding from mucous membranes)
  Renal: nephrosis (test for albuminuria)

- *The Succinimides: Ethosuximide, etc.*
  Central nervous system: headaches, dizziness, drowsiness, insomnia, restlessness, confusion
  Gastrointestinal: anorexia, nausea, and vomiting

Hypersensitivity reactions: skin eruptions, fever, sweating, hiccup
Dangerous reactions: blood dyscrasias (e.g., pancytopenia), renal and liver damage

- *Miscellaneous*
  Bromides: Acnelike skin rash; common-cold type symptoms, including running nose and eyes; gastrointestinal upset; possible toxic psychosis with delirium, delusions, hallucinations, and alteration in personality
  Phenacemide: Bone marrow changes leading to leukopenia, agranulocytosis, and aplastic anemia; liver damage marked by anorexia, nausea, vomiting, fever, general malaise and jaundice; psychological changes, including insomnia, restlessness, and possible apathy and withdrawal, leading to mental depression
  Primidone: Occasional acute gastroenteric syndrome marked by severe nausea, vomiting, dizziness, drowsiness, headache, fatigue, and general malaise; rarely, megaloblastic anemia, and leukopenia; morbilliform skin rash and edema of eyelids

ANTIPARKINSONISM AGENTS

The Nature of Parkinson's Disease

Parkinson's disease, or paralysis agitans, is a chronic, progressive motor disorder, resulting from damage to cells of the basal ganglia. Unlike the convulsive conditions, which afflict mostly children and young adults,

parkinsonism is seen mainly in people past middle life. Despite recent statistics indicating a decline in new cases, this condition is still second in numbers only to the epilepsies, among the neurological ailments.

The signs of parkinsonism are insidious in onset; at first barely perceptible, the patient's movement difficulties slowly become more pronounced. Some muscle groups grow weak; others become rigid or are subject to rhythmic tremors. Thus, the patient tends to move slowly and stiffly and to tremble when he is not moving. (A characteristic example is the so-called "pill rolling" motion seen in his hands when they are at rest.)

In advanced stages, the patient may drool, his speech becomes slurred, and his face assumes a masklike expression. He tends to shuffle along with his upper body bent and may seem sudenly to be propelled forward into a fall, because of his markedly impaired balance. All this sometimes leads some people to believe that the patient is mentally defective, when actually he is usually intellectually unimpaired and completely aware, to his embarrassment, of the reactions of other people to his appearance and behavior. Thus, the patient needs moral support to prevent discouragement and mental depression.

The Management of Parkinsonism

Although we are concerned primarily with the antiparkinsonism agents, drugs are only one aspect of the total care these patients require. Drugs cannot, of course, cure a condition caused by damage and death of motor neurons deep in the brain, but they can relieve some of the distressing symptoms of this condition in many cases. Employed together with massage and other physical therapy measures, drugs may help to delay development of crippling deformities.

Care of parkinsonism patients presents a challenge to even the most skilled and experienced nurse. Her duties include: assisting the patient with exercises prescribed for preventing deformity; encouraging him to take care of his personal needs himself; and instructing the patient and his family in administration of drugs for maximal effectiveness and minimal reaction discomfort. All these measures help the patient maintain his will to keep active despite his illness. This is very desirable, for feelings of independence tend to counteract the despair that often assails people with this chronic neurological condition.

The Older Antiparkinson Drugs

The first drugs introduced for relaxing muscle rigidity and relieving the other symptoms of Parkinson's disease were derivatives of plants of the deadly nightshade family, such as hyoscyamus and belladonna. More or less accidentally, the alkaloids atropine and scopolamine (Chap. 17) were found to help many patients. These anticholinergic agents are thought to act centrally to reduce the disorderly transmission of the impulses that are passing out to the skeletal muscles by way of extrapyramidal nerve tracts. Unfortunately, these drugs also have many undesirable peripheral actions, which are the result of blockade of parasympathetic nerve impulses to smooth muscles and glands. This results in many discomforting and even dangerous side effects (see Summary, p. 140).

Newer Antiparkinsonism Agents

In recent years a number of new synthetic chemicals (see Table 8-2 and the Drug Digests) have been developed for relaxing rigidity and reducing the tremors of parkinsonism. Like the natural substances, these somewhat safer antispasmodics bring about their therapeutically desired effects through their central action. In fact, they have an even greater affinity for these central sites. Thus, their main advantage is that

TABLE 8-2
SYNTHETIC ANTIPARKINSONISM AGENTS

Nonproprietary Name	Trade Name or Synonym	Usual Dosage Range (in Mg.)
* Benztropine Mesylate N.F.	Cogentin	0.5–6
Biperiden HCl & Lactate	Akineton	2–5
Caramiphen HCl	Panparnit	12.5–50
Chlorphenoxamine HCl	Phenoxene	50–150
Cycrimine HCl N.F.	Pagitane	1.25–5
Diphenhydramine HCl U.S.P.	Benadryl	25–50
Ethopropazine HCl	Parsidol	10–50
* Orphenadrine HCl	Disipal	50–100
Procyclidine HCl	Kemadrin	2.5–5
* Trihexyphenidyl HCl U.S.P.	Artane; Tremin	6–10

* See also Drug Digests.

they are less likely to cause the undesired peripheral effects of atropine-type alkaloids. Nonetheless, these synthetics are themselves not entirely free of peripheral side effects similar to those of atropine.

Side Effects. Atropinelike side effects include dryness of the skin and mouth, constipation, dysuria, and blurring of vision. Some of these secondary actions may actually be beneficial for some patients. For example, the secretion-drying effect may be desirable for patients with postencephalitic parkinsonism who often tend to drool and sweat excessively. In other patients, however, atropinelike side effects may precipitate severe reactions, including attacks of glaucoma and tachycardia. Elderly men, who often have an enlarged prostate gland that presses on the neck of the bladder, should be watched for signs of difficulty in urination brought on by the adverse effects that these drugs sometimes have on bladder function.

Behavioral Changes. Certain of these synthetic antispasmodic agents are capable of producing behavioral changes. In some cases, these psychopharmacological effects may be beneficial; in others, they may be harmful. For example, patients who tend to be tense and nervous may be calmed by the sedative action sometimes found when *diphenhydramine* (Benadryl), *benztropine* (Cogentin), or the natural substance, *scopolamine* (hyoscine), are being used to treat their tremors. On the other hand, patients whose illness is marked by excessive sluggishness may do better when taking an antispasmodic drug such as *orphenadrine* (Disipal) which has, in addition, a mild

central stimulating effect. (Amphetamine-type agents are also sometimes used to help overcome drowsiness and lethargy in parkinsonian patients with such symptoms.)

Obviously, these depressant and stimulating actions on the nervous system can be dangerous if they are allowed to go too far. Mental confusion, loss of memory, and disorientation may develop, especially in elderly patients with the atherosclerotic form of parkinsonism. The development of such signs should be watched for and reported to the doctor. They are usually relieved by a reduction in dosage. If, on the other hand, such drug-induced effects are assumed to be mere signs of the patient's illness or of his advanced age and are not mentioned in the nurses' notes, the continued administration of these drugs may lead to delirium and toxic psychosis.

Use in Tranquilizer Therapy. The antiparkinson agents have been found useful recently as adjuncts to the tranquilizer therapy of mental patients. The administration of phenothiazine and rauwolfia-type tranquilizers sometimes causes parkinsonlike muscle spasms and motor restlessness (See Chap. 7). These signs of drug-induced stimulation of the extrapyramidal system often can be controlled by the simultaneous use of a synthetic centrally acting antispasmodic such as *trihexyphenidyl* (Artane; Tremin), *benztropine* (Cogentin), and *biperiden* (Akineton). In this way, usually the patient is able to continue to take large doses of the psychotropic drugs without undue discomfort.

SUMMARY OF SIDE EFFECTS, CAUTIONS, AND CONTRAINDICATIONS OF ANTIPARKINSON DRUGS

- Mouth dryness or xerostomia

- Blurring of vision: this is due to cycloplegia and may be dangerous for people with glaucoma

- Skin dryness or anhidrosis: may lead to fever in warm weather

- Cardiac palpitations and tachycardia

- Constipation and, occasionally, nausea and vomiting

- Urinary retention: may be dangerous for elderly males with enlarged prostate gland

- Headache, dizziness, drowsiness, mental confusion

CENTRALLY ACTING SKELETAL MUSCLE ANTISPASMODICS

The Nature of Muscular Spasm and Spasticity

Painful muscular contractions occur in many musculoskeletal and neurological disorders. Acute muscle injuries and chronic connective tissue irritation are

often followed by involuntary muscle spasms. Damage to the nervous system that interferes with central control of motor reflexes is a cause of severe spasticity. In situations of both types, the objective of treatment is to bring about relaxation of the patient's "knotted" muscles. This is important, not only to relieve the pain, but also to permit the muscles to be exercised and thus prevent deformity and permanent loss of motion.

Actually, the excessive muscular contraction that is set off by trauma is part of a protective reflex mechanism intended to forestall further injury. Yet, this "muscle-splinting" action in response to painful injury is itself the source of still more pain and further spasm. Sometimes the application of heat will serve to terminate the vicious cycle of pain-spasm-increased pain. Usually, however, such conditions require the use of drug therapy to reduce muscle spasm.

Among the drugs sometimes employed for this purpose are local anesthetics (e.g., the spraying of ethyl chloride or the injection of procaine solution at certain pain spots). Sometimes, heavy sedation will produce the desired effect. Most commonly employed for this purpose are the skeletal muscle antispasmodics. Occasionally, especially in the hospital operating room, the peripherally acting curariform compounds (Chap. 17), which may actually paralyze skeletal muscles, may be preferred. However, in everyday practice the safer centrally acting antispasmodics (Table 8-3) have come into increasing use recently.

Manner of Action

This class of compounds, sometimes called *lissives* or *neurospasmolytics*, do not act on the muscles themselves. Instead, they tend to depress certain nerve cells that are involved in spinal and other motor reflexes. These are the connecting, or *internuncial*, neurons, which act as links between sensory neurons and the motor nerves that finally activate skeletal muscles. (Fig. 8-1).

In many spinal reflexes, for example, the sensory impulses streaming into the nervous system from the periphery do not pass directly to the motor neurons. They are, instead, relayed there by way of a complex chain of connecting neurons. Similarly, messages from upper motor neurons in the cerebral cortex are modified by the activity of motor neurons in the basal ganglia, reticular formation, etc. (Chap. 5), as they pass down to the lower motor neurons in the spinal cord.

When injury to muscles or to upper motor neurons makes these *polysynaptic reflexes* hyperactive, the muscles are twisted into spasm. Thus, by raising the resistance of such central synapses, these depressant drugs help to dam some of the stream of stimuli that are keeping the muscles contracted. Most important is their ability to reduce *excessive* reflex excitability without any significant reduction of the constant flow of *tonic* motor impulses needed for normal function.

At their best, the lissive drugs can, in this way, eliminate cramps and contractures without weakening

TABLE 8-3

CENTRALLY ACTING ANTISPASMODICS (LISSIVES OR NEUROSPASMOLYTICS)

Nonproprietary Name	Trade Name	Usual Dose (in Mg.)
Carisoprodol	Rela: Soma	250–350
Chlormezanone	Trancopal	100–200
Chlorphenesin carbamate	Maolate	400–800
Chlorzoxazone	Paraflex	250–750
Diazepam	Valium	2–10
Emylcamate	Striatran	200
Mephenesin N.F.	Dioloxol, Myanesin, Oranixon, Relaxar, Tolserol, etc.	2000–3000
Mephenesin carbamate	Tolseram	1000–3000
Meprobamate N.F.	Equanil, Miltown	400–800
Metaxalone	Skelaxin	800
Methocarbamol	Robaxin	750–1500
Orphenadrine citrate	Norflex	60–100
Phenaglycodol	Ultran	200–400
Phenyramidol HCl	Analexin	200–400
Promoxolane	Dimethylane	750–1000
Styramate	Sinaxar	200–400

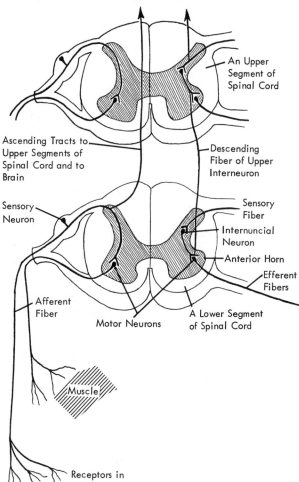

Ascending Tracts to Upper Segments of Spinal Cord and to Brain

An Upper Segment of Spinal Cord

Descending Fiber of Upper Interneuron

Sensory Neuron

Sensory Fiber

Internuncial Neuron

Anterior Horn

Efferent Fibers

Afferent Fiber

Motor Neurons

A Lower Segment of Spinal Cord

Muscle

Receptors in Muscle, Skin, etc.

Fig. 8-1. Polysynaptic reflex arc pathways. The neurospasmolytic drugs depress the internuncial neurons in hyperactive reflex pathways (hyperreflexia). This reduces excessive reflex excitability and muscle spasm without affecting normal muscle tone.

normal muscular activity. Such ideal action is best achieved with high doses of these drugs given by injection. Oral dosage is much less effective for relaxing spastic muscles.

Clinical Uses

These drugs are used in situations of the following general types: (1) *musculoskeletal conditions,* in which spasm is the result of *peripheral* injury or inflammation, and (2) *neurological conditions* in which muscles become spastic because of *central* nervous system disorders that interfere with control of reflex activity. Best results have been obtained in spasm resulting from acute muscle injuries; the drugs are

relatively ineffective against the muscle contractures that develop in chronic nervous diseases.

Musculoskeletal Conditions. This group of conditions includes the common low-back syndrome, strains, sprains, arthritis, bursitis, fibrositis, and myositis. In these conditions the antispasmodics are commonly combined with anti-inflammatory and analgesic drugs, such as the corticosteroids and salicylates. Some of the lissive drugs, such as *carisoprodol* * (Rela, Soma) and *phenyramidol* (Analexin), are claimed to possess analgesic activity also. That is, they seem to dull pain perception as well as reduce muscle spasm directly. Other agents have a desirable sedative or tranquilizing action that is said to add to their effectiveness. The minor tranquilizers *meprobamate* (Equanil, Miltown) and *diazepam* * (Valium) and such newer "tranquilaxant" drugs as *chlormezanone* (Trancopal) and *emylcamate* (Striatran) tend to reduce the emotional tension that often accompanies muscular disorders. This tranquilizing action may be more important than actual muscular relaxation in helping patients—especially those with nerve damage—move more efficiently.

Neurological Conditions. Conditions of the second class include cerebral palsy, multiple sclerosis, hemiplegia, poliomyelitis, and parkinsonism. The rigidity of parkinsonism is rarely overcome by these muscle relaxants; however, the drugs seem to have a place in the management of some phases of the other chronic neurological disorders.

Children with cerebral palsy, for example, are said to have benefited from *methocarbamol* * (Robaxin) given in large oral doses and by injection. The drug's dampening action on the overstimulated nerve cells connecting upper and lower motor neurons is claimed to have helped these children gain greater control over their movements, so that they become better able to sit up, walk, and bathe and dress themselves. In multiple sclerosis and poliomyelitis, these drugs may help the patients perform the guided exercises that they must do to prevent permanent contractures. By reducing the painful cramps caused when spastic muscles are stretched, the antispasmodics make it possible for the patients to keep moving and, thus, prevent crippling.

Side Effects and Disadvantages

Drugs of this group are not notably toxic. However, the need to use large oral doses or injections in order to get good results, sometimes results in side effects. For example, *mephenesin,* the first drug of this class frequently caused gastrointestinal upset. These occurred because the drug was eliminated rapidly and was transient in its action, so that often the patient was subjected to frequent massive amounts by mouth.

* See also Drug Digests.

The more recently developed derivatives that are more potent and prolonged in their action can be given in smaller doses with minimal digestive disturbances. However, the strong sedative component of some of the newer central antispasmodic-depressants may make some patients drowsy, dizzy, and lightheaded. Thus, ambulatory patients requiring high doses should be warned not to drive or attempt other potentially hazardous activities requiring motor coordination, skill, and judgment.

In general, these drugs are least successful in ambulatory patients taking oral dosage. Best results follow parenteral administration, but this involves a somewhat greater risk of toxicity. The saturated solution of *mephenesin* has caused the rupture of red blood cells when given by vein. The hemoglobin released by such hemolytic reactions may then clog kidney tubules and cause hematuria. Overly rapid administration of *methocarbamol* (Robaxin) solution occasionally causes vertigo and syncope. It must be used with caution in epileptic patients and is contraindicated in patients with kidney disease. Thrombophlebitis may follow leakage of the solution through the venous wall, and burning at the injection site is an occasional complaint after intramuscular administration.

Recently, two more of the centrally acting antispasmodics have become available in parenteral form. One of these, meprobamate (Intramuscular Miltown), is used mainly in the management of tetanus, along with other measures such as administration of tetanus antitoxin (Chap. 45), antibiotics, fluids and electrolytes, etc. This solution should never be injected intravenously, since it may cause venous thrombosis and hemolysis. One of the solvents for meprobamate, polyethylene glycol, is contraindicated for patients with kidney damage. The administration of intramuscular meprobamate must be discontinued if signs of hypersensitivity such as skin eruptions and bronchial spasm appear.

The injectable form of diazepam (Valium Injectable) may be administered by vein as well as intramuscularly. Although employed mainly for its mental effects in reducing apprehension and agitation in acute alcoholic withdrawal (Chap. 12) and severe psychoneurotic reaction, this parenteral form of the anti-anxiety-neurospasmolytic agent is also often rapidly effective for counteracting massive muscular spasm associated with cerebral palsy, athetosis and even epilepsy. (Although this drug is currently considered contraindicated for routine use in the management of seizure states, some neurologists have found the injectable form of diazepam very valuable for bringing the continuous convulsions of status epilepticus under quick control.) Injections should be made slowly to avoid hypotension and other adverse effects.

SUMMARY OF SIDE EFFECTS AND TOXICITY OF CENTRALLY ACTING SKELETAL MUSCLE ANTISPASMODICS

- Gastrointestinal upset: nausea, vomiting, diarrhea

- Central depression: drowsiness, dizziness, lightheadedness; *warning*—ambulatory patients should not drive or operate dangerous machinery.

- Skin reactions of hypersensitivity type: rash, redness, itching

- Blood cell damage: mephenesin may cause hemolysis of red blood cells and possible hematuria upon intravenous injection; parenteral methocarbamol does not do this but may cause thrombophlebitis, burning, and other reactions when injected.

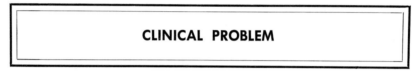

SUMMARY OF POINTS FOR NURSE TO REMEMBER ABOUT ANTICONVULSANT AND ANTISPASMODIC DRUGS

• The nurse must make the patient with a chronic neurological disease (e.g., epilepsy; Parkinson's disease) aware of the need to continue with the prescribed treatment. If she finds that the patient's personal problems are making him neglect his medication, she should inform the doctor.

• The patient and his family should be made to recognize the need to return to the physician for frequent studies of blood, urine, and so forth, in order to detect early signs of toxicity caused by long-term medication for chronic neuromuscular illnesses.

• Patients should be assisted with exercises but encouraged to take care of their personal needs, because physical and emotional factors are as important as drug therapy in slowing progressive deterioration in neurological diseases such as parkinsonism.

CLINICAL PROBLEM

Linda is a nine-year-old girl who has petit mal seizures. She is being treated with Tridione 0.3 Gm., b.i.d. What instructions would you, the clinic nurse, give Linda's mother about symptoms to observe and report to the physician?

REVIEW QUESTIONS

1. (a) What is the goal of drug treatment in epilepsy?
(b) What are some of the ways in which the nurse can cooperate with the doctor and patient to attain the objectives of drug therapy?

2. List several specific kinds of epileptic seizures and indicate the anticonvulsant drugs best suited for treating each type.

3. List the unusual side effects that are sometimes seen with (a) diphenylhydantoin, (b) trimethadione, and (c) primidone. Indicate other potentially dangerous reactions which may develop during treatment with these drugs.

4. What kinds of laboratory tests are required during long-term treatment with antiepileptic drugs such as *trimethadione, phenacemide*, etc., and what are some of the serious toxic reactions which may develop if these drugs are not discontinued when early signs are detected?

5. List several adjunctive drugs sometimes employed in the treatment regimen of epilepsy patients and indicate how they may act to increase anti-seizure activity.

6. What possible advantages may be claimed for each of the following:
(a) Diphenylhydantoin over phenobarbital

(b) Ethosuximide over trimethadione
(c) Primidone over phenacemide

7. What are some of the nurse's responsibilities in the management of patients with Parkinson's disease?

8. (a) What general advantage is claimed for the synthetic antispasmodics over the natural belladonna alkaloids in the treatment of parkinsonism?

(b) What are some of the peripheral side effects sometimes seen with the synthetic antiparkinsonism drugs and some central side effects?

9. (a) List some secondary effects of the synthetic antispasmodics which may favorably affect certain symptoms of parkinsonism other than muscular rigidity and tremor.

(b) List several conditions in which antiparkinson drugs must be employed with caution or in which these agents may be contraindicated.

10. (a) What are the site and the manner of action of the lissive, or neurospasmolytic, drugs?

(b) At what other site may certain skeletal muscle spasmolytics act to overcome spasticity and even to *paralyze* skeletal muscles?

11. (a) List several musculoskeletal conditions in which the centrally acting antispasmodics are employed.

(b) List several neurological conditions in which these drugs are employed.

12. Compare the newer spasmolytic agent *methocarbamol* with its predecessor of this class, *mephenesin*, in terms of efficacy and safety when each is administered orally or parenterally.

13. List the most common side effects of the centrally acting antispasmodics (lissives or neurospasmolytics) and indicate what warning is often given to ambulatory patients taking these drugs.

BIBLIOGRAPHY

Anticonvulsant Drugs in Epilepsy

Bray, P. F.: Diphenylhydantoin (Dilantin) After twenty years. Pediatrics, 23:151, 1959.

Currier, R. D.: Hints on seizure management. G.P., 30: 125, 1964.

Forster, F. M.: Management of the epileptic patient. Med. Clin. North Amer., 47:1579, 1963.

Gunn, C. G., Gogerty, J., and Wolf, S.: Clinical pharmacology of anticonvulsant compounds. Clin. Pharmacol. Ther., 2:733, 1961.

Lennox, W. G.: The petit mal epilepsies: their treatment with tridione. J.A.M.A., 120:1069, 1945.

Lennox, W. G., and Lennox, M. A.: Epilepsy and Related Disorders. Boston, Little, Brown & Co., 1960.

Rodman, M. J.: Epilepsy—advances in diagnosis and treatment. R.N., 17:44, 1954 (Dec.).

Yahraes, H.: Epilepsy—The ghost is out of the closet. Public Affairs Pamphlet No. 98, Public Affairs Committee, 1951.

Zimmerman, F. T., and Burgenmeister, B. B.: Drugs used in treatment of patients with petit mal epilepsy. J.A.M.A., 157:1194, 1955.

Antiparkinson Agents

Doshay, L. J.: Parkinson's disease. J.A.M.A., 174:1962, 1960.

Doshay, L. J., and Constable, K.: Treatment of paralysis agitans with orphenadrine (Disipal). J.A.M.A., 163: 1352, 1957.

England, A. C., Jr., and Schwab, R. S.: Parkinson's syndrome. New Eng. J. Med., 265:785, 1961.

————: Management of parkinson's disease. Arch. Int. Med., 104:439, 1959.

Friend, D.: Anti-parkinsonism drug therapy. Clin. Pharmacol. Ther., 4:815, 1963.

Magee, K. R.: The treatment of parkinsonism. G.P., 18: 139, 1958.

Markham, C. H.: Medical and surgical treatment of parkinson's disease. Med. Clin. North Amer., 47:1591, 1963.

Rabiner, A. M., and Frugh, A.: The treatment of parkinsonism. Med. Clin. North Amer., 641:1958.

Rodman, M. J.: Drugs for neuromuscular disorders. R.N., 25:67, 1962 (Jan.).

Centrally Acting Antispasmodics

Abrahamsen, E. H., and Baird, H. W.: Use of zoxazolamine (Flexin) * in children with cerebral palsy. J.A.M.A., 160:749, 1956.

Amols, W.: Clinical experience with a new muscle relaxant, Zoxazolamine.* J.A.M.A., 160:742, 1956.

Forsyth, H. F.: Methocarbamol (Robaxin) in orthopedic conditions. J.A.M.A., 168:163, 1958.

Friend, D. G.: Pharmacology of muscle relaxants. Clin. Pharmacol. Ther., 5:871, 1964.

Marsh, H. O.: Diazepam in incapacitated cerebral palsied children. J.A.M.A., 191:797, 1965.

O'Doherty, D. S., and Shields, C. D.: Methocarbamol—new agent in treatment of neurological and neuromuscular disease. J.A.M.A., 167:160, 1958.

Rodman, M. J.: Drugs for neuromuscular pain and spasm. R.N., 29:62, 1966 (May).

————: The muscle relaxants. R.N., 27:59, 1964 (Aug.).

Vazuka, F. A.: Comparative effects of relaxant drugs on human skeletal muscle hyperactivity. Neurology, 8:446, 1958.

* Although the drug zoxazolamine has been withdrawn from the market because of toxicity, these papers are included because they offer insights into the clinical use of all drugs of this class.

The Narcotic Analgesics

PAIN AND ITS RELIEF

Pain is the most common complaint of people seeking medical care. By depriving the patient of rest, sleep, and appetite, pain may undermine his strength and morale. Long continued severe pain may even set off a cycle of disastrous reactions that can endanger the patient's life. Thus, relieving pain is one of the most important services that doctors and nurses perform for their patients.

Actually, pain signals are part of a protective mechanism designed to indicate the presence of a potentially dangerous condition. Pain is useful if it forces a person to seek medical aid and when it helps the doctor to diagnose the disorder. However, once it has served this purpose, there is no reason why pain should not be relieved by drugs or other means. Indeed, stopping pain is more than just a humane measure; by promoting rest and reducing apprehension, it helps to speed the patient's recovery during convalescence.

Relief of pain may be accomplished by drugs that act at any of several sites along the pathway by which pain impulses travel from the periphery to the highest integrative levels of the central nervous system. (Fig. 9-1.) Thus, some drugs, such as the antispasmodics (Chap. 8) may stop pain by relaxing smooth or skeletal muscles in which the pain stimulus originates.

Other drugs, like the local anesthetics (Chap. 11), may act to dull peripheral pain receptors or the sensory fibers of spinal nerves carrying afferent impulses toward the dorsal root ganglia and spinal cord. However, the most important pain relievers are those that act within the central nervous system. These include the general anesthetics (Chap. 11), which suppress not only pain but all other sensations too. The true analgesics, on the other hand, are drugs which act centrally to relieve pain, but without causing loss of consciousness.

Analgesic Agents. Analgesics are often capable of reducing perception so specifically that they hardly affect other nervous system functions at all. They are thought to act, in part, by depressing the thalamus, which serves as a relay station for sensory impulses passing from the periphery to the cerebral cortex. These drugs may also raise the threshold, or responsiveness, of sensory cortex cells to incoming pain signals. The frontal lobes of the brain, which play a part in interpreting pain messages, may also be affected.

Analgesic drugs may be divided into two classes: (1) those that relieve only mild to moderate degrees of pain and (2) more potent agents which are capable of overcoming very severe pain. Drugs of the first class, the non-narcotic analgesics, are discussed in the next chapter. They include the salicylates and related coal-tar derivatives, which are most effective against pain arising in muscles, joints, and bones.

In this chapter, we shall take up the potent pain relievers that are often called narcotic analgesics. The term "narcotic" means merely that these drugs are capable of causing depression. In that sense, all central nervous system depressants, which, like these analgesics, can cause drowsiness, sleep, stupor, and coma, are narcotics. However, because these potent pain relievers are potentially addicting drugs, and their use is restricted under the provisions of the Harrison Narcotic Act (Chap. 4), the public has come to think of narcotics only as harmful drugs that are used for illicit purposes. Actually, these so-called narcotic analgesics need not cause addiction when they are properly employed. They are among the most valuable of all the drugs in the doctor's armamentarium. In fact, they are so useful that the doctor may even go on giving them despite the danger of addiction—in patients in the terminal stages of malignant diseases, for example.

These potent analgesics can be broadly subdivided into (1) the *opiates*, of which morphine is the main prototype and (2) the *synthetic* opiate-like, or opioid, narcotic analgesics. The student who learns the actions and uses of *morphine* will be able to understand the advantages and limitations of any new synthetic analgesics that may be introduced.

THE OPIATE-TYPE ANALGESICS

The poppy plant, *Papaver Somniferum*, is the source of opium, a substance used since ancient times for relieving pain. However, the effects of powdered opium and of liquid preparations such as laudanum and paregoric were often undependable because of differences in the alkaloidal content of the crude plant extracts. Then, early in the last century, a young German pharmacist, Friedrich Serturner, succeeded in isolating a pure plant principle which he called *morphine,* for Morpheus, the Greek god of dreams. This discovery led to the extraction of other crystalline opium alkaloids including *codeine,* and to the preparation of substances such as *heroin* and other semisynthetic derivatives, drugs made by chemically treating the natural opiate alkaloids.

Morphine Analgesia

Despite the recent development of various synthetic analgesics, morphine is still the most widely employed agent for relief of severe pain. It acts in several ways to bring about its desirable effects: (1) It raises the patient's pain perception threshold; (2) it reduces the anxiety and fear that are natural emotional reactions to painful stimuli and are largely responsible for the unpleasantness of the pain experience, and (3) it can produce sleep even in the presence of severe pain.

Relatively small doses of morphine are capable of dulling the ability to perceive pain. The drug may depress nerve cells in the thalamus and sensory cortex, so that fewer pain signals from the periphery break through into consciousness. It is especially effective against continuous dull pain of moderate intensity originating in the smooth muscles of the internal hollow organs.

Despite the effect of morphine on pain perception, the patient is still capable of feeling sharp, stabbing pain following fractures, extensive burns, and other traumata. However, the patient who is under the influence of morphine may not mind this pain even when he is aware of it. This alteration in the patient's response to pain is one of the most characteristic and important effects of morphine and other potent analgesics.

Just how morphine eliminates the disagreeable emotional reaction to pain is still obscure. It may affect transmission of nerve impulses between the frontal lobes of the cortex, which regulate learned or conditioned behavior, and the lower centers that influence emotional responses (see Chap. 5). This

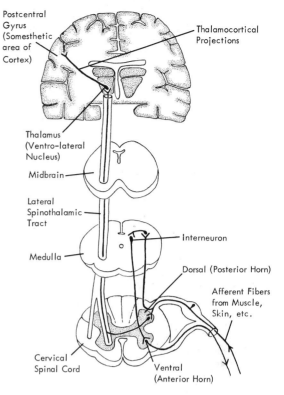

FIG. 9-1. Pain pathways. Afferent fibers carry impulses to dorsal horn of spinal cord. Connections with interneurons and motor neurons permit reflex motor responses. Impulses must be transmitted to higher centers in the thalamus and cerebral cortex for pain perception and reaction. Drugs act at various levels of these pathways to block transmission of impulses.

action of morphine so resembles that of the psychosurgical operation, prefrontal lobotomy, that it has been called a chemical lobotomy—a temporary cutting off of the nervous pathways that participate in the behavioral patterns by which people respond with alarm to volleys of pain stimuli.

Although morphine analgesia is not necessarily accompanied by drowsiness, the drug does often have a hypnotic action. Such a sleep-producing effect is sometimes desirable for patients whose rest is disturbed by their pain. It is especially important for some pain-tossed patients, such as those who have suffered a coronary occlusion or other condition which requires complete rest and relaxation. On the other hand, excessive drug-induced sedation is undesirable in patients who should remain ambulatory and active in spite of pain.

Other Actions of Morphine

In addition to their analgesic action, morphine and other narcotic opiates and opioids have various other central and peripheral effects. The latter pharmacological actions account both for their therapeutic usefulness in certain non-painful conditions and for the side effects and toxicity sometimes seen during their administration. Although the many natural, semisynthetic, and synthetic narcotic analgesics differ in the degree to which therapeutic doses produce these other actions, all share these properties to some extent at least. Thus, a description of some of the many pharmacological properties of morphine can serve to explain the effects sometimes seen with most other drugs of this class.

Subcortical and spinal centers seem to be both depressed and stimulated in ways that produce characteristic effects. Small doses of morphine, for example, depress the medullary cough center. Consequently, morphine is sometimes employed to suppress coughing. Doctors usually prefer, however, to use related drugs that are less likely to depress the closely related respiratory center. The more commonly used antitussive agents, including codeine * and hydrocodone, are also considered less likely to cause strong dependence and addiction if abused. However, morphine or its semisynthetic derivative *dihydromorphinone* * (Dilaudid) may be the doctor's choice following rib fractures or in bronchial carcinoma and other conditions in which coughing and pain occur together.

The emetic mechanism is sometimes stimulated by morphine and related drugs, so that nausea and vomiting often occur, especially in ambulatory patients. This action on the chemoreceptor trigger zone in the medulla (Chap. 38) is most marked with the alkaloid *apomorphine*, which is used clinically to induce vomiting deliberately, and not as an analgesic at all.

The gastrointestinal effects of morphine are the result of complex effects directly on the smooth muscles and glands of the digestive tract. The combination of decreased peristaltic motility, increased spasticity of sphincters and other bowel sections, together with lessened glandular secretion, often results in constipation. Actually, of course, this "side effect" is desirable for treating diarrhea. Thus, *Paregoric* (Camphorated Tincture of Opium) is commonly employed for this purpose.

The *biliary tract* pressure may actually be increased when morphine is administered for relief of spastic pain caused by gallstones blocking the biliary duct. Thus, morphine is commonly combined with an antispasmodic in treating biliary colic. The opium alkaloid, *papaverine*, which is not an analgesic and also not capable of causing addiction, is often used for its direct relaxing effect on the spastic smooth muscle. (Atropine also is employed to counteract the natural and morphine-induced smooth muscle spasm in this condition, as well as in renal colic caused by stones in the urinary tract.)

* See Drug Digests.

The pharmacological effects of morphine on the bronchial smooth muscle, the iris muscle of the eye, and the cardiovascular system will be mentioned in the discussion of the side effects and toxicity of the opiates.

Side Effects and Contraindications

In addition to the drowsiness, nausea and vomiting, and constipation commonly encountered with morphine, a number of other side effects are seen, especially in people who are hypersensitive to opiates. Patients often feel flushed, warm, dizzy and lightheaded. Some occasionally become excited, restless, and even delirious, instead of calm and sedated. This paradoxical reaction seems more common in women and elderly patients.

Older patients and those debilitated by chronic diseases may be more sensitive to the depressant effects of morphine and thus require relatively small doses. Also, patients with breathing difficulties are given smaller amounts of morphine. In bronchial asthma, emphysema, and other lung disorders, morphine may cause contractions of the muscles of the respiratory tree. This, together with the drug's depressant effect on the respiratory center, may tend to reduce pulmonary ventilation to dangerously low levels.

Morphine is undesirable in patients with head injuries, because it tends to increase intracranial pressure and mask signs of this complication. For the same reason, it is usually withheld from patients who have been injured during a bout of acute alcoholic intoxication, because its use may precipitate delirium tremens and "wet brain" (Chap. 12). Similarly, patients in a state of shock should not receive narcotics, because these drugs may cause a further drop in cardiac output and blood pressure.

Acute Toxicity

Morphine overdosage produces deep depression of respiration. Breathing becomes markedly slowed, shallow, and irregular as the respiratory center fails to respond to relatively high blood concentrations of carbon dioxide. Respirations may slow to only four per minute or may be characterized by alternating periods of apnea and hyperpnea (Cheyne-Stokes breathing).

The nurse, of course, should note any unusual decrease in the depth and rate of respiration before breathing difficulties become very advanced. Other early signs of opiate poisoning include constriction of the pupil to pinpoint size and deep sleep or stupor. Later, the patient may pass into coma, and, as his hypoxia becomes more severe, asphyxial dilation of the pupils may develop. The progressive anoxia causes the skin, which is at first flushed, warm and wet with sweat, to become cyanotic or lividly mottled, cold and clammy. Death is usually the result of respiratory failure. Occasionally, circulatory collapse develops before breathing stops, and, rarely, terminal convulsions occur.

Treatment of Acute Toxicity. In the relatively rare cases of oral overdosage, it may be desirable to wash the stomach with solutions of alkaloidal precipitants (e.g., tannic acid) or oxidizers (e.g., potassium permanganate, 1:5000 dilution). If a dosage error is discovered shortly after subcutaneous injection, the application of a tourniquet or of ice may delay full absorption of the drug long enough for the body's detoxifying mechanisms to destroy a good part of the overdose.

In actual practice, however, most measures are directed at combating advancing respiratory depression. Analeptics such as caffeine and amphetamine may be useful against relatively minor degrees of depression. Stronger stimulants, such as pentylenetetrazole, nikethamide, and even strychnine (Chap. 13) have also been advocated. However, these drugs are dangerous, since they may trigger tonic convulsive spasms. (Morphine tends to stimulate the spinal cord, an effect not usually apparent in humans except when unmasked by injudicious administration of strong central stimulants.)

The best specific antidotes available for counteracting opiate narcosis are the narcotic antagonists, *nalorphine* * (Nalline) and *levallorphan* (Lorfan). These remarkably effective agents are not stimulants, unlike the ordinary analeptics. They act instead by competing with morphine molecules for cellular receptors in the drug-depressed neurons. By displacing narcotic drugs from their cellular attachment sites, these narcotic antagonists quickly restore normal respiration and arouse the poison victim from his stupor or coma.

Chronic Toxicity or Opiate Addiction

Addiction to narcotic analgesics is commonly considered the most serious form of drug abuse. *Heroin* is the opiate alkaloid with the widest illicit use. *Morphine* and the synthetic analgesic *meperidine* (Demerol) are sometimes used by persons—including doctors, nurses, and pharmacists—who have ready access to medical supplies. Recently, there has been a rise in the abuse of cough medicines containing *codeine* and related antitussives by youths seeking "kicks."

Opiate abuse leads to all the phenomena that characterize addiction, including the development of tolerance and of psychological and physical dependence. Addicts often develop a relatively high level of resistance to the effects of opiates compared to the only moderate tolerance found when alcohol or barbiturates are chronically abused. Whereas 60 milligrams of morphine may prove toxic to most normal people, addicts are capable of taking several grams of opium alkaloids daily without suffering from severe

* See Drug Digest.

toxicity. Presumably, the cells of their central nervous systems undergo adaptive biochemical changes that enable them to withstand huge amounts of narcotics. It is, however, possible for the addict to kill himself by administering doses of these drugs that exceed even his high degree of tolerance.

The main effects sought by people who take opiates to excess is a drowsy relaxed feeling frequently called "goofing off," "getting high" or "going on the nod." Shortly after taking a subcutaneous injection ("skin-popping" or "joypopping"), the heroin addict "takes off" and drifts dreamily in a state between sleep and waking. His personal problems and conflicts seem to cease to exist, as the drug deadens his anxieties. This euphoria is one of the factors leading to psychological dependence, the powerful craving for the drug that develops in some individuals who find it difficult to cope with life's realities.

Unfortunately, as tolerance to the drug's effects develops, it becomes more difficult to maintain the desired effects, and he finds it necessary to raise the dose. This is true also of another effect commonly sought by addicts—the brief feeling of physical ecstasy that follows the intravenous injection, or "mainlining," of heroin. As a result of the need to take larger and larger doses more and more frequently, the opiate abuser finally becomes "hooked" or physically dependent upon the drug.

The cells of the central nervous system of such a person apparently require the presence of the drug, in order to function normally. If deprived of the drug, the addict suffers severe discomfort. The withdrawal or abstinence syndrome which begins to come on within a few hours of the last "fix" (or within minutes after injection of a diagnostic dose of the narcotic antagonists, nalorphine and levallorphan) is quite characteristic. The effects of withdrawal (See Summary, p. 156) are somewhat stereotyped and vary mainly in their degree of severity. This, in turn depends upon how much drug the addict had been taking daily, that is, on the degree to which he had become physically dependent on the drug.

Diagnosis of Addiction. The best evidence of narcotic addiction is of course the appearance of the pattern of signs and symptoms typical of abstinence (Summary, p. 156), when the addict is deprived of the drug upon which he is dependent. This begins about 12 to 18 hours after the last dose during "cold turkey" treatment—abrupt abstinence without the aid of any medication.

The use of nalorphine in the Nalline Test offers a more rapid means of determining whether a person is under the influence of a narcotic. However, the sudden precipitation of the abstinence syndrome in this way may be dangerous and needlessly cruel.

Thus, to detect individuals who have narcotic drugs in their systems as a result of a recent "fix," nalorphine is administered only in a relatively minute dose. This is enough, however, to bring about a characteristic pupillary dilatation in those whose pupils are even slightly constricted from a previously self-administered narcotic drug. Actually, the presence of pinpoint pupils alone, the result of the central miotic action of morphine and heroin, is by itself a conspicuous sign of the presence of opiates. The skin on the inner aspect of the arms of "mainlining" addicts is usually marked by "tracks." These raised and discolored areas running along the course of the veins are the scars of old sores and abscesses. The presence of fresh punctures is, of course, a sign that the person has taken a "fix" fairly recently. This can be confirmed by positive tests for opiates in the person's urine.

Treatment of Addiction. The medical management of addiction is best begun in a hospital staffed by specially trained physicians, psychiatrists, and nurses, where withdrawal can be conducted with confidence that the patient cannot get any drugs. The U. S. Public Service operates two such hospitals at Lexington, Kentucky and Fort Worth, Texas. The current drug withdrawal procedure at these institutions requires rapid elimination of the drug to which the patient is addicted. However, for a while, the synthetic narcotic, *methadone* (Dolophine), is substituted in doses intended to minimize the patient's discomfort. Finally, even this addicting drug, which causes a much milder abstinence syndrome than morphine or heroin, is stopped. Sedatives such as phenobarbital may be given at bedtime for a few days during withdrawal; salicylates help to control muscle aches. Good nursing care and physical measures such as massage, warm flow baths, and ice collars also help ease the patient through this trying period.

Actually, this detoxifying or "drying out" procedure for breaking the patient's physical dependence on drugs is the most successful aspect of addiction treatment. Much more difficult is the task of coping with the patient's underlying emotional difficulties. Most voluntary patients stay at Lexington, for example, just long enough to lose their tolerance to drugs. Then, they leave to seek again the gratification that taking drugs gives them. Some doctors feel that patients should be treated in a drug-free environment for four to six months. During that time, those who are amenable to psychotherapy may profit from it. They then also receive valuable vocational training, participate in recreational activities and other rehabilitative measures. Recently, communities in which addiction is relatively common have been setting up local facilities for following up the addict who returns after withdrawal. Attempts are being made to make available the strong psychological support he needs and to help him get work that will enable him to earn a living in the hope that this will reduce the high rate of relapse in this condition.

Methadone Maintenance. Methadone has recently been employed in a research program in a manner different from that described above and for a different purpose. Once the addict has been switched from heroin to the milder but longer-acting drug, methadone, he receives daily doses of the latter drug indefinitely instead of having it gradually discontinued. Daily administration of methadone in this way is said to remove the addict's hunger for heroin. In addition, the patient who has taken methadone is unable to attain his typical heroin "high" for about 24 hours; thus, it is claimed that he both has no craving for heroin and no reason for seeking it.

Some authorities disapprove of the idea of substituting methadone addiction for heroin addiction. The opponents of the methadone-maintenance plan argue that the addict *cannot* be compared to the diabetic who requires insulin or the heart patient who needs to take digitalis indefinitely. They claim that the addict's personality problems are only perpetuated by methadone maintenance therapy.

Nevertheless, this experiment employing methadone has created considerable interest, because it has worked for some addicts who seem to need a drug of this kind in order to function normally. Many appear to have been aided in their efforts to rehabilitate themselves; they have left the streets and have become self-supporting members of the community or students at colleges or vocational schools. Another drug that is being tried in similar programs is the experimental narcotic antagonist *cyclazocine*, which also has a long-lasting antinarcotic activity that keeps addicts from feeling the desired effects of heroin. Of course, both methadone and cyclazocine sometimes cause side effects; and treatment failures occur in a significant number of addict patients.

Preventing Addiction. Relatively few addicts become dependent upon drugs as a result of medical treatment with analgesic drugs for painful conditions. Most addiction is the result of a combination of unfavorable social and personality factors. That is, youngsters growing up in an environment in which illicit drugs are readily available are tempted to experiment with them. Some may find drug-taking distasteful and suffer dysphoria, rather than attaining the desired euphoric state; but those who are looking for a way to avoid facing up to their problems may find it in narcotic drugs and soon become dependent upon them.

Although the social and psychiatric approaches to addiction prevention are beyond the scope of this discussion, the nurse should know how to minimize the danger of addiction in the medical use of drugs. Thus, for example, the nurse may often be charged with determining when to give a potent analgesic to a patient in chronic pain. In such cases, various measures may be employed to delay development of dependence.

Pain often can be adequately controlled with non-narcotic analgesics, sedatives, tranquilizers, or oral doses of codeine, which has a relatively low addiction liability. If the nurse has a choice, she should alternate such agents with the more potent analgesics. In any case, it is desirable to give opiates in the smallest dose that will produce the desired degree of relief and at irregular intervals rather than on a regular schedule. Narcotics should, of course, never be administered routinely merely to keep the patient comfortably sedated, so that he will keep quiet and make few demands for nursing care!

On the other hand, analgesic drugs should not be withheld for fear of causing addiction if the patient's condition indicates the need for these drugs. Thus, narcotics should be avoided in such chronic conditions as arthritis, but their long-term use in patients with severe pain from terminal cancer is completely justified despite the danger of addiction. The nurse should not withhold "p.r.n." narcotics when such patients experience excruciating pain but should administer them at the intervals specified by the physician.

The nurse should be able to recognize the patient who typically tends to rely upon potent analgesics for relief of anxiety rather than actual pain. Such a patient may, for example, complain of pain in his incision postoperatively long after most other patients with similar conditions no longer require analgesics. The nurse, on perceiving such a reaction, should bring it to the physician's attention, since continued administration of narcotics to such patients could lead to addiction. Counseling by the physician and the nurse, or in some instances by a psychiatrist, may be desirable to help the patient become aware of his anxiety and develop insight. By helping the patient deal more effectively with his problems, such aid may reduce his desire for medication.

The nurse also has the responsibility of seeing that narcotic drugs, hypodermic syringes, and needles do not fall into the hands of addicts. Drugs which cannot for some reason be used (e.g., because of contamination) must be disposed of, after making a notation in the narcotic record and usually having it signed by two staff members. Disposable needles and syringes should be rendered unusable before being discarded and not simply thrown into the trash where they can be readily picked up by addicts.

The need for nurses and other medical personnel to guard themselves against the dangers of drug abuse and addiction has already been discussed (Chap. 3).

THE SYNTHETIC NARCOTIC ANALGESICS OR OPIOIDS

As we have seen, morphine and codeine and the semisynthetic agents prepared by chemically altering these natural opiate alkaloids have various disadvantages. Their adverse effects on the nervous system and gastrointestinal tract often limit the utility of these drugs. The constant need to consider the danger of addiction is another drawback.

Consequently, chemists have for some time been searching for safer analgesics, which would be equally effective against severe pain but free of the limitations and dangers of the older drugs. Several classes of synthetic analgesics have been prepared. Although no highly potent pain-relieving agent had previously proved entirely free of addiction liability, recent advances indicate that the chemists may have reached this goal at last. In any case, various of the synthetic narcotic analgesics now available possess some advantages which may make them more desirable than morphine for some patients. (See Drug Digests.)

In the following discussion, the advantages claimed for some of these synthetic analgesics will be emphasized. Actually, however, all of these drugs are capable of causing side effects and toxic reactions similar to those of morphine and all are addicting drugs. Thus, the nurse should remember that no potent pain reliever can ever be considered free of potential toxicity. The nurse should carefully observe patients who have received any of these opioids and report the patient's response. This may help the doctor select the drug most likely to provide pain relief for a particular patient with the least discomfort or danger.

Central Nervous System Side Effects and Toxicity

An advantage claimed for several of the synthetic agents is their ability to produce analgesia with less of the drowsiness, dizziness, and disorientation sometimes seen when morphine is employed. This may make the less-sedative synthetics *meperidine* * (Demerol) and *phenazocine* * (Prinadol), for example, better for the management of pain in patients whose treatment requires that they walk about.

Actually, whether these side effects and others such as *nausea* and *vomiting* occur depends more on the patient's physical condition than on the particular drug employed. Thus, it is well to remember that postoperative patients are likely to experience faintness, dizziness, and nausea upon early ambulation. This may be due not only to analgesic medication but also to the physical and emotional effects of surgery. The patient should be assisted when getting out of bed and carefully observed while he is walking, so that he can be aided, if necessary, in order to prevent fainting and injuries from falls.

Some sedative and somnifacient action may, of course, be desirable in certain painful situations. Thus, when meperidine and phenazocine are employed as adjuncts to anesthesia, the doctor often finds it necessary to reinforce these synthetic analgesics with promethazine (Phenergan), barbiturates or other

* See Drug Digests.

tranquilizers and sedative-hypnotics, in order to allay apprehension before the operation and reduce restlessness after it.

The respiratory depression produced by morphine is often undesirable, and most of the newer synthetic analgesics have been introduced with claims for superiority in this respect. Here too, however, any advantage of this type is relatively limited, and caution is required to prevent respiratory depression with all these drugs. In general, the more potent a drug is as an analgesic, the greater is its capacity to reduce the rate and depth of the patient's respiration. (That is, all share similar margins of safety, despite differences in their milligram for milligram potency.)

The shorter-acting synthetic analgesics, such as *alphaprodine** (Nisentil), may be less likely to depress respiration markedly in some situations marked by sudden sharp pain that subsides suddenly. For example, when a long-acting analgesic has been employed prior to the setting of a fracture or the passing of a cystoscope, the drug's action continues long after the painful manipulation has been completed and deep depression may develop.

On the other hand, with a drug that wears off comparatively quickly, such as alphaprodine, the patient's respiration tends to return to normal more rapidly. Similarly, in the event of overdosage requiring treatment with narcotic antagonists, respiratory depression can be overcome more readily when the analgesic employed was one of short duration of action. (Of course, for pain that is steady and long-continued—as in patients with malignancies and other chronically painful conditions, analgesics of the longest possible duration are preferred. *Levorphanol* (Levo-Dromoran) and *methadone* (Dolophine) are synthetic analgesics suitable for such situations (see Drug Digests).

Gastrointestinal Side Effects

Several of the synthetic analgesics are said to produce fewer of the undesirable digestive-tract effects of the opiates. Constipation, for example, is claimed to be less frequent following administration of phenazocine and *piminodine* (Alvodine). The same is said to be true of the related semisynthetic agents *dihydromorphinone* (Dilaudid) and *oxymorphone** (Numorphan), which have been claimed to be better than the parent opiate for bedridden patients.

The first of the synthetic drugs to be developed, *meperidine** (Demerol), was found in the course of a search for drugs capable of relaxing smooth muscles. The drug is said to exert an antispasmodic action, but this effect is not dependable enough to make meperidine especially useful for patients with biliary

* See Drug Digests.

or renal colic. Although the drug may be somewhat less spasmogenic—and, thus, less constipating—than morphine it must be supplemented with more potent spasmolytics such as atropine and papaverine when used as an analgesic in these conditions. (Similarly, the spasmolytic action of meperidine on the bronchial smooth muscle is probably too slight to give it any real advantage over morphine in patients with asthma and other pulmonary difficulties.)

Addiction

Most of the newer synthetic analgesics were prepared with the hope that they would prove less likely to cause dependence and addiction. Yet all are capable of being abused by people whose personalities predispose them to addiction. All require the precautions previously discussed if addiction is to be prevented during their prolonged use in chronically painful conditions.

Some authorities have expressed doubt that the chemists who are trying to develop better synthetic analgesics can ever succeed in separating analgesic potency from addiction liability. They claim that any drug that is capable of making the pain experience acceptable to suffering patients is also bound to be abused by people who want to escape from their psychic pain in coping unsuccessfully with life's harsh realities.

Other scientists are more optimistic. They believe that analgesia and addiction need not be related properties. The first indication of this was the development of *propoxyphene* (Darvon) and *ethoheptazine* (Zactane). These and other new non-addicting analgesics, which are discussed in the next chapter, possess about the same degree of pain-relieving activity as codeine and apparently offer so little euphoric satisfaction that they are very rarely taken to excess.

Obviously, however, non-addicting analgesics with potency no greater than that of codeine still fall short of the ideal. Thus, the recent introduction of two drugs with high pain-relieving ability and lack of addiction liability—pentazocine (Talwin) and methotrimeprazine (Levoprome)—has aroused considerable interest.

NON-ADDICTING POTENT ANALGESICS

Pentazocine (Talwin), one of a family of potent analgesic compounds derived from the synthetic opioid phenazocine, has the ability to relieve severe pain of all the types encountered in acute and chronic medical disorders and after surgical procedures. Administered parenterally in doses of 30 mg., pentazocine appears as effective as 10 mg. of morphine. Yet, in contrast to morphine and other opiates and opioids, including phenazocine, tolerance or drug dependence does *not* develop during prolonged use of this drug.

Pentazocine is also relatively free of the constipation and urinary retention often brought about by morphine, and it is said to cause less nausea, vomiting, sweating and dizziness than meperidine. It is also less likely to produce severe degrees of respiratory depression. However, it is administered only cautiously and in low doses to patients with bronchial asthma and other obstructive respiratory disorders or with respiratory depression from any cause. If moderate respiratory embarrassment develops in such patients, oxygen should be administered, together with an analeptic such as methylphenidate (Chap. 13). Nalorphine and other narcotic antagonists are not effective for treating depression produced by overdosage with this non-narcotic analgesic.

Pentazocine is, itself, a narcotic antagonist which was synthesized in a search for drugs that, like nalorphine, would have *both* potent analgesic properties and lack of addiction liability. Unlike nalorphine, a drug not clinically useful as a pain reliever because of the bizarre mental effects that often accompany its analgesic action, pentazocine very rarely causes confusion, disorientation or hallucinations. Nausea, lightheadedness, drowsiness, vertigo and vomiting are this drug's most frequent side effects.

Cyclazocine, another member of the same family of narcotic antagonists, has also been tested as a non-addicting analgesic. It is said to be 40 times as potent as morphine as a pain-reliever. However, certain side effects and withdrawal discomforts of a kind different from those characteristic of the opiates appear to be disadvantages. This drug is also being tried as a pharmacological adjunct in experimental programs for rehabilitating narcotics addicts (p. 150).

Methotrimeprazine (Levoprome), a member of the phenothiazine family, shares the tranquilizing and anti-emetic actions of the drugs of that class (Chap. 7). In addition, it has the capacity to relieve moderate-to-severe pain when injected intramuscularly. Unlike morphine and other opiates and opioids, this drug does not produce severe respiratory depression; nor do tolerance and dependence develop when methotrimeprazine is employed for prolonged periods to control pain in cancer patients and those with chronic painful conditions such as arthritis and neuralgia. However, this potent non-addicting analgesic is best limited to patients who are not ambulatory, because it often produces drowsiness, dizziness and faintness in those who try to stay active after receiving an injection. Dryness of the mouth, nasal congestion and constipation are other minor side effects.

THE ADMINISTRATION OF NARCOTIC ANALGESICS

The doctor often leaves the administration of pain-relieving medication to the nurse's discretion. The proper use of these drugs requires very astute judgment, if the best interests of the patient are to be served. The responses of patients to analgesics is very variable; so they should be carefully observed and the drug administered in accordance with these responses.

When medication is ordered, it should be given promptly; minutes can seem like hours to the patient in pain. If the dose ordered by the doctor does not relieve the patient's pain, the nurse should let the physician know this. Similarly, if the medication makes the patient so somnolent that he can not be readily aroused, this too should be reported to the doctor so that he can order a reduction in dosage. Idiosyncrasy to narcotics is not uncommon; therefore, patients receiving analgesics should be closely observed for any unusual reactions.

The patient's response to analgesic drugs should be charted. Before administering any analgesic, the chart should be checked to see when the last dose was given, so that the medication is not given any more frequently than the doctor had specified. The intervals (e.g., "q. 4 h. & p.r.n.") are based both on the drug's expected duration of action and the particular patient's response.

The physician, of course, orders potent analgesics only after the diagnosis has been established. It would not, for example, be desirable to relieve gastrointestinal pain with opiates, only to have the patient suffer a ruptured appendix because his true condition was masked by the drugs. It is equally undesirable to administer analgesic drugs that have been ordered for one painful condition in order to relieve pain that may develop suddenly from another source.

Thus, for example, if a patient for whom analgesic drugs were ordered during the postoperative period after abdominal surgery were to develop severe pain in a leg, the previously ordered drugs should not be routinely administered. Instead the physician should be notified, so that he can determine the reason for the pain in the extremity. This could be the result of a developing thrombophlebitis, which requires specific therapy rather than mere pain relief.

Medication ordered for pain should be administered promptly, because pain can often be relieved more effectively before it has fully developed. The nurse should be alert for signs of strain and tension and ask the patient whether he is experiencing pain. Some stoical patients pride themselves on never complaining. However, the skilled nurse recognizes their discomfort from such clues as a slight frown or tightness of the lips and takes prompt action to relieve it.

Some patients are so fearful of becoming addicted that they will refuse even a single dose of analgesic medication. The nurse should try to discuss the patient's fears with him in order to help him accept the drugs the doctor ordered. On the other hand, medication should not be forced on a patient who refuses it despite explanation and reassurance. The patient may once have been addicted to narcotics and consequently be rightly fearful of reactivating that condition. The physician should be notified so that he may discuss the situation with the patient.

The need for narcotic analgesics can often be reduced by offering the patient psychological support and attending to his physical comfort. A personal word of reassurance and such measures as a soothing backrub, a change of position, or even straightening the patient's bedclothes may help to lessen his pain. Instituting a program of counseling and diversional activities has also been found to reduce markedly the amount of narcotics required by ward patients with cancer.

The nurse should make every effort to keep her patient from being disturbed. Hospitalized patients in pain often say that they wish they could go home where it is quiet, so that they could rest. While the ward may not seem noisy to the busy staff, it may be bedlam for the suffering patient. Thus, a quiet environment, which encourages the patient to rest, may reduce his need for narcotic analgesics.

The route by which a potent analgesic is administered is often important in determining its efficacy or toxicity. For example, morphine, generally, is much more effective when given subcutaneously than it is when given by mouth. The intravenous route is preferred for patients in shock, because absorption from subcutaneous sites is poor when the peripheral circulation is sluggish. The patient may not respond to several subcutaneous doses; then, if blood pressure is brought back to normal by other therapeutic measures, several doses of the potent analgesic drug may be rapidly absorbed at once and send the patient into deep depression. Thus, for prompt pain relief without the danger of delayed toxicity, the doctor may give the drug by slow injection into a vein in such cases.

TABLE 9-1
NARCOTIC ANALGESICS

		Usual Dose Range (in Mg.)
Natural Alkaloids of Opium		
Codeine N.F. and its salts	methylmorphine	15–60
Morphine U.S.P. and its salts	–	5–20
Pantopium	Pantopon	5–20
Semi-synthetic Opiates		
Diamorphine	diacetylmorphine; heroin	2–5
Hydrocodone bitartrate N.F.	dihydrocodeinone	5–15
Dihydrocodeine	Drocode; Paracodin; Rapacodin	10–30
Hydromorphone N.F.	Dihydromorphinone HCl; Dilaudid; Hymorphan	1–3
Metopon HCl	methyldihydromorphinone	2–7
Oxycodone HCl	dihydrohydroxycodeinone (in Percodan)	2.5–5
Oxymorphone HCl	Numorphan	0.75–10
Entirely Synthetic Compounds or Opioids		
Alphaprodine HCl N.F.	Nisentil	20–40
Anileridine HCl N.F. and phosphate	Leritine	25–100
Dextromoramide tartrate	Palfium	2–5
Levorphanol tartrate N.F.	Levo-Dromoran	2–3
Meperidine HCl N.F.	Demerol; Dolantin; Isonipecaine; Pethidine	50–100
Methadone HCl U.S.P.	Adanon; Amidone; Dolophine	5–15
Phenazocine HBr	Prinadol	0.5–2
Piminodine ethanesulfonate	Alvodine	10–50
Non-addicting Potent Analgesics		
Methotrimeprazine	Levoprome; Nozinan; levopromazine	10–30
Pentazocine lactate	Talwin	20–30

SUMMARY OF MAIN PHARMACOLOGIC ACTIONS AND THERAPEUTIC USES OF OPIATES AND OPIOIDS

- *Analgesic, Sedative, Tranquilizer, Hypnotic*

  These C.N.S. actions account for the effectiveness of these drugs against even very severe pain including that caused by acute smooth muscle spasm and chronic bone disease. Among the conditions in which potent analgesics are employed are: acute coronary attacks; biliary and renal colic; trauma caused by fractures or extensive burns; intractable pain of malignancies; control of post-operative pain; preanesthetic sedation; short diagnostic and operative procedures in orthopedics, urology, ophthalmology, rhinology, and laryngology; obstetrical analgesia.

- *Antiperistaltic, Antisecretory, and Spasmogenic*

  These peripheral actions on gastrointestinal muscles and glands account for the usefulness of opiate alkaloids in diarrhea, dysentery, and various other gastrointestinal conditions including peritonitis.

- *Antitussive*

  The depressant action of many of these drugs on the medullary cough center mechanism accounts for their usefulness for decreasing the frequency of coughing. Morphine, methadone, and dihydromophinone are preferred for coughs accompanied by pain, following rib fractures, or in lung cancer, or tuberculosis. Less addicting and less depressant antitussives such as codeine and hydrocodone can control lesser coughs, including those caused by dryness and irritation of the respiratory tract mucosa in the common cold.

SUMMARY OF OPIATE SIDE EFFECTS, CONTRAINDICATIONS AND TOXICITY

- *Central Nervous System Side Effects and Toxicity*

  Drowsiness, clouding of consciousness, and inability to concentrate; occasionally, especially in women or elderly patients, paradoxical excitement marked by nervousness, restlessness, and even mania may develop. (Excitement is more common with codeine or meperidine overdosage and may progress to convulsions or to disorientation, delirium, or hallucinations.)

  Lightheadedness, dizziness, nausea, and vomiting are central in origin and more common when patients are ambulatory. Skin may become warm, flushed, and itchy.

  Respiratory depression, especially in elderly and debilitated patients and in those with certain pre-existing disorders. Among the conditions in which opiate administration requires caution or in which these depressants may be contraindicated, lest they cause apnea and coma, are:

  (1) Head injuries, delirium tremens, increased intracranial pressure
  (2) Severe bronchial asthma, emphysema, and other pulmonary diseases
  (3) Metabolic disorders, including myxedema, Addison's disease, hepatic cirrhosis, and renal failure.

  Circulatory collapse may be the result of severe hypoxia, or direct central and peripheral vasomotor depression. These drugs should be given only very cautiously to patients in shock, and preferably by vein in small fractional doses, because absorption from subcutaneous sites may be poor. Several subcutaneous doses might be absorbed at once if other measures bring blood pressure back to normal.

- *Peripheral Side Effects*

  Gastrointestinal tract smooth muscle movements are slowed and muscle tone is increased to the point of spasm. These actions and others, including reduced secretions, lead to constipation, a side effect to which the addict does not develop tolerance.

  Biliary and urinary tract muscle is also made spastic, increased choledochal pressure may lead to rupture of *diseased* gallbladder and duct tissues; spasm of the bladder sphincter may act to interfere with urinary flow.

  Bronchiolar constriction by morphine is undesirable for asthmatic patients; small doses of meperidine are less likely to cause contraction of bronchial muscles.

SUMMARY OF SIGNS AND SYMPTOMS OF OPIATE WITHDRAWAL. THE ABSTINENCE SYNDROME *

- *Early (after 10–12 hours): Mild Reactions*
    Rhinorrhea—nose running, reddened, swollen
    Perspiration—heavy sweating of face and body
    Lacrimation—eyes reddened and running with tears
    Yawning—frequent gaping and stretching

- *Later (18–24 hours): Moderate Reactions*
    Mydriasis—pupils widely dilated
    Piloerection—gooseflesh or "cold turkey"
    Anorexia—loss of interest in eating
    Muscular contractions—twitching, tremors, pain

    * The full blown syndrome described here is seldom seen today, possibly because the heroin obtainable by addicts is highly diluted. Withdrawal after substitution of methadone for heroin is milder but more prolonged.

- *Peak (36–72 hours): Marked Reactions*
    Restlessness, Insomnia—constant movement in bed may chafe skin of knees and elbows raw.
    Vasomotor Disturbances—hot flashes alternating with feeling cold and shivering
    Cardiovascular—rise in blood pressure of 15 to 30 mm. Hg; increased heart rate
    Respiration—breathing increased in rate and depth
    Body Temperature—fever of 1 degree or more
    Gastrointestinal—nausea, retching, vomiting, and diarrhea

- *Late Effects (7–10 days or many weeks or months)*
    Insomnia, nervousness, weakness, muscular aches, and poor appetite may persist but in a less acute form.

SUMMARY OF SOME POINTS FOR THE NURSE TO REMEMBER IN DEALING WITH NARCOTIC ANALGESIC DRUGS

- Remember that analgesic drugs, like all others, require the doctor's order before they may be administered to patients. Administer ordered analgesics promptly.

- Be alert to the patient's physical and emotional responses to analgesics and report any unusual response to the doctor, including any indications of beginning addiction.

- Never give narcotics as a substitute for nursing care or merely to keep the patient quiet.

- Let the patient know that the medicine you are giving him is for his pain, because the psychological effect of this and other actions on your part, such as reassuring him and making him comfortable, tend to increase the effectiveness of analgesics.

- Damage or destroy used disposable syringes and needles before discarding, so that the possibility of their being picked up and used by addicts will be eliminated.

- Make it a rule never to take any medication, and especially narcotic analgesics, without getting the advice of your doctor and a prescription from him.

+------------------------------------+
| **CLINICAL PROBLEMS** |
+------------------------------------+

This is Mrs. Wallenstein's third hospital admission. Her diagnosis is metastatic cancer of the breast. She is experiencing considerable pain, and her physician has indicated that her condition is worsening rapidly. At the beginning of her third stay in the hospital, Mrs. Wallenstein's pain was controlled with 50 mg. of Demerol q. 4 h., p.r.n. The amount later had to be increased to 100 mg. q. 4 h. At present, Mrs. Wallenstein is receiving 15 mg. of morphine sulfate q. 4 h., p.r.n. Her nurses have noted that Mrs. Wallenstein now requests the morphine regularly every four hours. The drug relieves her pain for about three hours after the injection. During the hour before her next injection can be given, the pain gradually returns.

- How would you respond to Mr. Wallenstein's question, "Is my wife addicted to narcotics?"

- What side effects of morphine would you watch for particularly, when caring for Mrs. Wallenstein?

- What nursing actions could you take to make Mrs. Wallenstein more comfortable and to help her tolerate the recurrence of pain before her next injection of morphine can be given?

REVIEW QUESTIONS

1. (a) What is one reason for justifiably delaying the administration of drugs for relieving pain?

(b) What is a good medical reason for relieving pain? (i.e., what factors beside humanitarian reasons make it desirable to keep the patient comfortable by reducing pain?)

2. (a) List several non-analgesic drugs that are commonly used to relieve pain.

(b) How do the true analgesic drugs differ from the other pain-relieving agents?

3. (a) What is the real meaning of the term *narcotic?*

(b) What does this word signify for most people?

(c) How do the narcotic analgesics differ from the *non*-narcotic analgesics in terms of relative pain-relieving potency and potential addiction liability?

4. (a) At what central sites are the analgesic drugs believed to act?

(b) In what three ways do potent analgesics, such as morphine, act to relieve severe pain?

5. (a) List several clinical situations in which morphine and other potent opiates and opioids are used for their analgesic, sedative, and hypnotic effects.

(b) List several other clinical uses of these drugs, which depend upon pharmacological effects other than analgesia.

6. (a) List some of the main side effects caused by therapeutic doses of morphine.

(b) In patients of what type is morphine given with caution, if at all?

7. (a) Describe the signs and symptoms of acute toxicity which may develop after an overdose of morphine or other potent narcotic analgesics.

(b) What measures may be used to counteract opiate toxicity?

8. (a) What psychopharmacological effects are desired by many individuals who abuse narcotic drugs?

(b) What factors besides craving or strong psychological dependence operate to produce addiction to opiates?

9. (a) What are some common signs which may indicate that an individual is a user of narcotics or under their influence?

(b) List some of the signs and symptoms of the abstinence syndrome seen upon withdrawal of opiates from a person who has been taking large amounts for long periods.

10. (a) Describe one type of procedure used in withdrawing drugs in order to detoxify addicted patients.

(b) What other measures are desirable in long-range attempts to keep the addict from going back to drugs after withdrawal has been accomplished?

11. (a) List some measures that the nurse may take to minimize the possible misuse of narcotics.

(b) List some measures that the nurse should take in administering narcotic analgesic drugs to patients in pain.

12. List the advantages claimed for each of the following opioids or synthetic narcotic analgesic drugs:

(a) Meperidine (Demerol)

(b) Alphaprodine (Nisentil)

(c) Levorphanol (Levo-Dromoran)

(d) Dihydromorphinone (Dilaudid)

13. Explain how each of the following drugs is used in the diagnosis or treatment of addiction:

(a) Methadone (Dolantin)

(b) Nallorphine (Nalline)

14. (a) List some side effects, potential toxicity, and limitations of the presently available synthetic narcotic drugs or opioids.

(b) What possible significant advantages may the new synthetic analgesics pentazocine and methotrimeprazine possess?

BIBLIOGRAPHY

Bonica, J. J.: The Management of Pain. Philadelphia, Lea and Febiger, 1953.

Dole, V. P., and Nyswander, M.: A medical treatment for diacetylmorphine (heroin) addiction. J.A.M.A., *193:* 646, 1965.

Eckenhoff, J. E., and Oech, S. R.: The effects of narcotics and antagonists upon respiration and circulation in man. Clin. Pharmacol. Ther., *1:*483, 1960.

Fraser, H. F.: Human pharmacology and clinical uses of nalorphine. Med. Clin. N. Amer., *41:*393, 1957.

Freedman, A. M., *et al.:* Cyclazocine and methadone in narcotic addiction. J.A.M.A., *202:*119, 1967.

Grimm, E. L.: Narcotics control in the hospital. Am. J. Nursing, *54:*862, 1954.

Isbell, H.: The search for a non-addicting analgesic. J.A.M.A., *161:*1254, 1956.

Isbell, H., and Fraser, H. F.: Addiction to analgesics and barbiturates. Pharmacol. Rev., *2:*355, 1950.

Kaufmann, M. A., and Brown, D. E.: Pain wears many faces. Am. J. Nursing, *61:*48, 1961.

Koch, D. M.: A personal experience with pain. Am. J. Nursing, *59:*1434, 1959.

Lasagna, L., and Beecher, H. K.: The optimal dose of morphine. J.A.M.A., *156:*230, 1954.

Lasagna, L., and De Kornfeld, T. J.: Methotrimeprazine, a new phenothiazine derivative with analgesic properties. J.A.M.A., *178:*887, 1961.

Martin, W. R., *et al.:* An experimental study in the treatment of narcotic addicts with cyclazocine. Clin. Pharmacol. Ther., *7:*455, 1966.

Mullen, J. F., and Van Schoick, M. R.: Intractable pain. Am. J. Nursing, *58:*228, 1958.

Murphree, H. B.: Clinical pharmacology of potent analgesics. Clin. Pharmacol. Ther., *3:*473, 1962.

Rodman, M. J.: Newer drugs for the control of pain. R.N., *26:*65, 1963 (Aug.).

————: The narcotic analgesics. R.N., *24:*49, 1961 (Feb.).

Sadove, M., *et al.:* Pentazocine—a new nonaddicting analgesic. J.A.M.A., *189:*199, 1964.

Wikler, A.: Sites and mechanisms of action of morphine and related drugs in the central nervous system. Pharmacol. Rev., *2:*435, 1950.

Analgesic-Antipyretics and Other Non-Addicting Drugs for Pain

SELF-PRESCRIBING OF DRUGS FOR RELIEF OF PAIN

Aspirin and related pain-relieving drugs are produced and consumed in tremendous amounts. This form of salicylate and similar non-addicting analgesics are often administered in hospitals and elsewhere by nurses acting on a doctor's order. Much more commonly, however, aspirin-containing tablets are taken by people who have bought a non-prescription product on the basis of advertisements that they have seen or heard on television, radio, and in the press.

Experience has proved that such self-administration of salicylate anti-pain products is not ordinarily dangerous or addicting; however, these non-narcotic analgesics are commonly misused in various ways. Sometimes patients resort to self-medication for chronic pain, instead of going to the doctor to have the condition diagnosed. Others continue to take these drugs for prolonged periods and in excessive amounts in ways that can eventually cause chronic toxicity or lead to other drug-abuse difficulties.

Nurses should be alert for such situations and for others in which these seemingly safe substances are being unwisely used or stored. Aspirin, for example, is the chemical most commonly involved in the accidental poisoning of children in this country. Thus, a thorough understanding of the usefulness and limitations of the salicylates and other non-addicting analgesic and antipyretic (fever-reducing) drugs will help nurses meet their responsibilities as health teachers.

Non-narcotic Drugs for Relief of Pain

Potent analgesics of the opiate-opioid type, which were discussed in Chapter 9, are capable of relieving severe pain. However, in doing so, even single small doses of these drugs usually produce some change in the patient's mental state and behavior. Larger doses taken over a period of time lead to tolerance, physical dependence, and other addiction phenomena. The drugs which we shall discuss in this chapter are not nearly as effective as the natural and synthetic opiates against acute pain. They are not, for example, very useful against the severe pain that stems from sudden spasms of visceral smooth muscles (e.g., in renal and biliary colic).

This does not mean, however, that these non-narcotic drugs are used only in minor illnesses or that the patient for whom they are ordered is not suffering. The doctor may even use these analgesics to manage pain in cancer patients before reluctantly turning to codeine, meperidine (Demerol), or morphine, etc. Likewise, in chronically painful conditions such as Buerger's disease and rheumatoid arthritis, the doctor relies upon salicylates and similar agents to provide pain relief, because these drugs can be taken indefinitely without affecting the patient's mental and physical functioning or requiring a rise in dosage because of developing tolerance or physical dependence. Thus, the nurse should never belittle the patient's pain, because the doctor ordered "only aspirin." This and the other non-narcotic analgesics used in chronically painful conditions should be given with the same care and concern for the patient's comfort that prevails when opiates are ordered for acute pain.

Sites of Action. The absence of addictive properties in these pain relievers is probably related to the sites and manner of action. These drugs do not seem to affect the cerebral cortex directly but are believed to dull pain perception by a combination of subcortical and peripheral effects. The central subcortical site of action is thought to be the thalamus, the group of nerve nuclei that serve as a relay station in the transmission of all sorts of sensory impulses between the periphery and the cortex. These analgesics are said to raise the threshold to pain impulses reaching the thalamus by way of the lateral spinothalamic tract. Thus, even though other aspects of consciousness are not at all affected, fewer pain messages are passed on to the sensory cortex and its associative areas to be perceived and interpreted as pain.

Recent evidence indicates that the salicylates may relieve pain of some types by a peripheral as well as a central action. Scientists studying the biochemistry of inflammation have found that salicylates antagonize the effects of certain natural chemicals that are released when tissues are injured. These products of tissue protein breakdown are believed to cause an increase in capillary permeability. Fluids then exude out of these tiny blood vessels, stretching the tissues and setting off pain impulses before any other signs of actual inflammation appear.

Thus, some of these scientists have suggested that small doses of salicylates may exert part of their pain-relieving action by a peripheral anti*pre*inflammatory effect. The drugs, it is said, may reduce vascular permeability and thus lessen the pressure of these fluid exudates on pain-sensitive nerve endings. Others think that the salicylates may directly antagonize the effects of certain pain-producing chemicals that are released by body tissues as a result of irritation or injury. Among the autopharmacological agents * of this kind that have recently been suggested as sources of pain in joints and other integumental tissues are the polypeptide, *bradykinin,* and a still chemically unidentified substance called *"slow-reacting substance A,"* or *SRS-A.* It is thought that aspirin somehow counteracts the actions of these substances on sensory nerve endings, muscles, and other tissues.

In any case, two facts about salicylates seem to have been established by everyday clinical experience: (1) Small doses of salicylates seem especially effective against mild to moderate degrees of pain originating in the skin, muscles, connective tissues in the joint and elsewhere, and in the teeth and other structures in the head, and (2) large doses often produce dramatic anti-inflammatory effects in rheumatic or arthritic conditions, as is indicated in the discussion on page 162.

The Salicylates

The salicylates, the most important group of non-addicting analgesic-antipyretic drugs, are derivatives

---

* The term, *autocoid* (Greek *autos*—"self"—and *akos*—"remedy"), has been coined to describe this class of locally released body chemicals with powerful pharmacological activity, which includes *histamine, serotonin,* etc. (Chap. 40).

of salicylic acid and include acetylsalicylic acid (aspirin), sodium salicylate, salicylamide, methyl salicylate, and many others (Table 10-1). Salicylate production has risen to about 30 million pounds annually, and Americans are said to take over 35 tons of salicylates daily, mostly in the form of billions of aspirin tablets.

Hippocrates and other ancient physicians employed plants now known to contain natural salicylates. These include species of willow and poplar, and a species of Gaultheria, from which oil of wintergreen (methyl salicylate) is obtained. Extracts of willow bark came back into use for treating fevers late in the eighteenth century (the word *salicylate* is derived from *Salix,* the Latin name for the willow tree). Synthetic salicylates were first prepared about a hundred years ago. Aspirin itself was introduced at the turn of this century as a substitute for sodium salicylate which has a disagreeable taste and caused a high incidence of gastrointestinal disturbance. It is interesting to speculate whether this, the most widely used of all analgesics, would have been discovered by today's drug screening methods in animals. In fact, the ordinary tests for analgesic activity in human subjects do not reveal any consistently significant rise in the pain perception threshold after administration of salicylates. Although common experience seems to have confirmed the presence in salicylates of a pain-relieving property that science cannot demonstrate, we are still not at all sure of how salicylates produce their various clinically useful pharmacological effects.

Pharmacological Effects. The salicylates act both centrally and peripherally to produce their varied therapeutic and toxic effects. Those most useful in treatment are: the *analgesic-antipyretic* actions, the *anti-inflammatory-antirheumatic* effects, and the *uricosuric* (uric-acid excreting) properties. The results of salicylate administration are dose-related to a large extent. Their pain-relieving and fever-reducing actions are readily brought about by administration of low doses. Moderate amounts of salicylates help to lower plasma levels of uric acid in gout. Relatively large doses are required to bring about the anti-inflammatory action desired in rheumatic conditions. Massive overdosage causes complex and potentially dangerous metabolic effects.

Analgesia of the kind and degree produced by salicylates and other non-addicting analgesics is usually achieved with about 600 mg. of aspirin, the amount contained in two tablets. This amount is readily absorbed from the upper gastrointestinal tract to produce peak plasma levels in about half an hour. Symptomatic relief of pain originating in joints, muscles, skin and connective tissues can be maintained by repeating this small dose every two to four hours.

The ease and safety with which such minor pains

TABLE 10-1

NON-NARCOTIC ANALGESICS AND ANTIPYRETICS

OFFICIAL OR GENERIC NAME	SYNONYM OR TRADE NAME	DOSE
Salicylates and related drugs		
Aluminum Aspirin N.F.	Aluminum acetylsalicylate	670 mg.
Aspirin U.S.P.	Acetylsalicylic acid	300–1000 mg.
Calcium acetylsalicylate carbimide	Calurin	300–600 mg.
Choline salicylate	Arthropan Liquid	870 mg.
Methyl salicylate U.S.P.	Oil of wintergreen	Topical
Salicylamide N.F.	o-Hydroxybenzamide	300 mg.
Salicylsalicylic acid	Salysal	
	ingredient of Persistin	300 mg.
Salicylic acid U.S.P.	o-Hydroxybenzoic acid	Topical
Sodium salicylate U.S.P.	—	300–1000 mg.
Para-aminophenol, coal tar, or		
aniline derivatives		
Acetanilid	Antifebrin	200–300 mg.
Acetaminophen N.F.	N-acetyl-p-aminophenol	650 mg.
Phenacetin U.S.P.	Acetophenetidin	300–600 mg.
Pyrazolon derivatives		
Aminopyrine	Pyramidon	300–600 mg.
Antipyrine N.F.	Phenazone	300–600 mg.
Dipyrone	Methampyrone	300–600 mg.
Oxyphenbutazone	Tandearil	300–400 mg. per day
Phenylbutazone N.F.	Butazolidin	300–600 mg. per day (100-mg. tablets)
Newer non-addicting agents of		
codeine-like action		
Ethoheptazine citrate	Zactane (also in Zactirin)	75–150 mg.
Propoxyphene HCl U.S.P.	Darvon	32–65 mg.

are relieved accounts for the very wide use of the salicylates in self-medication of common conditions such as headaches, arthritis and related musculoskeletal conditions, the general malaise of respiratory viral illnesses, and other ailments ranging from dental discomfort to dysmenorrhea.

Occasionally nurses may be asked which of the various heavily advertised analgesic products acts most rapidly and effectively. Despite the loud and conflicting claims that one or another headache remedy is most rapidly absorbed, the question of which one acts "*fast, faster* or *fastest*" is of no real clinical significance. When small doses of aspirin are being employed for relief of minor pain, as in most conditions, it matters little whether the salicylate is in solid or liquid form or whether it is administered alone or combined with other substances, including so-called buffer systems.* All produce the desired pain relief in essentially the same relatively short time, and therefore the nurse is justified in recommending to almost all people the purchase of the least expensive product available—preferably, plain aspirin U.S.P.

* Nurses, as well as doctors and pharmacologists, may well be confused by claims and counterclaims concerning over-the-counter pain products, especially when each of the competing pharmaceutical companies backs up its claims by pointing with pride to the published reports of reputable medical scientists. It may help to remember that scientists are only human and may err both in collecting data and in interpreting their findings. Unfortunately, some investigators seem remarkably prone to err in the direction of the desires of the companies that are supporting their research. The advertisers are then quick to pounce upon any crumb of data that they can distort into a half-truth—or even smaller fractional truth—in order to exploit a possible advantage in the fight for a larger share of the multimillion dollar proprietary drug product market. The unbiased consensus on this matter of relative efficacy of proprietary analgesic products is that the superiority of one product over another exists mainly in the imaginations of the Madison Avenue script writers of "commercials."

The antipyretic (or fever-reducing) *effect* of the salicylates is often useful for making a febrile patient more comfortable. The doctor will try primarily to determine what is causing the fever in order to treat the patient with specific anti-infective drugs; however, he may also order salicylates and other measures for symptomatic relief. This is especially true in young children who sometimes run very high temperatures that make them excessively restless and irritable. Often, after an antipyretic dose of aspirin has brought the temperature down a couple of degrees, the sick child stops tossing and thrashing about and falls asleep.

The antipyretic effect of the salicylates helps the body rid itself of the excess internal heat which has accumulated in hyperpyrexia. Normally, body temperature remains remarkably constant as the result of a delicate balance between the amount of heat being produced and the amount being lost by the body. This dynamic equilibrium is under the control of heat-regulating centers located in the hypothalamus, which transmit impulses to cutaneous blood vessels, sweat glands, and other peripheral structures. Infections and other illnesses may interfere with the functioning of these thermoregulatory centers in ways that let enough heat build up in the body to cause fever.

The salicylates and other antipyretics—which do not have any effect on normal body temperature—are thought to make this central thermostat more responsive to the high internal heat of fever. As a result, this hypothalamic center then sends out more messages of a kind that leads to dilatation of cutaneous blood vessels and increased sweat gland activity. The excess heat is then removed by radiation, conduction, evaporation, and other physical means. Just how the salicylates do this is still not well understood. Some scientists believe that aspirin acts directly upon the subcortical thermoregulatory center to reset it when an infection has caused it to be set too high. Others think that the drug may act by protecting the center from circulating pyrogenic (fever-producing) substances or by preventing the release of such chemicals by the invading microorganisms or the defending leukocytes (white blood cells).

The nurse, of course, keeps a close watch on a feverish patient, both for the patient's comfort and safety and because accurate charting often helps the doctor to diagnose his condition. After salicylates are administered, the nurse checks the patient's temperature until it is stabilized—every half hour, or even more often if the doctor desires. Because the patient usually perspires profusely as his temperature falls after antipyretic therapy, his gown, and even his bedding, may have to be changed to keep him comfortable and prevent chilling. Other measures for removing excessive body heat may be ordered, including alcohol sponge baths and application of cool, wet cloths.

Skill and gentleness are needed in administering salicylates to an irritable, feverish child. Brusquely forcing the medication down his throat while he struggles against it may only make him throw it up. If so, more may be lost than the dose of the drug alone. For as we have seen (Chapter 4), a child's trust in those caring for him is an important part of his total treatment. Any approach that disregards his needs and reactions is likely to make him react poorly to other forms of treatment also.

Thus, the child should not be tricked into accepting a salicylate by telling him, "it tastes like candy." If the tablets that have to be swallowed leave an unpleasant aftertaste, it is best to admit this and take steps to counteract it by offering the child a spoonful of jelly afterward. Crushing the tablets and mixing them with strained fruits or juices is another way to held the child accept salicylates. Flavored or "baby" aspirin may also be useful, but mothers should be advised never to call it "candy." For if a child in that household later eats the entire contents of the bottle, the disastrous results are not "accidental" but really the natural outcome of this form of trickery.

Anti-inflammatory Antirheumatic Action. Large doses of salicylates are often remarkably effective for controlling many of the manifestations of acute and chronic connective tissue inflammatory disorders. In acute rheumatic fever the response to salicylates is sometimes quite dramatic. Not only are pain and fever relieved, but the inflamed joints are also benefited. Heat, redness and swelling are reduced, and the patient can move his limbs more readily. Restoration of mobility helps prevent or delay crippling, even though the salicylates do not actually halt the underlying disease process, and doctors doubt that these drugs prevent cardiac damage. (The place of salicylates in the management of acute and chronic rheumatic conditions is discussed further in Chapter 41.)

Despite considerable study, the mechanism by which salicylates ease rheumatic joint symptoms is still not well understood. Some have suggested that the salicylates stimulate production of the adrenal cortex hormones *cortisone* and *hydrocortisone,* which have potent anti-inflammatory effects (Chapters 28 and 41). Large doses of salicylates and the adrenal-cortex-stimulating hormone of the pituitary gland (*corticotropin,* or *ACTH*) act alike in one respect. Both are known to reduce the amount of ascorbic acid (Vitamin C) in the adrenal cortices. Since the drop in adrenal ascorbic acid upon ACTH administration is accompanied by a rise in corticosteroid production, scientists reasoned that the salicylates also were acting to stimulate the pituitary-adrenal system to produce additional anti-inflammatory hormones.

Although salicylates are still commonly combined with corticosteroids and vitamin C in arthritis remedies, the theory mentioned above has lost favor in the light of recent evidence. It is thought, instead, that the salicylates themselves may act directly in some way to counteract local inflammation. For example, aspirin may act by suppressing the response of capillaries in connective tissues to chemical substances released in these tissues by irritation or injury. This, in turn, may tend to reduce the amount of fluid exudates formed in the joints and thus suppress the signs of acute arthritis. It does not, however, prevent late tissue damage by altering the underlying pathological processes in rheumatic fever and rheumatoid arthritis in any way.

Adverse Effects. The salicylates cause few ill effects when taken in the small doses usually employed for relief of minor pain. The much larger doses administered in acute rheumatic fever and chronic rheumatoid arthritis almost invariably cause discomfort that must be counteracted in various ways. Massive overdosage results in severe salicylate toxicity, which is often difficult to treat successfully and sometimes ends fatally.

The usual analgesic dosage of aspirin is well tolerated by most people. However, allergic hypersensitivity is not uncommon and may lead to skin and gastrointestinal disturbances of some severity. Skin symptoms include redness, rashes, and urticarial (hives) type reactions. Such edematous swellings can be extremely dangerous when they develop in respiratory tract mucous membranes. Asthmatic patients are especially susceptible to edema of the pharynx and larynx, and death from asphyxia has been reported in patients taking a single aspirin tablet.

Thus, although such catastrophic reactions are rare, the nurse should pay attention to the patient who volunteers the information, "I can't take aspirin," and report this to the doctor before administering any product containing salicylates that may have been ordered. The occurrence of such severe reactions from so commonplace a substance as aspirin also shows why the nurse should never administer an unordered drug. It may seem only sensible to give two aspirin tablets to the patient who demands them for a headache during the night, rather than annoy the on-call doctor by waking him. Yet, it is best to avoid prescribing aspirin or any other drug. This holds true even when the patient tries to apply pressure with comments such as, "If I were home, I'd take it without a doctor's advice, so what's the difference."

Gastrointestinal disturbances may be more common after even small doses of salicylates than was once suspected. Most people seem able to take a couple of aspirins occasionally without any apparent stomach upset. Yet recent reports by gastroenterologists indicate that gastric bleeding from aspirin is fairly common. Hemorrhage may be heavy enough to require hospitalization, or it may be chronic and remain hidden until discovered in a search for the cause of an iron deficiency anemia. Thus, patients with peptic ulcer or a history of heartburn and hematemesis after previous salicylate therapy should be carefully watched while taking these analgesics.

To reduce such gastric irritation, salicylates are sometimes administered in enteric-coated tablets and in solubilized form. Most commonly, aspirin is combined with buffering agents such as aluminum glycinate and magnesium carbonate—the Di-Alminate of the proprietary product Bufferin. Some studies indicate that such buffering has reduced the frequency and severity of gastric distress in patients who had previously reacted adversely to straight aspirin products. Other medical scientists say that the addition of such buffering substances to aspirin serves no useful purpose. They claim that incorporating a tiny amount of alkali into an aspirin tablet does little to prevent stomach pain or bleeding in salicylate-sensitive patients.

Gastrointestinal distress is most likely to occur in patients receiving the very large daily doses of aspirin or sodium salicylate required for symptomatic relief of acute rheumatic fever and rheumatoid arthritis. Five to 10 grams are usually administered in 6 daily doses of about 1 to 1½ Gm. each. Directions for spacing salicylate dosage at 4-hour intervals day and night should be carefully followed to keep the drug at plasma levels that are effective yet not toxic. Sometimes a patient forgets to take a dose and then tries to make it up with extra medication, only to suffer stomach pain, nausea and vomiting. Such symptoms can largely be avoided by taking the medication after meals or with milk and crackers rather than with water. Moderate amounts of sodium bicarbonate taken with the salicylates also help to allay stomach irritation.

Patients in whom dosage is being deliberately pushed to achieve effective antirheumatic plasma levels should be carefully watched for other signs of *salicylism.* Dosage is usually raised until tinnitus (a ringing and roaring in the ears) occurs. When this toxic sign appears, the daily dosage is reduced—by about 10 grains (600 mg.) usually—to a level that is effective yet tolerable. Continued administration of excessive salicylate dosage could lead to deafness and to blurring and dimness of vision, diplopia, and other signs of auditory and optic nerve damage resembling cinchonism, the syndrome caused by quinine and quinidine overdosage (Chap. 36).

Salicylate poisoning occurs most commonly in preschool children who are both most prone to take massive accidental overdoses and most susceptible to dangerous drug-induced metabolic derangements. Acute intoxication is manifested by early signs of central nervous system stimulation including a characteristically rapid respiration; later, complex acid-base imbalances and possible petechial bleeding may develop.

HEMORRHAGING into the skin is due in part to the anticoagulant action of salicylates, which act in this case like the coumarin-type drugs (Chap. 24) to reduce plasma prothrombin levels. (This is why patients on long-term anticoagulant therapy should be advised to consult their doctors before taking salicylates.) As in overdosage of coumarin compounds, the antidote for hypoprothrombinemia is vitamin K. Thus, signs of bleeding may call for administration of phytonadione or one of the synthetic hemostatic substances with vitamin-K activity.

ACID-BASE IMBALANCE. Much more difficult to treat are the complex biochemical imbalances that develop from salicylate overdosage. Most common in older children and adults is respiratory alkalosis. Infants, on the other hand, are very vulnerable to metabolic acidosis. Sometimes, the patient swings between the two states or suffers from both simultaneously, and the doctor must try to keep track of the patient's fluid and electrolyte status by having frequent laboratory studies done.

TREATMENT. The doctor often orders the injection of fluids by vein to correct acid-base imbalances and to keep the patient adequately hydrated. Parenteral solutions containing mixtures of physiological saline, sodium bicarbonate, and dextrose are first administered to get the patient's urine flow started. Then, solutions containing potassium and other electrolytes are given as needed to restore ionic and acid-base equilibria.

Patients with severe acidosis may get systemic alkalinizers such as sodium bicarbonate or sodium lactate solutions. These alkalinizers also increase the rate of renal excretion of salicylates. However, the sodium content of these solutions may be undesirable for patients with signs of heart failure. Thus, especially when hypokalemia is present, potassium salts may be used to alkalinize the urine.

An amine buffer, tromethamine (Talatrol; THAM; Trizma) is also said to speed salicylate elimination and correct acidosis without adding sodium to the patient's system. Sometimes hemodialysis (i.e., the "artificial kidney") is used to lower dangerously high salicylate levels. When this equipment is not available, peritoneal dialysis with buffered, isosmotic solutions of human albumin may be employed.

Other treatment measures include the use of vitamin K products to counteract hypoprothrombinemic bleeding and calcium gluconate solution to stop tetanic spasms. Short-acting barbiturates may be given cautiously if convulsions occur. Respiratory depression may require artificial respiration and oxygen, but ana-

leptics are not administered because such stimulants are ineffectual and may cause convulsions.

PREVENTION. Obviously, prevention of salicylate poisoning is better than undertaking its difficult treatment. Public health nurses and those working in schools and elsewhere should take every opportunity to tell parents and older children that aspirin should not be given to small children without a doctor's advice. The need to store salicylates properly should also be emphasized, and people with young children in the house should be advised to get rid of liniments containing oil of wintergreen, as methyl salicylate is the most toxic form of salicylate.

Severe systemic effects of salicylates often can be prevented by emptying the patient's stomach as soon as possible. This may be done at home by inducing vomiting mechanically or with an emetic such as syrup of ipecac. If this fails, a doctor may do a gastric lavage or administer apomorphine subcutaneously.

Non-Salicylate Analgesics

Other substances besides the salicylates possess properties that make them useful for relief of mild to moderate degrees of pain. Two of the earliest classes of chemicals synthesized—the para-aminophenols, or anilines, and the pyrazolons (Table 10-1)—were, like the salicylates, introduced as antipyretics late in the last century. Later, their analgesic action was recognized, and it is mainly for this purpose that some of them are still employed, either alone or, more commonly, in combination with salicylates.

Para-aminophenol Derivatives (Acetaminophen; Phenacetin; Acetanilid). These drugs, sometimes called coal-tar or aniline derivatives, do not possess the anti-inflammatory, or antirheumatic, actions of the salicylates. On the other hand, they seem less likely to cause gastric irritation or some of the other side effects sometimes seen with salicylates. They are probably best employed as analgesic-antipyretics for patients who cannot tolerate salicylates.

Acetaminophen, the safest of these agents, is sometimes employed alone for relief of pain and fever in children and others. *Phenacetin* (acetophenetidin) is found more frequently, in combination with aspirin in proprietary remedies widely used by the public for relief of head, joint, and muscle pains and for dysmenorrhea. Despite theoretical advantages claimed for such combinations, reducing the dose of a five-grain aspirin tablet by replacing a couple of grains of the salicylate with an equal quantity of phenacetin does not really reduce side effects of either drug significantly. In fact, it may actually expose sensitive individuals or those who take massive amounts of such analgesic combinations to two types of toxicity!

Potential Toxicity. Clinical experience indicates that these drugs are harmless for most people when taken occasionally in the small amounts contained in proprietary analgesic products. However, chronic toxicity can and does develop in people who become habituated to headache remedies and continue to take large amounts for long periods. The toxic effects most commonly observed are those involving the blood and the kidneys.

METHEMOGLOBINEMIA sometimes occurs when some part of the blood pigment hemoglobin is converted to methemoglobin by the oxidizing action of these drugs, especially *acetanilid,* the most toxic of the three. Because this abnormal blood pigment cannot carry oxygen to the tissues, the patient may suffer symptoms similar to those of anemia. The person's skin and fingernails may become bluish in color (cyanosis), and he may complain of dyspnea and chest pains. Sometimes, persons habituated to headache remedies containing acetanilid keep taking the product to relieve head pain which is actually being *caused* by the drug-induced hypoxia!

The condition is readily reversed, if it is detected early enough, and the drug is withdrawn. Thus, the nurse should look for signs of cyanosis in patients who have a history of taking self-prescribed analgesics for pain. An ashen-grey color of the skin, lips, and nail beds should be grounds for suspicion. The doctor may then have the laboratory do a spectroscopic examination of the patient's blood to confirm the diagnosis.

HEMOLYTIC ANEMIA is another blood dyscrasia sometimes seen in patients using acetanilid and phenacetin. This condition, in which red cells are destroyed and release their hemoglobin, may lead to acute kidney failure. It usually results from prolonged overdosage of these drugs. However, hemolytic anemia may occur when sensitive people take only small amounts of headache remedies containing phenacetin and other drugs. (See Chap. 3, Adverse Drug Reactions.) The condition is best treated by having the patient stop taking all drugs and by infusing fresh whole blood containing undamaged erythrocytes to replace those destroyed by phenacetin.

NEPHRITIS with papillary necrosis recently has been linked with the abuse of proprietary pain-relieving products containing phenacetin. It is thought that the chronic abuse of this drug may damage the kidneys directly or as the result of its adverse effects upon the blood. For this reason, the Food and Drug Administration now requires the labels of such products to bear a warning against taking them for longer than ten days or in doses larger than are recommended.

ACETAMINOPHEN appears to be the safest drug of this class. It seems much less likely than acetanilid or phenacetin to convert hemoglobin to methemoglobin or to cause hemolytic anemia. Many manufacturers have quietly replaced the phenacetin component of their mixtures with acetaminophen. Actually, however, there is as yet no proof that this drug may not also cause kidney damage if it is chronically abused.

A more realistic advantage of acetaminophen is its water solubility, which permits its use for preparing palatable liquid preparations for pediatric use.

Acetaminophen may be especially suitable for pain relief after tonsillectomies and extraction of teeth in patients susceptible to the hemorrhagic effects of salicylates. Its analgesic action is rapid in onset, and the drug does not cause the capillary bleeding sometimes seen with salicylates. However, this drug cannot replace salicylates in treating acute rheumatic fever, because it lacks an adequate anti-inflammatory action.

Similarly, phenacetin cannot be used to replace part of the high salicylate regimen in rheumatic fever, although this would undoubtedly reduce the danger of salicylism. Combining much smaller amounts of phenacetin with aspirin and caffeine—as in the common APC formulation—does not offer any real advantage to the person who takes a couple of tablets occasionally for a headache or other minor aches and pains. The small caffeine content has no pain-relieving property, and the phenacetin—despite advertising implications that its addition helps to "calm jittery nerves"—is no tranquilizer. Thus such combinations accomplish nothing which cannot be achieved by taking a full therapeutic dose of aspirin alone.

Pyrazolon Derivatives. This group includes the analgesic-antipyretics *antipyrine* and *aminopyrine* (see also Drug Digests), which were introduced late in the last century, and *phenylbutazone* (Butazolidin), which was prepared only a few years ago. These agents all exert excellent anti-inflammatory effects. However, because of their reputation for causing severe toxic reactions occasionally, these drugs, unlike the agents discussed earlier, are not widely used in this country for relief of minor pain in products available for self-medication.

Aminopyrine has been the cause of cases of agranulocytosis that have ended fatally. Sensitized individuals who take even a small dose of this drug may suffer a sharp drop in leukocyte count, which exposes them to fulminating infections. These usually begin with a severe sore throat characterized by breakdown of the mucous membranes and ulcerations. The number of patients hypersensitive to aminopyrine is statistically small. However, if the drug were as widely available as aspirin, the incidence of drug-induced agranulocytosis would be alarmingly high. Thus, it may not be dispensed without a prescription in the United States, and few American physicians care to prescribe the drug.

Unlike aminopyrine, which rarely offers any advantage over aspirin, the related compound phenylbutazone sometimes benefits some patients with chronic joint disorders that have not responded to salicylates. The use of phenylbutazone in such cases of gout, rheumatoid spondylitis, and arthritis is discussed in Chapter 41.

Newer Non-narcotic Analgesics. Recently, a number of analgesics claimed equal to codeine in pain-relieving potency have been introduced for the relief of mild to moderate degrees of pain. The most popular of these, *propoxyphene* (Darvon), is commonly prescribed in combination with aspirin and phenacetin, because it has little anti-inflammatory action of its own. Although propoxyphene is a relative of the narcotic analgesic methadone, it has rarely been abused and does not require a narcotic order. It is said to be relatively free of the gastrointestinal side effects of opiates such as codeine, including nausea, vomiting, and constipation. However, patients sometimes complain of abdominal pain when the larger of the two available doses is taken.

Ethoheptazine citrate (Zactane), a derivative of meperidine (p. 152) that does not share the potential addictive properties of that opioid, is also available in combination with aspirin and phenacetin for treating many conditions characterized by mild to moderate pain. This drug also is claimed not to cause the drowsiness and gastrointestinal upset sometimes seen with codeine. Also claimed to exert an analgesic action are the centrally acting skeletal muscle antispasmodics, *phenyramidol* (Analexin) and *orphenadrine citrate* (Norflex). These drugs, because of their combined analgesic and muscle relaxant effects, are said to be superior to other analgesics for relief of painful musculoskeletal conditions. However, in view of the difficulty in evaluating pain-relieving drugs of this kind, such claims cannot yet be considered to have been established. Both drugs are available in combination with aspirin, etc.

Some of the newer non-addicting analgesics resemble aspirin and phenylbutazone rather than codeine. Mefenamic acid (Ponstel), for example, possesses peripheral anti-inflammatory activity and is employed for pain relief in rheumatoid arthritis, bursitis, myositis and similar disorders. An analogue, flufenamic acid (Arlef), is also being tested clinically in similar conditions. Other on-trial agents of this type include prodilidine (Cogesic) and namoxyrate.

TABLE 10-2

PHARMACOLOGICAL ACTIONS AND THERAPEUTIC USES
OF THE SALICYLATES

Pharmacological Action	Clinical Uses
Analgesic: especially useful vs. pain originating in the joints, muscles, teeth, head, skin and connective tissues	Headache, toothache, arthritis and related musculoskeletal conditions, general malaise, dysmenorrhea, etc.
Antipyretic: to reduce fever	Respiratory viral illnesses, such as influenza and the common cold
Anti-inflammatory or antirheumatic	Acute rheumatic fever, acute and chronic rheumatoid and osteoarthritis and related rheumatic disorders
Uricosuric: increased excretion of uric acid	Chronic gout management

SUMMARY OF POINTS FOR THE NURSE TO REMEMBER ABOUT SALICYLATES AND SIMILAR ANALGESICS

• Aspirin and similar drugs should be administered as promptly as the more potent narcotic analgesics and with as much care and concern for other comfort-promoting measures. (The fact that these drugs are somewhat less potent does not mean that the patient's pain may not be severe or that his illness is not serious.)

• Do not give in to the temptation to administer non-addicting analgesics without a doctor's order, even when the patient demands them and points out that these drugs do not require a prescription. Remember that despite their ready availability, these drugs can cause severe and even fatal reactions in some patients and that the prescription of all drugs is legally the responsibility of the physician.

- Be prepared to answer the questions that the layman may ask you about the conflicting advertising claims made for the various types of products available for self-medication of conditions marked by mild to moderate pain.

- Remember that when the patient who must take large doses of salicylates complains of gastric distress, this may often be lessened by giving the drugs after the patient has taken some food. The doctor should be informed of persistent stomach pain complaints, so that he can decide whether to reduce dosage, order antacid medications such as sodium bicarbonate, or otherwise deal with this symptom.

- Pay attention when a patient volunteers the information that he is sensitive to aspirin. This should be reported to the doctor before administering any salicylate-containing product, in view of the hazard of severe allergic reactions.

- When salicylates are being administered for their analgesic effect, note the time required for response and the degree to which the drugs relieve the patient's pain and record this information on his chart.

- Note and record the temperature of patients receiving salicylates for their antipyretic effects. Because the patient may perspire profusely, be prepared to change the patient's gown and bedding when necessary. See that the patient maintains an adequate fluid intake. Be tactful and helpful in persuading feverish, irritable children to accept salicylates.

- Remember that salicylates are the most common cause of accidental poisoning among children. Instruct parents in the safe use and storage of salicylates (and all other drugs) whenever you get an opportunity to do so.

- Remember that, although these drugs are not narcotics, some people may tend to take products containing them in excessive amounts and too frequently. Abuse of these drugs is a particular problem because of the ease with which salicylates and related drugs can be obtained without a prescription. If you note that a person is taking such products for treating symptoms which seem to require a physician's attention, help him to understand and accept the idea that he should consult his doctor.

SUMMARY OF THE SIDE EFFECTS AND TOXICITY OF SALICYLATES AND OTHER NON-NARCOTIC ANALGESICS

- *Salicylates*

  Allergic hypersensitivity. Skin, gastrointestinal and respiratory effects of varying severity may develop suddenly.

  Early salicylism. Gastrointestinal upset including nausea, vomiting, pain and gastric bleeding; tinnitus, partial deafness, diplopia, dizziness, drowsiness, lethargy, mental confusion.

  Salicylate poisoning. Central stimulation may lead to convulsions, followed by respiratory and cardiovascular failure. Stimulation of respiratory center causes hyperpnea, which in turn leads to respiratory alkalosis. Metabolic acidosis and disturbances such as *hyper* or *hypo*glycemia and hypokalemia may also occur. Bleeding disorders caused by hypoprothrombinemia or thrombocytopenia may develop.

- *Acetanilid, Phenacetin, etc.*

  Hematological effects include methemoglobinemia marked by cyanosis, headache, chest pain and dyspnea; also hemolytic anemia, which may lead to hematuria, anuria, and acute kidney failure.

  Nephritis with papillary necrosis may develop in patients who abuse these drugs.

- *Aminopyrine and Related Drugs*

  Agranulocytosis manifested by very low leukocyte counts, severe sore throat and fulminating infection.

- *Propoxyphene (Darvon)*

  Gastrointestinal upset—nausea, vomiting, gastric pain.

  Central nervous system depression (drowsiness and dizziness) and, with massive dosage, stimulation that may lead to convulsions.

CLINICAL PROBLEMS

Mary Austin, age 11, is being treated at home for acute rheumatic fever. In addition to bed rest, her physician has ordered aspirin 0.6 Gm. given five times daily. Salicylate therapy resulted in marked relief of the painful inflammation of Mary's joints. It also resulted in profuse perspiration and relief of fever. How would you, as the public health nurse, reply to the following questions raised by Mrs. Austin?

• "Mary feels so much better, and she doesn't want to stay in bed any more. Do you think she could get up and sit in the chair?"

• "Mary says the aspirin upsets her stomach. Is there anything I can do to relieve this?"

• "Why does Mary perspire so much? I have to change her pajamas and her sheets several times a day."

• "That seems like an awful lot of aspirin for a child to take every day. Isn't it dangerous? How would I know if she is getting bad effects from it?"

REVIEW QUESTIONS

1. (a) How do the salicylates and other non-addicting analgesics differ from the opiates and opioids in the types of pain best relieved by each?

(b) What should be the nurse's attitude toward the doctor's orders for these drugs and the patient's requests for them?

2. (a) List the various actions of the salicylates that play a part in their therapeutic effectiveness.

(b) List various clinical conditions in which these actions of the salicylates are considered especially desirable.

3. Discuss briefly the combination of central and peripheral actions by which the salicylates are believed to produce their pain-relieving and anti-inflammatory effects.

4. How might you answer the following questions from laymen concerning analgesic products for self-medication?

(a) Which type of product will give me *fastest relief* of a headache—plain aspirin, buffered aspirin, or APC?

(b) What should I do to keep from getting an upset stomach when I take such products for relief of headache or arthritis pain?

5. (a) How do salicylates and other antipyretics act to reduce fever?

(b) What measures should the nurse take when administering salicylates to feverish children?

6. (a) What should be done when a patient advises you that he can't take aspirin because he is allergic to it?

(b) What measures may be taken to reduce gastric irritation in patients who have to take large doses of salicylates?

7. (a) What are some of the early signs of salicylism and some of the manifestations of severe poisoning by salicylates?

(b) What are some of the substances and measures employed in the management of acute salicylate poisoning?

(c) What advice may the nurse give to help prevent acute salicylate poisoning and the chronic abuse of proprietary analgesic products?

8. (a) Compare the pharmacological actions of phenacetin with those of aspirin.

(b) Does combining small fractional doses of aspirin and of phenacetin (e.g., 3 gr. to 2 gr.) offer any significant practical advantage over a full analgesic dose of aspirin alone (e.g., 5 gr.)?

9. (a) List the kinds of toxic effects that may appear in people who become habituated to headache remedies containing analgesics of the acetanilid and phenacetin types.

(b) Describe briefly the signs and symptoms of the two types of blood cell toxicity sometimes caused by these drugs.

10. (a) What advantages may acetaminophen have over the salicylates in certain clinical situations and over the other analgesic compounds of its chemical class?

(b) What important action of the salicylates is lacking in acetaminophen, and in what clinical condition can it *not* be used as a substitute for salicylates?

11. (a) What is the chief danger in the use of aminopyrine and what is an early clinical sign of drug-induced toxicity of this type?

(b) What precaution does the doctor take if he decides that the risk of using aminopyrine rather than salicylates is warranted?

12. (a) What advantages are claimed for propoxyphene (Darvon) and other drugs with similar properties?

(b) What advantage is gained by combining propoxyphene and similar drugs with aspirin and phenacetin?

BIBLIOGRAPHY

Alvarez, A. S., and Summerskill, W. H. J.: Gastrointestinal hemorrhage and salicylates. Lancet, *2*:920, 1958.

De Kornfeld, T. S.: Aspirin. Am. J. Nursing, *64*:60, 1964.

Dixon, A., *et al.* (eds.): Symposium. Salicylates. London, J. & A. Churchill, 1963.

Done, A. K.: The nature of the antirheumatic action of salicylates. Clin. Pharmacol. Ther., *1*:141, 1960.

————: Salicylate poisoning. J.A.M.A., *192*:770, 1965.

Gilman, A.: Analgesic nephrotoxicity. Am. J. Med., *36*: 167, 1964.

Gross, M.: The salicylates. Am. J. Nursing, *55*:1372, 1955.

Prickman, L. E., and Buchstein, H. F.: Hypersensitivity to acetylsalicylic acid (aspirin). J.A.M.A., *108*:445, 1937.

Rodman, M. J.: Drugs for the "aspirin age." R.N., *20*:50, 1957 (Dec.).

————: Fever—friend or foe. R.N., *18*:42, 1955 (April).

————: Newer drugs for the control of pain. R.N., *26*:65, 1963 (Aug.).

Schreiner, G. E.: The nephrotoxicity of analgesic abuse. Ann. Intern. Med., *57*:1047, 1962.

Singer, R. B.: The acid-base disturbance in salicylate intoxication. Medicine, *33*:1, 1954.

Smith, P. K.: The pharmacology of salicylates and related compounds. Ann. N. Y. Acad. Sci., *86*:38, 1960.

Tschetter, P. N.: Salicylism. Am. J. Dis. Child., *19*:498, 1955.

Wintrobe, M. M.: Toxicity of aminopyrine. J.A.M.A., *178*: 1051, 1961.

· 11 ·

General and Local Anesthetics

Anesthesia means, literally, the absence of sensation. Of the various kinds of sensation abolished by the drugs that are classed as anesthetics the most important is pain, including the very severe degrees of pain caused by surgical procedures.

The anesthetics commonly employed in patients who are about to undergo surgery may be classified as *general*, and *local*. General anesthetics are usually given in doses that depress the central nervous system to a degree that causes unconsciousness as well as analgesia. Local anesthetics are used for their effects on peripheral nerves. They block conduction of pain impulses passing toward the central nervous system from various parts of the body without necessarily reducing the patient's awareness of his surroundings or affecting his behavior.

Historical Aspects. Before the first general anesthetics came into use about 125 years ago, the only agents available for alleviating the pain of the surgeon's knife were opium extracts, alcoholic beverages, and various plant products with only weak central depressant effects.

These substances were neither safe nor effective. Their safety margin was so slim that the patient's respiration might readily fail if he were given amounts large enough to keep him unconscious all through the operation. Smaller, safer doses of opiate-alcohol-belladonna mixtures might succeed only in putting the patient into a stuporous fog from which the painful stimuli of surgery readily aroused him. Often, it took several husky assistants to hold down the struggling delirious patient, while the surgeon worked as swiftly as he could to complete his painful task.

Then, in the decade 1840–1850, several simple organic chemicals came into use for the relief of surgical and obstetrical pain. First, nitrous oxide, an inorganic gas first prepared in the previous century, was shown to induce analgesia deep enough to permit painless dental surgery. (The substance, also called "laughing gas," had previously been used only to amuse the public, because inhaling small amounts often caused delirium.)

At about the same time, inhalation of the vapors of two volatile liquids, ethyl ether and chloroform, was proved capable of producing a state of unconsciousness deep enough to block out the pain of extensive surgical procedures. For the first time, patients could be kept completely free of pain for as long a time as the surgeon needed for performing a lengthy, complicated operation.

Late in the last century, cocaine, an alkaloid extracted from the leaves of various species of *coca,* a South American plant, came into use as a local anesthetic in eye surgery. Doctors, noting that chewing the leaves deadened the sense of taste, began to use solutions of the crystalline alkaloid for its blocking effects on sensory nerve endings in the cornea and conjunctiva. Later, cocaine and synthetically prepared successors such as procaine were injected for blocking spinal and other nerves.

Anesthesiologists have continued to search for safer and more effective anesthetic substances. For a while, ultra-short acting barbiturates such as thiopental were favored for their rapid sleep-inducing effects. More recently, the fluorinated hydrocarbons of the halothane type have been touted for their potency. Actually, however, ether is still the most widely used general anesthetic. Cocaine, on the other hand, rarely is injected for local anesthesia, because it largely has been replaced by safer and more versatile regional anesthetics, such as lidocaine.

GENERAL ANESTHETICS AND ADJUNCTIVE DRUGS

The Objectives of General Anesthesia

We have defined anesthesia as the absence of sensation. Actually, the anesthesiologist usually has other aims as well, when he administers a powerful general anesthetic such as ether, cyclopropane, or halothane. He tries to use these drugs in ways that will produce pharmacological effects that both preserve the safety, comfort, and emotional well-being of the patient and suit the convenience of the surgeon.

Thus, the goals of general anesthesia are the safe achievement of the following effects:

1. *Analgesia*, the loss of pain perception.

2. *Complete loss of consciousness* of what is going on; later, *amnesia*, or loss of memory of what went on during the operative procedure. (The purpose is to provide the patient with protection from anxiety, fear, and anguish by blocking out undesirable mental-emotional activity.)

3. *Hyporeflexia*, a reduction in reflex actions that might adversely affect the patient's breathing and cardiovascular function. (Efforts are made, for example, to minimize involuntary breath holding, laryngospasm, and cardiac irregularities during anesthesia.)

4. *Skeletal muscle relaxation*—desirable from the surgeon's point of view, since reflex muscular contractions in the operative area tend to make his task more difficult. Thus, general anesthetics may be administered in amounts that produce motor block by interfering with the spinal reflexes that maintain muscle tone in the abdominal wall as well as the extremities.

In actual practice, no one general anesthetic provides all four of these pharmacological objectives with complete safety and effectiveness. Consequently, the anesthesiologist customarily employs balanced combinations of several kinds of drugs. In addition, it is necessary to prepare the patient mentally for anesthesia and surgery.

Preparing the Patient

The thought of going under anesthesia makes many people very fearful. Many patients, although they prefer to be unconscious during the surgical procedure and unaware of what is being done to them, dislike the thought of losing consciousness—perhaps because "passing out" arouses fears of death. Others are concerned about losing control of themselves while under the influence of the anesthetic.

People vary in their willingness to discuss such matters. Therefore, the nurse should adopt an approach to the patient that will leave the way open for him to express his concerns about the pending anesthesia and surgery, if he so desires. By being aware that such unexpressed fears exist, the nurse can often help to allay them.

In many hospitals, the anesthetist visits the patient the night before surgery and lets him have some idea of what to expect. He may tell him what type of anesthesia he will receive and how it will be administered. In addition to learning these facts, the patient gets an opportunity to meet the anesthetist in person, instead of seeing him for the first time as a pair of eyes peering over a mask in the operating room. This helps to develop the patient's confidence in the surgical team.

The nurse also plays a part in preparing the patient for anesthesia by answering his questions and reassuring him. She tries to work together with the anesthetist in easing the patient's fear of the unknown. If she practices nursing in a situation that does not permit preoperative visits by the anesthetist, the nurse must be especially alert for the patient's queries about anesthesia. If she cannot give him the necessary information, she should discuss the situation with the patient's doctor, who can then answer his questions.

Balanced Anesthesia

The lack of any single anesthetic ideally suited to every patient and all surgical situations has led to development of the concept called "balanced anesthesia." This involves the selection and administration of two or more general or regional (local) anesthetics together with several other drugs that need not be anesthetics at all. The purpose of selecting such combinations of anesthetics and adjunctive drugs is to make maximal use of their synergistic actions and to antagonize various undesirable actions of the anesthetics. This, of course, leads to increased effectiveness and reduced toxicity.

It is common practice, for example, to induce a state of basal anesthesia by the use of certain drugs, such as pentothal sodium and nitrous oxide. These depressants produce loss of consciousness rather rapidly and pleasantly, but safe doses rarely bring about adequate muscular relaxation. However, such skeletal muscle flaccidity can be attained by then having the unconscious patient inhale a relatively small amount of a more potent anesthetic such as ethyl ether or cyclopropane, which will then readily bring him down to deeper planes of surgical anesthesia. Thus, the patient benefits from the most useful properties of the two anesthetic agents of different types, without encountering the difficulties which might develop if either agent were to be administered alone in the relatively large amount needed to produce full general anesthesia.

Adjunctive Drugs

Several classes of *non*-anesthetic drugs are commonly administered before, during, and after surgery to prevent or overcome the various adverse effects of anesthesia. Proper premedication with some of these supplementary agents induces anesthesia more smoothly and with smaller amounts of anesthetics. Other adjunctive drugs tend to minimize postoperative pain and discomfort. The uses of these drugs, which are discussed in more detail elsewhere, will be briefly summarized here, because the nurse is usually charged with having these adjuncts to anesthesia ready when they are needed, and, often, she administers them herself.

Because the fearful, apprehensive patient tends to struggle against going under anesthesia, it is important to help him become as calm and relaxed as possible. The nurse can help do this both by her personal approach to the patient and by administering ordered preanesthetic depressant drugs at the time when they do the patient the most good. Administration of barbiturates or other hypnotic drugs in the evening before the scheduled operation assures the patient a good night's rest. (See Chap. 6.)

Short-acting barbiturates or other sedatives and tranquilizers are given shortly before the operation. The patient who has been properly premedicated with these drugs (or with a morphine-scopolamine mixture) and who has been helped to understand and accept the surgery, is drowsy and relaxed at the time the anesthetic itself is administered. Thus the presedated patient tends to slip more smoothly into a state of surgical anesthesia with relatively small amounts of anesthetic.

The phenothiazine-type tranquilizers (Chap. 7), and the opiates such as morphine, meperidine, and levorphanol (Chap. 9) may also have desirable postoperative effects. The opiate analgesics reduce the patient's pain and restlessness after the operation; the phenothiazines reduce the vomiting which sometimes follows anesthesia and surgery. Drugs of both of these types tend to depress respiration; therefore it is important that they be given in proper dosage and at a time when the depressant effects of the anesthetic have nearly worn off.

Atropine-type drugs (Chap. 17) are given mainly to reduce reflexly stimulated salivary and bronchial secretions. By keeping the respiratory passages dry and unclogged, these antisecretory agents make the inhalation of anesthetic vapors easier and reduce the danger of postoperative complications such as atelectasis. In addition, these anticholinergic agents have other actions which may be desirable during anesthesia. Atropine, for example, blocks the increase in heart-slowing impulses from the vagus nerve which is a common reaction to the inhalation of certain anesthetics. Scopolamine, as has been mentioned, has a desirable preanesthetic sedative effect; administered with morphine or meperidine, its amnesic action blots out remembrance of any pain and discomfort felt before the anesthesia takes full effect.

Peripherally acting skeletal-muscle-paralyzing drugs (e.g., tubocurarine, Chap. 17) are often used during the operation to bring about muscular relaxation while the patient is still at relatively light levels of anesthesia. This, of course, permits reduction of the amount of general anesthetic to be inhaled or injected and thus tends to lessen the ill-effects of anesthesia. However, these drugs may themselves dangerously depress respiration by keeping the intercostal muscles and the diaphragm from contracting fully during breathing movements.

In the hands of an experienced anesthetist, these drugs can be used to produce maximum relaxation of the abdominal muscles with minimal interference with respiration. If the patient should stop breathing, the anesthetist can support respiration, manually or with resuscitative apparatus, until the drug's effects wear off. Overdosage with the curare-type neuromuscular blocking agents may be counteracted by oxygenating the patient under positive pressure and by injecting neostigmine or related anticholinesterase agents as antidotes.

Neostigmine and other cholinesterase inhibitors (Chap. 15) may be useful postoperatively for overcoming weakness of certain visceral smooth muscles. These and other cholinergic stimulants are sometimes administered to patients suffering from abdominal distention and urinary retention. By stimulating the smooth muscles of the intestine and the urinary bladder to resume their stalled peristaltic activity, these drugs help to relieve the discomfort caused by retained gases and wastes.

The frequency of these complications can be reduced by various nursing measures administered within the framework of the doctor's orders. For example, helping the patient to turn and walk about can help to relieve such discomforts as distention with flatus. It is also important to provide the patient with privacy and the opportunity to assume a normal position while he is attempting to void or defecate.

If these often overlooked measures fail to relieve the patient's discomfort promptly, the physician should be consulted. He may then suggest the use of physical measures such as application of heat to the abdomen or prescribe adjunctive medication such as neostigmine in an effort to bring about the return of normal visceral function.

(For fuller discussions of each kind of adjunctive drug described above see the appropriate chapter elsewhere in the text.)

Methods of Administration

The volatile-type general anesthetics are best administered by inhalation. Various systems have been devised for delivering anesthetic vapors into the respiratory tract along with adequate amounts of oxygen; equally important, of course, is the way in which the drug and the waste gas, carbon dioxide, are removed from the lungs.

Open systems are the simplest means of giving an anesthetic. Liquids, such as ethyl ether or vinyl ether, are sometimes dropped from containers directly onto a gauze-covered mask, or cone, which is held over the patient's nose or mouth. The vaporized liquid is then drawn into the patient's lungs along with the air that he inhales through the porous mask.

Semi-open systems are similar except that the mask is better sealed to retain the anesthetic vapors. This permits a higher concentration to build up more rapidly. However, valves or T-tubes are arranged in the system to allow the rapid removal of excess gases. This method is used mainly for inducing rapid anesthesia in infants and young children.

Closed systems deliver mixtures of anesthetic and oxygen in a controlled flow from gas tanks and vaporizers to a rebreathing bag. This is the most economical method of administration, because the exhaled anesthetic is retained and rebreathed. Control of the flow rate of anesthetic and oxygen and removal of carbon dioxide require the highest degree of skill.

The semiclosed system is similarly enclosed in a way that keeps the inhaled gases from being diluted by outside air. However, the system is provided with valves to allow the escape of excess gases during exhalation. Nitrous oxide is often administered in this way.

The Pharmacology of the Inhalation Anesthetics

The general anesthetics act mainly by depressing the activity of the cells of the central nervous system. The degree of depression produced at any time after administration of a volatile anesthetic is started depends largely on the concentration that the depressant drug has reached in the different parts of the nervous system. This, in turn, is the result of a dynamic balance between the rates at which the anesthetic (1) enters the lungs and the blood stream, (2) is transported to the central nervous system, and (3) leaves the brain and is eliminated by the lungs.

Absorption, Distribution, and Excretion. As soon as the first breath of volatile anesthetic reaches the bronchioles and alveoli, it begins to pass into the capillaries lining the pulmonary membranes in this, the terminal portion of the respiratory tree. This transport from lungs to blood stream occurs because gases tend to diffuse from areas of higher concentration (e.g., the alveoli) into those in which their concentration is lower (e.g., the arterial capillaries). When continuous administration of volatile vapors keeps the partial pressure of the anesthetic in the lungs at a high level, the amount of the drug in the arterial blood leaving the lungs for the heart, brain, and other organs rises rapidly.

The drug's concentration in the brain builds up quickly because of the abundant blood supply and the high affinity of anesthetics for fatty tissues, including the lipoids of the nervous system. Even in concentrations too low to affect the functioning of other organs, these depressants begin to disrupt the highly sensitive neuronal pathways and the activities that these nerve cells control.

Each portion of anesthetic carried to the brain by the arterial circulation soon leaves it by way of the venous blood, which redistributes the drug to other body organs. Some is stored temporarily in the body's fat stores, but almost all of the volatile anesthetic is eventually excreted in the exhaled air. By balancing the amount of anesthetic that is entering the patient's lungs from an outside source against the quantity of anesthetic that the venous blood is delivering to the lungs for elimination, the anesthetist can control the drug's concentration in the brain and consequently keep the patient at any desired level of anesthesia.

When he wants to lighten the plane of anesthesia, or terminate it entirely, the anesthetist simply stops the flow of vapor into the patient's lungs. This leads to a reversal of the diffusion gradient and a lightening of the anesthesia. That is, the anesthetic moving "downhill" from the brain into the venous blood is no longer being replaced by new increments coming in via the lungs and arteries. The level of depressant drug in the nervous system drops, the neurons recover from their reversible narcosis, and the functions that these nerves control begin to return. The emergence from anesthesia may be slow or rapid, depending upon how much of a particular anesthetic had been administered and how long and how deeply the patient had been anesthetized.

The volatile anesthetics are considered safer than those that are given by vein, because the anesthetist can more readily control the elimination of any excess drug. As soon as he recognizes signs of overdosage, he removes the mask from the patient's face. As long as the patient is still breathing and his blood is circulating, each exhaled breath rids the body of some of the anesthetic, and the amount in the brain begins to fall promptly to safer levels. Unlike the volatile anesthetics, which are almost always excreted chemically intact, the injectable or "fixed" anesthetics must be broken down by the body's own detoxifying mechanisms. Thus, the elimination of an overdose cannot be influenced by the anesthetist and takes much longer than the exhalation of volatile substances through the lungs.

Sites and Mechanism of Action. Exactly how the anesthetics arriving at the brain depress neuronal function has not yet been determined. We know that lipoid-soluble substances tend to reach the nervous tissues most readily, but this does not tell us what they do there to disrupt nerve cell activity.

We shall not try to discuss the many theories that have been proposed, except to say that the various anesthetics probably attack several different enzyme systems in ways that somehow interfere with normal nervous system metabolism and activity.

The part of the brain most sensitive to anesthetics is the reticular activating system (R.A.S.), the midbrain neuronal network that relays sensory impulses to all parts of the cerebral cortex, thus maintaining consciousness (Chap. 5). Doses of anesthetics too small to exert any direct depressant effect on other parts of the nervous system disrupt the stream of impulses that ascend constantly from this area to the cerebral cortex. This interferes with the functioning of the higher centers; awareness of sensory perceptions is diminished and distorted and, finally, consciousness is lost.

As the concentration of anesthetic rises, other areas of the nervous system are progressively depressed. This produces a characteristic pattern of altered reflex activity because first the higher and then the lower nervous centers are knocked out. However, the depression from above downward temporarily bypasses the medulla oblongata to first affect the reflex centers in the spinal cord, which lies beneath it. This "irregularity" in the pattern of descending depression is what makes it possible for the anesthetic to bring about profound muscular relaxation without paralyzing the vital respiratory and cardiovascular centers of the medulla.

As each succeeding area becomes depressed, certain signs and symptoms—the "anesthetic syndrome"—appear. These have been grouped arbitrarily in ways that help the anesthesiologist determine how deeply depressed the patient is at any time. Nurses, too, should know these signs so that they know what the patient's condition is as they observe it during induction, in the operating room, and in the recovery room, where the nurse's care of the patient during the immediate postoperative period is so important.

The anesthetic syndrome described in the following section is based upon what commonly occurs when ethyl ether is employed. The pattern of stages and planes varies somewhat when various other anesthetics are used, and the picture may be altered in various ways by the administration of preanesthetic medication as part of a balanced anesthesia procedure.

The Stages and Planes of General Anesthesia

The anesthetic pattern is commonly broken into four stages that reflect fairly clear-cut differences in the patient's condition. The third stage, and sometimes the first, are further subdivided into "planes," based on finer distinctions in the patient's state. The first two stages comprise the induction period; the third stage is the one in which most surgical procedures requiring muscle relaxation may best be performed; the fourth is a stage of undesirably deep depression.

When basal anesthesia with rapid-acting barbiturates is employed, induction may occur so quickly that signs of the first two stages are scarcely seen. During recovery from deep anesthesia, reflex activities return in reverse order from that in which they were lost. (The effects of ether anesthesia on respiration, pupil size, eyeball activity and other important reflex signs are summarized in Figure 11-1.)

Stage I: Early Induction. This stage extends from inhalation of the first breath of anesthetic vapor until the patient loses consciousness. Progressive disruption of higher cortical activities causes a clouding of consciousness marked by feelings of floating, numbness, and the loss of pain sensation. This analgesic state has long been considered adequate for dental surgery and obstetrical procedures, but it was, until recently, deemed dangerous to do more extensive surgery at this level because of the possibility that the patient might pass from this stage with its dreamlike disorders of sight and hearing (visual and auditory hallucinations) into the delirium and excitement of stage II (see following section). Lately, however, various major operations, including cardiac surgery, have been performed under first stage ether analgesia. The patient, properly premedicated to minimize the danger of delirium, is first taken down to a deeper level of anesthesia, which is then gradually lightened until he can hear and respond to commands. Yet he feels no pain during the operation and remembers nothing of it later.

Stage II: Delirium or Excitement. No surgery is ever attempted in this stage of anesthesia. Instead, every effort is made to help the patient pass as quickly as possible through this dangerous stage and down to the deeper planes of surgical anesthesia. Many of the mechanical, pharmacological and nursing measures that are employed preoperatively are intended to help ease the patient through this period.

Thus, for instance, the anesthetist sees to it that the patient is secured by straps, even before anesthesia is begun, so that he will not harm himself by becoming restless and thrashing about during this stage. Similarly, the patient's stomach must be empty when he comes to the anesthesia room, because all his reflexes including the gag reflex become hyperactive during induction, and it is at this time that he is most likely to vomit and aspirate food particles. (The chances of inhaling gastric contents are increased during recovery also, when swallowing and cough reflexes are returning, but the proper positioning of the patient for emesis minimizes this danger.)

Administration of the phenothiazine-type of antiemetic drugs preoperatively may prevent vomiting at this stage. However, because of their possible adverse effects on blood pressure and breathing during induction, some anesthesiologists prefer to reserve these potent drugs for use only against persistent postoperative vomiting.

Among the other preanesthetic medications which reduce the dangers of the delirium stage are the anti-

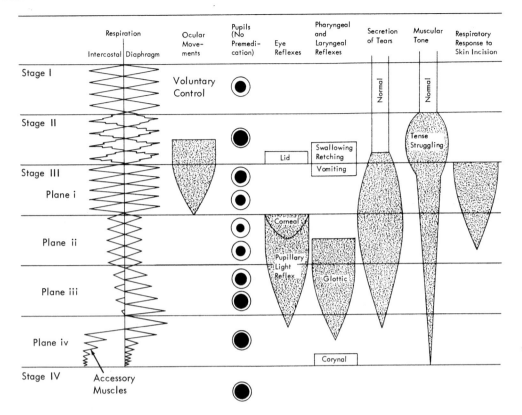

Fig. 11-1. The signs and reflex reactions of the stages of anesthesia. The wedge-shaped areas indicate (1) the variability from individual to individual and (2) the variability of the disappearance of the signs in the several planes of anesthesia. (Gillespie, N. A.: Curr. Res. Anesth. Analg., 22:275, 1943)

cholinergic drugs (e.g., atropine and scopolamine) and the sedatives and tranquilizers discussed previously. However, as we have indicated earlier, preparation of the patient emotionally is as important as the administration of drugs. The patient who has been helped to understand what to expect and has had a chance to express and explore his doubts and fears is likely to go through this stage quickly and with a minimum of excitement.

It is important to remember that the patient is not responsible for what he says or does in the excitement stage because he is actually unconscious. Thus, when a patient laughs, cries, swears, or tries to strike out, this is the result of the release of lower motor and emotional centers from normal inhibitory control by the higher cortical centers, which have been depressed by the anesthetic.

Some patients, who have heard that they may behave like a person acutely intoxicated by alcohol, are alarmed at the prospect of acting in ways not in keeping with their standards of proper conduct. They may also fear that they will disclose all the secrets of their past lives. If such patients express these concerns, they should be assured that, contrary to popu-

lar belief, most people who have been adequately sedated preoperatively show only brief restlessness and usually only mumble to themselves in a way not understandable to others.

Even if the patient does swear at the anesthetist or says something funny, he should not be told about it later in reprimand or in jest. The nurse holds in confidence anything she hears the patient say during the delirium stage of anesthesia. She knows that such behavior is understandable and that the patient might be deeply embarrassed to learn that he had acted in ways that do not conform to his usual standards. In any case, in caring for people during periods when they are helpless or have lost control, we always try to understand the reasons behind their behavior. Knowing the nature of the condition—drug-induced delirium, in this case—helps us accept uncontrolled behavior.

Stage III: Surgical Anesthesia. The third stage of anesthesia begins when the patient stops struggling and his breathing becomes regular again in rhythm and depth. It may be artificially divided into four planes, based on changes that can be detected in the patient's respiration, pupillary and eyeball movements, and reflex muscular responses, as the degree of anesthesia deepens.

Respiration changes are most informative and important to the anesthetist. Breathing is most nearly normal in the first two planes. Increasingly shallow breathing, caused by depression of the spinal nerves that control the muscles of the rib cage, marks entrance into the third plane of Stage III. The diaphragm contracts more strongly to compensate for the failing intercostal muscles; its downward pressure makes the abdomen heave heavily, and, at the same time, the movements of the patient's chest, or thorax, are diminishing. When thoracic breathing ceases entirely and even abdominal breathing begins to grow shallow and irregular, the patient has descended to the dangerous fourth plane of surgical anesthesia.

Eye signs are also informative to the anesthetist. The eyeballs, which roll or "rove" about as the patient is entering Plane 1, grow gradually less active until they finally become fixed and motionless at the top of Plane 2. (This diminishing eyeball activity reflects increasing depression of the midbrain's oculomotor center.)

The pupils, which were widely dilated during the excitement stage, return to normal in the first plane of this stage. They tend to contract in Plane 2 but then dilate progressively as inadequate pulmonary ventilation in the lower plane of this stage causes an asphyxial oxygen lack. (Premedication with atropine and morphine alters these pupillary responses, but the experienced anesthetist can, of course, still learn something of the patient's status from the eye signs.)

By the bottom of Plane 2 or early in Plane 3, the eyelid no longer contracts in a wink when the cornea is touched, and, a little later, light flashed in the patient's eye fails to cause pupillary constriction. Loss of these reflex signs indicates that the patient is down deep enough for any procedure and should be taken no deeper.

The skeletal muscles of the extremities and, later, of the abdomen become increasingly relaxed as spinal reflex centers no longer react to the stimuli that normally set off tonic contractions. By the bottom of Plane 2, cutting through the skin and into the muscles of the abdomen no longer elicits powerful reflex abdominal wall contractions. The paralysis of these muscles facilitates abdominal exploratory and surgical procedures. Such softening can be achieved at higher planes of anesthesia if a peripherally acting skeletal muscle relaxant is first administered (see p. 172).

Stage IV: Medullary Paralysis. This stage is marked by the complete cessation of breathing. Unless the anesthetic is withdrawn and resuscitative measures applied, the heart soon fails, blood pressure falls from shock level to zero, and the patient dies. Deaths of this kind need never occur; attention to the signs of anesthesia should keep the patient from ever being carried below the third plane of the previous stage. When volatile agents are employed, the still-functioning circulation will carry the anesthetic from the brain to the lungs, from which it may be removed by artificial respiration. Administration of oxygen by mechanical means may then help revive the patient. Overdoses of fixed anesthetics are not so readily removed, but the paralyzed medullary centers may sometimes be reactivated by prompt and vigorous analeptic therapy.

The Various Individual Anesthetics

No anesthetic drug is ideally suited for all patients and every clinical situation. Each agent has properties that make it desirable in some cases, but these are usually coupled with other actions considered disadvantageous. The following brief discussions emphasize the advantages and drawbacks of each agent. Some ways in which several drugs may be combined to counteract the undesired effects of certain anesthetics are also indicated.

The Potent Volatile Anesthetics. Those few substances that can by themselves produce complete anesthesia and keep patients in the deeper planes of the surgical stage for long periods with relative safety are considered potent. This term is applied to certain volatile liquids (e.g., ether, etc.) and gases (e.g., cyclopropane) with vapors that produce unconsciousness and good muscular relaxation when inhaled in very low concentrations, mixed with amounts of oxygen varying from 20 per cent (the content in air) to 95 per cent or more. (Other depressants also may be capable of producing full surgical anesthesia for short periods but only at great risk to the patient's safety. Such agents, which are not used alone for surgical anesthesia, are considered in the section on the Less Potent and Basal Anesthetics, p. 178.)

Ethyl Ether. Ether is considered the safest single all-purpose anesthetic. This is due in part to the potency of its vapors, which produce full anesthesia even when inhaled in low concentrations that permit administration of oxygen in amounts making up as much as 95 per cent of the mixture. Another factor in its relatively wide safety margin is the fact that its irritating action on the respiratory tract mucosa causes a reflex stimulation of the respiratory center. Ether is also unique in possessing a peripheral curare-like blocking effect on skeletal muscle, which helps to produce excellent abdominal relaxation. Most important is the fact that, even when patients are maintained in deep anesthesia during prolonged operations, ether causes relatively little harm to non-nervous tissues including the liver, kidneys, and heart.

Gastrointestinal disturbances are fairly common after operations in which large amounts of ether are employed. Postoperative nausea and vomiting occur in a high percentage of such cases. Such upsets are said to be less frequent when the patient has inhaled high oxygen concentrations simultaneously; when it seems severe enough to endanger the patient, vomiting may be counteracted by administration of one of the potent phenothiazine-type antiemetics. Postoperative distress from retention of gastrointestinal fluids and gases is sometimes blamed on ether's antiperistaltic effects, but such intestinal stasis may actually be the result of prolonged surgery, especially when the abdomen has been opened and the intestines handled during laparotomy. Paralytic ileus is treated by administration of peristaltic stimulants such as neostigmine or pitressin and by physical measures such as application of heat to the abdomen.

Ether is inexpensive and easy to use by the open drop method. Its vaporous mixture with air or oxygen is, however, flammable, and the danger of ignition limits its utility in some situations.

Chloroform. This potent anesthetic, introduced at about the same time as ether, is neither flammable nor irritating to the respiratory mucosa. Yet chloroform, unlike ether, is rarely used today despite these and other advantages. Its reputation for producing dangerous cardiac arrhythmias and hepatic necrosis has turned anesthesiologists and surgeons away from its use.

Deaths have occurred during induction of anesthesia with chloroform as a result of sudden cardiac arrest. Excessive vagal slowing can be counteracted by atropine premedication, but this does not prevent the direct depressant effects of high concentration of chloroform on the heart. Breathholding followed by deep gasping respiration may carry such concentrations directly to the myocardium and cause cardiac syncope even before the patient is fully anesthetized.

Chloroform, like the drycleaning chemical carbon tetrachloride to which it is closely related, has the capacity to cause late liver damage. Some anesthesiologists have recently suggested that this can be prevented by keeping the patient well oxygenated and by preventing carbon dioxide from accumulating, but fear of the hepatotoxicity of this halogenated hydrocarbon still persists.

Cyclopropane. This potent anesthetic gas is administered together with adequate amounts of oxygen by means of the closed system method. Inhalation of the gas for only two or three minutes induces surgical anesthesia with minimal struggling. Muscular relaxation is good but may require supplementation with neuromuscular blocking drugs in some cases. It does not cause nearly as much nausea as ether postoperatively, nor does it irritate the lining of the respiratory tract during induction.

Although cyclopropane does not poison the heart muscle as chloroform does, it often causes cardiac irregularities. These arrhythmias are believed to result from the drug's sensitization of the heart to circulating sympathomimetic substances released in the body during the excitement and stress of anesthesia and surgery. In any case, injection of epinephrine during cyclopropane anesthesia may set off ventricular tachycardia, and, therefore, such sympathomimetic drugs should not be employed simultaneously. Such rhythmic disturbances may be counteracted by administration of the antifibrillatory agent procainamide hydrochloride. The safe use of cyclopropane requires special precautions against sparks from static electricity, because it is highly flammable, and mixtures with oxygen contained within an enclosed circuit are potentially explosive.

The Fluorinated Anesthetics. Recently, several new anesthetic chemicals containing fluorine atoms have come into use. These substances—halothane, methoxyflurane, and fluroxene—possess high chemical stability, which makes them nonflammable and nonexplosive. The fluorinated compounds differ from each other somewhat in their pharmacological properties, but they are all potent analgesics.

Halothane (Fluothane), the most widely used of these drugs, has now been employed in millions of surgical procedures. Halothane vapors produce very rapid, pleasant induction of anesthesia, without irritating the respiratory mucosa or increasing secretions. Recovery is fast and free of nausea, vomiting, or residual depression. Cyclopropane-type ventricular arrhythmias do not ordinarily occur with halothane, and atropine premedication prevents the bradycardia, or slowing of the heart, which is sometimes otherwise observed in deep anesthesia. Skeletal muscle relaxation is fairly good but may be improved by administration of succinylcholine as a neuromuscular blocking adjunct.

The potency of halothane is so great that patients may pass quickly into states of very deep depression. Thus, a specially calibrated vaporizer is employed to keep the concentration of vapor being delivered to the patient within safe limits. Further, the anesthesiologist should have thorough training in the measures necessary to minimize potential toxicity, including the sharp sudden drops in blood pressure that sometimes develop. A couple of dozen deaths from toxic hepatitis have been reported, following surgery under anesthesia with halothane. The responsibility of halothane for these postoperative deaths has not been proved, but the possible role of halothane or impurities formed from it within the vaporizer is being intensively studied by government-sponsored scientists.*

Methoxyflurane (Penthrane) produces profound muscular relaxation and a prolonged period of postoperative freedom from pain, which may be desirable

* Halothane Study Subcommittee of the Committee on Anesthesia of the National Academy of Sciences, National Research Council.

for some patients including those who have undergone extensive abdominal surgery. However, the slow recovery from anesthesia requires close supervision of the patient by the recovery room nurse.

Induction of anesthesia also is slow, and basal narcosis may first be induced with a more rapidly effective agent. *Fluroxene* (Fluomar), which produces rapid, pleasant induction of analgesia and anesthesia, has recently been suggested for this purpose.

The Less Potent and Basal Anesthetics. Various powerful depressants have drawbacks that prevent their being used alone in full doses for achieving and maintaining deep, prolonged anesthesia. Some volatile agents, such as ethyl chloride, vinyl ether, and trichlorethylene, are powerful enough to produce complete anesthesia but are considered too dangerous to be used in this way. Others, such as the barbiturates and tribromoethanol, which are administered by vein or rectum, cause rapid loss of consciousness but do not produce adequate muscle relaxation or freedom from reflex responses to painful stimuli.

These drugs are used clinically:

1. As *basal anesthetics*, to bring patients down to the first plane of the third (the surgical) stage rapidly and pleasantly. They are then followed by potent anesthetics (e.g., ether, cyclopropane), relatively small amounts of which are then able to take the patient down from this state of basal narcosis to the deeper planes of anesthesia.

2. As *analgesics*, to relieve severe pain without bringing the patient down beyond Stage I of the anesthesia syndrome. Some of these drugs are used alone in small, safe amounts to relieve the pain of various minor surgical, obstetrical, orthopedic and dental procedures. For example, trichlorethylene may be used for relief of labor pains, nitrous oxide for brief dental operations, and thiopental or vinyl ether for setting a fractured bone or prior to passage of a cystoscope.

Some major points of interest concerning the various volatile and fixed anesthetics of this kind are briefly discussed below.

Nitrous oxide has to be inhaled in very high concentrations (85 to 100%) for full anesthesia. Obviously, this would keep the patient from getting enough oxygen, so that death from asphyxia would rapidly result. Therefore, this gas is never given alone for producing surgical anesthesia but is combined with other agents. For example, it is administered with oxygen (N_2O 80%, with O_2 20%) for rapid induction and then followed by ether; or it may be combined with preanesthetic sedation, skeletal muscle relaxants, and Pentothal, or spinal anesthesia to keep patients in a light, pain-free sleep state.

Vinyl ether (Vinethene) has a much shorter induction period than ethyl ether but, because it wears off very rapidly, the vapors must be kept flowing continuously to maintain deep anesthesia. When this is done for prolonged periods, the danger of liver and kidney damage rises. Hepatic toxicity has been claimed to be the result of hypoventilation and preventable if oxygen is supplied simultaneously in adequate amounts. Nonetheless, this anesthetic is recommended only for induction and for minor operations of short duration.

Trichlorethylene (Trilene) can produce surgical levels of anesthesia, but, because the required concentrations tend to cause cardiac arrhythmias, it is rarely used in this way. Instead, obstetricians often take advantage of its potent pain-relieving properties. A few inhalations—often self-administered by the patient—are usually enough to produce analgesia adequate for relief of labor pangs, without causing complete loss of consciousness. Such low concentrations are safe for the heart and harmless to the liver and kidneys.

Ethylene has a wide safety margin and other properties (e.g., rapid, pleasant induction and recovery) that make it especially suitable for use in poor-risk patients. Today, ethylene is employed mainly for obstetrical analgesia, but it has few if any advantages over nitrous oxide and the distinct disadvantage of being explosive in the concentrations used in closed systems. Special measures must be employed to prevent production of static electricity and other sources of sparks that might explode ethylene-oxygen mixtures.

Ethyl chloride is today used mainly as a local anesthetic for minor skin operations. Sprayed on a boil or carbuncle, for example, it evaporates rapidly and freezes the area, so that the doctor can make a quick, painless incision. When inhaled, the vapors of ethyl chloride cause rapid general anesthesia. However, a history of fatal accidents from heart stoppage has dampened enthusiasm for this agent.

The ultra-short-acting barbiturates—thiopental (Pentothal), hexobarbital (Evipal) methohexital (Brevital), etc.—cause loss of consciousness within seconds after injection into a vein or very shortly after instillation into the rectum. These drugs are widely used to induce quick, pleasant narcosis prior to administration of a more potent inhalation anesthetic or during prolonged operations performed under spinal or other forms of regional anesthesia. These barbiturates are rarely used by themselves, because the doses required for muscular relaxation cause marked depression of the medullary respiratory and circulatory centers. However, smaller doses of thiopental are commonly combined with a peripheral muscle relaxant and nitrous oxide–oxygen mixtures in many kinds of minor and even some major operations. Such a combination provides all the desired objectives of clinical anesthesia (pp. 170–171).

The rapidity with which these ultra-short-acting barbiturates take effect also makes them valuable in the emergency treatment of acute convulsive states. Convulsions caused by overdoses of C.N.S. stimulating drugs such as strychnine or of the local anesthetics can often be brought to a quick halt by the careful intravenous administration of thiopental-type agents.

These drugs are also occasionally used in psychiatry as disinhibiting drugs in the interviewing procedures known as "narcoanalysis" and "narcosynthesis." These are methods sometimes employed in psychiatric emergencies such as conversion hysteria to facilitate reaching the roots of a patient's emotional difficulties and to help him deal more effectively with them. Patients are carried to a state of very light anesthesia by slowly administered intravenous barbiturates. As the effects of the drug wear off, the drowsy patient becomes able to understand and respond to questions and, because his defenses are down, he may say things that he usually suppresses. The interviewing psychiatrist tries to uncover previously hidden material which will help him in making a diagnosis and in deciding on the direction that further psychotherapy should take.

Despite their wide utility, it is important to remember that these rapid-acting barbiturates are potentially dangerous drugs. They should never be used in dentistry or psychiatry unless resuscitative equipment similar to that found in a well equipped anesthesia room is available. This should include an endotracheal tube to counteract the danger of laryngospasm sometimes caused by these drugs and mechanical apparatus for administering oxygen under pressure, should sudden overdosage cause depression of the vital medullary centers. (See Chap. 6 for discussion of acute barbiturate toxicity treatment.)

Tribromoethanol (Avertin) was one of the first of the drugs to be used as a basal anesthetic. Administered by retention enema, it rapidly induces sleep, which state can be used as the base for deeper depression with other anesthetics. This depressant has been used for overcoming drug-induced convulsions and the seizures of status epilepticus, tetanus, and eclampsia. In recent years, tribromoethanol has been largely replaced by thiopental and the other ultra-short-acting barbiturates.

The steroid drug hydroxydione (Viadril) is capable of producing basal narcosis when administered by vein. However, such injections have been followed by thrombophlebitis and, since the drug has other disadvantages, it appears to be inferior to the ultra-short-acting barbiturates.

The Ideal General Anesthetic

It is obvious from our discussion of the various volatile and fixed anesthetics that there is at present no one drug that meets all the requirements for ideal

TABLE 11-1

GENERAL ANESTHETICS

NONPROPRIETARY NAME	TRADE NAME OR SYNONYM
Chloroform N.F.	Trichloromethane
Cyclopropane U.S.P.	Trimethylene
Ether U.S.P.	Ethyl ether; diethyl ether; diethyl oxide
Ethylene N.F.	Ethene
Ethyl vinyl ether	Vinamar
Fluroxene	Fluoromar; trifluoroethyl vinyl ether
Halothane U.S.P.	Fluothane
Hexobarbital sodium N.F.	Evipal
Hydroxydione sodium succinate	Viadril
Methitural sodium	Neraval Sodium
Methohexital sodium N.F.	Brevital Sodium
Methoxyflurane	Penthrane
Nitrous oxide U.S.P.	Nitrogen monoxide; "laughing gas"
Thiamylal sodium N.F.	Surital Sodium
Thiobarbitone sodium	Kemithal Sodium
Thiopental sodium U.S.P.	Pentothal Sodium
Tribromoethanol solution N.F.	Avertin Fluid
Thichloroethylene U.S.P.	Trilene
Vinyl ether N.F.	Divinyl oxide; Vinethene

anesthesia. These desirable properties can now be summarized as follows:

1. Induction of anesthesia should be rapid and pleasant, and recovery also should be quick and comfortable (e.g., the anesthetic should not irritate the patient's skin or mucous membranes or have an unpleasant odor; emergence from anesthesia should occur without nausea and vomiting, or excitement and restlessness; and analgesic and calmative actions should be prolonged).

2. Skeletal muscle relaxation should be good, but the respiratory muscles should not be impeded in their work of maintaining adequate ventilation of the lungs.

3. The substance should be nonexplosive, nonflammable and inexpensive.

4. Above all, the ideal anesthetic should have a wide margin of safety. This means not only that the planes of deep surgical anesthesia should be attained at doses well below those that depress the medullary vital centers, but that the drug should also have no

adverse effects on the functioning of the cardiovascular, renal, and hepatic systems.

Although no such paragon presently exists, it is not impossible that a single such drug may eventually be devised. Meanwhile, the application of the principles of balanced anesthesia—i.e., the administration of several anesthetic and nonanesthetic adjunctive substances so that they supplement one another synergistically—seems to be the best way to cope with the many different kinds of problems that arise during general anesthesia.

LOCAL ANESTHETICS

Local anesthetics are drugs that produce insensibility to pain by their depressant effects upon the peripheral nerves rather than the central nervous system. These drugs are often used, like the general anesthetics, to prepare the patient for painless surgery and are often employed in the diagnosis and treatment of various medical disorders.

Manner of Action. The local anesthetics act by temporarily blocking the conduction of nerve impulses. Applied in high enough concentration, these chemicals can stop conduction in any kind of nervous tissue. In practice, they are used mainly to interfere with passage of pain impulses, by way of sensory nervous pathways, from the periphery toward the central nervous system. However, the motor and sympathetic fibers of mixed spinal nerves may also be blocked, either deliberately to achieve certain desired ends, or as an unwanted side effect of the attempt to produce loss of sensation.

The reversible depression of conduction brought about by these drugs is the result of their action at the surface of the nerve fiber. Molecules of certain kinds keep sodium ions from flowing into the nerve cell through its outer membrane. As a result, the membrane remains stabilized in its resting condition and fails to respond to stimuli that usually set off nerve impulses. The exact way in which local anesthetic molecules do this is still not well understood.

Methods of Administration

In order to produce their effects, local anesthetics must be brought into direct contact with nervous tissues. Depending on how and where they are applied, these locally acting agents can produce a deadening of sensation in either small, discrete areas or large portions of the body.

Local anesthetics are usually administered in the following ways:

1. By topical application to mucous membranes or to broken skin. Such surface anesthetics penetrate to the sensory nerve endings and reduce their responsiveness to sensory stimuli.

2. By infiltration into tissues containing fine nerve fibers. Injection into intracutaneous, subcutaneous, and intramuscular sites anesthetizes the terminal portion of the nerve fibers in these tissues.

3. By injection close to the nerve roots near the spinal cord most impulses entering or leaving the cord at selected sites can be cut off. This conduction, or regional, type of nerve block includes such special techniques as spinal anesthesia and epidural (e.g., caudal) anesthesia.

It is vitally important to understand that the effects of local anesthetics need not be limited to the site of local application. Like other chemicals that are injected, applied, or inhaled, these drugs can be absorbed into the blood stream and carried to all parts of the body. Rapid systemic absorption may lead to high levels of the local anesthetics in the heart and brain, for example, with resultant toxic reactions involving the cardiovascular and nervous systems.

Topical or surface anesthesia is of two types, one involving application of insoluble compounds to the broken skin and the other the dropping or spraying of soluble substances on the mucous membranes of the eye, nose, throat, etc.

Application to Traumatized Skin. Applied to torn or ulcerated skin surfaces, anesthetics such as *ethyl aminobenzoate* (benzocaine) and *butamben picrate* (Butesin) give relatively long-lasting relief of pain and itching. Because absorption of these poorly soluble substances is very slow when they are spread over abraded skin as lotions, creams or ointments, systemic toxicity does not occur. However, topical application can cause sensitization and the development of allergic skin reactions. Certain newer topical anesthetics such as *pramoxine* (Tronothane) and *dimethisoquin* (Quotane), which differ chemically from the older agents, are claimed to be less likely to cause allergic reactions. (See Chap. 43 for further discussion of the clinical uses of local anesthetics on the skin.)

Application to Mucous Membrane. THE EYE. Applied to the mucous membranes of the eye, certain agents, including *cocaine, butacaine* (Butyn) and *proparacaine* (Ophthaine), provide anesthesia adequate for removal of foreign bodies or as an adjunct to infiltration with other anesthetics in various surgical procedures (e.g., extraction of cataracts). Cocaine, which was once widely used for this purpose, has drawbacks which have led to its being replaced by safer local anesthetics. For example, cocaine often causes initial irritation marked by a burning or stinging sensation before anesthesia sets in. Later, such irritation may lead to redness, dryness and other damage to the corneal epithelium. (See Chap. 42 for further discussion of the use of local anesthetics in the eye.)

BRONCHOTRACHEAL MUCOSA. Cocaine is still commonly sprayed into the tracheobronchial tree to deaden nerve endings in the mucosa before bronchoscopy or prior to passage of an endotracheal tube down into the throat of an anesthetized patient who requires extra respiratory support. Cocaine and other topically acting agents such as *tetracaine* (Pontocaine), *lidocaine* (Xylocaine) and *hexylcaine* (Cyclaine) eliminate coughing, gagging, and bucking, as well as the dangerous heart-slowing tracheal reflexes that are sometimes set off by the introduction of a tube into the throat.

When such solutions, which are sometimes sprayed liberally into the respiratory tract, are used, precautions must be taken to prevent excessive systemic absorption from mucosal surfaces. The local anesthetic solution should be made up in the lowest concentration capable of producing anesthesia and applied in a fine spray. The anesthesiologist then tries to keep a continuous record of the amount (in mg.) that has been administered, in order not to exceed the total dose that is considered safe. Sometimes he may have the nurse keep note of the amount that the patient has received internally.

Infiltration anesthesia also calls for precautions to avoid injecting excessive doses. This procedure sometimes requires relatively small amounts of solution (e.g., for the block of specific nerves in dentistry or in the paracervical-pudendal blocks now being employed increasingly in obstetrics). On the other hand, depending on the nature of the operative field, much larger amounts of dilute local anesthetic solutions may be needed to deaden all the sensory nerves supplying the skin, subcutaneous tissues, and muscles.

To keep the volume and the quantity of local anesthetic solution as low as possible it is commonly combined with a small quantity of a vasoconstrictor drug such as epinephrine. Epinephrine reduces the rate at which the locally injected drug is absorbed into the blood stream. This serves a double purpose: (1) It prolongs the local anesthetic action on the nerve fibers in the area of the operation, thus lessening the need for further injections during a prolonged operation, and (2) it slows down systemic absorption of the drug, so that the body's own detoxifying processes can eliminate it before toxic levels are reached. Epinephrine should not be added to solutions for use in areas of relatively restricted circulation, such as the fingers, toes, or ears, in order to avoid producing extensive vasoconstriction and ischemia.

In performing field blocks, local anesthetic solutions should not be injected into an infected area. The injections should be made slowly and cautiously in the minimal amounts needed to produce the desired degree of nerve block. It is important for the doctor to aspirate before each injection to avoid inadvertent intravenous injection of the local anesthetic solution. Procaine, for example, is sometimes given purposely by vein in low concentrations to produce generalized analgesia, but the more concentrated solutions used

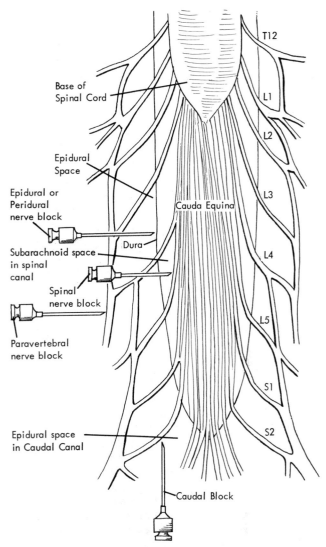

Fig. 11-2. Sites of injection for spinal anesthesia, showing position of needle for spinal and epidural types. Letters indicate vertebral level of injection.

for infiltration may be dangerous if accidentally injected directly into the blood stream. Procaine is a relatively safe drug because of the rapidity with which it is broken down in the body. However, large doses that enter the blood stream abruptly may overwhelm the body's capacity to destroy the drug before it exerts its dangerous effects on cardiovascular and nervous tissues.

Conduction Anesthesia. *The spinal type* does not actually affect the spinal cord itself but blocks the roots of mixed spinal nerves in the subarachnoid space (Fig. 11-2). First the sensory fibers are affected and later the motor fibers. The result of an injection into the spinal fluid in the lumbar portion of the spine is first the loss of all sensation in the lower half of the body and, a little later, the relaxation of the skeletal muscles of this large area. Muscle tone and sensation return in reverse order as the drug's effects wear off.

Spinal anesthesia is most useful for surgery of the lower extremities and the lower abdomen. It is preferred to inhalation anesthesia for patients with asthma, emphysema, and other pulmonary diseases which might be made worse by the irritating action of some volatile agents. Elderly patients with cardiac or renal disease and, also, diabetics may do better with spinal rather than general anesthesia. For emergency surgery in patients who have eaten recently and have a full stomach, spinal anesthesia is indicated.

COMPLICATIONS. Spinal anesthesia requires strict adherence to a careful routine in order to avoid complications during and after the procedure. For example, the patient must be carefully positioned so that the injected local anesthetic solution does not diffuse upward to block the medullary respiratory center or the roots of the phrenic and intercostal nerves, which control the movements of the diaphragm and other respiratory muscles.

In addition to possible respiratory complications, spinal anesthesia is often accompanied by sharp drops in blood pressure. Hypotension is, in part, the result of blockade of sympathetic vasomotor nerve fibers in the spinal nerves. Reduction in the flow of vasoconstrictor impulses to the arterioles leads to dilatation of these blood vessels and a steady fall in pressure. Other factors, including muscular relaxation and cardiac slowing, contribute to this hypotensive reaction to spinal anesthesia. Blood pressure falls may be prevented or counteracted by the prior administration of long-acting vasopressor amines such as ephedrine, phenylephrine, and methoxamine. (See Chap. 16.)

It is usually necessary to give the patient sedative premedication to prevent the natural anxiety he may feel when fully awake during procedures carried out under regional anesthesia. Of course, patients who would be extremely apprehensive should be given general anesthesia; or, if the potent inhalation anesthetics are contraindicated, basal anesthesia with a barbiturate may be employed prior to spinal anesthesia. If the patient is only lightly sedated, all operating room personnel should be careful not to say anything that might upset him.

POSTSPINAL AFTEREFFECTS. Neurological complications occur only rarely today and then mostly in people for whom spinal anesthesia was undesirable because of some pre-existing vertebral or spinal nerve abnormality. However, patients often fear that they have suffered a spinal injury when they find themselves unable to move their legs after spinal anesthesia. Therefore, it is important to explain in advance that this will occur and will last a short while only. Similarly, patients should also be told to expect feelings of numbness and "pins and needles" as sensation returns and that this will shortly disappear. Some-

times nerve palsies and paresthesias of longer duration occur, but even these are usually minor and transient.

A more common occurrence is postspinal headache, which develops in about ten per cent of cases, with a somewhat higher incidence in women patients. Some doctors believe that these are caused by a reduction in cerebrospinal fluid pressure. They suggest the use of needles of narrow diameter for spinal puncture in order to minimize fluid leakage through the hole made in the dural membrane. They also advise hydrating the patient with saline solution to keep his cerebrospinal fluid pressure up.

A measure commonly employed to reduce the chances that headache will occur is to keep the patient flat on his back for 6 to 12 hours after spinal procedures. Patients should be told that their doctor wants them to lie flat for a specific number of hours. They should not, however, be warned that this is to prevent headache, because such suggestion may only help to bring on this symptom.

The patient is permitted to turn from side to side, if he so desires, without raising his head. The use of siderails is desirable in the care of these patients, who may be drowsy because of barbiturates and other adjunctive medications; yet this detail of postoperative care may be overlooked because the patient under conduction anesthesia has not lost consciousness.

Epidural (Peridural) anesthesia is brought about by inserting the needle, not under the dural membrane but above it, so that the local anesthetic stays out of the spinal canal but still blocks the spinal nerve trunks close to where they emerge from the cord. This lessens the likelihood of postoperative headache and intrathecal infections, but still produces widespread anesthesia when the needle is correctly positioned.

CAUDAL, OR SACRAL, BLOCK (Fig. 11-2). The solution is placed in the extradural space at the base of the spine. Caudal anesthesia is commonly employed in obstetrical procedures and for surgery of the anus, rectum, and prostate.

SADDLE BLOCK anesthesia, which affects sensation in the perineum, buttocks, and thighs has somewhat similar uses.

Systemic Toxic Reactions

Toxic reactions from abrupt rises in the level of local anesthetics in the systemic circulation are of two types: (1) central nervous system overstimulation and depression, and (2) cardiovascular depression.

Central Nervous System Reactions. Overdoses reaching the brain by way of the blood stream may make the patient nervous, confused, and disoriented; he may begin to tremble and then develop convulsive spasms. Such motor stimulation is best counteracted by the careful intravenous administration of an ultra-

TABLE 11-2
DRUGS USED FOR LOCAL ANESTHESIA

Nonproprietary Name	Trade Name or Synonym	Main Use * Maximal Dose †
Benoxinate HCl	Dorsacaine	Topical
Benzocaine N.F.	Ethyl aminobenzoate; Anesthesin; etc.	Topical
Butacaine sulfate	Butyn sulfate	Topical
Butamben picrate	Butesin picrate	Topical
Butethamine HCl N.F.	Monocaine	Infiltration and Conduction 100–150 mg.
Butyl Aminobenzoate N.F.	Butesin	Topical
Chloroprocaine HCl U.S.P.	Nesacaine	Infiltration and Conduction 75–100 mg.
Cocaine & Cocaine HCl N.F.	—	Topical 150 mg.
Cyclomethycaine sulfate	Surfacaine	Topical 750 mg.
Dibucaine N.F.	Nupercainal; etc.	Topical
Dibucaine HCl	Nupercaine HCl	Infiltration and Conduction 7.5 mg.–100 mg.
Dimethisoquin HCl N.F.	Quotane	Topical
Diperodon	Diothane	Topical
Ethyl Chloride U.S.P.	Monochloroethane; Kelene	Topical
Hexylcaine HCl N.F.	Cyclaine	Infiltration and Conduction 250–500 mg.
Isobucaine HCl N.F.	Kincaine	Infiltration and Conduction
Lidocaine HCl U.S.P.	Xylocaine	Infiltration and Conduction 200–500 mg.
Mepivacaine HCl N.F.	Carbocaine	Infiltration and Conduction 100–400 mg.
Metabutethamine HCl N.F.	Unacaine	Infiltration and Conduction
Metabutoxycaine HCl N.F.	Primacaine	Infiltration and Conduction
Oxethazaine	Oxaine	Topical
Phenacaine HCl N.F.	Holocaine	Topical
Piperocaine HCl	Metycaine	Topical and Infiltration 50–300 mg.
Pramoxine HCl N.F.	Tronothane	Topical
Procaine HCl U.S.P.	Novocain	Infiltration and Conduction 150–1000 mg.
Proparacaine HCl	Ophthaine	Topical
Propoxycaine HCl N.F.	Ravocaine	Infiltration and Conduction 20–200 mg.
Tetracaine HCl U.S.P.	Pontocaine	Infiltration and Conduction 4–100 mg.

* Agents for topical use may, in some cases, be applied only to the eye or only to the skin; in other cases, these agents are also administered by injection.

† Lower doses apply usually to concentrated solutions for conduction anesthesia or application to respiratory and urethral mucosa; higher doses apply to infiltration of tissues with much more dilute solutions.

fast-acting barbiturate such as thiopental. The antidote is best given repeatedly in small doses that control the convulsions but do not depress respiration.

Barbiturates sometimes tend to intensify the C.N.S. depression that often follows initial nervous system stimulation by local anesthetics. Such a double depressant action could result in coma and respiratory failure. Consequently, facilities and equipment for administering oxygen should always be available when local anesthetics are employed in infiltration, conduction, and respiratory tract spraying procedures.

Cardiovascular Reactions. Administration of oxygen and manual massage of the heart may revive the rare patient who suffers *cardiac arrest* from rapid delivery to the myocardium of a large dose of an absorbed anesthetic. In such cases, cardiac standstill may occur with dramatic suddenness and require the use of immediate heroic measures. (See Chap. 21.)

Other *circulatory collapse,* caused more by vasodilatation than by myocardial depression, is slower in onset and easier to correct when the warning signs are noted in time. The patient, in these cases, may turn pale and get drowsy or dizzy; his heart may race, but the beats become progressively fainter until finally the pulse cannot be felt, and he becomes comatose. This vascular reaction—the result of direct depression of arteriolar smooth muscle—is best treated in the same way as the hypotensive reactions of spinal anesthesia, i.e., by parenteral administration of sympathomimetic vasopressor substances, such as ephedrine, phenylephrine, or methoxamine.

Types of Local Anesthetics

Cocaine, the first important local anesthetic, is a natural substance—an alkaloid extracted from the leaves of the South American coca plant. Its toxicity limited its usefulness, and this led to the synthesis of very many substances of similar chemical structure, which it was hoped would be safer to use.

Procaine (Novocain) one of the first synthetic local anesthetics, is still commonly employed because of its relatively low toxicity. However, its somewhat short duration of action and poor absorption from membrane surfaces (e.g., the eye) has led to a search for longer-lasting drugs of wider utility.

Tetracaine (Pontocaine, etc.) and *dibucaine* (Nupercaine), which have an exceptionally long duration of action, have been preferred for prolonged operations under spinal anesthesia. Recently, however, *lidocaine* (Xylocaine) has come into common use for procedures of all types, including the various kinds of conduction block. Another new agent, *mepivacaine* (Carbocaine), is proving valuable for infiltration, topical and regional administration.

The physical, as well as pharmacological, properties of various local anesthetics limit their utility to some extent. The slightly soluble agents such as *benzocaine* (ethyl aminobenzoate) are used only on the abraded skin or on mucous membranes and are never injected. Cocaine, though readily soluble, is considered too toxic for injection and is used mainly to anesthetize mucous membranes. Procaine, on the other hand, does not penetrate readily to nerve endings when it is applied topically; therefore it is not usually employed for surface anesthesia but is given by injection for field and regional blocks.

The characteristics of several local anesthetics of different types are taken up in the Drug Digests discussing these drugs.

SUMMARY OF TOXIC REACTIONS TO LOCAL ANESTHETIC DRUGS

- *Central Nervous System Reactions*
  1. *Stimulation.* Excitement marked by nervousness, apprehension, disorientation, confusion, and, possibly, dizziness, vertigo, nausea and vomiting. This may be followed by tremors and tonic-clonic convulsions.
  2. *Depression.* Convulsions may be quickly followed by loss of reflexes, coma, and respiratory depression and failure.

- *Cardiovascular Reactions*
  1. *Hypotensive Reaction.* Blood pressure falls gradually or abruptly. Patient shows pallor and may complain

of feeling faint and dizzy; cardiac palpitations occur when the heart reflexly speeds up. Patient may become drowsy and pass into comatose state as blood pressure falls to shock levels.
  2. *Cardiac Reaction.* Heart rate may slow down markedly; pulse pressure is reduced. Cardiac standstill or ventricular fibrillation may develop suddenly.

- *Miscellaneous Reactions*
  1. *Allergic Reactions.* Skin rashes, urticaria, bronchospasm and laryngeal edema may develop in sensitized individuals.

2. *Local Tissue Damage.* Application of cocaine and other topical anesthetics may cause itching, burning, redness, and possible corneal ulcerations.

3. *Post-Spinal Sequelae.* Headaches and, occasionally, paresthesias (numbness and tingling), palsies, and paraplegia.

SUMMARY OF CAUTIONS AND CONTRAINDICATIONS IN THE ADMINISTRATION OF LOCAL ANESTHETICS

- Local anesthetics should be used in the lowest concentration and amount of solution that will produce the desired degree of blockade.

- The total amount of the local anesthetic agent (in mg.) should be recorded each time a solution is injected or applied, and the maximum safe dose for each agent should not be exceeded.

- Local anesthetic solutions should not be injected into areas of infection or applied to traumatized mucous membranes.

- Injections of local anesthetics should always be made slowly and cautiously and the syringe plunger should be pulled back periodically. If blood is aspirated, the needle should be withdrawn and the injection made in another area.

- Epinephrine or a similar sympathomimetic vasoconstrictor drug should be added to delay systemic absorption of the local anesthetic, except when patients are known to react adversely to epinephrine-type agents (e.g., severe cardiovascular disease), or in areas with relatively restricted circulation.

- Patients should be placed in proper position for injection of spinal anesthetics to avoid upward diffusion of the anesthetic in the spinal fluid.

- Patients should be kept lying flat or with head down (Trendelenburg position) after spinal anesthesia. (This and the use of a narrow gauge needle may minimize postspinal headache.)

- Oxygen, rapid-acting barbiturates, and vasopressor drugs, together with apparatus for their proper administration, should be readily available whenever any procedure utilizing local anesthetics is to be carried out.

SUMMARY OF POINTS FOR THE NURSE TO REMEMBER ABOUT ADMINISTRATION OF ANESTHETICS AND ADJUNCTIVE MEDICATIONS

- *In the Pre-Anesthesia Period*

1. Encourage your patient to ask questions and express his concern about the forthcoming anesthesia and surgery. Let him know that you will take the time to listen and that you want to help him learn what to expect.

2. Show your concern for your patient's welfare by paying attention to his physical comfort, as well as by talking to him. A soothing backrub, for instance, can promote relaxation.

3. Encourage your patient to be as self-reliant as possible before the operation. Thus, if he is able to bathe himself, allow him to do so. Allowing him to stay active and help himself can help reduce his anxiety about undergoing surgery. Diversions such as reading, watching television, and listening to the radio are desirable for the same reason.

4. Administer all preoperative medications at the times specified by the doctor and observe your patient's reactions to drugs.

5. If the patient is unable to sleep the night before surgery, try nursing measures before asking the physician to order more sedation. Spend some time with the patient to give him an opportunity to talk about the

experience. This and such measures as straightening the bed and rubbing his back may help him fall asleep.

6. Make certain that you have completed all the details of preoperative care before administering the preoperative sedative, so that the patient can rest undisturbed. Explain that he should not get out of bed without assistance, or smoke while unattended, once he has been given the preanesthetic medication.

• *In the Post-Anesthesia Period*

1. Follow the physician's orders as to positioning the patient. If no specific orders were left, the patient is usually positioned on his side with the head of the bed flat and with no pillow provided. This position helps prevent aspiration of respiratory secretions and vomitus. Suction the patient as necessary.

2. Observe the patient's vital signs as ordered. If no specific orders were given, the blood pressure, pulse, and respiration are usually recorded every fifteen minutes until stabilized.

3. Observe the patient for any evidence of hemorrhage or signs of inadequate pulmonary ventilation.

4. Speak to the patient calmly and quietly as he regains consciousness, thus helping him to orient himself to his surroundings.

CLINICAL PROBLEM

Mr. Robertson had an appendectomy performed under spinal anesthesia. Approximately two hours after the operation, Mr. Robertson asked, "May I have the head of my bed rolled up?", and "Why do my legs feel numb?" How would you answer each of his questions?

REVIEW QUESTIONS

General Anesthetics

1. (a) List four goals, or objectives, which the anesthesiologist seeks to achieve in administering an anesthetic.

(b) How does he try to gain these goals with minimal danger to the patient?

2. (a) What is meant by *balanced anesthesia* and how does it differ from *basal anesthesia* and from *adjunctive premedication?*

(b) List three types of non-anesthetic *depressant* drugs and three other kinds of drugs which are used as adjuncts to anesthesia and indicate the purposes for which these agents are administered.

3. (a) What three processes determine the concentration of a volatile anesthetic in the nervous system at any time after administration is begun?

(b) Explain briefly how the anesthetist can control the drug's concentration in the brain to (1) induce rapid anesthesia, (2) maintain a patient at a desired level for a long period, and (3) bring about recovery from anesthesia.

4. (a) Which part of the brain is most sensitive to the action of anesthetics and what is the effect on the patient when small amounts of anesthetic drugs depress this area during the first stage of anesthesia?

(b) What "irregularity" in the pattern of downward depression of the nervous system by anesthetic drugs makes safe anesthesia possible?

5. (a) Indicate the chief effect on the patient which characterizes each of the four stages of the anesthetic syndrome.

(b) What can the nurse do to make the induction of anesthesia easier and safer for the patient?

6. (a) What signs in the patient's breathing, eyes, and neuromuscular responsiveness serve to warn the anesthetist that the patient has descended to the deeper, dangerous planes of anesthesia?

(b) What general measures are employed to resuscitate a too deeply anesthetized patient, and why are the volatile agents safer than the "fixed" anesthetics in this respect?

7. (a) List the properties of ethyl ether that are advantageous and those that are undesirable.

(b) How may the disadvantages of ether be minimized by adjunctive drugs, administration measures, and nursing skills?

8. (a) What disadvantages of chloroform, vinyl ether, and trichloroethylene limit their utility?

(b) How may these drugs best be administered to take advantage of their desirable properties, while minimizing their dangers?

9. (a) What are some of the advantages of cyclopropane anesthesia and for what surgical purposes is it preferred?

(b) What is a possible danger in cyclopropane anesthesia and how may it best be prevented or counteracted?

10. (a) What are some of the advantages of halothane anesthesia and what are its possible disadvantages?

(b) How may the adverse cardiovascular effects of halothane best be prevented or overcome?

11. (a) Why are (1) nitrous oxide and (2) thiopental not used alone for producing full surgical anesthesia?

(b) What are the two procedures in which these depressant drugs are mainly employed?

12. (a) List the properties of an "ideal" general anesthetic.

(b) In the absence of such an "ideal" drug, what general procedure do anesthesiologists try to follow for attaining full anesthesia safely?

Local Anesthetics

1. (a) List the three methods by which local anesthetics mainly are administered and indicate which portions of the nerve fiber are affected by application of the drug in each case.

(b) At what specific site in the nerve cell do these drugs exert their action?

2. (a) List at least four anesthetics that are applied topically and indicate some dosage forms in which they are administered.

(b) What drawbacks prevent the routine use in topical anesthesia of the eye of (1) cocaine and (2) procaine?

3. (a) What are two reasons for the addition of small amounts of epinephrine to local anesthetic solutions?

(b) What happens to local anesthetics after they leave the site of their application?

4. (a) In patients of what types may spinal anesthesia be indicated, or even preferred to general anesthesia?

(b) For patients of what types is caudal anesthesia commonly employed?

5. (a) Toxic reactions of what two types mainly may occur during spinal anesthesia, and how may these be prevented or counteracted?

(b) What is a common aftereffect of spinal anesthesia and how may it be prevented or overcome?

6. (a) What two measures are most important for controlling toxic central effects of local anesthetic overdosage?

(b) What measures are best for treating toxic myocardial and vascular reactions to rapidly absorbed local anesthetics?

7. (a) In what way does cocaine differ from other local anesthetics in its *acute* pharmacological effects?

(b) In what way does cocaine differ from other local anesthetics in its *chronic* pharmacological effects?

8. (a) What factor accounts for the prolonged activity and potential toxicity of tetracaine?

(b) What precautions are especially necessary in spraying or injecting tetracaine solutions locally?

BIBLIOGRAPHY

General Anesthesia

Abajian, J., Brazell, E. H., and Dente, G. A.: Experiences with halothane in more than five thousand cases. J.A.M.A., *171*:535, 1959.

Adriani, J.: Some newer anesthetic agents. Am. J. Nursing, *61*:60, 1961.

Adriani, J., and Zepernick, R.: Anesthesia for infants and children. Am. J. Nursing, *64*:107, 1964.

Alper, M. H.: New halogenated hydrocarbon anesthetics. G.P., *27*:123, 1963.

Beecher, H. K.: Anesthesia. Scientific Amer., *196*:70, 1957 (Jan.).

Council Statement: Liver necrosis after halothane anesthesia; post hoc, ergo propter hoc? J.A.M.A., *185*:204, 1963.

Little, D. M., and Stephan, C. R.: Modern balanced anesthesia. Anesthesiology, *15*:246, 1954.

Lundy, J. S.: New drugs for analgesia and amnesia. J.A.M.A., *162*:97, 1956.

Quastel, J. H.: Biochemical aspects of narcosis. Anesth. Analg., *31*:151, 1952.

Rapper, E. M.: The pharmacologic basis of anesthesiology. Clin. Pharmacol. Ther., *2*:141, 1961.

Rodman, M. J.: The newer anesthetics and adjunctive drugs. R.N., *25*:45, 1962 (Sept.).

———: New drugs for anesthesia. R.N., *27*:69, 1964 (Feb.).

Weaver, D. C.: Preventing aspiration deaths during anesthesia. J.A.M.A., *188*:971, 1964.

Woolbridge, P. D.: The components of general anesthesia. J.A.M.A., *186*:641, 1963.

Local Anesthesia

Adriani, J.: Clinical effectiveness of drugs used for topical anesthesia. J.A.M.A., *188*:711, 1964.

———: Absorption and systemic toxicity of local anesthetics. G.P., *25*:82, 1962.

———: The clinical pharmacology of local anesthetics. Clin. Pharmacol. Exp. Ther., *1*:645, 1960.

———: Local anesthetics. Am. J. Nursing, *59*:86, 1959.

Bell, H. M., *et al.*: Regional anesthesia with intravenous lidocaine. J.A.M.A., *186*:544, 1963.

Featherstone, R. M.: Pharmacology of compounds used to produce spinal anesthesia. J.A.M.A., *168*:1327, 1958.

Greene, N. M.: Local anesthetic agents with special reference to spinal anesthesia. Anesthesiology, *16*:573, 1955.

Moore, D. C., and Bridenburgh, L. D.: Oxygen: the antidote for systemic toxic reactions from local anesthetic drugs. J.A.M.A., *174*:842, 1960.

Rodman, M. J.: Local anesthesia. R.N., *24*:47, 1961 (Jan.).

———: Pain-relieving drugs in labor and delivery. R.N., *27*:95, 1964 (Sept.).

Steinhaus, J. E.: Local anesthetic toxicity. Anesthesiology, *18*:275, 1957.

The Pharmacology of Ethyl Alcohol

DRINKING AND THE PUBLIC HEALTH

Our concern with understanding the pharmacology of ethyl alcohol stems primarily not from its usefulness in drug therapy, but from the social consequences of the widespread use of alcoholic beverages. These are evident, not only among chronic abusers of alcohol but also in the behavior of people who are not yet compulsive drinkers. Drinking by the ordinary individual, who is also a driver, creates an ever-present danger to life and limb in our mobile society.

According to the National Council on Alcoholism, an estimated 70 million Americans drink alcohol in one form or another. Most of these people drink in a way that has no serious adverse effects. However, about five million drinkers have lost the ability to keep their intake of alcohol under control. The mental and physical consequences of their uncontrolled drinking makes alcoholism a major health problem.

The nurse, of course, knows how harmful excessive drinking can be both to the health of the drinker and to the well-being of his family and friends. Both in her professional contacts and in everyday life, she sees the harm done by alcoholism in terms of human unhappiness. The social cost of alcoholism is counted not only in deaths due to alcohol-induced disease, accidents, and crimes of violence, but also in disrupted family units. For, contrary to what was once commonly believed, alcoholism is not restricted to a relatively few "skid row" derelicts.

Problem drinking is now known to exist at every level of society. It has also recently become increasingly clear that there are probably as many women as men who drink to excess. Women with drinking difficulties may keep their secret hidden within the household for longer periods, but the consequences of a mother's alcoholism may be even more devastating to a family's stability than drinking by the father.

Of course, most of the social aspects of alcoholism are beyond the scope of this book. However, since the nurse's attitudes toward drinking and the problem drinker should be based upon facts rather than myth, she needs to know exactly what effects alcohol has on the brain and body, both when taken only occasionally and after its chronic abuse. Thus, we shall study alcohol as we do other biologically active chemicals —in terms of what it does to the functioning of susceptible cells and of how the body, in turn, handles the alcohol that reaches its tissues.

THE IMMEDIATE EFFECTS OF INCREASING CONCENTRATIONS OF ALCOHOL ON THE CENTRAL NERVOUS SYSTEM

The immediate actions of alcohol as a drug are exerted mainly upon the central nervous system. As with other general depressant drugs, the effects of alcohol follow a pattern in which the highest intellectual functions of the C.N.S. are the first to be interfered with and those vital functions that are under the control of brain stem regulatory centers are the last to go. The pattern of alcoholic depression of the C.N.S. is characterized by a particularly long excitement, or delirium, stage. This prolonged hyperactivity is actually the result of the depression of the inhibitory areas of the brain which normally keep the more primitive parts of the C.N.S. under control (Chap. 5). Later, as the released areas are themselves depressed, the drinker falls into a stupor and may become comatose.

Thus, contrary to the belief that still persists among many people, alcohol is *not* a stimulant. It was, in fact, once employed in preparing patients for surgery (Chap. 11). However, although it can help to put a patient to sleep, raise his pain threshold and finally produce unconsciousness, alcohol is not used as a general anesthetic in modern clinical practice. As we have seen (Chap. 11), the anesthetist tries to minimize the excitement stage of anesthesia, and he always wants to maintain the widest possible margin of safety. Alcohol, on the other hand, has a narrow safety margin between the amount needed to bring about skeletal muscle relaxation and that which may impair the medullary respiratory and cardiovascular control mechanisms; and, as indicated above, large doses of alcohol produce prolonged delirium.

The effects of alcohol on the functioning of the C.N.S. are related largely to the level of alcohol in the blood and brain. Individuals, of course, differ to some degree in their reactions to the same concentration of alcohol in the C.N.S. However, it is certainly true that the lower the level of alcohol in a person's blood, the less the extent of nervous function impairment; and the higher its concentration in the blood and brain, the more profound and widespread the degree of C.N.S. depression. As is true with other drugs (Chap. 2), the concentration of alcohol in the brain at any given moment after ingestion depends upon its rates of absorption, distribution and elimination—that is, to use the term broadly, upon its metabolism.

ALCOHOL METABOLISM

Before we discuss the effects of various blood concentrations of alcohol upon the functioning of the central nervous system, let us look at a few recent scientific findings concerning some of the factors involved in its absorption from the G.I. tract, transport to the tissues and final fate. Knowledge of these factors, which determine how quickly alcohol gets into the blood, how it is carried to the brain, and how it disappears from the body, will add to our understanding of the effects of the consumption of alcohol upon behavior. Also, it will give us the theoretical basis for some of the practical measures employed in the management of acutely intoxicated patients and of chronic alcoholics.

Absorption. Alcohol is a rapidly absorbed substance, because it requires no digestion and diffuses readily through the G.I. mucosa. About 20 per cent of the ingested alcohol is absorbed from the stomach, but the bulk of any drink makes its way into the blood stream only after it enters the small intestine. The C.N.S. effects of a concentrated alcoholic drink can often be felt very quickly when it is taken on an empty stomach, because absorption begins immediately and reaches a peak in as little as twenty minutes.

The period required for absorption may, however, be considerably delayed when the stomach contains a moderate amount of food. The presence of food tends to dilute the alcohol in the stomach and interfere with its absorption from that site. In addition, milk or other fat-containing foods tend to slow the rate at which the stomach empties into the first foot of the small intestine, from which most of the alcohol

is ordinarily absorbed. Since more of the alcohol can be detoxified (see Chap. 2) during such delayed absorption, its concentration in the blood and brain remains relatively low, and its effects on the C.N.S. are less marked. Similarly, sipping a drink over a period of time results in lower blood alcohol concentrations and fewer C.N.S. effects than are likely to occur when the same amount of alcohol is downed all in one gulp.

Distribution. Once the alcohol enters the capillaries it diffuses from the blood into all the body's tissues where it mixes with their water content. The better a tissue's blood supply, the more rapidly does its concentration of alcohol build up. Thus, the level of alcohol in the brain quickly comes into balance with that of the blood. Later, tissues that receive proportionally less blood or contain less water, finally take up their full share of the alcohol. Redistribution to secondary storage sites tends to draw some of the alcohol away from the brain and thus aids in the sobering-up process, provided that no further drinking is done.

Final Fate. By far the most important factor in the reduction of brain levels of alcohol is the body's ability to burn up, or oxidize, the alcohol, in the tissues. Between 90 and 95 per cent of all the alcohol that is absorbed is broken down to carbon dioxide and water in a series of three enzymatically catalyzed steps. Most of the remaining alcohol leaves the body unchanged by way of the breath and urine.

The first steps in the metabolic breakdown of alcohol take place largely in the liver. Two enzymes catalyze the conversion of alcohol, first to *acetaldehyde* and then to *acetate*. Ordinarily, the second step immediately follows the first, so that there is little or no accumulation of acetaldehyde. However, sometimes—e.g., after the prior administration of certain drugs that suppress the activity of the oxidative enzymes (p. 196)—acetaldehyde may build up to toxic levels.

The final step in the metabolism of alcohol takes place in all the cells of the body. Here, the acetate derived from alcohol is fed into the cellular system for obtaining energy from foodstuffs. This is the Krebs tricarboxylic acid cycle, the main chemical pathway used by the body's cells to burn the acetate fragments from foods, producing energy and giving off water and carbon dioxide as waste products.

Caloric Value of Alcohol. The third and final step in the complete oxidation of alcohol produces seven calories for every gram that is oxidized in the tissues. This is more energy than is obtained from an equal weight of carbohydrate or protein food and nearly as much as is obtainable from fat. Thus, alcohol can—up to a point—take the place of food as a source of energy. It does not, however, contain other essential food factors such as vitamins, minerals or amino acids

—a fact that often has serious consequences for the health of alcoholics who fail to eat even a minimally adequate diet while drinking large quantities of distilled spirits.

Thus, although the heavy drinker can satisfy a large part of his daily energy requirements by his alcohol intake alone, the nutritional result may be compared with that of trying to subsist solely on pure cane sugar, which also is a source of calories only. Thus many of the chronic alcoholic's ailments (p. 196) are the result of prolonged malnutrition and a consequent lack of the food factors that are needed to keep liver, nerve and other body tissue in good health.

Another consequence of practical significance is the development of obesity in some drinkers. Those who drink even moderately *without reducing normal food intake* are likely to put on weight, because the calories from alcohol are added to those derived from dietary carbohydrates, fats and protein. Certain beverages—beer, for example—contain substances with food value, besides their alcohol content. Thus, obesity is all the more likely in people who consume large quantities of such beverages and eat heartily at the same time.

Rate of Oxidation. The speed of oxidation of alcohol to acetaldehyde—the first step in the metabolic series—determines the rapidity with which alcohol disappears from the body. The rate of this reaction, which may vary from person to person and even in the same person at different times, has been calculated for the average man weighing 150 lbs. to dispose of about only 7 Gm. of alcohol per hour. (This is the quantity of pure alcohol in about ⅔ oz. of whiskey, 3 to 4 oz. of a light wine, or 8 to 10 oz. of light beer.)

The fact that alcohol, no matter how much is in the body, is metabolized at the same slow, steady rate is of some practical importance in the treatment of acute alcoholic intoxication (p. 194). In such patients it would, of course, be desirable to speed the destruction of the alcohol in the body and thus lower its level in the blood and brain. Doctors have often attempted to hasten the disappearance of alcohol in these patients by administering various hormones and other substances which increase the rate of cellular oxidation processes. However, reports of the results of such treatment have been conflicting. For example, some reports indicate that the administration of insulin together with glucose and B complex vitamins accelerates the elimination of alcohol, whereas other writers deny this. Similarly, although some scientific papers reporting the sobering effect of the thyroid hormones thyroxine and triiodothyronine have been favorable, the effectiveness of this treatment for speeding alcohol metabolism has not been proved.

An explanation of these conflicting results may be that such substances stimulate the rate of alcohol destruction when it is abnormally sluggish, but have little if any such effect when the body is already metabolizing alcohol at the maximal possible rate. For example, if a person's tissues are capable of consuming 7 Gm. of alcohol per hour but are burning only 4 Gm. for some reason, it may be possible to raise the rate of metabolism by administering metabolic stimulants, but if he is already removing 7 Gm. per hour, such drug treatment would do no good.

RELATIONSHIP OF BLOOD ALCOHOL LEVELS TO BEHAVIOR

When a person drinks more of an alcoholic beverage than his body can burn, the excess alcohol accumulates in his blood and brain. The rising levels of

---

ALCOHOL BLOOD LEVELS RELATED TO FITNESS TO DRIVE

- Category 1. Blood alcohol *under 50 mg.%* (*below 0.05%*) Considered *proof* that person was *not* driving "*under the influence*" of alcohol.*

- Category 2. Blood alcohol *between 50–150 mg.%* (*0.05–0.15%*) Safety as a driver is *questionable*. This blood alcohol level is not prima facie evidence of intoxica-

* A person with between 20–50 mg.% alcohol may nevertheless not possess his normal judgment and motor coordination and may consequently not be as "safe" a driver as he seems. This is the basis for the much lower legal limits set by statute in several European countries. West Germany, Czechoslovakia

tion; however, it may be weighed with other facts in determining whether a person was driving while intoxicated.

- Category 3. Blood alcohol *above 150 mg.%* (*above 0.15%*) Considered *proof* that person was driving "*under the influence*" of alcohol.

and Bulgaria, for example, allow only 30 milligrams of alcohol per 100 milliliters of blood. In Sweden, Norway and Poland, the limit is 50 mg. In Austria—and in Britain where a 1967 law permits the police to stop drivers for tests with the Breathalyzer device—the limit is put at 80 mg. per 100 ml. of blood.

alcohol bring about behavioral changes that—within limits—can be correlated with the concentration of blood alcohol. The most important application of this principle has been in determining a person's fitness to drive a motor vehicle.

Chemists have devised many tests for estimating the amount of alcohol in a person's brain by analyzing his blood, urine, or breath. Analysis of a person's breath is the basis for the Drunkometer and similar tests that drivers are sometimes required to take. Such tests have nothing to do with the *odor* of a person's breath, which is caused not by alcohol itself but by other substances contained in alcoholic beverages. The breath serves instead as an index of the amount of alcohol in the patient's blood, because the alcohol in the arteries is in balance with that of the air in the alveoli of the lungs.

Individuals vary in their ability to tolerate, or withstand, similar levels of alcohol in their brains; however, blood alcohol levels correlate well with the expected impairment in the driving ability of the vast majority of people. For such purposes, blood alcohol levels expressed in milligrams of alcohol per 100 milliliters of blood—that is, in *mg.%*—are related to probable fitness to drive on the basis of several broad categories, or zones (see summary of Alcohol Blood Levels Related to Fitness to Drive).

In the following discussion, we shall employ a somewhat similar scale as a means of correlating the effects of blood alcohol concentrations with probable changes in centrally controlled functions. In addition to discussion of the effects of various levels of alcohol on driving ability, we shall indicate the concentrations of alcohol that appear to produce those pharmacological effects that may be useful in therapeutics. Also, because of its intrinsic interest, we shall try to point out the possible effects of alcohol upon an average person's behavior during social drinking.

In the latter respect, however, the student must leave a considerable margin for error, because the effects of any psychopharmacological agent upon human intellectual processes and emotional responses are much less measurable or predictable than are its effects on motor coordination, reflex responses and reaction times. We may also note that, beyond an initial statement for use as a rough guide, no attempt will be made to correlate the alcohol blood levels that are mentioned with the amount of alcohol the person would have to drink to attain that level. Very many and varied factors are involved in determining how much alcohol from any drink of alcoholic beverage—beer, wine, whiskey, etc.—reaches the brain under the many different circumstances in which drinking may be done. Thus, it is not feasible to try to predict precisely what concentrations would be attained in various specific situations.

Levels of 20 to 30 mg.% of Alcohol (0.02–0.03%). This amount of alcohol may be measurable in the

TABLE 12-1

ALCOHOL CONTENT OF BEVERAGES *

BEVERAGE AND TYPE OR SOURCE	PER CENT ALCOHOL BY VOLUME	PROOF †
Neutral spirits	90–95	180–190
Vodka (from neutral spirits)	40–55	80–110
Gin (from neutral spirits)	40–45	80–110
Whiskey (from cereal grains)	40–45	80–110
Rum (from molasses)	40–55	80–110
Brandy (from wine)	40–55	80–110
Wine (table, light)	10–12	—
Wine (dessert)	15–22	—
Beer (light)	3–6	—
Ale	6–8	—
Cider (hard)	8–12	—

* The amount of a beverage taken within a brief period of time can be related within limits to the level of alcohol likely to be attained in the blood and brain and to the probable behavior of the individual.

For example, one ounce of a concentrated beverage such as 100 proof whiskey, taken all at once on an empty stomach, might produce an alcohol blood level of 20 mg.% (0.02%) within half an hour. Similarly, two to three ounces of whiskey could produce a blood level of 0.05% alcohol; 8 oz. (half a pint) 0.15%; 16 oz. (one pint) 0.300%, etc.

However, many factors might alter these relationships, including individual variation in tolerance, the amount of food taken before or during drinking, and the circumstances in which the drinking is done (e.g., with friends or alone, etc.).

† *Proof* is the standard of strength for alcoholic liquors. The proof figure in this country is always twice the percentage of alcohol by volume. The term is said to stem from an old test for the alcohol content of whiskey. If gunpowder on which the whiskey was poured ignited, this was "proof" that the whiskey contained at least 50 per cent alcohol.

blood in as little as 20 minutes after a man has downed a cocktail or highball containing a jigger (1½ oz.) of 100 proof whiskey on an empty stomach. Although it is highly unlikely that this much alcohol significantly impairs the driving ability of an average man, psychological tests and common experience indicate that one drink of this kind can affect certain C.N.S. functions. For example, a psychosensory function such as visual acuity may be shown to be slightly impaired. Mental activity also may be altered in the direction of reduced judgment and self-concern—an effect that is intensified by taking a second drink at about the time the first is reaching its peak effects.

Levels of 30 to 50 mg.% of Alcohol (0.03–0.05%). With this amount of alcohol in their blood, most people tend to feel somewhat relaxed and at ease in social situations. In neurological terms, we may say that this sedative effect reflects the action of alcohol on the reticular activating system (RAS; see Chap. 5), with a resulting release of some aspects of behavior from the inhibitory control of the cerebral cortex. More practically, the person so affected may talk more freely, fluently—and loudly—than he ordinarily would.

Psychologists suggest that people drink socially because alcohol helps to reduce self-consciousness and relieve feelings of inner tension. As a result of his increased self-confidence, a person with an alcohol blood level approaching 50 mg.% often tends to lower some of his socially acquired defenses. This may be psychologically healthful for him and also serve a useful social function.

Ordinarily, in our society people tend to be rather shy and subdued when thrown into the company of strangers. This is because we have learned to inhibit our natural drives, in response to the demands of society. When the effects of this blood level of alcohol upon the brain begin to appear, the normally or excessively inhibited person tends to lose some of his capacity for critically evaluating himself and his relationships with others. This, of course, makes it easier for casual acquaintances to communicate. (This action of alcohol as a social lubricant may be as beneficial as sociologists say, but alcohol-released social spouting can also be a bore—especially to those whose blood alcohol content is still at a substantially lower level.)

We must, of course, be cautious in attempting to predict changes in human behavior at this low level of alcohol, as circumstances may alter cases. For example, environmental factors—what psychologists call the "setting"—may make the same person react differently at various times. When partying with jovial companions, the imbiber may be gay and a bit boisterous. In boring company, or when alone, the same person may merely become sedated to the point of drowsiness from the same amount of alcohol. However, we may hazard one broad generalization about the psychological effects of 50 mg.% of alcohol in the blood—that is, the feeling that is elicited is the one that makes alcohol so attractive to many people in our society. This euphoric sedation is also the effect that may make alcohol medically useful in the management of some clinical conditions.

The medical uses of alcoholic beverages depend largely upon the ability of alcohol to relieve feelings of inner tension—that is, its *sedative* or *tranquilizing* effect. This, together with the *analgesic* action of alcohol which is also apparent when it reaches this blood level, accounts for its usefulness in certain conditions. Thus, in various cardiovascular disorders, it

is these C.N.S. effects of alcohol rather than any direct action on the heart or blood vessels that may be beneficial.

Whiskey has, for example, been commonly prescribed in the past for patients with angina pectoris and peripheral vascular diseases (Chaps. 22, 26). The basis for its use was the observation that a person's face often becomes flushed and warm following a couple of drinks. However, alcohol does not actually seem able to bring about any measurable increase in blood flow through the coronary circulation or in ischemic skeletal muscles. Its benefits are probably the result of its ability to reduce the patient's anxiety and to raise his threshold of pain perception.

The same sedative and analgesic effects are also sometimes obtained by infusing a 5 per cent solution of alcohol intravenously at a rate which maintains the patient's blood level at about 50 mg.%. Such parenteral administration of alcohol has been used in elderly patients debilitated by painful disorders including cancer. In such cases, and when used during convalescence after surgery, alcohol is claimed to offer the added benefit of its nutritive value—that is, it serves as a source of energy.

Alcoholic beverages are also said to stimulate the appetite and aid the digestion of patients with poor appetite. Alcohol in dilute solution does cause an increase in gastric secretions. However, it is probably its tranquilizing central action rather than its direct local actions that accounts for any increase in the anorexic patient's interest in food. Similarly, this sedative effect is what people are really seeking when they take a couple of cocktails before dinner. Such preprandial drinks may give a tense, nervous person more zest for eating a meal by relieving feelings of anxiety and fatigue.

The use of alcohol as a "nightcap" may help a restless person to fall asleep. However, its habitual use as a *hypnotic* in this manner may be harmful to people prone to abuse depressant drugs. Of course, alcohol is safe enough when used only occasionally for this purpose. For example, a person suffering from a heavy cold does himself no harm when he follows the time-worn practice of getting into bed after taking a warm alcoholic drink and a couple of aspirin tablets. The *diaphoretic* (sweat-inducing) action of the combination may help to lower a mild fever, though alcoholic sponge baths—applied *externally*—are better for this purpose. Actually, the main advantage of the alcoholic drink is that it makes the head-cold patient drowsy and so keeps him in bed where he belongs.

Levels of 50 to 100 mg.% of Alcohol (0.05–0.1%). As we have seen, when a patient takes a little alcohol, he may feel better as a result of its relaxant action. However, when alcohol is ingested in amounts that make the blood and brain concentrations rise rapidly to still higher levels, its beneficial effects begin to be outweighed by its definitely adverse effects. With rising blood alcohol levels, the drinker's judgment becomes increasingly blurred, and his ability to perform finely coordinated movements is diminished.

At first, these effects may be manifested merely by an excessive increase in self-confidence and by signs such as a seemingly accidental difficulty in lighting and holding a cigarette. Later, as blood alcohol levels rise toward 100 mg.%, the drinker's weakened ability to evaluate reality and restrain his impulses, coupled with his increasing clumsiness, may make it dangerous for him to drive a motor vehicle. At an alcohol blood level of 0.1%, most people can be considered mildly intoxicated and unfit to drive. Actually, *much lower levels* of alcohol can cause enough reduction in judgment and skilled motor abilities to make it unsafe for a person to drive. Thus, in view of the disrupting effects of alcohol on these important C.N.S. functions, *no one should attempt to drive while he still feels any effect at all from even moderate drinking.*

Levels of 100 to 150 mg.% of Alcohol (0.1–0.15%). Blood alcohol levels below 150 mg.% are not by themselves considered legal evidence of "driving under the influence of alcohol" in most states of this country. Drivers with blood alcohol levels between 50 and 150 mg.% may, however, be required to demonstrate their ability to pass certain simple tests of their motor coordination, and the results of these tests, taken together with the evidence from the chemical tests, may be the basis for indictment and conviction for driving while intoxicated.

The extent of a person's motor impairment with this level of blood alcohol may not be very great. It may be manifested only by slightly slurred speech and by a tendency to bump into things while brushing by them, rather than by overt staggering. Yet, when combined with the drinker's tendency to act impulsively or foolishly, and his delayed reaction times, motor incoordination of this degree markedly increases his chances of being involved in an accident. Thus, unwise drinking is the cause of serious injury and death as a result of falls, fires and industrial accidents, as well as those involving drivers and pedestrians who have been drinking.

Levels of 150 to 300 mg.% of Alcohol (0.15–0.30%). Most people with 150 mg.% blood alcohol, and just about all people with 200 mg.%, may be considered moderately intoxicated, and those with 300 mg.% are markedly intoxicated. People who have ingested enough alcohol to have blood levels this high show many signs of rapidly progressive deterioration of higher cortical functions. This appears in the form of increasingly uncontrolled behavior, as a result of the release from both emotional and motor inhibitory controls. The person at this stage of an alcoholic episode may become belligerent and pugnacious, or he may have a crying or laughing "jag." At the same time, he tends to have increasing difficulty in locomotion, marked at first by a staggering gait, then by trouble in simply trying to stand and, finally, by his falling and being unable to get up.

The drinker's uninhibited behavior may lead to his involvement in violence, in which *he* is the one likely to be injured because of his inability to defend himself. When the blood level of alcohol is at around 300 mg.%, the person's state of excitement may be similar to that of a patient in the second stage of anesthesia (Chap. 11), in the sense that he, too, is not truly conscious of what is going on and is really not responsible for his words and actions. Thus, it does little good to reason with the acutely intoxicated person, because he is not likely to understand. Instead, he should be kept from harming himself until he can be hospitalized and treated with tranquilizing medication and other medical measures (see p. 194).

Levels of 400 to 600 mg.% of Alcohol (0.4–0.6%). People with blood alcohol concentrations of 400 mg.% are no longer a behavioral problem; they have sunk into a stuporous state from which they cannot be readily aroused. Although the drinker can no longer bend an elbow to take in any more liquor, the continuing absorption from the G.I. tract of alcohol ingested earlier may cause him to lapse into coma. As his blood level rises above 500 mg.%, the alcoholic's breathing becomes shallow and slow, and his circulation may come close to collapse. Death from respiratory paralysis and shock usually occurs with blood levels of 600 mg.% and above.

However, unless the person has been taking other depressant drugs at the same time, the alcoholic patient ordinarily does not remain in prolonged coma. Instead, the body's slow but steady detoxifying mechanisms tend to lower blood and brain alcohol levels, once the patient is no longer capable of continuing his drinking. On the other hand, a person with a relatively low blood alcohol level—300 mg.%, for instance—may die of respiratory failure and circulatory collapse if he has also been taking moderate doses of a barbiturate, or of a non-barbiturate hypnotic such as glutethimide (Chap. 6), or a minor tranquilizer such as meprobamate (Chap. 7).

A person who collapses in an alcoholic stupor outdoors in winter may freeze to death, if he is not found. This is, in part, because alcohol depresses the brain's centers for regulating body temperature. Body heat is then rapidly lost, because the vessels of the skin tend to remain dilated instead of constricting reflexly. Even if found in time, the stuporous or comatose alcoholic may die of hypostatic pneumonia or as a result of a severe complicating bronchopulmonary infection. Also, head injuries or cerebral edema as a result of brain hypoxia may sometimes prove fatal.

THE MANAGEMENT OF ACUTELY INTOXICATED PATIENTS

Patients who require treatment may be in any of the following states at the time of admission: (1) stuporous or comatose; (2) excited or combative; (3) suffering the various effects of the withdrawal of alcohol after prolonged drinking. The management of each of these phases of acute alcoholism is, of course, quite different.

Acute Alcoholic Coma. As we have already indicated, such a stuporous or comatose state may need little treatment beyond letting the patient sleep off the effects of his excessive alcohol intake. On the other hand, if the coma is unusually deep, the doctor may want to take measures intended to rouse the patient more rapidly, in order to prevent development of hypostatic pneumonia and other complications. To reduce the depth of the patient's depression he may attempt the careful use of C.N.S. stimulants, or analeptics (Chap. 13), and try various measures for increasing the rate of metabolism of the alcohol. Neither of these treatments has proved very useful, however, and supportive measures for assuring adequate respiratory exchange and for combating shock are probably the most useful measures that can be employed, as is the case in overdosage by barbiturates and other general depressants. (See p. 199 for a summary of treatment measures for alcoholic coma.)

Acute Alcoholic Excitement. The noisy, combative alcoholic is a trial to those who have to care for him. However, the nurse's attitude toward him should be no different from her attitude toward her other patients as she follows the doctor's orders for keeping him under the sedation that he requires. Phenothiazine-type tranquilizers such as promazine (Sparine) are presently considered especially desirable for counteracting both restlessness and nausea. However, care is required in administering these drugs, because they may potentiate the depressant and hypotensive effects of alcohol. For example, intramuscular injections of promazine should be made with the patient recumbent, and he should be kept lying down in order to prevent dizziness and fainting leading to possible injury. Parenteral forms of the minor tranquilizers chlordiazepoxide (Librium) and diazepam (Valium) are now available and may be preferred by some physicians. (See Chapter 7 for discussion of the tranquilizers.)

Acute Withdrawal Syndromes. Many of the difficulties that occur after drinking are now recognized to be the result of its withdrawal. Symptoms may range in severity from an ordinary "hangover" to acute and possibly fatal delirium tremens. The degree of severity of the patient's illness depends mainly upon how much and how long he has been drinking. The doctor tries to fit the patient's treatment to the particular symptom complex that appears to be predominant.

Patients with a relatively mild withdrawal syndrome may suffer only from what they call "the shakes," a state of tremulousness and relatively slight agitation. This is commonly managed by the parenteral administration of chlordiazepoxide (Librium), which reduces the patient's psychomotor hyperactivity and tremors. The continued use of this minor tranquilizer during long-term convalescence may, however, be undesirable in alcoholic patients, because such people are prone to abuse general depressant drugs. Thus, in the past some alcoholics became addicted to the barbiturates, paraldehyde, chloral hydrate and other sedative-hypnotics with which they were being treated. Today, addiction to meprobamate, glutethimide and other modern tranquilizers and sedatives is common among former alcoholics.

The phenothiazine-type tranquilizers, which have relatively little abuse and addiction potential are preferred for the long-term treatment of patients with a history of alcoholism, as well as for coping with the more severe syndromes brought about by the withdrawal of alcohol from patients who have been drinking heavily. In the complication that alcoholics call "the horrors" and psychiatrists call *alcoholic hallucinosis*, some physicians now prefer to begin treatment with the less sedating phenothiazine derivatives such as trifluoperazine (Stelazine). Drugs of this kind are claimed capable of reducing the patient's terror in the face of frightening hallucinations without producing excessive C.N.S. depression or precipitating hypotensive episodes.

Delirium tremens ("D.T.'s"), on the other hand, requires deeper sedation in order to control the patient's extreme restlessness and prevent dangerous convulsive seizures. This condition, which usually develops after several weeks of heavy drinking, seems to be precipitated when the patient can no longer keep his blood alcohol up to the accustomed level. This falling off of blood alcohol may occur as a result of persistent vomiting or other conditions that keep the patient from continuing to drink. Patients who are hospitalized for acute alcoholic intoxication, or alcoholics who are hospitalized for treatment of pneumonia or other conditions, may, of course, develop delirium tremens after a day or two of treatment, during which they have had no alcohol.

Such a patient may no longer respond to the doses of the tranquilizing drugs which had at first quieted him. He may then become increasingly restless and disoriented, and, when terrified by his visual hallucinations, the patient may try to flee from his room. Treatment is aimed at sedating the patient so deeply that he cannot offer resistance to the medical and nursing care that he so desperately needs.

Phenobarbital, administered parenterally in large

doses, is still employed for keeping the patient deeply sedated during the couple of days when his delirium would otherwise be at its height. The anticonvulsant drug, diphenylhydantoin (Dilantin) may also be administered to control convulsive seizures. If increased intracranial pressure is present as a result of cerebral edema, the patient may also receive infusions of osmotic diuretics such as urea or mannitol (Chap. 20). Other measures often used in this dangerous disorder include the administration of intravenous fluids containing vitamins and electrolytes to counteract dehydration resulting from heavy sweating and vomiting and to correct the avitaminosis which is so common in chronic alcoholics.

THE MANAGEMENT OF THE CHRONIC ALCOHOLIC PATIENT

As with other addictions, getting the patient "dried out" and stabilized after a prolonged drinking bout is only the beginning of his treatment. When an acutely intoxicated patient is hospitalized, the patient's sobriety is brought about by others. However, to stay sober, the patient alone must take the responsibility for abstaining from alcohol. Helping him to do so is the most difficult and, in the long run, the most decisive aspect of treatment.

The alcoholic cannot be forced to stop drinking. He must himself be convinced that he can never take alcohol in any form. Once he has accepted this idea and stays away from liquor, he may undertake psychotherapy or other supportive treatment with some hope of success. In such cases, his earnest desire to keep from drinking can often be reinforced by the daily self-administration of certain drugs that help deter him from drinking.

Deterrent Drugs. The available deterrent drugs are agents that react with alcohol in the body to produce a very unpleasant reaction. The deterrent drug most commonly employed is disulfiram (see also Drug Digest); another agent, used in Canada and elsewhere abroad, is citrated calcium carbimide (Temposil). Both drugs are believed to act in the same way when the patient takes a drink after having earlier ingested a dose. Within a few minutes, the patient's skin turns bright red and warm as a result of peripheral vasodilation. The vasodilation sets off a pounding vasodilator-type headache, and, as his blood pressure drops, the patient feels faint, weak and dizzy and becomes nauseated. Violent vomiting, heart palpitations, chest pains and dyspnea may develop. Sometimes, the cardiovascular complications have proved fatal to patients with myocardial disease or cerebral damage who have begun to drink while under treatment with disulfiram.

Treatment Considerations and Contraindications. The doctor, of course, warns the patient of the dis-

comfort, and even danger, which will develop if he drinks while taking the drug. Occasionally the physician may let him learn at first hand what may happen. This is done by giving him half an ounce of whiskey some time after he has taken the deterrent drug. The reaction that follows is supposed to prove to the patient that it is pointless for him to drink once he has taken his daily tablet. However, most doctors would now rather withhold the drug from patients whose motivation does not seem strong rather than subject them to this "test dose" experience. Other patients not considered good risks for deterrent drug therapy include the ten per cent (roughly) of alcoholics who are considered psychopathic. These drugs are also contraindicated for patients with heart, liver or kidney damage, diabetes, epilepsy, asthma, and in pregnancy.

The use of deterrent drugs in properly selected patients has proved desirable in various ways. The patient's willingness to take a daily tablet is itself an indication that he really wants to stop drinking. Moreover, those who decide to take the drug each morning are relieved of the need to make countless decisions as to whether or not to take a drink that day. Then, as the days of abstinence lengthen into weeks and months, the patient realizes that he can, after all, get along without drinking. This often serves to reinforce his motivation and increases the likelihood of his profiting from concurrent psychotherapy.

Patients who backslide and drink, and become ill because of a reaction between the alcohol and residual disulfiram in the body, may require no treatment if the effects are merely unpleasant. However, more severe reactions may be treated by intravenous administration of massive doses of ascorbic acid (Vitamin C) and an antihistaminic drug such as diphenhydramine * (Benadryl). It may be necessary to treat shock by infusing saline and dextrose solution and by administering an adrenergic vasopressor drug such as ephedrine. Inhalation of oxygen is recommended, as is the administration of sedating phenothiazine tranquilizers such as promazine (Sparine) or chlorpromazine * (Thorazine), which help to put the patient to sleep. Ordinarily, he is fully recovered and has no further symptoms when he awakens.

Other Deterrent Drugs. Citrated calcium carbimide (CCC) is reported to possess several advantages over disulfiram. These include a lower incidence of side effects such as stomach upset, headache, drowsiness and dermatitis. Also, it acts more rapidly than disulfiram, which must be given for several days before it accumulates to levels that bring about the typical reaction if alcohol is taken. On the other hand, CCC has only a relatively short duration of action compared to disulfiram, which stays in the body for several days

---

* See Drug Digests.

after the last dose. This means that a patient may be able to drink without a reaction later in the day after a morning dose of CCC, whereas disulfiram would still have the desired effect—that is, of making him feel ill. Thus, a second daily dose of CCC is often necessary.

Various other drugs have been tried as aids in helping alcoholic patients abstain from drinking. The synthetic hypoglycemic drugs that are used in treating diabetes (Chap. 32) can cause a reaction similar to that seen with disulfiram and CCC. Like the latter agents, the antidiabetic sulfonamide drugs are thought to inhibit the enzymes responsible for the complete metabolic breakdown of ethyl alcohol. As a result, the intermediate metabolite, acetaldehyde, accumulates to levels that cause the pharmacological effects responsible for the reaction. Other drugs act in different ways to reduce the patient's desire to drink. The emetic drug apomorphine, for example, is still used in conditioned aversion therapy to make the patient nauseated soon after he has taken a drink of an alcoholic beverage, until, finally, he associates drinking with nausea. Recent reports indicate that patients taking the antitrichomonal drug metronidazole (Flagyl) also lose their interest in drinking alcoholic beverages.

The Pathological Effects of Chronic Alcoholism

Some alcoholics fail to respond to any known treatment program, including psychotherapy combined with the use of tranquilizing, antidepressant and deterrent drugs. Their continued heavy drinking leads almost inevitably to damage to various vital organs, including the liver and the central and peripheral nervous systems. Some of the tissue damage seen in chronic alcoholics is thought to be due to the direct action of alcohol; other difficulties are caused by malnutrition. Some syndromes appear to be caused by a combination of both the direct and the indirect effects of excessive drinking.

We shall briefly discuss some of the pathological effects commonly seen in far-advanced alcoholics and indicate at the same time the types of treatment that are employed in efforts to alleviate such tissue damage.

Gastrointestinal Tract. High concentrations of alcohol are directly irritating to the mucosal lining of the stomach. Thus, acute and chronic gastritis are quite common in heavy drinkers of concentrated alcoholic beverages such as "straight" whiskey. The nausea and vomiting caused by this inflammatory reaction often keep the drinker from satisfying the requirements of his physical dependence on alcohol, thus precipitating withdrawal symptoms. Ordinarily, acute gastritis is relieved when the alcoholic stops drinking and begins to eat again. Meanwhile, his symptoms usually respond to treatment with antacids

and antispasmodics, and to phenothiazine-type antiemetics (Chap. 38). Although alcohol has not been proved to cause peptic ulcer, alcohol does stimulate gastric acid secretion and is thus undesirable in patients who already have ulcers. Gastric bleeding is common in alcoholic patients with ulcers.

Effects of Alcohol on the Liver. Acute and chronic liver disease are commonly seen in people who have been drinking large amounts of alcohol for a long time. Acute alcoholic hepatitis, a condition resembling infectious hepatitis, sometimes develops during a drinking bout. It is characterized by anorexia, nausea, vomiting, abdominal pain, jaundice and an enlarged liver. The incidence of chronic hepatic disorders such as fatty liver and cirrhosis is much higher in chronic alcoholics than in the general population. However, not all heavy drinkers—and, indeed, only a small proportion of them—develop cirrhosis of the liver.

Although the drinker's faulty dietary habits undoubtedly play an important part in his developing serious liver disease, recent evidence indicates that alcohol itself has adverse effects upon hepatic function when taken in immoderate amounts for prolonged periods. It has been suggested that, in addition to inducing deficiencies of nutrients necessary for keeping the liver healthy, alcohol may affect the liver in several subtle ways by interfering with the activity of its enzyme systems. Such metabolic defects may account, in part, for the gradual fatty infiltration and proliferation of fibrous tissue which finally destroys functional liver tissue.

If the alcoholic can be helped to stop drinking before the degenerative process has gone too far, the liver's remarkable regenerative properties can come into play. Recovery is often rapid when the alcoholic begins to eat again. The nurse encourages the patient to eat the diet prescribed by the doctor, which is high in proteins, in lipotropic substances such as choline and methionine, and B complex vitamins such as folic acid and cyanocobalamin.

Alcoholism and the Nervous System. We have discussed in detail the progressive disturbance in neurological function that occurs as a result of an episode of acute alcoholic intoxication, or drunkenness. Also, we have seen that the withdrawal of alcohol from a person who has been drinking heavily for some time may set off a variety of nervous system disturbances, including delirium and convulsions. Here, we shall briefly discuss certain neurological complications which show up only after many months or even years of uncontrolled drinking.

In some of these disorders, the damage is due mainly to malnutrition rather than to the direct effects of alcohol. Such nutritional disorders include Wernicke's encephalopathy, Korsakoff's psychosis, and alcoholic polyneuropathy.

Wernicke's disease is marked by the sudden onset of clinical signs of three kinds—ocular muscle paralysis, ataxia, and mental confusion. Once the disease is recognized and treated with massive doses of *thiamine*, the eye signs and muscular incoordination clear up quickly and the patient becomes more alert and responsive.

Korsakoff's Psychosis. Some patients continue to show mental symptoms even after they have recovered from the acute phase. These alcoholics are suffering from a peculiar kind of intellectual impairment called Korsakoff's psychosis. This is characterized by a disturbance in memory, especially the memory of recent events, as well as an inability to learn new material. Even when the patient has improved after several months of hospitalization, he still has difficulty in putting past events into their proper sequence. Most victims of this amnesia-type psychosis are unable to function in society and have to be institutionalized. Apparently, in such cases, the severe thiamine deficiency has caused neuropathological lesions in the thalamus that have gone too far to be corrected in the same manner as can the cerebellar lesions of Wernicke's disease.

Alcoholic Polyneuropathy. Many patients show signs of damage to the motor and sensory fibers of peripheral nerves. Most complain of muscle weakness of the legs and arms or numbness and tingling of the skin. A few suffer from burning pain in the feet or hands or deep aching of the legs. Such polyneuropathy is thought to be the result of a multiple vitamin deficiency resulting from a state of semistarvation. Treatment involves mainly the daily administration of large doses of thiamine, pyridoxine, pantothenic acid, riboflavin and other vitamins. These may have to be given by injection because of the patient's persistent vomiting or other G.I. complications. Salicylates, and occasionally codeine, may be ordered for relief of the patient's muscle pains during his long weeks of convalescence. He should be encouraged to consume the ordered diet, which is high in calories from protein and supplemented by multiple vitamins.

Cardiac Complications of Alcoholism. Ordinary doses of alcohol have few, if any, direct effects upon the heart. As we have previously indicated, the sedative and analgesic actions of alcohol may even be beneficial for some patients with pain from coronary insufficiency. However, excessive drinking can adversely affect cardiac function in various ways. Acute intoxication may set off transient cardiac irregularities that can usually be relieved by sedation with a barbiturate or with a minor tranquilizer such as hydroxyzine (Chap. 7). Chronic alcoholics sometimes suffer from myocardial damage that may lead to congestive heart failure. Such myocardopathy may be a manifestation of beriberi, a disease resulting from a deficiency of vitamin B-1. In addition, recent evidence indicates that a prolonged excessive alcohol intake may have a directly toxic effect upon the heart muscle.

Alcohol and the Kidneys. Despite former claims that alcohol was a cause of nephritis, there seems to be no evidence that alcohol damages the kidneys or even that its use is harmful to patients who have nephritis. Drinking is, however, undesirable for patients with genitourinary tract infections. The increased urinary output induced by drinking alcoholic beverages may cause urgency and frequency in patients with enlargement of the prostate gland.

The diuretic effect of drinking is due only in part to the large quantities of fluid that drinkers often ingest. Recent evidence indicates that alcohol depresses the brain–posterior pituitary gland mechanism that controls the release of the antidiuretic hormone (ADH, see Chap. 27). As a result of reduced ADH secretion, the renal tubules reabsorb a smaller proportion of the glomerular filtrate, and the volume of urine produced by the kidneys is consequently increased.

Alcoholism and Respiratory Tract Infections. Before the advent of the antibiotic era, many alcoholics died of pneumonia, and even today alcoholics suffer frequent acute bronchopulmonary infections. Recent evidence indicates that the presence of alcohol in the blood, even of *non*-alcoholics, may interfere with the migration of macrophages from the blood into tissues that are being invaded by infectious organisms. This effect of alcohol in inhibiting one of the body's main defense mechanisms against infection may account for the alcoholic's low resistance. In any case, the incidence of pulmonary tuberculosis among alcoholics is very much higher than in the general population, presumably because of the alcoholic's neglect of himself and the unsanitary conditions in which he may be forced to live.

The incidence of acute and chronic bronchitis also is high in alcoholics. This may be because drinking reduces the production of the respiratory tract fluids (RTF, Chap. 40) that act as a natural protective covering to the mucosa, and mucous secretions tend to accumulate in the lungs during drinking bouts. Alcoholics are often heavy smokers—and smoke more heavily when drinking—and commonly suffer from pulmonary fibrosis and emphysema. Finally, prolonged alcoholic stupor may lead to hypostatic pneumonia, and the alcoholic may aspirate vomitus while recovering consciousness.

OTHER ALCOHOLS

Ethyl alcohol (ethanol) is one of a series of alcohols containing a single hydroxyl (—OH) group. The other monohydric alcohols are never sold for beverage purposes; they are too toxic to be taken internally. However, some of them are occasionally mis-used in ways that may bring the drinker to medical attention.

One type of toxicity of this series of alcohols is similar to that which we have already discussed in dealing with the pharmacology of ethyl alcohol—that is, central nervous system depression. In this re-gard, an interesting relationship exists between the chemical structure, physical properties, and pharma-cological actions. These compounds contain varied numbers of carbon atoms linked together in an open chain. As the length of the chain of carbons in this series of compounds is increased, there is a corre-sponding intensification of the depressant action, pre-sumably because of the increased solubility in the lipids of the C.N.S. Thus, ethyl alcohol, a two-carbon alcohol, is a more potent depressant than the single-carbon methyl alcohol. The three-carbon compound, isopropyl alcohol, is even more potent in its central action, and the next higher homologues, butyl al-cohol and amyl alcohol, cause still greater depres-sion.

Isopropyl alcohol is the principal ingredient of rubbing alcohol compounds, which, therefore, can cause intoxication quickly when taken internally. However, the most toxic of these alcohols is *methyl alcohol*, the lowest member of the series and the least depressant of the group. Methanol is metabolized in the body to formaldehyde and formic acid, and it is these toxic metabolites, rather than the alcohol itself, that can cause severe poisoning.

Because of the frequency of cases of mass poisoning caused by the drinking of methyl, or wood, alcohol, we shall discuss the nature and treatment of methanol intoxication.

Methyl Alcohol Poisoning. Cases of poisoning ordinarily occur among derelicts who drink paint removers or antifreeze fluid despite the presence on the container of a label indicating the danger of their methanol content when taken internally. The depres-sant effect of the wood alcohol is relatively weak and is masked by that of the ethyl alcohol in the mixture. However, after a delay of 6 to 36 hours, during which the metabolites of this slowly oxidized compound are building up in the body, signs and symptoms of poisoning may develop quite suddenly.

The patient complains of severe headache, dizzi-ness, blurred vision, nausea, vomiting and severe ab-dominal pain. Later the patient's dilated pupils may fail to react to light, his vision is blurred, and finally he becomes blind. In the more severe cases, delirium and then coma develop rapidly and the patient dies of respiratory failure after a brief period of severe con-vulsive spasms. Most of these severe symptoms are the result of acidosis, pancreatitis, and the effects of formaldehyde on the cells of the retina.

Treatment requires prompt correction of the acidosis by the intravenous infusion of a solution of sodium bicarbonate and glucose or of sodium lactate solution. The results of treatment with these alkali solutions are often dramatic. However, the infusion is not stopped as soon as the symptoms vanish, be-cause the continued slow oxidation of the methanol results in the production of still more formic acid, which may cause a late relapse into the acidotic state. Thus the alkali treatment is continued for several days, with frequent laboratory monitoring to avoid development of alkalosis, which can be equally dan-gerous. Unfortunately, permanent blindness may re-sult despite quick correction of the acidosis by bi-carbonate treatment and the use of such measures as keeping the patient's eyes covered.

Ethyl alcohol is also sometimes administered as an antidote in amounts calculated to maintain a blood level of about 100 mg.%. The basis for this treatment is experimental evidence indicating that the presence of ethanol in the body delays the metabolism of methanol by inhibiting the enzymes responsible for converting it to its toxic metabolites. Thus, it has been suggested that giving small doses of ethanol repeat-edly will reduce the rate at which formaldehyde and formic acid are formed and so prevent relapse.

SUMMARY OF NURSING POINTS

- When caring for the acutely intoxicated patient, the nurse must remember that his behavior is due to ill-ness and not to willful disregard of the needs of others. The alcoholic patient's family often require special consideration and thoughtful explanations con-cerning the patient's condition and treatment, be-cause they may feel that they, as well as the patient, are not accepted by nurses and physicians.

- Safety is a paramount consideration when working with a patient who is acutely intoxicated, or with a pa-tient with delirium tremens. Measures that help the patient orient himself to his surroundings and assure him of the presence and concern of those who care for him are essential.

- The nurse must be alert to symptoms of the varied complications that can result from alcoholism. For example, nausea and vomiting may indicate gastritis and should be promptly reported to the physician.

- The nurse must be prepared to answer questions concerning alcohol and its effects—whether she works in school, hospital or industry. (For example, many people still believe that alcohol is a stimulant and should be administered for fainting spells.) The public health nurse, particularly, can play an important role in encouraging alcoholics in the community to seek treatment.

- Therapeutic measures designed to improve the patient's nutrition and to keep him comfortable should be administered conscientiously. Not only are such measures essential in combating the physical ravages of alcoholism; also they convey the nurse's personal concern for the patient's welfare and her hopeful attitude toward his eventual recovery.

- Care of the alcoholic who is repeatedly re-admitted presents a particular challenge, because it is easy for the nurse to lose hope for the patient's recovery. The nurse should be quick to recognize and correct any attitudes of her own toward the alcoholic patient that might adversely affect the quality of the patient's care.

SUMMARY OF TREATMENT MEASURES IN ACUTE ALCOHOLIC COMA

- The patient's stomach is emptied by gastric lavage if the doctor believes that it still contains large amounts of unabsorbed alcohol. Care is, of course, taken to prevent aspiration of the gastric contents.

- Analeptics are occasionally employed parenterally to help the patient's respiration and to reduce the depth of depression. Caffeine sodium benzoate (0.5 Gm.) may be administered parenterally, or the doctor may prefer pentylenetetrazol or one of the other analeptics that are used for barbiturate poisoning.

- Attempts may be made to hasten the rate of alcohol metabolism. Among the measures employed for this purpose have been the administration of hormones such as thyroxin and insulin. The value of such meas-

ures is considered doubtful and even dangerous in some circumstances. The removal of alcohol from the body by hemodialysis or by the administration of diuretics to increase urinary flow has recently been recommended.

- Artificial respiration with oxygen may be desirable. Maintenance of an open airway by suctioning of secretions or by performing a tracheotomy is important in maintaining respiratory exchange.

- Injection of intravenous fluids for combating shock and overcoming the effects of dehydration and malnutrition is desirable. Various vitamins and electrolytes are commonly added to dextrose solutions for intravenous infusion.

SUMMARY OF DRUG TREATMENT OF ALCOHOLIC EXCITEMENT AND MILD TO MODERATELY SEVERE ALCOHOL WITHDRAWAL SYNDROMES

- *Acute Alcoholic Excitement*
  Phenothiazine tranquilizers with sedative and antiemetic components, such as promazine (Sparine) and

chlorpromazine (Thorazine), are administered parenterally to control hyperexcitability, nausea and vomiting. The minor tranquilizers, chlordiazepoxide (Librium), diazepam (Valium), and hydroxyzine (Atarax), are sometimes preferred for this purpose.

- *Mild to Moderate Alcohol Withdrawal Syndrome*

    Ethyl alcohol, itself, is *not* ordinarily administered in an attempt to ease the patient's tremulousness and anxiety. Instead, sedative and tranquilizing general depressant drugs may be administered to substitute for the sedative effect of alcohol. Pentobarbital (Nembutal), which is commonly employed for treating withdrawal symptoms due to abuse of other general depressant drugs, may be used here also. Other physicians prefer parenteral chlordiazepoxide (Librium) for its prolonged duration of action and relative safety. Meprobamate

(Miltown; Equanil) also may be employed for this purpose.

- *Alcoholic Hallucinosis Phase of Withdrawal*

    Signs of toxic psychosis which sometimes appear on about the second or third day of withdrawal, including auditory hallucinations, confusion, disorientation and agitation, are best counteracted with increased doses of phenothiazine-type tranquilizers. Some doctors prefer to raise the dosage of promazine and chlorpromazine (see above) to keep patients deeply sedated and prevent development of delirium. Others employ phenothiazines such as trifluoperazine (Stelazine) and other less sedating antipsychotic agents.

SUMMARY OF TREATMENT MEASURES IN DELIRIUM TREMENS

- *Sedation* of a greater degree than that obtainable with phenothiazines alone may be required for control of extreme agitation. Thus, hypnotic doses of medium- to long-acting barbiturates, such as amobarbital and phenobarbital, or of paraldehyde may be administered frequently in addition to full doses of the more sedating phenothiazines, such as promazine and chlorpromazine.

- *Anticonvulsants,* such as I.V. diphenylhydantoin (Dilantin) and I.M. phenobarbital, may be administered for the prevention or treatment of withdrawal seizures or "rum fits."

- *Fluids and electrolytes* are administered parenterally to replace the patient's large fluid losses from fever, severe sweating, vomiting, and hyperventilation. A 5 or 10 per cent dextrose in saline solution is infused, and potassium, sodium, chloride or bicarbonate added as required, in accordance with the result of frequent checks of the patient's serum electrolyte levels. B-complex vitamins may also be administered I.M., or by addition to the infusion fluid, in order to make up for the depletion of these nutrients during the period of drinking.

- *Osmotic diuretics* such as urea or mannitol may be administered by intravenous drip to reduce intracranial

pressure, if cerebral edema or "wet brain" develops, or to counteract circulatory overload by parenteral fluids.

- *Nursing care* should be especially sympathetic and understanding. The nurse recognizes the patient's need for care and is aware that his hostile, and even combative, behavior is the result of his illness. Patients should not be restrained, if this can be avoided, and measures for increasing the patient's orientation to his surroundings should be employed. For example, concrete statements telling the patient where he is should be made repeatedly and spoken slowly.

    The nurse should always carefully explain what she is about to do before undertaking any procedure, because the patient, reacting in fear to visual, auditory, and tactile hallucinations, may struggle against attempts to feed and bathe him as well as against potentially painful procedures such as blood taking or spinal punctures.

    It is desirable to keep the room lighted at night and not to leave the patient unattended. The calm and reassuring presence of the nurse and her firm but gentle manner are most important for keeping the patient relatively quiet. However, if the nurse cannot stay with the patient, it may be permissible to let understanding friends or relatives remain with him to calm him and allay his fears.

REVIEW QUESTIONS

1. (a) What, in general, is the pattern of C.N.S. depression produced by increasing concentrations of alcohol?

(b) What actions of alcohol might make it useful in preparing a patient for surgery, and which of its properties make it undesirable for use in modern clinical anesthesia?

2. (a) How does the presence of food in the stomach affect the absorption of ingested alcohol?

(b) Why does a slow rate of absorption result in a lower blood level of alcohol than would be reached if the same amount of alcohol were rapidly absorbed?

3. (a) What factors in the distribution of alcohol account for the rapid build-up of alcohol in the brain and the tendency for this concentration to drop after the person stops drinking?

(b) What proportion of absorbed alcohol is removed from the body by oxidation, and what are some other routes by which it may be eliminated?

4. (a) What are the metabolites and final end products formed in the oxidation of alcohol?

(b) What are some points of practical significance in the fact that alcohol furnishes a source of energy to the body when it is burned?

5. (a) What are the probable effects on an average person's ability to drive a motor vehicle when his alcohol blood level is in each of the following ranges: 0–50 mg.%; 50–150 mg.%; 150–250 mg.%?

(b) What other tests may be made to determine a person's fitness to drive when his blood contains alcohol?

6. (a) What two pharmacological actions of alcohol blood levels of 50 mg.% appear to account for some of its main medical uses?

(b) What are some of the medical conditions in which alcohol has been employed?

7. (a) What are some nursing measures that can help the acutely intoxicated patient or one who is suffering from alcohol withdrawal, while drug therapy is taking effect?

(b) What observations should the nurse make of the chronic alcoholic patient who is brought to the hospital in a state of acute alcoholic intoxication?

8. (a) List some measures that may be employed in the management of acutely intoxicated patients in alcoholic coma.

(b) List some major and minor tranquilizers, sedative-hypnotics, and anticonvulsants that are used in the management of excitement stages of alcoholism and in alcoholic withdrawal syndromes.

(c) List some other medical and nursing measures employed in the management of delirium tremens.

9. (a) What is the rationale for the use of deterrent drugs such as disulfiram (Antabuse) in the management of chronic alcoholism?

(b) What are some of the signs and symptoms that result when a person drinks alcohol while under treatment with disulfiram, and what is the biochemical cause of this reaction?

10. (a) What types of patients are not considered good risks of treatment with deterrent drugs?

(b) What measures are employed for treating patients who have suffered an alcohol-disulfiram reaction?

11. (a) Of what types are the drugs used for relief of symptoms of gastritis in chronic alcoholic patients?

(b) What are some of the drugs and dietary measures that are commonly employed in attempts to overcome the effects of liver damage in chronic alcoholic patients?

12. (a) What are the signs of Wernicke's disease and by what treatment may they be reversed?

(b) What vitamins are employed in treating alcoholic polyneuropathy, and what other drugs and measures may be employed to relieve muscular pain?

13. (a) What circumstances may make the chronic alcoholic more susceptible to cardiac and respiratory diseases?

(b) What is the likely effect of drinking upon the renal tubular reabsorption of the glomerular filtrate and how is this effect brought about?

14. (a) What are the major pathological changes that occur in methyl alcohol poisoning, and which metabolites of methyl alcohol are believed responsible for these ill effects?

(b) Treatment measures of what two types mainly are employed to counteract the toxicity of methyl alcohol?

BIBLIOGRAPHY

Block, M. A.: Medical treatment of alcoholism. J.A.M.A., *162*:1610, 1956.

———: Preventive treatment of alcoholism. *In* Symposium on the treatment of alcoholism. Modern Treatment, *3*:450, 1966 (May).

Campbell, H. E.: Traffic deaths go up again. J.A.M.A., *201*:861, 1967.

Gitlow, S. E.: Treatment of the reversible acute complications of alcoholism. *In* Symposium on the treatment of alcoholism. Modern Treatment, *3*:472, 1966 (May).

Golder, G. M.: The nurse and the alcoholic patient. Am. J. Nurs., *56*:436, 1956.

Himwich, H. E.: The physiology of alcohol. J.A.M.A., *163*:545, 1957.

Klatskin, G.: Effect of alcohol on the liver. J.A.M.A., *170*: 1671, 1959.

McCarthy, R. G.: Alcoholism. Am. J. Nurs., 59:203, 1959.

Morton, E. L.: Nursing care in an alcoholic unit. Nursing Outlook, 14:45, 1966 (Oct.).

Quiros, A.: Adjusting nursing techniques to the treatment of alcoholic patients. Nursing Outlook, 5:276, 1957.

Rodman, M. J.: Alcohol: food, drug, and poison. R.N., 20:70, 1957 (May).

Smith, D. W., and Gips, C. D.: Care of the Adult Patient. Chapter 5, ed. 2. Philadelphia, J. B. Lippincott, 1966.

Victor, M.: Alcohol and nutritional diseases of the nervous system. J.A.M.A., 167:65, 1958.

———: Treatment of the neurologic complications of alcoholism. *In* Symposium on the treatment of alcoholism. Modern Treatment, 3:491, 1966 (May).

· 13 ·

Central Nervous System Stimulants

Many natural and synthetic substances can excite central nervous system cells into increased activity. Such drug-induced central stimulation is manifested in many ways. Excitation of some brain stem cells results only in an increase in alertness; on the other hand, stronger central stimulation may trigger massive convulsive spasms, followed by a period of postconvulsive depression.

Relatively few of the substances known to stimulate central activity have found a place in the therapy of illnesses in which central function is undesirably depressed. This is so mainly because only a few of these drugs can be used in ways which allow stimulation of neuronal activity of a single type, without setting off undesirable secondary side effects at the same time. Thus, some stimulants are capable of producing a desirable increase in the activity of the depressed respiratory center; however, at the doses that do so, the drugs may, at the same time, overstimulate other groups of nerve cells and thus cause harmful effects.

Similarly, other drugs can sometimes stimulate sluggish cerebral cortical functions. However, these agents may simultaneously act outside the C.N.S. to affect the functioning of the cardiovascular system adversely. Peripheral effects may, in fact, so outweigh the central ones that we do not even classify the drugs that cause them as C.N.S. stimulants. Ephedrine, for example, is a drug with stimulating action on the C.N.S. Yet, we shall discuss it under another heading (see Chap. 16), and there we look upon its central effects as adverse ones which interfere with the usefulness of ephedrine in the management of bronchial asthma, etc.

The classification of C.N.S. stimulants (Table 13-1) has never been put upon an entirely satisfactory basis. They are most commonly grouped on the basis of their primary sites of central action. However, when we classify C.N.S. stimulants in this way as *cerebral, brain stem,* and *spinal* agents, we may give the mis-

leading impression that these drugs possess more selectivity of action than they actually do. For, although small doses of these drugs may stimulate some cells before they affect others, their actions tend to spread swiftly to nearby, and even distant, parts of the neuraxis. Besides, drug-induced changes in the functions of one area of the C.N.S. may actually be brought about by pharmacological activity at another site. So-called cerebral stimulants such as the amphetamines may actually act mainly at certain subcortical centers. These areas then send impulses upward to activate cerebral cortical functions.

The best way of classifying the C.N.S. stimulants would be on the basis of their manner of action—that is, in terms of *how* they excite neuronal function, rather than *where.* Neuropharmacologists have recently learned a great deal about the intimate actions of these drugs on cellular function; however, we are not yet ready for such a way of categorizing these drugs. Here, we shall discuss the various kinds of central stimulants mainly on the basis of the several types of clinically significant activity that they tend to promote most prominently. Thus, we shall group these drugs as: (1) those that stimulate *psychomotor activity*—that is, various kinds of cerebral cortical functions; (2) those that act mainly as respiratory stimulants—the so-called *analeptics,* and (3) those that cause convulsive activity—the *convulsants.*

As we shall see, these categories cannot be adhered to rigidly. Thus, drugs classified as psychomotor or cerebral stimulants (amphetamine and caffeine, for example) may sometimes be used to stimulate the brain stem respiratory control centers; and the effects of analeptics such as pentylenetetrazol may spread from the brain stem to set off spinal convulsions. On the other hand, small doses of a so-called spinal convulsant such as strychnine can, in some circumstances, stimulate respiration *without* causing convulsions.

PSYCHOMOTOR STIMULANTS
(TABLE 13-1)

Caffeine (See Drug Digest)

Caffeine is the oldest of the drugs that primarily stimulate the mental and motor activities of the cerebral cortex. This alkaloid, which is found in coffee beans, tea leaves and kola nuts, produces mild mental stimulation and helps to overcome drowsiness and feelings of fatigue. These alerting and antidepressant actions probably account for the popularity of caffeine-containing beverages, and they play an important part in the few therapeutic applications of caffeine in medical practice.

Caffeine is capable of stimulating all parts of the C.N.S. However, the amounts taken in during ordinary drinking of the beverages containing it affect mainly the mental functions of the cerebral cortex. The effects of drinking coffee and tea have been extensively studied by psychologists. They have shown that small doses of caffeine increase the ability to maintain intellectual effort in the face of weariness. This is probably the result of the psychic effect of caffeine in counteracting fatigue, boredom and drowsiness. Although people seem somewhat more alert to sensory stimuli and react more rapidly and with a freer flow of ideas, it is doubtful that caffeine improves learning ability and memory. Caffeine-induced tremors may actually interfere with the efficiency of motor performance requiring coordinated muscular activity.

The Coffee Habit. *Coffee* is, of course, drunk in enormous quantities in this country. It is hard to think of this dietary beverage as the cause of a "drug habit,"

TABLE 13-1
CENTRAL NERVOUS SYSTEM STIMULANTS

Official or Nonproprietary Name	Proprietary Name (or Synonym)	Usual Dosage
Psychomotor (Cerebral) Stimulants		
Amphetamine phosphate N.F.	Raphetamine	5 mg. t.i.d.
Amphetamine sulfate N.F.	Benzedrine	10 mg. b.i.d.
Dextroamphetamine sulfate U.S.P.	Dexedrine	5 mg. q. 4 to 6 hrs.
Methamphetamine HCl U.S.P.	Desoxyn; desoxyephedrine, Methedrine, etc.	2.5 to 5 mg. t.i.d.
Methylphenidate HCl N.F.	Ritalin	10 mg. t.i.d.
Pipradrol HCl N.F.	Meratran	2.5 mg. b.i.d.
Caffeine U.S.P.		200 mg.
Caffeine and Sodium Benzoate U.S.P.		500 mg. I.M. or S.C.
Citrated Caffeine N.F.		60 to 120 mg.
Analeptic Agents (Brain Stem Stimulants)		
Bemegride U.S.P.	Megimide	50 mg. I.V.
Doxapram	Dopram	0.5 to 1.5 mg./Kg., I.V.
Ethamivan	Emivan	0.5 to 5 mg./Kg., I.V. or 20 to 60 mg. orally 2 to 4 times daily
Nikethamide N.F.	Coramine	1 ml. of a 25% sol. I.M. or I.V.
Pentylenetetrazol N.F.	Metrazol	100 mg. I.V. or S.C.
Picrotoxin N.F.		3 mg. (1 ml.) I.V.
Convulsant Poisons and Drugs (Brain Stem and Spinal Stimulants)		
1. *Poisons.* Brucine, Camphor, Cocaine, Strychnine, etc.		
2. *Pharmacoconvulsants*		
Flurothyl	Indoklon	2 to 5 ml. by inhalation
Pentylenetetrazol	Metrazol	500 mg. I.V.

and, indeed, for most people the degree of habituation, or psychic dependence, is so mild as to constitute no real problem. On the other hand, the adverse effects of overindulgence may be more common than is generally suspected. People who habitually drink too much coffee may suffer from cardiac irregularities and gastrointestinal upset as well as restlessness. There is also evidence that they may often be irritable and have headaches when forced to go without their usual amounts of coffee.

Coffee and Fatigue. Perhaps the worst result from the habitual overuse of coffee is that many people who drink it in order to keep awake often deprive themselves of much needed rest. The kind of physical fatigue that ordinarily forces us to stop working is actually a warning signal intended to keep us from unwisely using up our energy reserves. Drugs such as caffeine and amphetamine make it easy to ignore the sensation of tiredness but do nothing to replenish our low energy stores. Thus, their habitual use may set up a vicious cycle marked by the various adverse effects mentioned above superimposed upon those of physical exhaustion.

Fatigue is, of course, often emotional in origin. That is, anxiety and tension, or feelings of futility, boredom and aimlessness may be the most significant source of a person's habitual weariness. However, when a person's chronic fatigue is fundamentally psychosomatic in nature, it will not be allayed by an endless round of coffee drinking or by taking tablets or capsules of caffeine or the amphetamines.

The nurse may be able tactfully to guide such people to a good doctor. He will seek the sources of emotional tension or maladjustment responsible for the patient's fatigue. If he finds the underlying emotional causes, psychotherapy may succeed in re-educating the patient, so that he may rechannel his energy into constructive activity. Such "dead tired" or "totally exhausted" patients then often find that they have hidden reserves of vigor. (The nurse, we may note, is not immune to fatigue, and the nature of her work may, in fact, make her more prone than other people to both physical and emotional weariness. *She* should certainly understand that coffee, drunk "by the gallon," is an unwholesome stopgap remedy for dealing with fatigue, as is the habitual use of amphetamine-type "pep pills.")

Therapeutic Uses of Caffeine. Caffeine possesses some of the peripheral actions of the other xanthine derivatives such as theophylline and theobromine. However, its effects upon the heart, kidneys and bronchial smooth muscle are relatively weak, whereas its central stimulating action is stronger than that of its relatives. Thus, unlike aminophylline (Chaps. 19 and 40), it is not used in treating bronchial asthma or congestive heart failure, and its effects upon the heart are considered undesirable when they occur.

Caffeine is often combined with aspirin, phenacetin and other analgesics in many headache remedies. (The "C" in APC stands for caffeine.) It is also sometimes administered in combination with ergotamine for treating migraine headaches. The small doses of caffeine employed for this purpose are believed to help relieve pain, not by producing significant central stimulation, but by a peripheral effect. Caffeine is said to constrict cerebral blood vessels and thus to reduce the painful pulsations of vascular headaches, including those that often develop in patients with high blood pressure (hypertension headache).

Caffeine is also the main ingredient of various proprietary products that are promoted for allaying drowsiness. It seems wasteful for people to purchase such preparations for keeping themselves from dozing, when they can get at least as much caffeine in a cup of coffee. Unless one is sensitive to the volatile oils in coffee or the tannins in tea, it would seem more sensible to drink one of these beverages (while taking a break from work or driving) rather than pay the cost of caffeine in tablet or capsule form.

People who have been drinking alcoholic beverages are sometimes urged to drink a cup of coffee before attempting to drive. Although the advice to make the "one for the road" coffee instead of alcohol is well-intentioned, it is probably unwise. Coffee is unlikely to sober an unfit driver sufficiently to make it safe for him to operate a motor vehicle. He might better be urged not to start out at all, until the effects of the alcohol he has imbibed are entirely dissipated.

Caffeine has, however, been used in the treatment of acute alcoholic intoxication to stimulate the patient's depressed respiration and speed his arousal. Caffeine sodium benzoate is sometimes administered intramuscularly for this purpose. If this parenteral product is unavailable, an infusion of coffee may be prepared which, after cooling to body temperature, may be instilled as a retention enema.

The Amphetamines (See Drug Digests)

The drugs of this chemical class were first synthesized in a search for safer sympathomimetic drugs (Chap. 16). Scientists attempting to discover a substitute for the natural vasoconstrictor adrenergic drug ephedrine developed a series of related compounds that included amphetamine (Benzedrine), dextroamphetamine (Dexedrine) and methamphetamine (desoxyephedrine; Desoxyn, Methedrine, etc.). When these drugs were tested in laboratory animals and clinically, their peripheral effects upon blood vessels and bronchial smooth muscles turned out to be less powerful than their stimulating effect upon the central nervous system. That is, although the amphetamines proved less potent than ephedrine for constricting dilated blood vessels or for relaxing constricted bronchial tubes, these compounds caused an even greater degree of central stimulation than the natural plant alkaloid upon which the shape of their molecules had been modeled.

This was first seen when amphetamine tended to rouse anesthetized animals to which it was administered in laboratory experiments. Later, when amphetamine was tried out clinically in nose drops for shrinking swollen nasal tissues, patients complained that, although the test product worked well enough, they had trouble falling asleep when they used the drops at night. A final indication of the central activity of these drugs was the discovery that some people were removing the drug-impregnated paper from nasal inhalers and chewing it in order to get "high"—that is, for the euphoria induced by the drug's central effects.

Pharmacological Effects. All of the amphetamines possess certain central actions that form the basis for their use clinically in the management of many conditions. However, all also act peripherally to varying degrees to bring about side effects which are ordinarily considered undesirable. The doctor tries to use these drugs in small doses that are intended to produce the desired primary effects upon the C.N.S. without adversely affecting cardiovascular function. Dextroamphetamine and methamphetamine are preferred to amphetamine because their ratio of desired central to undesired peripheral effects is more favorable. However, *all* of these drugs are capable of causing sympathomimetic actions when administered in excessive doses; and some sensitive patients are discomforted by the peripheral effects of even small doses administered for mild central stimulation.

Psychopharmacological effects of two types form the basis for the various clinical uses of these drugs and for most of the *central* side effects that are seen when they are taken in excessive amounts. One of these effects is an *increase* in alertness and wakefulness. The other action is manifested by a *mood-elevating,* or *euphorigenic,* effect. Both effects are dose-related, in the sense that they become progressively more marked as the dosage of these drugs is raised. We shall describe each of these actions in further detail. However, we must remember that, with drugs that exert psychopharmacological effects, the nature of a particular patient's response depends in large part upon his underlying personality, his mental state at the time he takes the drug, and the setting, or circumstances, in which the drug is taken.

THE INCREASE IN ALERTNESS produced by small doses of amphetamines is believed (on the basis of electroencephalographic (EEG) evidence) to stem from the stimulating action upon the reticular activating system (RAS). The evidence that appears on the EEG record of increased activity at this cortical site manifests itself clinically in signs of stimulation of certain cerebral cortical functions. Thus, a person who might expect to feel sleepy and fatigued some-

times finds himself wakeful and willing to keep on working because he does not feel at all tired. If he is engaged in intellectual activity, his ideas may seem to come more freely and he may express these thoughts with more than ordinary ease. Some types of athletic performances are also reported to be improved by small doses of amphetamines.

As the dose of these drugs is raised, the mild alerting and fatigue-fighting effect is replaced by less desirable signs of excessive cortical activity. The patient may become aware of an inner tension or irritability which is somewhat discomforting. He may find himself restless, nervous and "jittery"—a term that he uses to describe his awareness of tremulousness caused by muscular as well as emotional tension. His earlier increased ability to concentrate and to express himself may give way to easy distractibility and a sense of confusion. Thus, although he may be even more talkative than before, the patient's increased loquacity may be marked by a flight of ideas that do not quite make good sense.

With still higher doses of these drugs, the patient suffers from insomnia, headache, dizziness and a variety of side effects (see Summary) that are the result of the peripheral actions of these drugs on adrenergic neuroeffectors rather than on extension of their central stimulating action. On the other hand, with continued abuse of amphetamine-type drugs, their adverse effects on brain function are seen, first, in signs of marked agitation and apprehension and, later, in states of panic that may end in a toxic psychosis marked by delirium and visual and auditory hallucinations which elicit paranoid delusions.

THE EUPHORIC, OR MOOD-ELEVATING, EFFECT is also one which is best elicited by doses of the amphetamines so small that the patient hardly realizes that his feeling of well-being is drug-induced. That is, these drugs are acting desirably when they gently evoke favorable attitudes toward tasks that need to be done, bring about an increase in a depressed and apathetic patient's self-confidence and initiative, and foster in the somewhat withdrawn person a tendency to become more outgoing in his human relationships. The extension of this action to a point at which the patient feels excessively elated and so sanguine about his abilities and prospects that he gets grandiose ideas and expresses them with great garrulity is undesirable.

Clinical Uses of the Amphetamines. The uses to which the amphetamines have been put clinically in neurology, psychiatry and general medicine are based mainly upon the ability of small doses to produce one or both of the psychopharmacological effects described above. Thus, the *alerting action* is sought in treating patients suffering from narcolepsy, postencephalitic parkinsonism, or the effects of depressant drugs. The *mood-elevating effect* makes the amphetamines useful in the treatment of mild mental depression. It is also probably responsible for whatever usefulness these drugs possess when employed as an adjunct to low-calorie diets in the management of obesity. Similarly, the effect of amphetamines upon the mental state of patients who are in pain accounts for their use in combination with analgesic drugs. Let us examine the current status of these drugs in the management of these clinical conditions.

Narcolepsy is a neurological condition in which the patient is periodically overcome by uncontrollable drowsiness. Patients may be overwhelmed by a sudden desire to sleep anywhere and at any time. Such "sleep attacks" occur most commonly during an emotional reaction marked by surprise, anger, or laughter. Discovery of the alerting action of amphetamine led to its use in this embarrassing and potentially dangerous condition. Large doses—25 to 50 mg., or more, daily—are required to prevent narcoleptic sleep paroxysms. However, the results seem to make such treatment worthwhile, since most patients are able to remain awake all day—a response to drug therapy that often converts them from social and occupational misfits into useful, productive citizens.

Epilepsy, unlike narcolepsy, is only rarely responsive to the central stimulating action of the amphetamines. However, these drugs are commonly combined with antiepileptic drugs, mainly to counteract their tendency to cause drowsiness. Thus, in the management of grand mal epilepsy, methamphetamine is often added to phenobarbital and diphenylhydantoin mixtures. Similarly, small doses are administered together with trimethadione to counteract the sedation which that drug occasionally produces in patients with petit mal epilepsy. Some children with petit mal or with behavioral disorders are even said to improve when treated only with dextroamphetamine.

Postencephalitic parkinsonism, a neurological disorder that sometimes follows so-called sleeping sickness, often responds to treatment with amphetamines. These drugs sometimes relieve other symptoms besides the patient's lethargy. Thus, the characteristic tremors—but not the rigidity—of parkinsonism are often relieved. Similarly, the distressing complication called oculogyric crisis, in which the patient's head is pulled back by neck muscle contractions and his eyes deviate upward in their orbits, frequently responds to amphetamine drug treatment. In parkinsonism of other types, the amphetamines often help to counteract both the physical depression produced by some of the antiparkinsonism drugs (Chap. 8) and the mental depression that afflicts many of these patients.

Depressant drug overdosage is sometimes treated with injections of various amphetamines. In alcohol or barbiturate intoxication these drugs may be useful not only for reducing the depth of psychomotor and respiratory depression but also for their peripheral effects upon the patient's circulation (see Chap. 16

for a further discussion of the use of *adrenergic vasopressor* drugs in the management of states of shock). The desirability of the use of amphetamines for this purpose is in dispute, as is, indeed, the entire concept of analeptic drug therapy (discussed later in this chapter). There is, however, no controversy concerning the rationale for the addition of small doses of amphetamines to products containing C.N.S. depressants capable of causing undesirable degrees of drowsiness. A common example of such combinations —in addition to the antiepileptic and antiparkinsonism medications mentioned above—is seen in products for the treatment of allergy, which often contain amphetamines to counteract drowsiness induced by the central depressant action of certain antihistaminic drugs (Chap. 40).

Mentally depressed patients with relatively mild and temporary mood disturbances are often benefited by administration of amphetamines as an adjunct to psychotherapeutic support. Such patients, reacting to distressing events such as a death in the family, marital unhappiness or divorce, financial loss, or prolonged unemployment, seem to lose their zest for life and their interest in their former goals. Often, suffering from so-called "morning melancholia," they feel fatigued even after a night's sleep and seem unable or unwilling to rouse themselves to face another day.

Somehow, in such cases of mild "reactive" depression, small daily doses of the amphetamines tend to speed the patient's recovery, especially if he has the help of people—whether professional, or friends and family—who are willing to listen to him to offer him sympathetic understanding. The drugs then seem to help make the patient brighter and more alert and attentive. His depressive apathy, listness and lethargy are gradually overcome, and he regains his interest in participating in the normal activities of daily living.

Patients with more severe degrees of mental depression are not ordinarily helped by amphetamine therapy and may even be harmed by these drugs. These psychomotor stimulants tend to increase the insomnia and appetite-loss of people who are already sleeping and eating poorly. Thus, they are not employed for the more severe neurotic and psychotic depressive symptoms, which require the more potent antidepressant drugs (Chap. 7), electroshock therapy, and intensive psychotherapy.

The mood-elevating effect of the amphetamines is sometimes helpful to patients suffering from various painful or disabling organic ailments. People with arthritis, for example, may be aided by the addition of small doses of amphetamines to their regimen of salicylates, rest, special exercises and physical therapy. Although the amphetamines are neither analgesic nor anti-inflammatory, their favorable effects on the patient's emotional state makes him better able to bear discomfort. Similarly, women with dysmenorrhea or other menstrual disturbances often do better when an amphetamine is added to their antispasmodic, analgesic or hormone medication.

Non-amphetamine psychomotor stimulants that are promoted for the management of mildly depressed patients are claimed to be free of the limiting side effects of the amphetamines. Methylphenidate (Ritalin) and pipradrol (Meratran), for example, are said not to overstimulate cardiovascular activity nor to suppress the appetite, as the amphetamines do. These drugs and pentylenetetrazol (Metrazol) are available in geriatric tonic products that also contain vitamins, minerals and, sometimes, male and female sex hormones.

The rationale of their use in such metabolic-aid products is that these stimulants are well tolerated by elderly patients and favorably affect the appetite of the patient who may be losing his interest in food along with his other drives. However, although they may occasionally help to overcome functional fatigue and briefly restore some of the patient's lost zest for living, these drugs are no more effective than the amphetamines for major depressions and are not recommended for use in such cases.

Amphetamines as Appetite Suppressants. The amphetamines are widely employed in products advocated for use as adjuncts to low-calorie diets in the weight-reducing programs of obese patients and other dieters. These drugs tend, temporarily, at least, to lessen the patient's desire to eat. The way exactly in which the amphetamines exert this so-called anorexiant action is disputed, but there seems no doubt that the appetite suppression that they produce is mainly central in origin rather than the result of their peripheral effects upon the G.I. tract. Most authorities feel that the anorectic effect of the amphetamines is related to their mood-elevating action. That is, these drugs are thought to help people stick to a low-calorie diet, despite its discomforts, by making the patient feel better mentally.

The usefulness of this psychopharmacological effect is limited at best. Most patients soon tend to develop tolerance to the psychological lift that the amphetamines offered them at first. Truly compulsive overeaters do not seem to respond at all to these appetite suppressant drugs, possibly because they eat, not just to satisfy appetite but for the more complex psychological satisfactions that they gain from stuffing themselves and even from being obese. Such patients are not likely to benefit from *any* drug and dietary regimen without simultaneous psychotherapy. They may, in fact, suffer severe emotional disturbances that are not drug-induced but the result of failure to provide them with a substitute for the satisfactions that they ordinarily derive from overeating.

The amphetamines sometimes cause central and peripheral side effects that limit their utility. Thus, the obese patient with a history of hypertension or coronary disease may be unable to take these drugs because of their tendency to raise blood pressure or speed the heart rate. Other patients are sometimes overstimulated and may feel uncomfortably jittery during the day and find it difficult to fall asleep at night. Doctors try to get around this drawback by prescribing amphetamines in combination with barbiturates and minor tranquilizers and by having patients take their last dose in the late afternoon rather than at night. This, however, makes the drugs less useful for people with the so-called "night eating syndrome"—a pattern of food intake marked by insomnia and a desire to eat heavily at night.

The inadequacies and disadvantages of the more commonly employed amphetamines have led to the synthesis and introduction of many newer anorexigenic drugs (Table 13-2). All these compounds are

TABLE 13-2

ANOREXIANT AGENTS

Official or Generic Name	Proprietary Name	Usual Dose
Amphetamines (see Table 13-1)		
Benzphetamine HCl	Didrex	25 to 50 mg. 1 to 3 times daily
Chlorphentermine HCl	Pre-Sate	65 mg. daily
Diethylpropion HCl	Tenuate; Tepanil	25 mg. t.i.d.
Phendimetrazine tartrate	Plegine	17.5 to 70 mg. 2 to 3 times daily
Phenmetrazine HCl, N.F.	Preludin	25 mg. 2 to 3 times daily
Phentermine Resin	Ionamin	15 to 30 mg. once daily
Phentermine HCl	Wilpo	8 mg. t.i.d.

congeners of amphetamine that are claimed not to cause nervousness, because of their ability to act specifically upon a special appetite control center in the brain without, at the same time, acting elsewhere to stimuate undesirable central and sympathetic nervous system activity.

Actually, there is at present no reliable evidence to indicate that these drugs act specifically at the hypothalamic centers that regulate food intake in humans —that is, at a so-called subcortical "appestat." Like the amphetamines, these newer anorectics probably affect cerebral cortical function; and, although this may well act, in turn, to affect the functioning of the hypothalamic "feeding" and "satiety" centers, it is thought unlikely that these drugs can do this without causing C.N.S. stimulation simultaneously.

It is, of course, entirely possible that some small change in molecular structure may make a particular drug more or less potent in its central action. So far, however, drugs that produce fewer C.N.S. side effects than dextroamphetamine and methamphetamine also seem to be weaker than these drugs in their appetite suppressant activity. That is, there seems to be a relationship between a drug's ability to give the dieting patient a sense of well being and its tendency to cause nervousness and insomnia when taken in excessive amounts. In any case, a practical point to remember about all these drugs (regardless of their claims) is this: *All* are capable of causing *any* of the central or peripheral side effects listed in the Summary on page 215, and, consequently, all of these drugs must be used with caution in patients with hypertension, heart disease or hyperthyroidism and in those whose history indicates that they may be prone to abuse C.N.S. stimulants in order to gain their euphoric effects.

The Abuse of Amphetamine-Type Drugs. The amphetamines seem to be widely available to people who use them without medical supervision. College students studying for examinations, for example, appear to have no difficulty in supplying themselves with amphetamine tablets for use in staying awake while cramming. Other individuals are said to misuse amphetamines in order to keep themselves awake— long-distance truckers (and other drivers), during long hauls; writers, for meeting looming deadlines.

Such unsupervised use of the amphetamines is undesirable for various reasons. For one thing, when a person takes amphetamines to stay awake and keep working when he should be resting, he runs the risk of pushing himself past the limits of his physical endurance without realizing it. Although the amphetamines effectively mask the signs of fatigue, they in no way reduce the body's natural need for rest. All that these drugs do is postpone payment of the debt that is owed to the body's energy stores. Thus, the use of these drugs is commonly followed by a let-

down that is manifested by mental and physical fatigue.

This, in itself, need not be serious if the person who has relied on these drugs to help him through an emergency period then goes to bed and makes up for the rest that he has lost. Sometimes, however, either because of continuing pressure or a deliberate seeking of "kicks," individuals may continue taking amphetamines in order to keep active instead of going to sleep. Occasionally, for instance, students may try to stay "high" during an entire examination period. Some may even have the mistaken notion that the drugs will help them make up for a lack of factual knowledge. Not only does continued taking of these drugs not aid learning or memory, but the confusion that they often cause actually tends to reduce the quality of intellectual performance. Much more serious is the possibility that the misuse of these drugs in this manner may lead to collapse. Such a reaction is usually the result of simple exhaustion, upon which may be imposed the adverse central and cardiovascular effects of these drugs.

A different kind of abuse pattern is sometimes seen in individuals with psychopathic personalities. These people do not take amphetamines merely to stay awake, but rather for their euphoric effects. They may, for example, go on periodic sprees during which they take hundreds of milligrams daily for days or weeks, in order to stay at a hypomanic "high." As tolerance develops, the amphetamine abuser often begins to inject the drug intravenously in order to intensify its effects.

Pattern of Parenteral Abuse. Injection of a concentrated solution of methamphetamine into a vein is followed by an immediate "flash" or "rush"—an orgiastic feeling marked by increased sex drive and the illusion of increased physical and mental power. Because this feeling fades rapidly, the "meth head" or "speed freak" (as he is called in the drug subculture) must make injections every two hours in order to sustain the desired effect.

A "run" of this kind, during which the abuser stays continuously awake, usually lasts for three to six days. Groups of users gather together, talking incessantly, and making less and less sense. Finally, the hypomanic user often falls into an exhausted sleep that lasts 12 to 18 hours. Upon awakening, he may begin a new "run" with larger doses of the drug. After a series of such episodes, he suffers from severe physical and psychotoxic effects.

Physically, the amphetamine abuser shows the effects of malnutrition. Because appetite is completely suppressed, he loses 20 to 30 lbs. during a period of sustained intravenous use. Mentally, he becomes badly disorganized and uncomfortably tense and nervous. Often, barbiturates are taken to relieve these discomforts or in order to terminate the "run" and initiate sleep. Sometimes, amphetamines and barbiturates are taken in combination. This is similar to the manner in which other addicts alternate their use of the stimulant cocaine with the depressant heroin; or the way in which they often inject the two together in what is called a "speedball."

A toxic psychosis is often the end result of this kind of chronic overdosage with amphetamines, or rarely, the result of a single very large dose. Patients may then be hospitalized with signs and symptoms that very much resemble those of a schizophrenic reaction of the paranoid type. That is, the patient suffers visual, tactile, and auditory hallucinations to which he reacts with systematized delusions of persecution. As in the case of cocaine addiction, such paranoid thinking can trigger dangerous assaultive behavior. Unlike cocaine, however, the amphetamines rarely cause convulsions, and the psychotic symptoms are readily controlled by the administration of pheno-thiazine-type tranquilizers. Ordinarily, hospitalized patients become entirely rational during the first week or two of abstinence.

Withdrawal. The abrupt withdrawal of amphetamines does not, fortunately, set off an abstinence syndrome such as those seen with opiates, barbiturates, alcohol and other depressant drugs. Although the abuser of stimulants does not suffer the same kinds of dangerous and disabling reactions that follow the elimination of depressants, some authorities feel that the deep and prolonged sleep that follows the end of a sustained series of "runs" does actually represent an abstinence syndrome.

The doctors suggest that the semicomatose state that sometimes lasts three or four days and the lethargy and fatigue lasting several weeks are evidence of more than merely the unmasking of a state of exhaustion. They believe that it is, instead, the result of physiological and biochemical adaptations similar to those that occur with the chronic abuse of other drugs that cause physical dependence. Thus, the physical lethargy that follows the recovery sleep is said to reinforce the abuser's psychological craving and lead to his rapid return to amphetamine abuse. In any case, these drugs are correctly classified as "addictive" on the basis of the harm their abuse can do to the individual and to society.

The amphetamines also possess other abuse characteristics, such as the ability to create development of tolerance and compulsive behavior—that is, strong psychic dependence. In practice, this means that, even without the reinforcement of physical dependence, an individual may develop a craving for the amphetamine-induced euphoria. In pursuit of this euphoric effect in the face of increasing tolerance, he may build up to a daily intake of dozens of tablets. However, although he may become quite resistant to the adverse cardiovascular effects of these drugs, the amphetamine abuser is likely finally to suffer from the centrally induced psychotic reaction.

As a result of public alarm over the abuse of amphetamines and barbiturates, legislation passed in 1965 now makes mandatory closer control over the sale and distribution of these drugs. It remains to be seen, however, whether these Drug Abuse Amendments of 1965 will actually succeed in restricting illegal traffic in these drugs. Testimony before legislative committees concerning actually the *bootlegging* of "Bennies" (Benzedrine) led to passage of this legislation; however, the main effect of the law so far has been to cause complications for physicians and pharmacists. It would be most unfortunate if these "Dangerous Drug" laws made it more difficult for patients to get drugs that are relatively safe and effective when taken with a doctor's advice and guidance, without keeping the psychopaths and thrill seekers from having the same ready access to the "pep pills" that previously permitted their indiscriminate abuse.

Other Psychomotor Stimulants

New chemicals are constantly being subjected to psychological testing procedures intended to uncover the presence of brain-stimulating properties. One so-called "fatigue-fighter" is made up of the potassium and magnesium salts of an amino acid, aspartic acid (*Spartase*). Thus far, there is little valid evidence to indicate that the theoretical basis for the use of this substance to benefit vital metabolic processes has borne clinically useful fruit.

Another product, also studied originally for anti-fatigue activity, *pemoline with magnesium hydroxide* (Cylert), is claimed to possess a unique ability to enhance the learning ability and memory of rats. However, the ability of pemoline to improve such intellectual functions in humans has not yet been proved.

ANALEPTIC-TYPE C.N.S. STIMULANTS (SEE DRUG DIGESTS)

The Greek word analeptikos means *restorative*, and certain C.N.S. stimulants that have the capacity to restore consciousness to a patient deeply depressed by central depressant drugs are often classified as analeptics. Actually, such emphasis upon the capacity of these stimulants to bring about the arousal of patients from comatose states tends to distort the objectives of modern treatment with these agents and their true current status.

Actions. These drugs, which act mainly as brain stem stimulants, act primarily in two ways: (1) Small doses stimulate the vital centers located in the medulla oblongata. Thus, they tend to increase the sensitivity of the respiratory center neurons to the carbon dioxide that has built up to abnormal blood levels during the patient's period of depression. Similarly, the medullary vasomotor and cardiac centers tend to increase their output of efferent impulses under the influence of analeptic drugs. (2) Somewhat larger doses stimulate the reticular activating system (RAS) in a manner that results in both electroencephalographic (EEG) activation and in clinical arousal from states of drug-induced depression. That is, increased numbers of nerve impulses pass by way of ascending pathways to the cerebral cortex, thus stimulating various cortically influenced functions, including consciousness.

Unfortunately, the actions of the presently available analeptic agents are not limited to these specific sites. Thus, when the analeptics are administered in the doses often needed to produce arousal, the stimulating actions of these drugs spread to other parts of the neuraxis, including the spinal cord. Such nonspecific, or generalized, central stimulation can cause various adverse reactions. These include: (1) *respiratory difficulties* such as cough, hiccough, laryngospasm, bronchospasm, and dyspnea; (2) *cardiovascular complications* such as irregular heart rhythms and the elevation of blood pressure; (3) *motor system stimulation* marked by hyperreflexia, muscular twitching, and even massive convulsive spasms.

The possibility of the occurrence of these and other dangerous reactions has led various authorities to condemn the administration of analeptics under any circumstances. They have argued that giving these drugs to patients already in deep difficulty could very readily make their condition even worse. Other experts (anesthesiologists, particularly) have suggested that the judicious use of analeptics in carefully selected patients could be of value in various clinical situations. These physicians have attempted to determine the manner in which analeptics might be used with the greatest degree of safety and efficacy. As a result of their research, some new principles of analeptic therapy appear to be emerging at the present time. Perhaps these, together with the current trend toward the development of analeptic drugs with wider safety margins, may result in a more respectable status and wider use for these controversial agents.

Uses. In the following discussion of the various uses to which analeptics are presently being put, we shall attempt to make clear their limitations, the precautions that are required in their administration, and the advantages and disadvantages of the several drugs which are presently preferred for use in different clinical conditions or circumstances.

Depressant Drug Intoxication. The convulsant drugs *picrotoxin, nikethamide* and *pentylenetetrazol* have long been reserved largely for one clinical purpose—to counteract the effects of overdosage by barbiturates, alcohol and other C.N.S. depressant drugs. Although heated controversies have sometimes erupted concerning the desirability of employing these drugs for this purpose, there now seems to be general agreement on at least two points:

1. If analeptics are administered, they should be used only to stimulate depressed respiration and not with the intention of bringing about the rapid arousal of the unconscious patient.

2. Analeptics should never be used without at the same time applying every possible method for supporting the patient's respiration, circulation and other vital functions. (See Chaps. 3 and 6, and Summary, p. 108.)

Perhaps the most common error in the past was the administration of these drugs to patients who did not really require analeptic therapy. Patients who are in a relatively light stupor can be readily aroused by relatively weak analeptics such as caffeine and nikethamide. An acutely intoxicated alcoholic patient, for example, may waken very quickly and respond to questions quite coherently. However, such a dramatic arousal is not really necessary, and the patient would probably have been better off if simply allowed to sleep off his stuporous state. For one thing, these patients sometimes wake in a difficult-to-control delirium. Also, some chronically addicted patients may suffer a late psychotic reaction brought on by the sudden drug-induced withdrawal from barbiturate or alcohol depression.

There is also the danger that partial arousal of the patient may result in return of the vomiting reflexes. Stimulation of the vomiting mechanism may cause him to aspirate the gastric contents that he regurgitates. Most serious is the danger that administration of a potent motor-system stimulant to an only lightly depressed patient may precipitate convulsive activity. This may leave the patient in worse shape than before, because of the increased oxygen demands of the brain and muscles and the postconvulsive depression.

To avoid these dangers, some medical scientists have suggested that analeptic therapy be employed only after the patient has been proved actually to be in a state of deep depression. Patients who can be roused by physical stimulation, they point out, are not in need of analeptic drugs and should be managed supportively. Even among comatose patients, not all need repeated injections of analeptics.

Whether or not these deeply depressed patients really require analeptic treatment may sometimes be determined by administering a single intravenous dose (5 ml. of a 10% solution) of pentylenetetrazol (see Drug Digest). If the patient is readily aroused and his reflex activity returns, even temporarily, no further analeptic therapy is thought necessary. However, if the patient's depression is so deep that he fails to react at all to such an "orientation dose" of this short-acting analeptic, he is unlikely to be harmed by repeated injections of the same drug. In fact, according to the advocates of this treatment plan, intensive analeptic therapy may be essential for restoring respiratory activity in such cases.

As we have indicated, however, even those who believe that the use of analeptics is sometimes justified agree that it is essential that these patients receive both medical support of respiration and superior nursing care, in order to avoid complications such as atalectasis and hypostatic pneumonia. Among the measures employed are mechanical artificial respiration, oxygen inhalation through a nasal catheter or pharyngeal airway, and removal of secretions from the patient's tracheobronchial tree. The patient should be turned from side to side every few hours, and his tongue kept from falling back into the pharynx. Endotracheal intubation or even tracheotomy may be employed to maintain a patent airway.

Besides pentylenetetrazol, analeptics that are sometimes given by vein in such cases include: (1) *picrotoxin,* a drug of relatively slow onset and somewhat longer duration of action. Because of the narrow margin between respiratory stimulation and preconvulsive muscular twitching, it is infrequently administered today except in cases of very severe *barbiturate* depression that have failed to respond to treatment with safer, short-acting analeptics; (2) *bemegride* (see Drug Digest), an agent with properties similar to those of pentylenetetrazol; (3) *methylphenidate,* an agent midway between caffeine and amphetamine in psychomotor-analeptic stimulating activity; (4) *ethamivan,* an agent that is infused slowly over a period of several minutes, because rapid injection of a single dose tends to cause coughing, sneezing, tremors and chest muscle spasms.

Postanesthetic Respiratory Depression. Patients who have received various central and peripheral depressants before and during surgery sometimes suffer from drug-induced respiratory depression of varying degree postoperatively. Recovery room nurses try to encourage patients to breathe deeply as part of the so-called "stir up" regimen for preventing the development of atalectasis. Some anesthesiologists have recently suggested that respiratory stimulant drugs might be useful to produce deep breathing and physiological sighing and to hasten the return of the protective cough and swallowing reflexes of such patients. *Doxapram* (Dopram), the newest analeptic drug, has reportedly helped to prevent postoperative respiratory complications when infused intravenously for 30-minute periods in such situations.

Analeptics are *not* used routinely in the recovery room, either to hasten the recovery of pharyngeal and laryngeal reflexes, or to shorten postanesthetic recovery time in patients who have received barbiturates, narcotic analgesics, or long-lasting inhalation anesthetics such as methoxyflurane (Penthrane). However, some of the newer, more specific, respiratory stimulants such as doxapram and ethamivan may have a place in the diagnosis and treatment of postanesthetic apnea.

Patients sometimes fail to resume spontaneous respiration for quite some time after anesthesia has been discontinued. When patients have received a variety of central depressants together with a peripherally acting skeletal muscle relaxant, it is often very difficult for the doctors to determine which drug is responsible for the postanesthetic apnea. However, it has recently been suggested that the patient's response to a relatively specific respiratory-center stimulant such as doxapram may be an aid in differential diagnosis. Small doses of this drug usually bring about a prompt though transient increase in the rate of respiration and in the tidal volume (the air taken in with each breath) when the patient's poor breathing is due to central depression. In such cases, the drug may be injected repeatedly or continuously to sustain the desired effect.

On the other hand, when hypoventilation is the result of residual curarization—that is, persisting partial depression by neuromuscular blocking agents such as *curare* (Chap. 17)—injection of the central respiratory stimulant will increase the breathing rate but *not* the respiratory minute volume. In such cases, administration of the anticurare agent neostigmine is used to restore respiration by its peripheral action.

Chronic Obstructive Lung Diseases. Patients with chronic respiratory diseases such as pulmonary emphysema may occasionally benefit from very careful infusion of a respiratory stimulant. These drugs cannot, of course, reverse the underlying cause of the patient's hypoventilation. That is, they cannot correct the obstruction caused by the breakdown of the walls of the alveoli, the millions of tiny air sacs that have lost their elasticity and, with it, the ability to expand and contract. Drugs may, however, help to overcome some of the complications that have resulted from the patient's rapid, shallow, labored breathing.

Because of their decreased ability to expel air, patients with pulmonary emphysema tend to retain high levels of carbon dioxide in their blood. This end product of metabolism makes the patient drowsy and may even cause coma. Accumulation of this acid waste product also leads to respiratory acidosis and dyspnea. In such cases, some doctors have reported that administration of the relatively specific respiratory center stimulants ethamivan (Emivan) and doxapram (Dopram) has helped to increase the depth of the patient's respiration and improved the ventilation of the alveoli. The resulting decrease in arterial carbon dioxide levels is also said to help to rouse drowsy patients from their hypercapnic lethargy.

Patients must be attended constantly during the slow infusion of these respiratory stimulants, in order to avoid adverse effects. Although generalized stimulation of the C.N.S. is said to be less likely with the more recently introduced analeptics, their dosage must still be carefully controlled. Excessive stimulation of respiration may make the muscles used in breathing work *too* hard. This makes them use up too much oxygen and permits the accumulation of even more of the carbon dioxide by-product of muscular effort.

In addition to their direct action on the medullary respiratory center, some of the analeptics, including nikethamide (Coramine) and doxapram, stimulate respiration indirectly, by acting peripherally upon chemoreceptors located in the aorta and carotid arteries. These cells ordinarily respond to high levels of carbon dioxide, high blood acidity, and low blood oxygen by sending signals that stimulate respiratory center activity.

Such drug-induced reflex and central stimulation of respiration is particularly useful for patients with pulmonary emphysema or in status asthmaticus, who require oxygen therapy for correction of hypoxemia. Ordinarily, when oxygen inhalation raises blood oxygen levels, the chemoreceptors send fewer impulses centrally to stimulate respiration reflexly. Careful administration of nikethamide, doxapram, or ethamivan may prevent the alveolar hypoventilation that often occurs when oxygen is administered to these dyspneic patients.

The Neuropsychiatric Uses of Analeptic Drugs. Some of the analeptics are occasionally used in certain psychological and neurological conditions and procedures. Pentylenetetrazol, for example, is sometimes administered orally to elderly patients suffering from senile dementia or simply from functional fatigue and general depression. Although it is incorporated in many products, in combination with vitamins, minerals, etc., there is little evidence to indicate that it is even as effective as the psychomotor stimulants such as the amphetamines, methylphenidate, and pipradol for this purpose.

Pentylenetetrazol has also been employed as a pharmacoconvulsant. However, as indicated in the discussion of *flurothyl* later in this chapter, electroconvulsant therapy seems to be preferred to chemoshock therapy, at present, by psychiatrists. The slow infusion of subconvulsant doses of pentylenetetrazol is sometimes used in neurology for the diagnosis of epilepsy. Pentylenetetrazol brings about characteristic changes in the electroencephalographic pattern of epileptic patients after the infusion of relatively small amounts of solution, compared to the amounts that alter the normal EEG.

CONVULSANT DRUGS AND POISONS

Many natural and synthetic stimulants of the C.N.S. are capable of causing increased impulse transmission in motor pathways so marked that various of the patient's muscle groups are sent into violent involuntary contractions, or convulsions. These convulsions are typically *clonic* or *tonic*.

Clonic convulsive spasms are characterized by the occurrence of a quick series of alternating *contractions* and *relaxations,* first in one and then in another group of muscles. This *coordinated* muscular activity may give the appearance of being *purposeful,* or cortically directed. Actually, the individual reacting in this way has no control over the tics, twitches and spasms that seem to start in the muscles on one side of the body and move to the other—that is, in an *asymmetric* pattern. Clonic convulsions are seen most commonly with small overdoses of the stimulants—including picrotoxin and pentylenetetrazol—that act primarily at brain stem centers.

Tonic convulsive seizures are much more dramatic, and even fearful, to see. They are characterized by the *sustained rigidity* of all muscle groups. Actually, the action of the more powerful of two opposing muscle groups predominates, but, because the antagonists are also maximally contracted, coordinated muscular activity is impossible. Thus, in humans the *extensor* muscles of the legs, back and neck are the stronger and pull the person into a bowlike position, with his back arched and his body resting only on the head and heels (opisthotonus). Such tetanic spasms are *symmetrical*—that is, they occur in the muscles on both sides of the body simultaneously. Tonic muscular activity is also *uncoordinated*, so that no purposeful movements can be carried out. This happens because the opposing muscle groups (the *flexors,* for example) which would ordinarily be relaxed as a result of reciprocal inhibition, remain, instead, in a state of spasmodic contraction. Tonic convulsions are seen mainly following poisoning by spinal cord stimulants such as *strychnine,* but they may also occur with massive overdoses of brain stem stimulants such as pentylenetetrazol when the effects of these drugs spread to the spinal cord from their primary site of activity.

Not much is known about the exact biochemical mechanisms by which drugs cause convulsions. However, neurophysiologists have recently uncovered some of the complicated ways in which central stimulants may increase synaptic activity in motor pathways. *Strychnine,* for example, seems to remove some of the inhibitory influences normally impinging upon motoneurons. The postsynaptic neurons which are released in this way are then free to respond more fully to the excitatory stimuli that are reaching them by way of other synaptic connections (see Chap. 5). *Picrotoxin* acts in yet another complex way to block transmission at inhibitory synapses, and thus this drug indirectly increases the relative total amount of central excitatory activity. *Pentylenetetrazol*, on the other hand, probably acts by increasing the transmission of stimuli at excitatory synapses to a greater degree than it promotes activity at inhibitory synapses. As a result, the sum total of excitatory activity is such that it initiates enough motor neuron impulses to cause convulsions.

Clinical Uses of Convulsant Drugs

The drugs of this class have only limited clinical utility, since convulsions are generally considered a complication to be feared rather than a therapeutically desirable action. However, certain pharmacoconvulsants are occasionally employed in psychiatry and neurology.

Chemoshock is a rarely used alternative to electroshock therapy (EST or ECT) in the treatment of psychotic depressive states and certain schizophrenic reactions. Pentylenetetrazol was the convulsant first employed for this purpose. Injected rapidly by vein, a large dose (5 ml. of a 10% solution) produces clonic spasms, followed by a massive tonic convulsion. A series of such treatments often improves the patient's mental condition.

However, as indicated in Chapter 7, pentylenetetrazol proved to have various disadvantages that resulted in its being displaced by electroshock therapy, which can be carried out with less discomfort to the patient, greater predictability and reliability and, consequently, with increased safety and convenience. Among the drawbacks of drug-induced convulsions are: (1) a slow onset of activity, during which some patients often experience a feeling of great fear; (2) occasional failure of convulsive activity to occur at all, after which the patient may be left in a panic state for a day or more; and (3) occasional development of prolonged and repeated convulsive seizures.

Recently, inhalation of the volatile vapors of a drug have been used to produce convulsions in selected psychiatric patients. This convulsant agent, called flurothyl (Indoklon), has been employed in the treatment of the same kinds of cases in which pentylenetetrazol was previously thought indicated and for which EST is presently most commonly employed. These indications include: (1) patients who have not responded to courses of therapy by the major modern antidepressant drugs (Chap. 7), (2) those who are considered such high suicide risks that the doctor thinks it dangerous to temporize by waiting for the slow-acting antidepressant drugs to take effect, and (3) patients whose depression is diagnosed as schizo-affective, or whose withdrawal or agitation is judged to be catatonic and part of the picture of an acute schizophrenic reaction.

In such cases, however, the inhalation of flurothyl does not seem to offer any marked advantages over EST, despite various claims for its superiority that have been made by the sponsors of this pharmacoconvulsant agent. Both procedures require the use of premedication with other drugs to minimize complications. Adjunctive agents include the skeletal muscle relaxant, succinylcholine (Chap. 17), which is employed to prevent the fractures and dislocations that might otherwise be caused by the convulsions. Administration of atropine and thiopental is part of the pretreatment routine for flurothyl inhalation as well as EST. Thus, patients must be watched for signs of adverse reactions to these potent drugs as well as to flurothyl itself. Flurothyl is also no less likely than EST to cause prolonged apnea, cardiac arrest or vascular collapse. Thus, like EST, its use is contraindicated in patients with a history of cardiovascular disease and for others who might be endangered by seizure activity.

Pentylenetetrazol and bemegride are sometimes infused slowly in subconvulsant doses in a diagnostic procedure to uncover the presence of epilepsy. Both drugs then bring about electroencephalographic changes indicative of neurological abnormalities. Sometimes the I.V. infusion is accompanied by the use of a flickering light to speed the onset of abnormal EEG patterns. This combination of chemical and physical means is sometimes employed to produce an actual clinical convulsion, as this may aid the neurologist in determining the exact nature of the patient's illness and, consequently, in choosing the type of anticonvulsant drug best suited for control of his seizures.

Strychnine Poisoning. Strychnine is a drug that should have no place in modern therapy. It has been used as a respiratory stimulant, digestive tonic, and an ingredient of cathartic combinations. Its usefulness, if any, is far outweighed by the danger of poisoning from accidental ingestion. Similarly, the use of strychnine in so-called mouse "seeds" or rat "poison pellets" and as a bait for field rodents is unjustified in view of the present availability of safer substances.

The incidence of strychnine poisoning has declined as preparations containing it have deservedly lost popularity; however, cases are still reported in which children have died after swallowing a handful of candy-coated "tonic" or cathartic tablets. The quantity of strychnine in a single tablet of aloin, strychnine and belladonna (for example) is harmless—as well as useless—but the total alkaloid contained in several pills may be capable of causing fatal convulsions.

Signs and symptoms of strychnine overdosage come on quickly. Often, the patient begins to feel a tightness in the muscles of his face, neck, back and legs. He is alert, anxious and fearful, and his reflexes become hyperactive. Then, quite suddenly, a slight stimulus may set off a violent convulsion. In a characteristic full-blown tonic seizure, the patient's back is arched and his face contorted into what seems a smile. Actually, the patient, who does not usually lose consciousness until he becomes asphyxiated, is capable of fully feeling the extreme pain produced by the massive muscular spasms.

Treatment is intended primarily to control convulsions and prevent asphyxia. The patient quickly becomes hypoxic and cyanotic, as a result of the severe muscle spasm. Such muscular activity utilizes large quantities of oxygen at a time when spasticity of the diaphragm and chest muscles interferes with breathing. Thus, mechanical artificial respiration or the administration of oxygen by means of a nasal catheter may be needed. After the convulsions are controlled, an endotracheal tube may be inserted to protect the patient against regurgitation and aspiration of gastric contents.

CONTROL OF CONVULSIONS requires the careful administration of depressant drugs in doses that produce muscle relaxation and light sleep without impairing respiratory-center function. Intravenous injection of small doses of an ultra-short-acting barbiturate such as thiopental may be repeated as needed to keep muscular activity under control. This may be followed by intramuscular injection of the long-acting anticonvulsant, phenobarbital. Muscle relaxants such as mephenesin and d-tubocurarine have been found useful in the hands of anesthesiologists called in to aid in controlling the patient's convulsions.

REMOVAL OF THE POISON from the stomach is best delayed until the patient's hair-trigger hyperreflexia has been blunted with anticonvulsant drugs, because the attempt to pass a stomach tube may set off convulsive seizures. The gavage solution is used in copious quantities to wash out all traces of strychnine before it can be absorbed. A solution of 1:10,000 potassium permanganate (100 mg. per liter) is said to aid by destroying the poison chemically.

Induction of vomiting by means of drugs or otherwise is not considered desirable, since the procedure may precipitate convulsions. It is generally wise to try to keep all sensory stimulation to a minimum by putting the patient in a quiet, darkened, warm room. He should be constantly watched and protected from hurting himself in any way. If reflex activity begins to increase, the doctor is informed, as the patient may require more of the sedative-anticonvulsant.

Strychnine poisoning is fortunately seen less frequently today in this country. However, most of the measures described above for dealing with strychnine toxicity may, of course, be applied to the management of acute convulsions induced by other drugs. Various chemicals that are not classified as convulsants can, in some circumstances, set off seizures. Some of these agents may be categorized as peripherally acting drugs or even as central depressants. The antihistaminic agents, for example, act mainly outside the C.N.S. Yet children taking accidental overdoses (Chap. 40) sometimes suffer from sudden convulsions superimposed upon their initial drowsiness and depression. The use of barbiturates for controlling convulsions in such cases requires particular care, since these drugs may add to the patient's respiratory depression.

SUMMARY OF SIDE EFFECTS, TOXICITY, CAUTIONS AND CONTRAINDICATIONS OF AMPHETAMINE-TYPE DRUGS

- *Central Side Effects and Toxicity*

  Nervousness, restlessness, jitteriness, irritability, anorexia, insomnia, headache, dizziness; anxiety, tension, difficulty in concentrating; confusion, delirium, hallucinations, toxic psychosis with paranoid delusions.

- *Peripheral Side Effects and Toxicity*

  Cardiac palpitations and tachycardia, with possible chest pains and other heart-beat irregularities; elevation of both systolic and diastolic blood pressures; dryness of the mouth, constipation, nausea and vomiting, excessive sweating, dilated pupils.

- *Cautions and Contraindications*

  These drugs are administered with caution, if at all, to patients with advanced coronary or cerebral atherosclerotic disease or other cardiovascular disorders including severe hypertension, or in the presence of hyperthyroidism. They are not desirable for patients with depression marked by signs of agitation, severe sleeplessness and appetite loss, or for those who are already receiving antidepressants of the MAO inhibitor type (Chap. 7). These drugs are not desirable for individuals with a history of psychological instability, who may be prone to abuse these drugs—for example, patients with psychopathic personality or a history of homicidal or suicidal statements.

SUMMARY OF NURSING POINTS

• The nurse, particularly in industrial and school settings, has an opportunity to provide instruction concerning the misuse of caffeine and amphetamines; sometimes she observes individuals misusing these preparations. In the latter instance the individual should be advised to consult his physician, so that the reasons for his misuse of these agents can be explored, and he can be helped to find other ways of dealing with problems such as chronic fatigue.

• The depressed patient who is being treated with amphetamines should be carefully observed for insomnia, loss of appetite, restlessness, and agitation. These symptoms may be related to the patient's illness, but they also can be caused, or be made worse, by the use of amphetamines.

• When powerful central nervous system stimulants such as Metrazol and picrotoxin are used, the patient should be observed carefully for symptoms of hypoxia; preconvulsive muscular twitching; convulsions. Many of the patients who require these stimulants have attempted suicide by taking overdoses of barbiturates or other depressant drugs. As the patient regains consciousness he requires the nurse's careful observation and support, in an effort to prevent further suicide attempts.

REVIEW QUESTIONS

1. (a) What difficulties limit the clinical usefulness of the central nervous system stimulants?

(b) How may the C.N.S. stimulants be classified in terms of their main sites of central action and their clinically most significant pharmacological effects?

2. (a) What are the main effects of small doses of caffeine when it is taken orally in tablet form or in a beverage such as coffee?

(b) What are some of the central and peripheral side effects of caffeine in sensitive individuals?

3. (a) What advice might the nurse give to people who complain of chronic fatigue which they try to overcome by frequent drinking of coffee or other caffeine-containing beverages?

(b) What advice may the nurse give to a person who wishes to drink coffee in order to increase his ability to drive after drinking alcoholic beverages?

4. (a) How is the small amount of caffeine contained in various headache products thought to bring about its desirable effects?

(b) For what purpose are small doses of caffeine added to cold remedy products; for what purpose is caffeine sodium benzoate sometimes employed parenterally?

5. (a) What are the two main psychopharmacological effects of the amphetamine-type psychomotor stimulants?

(b) What are some of the clinical conditions in which these actions of the amphetamines may produce favorable effects?

6. (a) What are the chief central and peripheral side effects of the amphetamines?

(b) In patients of what types may the administration of the amphetamines be contraindicated?

7. (a) What advantages are claimed for the *nonam-phetamine* type stimulants, methylphenidate and pipradrol?

(b) What are the advantages over the amphetamines which the *newer* anorexiants are claimed to possess, and what is the true status of these drugs?

8. (a) Why is the unsupervised use of amphetamines for producing prolonged wakefulness in studying for examinations or to meet deadlines and other obligations considered undesirable?

(b) What may be the end result of continued abuse of the amphetamines by psychopathic individuals and thrill seekers?

9. (a) Of what two types mainly are the *desired actions* brought about by the actions of the analeptic drugs at certain specific central sites?

(b) What types of *adverse effects* may result from the spread of the actions of the analeptics to other central sites?

10. (a) What pharmacological test may be employed to determine whether a patient who has taken an overdose of a depressant drug really requires continued analeptic drug therapy?

(b) List some of the analeptics employed for this purpose and some of the supportive measures that are employed in treating patients suffering from depressant drug overdosage.

11. (a) What are some proposed diagnostic and therapeutic uses for analeptic drugs in anesthesiology?

(b) What are some chronic lung conditions for which the cautious use of analeptic drugs may sometimes be indicated?

12. (a) What are some diagnostic and therapeutic uses for certain analeptic and convulsant agents in neurology and psychiatry?

(b) What kinds of pharmaceutical preparations sometimes contain strychnine?

13. (a) What are some of the signs and symptoms of strychnine poisoning?

(b) What are some of the measures that are used in the management of strychnine poisoning and in the control of other kinds of drug-induced convulsions?

BIBLIOGRAPHY

Adriani, J.: Respiratory stimulants. G.P., 20:100, 1959.

Clemmesen, C., and Nilsson, E.: Therapeutic trends in the treatment of barbiturate poisoning. Clin. Pharmacol. Ther., 2:220, 1961.

Connel, P. H.: Clinical manifestations and treatment of amphetamine type dependence. J.A.M.A., 196:718, 1966.

Dulfano, J. J., and Segal, M. S.: Nikethamide as a respiratory analeptic. J.A.M.A., 185:69, 1963.

Elser, J. R.: Acute barbiturate poisoning. Am. J. Nurs., 60:1096, 1960.

Hawkins, G. F.: Two cases of strychnine poisoning in children. Brit. Med. J., 2:26, 1962.

Kramer, J. C., et al.: Amphetamine abuse. J.A.M.A., 201:305, 1967.

Modell, W.: Status and prospect of drugs for overeating. J.A.M.A., 173:1131, 1960.

Noe, F. E., et al.: Use of new analeptic, doxapram during general anesthesia and recovery. Anesth. Analg., 44:206, 1965 (Mar.–Apr.).

Rodman, M. J.: The central nervous system stimulants. R.N., 30:85, 1967 (Sept.).

———: Nervous system stimulants. R.N., 23:33, 1960 (Jan.).

———: Drugs for dealing with weight problems. R.N., 26:41, 1963 (May).

Smith, G. E., and Beecher, H. K.: Amphetamine sulfate and athletic performance. J.A.M.A., 170:542, 1959.

Swissman, N., and Jacoby, J.: Strychnine poisoning and its treatment. Clin. Pharmacol. Ther., 5:136, 1964.

Werner, G.: Clinical pharmacology of central stimulant and antidepressant drugs. Clin. Pharmacol. Ther., 3:59, 1962.

Wilson, C. W. M., and Huby, P. M.: An assessment of the responses to drugs acting on the central nervous system. Clin. Pharmacol. Ther., 2:587, 1961.

Drugs Acting on Autonomic Neuroeffectors

In this section we shall study the several classes of so-called autonomic drugs. These are agents that modify the functioning of various body organs and structures in much the same way as does an increase or a decrease in the number of nerve impulses reaching the cells of these structures by way of nerve fibers of the autonomic nervous system (the A.N.S.).

The autonomic drugs act mainly *not* on the autonomic nerves themselves, but upon the muscle and gland cells in which the nerve fibers end. Such cells, which respond to nerve impulses by *doing* something —that is, causing an effect—are called *effectors,* or *neuroeffectors.* Thus the autonomic drugs act to alter the rate at which autonomic neuroeffectors contract, relax, secrete, etc.

Students who are exposed for the first time to the complexities of autonomic pharmacology tend to find the study of this class of drugs unusually difficult. One reason for this is the large number of unfamiliar terms and difficult concepts that must be learned before one can begin to understand the actions of these drugs. Even after they have learned this "lingo," difficulties still abound for conscientious students. These stem largely from the fact that autonomic drugs generally act at many places in the body at once—resulting in a veritable three-ring circus of activity.

Yet the study of autonomic pharmacology is rewarding in many ways. Most important for the nurse, of course, is the fact that these are very potent drugs with a great potential for helping or harming patients. The better the nurse understands what these drugs are actually doing in the patient's body, the greater is the chance that she can play a useful role in helping the patient to gain the benefits of autonomic drug therapy while avoiding the adverse effects. In addition, many students may gain great satisfaction from successfully meeting the intellectual challenge posed by the need to apply one's reasoning powers to the study of these drugs.

Before beginning our study of the drugs themselves, we shall, in the first chapter of this section, review the anatomy and physiology of the autonomic nervous system. For once you really grasp the fundamental principles of how this system functions, you can very often apply *reason* rather than brute memory to the study of autonomic drugs. Also, we shall take up the specialized terminology of autonomic pharmacology in the next chapter. For here too, once the student has taken the trouble to learn the ground rules, the game becomes easier to play. Then, having suitably fastened our seat-belts (so to speak), we will take our plunge into the study of the several classes of autonomic stimulating and blocking drugs.

· 14 ·

The Autonomic Nervous System

DIFFERENCES BETWEEN AUTONOMIC AND SOMATIC NERVES

The autonomic nervous system is also called the *involuntary*, and the *visceral*, nervous system. These terms indicate a major functional difference between the A.N.S. and other nerves; that is, the A.N.S. regulates the functioning of organs and structures such as the viscera, or internal organs, the functions of which we *cannot* control by an act of the will. For example, the A.N.S. nerve fibers influence the functioning of the heart, the smooth muscle of the iris, the smooth muscles making up the walls of the blood vessels, gastrointestinal and genitourinary tracts, etc.

There is also a major *anatomical difference* between A.N.S. fibers and the so-called somatic fibers by which we send the voluntary nervous messages which make our skeletal muscles move. The nerve cell bodies of the *voluntary* system are located entirely within the central nervous system, from which they send out fibers that go directly to the skeletal muscles which they control. The A.N.S. also originates within the central nervous system, but the axonal fibers from its centrally located neurons do *not* pass directly to the organs which they innervate. Instead, these fibers end in *ganglia*, groups of nerve cell bodies packed together at various locations outside the cerebrospinal axis. At these *synaptic junctions* in the autonomic ganglia, the preganglionic nerve impulses are transmitted to a second neuron (or sometimes to as many as twenty or more ganglion cells). The postganglionic axonal fibers of the second neurons then relay the nervous signal to the neuroeffectors in the visceral and other organs that respond to A.N.S. impulses.

GENERAL FUNCTIONS OF THE AUTONOMIC NERVOUS SYSTEM

Although the A.N.S. exerts its regulatory functions automatically—that is, without our willing it and usually without our even being aware of the changes

taking place—we should not be misled into thinking that it works without relationship to the activity of the central nervous system. That is, although we tend to think of the A.N.S. as being made up solely of motor fibers, the efferent impulses that affect organ functioning are actually the end result of reflex activity. This means that, as with most *reflex arcs*, the motor or secretory response of the autonomic neuroeffector is initiated by a stimulus that sets off sensory impulses. These then travel via afferent fibers to regulatory centers within the central nervous system and influence their rates of nervous outflow to the visceral organs.

The nerve centers that integrate the activity of the A.N.S. are located largely in subcortical sites such as the hypothalamus and the medulla oblongata. These are the areas that regulate very important functions including, among other activities, blood pressure, respiration, body temperature and the metabolism of water, carbohydrates and fats. Thus, A.N.S. activity exerts a constant moment-to-moment control over those activities that keep the body's internal environment, within a narrow range, close to the requirements for optimal functioning of all its cells and tissues.

Such *homeostasis* results from the never-ending interplay of two opposing subdivisions of the A.N.S., which exert more or less mutually antagonistic effects on the functioning of the organs that are not under our voluntary control. Thus, these two subsystems adjust the activities of functions such as circulation and digestion to meet the needs of the moment, and each counteracts any tendency of the other to over-react to temporary environmental situations.

ANATOMY AND PHYSIOLOGY OF THE AUTONOMIC NERVOUS SYSTEM

The autonomic nervous system is made up of two major subdivisions. These are (1) the *sympathetic* and (2) the *parasympathetic* systems. These divisions of

221

the A.N.S. differ in (1) the location within the central nervous system of the first nerve cell body of the two neuron chain, (2) the location of the ganglia containing the second cells in the link, and (3) the relative lengths of the preganglionic and postganglionic nerve fibers that connect these subdivisions of the A.N.S. with the visceral organs which they innervate (see Table 14-1 and Fig. 14-1).

Anatomy of the Sympathetic System. This system is also called the *thoracolumbar system*, because the first nerve cell bodies are located in the part of the spinal cord that runs through the chest, or thorax, down into the lumbar region of the back. These centrally located cells send out relatively short *pre*ganglionic fibers that synapse with nerve cells in ganglia located mostly in chains that run like a paired string of beads just outside the spinal cord (Fig. 14-1). Relatively long *post*ganglionic fibers then make their way to the autonomically innervated visceral organs.

Anatomy of the Parasympathetic System. This system is also called the *craniosacral system*, because its cells of origin lie centrally at the two extreme ends of the cerebrospinal axis. Some are located at subcortical levels of the brain (i.e., within the cranium), while other nerve cell bodies are located in the sacral portion of the spinal cord. Thus, some parasympathetic fibers run in cranial nerves such as the facial and vagus nerves. Other axons, originating at lower levels of the spinal cord, form the pelvic nerves, which send branches to organs such as the urinary bladder and lower large intestine.

Comparison of Physiological Functions. The sympathetic system, working together with the adrenal medulla, which it innervates, tends to regulate the expenditure of energy, especially in times of stress. The parasympathetic system, on the other hand, mainly influences functions that help the body to store up and save energy.

Each system is organized anatomically and chemically in ways that serve these differing functions. Thus, the sympathetic system sends out numerous nerve fibers that synapse with many different ganglion cells. Its postganglionic fibers release sudden spurts of nerve-impulse-transmitting chemicals all at once at many different sites. These chemical substances and the related ones released by the adrenal medulla are relatively long-lasting in their effects. The parasympathetic system, on the other hand, discharges its impulses to specific organs in more narrow and localized a manner. Its neurochemical transmitter is more rapidly destroyed. Thus, the sympathetic system helps the organism to react vigorously to emergencies, whereas the parasympathetic helps to restore the expended energy gradually, through a series of separate but interrelated activities of various organs.

The opposing functions of the two divisions of the A.N.S. may be grasped by a thoughtful study of Table 14-2. A typically sympathetic response is the "fight or flight" reaction that occurs when the organism feels threatened and reacts with rage and fear: the heartbeat speeds up, blood pressure rises, blood leaves the constricted vessels of the skin and viscera and is shunted to the dilated arterioles in the hardworking heart and skeletal muscles; at the same time, the extra amounts of oxygen and glucose that these muscles require are supplied by liver glycogen breakdown and by rapid deep breathing to take in air through widely dilated lung bronchi.

The parasympathetic system, on the other hand, slows the heart, constricts the dilated pupils of the eyes to protect the retinas from excessive light, and restarts the temporarily stalled gastrointestinal movements and secretions so that digestion and assimilation of foodstuffs can once more proceed. It helps also to rid the urinary bladder and the rectum of body wastes.

We must not think of these systems only as emergency mechanisms, however; their work goes on continuously, making possible the delicate adjustments needed to keep up with the ever changing environment. It is perhaps better to think of the two systems as functioning like the handlebars of a bicycle, which helps the rider keep to a straight course when he automatically puts pressure on one handle or the other to correct any tendency of the bike to veer too far to either the right or left.

Actually, this picture is somewhat simplified. Both divisions of the A.N.S. do not exert equal control over all organs. For example, the parasympathetic system has greater influence on gastrointestinal tract function than does the sympathetic, whereas the latter regulates blood vessel tone and blood pressure to a much greater extent than does the parasympathetic system.

Nonetheless, the general concept of two opposing systems in a state of tonic, or continuous, activity designed to achieve an unstable, shifting functional balance is a useful one for helping us understand the actions of the various autonomic drugs. For, by acting at the same synapses and neuroeffectors as do the A.N.S. nerve impulses, these drugs tend to upset the temporary balance in one direction or another. Thus, some drugs may imitate, or *mimic*, the effects either of sympathetic or of parasympathetic stimulation in slowing down or speeding up a particular function. On the other hand, some drugs may keep nerve impulses from reaching the muscle or gland cells through one or the other division of the A.N.S. In that case, the still active division tends to exert a disproportionate influence upon the functioning of most of the organs, structures and systems that have had part of their tonic nervous control blocked out.

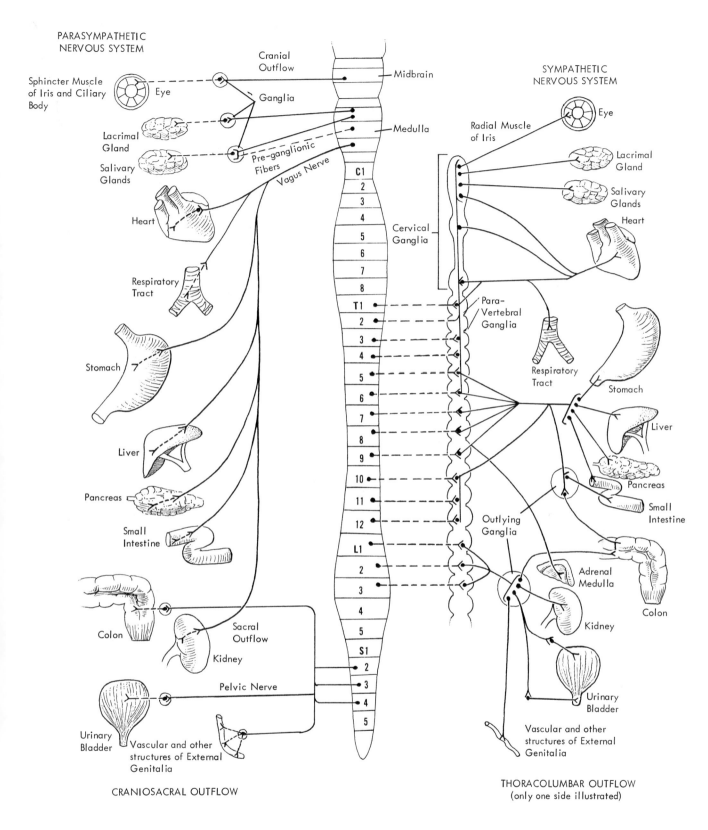

FIG. 14-1. The autonomic nervous system. Solid lines from cranial and sacral portions of the cerebrospinal axis indicate *pre*ganglionic fibers of the parasympathetic nervous system. Short broken lines within or just outside organs indicate *post*ganglionic fibers.

Short broken lines from thoracolumbar portions of the spinal cord to chain of paravertebral ganglia indicate *pre*-ganglionic fibers of the sympathetic nervous system. Long solid lines indicate *post*ganglionic fibers.

TABLE 14-1

ANATOMICAL AND PHYSIOLOGICAL CHARACTERISTICS OF SYMPATHETIC, PARASYMPATHETIC, AND SOMATIC NERVES

CHARACTERISTICS	SYMPATHETIC NERVOUS SYSTEM (INVOLUNTARY)	PARASYMPATHETIC NERVOUS SYSTEM (INVOLUNTARY)	SOMATIC MOTOR NEURONS (VOLUNTARY)
Structures innervated	Heart, smooth muscles of blood vessels, viscera, ocular structures, glands	Heart, smooth muscles of blood vessels, viscera, ocular structures, glands	Skeletal muscles
Origin of centrally located neuron	Thoracolumbar portion of spinal cord (i.e., lateral horn cells in T_1–T_{12}; L_1 & L_2)	Cranial and sacral portion of the cerebrospinal axis (i.e., cells in midbrain, medulla, and S_2, S_3, and S_4 of spinal cord)	Anterior horn of spinal cord at all levels, etc.
Axonal pathway from C.N.S. nerve cell body	Short, myelinated preganglionic fibers (e.g., white rami communicantes to vertebral ganglia), and other relatively short fibers	Relatively very long myelinated preganglionic fibers travel in cranial (e.g., facial; vagus) and spinal (e.g., pelvic) nerves.	Myelinated motoneuron axons lead directly to skeletal muscles, where they divide into many branches.
Final distribution of terminations of central neuron	Terminals in contact with *many neurons* in a single ganglion (i.e., preganglionic fiber may pass through many ganglia before synapsing with as many as 20 or more ganglionic neurons which also receive ends of other preganglionic fibers)	Terminals synapse with *only 1 or 2 neurons* of terminal ganglia lying near, or even in, the visceral or other organs usually (e.g., make contact with nerve cells in ganglia of abdominal, pelvic and thoracic organs).	Each axon makes contact with 100 or more muscle fibers (i.e., a motor unit is formed). Axon ending becomes *non*-myelinated to form nerve end plate, which comes in contact with muscle sole plate in invagination of muscle membrane, thus forming the motor end plate. Acetylcholine released by axon ending depolarizes the motor end plate (nicotinic type of cholinergic transmission). Impulses can be blocked by certain anticholinergic agents (e.g., *curare*).
Impulse transmission (*nicotinic* type of *cholinergic* transmission in *both* types of autonomic ganglia and at the myoneural junction of the skeletal muscle fibers)	*Acetylcholine* released at preganglionic nerve terminals stimulates neurons in ganglia located relatively *close to C.N.S.* Impulses can be blocked by certain anticholinergic agents (e.g., C_6).	*Acetylcholine* released at preganglionic nerve terminals stimulates neurons in ganglia located relatively *far from C.N.S.* Impulses can be blocked by certain anticholinergic agents (e.g., C_6).	
Postganglionic fiber distribution	Gray rami communicantes from ganglia join spinal nerves and travel to junctions in smooth muscle and gland cells.	Very short fibers from ganglia terminate in smooth muscle and gland cells (i.e., in neuroeffectors).	
Impulse transmission at postganglionic neuroeffectors (i.e., junction between terminations of nerve fibers and receptors of cardiac and smooth muscle and gland cells)	*Norepinephrine* released and stimulates neuroeffectors except in sweat glands and some blood vessels. Impulses can be blocked by alpha *or* beta blocking agents (e.g., alpha by phenoxybenzamine; beta by pronethalol, DCI, etc.)	*Acetylcholine* released to stimulate smooth muscle, cardiac and gland cells (i.e., *Muscarinic* type of cholinergic transmission). Impulses can be blocked by certain anticholinergic agents (e.g., *atropine*).	

TABLE 14-2
RESULTS OF AUTONOMIC NERVOUS STIMULATION
(Comparison of Responses to Sympathetic and Parasympathetic Nerve Impulses)

ORGANS AND STRUCTURES	SYMPATHETIC (ADRENERGIC) NERVE IMPULSES	TYPE OF ADRENERGIC RECEPTOR	PARASYMPATHETIC AND OTHER CHOLINERGIC NERVE IMPULSES
Heart	Increase in rate, contractility and conduction speed	Beta	Decrease in rate, contractility and A-V conduction
Blood Vessels			
1. Skin and mucous membrane	Constriction	Alpha	Dilatation
2. Skeletal muscle	Dilatation (usually)	Beta	Dilatation *
3. Coronary	Dilatation (may be due to indirect, metabolic effects)	(?)	Dilatation
Bronchial Muscle	Relaxation (lumen dilated)	Beta	Contraction (lumen constricted)
Gastrointestinal			
1. Muscle motility and tone	Decrease	Beta	Increase
2. Sphincters	Contraction (ordinarily)	Alpha	Relaxation (ordinarily)
3. Exocrine glands	Secretion reduced (?)	(?)	Secretion increased
4. Gallbladder	Relaxation	(?)	Contraction
Urinary Bladder			
1. Detrusor	Relaxation	Beta	Contraction
2. Trigone and sphincter	Contraction	Alpha	Relaxation
Ocular Structures			
1. Iris radial muscle	Contraction (pupil dilates)	Alpha	—
2. Iris sphincter muscle	—	—	Contraction (pupil constricts)
3. Ciliary muscle	Relaxation (but with relatively little effect on lens movement)	Beta	Contraction (lens adjusted for near vision)
Skin Structures			
1. Sweat glands	Increased palmar and other localized sweating	Alpha	Generalized increase *
2. Pilomotor muscles	Contracted (gooseflesh)	Alpha	—
Miscellaneous			
1. Salivary glands	Thick, viscid secretion	Alpha	Copious, watery secretion
2. Lacrimal and nasopharyngeal glands	—	—	Increased secretion
3. Liver	Glycogenolysis	—	—
4. Male sex organs	Ejaculation	—	Erection (vascular dilatation)

* Cholinergic transmission, but nerve cell chain originates in thoracolumbar portion of spinal cord and is, thus, sympathetic.

PHARMACOLOGICAL ACTIONS

When we have learned how the various organs and structures normally respond to the nerve impulses arriving by way of the two divisions of the A.N.S., we know in general what to expect from a drug that is classified as *sympathomimetic* or *parasympathomimetic*. For example, if we are told that a drug such as *epinephrine* is categorized as sympatho*mimetic*, we might predict that it will probably speed up the heart, constrict skin blood vessels (and thus stop local bleeding), and dilate the bronchial tubes of an asthmatic patient in a way that will be clinically useful.

Similarly, if we know that a drug—atropine, for example—is classified as a parasympathetic *blocking agent*, we can reasonably expect that it also will speed up the heart and that it will reduce gastrointestinal motility. Our reasoning runs something like this: (1) The vagus nerves send tonic parasympathetic impulses that tend to slow the heart and make the G.I. muscles contract; (2) a parasympathetic blocking agent keeps many of these messages from reaching the heart and the gut; (3) the balance between parasympathetic and sympathetic impulses is thus reset to favor the latter; (4) since the sympathetic impulses stimulate the heart and reduce intestinal motility, the parasympathetic blocking drug tends to bring about some of the same effects as sympathetic stimulation does.

Chemical Transmission of Nerve Impulses

The endings of nerve cell fibers do not come into direct contact with the processes of other neurons or with the muscle fibers and secretory cells to which they run. The electron microscope has shown that there is a microscopic gap at the synaptic connection between any two nerve cells and at the junctions between nerves and muscle or gland cells. It is now known that the nerve impulse bridges these spaces at synapses, myoneural junctions etc., by releasing minute amounts of chemicals from the nerve endings. When the amount of the chemical mediator (*neurohumor*, or *neurohormone*) that diffuses across the tiny junctional cleft is adequate, and enough of its molecules make contact with the membranes of the cells on the other side of the junction, the nerve impulse is transmitted to the second cell in the series. These stimulated muscle, gland, or nerve cells then respond to the chemical messages from the first nerve fibers in their characteristic ways—that is, by contracting, relaxing, secreting, or firing.

Several substances synthesized by nerve cells are thought to act as neurohumoral transmitters. The most thoroughly studied of the neurohormones secreted by peripheral nerves are acetylcholine (ACh) and norepinephrine (NE, formerly called sympathin). Most peripheral nerve fibers release ACh (see Cholinergic Transmission, below). The exceptional fibers are the postganglionic sympathetic axons, which originate in sympathetic ganglion cells that synapse with preganglionic fibers from the thoracolumbar levels of the spinal cord. These fibers are called *adrenergic*, because their terminals release the adrenalinelike catecholamine norepinephrine.

The complicated processes by which these nerve-impulse-transmitting substances are synthesized, stored, released and destroyed are very vulnerable to interference by foreign chemicals. Many drugs and poisons act in various ways, to (1) imitate or mimic the actions of the natural neurohormones, (2) intensify their activity or (3) impair it. Thus, in order to understand how drugs of the different types discussed in this section bring about their effects, we should first review some of the principles of the impulse transmission process. For, if we know something about how ACh and NE transfer the commands of the A.N.S. to effector cells, the many complex effects of autonomic drugs will become more clear.

Cholinergic Transmission. Acetylcholine, the chemical that is released from most peripheral nerve fiber endings, is an ester synthesized in the nerve terminals from acetic acid and the organic alcohol choline. Its molecules are then stored in a bound, or inactive, form in tiny storage sacs (the synaptic vessels), from which they are finally released into the junctional gap when the nerve impulse reaches the end of the cholinergic nerve fiber.

The freed acetylcholine molecules then pour out of the nerve terminals and cross the junction to make momentary contact with a chemically specialized spot on the postjunctional membrane. The combination of active acetylcholine with this cholinergic receptor, or *cholinoceptive site*, changes the permeability of the nerve, muscle, or gland cell membrane. This leads to leakage of ions in and out of these cells, with a resulting change in membrane polarity. *D*epolarization or *hyper*polarization of the nerve or muscle cell membrane then excites or inhibits cellular activity.

Once the second cell has reacted by sending along the nerve impulse (in the case of neurons), by secreting (in the case of exocrine gland cells), or by contracting or relaxing (in the case of muscle cells), it is essential that any remaining neurohormone at the junction be quickly destroyed. An excess of acetylcholine might keep the membrane from recovering its normal polarity and thus reduce its responsiveness to the next volley of nerve impulses.

The destruction of the excess acetylcholine is carried out almost instantly by an enzyme that is packed into the synaptic and neuromuscular junctions. This enzyme, *acetylcholinesterase (AChE)*, combines with the acetylcholine molecules and converts them into the neurochemically inactive compounds acetic acid and choline, the same metabolites from which it was made. Once the neurohormone is broken down—a matter of thousandths of a second—the membrane of the nerve, muscle or gland cell repolarizes and becomes ready to respond to the next nerve impulse.

Cholinergic Nerves. Acetylcholine is the mediator for the transmission of nerve impulses from several different kinds of peripheral nerve fibers. (It is also believed to act at certain central synapses, but this will not be discussed here.) These cholinergic fibers may be classified in terms of the neuroeffector and synaptic junctions to which they transmit their nerve impulses (see Table 14-1). The three major classes are:

1. *Postganglionic cholinergic fibers.* These include all the parasympathetic postganglionic fibers and a few exceptional sympathetic postganglionic fibers.

2. *Preganglionic cholinergic fibers.* All of the fibers of both sympathetic and parasympathetic preganglionic nerves release acetylcholine from their endings in autonomic ganglia.

3. *Somatic motor nerve fibers.* These *non*autonomic fibers also release acetylcholine at the myoneural junctions in skeletal muscles. The acetylcholine released here makes contact with specialized structures, called motor end plates, located on the muscle fiber membranes.

We may single out peripheral cholinergic nerves of two other types for special mention at this point. First, there are some postganglionic fibers that are classified anatomically as "sympathetic" because the two-cell chain of which they are a part originates in the thoracolumbar portion of the cord, but secrete acetylcholine rather than norepinephrine. The sweat glands and certain blood vessels are innervated by such exceptional "sympathetic cholinergic" nerves (see Table 14-2, footnote). These neuroeffectors react to cholinergic drugs (see below) rather than to adrenergic drugs.

The other cholinergic nerve fibers that need special mention are those that innervate the cells of the *adrenal medulla.* Impulses arriving at this endocrine gland cause its cells to release adrenergic chemicals into the blood stream. These, in turn, activate adrenergic neuroeffectors, which they reach by way of the blood stream. It may seem surprising, at first, for cholinergic nerves to bring about an increase in adrenergic activity. However, this is essentially not very different from what happens when acetylcholine is released from *pre*ganglionic fibers in sympathetic ganglia. The sympathetic nerve impulses that are discharged down the postganglionic adrenergic fibers also lead to increased adrenergic activity.

Cholinergic Receptors. All of the postjunctional cells that are innervated by cholinergic nerves contain chemical groupings that are specifically designed to combine with acetylcholine and with cholinomimetic

drugs. However, some cholinergic drugs that act at one cholinoceptive site fail to produce an effect when they come in contact with cholinergic receptors in the cells of other organs and structures. This may be because slight differences in the shapes of the cholinergic receptor complexes at different sites allow some drug molecules to approach and attach more readily than others (see Chap. 5, Receptor Theory). Thus, the structure of the *cholinoceptive complex* on the various cell membranes must differ to some extent, depending upon whether the postjunctional cells are autonomic effectors, skeletal muscle fibers, or ganglion nerve cells.

Cholinomimetic and Cholinergic Blocking Drugs (See also Drug Digests)

The actions of acetylcholine at the various peripheral junctions at which it is released are sometimes referred to as "muscarinic" and "nicotinic"—terms that refer to the plant alkaloids muscarine and nicotine, which were used in early studies of autonomic function.

Muscarine is a cholinomimetic drug, the actions of which are limited largely to the postganglionic cholinergic neuroeffectors. That is, this drug acts like acetylcholine by combining with receptors in smooth and cardiac muscles and in glands, but *not* at autonomic ganglia or in skeletal muscles. Nicotine, on the other hand, acts only at the latter sites and not on autonomic neuroeffectors that receive postganglionic fibers. Thus, we speak of the "muscarinic" and the "nicotinic" actions of acetylcholine (Table 14-1) and of the cholinergic drugs that act mainly on cholinoceptive sites of one or the other type.

Cholinergic drugs of the *anticholinesterase* class (Tables 14-3 and 15-1) have both muscarinic and nicotinic actions. These agents keep the enzyme that is responsible for the destruction of cholinesterase from doing its work. As a result, free acetylcholine accumulates at cholinergic junctions of all types. At first, this causes increased transmitter activity, but later the excess of ACh leads to lessened transmission at all sites as the postjunctional membrane fails to repolarize.

The cholinergic blocking drugs—agents that interfere with the action of acetylcholine by occupying cholinoceptive sites so that the neurohormone's molecules cannot make their normal contacts—also act more selectively at some junctions than at others. Thus, atropine, curare, hexamethonium and other cholinergic blockers all keep acetylcholine from activating cellular receptors, but they vary considerably in the degree of their specificity for particular cholinoceptive sites.

Atropine acts mainly on cholinergic receptors of autonomic postganglionic neuroeffectors such as cardiac and smooth muscle and exocrine glands—the *muscarinic* sites. Atropine is a much less effective blocker of the acetylcholine that is released by preganglionic nerve endings at synapses in both types of autonomic ganglia, and it does not block the other type of *nicotinic* sites (at the motor end plate junctions in skeletal muscle) at all.

Curare and its relatives block cholinergic transmission at the motor end plates in skeletal muscle. Higher doses of these drugs will also keep acetylcholine from triggering nerve impulses in the other nicotinic-type receptors in autonomic ganglia. However, no clinically practicable dose of curare will cut off cholinergic nervous transmission at the *post*ganglionic neuroeffectors in the heart, smooth muscles, and exocrine glands.

Hexamethonium and the other ganglion blockers are much less selective in their ability to block transmission at the other sites where acetylcholine is the nerve impulse transmitter. The relative selectivity of the three types of blocking drugs depends, presumably, upon differences in their molecular structures that allow each to fit more neatly than the others onto complementary chemical configurations in the slightly differing cholinoceptive complexes of postjunctional cells of the various types.

Adrenergic Transmission. *Norepinephrine (NE)*, the chemical released when nerve impulses pass down most postganglionic sympathetic fibers, is synthesized in the nerve endings in a series of enzymatically catalyzed reactions. Some of the NE made and stored there is chemically converted to epinephrine (also known as *adrenaline,* because its chief source is the medulla of the adrenal glands). Thus, stimulation of sympathetic nerves leads to the discharge of a mixture of norepinephrine and epinephrine.

When these stored catecholamines are released by nerve impulses, they react with receptor sites in the sympathetically innervated organs and thus activate the adrenergic neuroeffectors. The free NE molecules do so by simply crossing the synaptic gap and attaching themselves momentarily to the *adrenoceptive* substance, but most of the epinephrine that reaches such adrenergic receptors gets there from the adrenal glands by way of the blood stream.

The reaction between the released neurohormones and the adrenergic receptors on the membranes of smooth muscle and gland cells results in changes in their activity. That is, some muscles respond by contracting, others by relaxing, etc. (see Table 14-2). Whether the activity of a particular adrenergic neuroeffector increases or decreases in response to nerve stimulation depends largely upon the nature of the receptors in the particular organ or structure involved.

According to one theory, muscles and gland cells contain adrenergic receptors of two types, designated *alpha* and *beta*. The *alpha receptors* respond to natural and synthetic catecholamines and to sympathomimetic (adrenergic) drugs by setting off an increase in the activity of smooth muscle cells (i.e., an excitatory response). Thus, those smooth muscle cells in

which alpha receptors predominate respond to adrenergic stimulation by contracting. This is seen, for example, in the blood vessels of the skin and mucous membranes which are constricted by sympathetic stimulation (Table 14-2).

On the other hand, those smooth muscle cells that contain mainly *beta receptors* respond to adrenergic stimulation by a decrease in their contractile activity. For example, the smooth muscle walls of the bronchi relax, and the openings of those respiratory tubes become widely dilated. However, not all structures containing predominantly beta receptors respond with an inhibition or lessening of activity. The heart, which contains mainly beta type adrenergic receptors, reacts to sympathetic stimulation and to circulating epinephrine and other sympathomimetic substances by an increase in the rate and strength of its contractions (Table 14-2).

Once the catecholamines have completed the task of transmitting the impulses from their nerves to the alpha and beta receptors of the neuroeffectors, the excess of these chemicals leaves the vicinity of the myoneural junction. Some of the molecules simply diffuse away from the junction and enter the blood stream. Carried to the liver and other tissues that contain the catecholamine-destroying enzymes monoamine oxidase (MAO) and catechol o-methyl transferase (COMT), the excess catecholamines are converted into inactive metabolites that are then excreted in the urine.

Some of the free NE is not destroyed at all but makes its way back into the adrenergic nerve endings to be stored there until released again by more nerve impulses. In general, the adrenergic transmitters are much more slowly eliminated than is acetylcholine. This is one of the reasons for the relatively prolonged and widespread effects of sympathoadrenal discharge compared to parasympathetic system activity. Contrary to the case in cholinergic nerves, continued normal function of adrenergic nerves does not depend upon immediate destruction of the chemical transmitter, and drugs that tie up the enzymes involved in its destruction do not seriously affect the functioning of these nerves.

Adrenergic Stimulant and Blocking Drugs (See also Drug Digests)

A number of drugs that resemble the natural catecholamines in their chemical structures are capable of producing many of the effects typical of sympathetic nervous system stimulation. Such *sympathomimetic,* or *adrenergic,* drugs (Chap. 16) are thought to act in two ways: Some are similar enough in structure to norepinephrine to elicit the same effects when their molecules come in direct contact wtih adrenergic receptors; others, it is now known, act indirectly— that is, by increasing the rate at which the adrenergic

TABLE 14-3
AUTONOMIC DRUGS CLASSIFIED BY SITE AND TYPE OF ACTION

Site of Action	Stimulants	Blocking Agents
Cholinergic autonomic neuroeffectors (e.g., smooth and cardiac muscle; exocrine glands)	Parasympathomimetics * (Muscarinic type cholinergic agents) Acetylcholine and the synthetic choline esters (e.g., methacholine, etc.) Cholinomimetic alkaloids (e.g., muscarine; pilocarpine, etc.) Anticholinesterase agents (e.g., neostigmine, etc.)	*Antimuscarinic type cholinergic blockers* Natural solanaceous alkaloids † (e.g., atropine, etc.) Synthetic anticholinergic agents ‡ (e.g., methantheline bromide, etc.)
Autonomic ganglia (both sympathetic and parasympathetic)	Nicotinic type cholinergic agents (in low doses) Acetylcholine and certain synthetic choline esters * (e.g., carbachol, etc.) Anticholinesterase agents * (e.g., neostigmine, etc.) Nicotine Dimethylphenylpiperazinium (DMPP)	*Ganglion cell transmission blockers* Large doses of most of the nicotinic type stimulants listed at the left will interfere with impulse transmission Ganglionic blocking agents § (e.g., mecamylamine, etc.)
Somatic neuromuscular junctions ‖ (motor end plates of skeletal muscle fibers)	Acetylcholine * Anticholinesterase agents, low doses * (e.g., edrophonium, etc.) Phenyltrimethylammonium (PTMA)	*Neuromuscular blocking agents* ** Competitive type (e.g., curare, etc.) Depolarizing type (e.g., succinylcholine, etc.) Large doses of most of the nicotinic type stimulants listed at the left will interfere with impulse transmission.
Adrenergic neuroeffectors (e.g., in cardiac tissues, smooth muscle of blood vessels, bronchioles, etc.)	Sympathomimetics †† (Adrenergic receptor stimulants) Catecholamines (e.g., epinephrine, etc.) Aliphatic amines (e.g., phenylephrine, etc.)	*Adrenergic blocking agents* Alpha type blockers ‡‡ (e.g., tolazoline, etc.) Beta type blockers *** (e.g., dichloroisoproterenol (DCI), etc.)
Adrenergic nerve endings	Sympathomimetics (acting at nerve ending, rather than at postjunctional receptor) Tyramine, ephedrine, cocaine	*Adrenergic nerve transmission blockers* Reserpine, guanethidine, methyldopa

* See Table 15-1 for detailed listing.
† See Table 17-1 for detailed listing.
‡ See Table 17-3 for detailed listing.
§ See Table 23-2 for detailed listing.

** See Table 17-4 for detailed listing.
†† See Table 16-1 for detailed listing.
‡‡ See Table 26-1.
*** See list and discussion, Chapter 17.

‖ These are *not* autonomic sites but drugs acting at these sites are included here because some also act simultaneously (especially in large doses) at autonomic sites.

mediator (NE) is released from the nerve ending into the myoneural junction.

There are two classes of *adrenergic blocking drugs* also (Chap. 17). Drugs of one type suppress nerve impulse transmission to the *alpha* type adrenergic receptors by occupying these sites without interfering with the effects of norepinephrine or of adrenergic drugs upon receptors of the *beta* type. However, the latter receptors, including those in the heart, can be blocked by compounds of a new class which has little, if any, effect on transmission to alpha receptors. Thus, we see once more how receptors designed to react with a particular neurohormone—in this case, norepinephrine—differ enough in their chemical structure to react differently to various drugs. That is, although norepinephrine fits adrenergic receptors of both types, some synthetic drugs occupy and block only the alpha type, and others, of different structure, block only the beta type.

Sympathetic nervous system activity can also be suppressed by drugs that act not on the receptors of the neuroeffectors but on the adrenergic nerve endings. These adrenergic *neuron* blocking drugs are discussed in Section Four, Chap. 23, Drugs Used in Hypertension. The other classes of autonomic drugs listed in Table 14-3 are taken up in the remaining chapters of this section.

REVIEW QUESTIONS

1. (a) What is meant by the term *neuroeffector?*

(b) At what general sites mainly do the autonomic drugs act in producing their effects?

2. (a) List some organs and structures that are innervated by the autonomic nervous system and indicate how the control of these neuroeffectors differs in general from that of the structures innervated by somatic nerves.

(b) How do the autonomic and somatic nervous systems differ in the number and location of their motor neurons?

3. (a) In general, what sort of activities are regulated by the autonomic nervous system?

(b) Where are the nerve centers located that respond to sensory impulses by altering the outflow of motor impulses from autonomic efferent fibers?

4. (a) Compare the anatomical origins of the first neurons in the sympathetic and the parasympathetic chains.

(b) Compare the locations of sympathetic and parasympathetic ganglia and the nature and locations of their *pre*ganglionic and *post*ganglionic fibers.

5. (a) Indicate the opposing effects of sympathetic and parasympathetic stimulation upon the following organs: heart; blood vessels of the skin; bronchi of the lungs; iris of the eye; intestinal muscle; urinary bladder muscles.

(b) Predict the effects of a sympathomimetic drug or of a parasympathomimetic drug on the above organs. Can you anticipate how these organs might react to a drug that blocked out parasympathetic impulses to these organs, while the sympathetic nervous system continued to send impulses to each organ or structure?

6. (a) How, in general, are nerve impulses transmitted to the cells that the nerves innervate?

(b) How, in general, do autonomic and other drugs and poisons affect such transmission of impulses from nerve fibers to neuroeffectors?

7. Explain briefly the events that take place between the time that a nerve impulse reaches the terminals of a cholinergic nerve and the time that a neuroeffector responds and is ready to receive the next nerve impulse.

8. (a) List three main types of cholinergic nerves and the kinds of cells that they innervate.

(b) In what way are the nerves that innervate the sweat glands exceptional, and how does the response of the adrenal medulla to cholinergic stimulation differ from that of the autonomic ganglia?

9. (a) What is thought to account for the fact that different drugs that imitate the action of acetylcholine tend to act selectively, i.e., at some cholinoceptive sites and not at others?

(b) At cells of what type is a cholinomimetic drug acting when it is producing muscarinic effects?

(c) At cells of what two types may a cholinergic drug act to cause effects that we call nicotinic?

10. (a) At what particular cholinergic receptors do each of the following cholinergic blocking agents act most specifically: (1) atropine; (2) curare; (3) hexamethonium?

(b) What is thought to account for the fact that each of these drugs can block cholinergic activity at one particular site so much better than at other postjunctional cholinoceptive sites?

11. (a) What chemical substances are released by stimuli that set off sympathoadrenal discharge?

(b) How, in general, do the effects of these chemicals vary when they come in contact with adrenergic receptors of the *alpha* and of the *beta* type adrenergic receptors in smooth muscle?

(c) What is the result of their contact with beta receptors in the heart?

12. (a) In what two general ways are sympathomimetic (adrenergic) drugs thought to act?

(b) What two types of adrenergic blocking agents are now available?

Cholinergic (Parasympathomimetic) Drugs

GENERAL CONSIDERATIONS

The cholinergic drugs are chemicals that act at the same sites as the neurohormone *acetylcholine* to produce effects similar to those that occur when cholinergic nerves are stimulated. Since, as we have indicated (Chap. 14), there are several different kinds of cholinergic nerves innervating very many organs and structures, these drugs are capable of causing widespread effects throughout the body.

The difficulty of confining the effects of cholinergic drugs to specific sites severely limits their clinical utility. That is, their relative *lack of selective action* often leads to side effects that appear with the therapeutically desired effects for which the drug is administered. Nonetheless, these potent cholinergic agents produce such dramatic improvement in some clinical conditions that the doctor often orders them despite their adverse effects.

The patient for whom these medications are prescribed ought to be given some idea of what to expect in the way of discomforting side effects. He may tolerate their annoying effects better if he knows what to expect and is assured that there is no danger. However, it is not enough merely to admonish the patient to keep on taking his medication despite discomfort. The nurse should do what she can to minimize drug-induced unpleasant effects and to offer the patient relief. It often helps to accent the positive by showing the patient evidence of the progress he is making as a result of the drug treatment.

MANNER OF ACTION

Cholinergic drugs bring about their cholinomimetic effects in one of two main ways: (1) directly, and (2) indirectly.

The **direct-acting drugs** (Table 15-1) act like acetylcholine itself, because the chemical structure of their molecules is such that they can approach and occupy cholinoceptive sites on the membranes of the effector cells that receive the endings of cholinergic nerves. They then evoke effects similar to those produced by the acetylcholine molecules released by cholinergic nerve impulses.

The **indirect-acting drugs** (Table 15-1) produce their effects by bringing about an increase in the amount of acetylcholine in the junctional spaces between cholinergic nerve endings and cholinergic receptor sites on the neuroeffectors. That is, they have no direct action of their own on the cells that receive cholinergic nerve fibers. They act, instead, by occupying receptors on the surface of the enzyme acetylcholinesterase. This inhibitory action keeps the enzyme from performing its natural function (i.e., capturing acetylcholine molecules and destroying them within milliseconds after the free neurohormone has completed its impulse-transmitting action. This *anti-cholinesterase* activity results in an increase in the level of acetylcholine locally in the junction. Thus, the action of acetylcholine released by nerve impulses is intensified and lengthened by these indirect-acting drugs.

The main clinical advantage that both kinds of cholinergic drugs have over acetylcholine itself lies in their longer duration of action. Acetylcholine itself is destroyed so swiftly by the cholinesterase enzymes in the blood and at junctions when it is injected, that its action is too short to be clinically useful. Thus, the indirect-acting drugs, by slowing the destructive enzymatic action, permit acetylcholine to accumulate to levels that bring about clinically desirable effects. Similarly, the direct acting drugs, such as the synthetic choline esters (Table 15-1) are much more

231

TABLE 15-1

CHOLINERGIC DRUGS
(Cholinomimetics; Parasympathomimetics)

NONPROPRIETARY OR OFFICIAL NAME	TRADE NAME OR SYNONYM	DOSAGE
Direct-Acting Drugs		
Synthetic Choline Esters		
Bethanechol chloride U.S.P.	Urecholine	Oral 5 to 30 mg. S.C. 2.5 to 5 mg.
Carbachol U.S.P.	Carbamylcholine; Carcholin; Doryl	Topical only, for ophthalmic use
Methacholine bromide N.F.	Mecholyl Br	Oral 200 mg.
Methacholine chloride N.F.	Mecholyl Cl	S.C. 20 mg.
Cholinomimetic alkaloids		
Arecoline hydrobromide N.F.	—	Veterinary use only (e.g., horses, 30 mg. Dogs, 1.5 mg./Kg.)
Muscarine	—	—
Pilocarpine HCl U.S.P.	—	Topical, for ophthalmic use
Pilocarpine nitrate U.S.P.		
Indirect-Acting Drugs (Anticholinesterase agents)		
Quarternary Ammonium Compounds, etc.		
Ambenonium chloride	Mytelase	5 to 25 mg.
Benzpyrinium bromide N.F.	Stigmonene	2 mg. I.M.
Demecarium bromide	Humorsol	Topical ophthalmic
Edrophonium chloride U.S.P.	Tensilon	5 to 20 mg.
Neostigmine bromide U.S.P.	Prostigmin Br	10 to 30 mg., oral
Neostigmine methylsulfate U.S.P.	Prostigmin methylsulfate	0.25 to 1 mg. I.M. or S.C.
Physostigmine and its salicylate and sulfate salts U.S.P.	—	Topical, ophthalmic
Pyridostigmine bromide U.S.P.	Mestinon	180 to 600 mg. daily
Organophosphate Compounds		
Echothiophate iodide U.S.P.	Phospholine	Topical ophthalmic
Isoflurophate N.F.	Floropryl; DFP	Topical ophthalmic
Malathion	—	Insecticide
OMPA	—	Insecticide, etc.
Parathion	—	Insecticide
Sarin	—	Nerve gas
Soman	—	Nerve gas
Tabun	—	Nerve gas

resistant to enzymatic destruction and elimination than is the natural neurohormonal choline ester. Thus, their actions, unlike the action of acetylcholine, persist for long enough periods to become clinically useful.

Of all the junctions at which cholinergic nerves release acetylcholine (Chap. 14), the ones most sensitive to the actions of most cholinergic drugs are the *postganglionic cholinergic neuroeffectors.* These consist mainly of the cardiac and smooth muscle cells and the exocrine gland cells that receive their innervation via the parasympathetic nervous system. This is why these drugs are sometimes called *parasympathomimetic agents.* However, since some structures that are innervated by *sympathetic* cholinergic fibers (e.g., the sweat glands) and by *somatic* motor fibers (e.g., skeletal muscles) also respond to these drugs, the more inclusive terms *cholinergic* or *cholinomimetic* describe the broad scope of their actions more accurately.

As has been indicated in Chapter 14, the actions of cholinergic drugs at the autonomically innervated postganglionic neuroeffectors is called *muscarinic*. Drugs such as muscarine and pilocarpine (another alkaloid) exert their pharmacological actions primarily on these smooth muscle, cardiac and gland cells in ways that produce effects similar to those that are evoked by the continued stimulation of the cholinergic nerves that innervate these cells. The long-lasting effects of the synthetic choline esters bethanechol, carbachol and methacholine are mainly muscarinic.

On the other hand, the indirect-acting anticholinesterase drugs produce clinically useful effects not only at autonomic neuroeffectors but also at the motor end plates in skeletal muscle fibers (a "nicotinic" site). Unfortunately, the doses required to stimulate disease-weakened skeletal muscles often also trigger responses in other nerve, muscle and gland cells at which acetylcholine is released from nerve endings. Thus, these drugs commonly cause side effects that are the result of their actions at sites in various visceral organs. In addition, overdoses of these drugs cause complex toxic effects that are the result of their stimulating and depressant actions at the *ganglia* of both divisions of the autonomic nervous system (nicotinic sites of a different type) as well as upon certain cells of the central nervous system.

In this chapter, we shall first discuss the pharmacological effects of all the cholinergic drugs upon various smooth muscles and glands and the heart. We shall then take up the effects of the *anticholinesterase type* cholinergic drugs upon skeletal muscles, autonomic ganglia and the central nervous system. In each case, we shall point out, for each affected structure, the significance of the actions of various cholinergic drugs in terms of usefulness in the treatment of specific clinical conditions, side effects and toxicity, and the conditions in which their use requires caution or may be contraindicated.

CLINICAL PHARMACOLOGY

In treating disorders that are responsive to cholinergic drugs the doctor tries to choose the particular agent that experience has proved most likely to act primarily at the organ which he wants to influence. He also adjusts the drug's dosage carefully in an attempt to limit its actions as much as possible to these target tissues. Since the *selective affinity* of these drugs is limited at best, the occurrence simultaneously of some unwanted drug actions at other sites is almost inevitable. It often becomes necessary to turn to adjunctive drugs and measures for relief of discomforting side effects from the widespread systemic actions of the cholinergic agents. The nurse is sometimes asked to note such unusual reactions and to administer standby medications that are held in reserve on a p.r.n. basis.

Thus, although the clinically useful and the undesirable effects of the cholinergic drugs upon each of various organs, structures and systems will be discussed separately, it is well to remember that the effects of these agents sometimes appear at several cholinergically innervated organs at the same time.

Gastrointestinal Tract

As has been previously indicated, the parasympathetic system strongly influences the functioning of the gastrointestinal tract. If the physiological effects of parasympathetic actions are understood (Table 14-2), the effects of parasympatho*mimetic* drugs on G.I. smooth muscle and glands should be readily predictable. In general, the effects of cholinergic drugs on smooth muscle cells that are innervated by postganglionic fibers of the vagus and the pelvic nerves are manifested by an increase in the tone and motility of the musculature. These actions have a certain limited clinical utility in some patients with poor gastrointestinal tone and motility that is not responsive to the standard cathartics (Chap. 38). More commonly, the gastrointestinal actions of the cholinergic drugs are a source of discomforting side effects when these drugs are given primarily for their effects on structures other than the G.I. tract.

Clinical Indications. Among the clinical conditions in which the effects of cholinergic drugs on G.I. motility are considered desirable are *postoperative atony,* and *paralytic ileus*—conditions in which the patient's abdomen becomes bloated and distended with unremoved wastes and gases as a result of a *nonmechanical* obstruction due to bowel wall paralysis. Bethanecol (see Drug Digest), a choline ester with a relatively selective action on the G.I. tract, is often preferred for stimulating G.I. motility in such cases. It is given by mouth with meals, or subcutaneously when it cannot be readily absorbed by the oral route. The doctor may also order various physical and mechanical measures, including enemas, heat applications to the abdomen and the use of rectal tubes to aid removal of intestinal gases.

Patients sometimes treated with cholinergic drugs include those who, after surgical treatment of peptic ulcer by *bilateral vagotomy,* suffer from temporary paralysis of gastric motility; certain cases of *congenital megacolon;* and patients with essential hypertension who are being treated with *constipating ganglionic blocking agents* (Chap. 17).

Some doctors prefer to employ neostigmine (see Drug Digest) for these clinical actions on the gastrointestinal tract. However, the utility of this anticholin-esterase type cholinergic agent is somewhat limited because it acts at nicotinic sites (i.e., autonomic ganglia and skeletal muscles) as well as at the desired muscarinic sites of action in the gut. Widespread side effects also limit the utility of carbachol and pilocarpine against gastrointestinal atony, and these cholinergic drugs are now used mainly by topical administration in the eye.

The gastrointestinal side effects to be expected with the cholinergic drugs include intestinal cramps and diarrhea. In addition, the stimulation of gastric acid secretion often leads to heartburn and belching, nausea and vomiting, and other discomfort. The use of these drugs is undesirable in patients with peptic ulcer or with spastic or obstructive gastrointestinal disease.

When cholinergic drugs are given by injection in the treatment of other conditions, it is advisable to place the patient on a bedpan and to have ready a syringe containing an injectable solution of atropine, the specific antidote for the muscarinic effects of cholinergic drugs.

Genitourinary Tract

Cholinergic drugs cause the detrusor muscle of the urinary bladder to contract, at the same time relaxing the trigone and sphincter muscles. This simultaneous squeezing of the body of the bladder while the entrance into the urethra is opened results in the evacuation of retained urine. Such drug-induced stimulation of micturition is often desirable for patients with *postoperative* or *postpartum urinary retention* or in patients partially paralyzed by spinal cord injury or disease who suffer from a *neurogenic bladder.* The pharmacological "catheterization" that usually follows subcutaneous injection of one of these drugs often obviates the need for mechanical catheterization, with its attendant increased risk of urinary tract infection.

Among the cholinergic drugs which are said to have a relatively selective action on neuroeffectors in the urinary bladder is the direct-acting drug bethanechol and the indirect-acting anticholinesterase compounds benzpyrinium and neostigmine. The patient being treated with any of these drugs should have a bedpan or urinal handy and be given whatever assistance seems necessary. Since these drugs sometimes cause a sudden feeling of urgency to void, it is essential that the patient's call be answered quickly. Atropine should also be available for counteracting excessive cholinergic side effects.

The chief precaution prior to treating urinary bladder atony is the ruling out of the presence of any obstruction to the expected flow of urine in the neck of the bladder. In acute retention, the cholinergic drug is withdrawn once the patient voids spontaneously; in chronic cases, patients take the drug until automatic micturition becomes established, after which it is gradually discontinued.

Cardiovascular System

The heart responds directly to cholinergic drugs in much the same way as when the vagus nerves are stimulated—that is, it is markedly slowed. Sometimes, however, the heart rate may be reflexly speeded up—for example, when a drug-induced fall in blood pressure sets into motion compensatory cardioacceleratory and vasopressor mechanisms. Other unpredictable cardiac effects that occur occasionally range from heart block to atrial fibrillation.

The relatively long-lasting choline ester methacholin is the cholinergic drug most commonly employed in treating certain cardiac and vascular conditions. It is occasionally used, for example, to overcome attacks of *atrial tachycardia,* a condition marked by a sudden loss of vagal control over the atria. Methacholine sometimes brings about a return of vagal tone and returns the runaway heart to its normal rate and rhythm by its vagomimetic action upon cardiac neuroeffectors. It works best when combined with mechanical measures such as pressure on the eyeballs or massage of the carotid sinuses in the neck, maneuvers which reflexly increase vagal control over the heart.

Actually, methacholine's many side effects make it one of the last drugs the doctor turns to for treating attacks of paroxysmal atrial tachycardia. Most physicians tend to hold it in reserve for use in selected patients who have failed to respond to other standard measures, such as the use of phenylephrine, digitalis, quinidine, or emetic drugs such as ipecac which set off reflex vagal activity. Recently, the increasing use of *cardioversion* for coping with such refractory cases of tachycardia originating in the atria has further reduced the use of this cholinergic drug in the treatment of atrial arrhythmias (see Chap. 21).

Side Effects. The predictable cardiac side effect of cholinergic drugs is excessive slowing, but *bradycardia* is not the only arrhythmia produced by overdosage of these drugs or sensitivity to them. The drug may cause heart block and this, in turn, may predispose the patient to atrial fibrillation. Since this occurs most commonly in patients with hyperthyroidism, the administration of methacholine in an attempt to counteract tachycardia in such cases is contraindicated.

Methacholine is sometimes used for its effects on blood vessels. Like parasympathetic stimulation (see Table 14-2), this close relative of acetylcholine causes vasodilatation of various vascular beds, including those of the skin and muscles. The increased flow of blood to these areas is desirable in the treatment of peripheral vascular disorders such as Raynaud's disease and acrocyanosis, and to help the healing of chronic skin ulcers (see Chap. 43).

The systemic side effects of methacholine limit its utility here as elsewhere when it is given subcutaneously. However, the fact that this drug is a quarternary ammonium compound with the typical positive electric charge of such chemicals has led to its use locally by the method of administration called *iontophoresis*. This involves application of a methacholine solution to a positive electrode that is then placed upon the patient's skin in an area of poor circulation. The current is then turned on, driving the drug into the skin where it produces its vasodilating effects locally without being carried elsewhere in the body by the bloodstream.

Generalized vasodilatation as a result of overdosage with cholinergic drugs occasionally leads to episodes of hypotension. However, such falls in blood pressure are not ordinarily serious, because compensatory vasopressor reflexes quickly bring pressure back to normal. Actually, after overdosage with certain cholinergic drugs, the blood pressure may *rise* as a result of stimulation of the sympathetic ganglia and the adrenal medulla (i.e., nicotinic actions). In any case, the effects of cholinergic drugs on the systemic circulation are too complex and short-lived to be either seriously toxic or dependable enough to be of any use in the treatment of essential hypertension.

Skin

In addition to the flushing and feeling of warmth induced by certain cholinergic drugs, profuse sweating is a common occurrence. Such diaphoresis is most marked with pilocarpine (see Drug Digest), a drug that stimulates both the sweat gland cells and the sympathetic ganglia that send postganglionic cholinergic fibers to them. In the past, pilocarpine has sometimes been used to promote removal of retained wastes by way of the skin, in patients with acute renal failure.

However, the accompanying side effects, which are especially dangerous for patients with renal disease, have led to the abandonment of drug-induced sweat therapy in favor of more effective modern methods such as renal dialysis with the artificial kidney. Pilocarpine sweating is still sometimes used by neurologists for mapping the extent of injury to peripheral nerves. Failure of sweating in some skin areas in response to pilocarpine and heat helps to diagnose the degree of nerve fiber damage.

Other Glands and Smooth Muscles

Besides gland cells in the skin and stomach, others that are stimulated by cholinergic drugs include the mucus-secreting cells of the respiratory tract. The outpouring of such secretions, together with contraction of the bronchial smooth muscles, causes some patients to cough, choke and wheeze when these drugs are administered. Such side effects are especially likely in patients with a history of asthma, and thus, the use of methacholine, bethanechol, pilocarpine, etc., is avoided in such cases.

Salivation is a common side effect of cholinergic drugs. Stimulation of the salivary glands has little clinical utility. However, pilocarpine has occasionally been prescribed to counteract excessive dryness of the mouth, of which patients taking ganglionic blocking drugs for hypertension sometimes complain. However, the xerostomia resulting from overdosage with atropine and other anticholinergic drugs used in peptic ulcer treatment is best relieved by having the patient suck on hard candies, since administration of pilocarpine as a sialagogue may also increase the undesired secretion of gastric acid and enzymes.

The Eye. The smooth muscle structures of the eye, including the circular (or sphincter) muscle of the iris, and the ciliary body, which controls movements of the lens, are contracted by cholinergic drugs. The resulting pupillary constriction, or miosis, is therapeutically useful in ophthalmology. Physostigmine, for example, is often instilled in the eye to counteract the long-lasting mydriasis, or pupillary dilation, produced by atropine administration. Similarly, these two opposing drugs may be applied to the eye alternately to contract and relax the muscles of the iris. This form of forced exercise of ocular structures helps to break up adhesions forming between the iris and the lens. (See Chap. 42 for a fuller discussion of the use of various cholinergic drugs in the treatment of glaucoma and the adverse local ocular effects of these agents.)

Skeletal Muscle Effects and Myasthenia Gravis

Certain of the cholinergic drugs tend to act more or less selectively at the neuromuscular junctions in skeletal muscles. Small doses of these drugs stimulate nerve impulse transmission and increase muscular contractions; larger doses can lead to a later blockade of transmission and muscle paralysis. The initial drug-induced increase in muscle strength has been utilized clinically in the treatment of myasthenia gravis, a disease marked by muscle weakness. The secondary paralytic action is sometimes seen after overdoses of the cholinergic drugs that are used to treat myasthenia. Skeletal muscle paralysis after initial stimulation is also a factor in fatal accidental poisoning by certain insecticides and by the so-called "nerve gases." In all such cases of overdosage, the effects of the cholinergic chemicals at other sites besides the skeletal muscles are also seen.

Myasthenia gravis is a disease in which the patient's muscles quickly become fatigued. Yet there appears to be nothing wrong with the muscles themselves or with the motor nerves that innervate them. The patient's difficulties seem to stem from some abnormality in the junction between the motor axon terminals and the motor end plates on the skeletal muscle fiber membranes. The exact nature of the neuromuscular transmission defect at this junction is still unknown. However, the myasthenic's muscle weakness resembles that which develops in animals injected with curare, a chemical that interferes with impulse transmission by occupying the motor end plates and thus preventing acetylcholine from reaching its receptors (see Chap. 14).

It was the resemblance between the signs and symptoms of myasthenia gravis and those of curare poisoning that led doctors to try treating myasthenic patients with physostigmine (eserine), a drug long known to be an antidote to curare. This anticurare agent proved to have a remarkable ability to overcome the muscular fatigue of myasthenia. Shortly after taking the drug, the patient's ptosis—the drooping eyelids seen in most myasthenics—vanishes, as does the diplopia or double vision that stems from weakness of his extraocular muscles. Under the drug's influence, sufferers from dysphagia and dysarthria become able to chew, swallow and speak once more—at least, as long as the drug's action lasts.

Unfortunately, physostigmine, an anticholinesterase, causes widespread muscarinic side effects because its cholinesterase-inhibiting action is not limited to skeletal muscle myoneural junctions. This led scientists to search for chemically related drugs that would act selectively on skeletal muscle fibers only. A number of synthetic derivatives, including neostigmine, were developed, which do have a somewhat more selective action on the motor end plates in skeletal muscle. However, these safer antimyasthenia drugs, which have replaced physostigmine (which is now used only topically in ophthalmology), are themselves by no means free of adverse effects that stem from their actions at other sites.

Anticholinesterase Drugs vs. Myasthenia

Neostigmine (see Drug Digest) is the drug most commonly employed in the management of myasthenia gravis. It acts mainly by binding the enzyme acetylcholinesterase present at the myoneural junctions of the myasthenic patient's muscles. This keeps the enzyme from destroying the acetylcholine released by the nerve endings. When the neurohormone accumulates sufficiently to overcome the block in myasthenic muscle, motor impulses activate the weakened fibers and cause them to contract. Neostigmine, in addition to increasing the local concentration of acetylcholine, also acts directly on the motor end plates to depolarize them. This, of course, adds to the drug's muscle-strengthening effects.

Neostigmine has a relatively short duration of action, which makes frequent administration necessary.

Myasthenic patients often tend to become resistant to its action, so that the dose must be raised to high levels to maintain the muscle-strengthening effects. In such cases, the drug's action at autonomic neuroeffectors also increases. This causes a variety of muscarinic side effects, including abdominal cramps, diarrhea, nausea and vomiting, and increased secretion of sweat, saliva, tears and bronchial mucus.

Other drugs for treating myasthenia have been introduced, with claims that they have certain advantages over neostigmine. Pyridostigmine (see Drug Digest) has a somewhat longer duration of action, which is further increased by presenting it in a slow-release form. The main advantage is that patients taking the drug at bedtime need not be wakened during the night to take more medication. In addition, patients who used to waken too weak to swallow their morning dose of neostigmine, and, thus, had to receive their medication by injection, do not suffer from morning dysphagia when taking the sustained-action oral form of the longer-acting drug.

A further advantage claimed for this and another, newer, antimyasthenic drug, *ambenonium* (see Drug Digest), is that they cause fewer muscarinic effects. Pyridostigmine, for example, is said to cause much less gastrointestinal stimulation than neostigmine, a fact that might make it more desirable for myasthenics unable to take effective doses of the latter drug without suffering from severe cramps. Similarly, ambenonium may be better for myasthenics who are being maintained in a respirator, because this agent causes less bronchial secretions than the other anticholinesterase drugs.

Some authorities suggest that a reduction in muscarinic side effects, such as may be achieved with these newer drugs or by the simultaneous administration of atropine, is not always desirable. They argue that drug-induced gastrointestinal upset and glandular secretions of increasing severity serve as a useful warning against development of the much more dangerous nicotinic effects of overdosage, which may come on insidiously and can result in increasing skeletal muscle weakness and, finally, paralysis.

Because of the tendency of myasthenics to suffer from the effects of underdosage or overdosage of medication, they must be taught the importance of adjusting dosage to their individual needs and then maintaining their muscle strength at optimal levels by regular administration of the drug. Their families also should learn how to help the patient, in case he is left helpless either by waiting too long between doses or by taking too much medication. In either case, he may waken in the morning unable to move, swallow, or call for help. Thus, he has to arrange his living accommodations so that he can get assistance from another person when he requires it. Someone in the family, for example, should be able to administer a parenteral form of an antimyasthenic agent if the patient becomes unable to swallow his tablets.

Because the course of the disease is unpredictable, the patient's response to drug treatment must be observed often and with care. Any change in his condition must be reported to the doctor, who may then order a change in drug dosage. This is true not only for the patient who suffers a flare-up in intensity of the disease, requiring an upward adjustment of dosage. The patient in remission must reduce his dosage, lest maintenance of the same amount of medication result in overdosage and an insidious return of muscle weakness which is actually drug-induced. Raising the dosage in such circumstances can cause cholinergic crisis.

Cholinergic Crisis. Administration of overdoses of anticholinesterase-type medications to myasthenic patients sometimes sets off a serious cholinergic crisis. This is marked not only by muscarinic side effects that can be counteracted by atropine but also by skeletal muscle weakness and respiratory difficulties, which do not readily respond to treatment with this antimuscarinic antidote. This drug-induced muscle weakness stems from the accumulation of excessive amounts of acetylcholine at the motor end plates, with a resulting reduction in impulse transmission (Chap. 14).

It is often difficult to differentiate cholinergic crisis from *myasthenic crisis*, a situation in which, for poorly understood reasons, the patient suffers a sudden flare-up of his underlying disease. This, like cholinergic crisis, is manifested by respiratory muscle weakness. However, whereas cholinergic crisis calls for *withdrawal* of anticholinesterase drug therapy, patients in myasthenic crisis require *more* antimyasthenic medication.

It is, of course, essential for the nurse to recognize that, regardless of whether the crisis is cholinergic or myasthenic, this is an acute emergency requiring medical intervention and she should promptly call the physician to see his patient. The doctor, who then is faced with what has been called "a desperate dilemma" in deciding how to handle his rapidly weakening patient, now has available a useful drug to help determine the myasthenic patient's true status.

This drug, *edrophonium* (Tensilon, see Drug Digest) was developed during the search for safer antimyasthenic drugs. It is a rapidly effective cholinergic skeletal muscle stimulant. However, its action, which comes on within 30 seconds or so, also wears off within a few minutes. Thus, this drug proved of little use in the treatment of myasthenia, in which—as we have seen—drugs of long duration are desired. However, these properties, i.e., rapid onset and short duration, make edrophonium more useful than other anticholinesterase drugs for *diagnostic* purposes.

A small amount of this drug is injected into the vein of a myasthenic patient suffering from severe respiratory difficulties. If the patient's condition *improves* dramatically—even if for only a couple of minutes—he is probably suffering from *myasthenic* crisis and requires treatment with larger doses of one of the longer-acting anticholinesterase compounds. If, on the other hand, the edrophonium injection makes the myasthenic patient even *weaker*, this is an indication that all medication except atropine must be withdrawn and that he should be managed by mechanical and surgical measures such as endotracheal intubation, suction, tracheotomy and artificial respiration. Atropine is useful no matter what the diagnosis, and the nurse should always have it available both in oral and parenteral form when she is caring for any myasthenic patient. Small oral doses counteract the common G.I. discomforts; large parenteral doses of atropine aid the breathing of patients in cholinergic crisis, although mechanical measures are also often required.

Since the effects of edrophonium wear off so rapidly, the temporary exacerbation of the cholinergic crisis is not serious. This short action also makes the drug more desirable than longer-acting anticholinesterase drugs in the differential diagnosis of myasthenia gravis from other conditions in which the patient may complain of muscular weakness and fatigability. The drug's fleeting effects allow the physician to repeat the so-called Tensilon test several times in the course of a single visit and thus rule out false positive or negative responses.

POISONING BY ANTICHOLINESTERASE CHEMICALS

Certain cholinergic chemicals, especially those of the *organic phosphate* class (Table 15-1), are extremely potent and long-lasting inhibitors of the enzyme cholinesterase. Some of these substances have been tried in the treatment of myasthenia gravis and other conditions responsive to cholinergic drugs, but they are considered too toxic generally for routine clinical use, except by topical administration to the eye in glaucoma (Chap. 42). These chemicals are used mainly as insecticides and chemical warfare agents ("nerve gases").

Agricultural workers and others poisoned by coming in contact with *parathion* or other organophosphates may show signs and symptoms of the *muscarinic, nicotinic* and *central* types (see Summary of Side Effects). All such ill effects are caused by the acetylcholine which accumulates as a result of the inhibitory action of these chemicals upon plasma cholinesterases and upon the acetylcholinesterase found at *all* the junctions between cholinergic nerves and the peripheral and central cells that they innervate.

Prevention of poisoning by parathion-type insecticides is preferable to treating the complicated disorder that follows exposure to these chemicals. Thus, the public health nurse should help avert such poisoning by calling attention to the unwise use of such insecticides by individuals in her community, including those working in greenhouses as well as in the fields. Nurses in hospital emergency rooms should ask people who call about such accidents to bring in a sample of the material or the container in which it came. *Malathion,* the only organophosphorous compound permitted in household insecticides, is much less toxic than other chemicals of this class. However, carelessness in handling it could lead to toxic symptoms that require atropine treatment.

Treatment. *Atropine* is the specific antidote for the muscarinic and central toxic effects of the undestroyed acetylcholine that piles up at many sites following exposure to anticholinesterase-type insecticides. Administered in large doses, this antidotal drug protects smooth muscles, exocrine glands and central nerve cells from the excessive amounts of the neurohormone that accumulate at the peripheral neuroeffectors and central synapses. As a result, the patient may get dramatic relief from many disabling and dangerous symptoms (see Summary) including bronchial constriction and congestion, bradycardia and hypotension, and convulsions or coma.

Atropine does *not,* however, effectively combat the *nicotinic* actions of the anticholinesterase-type poisons. For example, respiratory muscle paralysis following overstimulation of the skeletal myoneural junctions by cholinergic chemicals cannot be counteracted by atropine. Treatment in such cases requires the administration of oxygen by artificial respiration after a clear airway has been established by suction and by tracheotomy if necessary. In addition, a recently introduced antidote called *pralidoxime* (Protopam) has sometimes helped save the lives of patients severely poisoned by cholinesterase inhibitors.

Pralidoxime brings about its antidotal effects by breaking the bond between the poisonous chemical and the molecular surface of the inhibited enzyme cholinesterase. Freed of the chemical that had been keeping it from reacting with its natural substrate the neurohormone acetylcholine, the reactivated enzyme becomes capable of carrying out its function once more. The excess of acetylcholine molecules that had accumulated at the myoneural junctions is then destroyed by the enzyme which is made available as a result of the antidotal action of pralidoxime.

Administered by vein in doses of 1 Gm. or more, after intravenous administration of 2 to 4 mg. of atropine, pralidoxime has helped to reduce muscular weakness, cramps and paralysis in patients poisoned by parathion and by the nerve gas, sarin. This antidote is less effective as an antagonist to *carbamate-type* cholinesterase inhibitors such as neostigmine, pyridostigmine and ambenonium, but it has sometimes been of value in counteracting the signs and symptoms of cholinergic crisis in myasthenia gravis patients suffering the effects of overdosage by these antimyasthenic agents.

SUMMARY OF THE PHARMACOLOGICAL ACTIONS AND THERAPEUTIC USES OF CHOLINERGIC DRUGS

Pharmacological Actions

- *Gastrointestinal*
  Increased tone and motility of musculature, leading to defecation; increased secretion of gastric and other glands

- *Genitourinary*
  Increased tone of detrusor muscle of bladder and relaxation of trigone and sphincter results in stimulation of micturition

- *Cardiac*
  Decrease in heart rate (bradycardia); decrease in atrial contractility, impulse formation and conductivity

- *Vascular*
  Vasodilation resulting in rise in skin temperature and local flushing

Therapeutic Uses

Relief or prevention of postoperative abdominal distention and of gastric atony following vagotomy; management of megacolon and of constipation induced by ganglionic blocking agents

Relief or prevention of postoperative and postpartum urinary retention; management of patients with neurogenic bladder

Arrest of attacks of atrial tachycardia, especially when combined with ocular pressure and carotid sinus massage

Relief of local pain, coldness and cyanosis in selected cases of peripheral vascular disease

- *Ocular*

    Contraction of sphincter muscle of iris causes miosis; contraction of ciliary body causes spasm of accommodation

- *Respiratory*

    Bronchial constriction and increased mucus secretion

- *Skeletal muscle*

    Stimulation of muscle fibers improves strength of abnormally weak motor units but causes fasciculation and weakness of normal muscles

- *Glandular effects*

    (1) *Diaphoresis*—profuse sweating with some drugs
    (2) *Sialagogue*—profuse salivary secretion with some drugs

Reduction of intraocular pressure in chronic simple wide-angle glaucoma. Alternated with mydriatics to break up adhesions between the iris and the lens.

Not a therapeutically useful action

Long-term relief of myasthenia gravis; emergency treatment of myasthenic crisis; differential diagnosis of myasthenia gravis and of myasthenic from cholinergic crisis; curare antidote

(1) Diagnosis of peripheral nerve injuries and, rarely, for removal of waste materials in acute renal failure
(2) Used to counteract xerostomia (mouth dryness) in some situations

---

SUMMARY OF THE SIDE EFFECTS, CAUTIONS AND CONTRAINDICATIONS OF CHOLINERGIC DRUGS

Side Effects

- *Muscarinic-Type*
- *G.I.:* Heartburn, belching, epigastric distress, abdominal cramps, tenesmus (painful anal spasms), diarrhea, nausea and vomiting.
- *G.U.:* Involuntary micturition; increased tone and motility of ureters.
- *Cardiovascular:* Bradycardia and hypotension usually but with reflex cardioacceleration and hypertension in some individuals exposed to overdoses of some agents.
- *Ocular:* Blurring of vision and miosis; aching of brow and eyes; photophobia, myopia, etc.
- *Respiratory:* Bronchoconstriction and increased bronchial mucus secretion may cause wheezing cough, feelings of tightness and pain in chest.
- *Glandular:* Profuse sweating, salivation, lacrimation.

- *Nicotinic-Type*

    Initial skeletal muscular fasciculations, twitching and cramps followed by fatigue, weakness and paralysis of all striated muscles including the diaphragm and intercostals, leading to respiratory distress and failure.

- *Central*

    The organic phosphate (*non*quaternary amine) compounds may cause anxiety, confusion, restlessness, disorientation, difficulty in concentrating, slurring of speech, apathy and drowsiness. Also ataxia, dizziness, headache, weakness, tremor and convulsions. Finally, depression of respiration with Cheyne-Stokes breathing, cyanosis, coma, cardiovascular collapse, areflexia, respiratory failure and death.

Contraindications

Contraindicated in patients with peptic ulcer or spastic or obstructive G.I. disturbances.

Contraindicated in patients with vesical neck obstruction.

Contraindicated in patients with vasomotor instability, recent myocardial infarction, or hyperthyroidism. Use with caution in patients being treated with ganglionic blocking agents.

Contraindicated in narrow angle glaucoma.

Contraindicated in patients with bronchial asthma and with pulmonary edema.

Possible loss of fluids and electrolytes undesirable in patients with acute renal failure.

Contraindicated in patients in cholinergic crisis. Possible sympathetic ganglionic and adrenal medullary stimulation may cause occasional cardioacceleration and elevation until counteracted by parasympathetic stimulation and late ganglionic depressant effects.

```
┌─────────────────────────────────────────────────────┐
│  SUMMARY OF POINTS FOR THE NURSE TO REMEMBER          │
│         CONCERNING CHOLINERGIC DRUGS                  │
└─────────────────────────────────────────────────────┘
```

- Cholinergic drugs have a wide range of effects. Note carefully the patient's response to therapy, both those that are desired and those that are unwanted.

- Emphasize the progress that the patient is making as a result of cholinergic drug therapy even though he may be experiencing some discomfort as a result of the medication. Make certain that distressing symptoms are brought to the attention of the physician so that the patient can benefit from any measures to minimize discomfort that may be available.

- Be alert for any comment by the patient concerning previous illnesses, such as asthma or peptic ulcer, that he may have neglected to mention to the physician. Report such information to the doctor, because it may mean that the patient should not receive a cholinergic drug.

- Remember that atropine is an antidote for cholinergic drugs, and make certain that a supply, along with equipment for parenteral injection, is available at all times.

- For patients with myasthenia gravis, stress the importance of regular timing of the medication, careful observation of symptomatic response, and the necessity of providing for assistance from others when the patient's symptoms result in sudden helplessness.

- Insecticides such as parathion can cause serious toxic effects. Be alert to the hazards of injudicious use of such chemicals and explain these to others in an effort to avert accidental poisoning.

REVIEW QUESTIONS

1. Explain briefly the manner in which the so-called *direct-acting* cholinergic drugs exert their cellular effects, and name some drugs of two *chemically different* subclasses of direct-acting agents.

2. Explain briefly the manner in which the *indirect-acting* cholinergic drugs exert their cellular effects and name some examples of two *chemically different* subclasses of indirect-acting agents.

3. (a) What difficulty tends to limit the clinical usefulness of the cholinergic drugs?

(b) What is the main advantage clinically of the synthetic choline esters over the natural neurohormonal choline ester, acetylcholine?

4. (a) At what sites of cholinergic transmission do the direct-acting cholinergic drugs exert their main effects, and what term describes this type of activity?

(b) At what additional sites do the indirect-acting (anticholinesterase-type) drugs act, and what terms describe these cholinergic actions?

5. (a) What are the predictable effects of cholinergic drugs upon gastrointestinal smooth muscles and glands?

(b) List several gastrointestinal conditions which may be benefited by treatment with these drugs.

(c) What gastrointestinal side effects may be expected from these drugs and what precautions should be taken when they are used? In what types of G.I. conditions is their use contraindicated?

6. (a) Indicate the effects of cholinergic drugs upon the urinary bladder and the clinical conditions in which these effects may be desirable.

(b) Which cholinergic drugs are most commonly employed for their effects on the bladder, and what adjunctive measures and precautions are employed?

7. (a) What is the direct effect of methacholine upon the heart and in what clinical condition is this effect considered desirable?

(b) In what patients is methacholine contraindicated because of its possible adverse cardiac effects?

8. (a) In what clinical conditions is the effect of methacholine upon blood vessels considered desirable and how is it best administered to limit its effects to local sites?

(b) What effect upon systemic blood pressure might be expected from methacholine overdosage, and what is the actual status of this drug insofar as its circulatory effects are concerned?

9. (a) What are the effects of cholinergic drugs upon exocrine gland structures such as the salivary, sweat, lacrimal, stomach and bronchial glands?

(b) What is the combined effect of the actions of cholinergic drugs upon bronchial muscles and glands, and in what patient may such actions be especially dangerous?

10. Explain briefly the main manner in which the anticholinesterase-type cholinergic drugs act to increase skeletal muscle strength in myasthenia gravis.

11. (a) What advantages are claimed for the antimyasthenic agents pyridostigmine and ambenonium over earlier agents such as physostigmine and neostigmine?

(b) Why is the relative lack of muscarinic side effects in some drugs sometimes considered undesirable, and why may the simultaneous administration of atropine to counteract such side effects be similarly undesirable, according to some authorities?

12. (a) What is the cause of cholinergic crisis and how are patients managed once this condition has been diagnosed?

(b) What treatment is required when myasthenic crisis is diagnosed?

13. (a) Explain briefly how edrophonium is employed to differentiate between myasthenic and cholinergic crisis.

(b) For what other purpose is the so-called Tensilon test employed?

14. (a) Explain briefly how *atropine* counteracts many but not all signs and symptoms of poisoning by anticholinesterase chemicals.

(b) Explain briefly how *pralidoxime* may help counteract toxic reactions that are not readily overcome by the administration of atropine alone.

BIBLIOGRAPHY

Clagett, O. T.: Myasthenia gravis. Am. J. Nurs., *51:*654, 1951.

Council on Drugs: An antidote of parathion poisoning. Pralidozime chloride. J.A.M.A., *192:*314, 1965.

Fleming, A. R.: The use of Urecholine in the prevention of postpartum urinary retention. Am. J. Obstet. Gynec., *74:*569, 1957.

Furman, R. H., and Geiger, J. A.: Use of cholinergic drugs in paroxysmal supraventricular tachycardia. Serious untoward reactions and fatality from treatment with methacholine and neostigmine. J.A.M.A., *149:*269, 1952.

Grob, D.: Myasthenia gravis. Arch. Int. Med., *108:*615, 1961.

Hayes, W. J.: Parathion poisoning and its treatment. J.A.M.A., *192:*49, 1965.

McGee, K. R.: Myasthenia gravis. Am. J. Nurs., *60:*336, 1960.

Osserman, K. E., and Shapiro, E. K.: Nursing care in myasthenia gravis. Nursing World, *130:*12, 1956.

Rodman, M. J.: Drugs for neuromuscular disorders. R.N., *25:*67, 1962 (Jan.).

———: Muscle relaxants and stimulants. R.N., *21:*54, 1958 (Feb.).

———: Muscle metabolism. R.N., *19:*52, 1956 (May).

Schwab, R. S.: The pharmacologic basis of the treatment of myasthenia gravis. Clin. Pharmacol. Ther., *1:*319, 1960.

Stein, I. F., Jr., and Meyer, K. A.: Effect of Urecholine on stomach, intestine and urinary bladder. J.A.M.A., *140:*522, 1949.

· 16 ·

Sympathomimetic (Adrenergic) Drugs

GENERAL CONSIDERATIONS

The physiological functions of the two natural cate-cholamines, epinephrine and norepinephrine, have been discussed in Chapter 14. In this chapter we shall take up some of the pharmacological actions of these substances and the clinical conditions in which they have proved useful. We shall also discuss the actions and uses of the *sympathomimetic amines*—synthetic substances of similar chemical structure which imitate many of the effects of the adrenergic neurohormones.

Like the natural substances, the synthetic adrenergic amines produce most of their effects by acting upon the alpha and beta receptors of effector cells—mainly smooth muscle structures innervated by post-ganglionic fibers of the sympathetic nervous system. Some (e.g., phenylephrine) are thought to act directly on the adrenergic receptors, as do epinephrine and norepinephrine themselves; others (e.g., amphetamine; ephedrine) act indirectly, by releasing the natural neurohormone from nerve endings and other tissues; still others exhibit a combination of such direct and indirect actions.

These synthetic drugs differ somewhat from one another in their chemical structures, and they vary also in their pharmacological properties. Thus, some drugs have a greater affinity for the adrenergic neuro-effectors of the blood vessels; others may act mainly on those of the smooth muscles of the bronchi. Some (e.g., ephedrine) may enter the central nervous system to produce excitatory effects; others may be almost purely peripheral in their actions. The chemical configuration of some sympathomimetic substances (e.g., ephedrine, phenylephrine, etc.) makes them stable in the gastrointestinal tract and permits their oral administration; others (e.g., epinephrine) are effective only when administered by injection, because they are destroyed in the gut. These differences in affinity for various sites largely determine the clinical conditions for which each of the numerous sympathomimetic drugs is best suited. Thus, in treating the various conditions for which these drugs are used, the doctor tries to select a sympathomimetic agent that exerts its predominant effects at the particular peripheral site that must most be affected to exert clinically desirable effects. Of course, because all of these agents act to varying degrees at secondary sites also, side effects occur fairly frequently during adrenergic drug therapy.

In the following section, the main pharmacological effects of various typically adrenergic drugs will be discussed together with the chief clinical conditions in which the drugs are used for these desirable actions. It will become apparent that an action that is clinically useful in some cases may constitute an undesired side effect in others. This is especially so in patients whose physical condition makes them especially susceptible to the adverse effects of adrenergic drugs, and so use of these drugs is contraindicated in such people.

Detailed information about the clinically most important adrenergic agents will be found in the Drug Digests. Detailed discussions of how these drugs are used and administered in various common clinical conditions appears usually in the chapter dealing with the management of each such condition (Section Seven and elsewhere, as indicated by cross references).

PHARMACOLOGICAL EFFECTS AND CLINICAL USES

The sympathomimetic amines are used in a wide variety of clinical situations. Their employment for therapeutic purposes is based mainly on their effects on the heart, and on the smooth muscle walls of the blood vessels and bronchi. These actions and uses will be taken up here (the adrenergic drugs that are used mainly for their central stimulating effects (e.g., the amphetamines) are discussed in Chapter 13).

242

Cardiovascular Effects

The actions of adrenergic drugs on the heart and blood vessels are extremely complex and variable. Although some effects can be predicted on the basis of what would be expected from sympathetic nervous system stimulation, the circulatory effects of these drugs may vary widely, depending upon many factors. We shall concern ourselves only with the main actions that occur when these drugs are given in clinically effective doses and by clinically practical means of administration.

Cardiac Effects of Adrenergic Drugs. These agents are capable of affecting the rate, rhythm, and strength of the heartbeat in ways which may be both desirable and dangerous. The main pharmacological effects of the prototype adrenergic drug, epinephrine, on the heart are the following: (1) an increase in contractile force; (2) an increase in coronary blood flow; (3) an increase in cardiac rate, although this may in some circumstances be masked by (4) a reflex slowing of the heart; and (5) an increase in cardiac irritability, which may lead to production of arrhythmias. Other adrenergic drugs often differ from epinephrine in the particular cardiac action that tends to be predominant.

Epinephrine (Adrenalin) is sometimes employed in cases of cardiac arrest in an attempt to resuscitate the victim of cardiac standstill. Injected directly into the heart, the drug may occasionally overcome asystole and stimulate spontaneous beating if the myocardium is simultaneously massaged to force the injected epinephrine through the coronary circulation.

Another adrenergic drug, *isoproterenol* (Isuprel), is preferred for treating Stokes-Adams seizures, a condition in which the heart may slow excessively or even stop temporarily. These attacks are marked by syncope (fainting) and may be fatal if the heart fails to begin beating again within a short time. Isoproterenol stimulates the ventricles to contract forcefully and is claimed less likely to cause ventricular fibrillation than epinephrine. The use of these drugs and of ephedrine in Stokes-Adams disease is more fully discussed in Chapter 21, Antiarrhythmic Agents.

Among the side effects that the adrenergic drugs commonly tend to cause are tachycardia and cardiac palpitations. Due to this action, the use of these drugs is contraindicated in patients with angina pectoris, hyperthyroidism, and other conditions in which an increase in the work load of the heart is undesirable. However, certain adrenergic drugs may actually be employed occasionally to terminate paroxysmal atrial tachycardia because, instead of accelerating the heart, they tend to slow it. *Methoxamine* (Vasoxyl), for example, has little or no direct stimulating effect on the heart. It acts mainly on the blood vessels, as described below, to bring about a rise in blood pressure. This, in turn, leads to reflex stimulation of the cardioinhibitory center. As a result, increased numbers of nerve impulses pass down the vagus nerve. This slows the heart and abolishes the attack of atrial tachycardia. The use of this agent and of phenylephrine (Neo-Synephrine) and other drugs, for this purpose, is also discussed in Chapter 21.

Vascular Effects of Adrenergic Drugs. The most common over-all vascular effect of a large dose of an adrenergic drug is a generalized vasoconstriction, which tends to raise diastolic blood pressure by increasing peripheral resistance to blood flow. However, the arterioles of certain tissues (e.g., heart and skeletal muscles) tend to dilate, even while the vessels of other vascular beds are being constricted. In fact, certain adrenergic drugs are used mainly for their ability to dilate constricted arterioles in skeletal muscles and elsewhere, in order to increase local blood flow to ischemic areas. The clinical use of *nylidrin* (Arlidin) and other vasodilator-type adrenergic drugs in treating certain peripheral vascular diseases is discussed in Chapter 26, Peripheral Vasodilator Drugs.

Local vasoconstriction is an adrenergic action which has more common clinical applications, the best known of which is for nasal decongestion—the main therapeutic application of drugs such as *phenylephrine* (Neo-Synephrine), *naphazoline* (Privine), *tetrahydrozoline* (Tyzine), *xylometazoline* (Otrivin), etc. These drugs are either applied topically—as nose drops or inhalants, for example—or administered by mouth and absorbed systemically so that they reach the nasal and sinus mucosa by way of the blood stream.

In either case, these adrenergic drugs constrict the dilated arterioles and capillaries that course through the mucous membranes covering the nasal turbinates and paranasal sinuses. This shrinks swollen membranes, tends to open clogged nasal passages, and promotes drainage through the ostia of the sinuses. The cold sufferer usually gets at least temporary relief from the discomfort of a blocked nose. The use of these decongestant drugs for the symptomatic relief of nasal obstruction is further discussed in Chapter 40. (For the use of some of these same agents as *ocular* decongestants and for reducing intraocular pressure, see Chap. 42.)

Topical application of epinephrine to the nasal membranes is also used to stop nosebleed. Insertion of tampons saturated with a 1:1,000 solution of the vasoconstrictor usually checks capillary oozing quickly in such cases of epistaxis. This hemostatic action of epinephrine is also utilized to stem local bleeding after tonsillectomy and other types of throat surgery. Occasionally, if clotting does not occur quickly, the early vasoconstrictor action of epinephrine may wear off, and a late vasodilator effect develops which may tend to dangerously prolong local bleeding.

Another clinical use of the local vasoconstrictor action of adrenergic drugs is seen in the addition of epinephrine, phenylephrine, and other sympathomimetic amines to local anesthetic solutions. These drugs, even in dilutions of 1:50,000 or 1:100,000, exert a local ischemic action which reduces the rate of absorption of the local anesthetic. This serves a twofold purpose: (1) It prolongs the desired local pain-preventing effect, and (2) it reduces the danger of systemic toxic reactions that might be caused by too high levels of the local anesthetic accumulating in the brain and heart. (Patients who are sensitive to even small amounts of sympathomimetic amines may complain of cardiac palpitations, nervousness, nausea, and tremor—side effects, not of the local anesthetic, but of the added adrenergic drugs.)

Epinephrine's local vasoconstrictor action in the skin and in mucous membranes of the respiratory tract is very valuable for counteracting certain severe allergic symptoms. For example, the drug is injected subcutaneously as an emergency measure in cases of acute urticaria and angioneurotic edema. It can sometimes save the life of a patient in whom sudden swelling in the larynx threatens to cut off the airway and cause asphyxia. In such cases, it is the drug's ability to constrict arterioles and decrease capillary permeability which is useful, as it prevents leakage of serum out of the vessels and consequent swelling of adjacent tissues. In anaphylactic shock, the bronchodilator and vasopressor effects of epinephrine (discussed below) are often lifesaving.

Systemic vasoconstriction produced by sympathomimetic drugs is often useful for helping to bring blood pressure back to normal in acute hypotensive states. These drugs act mainly by stimulating the smooth muscles of the splanchnic arterioles. However, some also have direct and indirect actions on the heart that may help to counteract circulatory collapse. These vasopressor agents, although they are no substitute for blood transfusions or replacement of plasma when blood volume is low, may often serve as a useful adjunct to these and other general measures. The employment of these potent adrenergic drugs for this purpose always constitutes a medical emergency and requires close observation of the patient, in order to prevent the development of dangerous toxic reactions.

Administration of adrenergic vasopressor agents seems especially useful for counteracting drug-induced hypotension caused by a reduction in sympathetic vasoconstrictor nerve impulses to the blood vessels. The loss of vasomotor tone produced by spinal anesthetics or by overdoses of ganglionic and adrenergic blocking drugs is best counteracted by parenteral administration of drugs such as *levarterenol* (Levophed), *metaraminol* (Aramine; Pressonex), and *methoxamine*

(Vasoxyl). Administration of longer-acting agents such as ephedrine and phenylephrine (Neo-Synephrine) is preferred for prophylaxis—for example, prior to surgery under spinal anesthesia.

Angiotensin amide (Hypertensin), a new *nonadrenergic* agent which acts directly on vascular smooth muscle, is the most potent agent available for raising peripheral resistance in patients who fail to respond to levarterenol and other adrenergic vasopressors. On the other hand, the reverse is sometimes true, and some patients react to levarterenol, after angiotensin amide has failed to raise their blood pressure from shock levels.

Cardiogenic Shock (see also Chap. 22). Of the various kinds of shock, one of the most difficult to treat is that which often follows a coronary attack and myocardial infarction. In such cases of severe cardiogenic shock, the best drugs are those that do not affect the heart adversely. Thus, epinephrine, which tends to increase the heart's work load and to set off cardiac arrhythmias, is considered undesirable in this condition. The adrenergic drugs that produce both a peripheral vasoconstrictive effect and a reflex slowing of the heart (e.g., levarterenol, methoxamine, and phenylephrine) are preferred. In addition to restoring the tone of the blood vessels, these drugs exert the following cardiac effects, considered desirable in coronary shock: (1) *bradycardia*, a slowing of the heartbeat that often increases cardiac efficiency; (2) *myocardial stimulation*, which strengthens the beat without excessively raising cardiac oxygen requirements, and (3) *coronary vasodilation*, which increases the flow of blood to the oxygen-starved myocardium.

The main danger in the use of potent vasopressors is that they may raise the blood pressure to too high levels. In cardiac shock, this could cause reflex arrhythmias that decrease myocardial efficiency, or precipitate fatal ventricular fibrillation. The latter condition has also occurred in patients receiving the general anesthetic, cyclopropane, which seems to sensitize the heart to sympathomimetic drugs in a way that tends to set off dangerous arrhythmias.

Severe pressor drug-induced hypertension is especially dangerous for patients with atherosclerotic cerebral arterioles, because a sudden rise in pressure may cause a cerebral vascular accident. The nurse should always watch the patient for signs of developing headache, during infusion of levarterenol, angiotensin amide and other powerful vasopressors. Projectile vomiting may be a sign of excessive pressure in the vascular bed of the brain.

To guard against excessive blood pressure rises, the patient receiving a pressor drug infusion should never be left unattended. Blood pressure should be checked every two minutes when the intravenous drip is first started. Later, after pressure has stabilized and is being maintained at the desired level, the nurse should continue to take the patient's blood pressure at intervals of no more than five minutes. The rate of flow of the infusion should be slowed, if necessary, to reduce a too rapidly rising pressure, or speeded up if the patient fails to respond at first.

It is also important to see that the needle or the plastic catheter through which the intravenous infusion of levarterenol is being made stays securely within the vein. Infiltration of the vasoconstrictor solution into the surrounding tissues can cause local ischemia, necrosis and sloughing. To avoid this, the infusion site should be inspected frequently and extra care taken when turning the patient to avoid dislodging the needle. If infiltration does occur, the infusion must be stopped immediately and the doctor promptly notified. He may then restart the infusion in another vein and inject an adrenergic blocking vasodilator drug such as *phentolamine* (Regitine) to counteract the local ischemia. The physician may sometimes order the nurse to apply hot packs to the new infusion area, in order to increase blood flow into collapsed peripheral veins and thus facilitate venipuncture.

With the longer acting vasopressors such as *metaraminol* (Aramine; Pressonex), *ephedrine* and *phenylephrine*, which are given mainly by intramuscular injection, blood pressure readings need not usually be taken as frequently. Nonetheless, skilled nursing care is always a prime requirement in shock treatment. This includes keeping the patient calm and quiet, since fright and anxiety add to his circulatory burden. The nurse should try to convey an attitude of calm competence while attending to the patient in shock. She should avoid saying anything that might alarm the patient, nor should she communicate dismay or apprehension to the patient by her actions or facial expression.

Bronchial Actions of Adrenergic Drugs

Certain sympathomimetic agents strongly stimulate the beta-type, or inhibitory, adrenergic receptors in the smooth muscles of the bronchi. This results in relaxation of the muscular walls and in dilation of the bronchial tubes—an action which is most desirable in patients with asthma, emphysema, and other conditions marked by bronchiolar constriction and congestion (see Chap. 40). This bronchospasmolytic effect, coupled with shrinkage of the swollen respiratory tract membranes and reduced mucus secretion, often offers rapid relief of asthmatic wheezing, coughing, and dyspnea.

Epinephrine is still the agent most widely used for relieving air hunger in acute allergic emergencies. It acts promptly to permit passage of air when inhaled as a fine mist from an oral nebulizer which releases an aerosol of a 1:100 concentration solution. Subcutaneous injection of a fraction of a milliliter of the 1:1,000 solution also provides prompt relief of bronchial congestion in most cases. However, these actions are of short duration, and repeated administration tends to produce tolerance to epinephrine.

Patients who become refractory to the bronchodilator action of epinephrine often continue to respond to the related adrenergic antiasthmatic agent, *isoproterenol* (Isuprel, Norisodrine, etc.). This drug is given sublingually as well as by inhalation; it is absorbed, though somewhat irregularly, when taken by mouth in cough medicines. Inhalation is the most rapid route for aborting an acute asthmatic attack; it is also the safest way to give this potent drug, since low concentrations acting locally in the respiratory tract do not tend to produce undue cardiac stimulation. (Systemic absorption from under the tongue or from subcutaneous sites is often followed by marked tachycardia and palpitations.) Isoproterenol tends to dilate blood vessels; thus, for counteracting bronchial congestion, it is best administered in combination with the vasoconstrictor phenylephrine. It is never combined with epinephrine, because the two drugs tend to overstimulate the heart.

Ephedrine is preferred for prophylaxis against asthmatic attacks in long-term treatment. It has the advantage of being fully effective when taken by mouth, producing a prolonged bronchodilator and decongestant action. Unfortunately, ephedrine often stimulates cerebral cortical activity, causing restlessness and insomnia. It is commonly given in combination with barbiturates or other sedatives to counteract the central side effects. Other adrenergic bronchodilators, including *methoxyphenamine* (Orthoxine) and *protokylol* (Caytine), which do not penetrate the blood-brain barrier as readily as ephedrine, are claimed to cause fewer central effects. However, these drugs have been known to cause both wakefulness and drowsiness in some patients.

Adrenergic Actions on Other Organ Systems

Adrenergic drugs act to varying degrees on other structures including the eye, gastrointestinal tract, uterus, and skeletal muscles. However, except for the ocular effects obtainable by topical application of ophthalmic solutions, few of the other actions are of clinical importance. This is because they are usually elicited only by relatively large doses which can also cause cardiovascular and central side effects.

The pupil of the eye is dilated by the stimulating action of adrenergic drugs on the radial muscle of the iris. This mydriatic effect produced by instillation of ephedrine (10% solution), *hydroxyamphetamine* (Paredrine 1%) and certain other sympathomimetic agents is employed for facilitating ophthalmoscopic examination of the eye grounds. These drugs do not cause cycloplegia, or paralysis of accommodation. Thus, for refraction, they must be combined with atropine-type agents; on the other hand, the lack of cycloplegic effects makes these drugs less likely to raise intraocular pressure and permits their use in treating some types of glaucoma (see Chap. 42).

Uterine responses to adrenergic drugs are very variable. Small doses of epinephrine injected subcutaneously are said to relax spasms of the uterus that develop during labor. However, the drug is rarely used for this purpose in obstetrics; when added to local anesthetic solutions, its presence may interfere with uterine contractions and, thus, slow labor.

Gastrointestinal smooth muscle in spasm occasionally is relaxed by epinephrine and ephedrine, as would be predicted from the effects of sympathetic nervous system stimulation on the gastrointestinal tract. However, the slight inhibitory action on the gut elicited by safe doses of these adrenergic drugs is of little clinical utility, compared to the gastrointestinal antispasmodic action of drugs that act by blocking parasympathetic motor activity (e.g., atropine, propantheline, etc., Chaps. 17 and 38).

Isometheptene (Octin), an adrenergic drug, has been employed clinically for relaxing smooth muscle spasm of the gastrointestinal, genitourinary, and biliary tracts. This drug is also sometimes used in treating migraine headache. In that condition, it is thought to act by constricting dilated cerebral blood vessels, thus reducing pulsations and pain (see Chap. 41).

TABLE 16-1
SOME SYMPATHOMIMETIC AMINES *

NONPROPRIETARY NAME	TRADE NAME	DOSE
Ephedrine (base, HCl and sulfate salts) U.S.P., N.F.		25 to 50 mg. oral
Epinephrine U.S.P.	Adrenalin; Suprarenin	0.5 mg. I.M repeated every 8 to 16 hours as necessary; 0.5 mg. S.C. repeated every 4 hours as necessary
Epinephrine Injection U.S.P.	Epinephrine HCl 1:1,000 solution	0.1 to 0.5 ml. S.C.; 0.1 to 0.2 ml. I.V., well diluted and injected very slowly
Sterile Epinephrine Suspension U.S.P.	Epinephrine in Oil 1:500 suspension	0.5 mg. I.M. repeated every 8 to 16 hours as necessary
Epinephrine Inhalation U.S.P.	Epinephrine HCl 1:100 solution	Oral inhalation of a fine mist as required. *Never* injected.
Epinephrine bitartrate U.S.P.	Epitrate; Mytrate	Topically applied to the conjunctiva: 0.1 ml. every 5 to 15 minutes for three applications
Isoproterenol HCl U.S.P. and sulfate	Isuprel; Isonorin; Norisodrine; etc.	10 to 20 mg., sublingual; 3 to 5 mg., oral and rectal; 0.02 to 0.15 mg., parenteral
Levarterenol bitartrate U.S.P.	Levophed	0.2% sol. I.V. dissolved in dextrose solution and administered at an average rate of 2 to 4 mcg. of base per minute
Mephentermine sulfate N.F.	Wyamine	12.5 to 25 mg. orally; 30 to 60 mg. I.V. or I.M. of 0.1% solution
Metaraminol bitartrate U.S.P.	Aramine; Pressonex	2 to 10 mg., S.C. or I.M.; 0.5 to 5 mg. I.V.
Methoxamine HCl U.S.P.	Vasoxyl	10 to 15 mg. I.M.; 5 to 10 mg. I.V.
Methoxyphenamine HCl	Orthoxine	50 to 100 mg. orally
Phenylephrine HCl U.S.P.	Neo-Synephrine	2.5 mg. S.C. or I.M.; 0.5 to 1 mg. I.V.
Phenylpropanolamine HCl	Propadrine	25 to 50 mg. orally
Protokylol HCl	Caytine	2 to 4 mg. orally; 0.1 to 0.5 mg. S.C. or I.M.

* Other adrenergic drugs are listed elsewhere (see Chaps. 26, 40, 42).

SUMMARY OF CHIEF PHARMACOLOGICAL ACTIONS AND CLINICAL USES OF ADRENERGIC DRUGS

Cardiac Actions and Uses

- *Increase in rate and strength of heartbeat:*
  Useful in treating cardiac slowing and heart block in Stokes-Adams disease and the carotid sinus syndrome; may help to resuscitate heart in cardiac standstill, or asystole, but not in ventricular fibrillation.

- *Decrease in heart rate as a result of reflex vagal stimulation:*
  May be useful for terminating paroxysmal atrial (supraventricular) tachycardia.

- *Strengthening and slowing of heart and coronary vasodilation:*
  These actions may be desirable in adrenergic drugs used in cardiogenic shock.

Vascular Actions and Uses

- *Local vasodilation* by some adrenergic drugs is useful for treating certain peripheral vascular diseases (see Chap. 26).

- *Local vasoconstriction* is useful in many circumstances:
  1. *Nasal decongestant* in acute and chronic inflammatory and allergic disorders, including the common cold, hay fever, vasomotor rhinitis, etc.
  2. *Ocular decongestant* in conjunctivitis and in some forms of glaucoma
  3. *Hemostatic* in epistaxis (nosebleed) and after tonsillectomy and other throat surgery
  4. *Additive to local anesthetic* solutions for reducing systemic absorption of these drugs
  5. *Antiallergic action* in urticaria, angioneurotic edema, and anaphylactoid reaction

- *Systemic vasoconstriction* to raise blood pressure, in:
  1. Acute hypotension caused by drug-induced reduction of sympathetic vasomotor tone (e.g., spinal and inhalation anesthetics, ganglionic and adrenergic blocking agents, etc.)

  2. Cardiogenic shock following myocardial infarction
  3. Circulatory collapse from other causes, including that resulting from severe hemorrhage (here, replacement of blood or restoration of blood volume with plasma or other fluids is the most important measure and the use of adrenergic vasopressors is only adjunctive)

Bronchial Muscle Actions and Uses

- Stimulation of beta type (inhibitory) receptors in smooth muscle of bronchi relaxes spasm and dilates bronchial tubes in the following conditions:
  1. Acute and chronic asthmatic states
  2. Pulmonary emphysema and fibrosis
  3. Chronic bronchitis and bronchiectasis

Miscellaneous Actions and Uses

- Stimulation of alpha type (motor) receptors in radial muscle of the iris results in mydriasis, which is useful for facilitating ophthalmological examinations.

- Gastrointestinal, genitourinary, and biliary tract musculature may occasionally be relaxed to relieve spasm of these viscera in ureteral and biliary colic and in dysmenorrhea and labor.

- Skeletal muscle is sometimes strengthened by ephedrine in myasthenia gravis.

- Dilated cerebral vessels are sometimes constricted by isometheptene in migraine headaches.

- Increased tone of trigone and sphincter of urinary bladder brought about by ephedrine may be helpful in nocturnal enuresis (bedwetting).

- Central stimulation by amphetamines and ephedrine, may be useful in narcolepsy, etc. (See Chap. 13.)

SUMMARY OF SIDE EFFECTS, TOXICITY AND CONTRAINDICATIONS OF ADRENERGIC DRUGS

Side Effects

- *Cardiovascular:* cardiac palpitations, possible precordial pain, pallor, headache, hypertension.

- *Nervous:* anxiety, nervousness, vertigo tremor, insomnia.

- *Other:* dilated pupils, nausea, vomiting, glycosuria.

Severe Toxicity

- Cardiac arrhythmias ranging from tachycardia to bradycardia and various other irregularities, including possible fatal ventricular fibrillation. Severe hypertension may result in cerebral hemorrhage, especially in patients with cerebral atherosclerosis. Cardiac dilata-

tion and pulmonary edema may also develop as a result of a sharp, sustained rise in blood pressure.

Cautions and Contraindications

- Give with extreme caution, if at all, to patients with coronary artery and other organic heart disease, hypertension, hyperthyroidism, and diabetes. These drugs are also undesirable for elderly patients and should not be employed during inhalation anesthesia with halogenated hydrocarbons (e.g., chloroform; trichlorethylene) and cyclopropane.

- Patients receiving intravenous infusions of potent vasopressors should not be left unattended; blood pressure should be taken frequently; the site of infusion should be frequently inspected for signs of extravasation and tissue infiltration.

SUMMARY OF SOME POINTS FOR NURSES TO REMEMBER IN ADMINISTERING ADRENERGIC VASOPRESSORS

- Adrenergic drugs are usually kept on emergency trays. Be sure that the solutions are in good condition (e.g., have not turned brown) and in ample supply. Check the tray frequently and replace used materials as soon as the emergency is over.

- Remember that these are very powerful drugs and that errors in dosage are especially serious. Take special note of the *strength* of the solution (is it 1:100 or 1:1,000?), the *dosage* (0.10 ml. or 1.0 ml.), and the *route* of administration (spray for inhalation; subcutaneous injection).

- When administering vasopressor infusions, take extra care in moving the patient to keep the needle from being dislodged. Check the injection site frequently for signs of leakage and tissue infiltration, which re-

quire that the flow of solution be stopped. Notify the physician so that the infusion can be restarted as soon as possible.

- During the administration of vasopressors, take the patient's blood pressure at the intervals specified by the physician. Be alert for signs of toxicity and notify the physician if these begin to appear.

- All general emergency nursing measures are applicable here both in regard to the patient and to his family. During the emergency, the patient's welfare requires the utmost devotion; after the emergency is over and to the extent that time permits, provide the patient and his family with opportunities to talk about the experience and their reactions to it.

REVIEW QUESTIONS

1. (a) At what specific cellular sites do adrenergic drugs act to produce their sympathomimetic effects?

(b) In what manner do the synthetic drugs act to produce effects that mimic those of the natural neurohormones, or sympathetic catecholamines?

2. (a) List two components of the cardiac actions of adrenergic drugs which may be beneficial in some cases, and indicate two clinical conditions in which these cardiac actions of certain sympathomimetic drugs may be useful.

(b) List two cardiac components which may have undesirable effects in some patients, and indicate patients of two types whose hearts may be adversely affected by adrenergic drugs (i.e., patients in whom adrenergic drugs are contraindicated).

(c) List several other situations in which adrenergic drugs are contraindicated or used only with great caution.

3. (a) List several adrenergic drugs used mainly as nasal decongestants, and indicate the manner in which they bring about their desirable effects.

(b) List several clinical situations in which the local vasoconstrictor action of epinephrine is useful, and indicate in each case what the drug does that is desirable.

4. (a) List several adrenergic drugs used mainly as vasopressor agents in treating acute hypotensive (shock) states, and indicate the main manner in which they raise blood pressure.

(b) Indicate additional actions which may make an adrenergic drug especially desirable or undesirable in shock following a heart attack and myocardial infarction.

5. (a) List several precautions which the nurse should take for the safety of the patient in shock who is receiving an infusion of the vasopressor drug levarterenol (Levophed).

(b) List some of the dangers of overdosage of levarterenol and epinephrine, and indicate some of the early signs and symptoms of toxic reaction.

6. (a) List two adrenergic drugs that are often rapidly effective for aborting an acute asthmatic attack, and state at least one disadvantage that tends to limit the usefulness of each drug for this purpose.

(b) List two adrenergic drugs that are preferred for the long-term treatment of bronchial asthma, and indicate a disadvantage of one drug which the other does not share.

7. (a) Indicate some miscellaneous actions and unusual clinical actions of the following adrenergic drugs: (1) *Ephedrine;* (2) *Isometheptene.*

(b) Name a potent *non*adrenergic vasopressor drug and indicate a possible advantage that it may have over levarterenol.

BIBLIOGRAPHY

Baker, A. G.: Sublingual treatment of bronchial asthma with a potentiated isoproterenol preparation. Ann. Allergy, *11*:49, 1953 (Jan.–Feb.).

Bradley, E. D., and Weil, M. H.: Vasopressor and vasodilator drugs in the treatment of shock. *In* Symposium on Treatment of Shock. Modern Treatment, *4*:243, 1967 (March).

Bresnick, E., *et al.*: Evaluation of therapeutic substances for relief of bronchospasm. V. Adrenergic Agents. J. Clin. Invest., *28*:1182, 1949.

Freedman, B. J.: Accidental adrenalin overdosage and its treatment. Lancet, *2*:575, 1955.

Gay, L. N., and Long, J. W.: Clinical evaluation of isopropyl epinephrine in management of bronchial asthma. J.A.M.A., *139*:452, 1949.

Haggerty, R. J.: Levarterenol for shock. Am. J. Nurs., *58*:1243, 1958.

Kuhn, L. A.: Treatment of cardiogenic shock. *In* Symposium on Treatment of Shock. Modern Treatment, *4*:299, 1967 (March).

Marshall, R. J., and Darby, T. D.: Newer agents in the treatment of shock. Med. Clin. N. Am., *48*:311, 1964 (March).

Miller, A. J., and Moser, E. A.: Arterenol therapy for shock after acute myocardial infarction and pulmonary embolization. J.A.M.A., *169*:2000, 1959.

Mills, L. C., *et al.*: Treatment of shock with sympathicomimetic drugs. Arch. Int. Med., *106*:816, 1960.

Page, I. H., and Bumpus, F. M.: A new hormone. Angiotensin. Clin. Pharmacol. Ther., *3*:758, 1962.

Rodman, M. J.: Drugs to treat shock. R.N., *28*:65, 1965 (March).

Simard, O. M.: Nursing care during levarterenol therapy. Am. J. Nurs., *58*:1244, 1958.

Von Euler, U. S.: Epinephrine and norepinephrine: actions and uses in man. Clin. Pharmacol. Ther., *1*:65, 1960.

Autonomic Blocking Agents

General Considerations. We have seen (Chap. 14) that certain natural and synthetic substances are able to interfere with the transmission of impulses from nerve endings to the cells that normally respond to such signals. When these cells, which may be other neurons, smooth or skeletal muscle fibers, or the secretory cells of exocrine glands, fail to receive the impulses which ordinarily activate them, their normal functioning is reduced.

Thus, blockade of synaptic transmission at autonomic ganglia leads to a reduction in the number of nerve impulses passing to peripheral effector cells by way of postganglionic nerve fibers. Similarly, inhibition of nerve impulse transmission to muscles makes them relax or become paralyzed, and cutting off the streams of nervous stimuli to gland cells reduces or stops their secretions.

In this chapter we shall take up four major classes of blocking agents:

1. Those that keep acetylcholine molecules from fulfilling their impulse-transmitting function at tissues and organs that are innervated by *postganglionic cholinergic nerve fibers* (i.e., so-called *anticholinergic* or *antimuscarinic agents*)

2. Those that interfere with cholinergic transmission from *somatic motor fibers* to *skeletal muscles* (i.e., the *neuromuscular blocking agents*)

3. Agents that keep acetylcholine from activating the neurons in *autonomic ganglia* (i.e., *ganglionic blocking agents*)

4. Drugs that act in various ways to reduce the transmission of nerve impulses to those tissues that are innervated by *sympathetic postganglionic fibers* (i.e., the *adrenergic blocking* or *antiadrenergic agents*)

ANTIMUSCARINIC-TYPE CHOLINERGIC BLOCKING DRUGS

The drugs discussed in this section act primarily by preventing acetylcholine from exerting its neuro-

transmitter action between postganglionic cholinergic nerves and the structures which they innervate—the autonomic neuroeffectors of *smooth* and *cardiac muscles* and of *exocrine glands*. The action of acetylcholine at these cholinotropic structures is called *muscarinic* because the mushroom alkaloid, muscarine, acts almost exclusively at cholinergic receptor sites of this particular type (Chap. 14).

Thus, these drugs, which interfere most markedly with cholinergic transmission at *postganglionic neuroeffectors* rather than at autonomic ganglia or at the neuromuscular junctions in skeletal muscles, are called *antimuscarinic* agents. The term *anticholinergic* also adequately describes this type of cholinergic blocking drug. Such agents are sometimes also referred to as *parasympatholytic*—a term that emphasizes their ability to prevent the effects of acetylcholine released by parasympathetic nerve endings—but this designation is not adequately inclusive. For, as indicated in Chapter 14, some *sympathetic* nerve endings release acetylcholine at postganglionic receptor sites, and the anticholinergic drugs of the antimuscarinic type are able to keep the neurohormone from exerting its effects at these *nonparasympathetically* innervated structures—for example, the sweat glands and certain blood vessel walls.

Mechanism of Action

The drugs of this class have a particular affinity for the cholinergic receptor sites of various visceral effector organs. However, when the molecules of one of these drugs (*atropine,* for example) combine with the receptor substance of muscle and gland cells, this reaction does not trigger the series of events which acetylcholine ordinarily sets off. On the contrary, because these blocking molecules keep the acetylcholine released by nerve endings from making the necessary attachment to the receptors, cellular function fails.

Thus, the action of these anticholinergic drugs is a prime example of how foreign chemicals often compete with natural substances to inhibit normal biochemical activity and physiological function (Chap. 2). Such *competitive inhibition* or *antagonism* can sometimes be overcome by raising the local level of acetylcholine at the postganglionic cholinergic receptor sites. Thus, the anticholinesterase agents (Chap. 15), which act indirectly to increase the concentration of acetylcholine, can sometimes counteract the actions of atropine; and of course, atropine is the antidote for overdosage of these cholinesterase-inhibiting chemicals.

Natural and Synthetic Anticholinergic Substances

The earliest (and still the most important) source of chemicals with cholinergic blocking action was the potato plant family, the Solanaceae. The alkaloids *atropine* (dl-hyoscyamine) and *scopolamine* (l-hyoscine) were extracted from plants such as deadly nightshade (*Atropa belladonna*), henbane (*Hyoscyamus niger*), and Jimson weed (*Datura stramonium*). They are available both as the purified plant princi-

ples and in the form of galenical preparations, including the tincture, extract, and fluidextract of Belladonna (Table 17-1).

Because of the many undesired secondary effects of these substances, chemists have long tried to synthesize drugs with an affinity greater than that of the natural alkaloids for specific sites, such as the gastrointestinal tract. At first, they tried to modify the plant derivatives themselves by treating them chemically. *Homatropine*, which is used mainly for its effects on the eye, is such a semisynthetic derivative. Later, they learned that when the nitrogen atom of the natural alkaloid was quaternized (i.e., altered so that it combines with four, rather than three, other chemical groups), these quaternary ammonium derivatives differed in some of their pharmacological properties.

For example, atropine *methylnitrate*, scopolamine *methylbromide*, and homatropine *methylbromide* (Table 17-1) have fewer C.N.S. side effects, since quaternization reduces a drug's ability to enter the central nervous system. At the same time, these drugs are

TABLE 17-1

NATURAL SOLANACEOUS ALKALOIDS, PREPARATIONS, AND DERIVATIVES

Nonproprietary Name (and Trade Name or Synonym)	Dose
Atropine N.F.	400 mcg.
Atropine methylnitrate (Eumydrin; etc.)	1 mg.
Atropine oxide HCl (genatropine)	0.2 mg.
Atropine sulfate U.S.P.	0.3 to 1.2 mg.
Atropine tannate (Atratan, tantropin)	1 mg.
Atropine tartrate	1 mg.
Belladonna Extract N.F.	15 mg.
Belladonna Leaf Fluidextract N.F.	0.06 ml.
Belladonna (Leaf) Tincture U.S.P.	0.3 to 2.4 ml.
Eucatropine HCl U.S.P.	Topically, 0.1 ml. of a 2 to 5% sol.
Homatropine hydrobromide U.S.P.	Topically, 0.1 ml. of a 1 to 2% sol.
Homatropine methylbromide N.F.	5 mg.
Hyoscyamine sulfate N.F.	250 mcg. to 1.0 mg.
Methscopolamine bromide N.F. (Lescopine; methylscopolammonium bromide; Pamine; scopolamine methylbromide)	2.5 mg. oral; 0.5 mg., parenteral
Methscopolamine nitrate (Skopalate; Skopyl)	2 to 4 mg. oral; 0.25 to 0.5 mg., parenteral; 300 to 800 mcg., oral or S.C.
Scopolamine hydrobromide U.S.P.	Topically, 0.1 ml. of a 0.2% sol.

TABLE 17-2

SYNTHETIC ANTISPASMODIC DRUGS *

Nonproprietary Name	Trade Name	Dosage
Adiphenine HCl	Trasentine	75 to 150 mg.
Alverine citrate	Spacolin	120 mg.
Amprotropine phosphate	Syntropan	50 to 100 mg.
Anisotropine methylbromide	Valpin	10 mg.
Carbofluorene HCl	Pavatrine	125 mg.
Dicyclomine HCl	Bentyl	10 to 20 mg.
Methixene HCl	Trest	1 mg.
Triphenamil HCl	Trocinate	100 to 400 mg.

* These drugs are claimed to act mainly by a *direct* action on the contractile mechanism of smooth muscle and only slightly by producing blockade of parasympathetic motor impulses. This is the basis for claims that they are likely to cause few atropinelike side effects. Nevertheless, caution is required in administering these drugs to patients for whom belladonna alkaloids and synthetic anticholinergic drugs would be contraindicated.

less readily absorbed when taken by mouth because quaternization interferes with absorption through the gastrointestinal mucosa. The highly ionized quaternary ammonium compounds penetrate cell membranes poorly (see Chap. 2).

Finally, the search for synthetic anticholinergic drugs led to the development of drugs quite different from the alkaloids in chemical structure. Some of these, such as *dicyclomine* (Bentyl), etc. (Table 17-2), are so different that they produce few of the desirable actions of atropine, as well as less of the side-effects typical of that alkaloid. Others are synthetic quaternary ammonium compounds that are claimed to have more potent gastrointestinal actions than the natural products. However, the advantages claimed for the prototype of this group, methantheline bromide (Banthine) and its successors (Table 17-3 and Chap. 38), are said by some authorities to be unimportant (see discussion below).

Pharmacological Actions and Their Clinical Significance

Atropine, the prototype anticholinergic agent, has many and varied peripheral and central actions. These make it potentially useful in the treatment of a large number of clinical conditions, but they also account for the numerous discomforting side effects that often accompany its use. Thus, when atropine-type drugs are employed clinically for treating gastrointestinal ailments, their effects are not limited to the G.I. tract. This relative lack of specificity results in the development of many undesirable secondary effects.

Atropine and related drugs do, however, seem to have a greater affinity for some sites than for others. The junctions between the postganglionic nerve endings and the salivary and sweat gland cells, for example, are blocked by much smaller doses than are needed to reduce secretion by the gastric glands. Similarly, the ocular effects of these drugs often come on before those on the smooth muscle of the gastrointestinal and genitourinary tracts.

What is the clinical significance of this pattern of relative selectivity? In practice, it means that doses of these drugs capable of relaxing gastrointestinal spasm and reducing gastric secretions will almost inevitably cause mouth dryness and blurring of vision. In addition, the development of these ocular effects in the ulcer patient who also happens to have narrow angle glaucoma is a special danger. On the other hand, such so-called side effects may, in some situations, be the main action that the doctor (e.g., the ophthalmologist) wants to elicit. Thus, atropine is a prime example of a drug with which one man's side effect is often another's therapeutic action!

In the following discussion of the pharmacological effects of atropinelike drugs on the various organs, structures, and systems, we shall proceed as follows: After indicating what atropine and its relatives do to alter the functioning of the particular tissue, we shall point out the clinically significant aspects of each particular action. Thus, we shall take up, together, both the therapeutic use of each action and also its undesirable aspects, particularly those that make atropine and similar drugs unsafe for patients with various pathological states that increase susceptibility to such adverse actions. All the therapeutic uses, side effects, cautions, and contraindications will be found summarized on pages 266 to 268.

Glandular Secretions. The effects of atropine, scopolamine, and other anticholinergic drugs on glandular secretion are probably less useful therapeutically than the relaxant action of these drugs on smooth muscle. However, since their effects on the salivary and certain other glands are seen with the smallest doses of these drugs and cause the side effects that the patient is most likely to complain about, we shall discuss them first.

Salivary gland secretion is readily reduced by atropine, which blocks transmission of the parasympathetic postganglionic impulses that ordinarily induce secretion of watery saliva. The patient's mouth becomes uncomfortably dry, and he may have difficulty in swallowing and talking. Such xerostomia may be useful for patients with parkinsonism who sometimes drool, but it is usually considered an undesirable side effect in most conditions for which these drugs are employed.

The patient who receives atropine preoperatively is especially likely to have a very dry mouth after surgery. Thus the nurse should see that he gets thorough mouth care, including frequent rinsings and cold drinks if oral fluids are permitted. Similar measures may be suggested to patients taking belladonna derivatives for gastrointestinal disorders or other conditions, and the patient should be told that sucking hard candies or chewing a stick of gum may stimulate some salivation when xerostomia is especially discomforting. It may help, too, to let him know that tablets containing these products are to be swallowed and not chewed. Methantheline (Banthine) is especially bitter, and the patient needn't add its bitterness to the dryness that the drug will induce anyway.

Respiratory tract gland secretion is also suppressed. The inhibition of nasal secretion is the basis for the use of belladonna alkaloids in various products sold to the public for treating symptoms of the common cold (e.g., Contac). One of the main reasons for administering atropine or scopolamine preoperatively is to reduce the likelihood that an inhalation anesthetic such as ether will stimulate an excessive flow of bronchial, nasal and salivary gland secretion, which might interfere with the patient's breathing. These drugs also tend to reduce the reflex laryngospasm which is sometimes set off by such secretions.

The reduction of bronchial gland secretions is occasionally useful in the treatment of an allergy-induced cough. More often, it is considered undesirable for patients with chronic respiratory difficulties, for, when respiratory tract fluids are reduced, they may thicken, harden and plug up narrow passages. Thus, though the solanaceous alkaloids can sometimes relax constricted bronchial muscles, and stramonium leaves are a constituent of so-called "asthma cigarettes," the usefulness of the mild bronchodilator action of atropine is outweighed by the danger that the drug may make the bronchial secretions too viscid to be readily removed by coughing. This is one reason why adrenergic drugs (Chap. 16) are preferred to anticholinergic agents for treating asthmatic patients. However, when excessive bronchosecretion and bronchoconstriction has been caused by overdosage of cholinergic drugs

TABLE 17-3
SYNTHETIC ANTICHOLINERGIC AGENTS USED IN TREATING PEPTIC ULCER *

Nonproprietary Name	Trade Name	Dosage
Aminopentamide	Centrine	0.5 mg.
Dibutoline sulfate	Dibuline	25 mg.
Diphemanil methylsulfate N.F.	Prantal	100 mg., oral; 25 mg., parenteral
Glycopyrrolate	Robinul	1 mg.
Hexocyclium methylsulfate	Tral	25 mg.
Isopropamide iodide	Darbid	5 mg.
Mepenzolate bromide	Cantil	25 mg.
Mepiperphenidol bromide	Darstine	50 to 100 mg.
Methantheline bromide N.F.	Banthine	50 mg.
Oxyphencyclimine HCl	Daricon	10 mg.
Oxyphenonium bromide	Antrenyl	10 mg., oral; 1 to 2 mg., parenteral
Penthienate bromide N.F.	Monodral	5 mg.
Pipenzolate bromide	Piptal	5 to 10 mg.
Piperidolate HCl	Dactil	50 mg.
Poldine methylsulfate	Nacton	5 to 10 mg.
Propantheline U.S.P.	Pro-Banthine	15 mg.
Tricyclamol chloride	Elorine; Tricoloid	50 mg.
Tridihexethyl chloride N.F.	Pathilon	25 to 50 mg.
Valethamate bromide	Murel	10 to 20 mg.

* See Chapter 38 for discussion of the use of these compounds in the management of peptic ulcer.

(as in the management of myasthenia gravis patients, or in poisoning by certain insecticides and the nerve gases), atropine is the antidote of choice.

The sweat glands, as we have seen, receive sympathetic postganglionic nerve fibers which release acetylcholine rather than the adrenergic transmitter. Anticholinergic drugs effectively keeping acetylcholine (and cholinergic drugs also) from reaching the cholinotropic receptors in sweat gland cells and setting off secretion of perspiration. This action has proved useful in some patients with hyperhidrosis. However, the possibility of systemic side effects prohibit its routine use for reducing perspiration. Attempts to apply anticholinergic drugs locally in the form of antiperspirant creams and lotions have not proved successful, despite occasional claims to the contrary, apparently because these potent drugs do not penetrate readily down to the secreting glands deep in the skin.

Infants and young children often become flushed after atropine has been administered preoperatively. The nurse should recognize that this is a common cutaneous side effect caused mainly by the drug's vasodilating action, and parents, if present, can be spared needless worry that the child has spiked a sudden fever, if this is explained to them.

On the other hand, atropine overdosage can cause an elevation of temperature. This is especially likely in warm weather when the body rids itself of excess heat mainly by evaporation of fluid (perspiration) from the skin. By causing cessation of sweating, atropine-type drugs may sometimes precipitate a dangerous hyperpyrexic reaction. The nurse should be alert to the possibility that a feverish patient with a hot, dry flushed skin or even a scarlatiniform rash may be suffering from atropine poisoning.

Cardiovascular Actions. The flushing mentioned above, which is the result of atropine-induced dilation of blood vessels in the skin, is one of the drug's few vascular effects. Atropine has little effect upon blood vessels in general, and consequently it does not affect blood pressure significantly. Its cardiac effects, on the other hand, are often quite marked.

Small doses of atropine tend to slow the heart somewhat—an effect attributed to mild stimulation of the medullary vagal nuclei, which then send their slowing impulses to the heart. With larger doses, however, this central action is counteracted by the peripheral effect of atropine at the vagal neuroeffectors in the sino-auricular (S-A) node. Blockade of the vagal impulses by atropine permits sympathetic cardioacceleratory impulses to predominate, and the heart rate speeds up.

Atropine-induced tachycardia is not in itself clinically useful. In fact, it is usually considered a side effect that is especially undesirable for patients with a history of heart disease. Thus, the nurse should always be alert to changes in pulse rate after atropine has been administered. Atropine and related drugs must be used cautiously, if at all, in patients with angina pectoris, because they may set off an episode of coronary insufficiency. Too rapid heart action may also cause cardiac decompensation in patients with heart failure, by interfering with diastolic filling of the heart's chambers and, thus, reducing cardiac output.

The vagal blocking action of atropine is, however, useful for treating cardiac conditions marked by excessive vagal tone. The marked slowing of the heart in patients with carotid sinus syndrome can often be prevented or counteracted with atropine. Such patients suffer from a hyperactive reflex, so that even a slight pressure on the neck sets off afferent impulses which bombard the vagal center. Atropine premedication keeps the resulting vagal efferent impulses from reaching the atrial pacemaker and slowing or stopping the heart. This protective effect against reflex vagal inhibition of the heart is another reason (besides the reduction of secretion) for the use of atropine prior to administration of inhalation anesthetics.

The ocular effects of atropinelike drugs are of considerable clinical importance. Atropine blocks the tonic impulses that pass by way of parasympathetic postganglionic (ciliary) nerve fibers to the sphincter muscle of the iris and to the ciliary muscles which control the movements of the lens. As a result of the loss of tone in these muscles, the pupil becomes widely dilated (mydriasis) and accommodation for near vision is lost (cycloplegia).

Mydriasis is in itself not usually serious. In fact, Italian ladies of Renaissance days used to put belladonna drops in their eyes to dilate their pupils for a desired cosmetic effect. (Belladonna means "beautiful lady," and the girl's date may have admired her luminous widely dilated pupils, but the dark-eyed beauty probably saw little of her escort because of the blurring of her own vision brought about by the drug's cycloplegic action.) However, if a patient in whose eyes an atropinelike drug was instilled complains of discomfort from the greater amount of light reaching the retina, the nurse should advise him to wear dark glasses to counteract the photophobia.

Mydriasis and the loss of the light reflex, which often also occurs, allow the ophthalmologist to examine the inner structures of the eye, including the retina and optic disk, more easily. Similarly, production of cycloplegia permits the doctor to examine the eye for refractive errors without interference by involuntary adjustments of the lens. Relaxation—even paralysis—of these smooth muscles of the eye is desirable in treating various inflammatory ocular disorders. (For a more detailed discussion, see Chap. 42.)

The ocular actions of atropinic drugs may be brought about inadvertently when the drugs are given orally or parenterally for other purposes. Blurring of vision because of partial cycloplegia is an annoyance for patients who wish to read or do other work requiring near vision. The thoughtful nurse can help the patient plan his work by letting him know when he can expect the effects of a topically applied drug to wear off. Elderly patients who may not be too steady on their feet should be warned to take special care in going down stairs, if their vision becomes blurred while taking belladonna-type drugs. In fact, the nurse should briefly mention the possible occurrence of blurred vision, mouth dryness and other atropine-type side effects to all patients taking such drugs, to prevent their becoming alarmed, thinking that these symptoms signal some serious disorder. They should also be told that, although such side effects are not usually serious, they should report any marked visual changes to the doctor.

More serious than mere discomfort is the danger that these drugs may precipitate an attack of glaucoma. This is not likely to happen to people with normal eyes. However, in those with a congenitally narrow angle in the anterior chamber of the eye, the effect of these drugs on ocular smooth muscle may lead to a sharp rise in intraocular pressure. The relaxing or paralyzing action of atropine upon the iris and ciliary bodies may make these structures crowd back into the angle. This may then block the canals through which the aqueous humor ordinarily drains, thus resulting in a build-up of hydrostatic pressure within the chamber. For this reason anticholinergic drugs are always contraindicated for patients with a history of glaucoma. Their use in patients over 40 years old also requires caution, since in most people ocular smooth muscles tend to undergo changes at around that age which make them more susceptible to attacks of glaucoma.

Smooth muscles of various visceral organs are relaxed by the antispasmodic action of atropine and related natural and synthetic drugs. This is especially desirable in conditions marked by painful hypertonicity and hypermotility of the gastrointestinal and genitourinary system smooth musculature.

The urinary bladder becomes irritable when infected, and reflex spasms then cause frequent painful micturition. Such frequency and urgency in cystitis may be reduced somewhat by administration of adequate doses of belladonna derivatives or of the synthetic anticholinergics. These drugs diminish the number of motor impulses that pass to the fundus of the bladder by way of parasympathetic (sacral) postganglionic nerve fibers. This quieting action on the detrusor muscle, together with the drug's ability to increase the tone of the trigone and vesical sphincter, is useful for increasing the capacity of the bladder—an effect desirable in paraplegics and others with urinary incontinence, and in treating children with nocturnal enuresis.

Atropine is often combined with morphine and meperidine (Demerol) in the treatment of patients with renal or biliary colic. The purpose is to bring about relaxation of the extremely painful reflex spasm set off by the presence of a stone in the ureter or bile duct. Actually, the relaxant action of atropine on these smooth muscles is not very strong. However, the atropine does, at least, help to counteract the spasmogenic effect of morphine. Morphine, which is often very effective for relieving pain by its central analgesic action, actually tends to increase muscle spasm by its peripheral action.

The loss of bladder tone produced by atropine may make micturition difficult in some cases. This is especially true in elderly men with an enlarged prostate gland which already partially obstructs urine flow. Thus, the drug is contraindicated in patients with prostatic hypertrophy, because its use may result in dysuria and urinary retention. If the nurse notes that a man of upper middle age who is receiving atropine for peptic ulcer tends to get up and go to the bathroom every two hours or so, she should report this to the doctor, who may not know that the patient has a voiding problem. Often the patient fails to tell the physician because he is embarrassed or does not understand the significance of this troubling symptom.

Uterine spasm is sometimes treated with belladonna derivatives. These drugs, which have little if any relaxant effect on the smooth muscle of this organ, are often prescribed for the treatment of dysmenorrhea. Some gynecologists think that the relief often reported is the result of a placebo effect or the presence of aspirin-type analgesics in the combination rather than by any atropine-induced uterine relaxation.

The gastrointestinal actions of the anticholinergic drugs are the ones of greatest clinical importance. Atropinelike drugs are used mainly to reduce gastrointestinal spasm and secretions in conditions marked by hypermotility, hypertonicity of smooth muscle and the hypersecretion of gastric acid. Among the disorders in which these drugs are employed are peptic ulcer, gastritis, cardiospasm, pylorospasm, ileitis, diverticulitis, ulcerative colitis and other functional and organic inflammatory and infectious diseases of the upper and lower gastrointestinal tract.

The use of anticholinergic drugs as adjuncts in the management of acid peptic disease is discussed in more detail in Chapter 38. We need only note here that none of these drugs is entirely satisfactory for this purpose. For although they reduce painful reflex spasms set off by the action of acid gastric secretions on naked nerve endings in the ulcer crater, their ability to inhibit production of the acid itself and to speed healing of the eroded mucosa is limited. The large doses of belladonna alkaloids required for adequate antisecretory action almost invariably cause dry mouth, blurred vision and other side effects.

Such adverse reactions also occur with the somewhat more potent synthetic quaternary ammonium antisecretory agents such as methantheline (Banthine) and propantheline (Pro-Banthine) (see Drug Digest) and their successors (Table 17-3). Drugs of this kind are said to produce their antisecretory effects by a double action—blockade of parasympathetic ganglia, as well as of the postganglionic sites; however, the undesired effects of adequate doses often run parallel with increased therapeutic activity.

Certain of the synthetic antispasmodics discovered in the search for safer and more effective belladonna-like drugs cause fewer atropine-type side effects. However, these drugs (dicyclomine (Bentyl) and the others listed in Table 17-2) are not as effective as the belladonna derivatives for relaxing spasm, and they are almost entirely lacking in antisecretory activity. Thus, these drugs are rarely used in peptic ulcer and are reserved instead for patients with intestinal hypermotility and spasm who cannot tolerate the belladonna alkaloids.

In such conditions, these spasmolytics and inhibitors of intestinal motility sometimes provide symptomatic relief of both diarrhea and constipation. Combined with opiates such as paregoric, these drugs often control the patient's cramps and reduce the number of loose bowel movements. On the other hand, combined with sedatives or tranquilizers, these antispasmodics sometimes help patients with constipation of the spastic type by relaxing the hypertonic intestinal segment. Generally, however, these drugs tend to *cause* constipation by reducing intestinal tone and motility. More serious than this side effect is the possibility of obstruction in patients in whom the G.I. tract has already been narrowed by disease. This is why anticholinergic drugs are contraindicated for peptic ulcer patients with pyloric stenosis.

Central Nervous System. In addition to their peripheral actions, the belladonna alkaloids possess central effects of clinical importance. Atropine and scopolamine both penetrate into the central nervous system, and both presumably block impulse transmission by acetylcholine at certain central synapses. However, the two alkaloids differ somewhat in their effects. Scopolamine produces mainly depressant effects; the actions of atropine on the cerebral centers and medulla are mainly those of a mild stimulant.

Scopolamine acts in relatively small doses to depress the reticular activating system (Chap. 5) and produce drowsiness. This action contributes to the calming and amnesic effects sought when this drug is administered alone or with morphine prior to anesthesia in surgery and obstetrics. However, scopolamine may cause considerable restlessness and even delirium, especially in patients who are in pain. Some doctors now prefer to use a phenothiazine tranquilizer preoperatively. These major tranquilizers have largely replaced scopolamine as a means of quieting agitated patients also.

Small oral doses of scopolamine, which are not nearly as effective for sedation as the parenterally administered drug, are often combined with centrally depressant drugs of the antihistamine class in nostrums sold directly to the public as "safe sleep" products, so-called and advertised on television. Similar mixtures are sometimes offered for sale as motion sickness preventives. Just how scopolamine exerts its prophylactic action in this condition is still uncertain. It may do so by blocking cholinergic transmission of nerve impulses originating in the inner ear. Atropine and the newer drugs such as dimenhydrinate (Dramamine) which are used for the same purpose also probably act by such a central anticholinergic mechanism (see the section on Antiemetic Drugs in Chap. 38).

The effectiveness of atropine in preventing convulsions and respiratory failure caused by organophosphate insecticides and the nerve gases (Chap. 15) stems from its central actions. Administration of massive doses of atropine may be employed for this purpose without danger, to counteract the high levels of acetylcholine that accumulate in the brain and elsewhere in poisoning by these chemicals. The bronchial actions of atropine are also useful for maintenance of normal breathing, but this drug does not counteract the paralysis of respiratory skeletal muscles that sometimes results from overdosage of anticholinesterase agents.

The central effects of the belladonna alkaloids become prominent when these drugs are taken in toxic amounts. These effects include restlessness, dizziness, disorientation and delirium. This syndrome together with the peripheral effects described previously has evoked the following descriptive diagnosis of atropine poisoning: "Hot as a hare, blind as a bat, dry as a bone, red as a beet, and mad as a hatter."

Such poisonings sometimes occur when children ingest Jimson weed seeds or people pick the leaves of a solanaceous plant and use them in preparing a salad. Infants given overdoses of belladonna preparations for colic or treated with eye drops which may be absorbed from the ocular and nasal mucosa, are sometimes the victims of atropine poisoning. Cholinergic drugs such as pilocarpine help to antagonize the discomforting peripheral actions of atropine on the eyes, the skin and mucous membranes, and the heart, but these antidotes do not readily counteract the more dangerous central effects of atropine toxicity. Death, when it occurs, is usually the result of respiratory center paralysis. Fortunately, the margin of safety is relatively wide, and patients usually respond to treatment with various supportive measures.

Fatal reactions to overdosage with atropine medication are rare despite the patient's great discomfort and the many alarming signs and symptoms which may occur. However, the drug is a potent one and is administered in very small dosage. Thus, the nurse should take special care to see that the patient is receiving the right dose. The small doses of this drug are sometimes ordered in the apothecary system and at other times in the metric system, which could lead to confusion and result in a child's getting a dangerous overdose. The nurse should be especially cautious when an atropine solution is to be mixed in the same syringe with a narcotic analgesic for preoperative administration.

One advantage of the quaternary-ammonium-type synthetic anticholinergic agents such as methantheline, propantheline and oxyphencyclimine, etc. (Chap. 38) is that they are relatively free of the central side effects seen with the natural belladonna alkaloids. On the other hand, another group of synthetic anticholinergic drugs, of which trihexyphenidyl (Artane, Tremin) is the prototype, are employed in Parkinson's disease mainly for their central antispasmodic actions. The use of these drugs and of the alkaloids atropine and scopolamine in the management of parkinsonism and related conditions is discussed in Chapter 8.

ADRENERGIC BLOCKING AGENTS

General Considerations

We have seen (Chap. 14) that nerve impulses are transmitted from the sympathetic nervous system to muscle and gland cells when the neurohormone *norepinephrine* is released from nerve endings and makes contact with specialized receptors on these effector cells. We have also noted that these sympathetically innervated neuroeffectors may contain adrenergic receptors of two types (termed *alpha* and *beta*) and that the way in which these cells respond to sympathetic nerve impulses and sympathomimetic drugs depends upon which receptors predominate in a particular tissue.

In this section, we shall discuss drugs that interfere with the transmission of nerve impulses to adrenergic neuroeffectors by their ability to occupy adrenoceptive sites of the alpha *or* the beta type. By attaching themselves to these receptors, without themselves evoking any response from muscle or gland cells, the molecules of these adrenergic blocking drugs keep the neurohormone norepinephrine from producing the effects typical of sympathetic nervous system stimulation. In addition, these blocking drugs prevent other sympathomimetic amines such as epinephrine (the adrenal medullary hormone) and isoproterenol (a synthetic catecholamine), and other adrenergic drugs from activating the receptors and calling forth the characteristic cellular responses. These blockers, in fact, prevent cells from responding to adrenergic drugs and circulating catecholamines even more effectively than they block the response to norepinephrine released by sympathetic nerve impulses.

Alpha-Type Adrenergic Blocking Agents

In theory, adrenergic blocking drugs should be just as effective in counteracting hyperactivity of the *sympathetic* nervous system as atropine and the other cholinergic blocking drugs have proved to be in overcoming the effects of excessive *para*sympathetic nervous system activity. In practice, this has not proved to be true, and the adrenergic blockers play only a minor role in clinical practice compared to the anticholinergic drugs discussed in the previous section of this chapter.

There are various reasons for this, but the most important is probably the relative lack of specificity of the currently available adrenergic blocking drugs. Not only do these drugs *not* block *all* adrenergic receptors, but the doses required to reduce transmission of sympathetic nervous impulses are often so high that the drugs act at various *non*adrenergic peripheral and central sites. This may cause unwanted *side effects* that make the physiological cost of using these drugs in clinical practice prohibitively high.

Most of these drugs are unable to prevent the effects of sympathetic stimulation of the heart. Most adrenergic blockers act *only* at the *alpha*-type receptors, and, since the cardiac receptors are of the *beta* type, these drugs do nothing to reduce the rate or alter the rhythm of a heart that is beating rapidly and irregularly, nor do they lessen the force of the heart that is working too hard. In fact, as we shall see, some adrenergic blocking drugs tend to make the heart beat even more inefficiently by their direct and indirect (reflex) actions. (For review of autonomic nervous stimulation see Table 14-2.)

Pharmacological Action. The most important blocking action of the drugs that more or less specifically block the alpha-type adrenergic receptors develops at the alpha receptors of *vascular smooth muscle* cells. By occupying these receptors, molecules of these drugs prevent the excitatory response to sympathetic stimulation and to adrenergic drugs, which, it will be recalled, results typically in tonic constriction of the blood vessels. Other excitatory effects of sympathetic stimulation (for example, contraction of the radial muscle of the iris) may also be blocked, but pharmacological effects of the alpha adrenergic blockers that affect the patient's blood vessels are by far the most clinically significant.

As you should be able to predict (Chap. 14), blockade of tonic sympathetic nerve impulses to a patient's arterioles results in relaxation of the smooth muscle walls. The resulting dilatation of the vessel should then lead to two effects: (1) an increased local flow of blood into the skin and other organs, and (2) a tendency for the patient's arterial blood pressure to fall as a result of reduced peripheral resistance. Thus, we should expect these drugs to be tried in clinical conditions marked by poor local circulation or by excessively high diastolic blood pressure. These conditions (peripheral vascular disease and hypertension, for instance) have, indeed, been the ones for which the alpha adrenergic blockers have been employed—but, unfortunately, with only indifferent success.

Clinical Uses. As indicated in Chapter 23, one of the most important ways by which today's antihypertensive drugs reduce the blood pressure of patients with *essential hypertension* is by reduction of the sympathetic nervous outflow to the blood vessels. Among the drugs that do this are the ganglionic blocking agents and the adrenergic neuron blocking agents (see below). One would assume that the alpha adrenergic blocking drugs would be at least equally effective, but this has not proved to be the case in clinical practice.

One of the main reasons for the disappointing performance of these drugs in most cases of high blood pressure is the fact that they often cause adverse cardiac effects. Thus, although their blockade of alpha adrenergic receptors in the patient's blood vessels brings about a drop in pressure (especially when he is in the standing position), their failure to block beta receptors in the heart results in reflex tachycardia. (Some adrenergic blockers such as *tolazoline* (see Drug Digest) also stimulate the heart directly.) Such an increase in the speed and work of the hypertensive patient's heart can cause coronary insufficiency and set off anginal attacks, or it may even throw the patient into heart failure. This is, of course, particularly likely in patients with a history of hypertensive heart disease.

Attempts have been made to overcome this difficulty by combining an alpha adrenergic blocker with antihypertensive drugs that slow the heart instead of speeding it up. For example, phenoxybenzamine (Dibenzyline; see Drug Digest and Table 26-1) is available in combination with rauwolfia and veratrum alkaloids—hypotensive drugs with a bradycrotic action. However, such combinations are not widely used, and the use of phenoxybenzamine alone in fully effective doses has the further drawback of frequently causing episodes of postural hypotension. (See Chap. 23 for a full discussion of the dangers of such orthostatic hypotensive episodes and the part that the nurse may play in helping the patient avoid this adverse effect.)

These and other side effects of the large doses needed to control the blood pressure of patients with essential, or primary, hypertension limit the usefulness of the alpha adrenergic blocking drugs. In addition, patients tend to become resistant to the hypotensive

action of these drugs. However, some of these drugs have proved useful for both treatment and diagnosis of a *secondary* hypertension which develops in patients with *pheochromocytomata*. These are chromaffin cell tumors of the adrenal glands and elsewhere which secrete excessive amounts of epinephrine and norepinephrine into the patient's blood stream. The abnormally high levels of these sympathomimetic substances cause chronically sustained high blood pressure in some patients and sudden attacks of paroxysmal hypertension in others.

Diagnosis and Treatment of Pheochromocytoma. The use of alpha-type adrenergic blocking agents in the diagnosis and treatment of chromaffin-cell-tumor hypertension is based upon the ability of even very small doses of these drugs to block the effects of circulating catecholamines upon the patient's arterioles. This adrenergic blocking action counteracts the tendency toward generalized vasoconstriction and the resulting rise in blood pressure which otherwise would be produced when epinephrine and norepinephrine released by the tumor tissues arrive by way of the blood stream at reactive adrenergic receptors in the vessels.

Administration of a long-acting adrenergic blocking agent such as phenoxybenzamine (Dibenzyline) is useful for controlling hypertension in the medical management of pheochromocytoma. However, the definitive treatment of this condition is not medical, since a complete cure can be achieved only by finding and surgically removing the secreting tumor masses. Thus, the adrenergic blocking drugs are used mainly as a stop-gap measure to control the patient's blood pressure in the interval between the time of discovery of the tumor and surgical excision.

During that time, oral doses of phenoxybenzamine or phentolamine hydrochloride may be administered daily to keep the patient's blood pressure at safe, stable levels (see Table 26-1 for usual dosage of these drugs). When the patient is being prepared for surgery, he may receive preoperative injections of phentolamine mesylate (Regitine; see Drug Digest) to reduce the danger from sudden spurts of epinephrine released from the tumor tissues during anesthesia and emotional excitement. Similarly, during the operation, when manipulation of the tumor may force jets of epinephrine into the patient's blood stream, phentolamine may again be injected by vein to control the adverse effects of high levels of circulating catecholamines on the patient's blood pressure, heart rate, and respiration.

There is some danger that the adrenergic blocking agent may make the patient's blood pressure fall too low, particularly in the period following removal of the tumor, at which time the patient's pressure tends to plummet, in any case. Phentolamine, a short-acting adrenergic blocker, is preferred for this reason. Since its effects tend to wear off rather rapidly, it does not cause prolonged hypotension. Similarly, since such postoperative shock states often require treatment with the adrenergic vasopressor drug levarterenol (Levophed), the doctor prefers to employ a transiently acting adrenergic blocker during the operation so that there will be no postoperative residual action to counteract adrenergic vasopressor drug treatment. Local infiltration of phentolamine is sometimes used to prevent necrosis, in cutaneous ischemia from levarterenol that has leaked into the tissues during intravenous administration (see Chap. 16).

The fact that phentolamine is a relatively weak blocker of sympathetic nerve impulses is also a factor in its efficacy when used for the differential diagnosis of pheochromocytoma. This screening test is based upon the fact that a dose of phentolamine, too small to lower blood pressure by blocking tonic vasoconstrictor nerve impulses, is able to prevent the adrenergic receptors from responding to circulating catecholamines, thus causing a sharp drop in blood pressure that had been elevated by abnormally high levels of these sympathomimetic substances.

A *positive* test is one in which the patient's blood pressure quickly falls more than 35 mm. systolic and 25 mm. diastolic. Such a response to the phentolamine screening test in a patient with sustained hypertension alerts the doctor to the possibility that his patient's high blood pressure may be the result of tumor-produced catecholamines. He then orders a battery of other studies, including so-called provocative tests employing histamine, methacholine or other drugs with a direct stimulating action on chromaffin tumor tissue. New methods for detecting excessive catecholamines and their metabolites in blood and urine are now available for confirming the diagnosis.

Patients whose high blood pressure stays steady or changes very little following a diagnostic injection of phentolamine are considered to have hypertension of other etiology. Because false negative and false positive tests sometimes occur in patients taking other drugs, patients should be told to take no medication for at least a day or two before being tested with phentolamine for pheochromocytoma.

Other Clinical Uses. The adrenergic blocking drugs have their greatest clinical utility in the management of certain peripheral vascular diseases, particularly those in which a strong vasospastic component is responsible for the patient's poor local blood flow. A discussion of the use of these drugs for this purpose appears in Chapter 26; see also Drug Digests for phenoxybenzamine, tolazoline, and azapetine, the adrenergic blockers most commonly used in these conditions.

Other circulatory conditions for which alpha adrenergic blocking agents are being tried experimentally include certain types of circulatory shock, some kinds

of cardiac arrhythmias, and pulmonary edema. In all these situations, it is the reduction in sympathetic vasoconstrictor impulses to the blood vessels that is believed responsible for the desirable hemodynamic effects that result from the administration of these drugs.

In *shock*, for example, even though the alpha adrenergic blockers reduce the blood pressure, they often bring about an increase in cardiac output and an improvement in the perfusion of vital tissues. Patients suffering from severe infection by gram-negative invaders of the blood stream are said to benefit from treatment with alpha adrenergic blockers, because shock caused by bacteremia (*endotoxin shock*) is marked by excessive reflex vasoconstriction.

In such cases, intravenous injection of *phentolamine* or *phenoxybenzamine*, after the blood volume has first been restored by the administration of appropriate fluids, is said to result in improved blood flow. Apparently, these drugs—by reducing peripheral resistance—decrease the heart's work load. Blood pooled in the veins is also then returned to the heart more readily, the cardiac output increases, and the systemic blood flow becomes better. Combined with massive doses of corticosteroids and antibiotics, this treatment with adrenergic blockers is claimed to have proved lifesaving in this particular shock syndrome.

The purported usefulness of these drugs in pulmonary edema is based upon their ability to bring about generalized vasodilatation, thus providing space in the systemic circulation for blood trapped in the pulmonary circulatory tree. Some irregularities of heart beat may also respond to treatment with these drugs. In such cases, the improvement is not the result of the drug's action on the heart but is secondary to the circulatory effects. That is, the drug-induced vasodilation and reduction of blood pressure tend to suppress the potentially dangerous cardiac reflexes thought to be responsible for setting off arrhythmias.

In *glaucoma*, reduction in intraocular pressure may be due, in part, to the miosis, or pupillary constriction, brought about by the blockade of sympathetic dilator impulses to the radial muscle of the iris (see Chap. 42). However, other mechanisms also have been suggested for the fall in intraocular pressure sometimes brought about in acute glaucoma by the administration of certain alpha adrenergic blocking agents.

Beta-Type Adrenergic Blocking Agents

Until recently, the term *adrenergic blocking agent* applied only to drugs that acted at alpha-type receptors. There were no drugs capable of blocking the beta adrenergic receptors in the heart and elsewhere when administered in safe doses. Now, however, a number of such drugs have been developed, some of which have proved effective for the treatment of cardiac arrhythmias and angina pectoris. Such beta adrenergic blockers include the experimental drugs *dichloroisoproterenol* (DCI) and *pronethalol* (nethalide, Alderlin), as well as *propranolol* (Inderal)—the first to be introduced into actual clinical use in this country.

By occupying beta receptors in the heart, these drugs reduce the excitatory responses of the myocardium to cardiac sympathetic nervous stimulation. They do so by keeping the released neurohormone norepinephrine from reaching these receptors and activating a cardioacceleratory or increased contractile response.

This blockade of catecholamines helps to protect the heart of patients with coronary insufficiency from the stimulating effects of excitement and physical stress. By keeping the ischemic heart from being overworked, the drugs often prevent chest pains in such patients. Patients with atrial fibrillation and other heart-speeding arrhythmias, including those caused by digitalis overdosage, have been helped by the ability of these experimental drugs to slow the heart. It must be remembered, however, that a large part of the cardiac reserve depends on the ability to respond to sympathetic stimulation. Thus, the use of drugs of this type, by keeping the heart from being able to react to nerve-released catecholamines, could lead to weakened myocardial contractions, steep drops in blood pressure, and even congestive heart failure. (Further discussion of the clinical indications and potential dangers of beta adrenergic blocking drugs appears in Chaps. 19, 21 and 22.)

Other Inhibitors of Sympathetic Hyperactivity

A number of other drugs act to reduce the effects of hyperactive sympathetic nervous system functioning upon the cardiovascular system. Unlike the adrenergic blocking agents, such drugs act upon the sympathetic nervous pathways rather than upon the receptors of the neuroeffectors or reacting muscle and gland cells. These *non*adrenergic blocking drugs (see Chap. 23) include the ganglionic blocking agents and a group which may be classified as adrenergic *neuron* blocking drugs.

The latter (e.g., *reserpine, guanethidine* and *methyldopa*, among others) also act at the junction between sympathetic postganglionic fibers and neuroeffector cells. However, they differ from the true adrenergic blocking agents in that they affect impulse transmission through their effects upon the *nerve endings* rather than on the responsive muscle or gland cells. That is, these neuron blocking drugs act in one way or another to interfere with the normal rate of release of the sympathetic neurohormone. They may do this by emptying the terminal reservoirs of catecholamines (e.g., the depleting effect of reserpine), or they may, in some cases, somehow keep the neurohormone from being released by the nerve impulses that reach the nerve endings.

GANGLIONIC STIMULANTS AND BLOCKERS

Ganglionic Stimulation and Blockade

We have seen (Chap. 14) that the neurohormone acetylcholine (ACh) is responsible for transmission of nerve impulses from preganglionic to postganglionic nerves in both divisions of the autonomic nervous system. When the neurotransmitter is released by preganglionic nerve impulses from storage sites in the nerve endings of the first neurons in the chain, it acts to depolarize the nerve cell bodies of the second neurons, located in the ganglia. This results in the propagation of nerve impulses that pass down the postganglionic parasympathetic and sympathetic fibers to the smooth muscle and gland cells which they innervate.

This stimulating action of acetylcholine on the ganglia is called nicotinic, because early investigators noted that the tobacco-alkaloid nicotine produced the same sort of stimulating effects as ACh at autonomic ganglia and on skeletal muscles. An excess of nicotine, however, can block ganglionic and skeletal muscle transmission by making the cells insensitive to ACh. Thus, the first stimulating effects of nicotine may be followed by depression and paralysis of the ganglia, if the amount administered is large enough.

Other drugs besides nicotine are able to stimulate or depress the autonomic ganglia. No drugs that act to *stimulate* the ganglia are presently employed clinically. However, when nicotine is inhaled in tobacco smoke it often produces effects on circulatory and gastrointestinal functions that are the result of stimulation of sympathetic and parasympathetic ganglia (see below).

The most important of the drugs with ganglionic effects are those that *block* transmission of nerve impulses through autonomic ganglia. These so-called *ganglionic blocking agents* are used clinically to reduce sympathetic nerve impulse transmission and thus produce effects considered beneficial in certain circulatory diseases. The ganglionic depression which these drugs cause is not preceded by an initial stimulation.

In this chapter, we shall first discuss some points of clinical interest concerning the actions of nicotine. Then, we shall summarize the most important aspects of the pharmacological actions and clinical uses of the ganglionic blocking agents. The details of how these drugs are employed in therapeutics will be discussed in Chapters 23 and 26.

Nicotine

This alkaloid of the tobacco plant causes complex stimulating and, later, depressant effects at many sites throughout the body. These varied actions on the central nervous system and skeletal muscles, as well as upon organs innervated by the autonomic nervous system, are of great interest to experimental pharmacologists and other biological scientists. In fact, much of what we know about autonomic nervous system function was first learned by physiologists who employed nicotine as a pharmacological tool for studying ganglionic transmission of nerve impulses.

Nicotine is not, however, used in medicine. Its potent effects are too widespread to be readily controlled and put to good use. Ganglionic blockade, for instance, can be achieved only after initial stimulation which would produce violent toxic effects. Thus, nicotine is of clinical interest in only two situations: (1) when the nicotine inhaled during smoking produces effects that are undesirable for patients with certain illnesses, and (2) in cases of acute accidental poisoning caused by insecticidal sprays that contain high concentrations of the alkaloid.

Smoking. The small amounts of nicotine absorbed from the lungs during smoking produces effects on the central nervous system which smokers find pleasurable. These effects, together with the complicated psychological effects of the smoking process itself, are thought to account for people's becoming habituated to tobacco. These same small quantities of nicotine also stimulate the autonomic ganglia to produce effects which can be harmful to people with certain diseases. It is these actions, rather than the possibly deleterious effects of other toxic substances in tobacco smoke, which we shall discuss here.*

Stimulation of sympathetic ganglia and of the adrenal medulla by the nicotine in tobacco smoke tends to produce the following effects upon circulation: (1) a moderate speeding up of the pulse rate; (2) a transient rise in systolic blood pressure; (3) constriction of the peripheral blood vessels, leading to a definite drop in skin temperature. Although these effects can be minimized by smoking tobacco low in nicotine content or by the use of an effective filter, doctors often feel that patients with certain conditions should stop smoking entirely.

Patients with thromboangiitis obliterans (Buerger's disease) should never use any form of tobacco. Even the transient vasoconstriction caused by nicotine increases the risk of still further reducing blood flow in the extremities. This not only increases the feeling of cold and the aching pain but speeds the thrombotic processes which lead to gangrene and the need to amputate necrotic tissues. Patients with other peripheral vascular diseases also—including Raynaud's disease—should not smoke.

The acceleratory effect of nicotine on the heart and the rise it causes in blood pressure are often

* Students interested in the current status of the controversy concerning smoking as a cause of bronchogenic cancer and also as a possible factor in increased mortality from other diseases should consult the U. S. Public Health Service report, *Smoking and Health*, 1964.

considered reason enough to urge patients with coronary conditions or high blood pressure not to smoke. This certainly seems a wise decision in the case of patients with active rheumatic heart disease, severe angina pectoris, hypertension with tachycardia, and in those recovering from an acute myocardial infarction. On the other hand, if the patient's cardiovascular condition is not very severe or acute and giving up smoking upsets him emotionally, the doctor and patient may make a decision in favor of continued smoking in an individual case.

The stimulating action of nicotine on the parasympathetic ganglia in the gut tends to cause increased secretion of stomach acid in some people. This and the local mucosal vasoconstriction that may result from sympathetic stimulation make smoking undesirable for patients with peptic ulcer. Similarly, the increased peristaltic activity caused by stimulation of parasympathetic ganglia in the intestinal walls may adversely affect the condition of patients with spastic colitis and other intestinal diseases. On the other hand, smoking may have a desirable laxative effect in some people. The nausea and vomiting sometimes suffered by novice smokers is probably not the result of nicotine stimulation of intestinal ganglia but stems instead from stimulation of the central vomiting mechanism.

In summary, the small amounts of nicotine inhaled in smoking produce definite pharmacological effects. These may not be harmful for most people; however, they may seriously impair the recovery of patients whose conditions make them especially sensitive to these actions of nicotine. In addition, other effects of smoking may make this habit an undesirable one even for people in good health.

Acute Poisoning. Poisoning by nicotine is relatively rare but can be very severe and difficult to treat. Illness has occurred when children have eaten tobacco products, but, usually, the stomach is emptied by spontaneous vomiting before enough of the alkaloid is absorbed to cause really serious effects. On the other hand, ingestion of the 40 per cent nicotine sulfate solution marketed as an insecticide, or systemic absorption of the liquid alkaloid accidentally spilled on the skin, has caused death in as little as five minutes.

Death results, generally, from paralysis of the respiratory muscles, the result of nicotinic blockade of nervous transmission. The medullary respiratory center may also be paralyzed after initial stimulation. Bronchial muscle constriction and glandular secretions may add to the patient's breathing difficulties. The complex pattern of stimulation and depression of autonomic ganglia of *both* types may be manifested by varied effects, such as a slowing *or* a speeding up of the heart rate; sharp rises *and* sharp falls in blood pressure; salivation, vomiting, and diarrhea.

Treatment is aimed mainly at keeping the patient

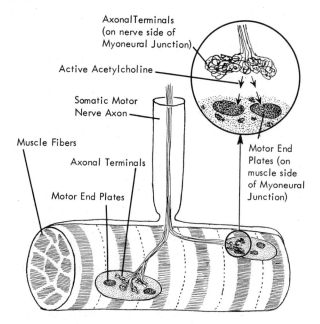

FIG. 17-1. Transmission of nerve impulses to skeletal muscle fibers at a myoneural junction. Fiber terminals release acetylcholine.

breathing by use of artificial respiration and oxygen inhalation. At the same time, the circulation must be supported—by external cardiac massage or intracardiac epinephrine injection, in the event of cardiac standstill. Small doses of short-acting barbiturates may be cautiously injected by vein to control the clonic-tonic convulsions that sometimes occur as a result of C.N.S. stimulation. Certain atropinelike drugs, including *caramiphen* (Panparnit) and *diethazine* (Diparcol), have been employed experimentally and are claimed to be effective for this purpose.

Ganglionic Blocking Agents

The drugs that are able to block autonomic ganglia without first stimulating them are used clinically for several purposes. Most of these agents, both the first to be introduced—*tetraethylammonium chloride* (Etamon) and *hexamethonium bromide* and *chloride* (Bistrium; Esomide; Methium)—and those currently employed, such as *pentolinium tartrate* (Ansolysen) and *chlorisondamine chloride* (Ecolid), are quaternary ammonium compounds.

Chemicals of this kind resemble acetylcholine structurally in possessing a nitrogen atom to which are attached four radicals. It is thought that this configuration accounts for the ability of these drugs to compete successfully with acetylcholine for cholinotropic receptor sites on autonomic ganglion cells and

thus prevent the neurohormone from transmitting preganglionic nerve impulses to ganglion cells and beyond. However, a quaternary nitrogen atom is not essential for producing ganglionic blockade, since the effective blocker *mecamylamine* (Inversine) is a *secondary*, rather than a quarternary, amine.

In any case, the therapeutic usefulness of all these drugs stems mainly from their ability to block transmission of tonic and reflexly stimulated nerve impulses passing through sympathetic ganglia to the blood vessels and the heart. The fall in blood pressure which often results from the circulatory changes set in motion by this action of these drugs accounts for their use in the treatment of moderate to severe cases of hypertension, or high blood pressure (see Chap. 23).

Reduction of excessive sympathetic vasoconstrictor impulses to the smooth muscle walls of the blood vessels causes them to relax. This dilates the vessels and leads to a local increase in blood flow, with flushing of the skin and a rise in the temperature of the area. These drugs have been used for this vasodilator effect in the treatment of peripheral vascular diseases (see Chap. 26).

The amount of blood flowing to any organ depends upon two factors: (1) the level of systemic blood pressure, and (2) the degree of resistance in the local arterioles. Thus, if the blood pressure falls *too* low, local flow may be *diminished* rather than increased. This tends to limit the usefulness of the ganglionic blocking agents in some situations. On the other hand, it also accounts for the occasional use of some of these drugs for reducing bleeding during surgery (see Drug Digest, *trimethaphan*).

NEUROMUSCULAR BLOCKING AGENTS

We have seen that skeletal muscle fibers contract in response to nerve impulses transmitted by the chemical mediator acetylcholine, which is released by the endings of somatic motor nerves (Chap. 14). We have also noted that a breakdown in neurohumoral transmission at this myoneural junction is responsible for the muscular weakness of patients suffering from myasthenia gravis and that certain drugs are able to overcome this disease-induced block to some extent (Chap. 15). We shall now discuss those drugs that are used clinically to relax or even paralyze voluntary muscles by interfering with cholinergic nerve impulse transmission at these same junctions between somatic axon terminals and the motor end-plates on skeletal muscle fiber membranes (Fig. 17-1).

History. *Curare*, a plant-derived substance now known to cause muscular paralysis in this manner, has been used for centuries by South American Indians in hunting small game. These primitive peoples learned to prepare crude extracts of certain tropical vines, which they then applied to the tips of their arrows, darts, and spears. Animals wounded even superficially by these poisoned points were unable to run far before collapsing, as a result of skeletal muscle paralysis. The flesh of small game immobilized or killed in this manner could be safely eaten, because the poison is not absorbed from the gastrointestinal tract.

Although crude curare was first studied scientifically more than a century ago, its composition and strength were, until rather recently, too variable and its action too uncertain to permit its safe use in clinical medicine. It was only after the purified alkaloid d-*tubocurarine* was isolated from the plant *Chondodendron tomentosum* in 1935 that physicians could begin to put these peripherally acting muscular relaxants to use.

Once the chemical structure of the natural alkaloid was known, chemists were able to synthesize substances of similar but simpler structure that also proved potent as neuromuscular blocking agents. Most of the natural and synthetic curarelike substances contain quarternary ammonium groups, as does acetylcholine, the neurohumoral transmitter, and they act in one way or another to block impulse transmission by the natural chemical mediator between motor nerve endings and skeletal muscle fibers.

Manner of Action. The neuromuscular blocking agents act in two main ways to interfere with cholinergic transmission of tonic motor impulses from somatic nerves to skeletal muscles: (1) by *competitive blockade,* in which acetylcholine is kept from depolarizing the muscle fiber membrane, and (2) by *depolarizing blockade,* in which the drugs act, like an excess of acetycholine (or like nicotine), to first stimulate and then depress transmission.

Competitive Blockade. One group of drugs (Table 17-4), of which *tubocurarine* (Drug Digest) is the prototype, acts by competing *with acetylcholine* for the cholinoceptive substance on the membrane of the motor end-plate, the specialized structure of the myoneural junction between somatic nerve fibers and striated muscle fibers. The bulky molecules of these drugs occupy the cholinergic receptors without activating the train of metabolic events that ordinarily occurs when acetylcholine molecules released by nerve endings reach these receptors. The continued presence of the blocking drug keeps acetylcholine from depolarizing the membrane and triggering contraction of the muscle fibers of the motor unit.

Depolarizing Blockade. Certain other drugs that prevent muscular contractions do so by producing a *persistent depolarization* of these structures. Molecules of *succinylcholine* (Drug Digest) and *decamethonium* (Table 17-4), for example, occupy the muscle membrane receptors much as acetylcholine does, and like the latter, they depolarize the membrane and thus set off muscular contractions. However, unlike the neurohormone, which is instantly destroyed by the enzyme acetylcholinesterase concentrated at the neuromuscular junction, the molecules of these drugs remain on the receptor until they diffuse away into the blood stream.

The continued presence of these depolarizing drugs at the junction keeps the muscle fiber from responding to further volleys of nerve impulses. The exact cause of this failure of the muscles to react to nerve-released acetylcholine is still uncertain. In any case, after the initially increased contractions, the muscles rapidly become weakened and, finally, a flaccid paralysis

TABLE 17-4
NEUROMUSCULAR BLOCKING DRUGS

NONPROPRIETARY OR OFFICIAL NAME	PROPRIETARY NAME OR SYNONYM	INTRAVENOUS DOSAGE RANGE
Competitive or NON-*Depolarizing Type*		
Benzoquinonium chloride	Mytolon	3–9 mg.
Chondodendron tomentosum extract, purified	Intocostrin	40–60 units
Dimethyl tubocurarine chloride	Mecostrin	2–3 mg.
Dimethyl tubocurarine iodide N.F.	Metubine	1.5–7 mg.
Gallamine triethiodide N.F.	Flaxedil	1.0 mg./Kg.
Hexafluorenium bromide	Mylaxen	0.4 mg./Kg.
Tubocurarine chloride U.S.P.	Tubarine; Tubadil	6–9 mg.
Depolarizing Type		
Succinylcholine chloride U.S.P.	Sucostrin; Anectine; Quelicin; etc.	10–40 mg.
Decamethonium bromide	Syncurine; C_{10}	0.5–3 mg.

develops that looks no different from that which is produced by the competitive blocking agents. One practical difference, however, is that the paralysis caused by the *competitive* blockers can sometimes be overcome by the anticholinesterase-type drugs that indirectly increase the local concentration of acetylcholine at the junctions, whereas the effects of the *depolarizing-type* blocking drugs cannot be counteracted in this way.

Pharmacological Effects. When administered in clinically practicable doses, the pharmacological effects of these drugs occur mainly in the skeletal muscles. Occasionally the curarelike compounds act at certain other sites to cause unwanted actions on other organs, but such side effects are rare with the depolarizing drugs. With blocking agents of both types, the sequence of progressive paralysis of various muscle groups is similar, except, of course, that the depolarizing drugs first produce a brief period of muscular twitching before the weakness and paralysis begin to develop.

The muscles first to show signs of weakness are those that are innervated by motor fibers of cranial nerves. Thus, the patient may first find it difficult to keep his eyelids up or his vision focused, and this is quickly followed by difficulty in swallowing and in talking. It is of interest that these small muscles are also often the first to show weakness when a patient develops myasthenia gravis and patients with this neuromuscular disorder are extremely sensitive to small doses of curariform drugs.

The muscles next to lose tone and relax, as a solution of one of these drugs is slowly infused, are those of the limbs, back and abdomen. Finally, if the infusion is continued only a bit beyond this point, the muscles that are responsible for respiratory movements become paralyzed (these are the *diaphragm*, which is made up of skeletal muscle sheets that separate the thoracic and abdominal cavities, and the *intercostal* muscles that control movements of the rib cage.

Clinically, these drugs are most often employed to produce relaxation of the muscles of the abdomen and the extremities. However, the dosage of these drugs that will bring about these desired effects is so close to the dose that will block the muscles of respiration that breathing difficulties are a common occurrence. This narrow safety margin, which makes some degree of respiratory embarrassment and even apnea almost unavoidable, makes it imperative to have readily available the necessary equipment for maintaining the patient's respiration artificially until the effects of the neuromuscular blocking agents wear off. In this respect, succinylcholine, a drug that is ordinarily rapidly destroyed, is superior to the relatively long-acting agent, tubocurarine.

Other Actions. Another advantage of succinylcholine is that its effects are largely limited to the muscle

end-plates, whereas tubocurarine and its relatives sometimes act at certain other sites also. This can result in undesired side effects, besides the respiratory depression that is common to both drugs.

Tubocurarine, for example, acts primarily at skeletal muscle end-plates, but it may sometimes cause some degree of blockade at the other kind of nicotinic site of cholinergic action—the autonomic ganglia. That is, the molecules of this drug may occasionally keep acetylcholine from transmitting nerve impulses at some of the synapses between preganglionic fibers and ganglionic neurons, as well as at the myoneural junctions in skeletal muscles. Such a partial blockade of the sympathetic ganglia, which relay tonic vasoconstrictor nerve impulses to the smooth muscle walls of the blood vessels, may lead to a loss of their tone. The resulting vasodilation is one cause of the circulatory collapse that sometimes occurs from overdosage with tubocurarine.

Another disadvantage of tubocurarine, compared to succinylcholine, is that the curare alkaloid sometimes causes some tissues to release *histamine*. The vasodilating effects of free histamine upon the arterioles and capillaries (Chap. 40) may add to the danger of circulatory depression from tubocurarine. Histamine freed by the curare alkaloid may also cause bronchial constriction, thus adding to the breathing difficulties the patient may be suffering. Since such reactions are especially undesirable in patients with bronchial asthma, succinylcholine, which does not cause histamine release, is the preferred muscle relaxant for these and other patients with respiratory diseases.

Generally, succinylcholine is considered safer than tubocurarine because of its lack of ganglionic-blocking and histamine-releasing effects and the short duration of its neuromuscular blocking action. However, it occasionally causes prolonged apnea in some patients, perhaps because they lack the plasma enzyme that ordinarily converts succinylcholine to inactive metabolites very rapidly.

Since this detoxifying enzyme is synthesized in the liver and then sent out into the blood stream with other plasma proteins, patients with a history of liver disease, malnutrition or anemia are considered poor candidates for succinylcholine administration. Others in whom the use of this agent is undesirable are those with a genetic defect that results in a lack of the enzyme required for eliminating this drug from the body (Chap. 2).

Clinical Uses. The most important use of the neuromuscular blocking agents is as an *adjunct to anesthesia* (Chap. 11). Administered as supplements to general anesthetics, these drugs—which are *not* themselves anesthetics—often allow abdominal and other major surgery to be carried out under relatively light anesthesia.

Ordinarily, large amounts of general anesthetics

are required to depress the spinal reflex centers which control muscle tone. The continued administration of high concentrations of such anesthetics in order to produce and maintain muscular relaxation may lead to various adverse reactions, ranging from postoperative vomiting to respiratory center depression. By bringing about relaxation of skeletal muscles through their *peripheral* blocking effects, drugs such as tubocurarine and succinylcholine permit a marked reduction in the amount of general anesthetic required, and this lessens the likelihood of anesthetic complications. Of course, the muscle relaxants are themselves often a cause of dangerous complications and must be employed with great caution if these are to be avoided.

The neuromuscular blocking agents are best employed in short surgical procedures that do not require the patient to be deeply anesthetized. For such operations, the patient readily can be rendered unconscious and unable to perceive pain through the use of thiopental injections or nitrous oxide-oxygen inhalation (Chap. 11). However, since these anesthetics do not give good muscle relaxation, they must be supplemented with one of the peripherally acting agents when the procedure is one that requires profound relaxation.

The amount of these muscle relaxant drugs that is needed is much lower when one of the more potent anesthetics such as ether is employed. In fact, ether has a curariform action of its own in addition to its spinal cord depressant effects. The dose of tubocurarine is often reduced to as little as one third of normal when it is given in combination with ether in longer procedures such as cholecystectomies which require deep relaxation of the abdominal wall muscles.

These drugs are best administered *after* the patient has been rendered unconscious by premedication and anesthesia so that motor reflex signs of central depression are not interfered with. In addition, the initial twitching caused by a depolarizing blocker such as succinylcholine can be quite painful to the unanesthetized patient. Such preliminary twitchings can be best reduced or prevented by infusing the drug very slowly or by pretreating the patient with a small amount of *hexafluorenium,* a *non*depolarizing relaxant.

When the patient has been taken down to the upper planes of Stage III anesthesia (see Chap. 11), the muscle relaxant may be administered. The resulting relaxation of the jaw then permits easy insertion of an endotracheal tube, if the doctor so desires. These relaxants reduce laryngospasm by blocking the motor portion of the reflex arc; to block out the sensory stimuli that set off the afferent impulses of the gag reflexes, the patient's throat is often sprayed with cocaine or some other topical anesthetic.

Other intubation procedures for which neuromuscular blocking drugs are often employed include laryngoscopy, bronchoscopy, esophagoscopy and sigmoidoscopy. Among orthopedic procedures said to be facilitated by prior curarization are the reduction of fractures and of dislocations of the jaw, the knee and the shoulder. In ophthalmological surgery, the relaxant effect of relatively small doses of these drugs on the muscles of the eye has been utilized to ease procedures such as the removal of cataracts.

Succinylcholine is commonly used today as part of the premedication of psychiatric patients prior to electroshock therapy. Its use helps to dampen the severity of the convulsive spasms set off by passage of the current through the brain. This lessens the likelihood of the massive muscular contractions that might otherwise occur and the consequent vertebral fractures or dislocations. Since the use of this drug together with thiopental increases the likelihood of post-seizure apnea, the patient is well oxygenated prior to the procedure and oxygen is kept readily available for administration through an endotracheal tube.

The use of curariform drugs has also been advocated for various acute and chronic conditions marked by muscle spasm and rigidity. Thus, these drugs have been used to relax the early muscle spasm of poliomyelitis and the convulsions of tetanus and for patients with cerebral palsy, hemiplegia and various chronic states of dystonia and athetosis.

These drugs have helped produce some degree of muscle relaxation and pain relief, but their use in these neuromuscular disorders has not proved very successful. This is due, in part, to their relatively brief duration of action, which makes frequent injections necessary. Attempts have been made to overcome this drawback by suspending tubocurarine in oil and injecting it intramuscularly.

Unfortunately, when administered in this way, the curariform drug is sometimes erratically absorbed. Too rapid absorption may cause muscular paralysis instead of merely the desired reduction in hyperreflexic spasm without loss of muscle strength. Thus, patients receiving repository dosage forms of these peripheral neuromuscular blockers must be closely watched to avoid overdosage and prevent muscle weakness and, possibly, paralysis. Recently, following the introduction of parenterally administered centrally-acting muscle relaxants such as *methocarbamol, meprobamate* and *diazepam* (Chap. 8), the use of curare-type drugs for the treatment of spastic and convulsive conditions has declined considerably.

Precautions and Treatment of Overdosage. The main danger in the use of blocking agents of both types is that paralysis of the diaphragm and chest muscles may cause respiratory difficulty and even apnea. For this reason, these drugs are never used when facilities for controlled respiration are unavailable, nor are they ever to be administered by individuals not completely skilled in their use. The occurrence of apnea following administration of these drugs is no great problem to the experienced anesthesiologist, who merely ventilates the patient artificially until the effects of the drug wear off—usually in a matter of minutes. Indeed, apnea is sometimes deliberately induced in chest and heart surgery without harm, as long as the patient continues to get oxygen by mechanical means.

Sometimes, however, spontaneous respiration may not be so readily re-established during drug-induced apnea. When the blocking drug is one of the *competitive*, or *non*depolarizing, type, the patient may be treated by administration of an anticholinesterase agent of the kind used in the diagnosis and treatment of myasthenia gravis such as edrophonium or neostigmine methylsulfate. These anticurare drugs act mainly by indirectly increasing the amount of endogenous acetylcholine at the myoneural junctions. That is, they prevent the enzymatic destruction of the nerve-released neurohormone by acetylcholinesterase. This helps the acetylcholine molecules to accumulate to levels at which they can compete successfully with the curariform compounds for the motor endplate receptors. Often this overcomes moderate degrees of curare block and restores the poisoned patient's muscle strength.

These anticholinesterase drugs do *not*, however, counteract the effects of overdosage with the *depolarizing*-type blocking agents. On the contrary, since neostigmine and edrophonium are themselves direct and indirect depolarizing agents, they may make a succinylcholine- or decamethonium-induced block even worse by their additive actions.

Although there is no pharmacological antidote for overdosage with a depolarizing-type blocker such as succinylcholine, its effects ordinarily are overcome rather readily by simply supplying the patient with oxygen under pressure—preferably through a previously-inserted airway—until the body's own detoxifying enzymes destroy the excess of the drug. In the relatively rare cases of prolonged apnea following succinylcholine, the administration of whole blood or plasma may be helpful. These fluids contain cholinesterases, the enzymes that account for the ordinarily short action of succinylcholine by their ability to convert it to inactive metabolites. (As has been indicated (see Chap. 2, p. 30), prolonged apnea following succinylcholine has been attributed to a lack of circulating cholinesterases.)

It is often important to maintain the patient's blood pressure at adequate levels. In cases of hypotension resulting from curare-induced histamine release and ganglionic blockade the administration of ephedrine or other adrenergic vasopressor drugs may prevent circulatory collapse. Atropine administration also is often desirable to counteract salivation, bronchial mucus secretion and other muscarinic side effects of curare-drug antidotes such as neostigmine.

SUMMARY OF THE PHARMACOLOGICAL ACTIONS AND THERAPEUTIC USES OF ATROPINE-TYPE DRUGS

Pharmacological Actions

- **Gastrointestinal**

    Smooth muscle. Antispasmodic and antiperistaltic actions reduce the tone and motility of the stomach and intestines.

    Gastric glands. Large doses reduce secretion of acid and of digestive enzymes.

- **Other Smooth Muscle**

    Urinary tract. Reduces tone and motility of ureters, fundus of the bladder, and possibly the uterus; increases tone of the bladder sphincter.

    Biliary tract. Weak antispasmodic action on gallbladder and bile ducts accounts for its use combined with morphine.

Therapeutic Uses

Used to reduce hypermotility and hypersecretory activity in such conditions as peptic ulcer, gastritis, cardiospasm, pylorospasm, regional enteritis (i.e., ileitis, ulcerative colitis, diverticulitis), and vs. diarrhea in mild dysentery and constipation of the hypertonic or spastic type.

Used to increase bladder capacity in children with nocturnal enuresis and in spastic paraplegics and others with urinary incontinence; in cystitis and other irritative conditions to relieve urinary urgency and frequency; as an antispasmodic in renal colic to relax ureters or to counteract added spasm caused by morphine; for relief of pain in dysmenorrhea.

For relief of biliary colic.

Pharmacological Actions (Cont'd)

Bronchial muscle is only slightly relaxed to cause relatively weak bronchodilation.

- **Cardiovascular System**

  Cardiac actions. Small doses of atropine slow the heart rate slightly and larger doses accelerate it markedly. The decrease in rate is more marked with scopolamine.

  Vascular. Local vasodilation often causes flushing of the face. Blood pressure is not much affected, except that the hypotension caused by cholinergic drugs can be prevented and counteracted.

- **Ocular Effects**

  Produce dilation of the pupil (mydriasis) and paralysis of accommodation (cycloplegia) by blocking tonic impulses to the sphincter muscle of the iris and to the ciliary muscles. This may raise the intraocular pressure in the eyes of patients with narrow angle glaucoma.

- **Glandular Secretions**

  Small doses markedly reduce sweating, salivation, and the secretions of the nose, throat, and bronchial glands.

- **Central Nervous System**

  Atropine, in therapeutic doses, has a slight excitatory action, whereas scopolamine, in equivalent amounts, causes depressant effects, including drowsiness, sleep, and amnesia. Both alkaloids depress motor mechanisms responsible for abnormal skeletal muscle tone. Toxic doses of atropine cause excitement, restlessness, disorientation and delirium.

Therapeutic Uses (Cont'd)

Although it is not very useful in bronchial asthma, this action is useful for counteracting bronchoconstriction caused by cholinergic drugs, including methacholine and the anticholinesterase insecticides and nerve gases.

Used to prevent or counteract reflex bradycardia caused by excessive vagal tone: in anesthesia (e.g., with Halothane); during certain surgical procedures; in the carotid sinus syndrome; and in certain kinds of heart block.

Used in ophthalmologic examinations of the retina and optic disk and for measuring refractive errors. Mydriasis alone or alternated with miosis is used to keep the lens from adhering to the iris in iritis. Also used to relax ocular muscles and reduce irritation in inflammatory conditions such as iridocyclitis and choroiditis.

Used prior to inhalation anesthesia to reduce respiratory tract secretions.

Used to reduce nasal secretions in acute rhinitis of the common cold and hay fever.

Used to reduce excessive sweating in hyperhidrosis and in the night sweats of tuberculosis.

Used to reduce tremor and rigidity in parkinsonism.

Used as prophylaxis against motion sickness.

Scopolamine is an ingredient of sleep-producing products advertised to the public for self-medication of insomnia.

Scopolamine was once widely used for its sedative and amnesic effects, when combined with opiates as a preoperative adjunct to general anesthesia. It has been largely replaced by phenothiazine-type tranquilizers for this purpose and for quieting manic patients and alcoholics with delirium tremens.

SUMMARY OF THE SIDE EFFECTS, CAUTIONS AND CONTRAINDICATIONS— ATROPINE-TYPE DRUGS

- *Mouth dryness,* due to reduced salivation: may make swallowing difficult; dryness of respiratory tract and hardening of reduced bronchial secretions may be *bad for patients with asthma and other chronic lung diseases.*

- *Skin dry, hot, red,* due to abolition of sweating, and vasodilation. The interference with heat loss may lead to *fever,* especially in infants and young children; patients may suffer *hyperpyrexia* in warm weather or hot climates.

- *Eyes:* possible photophobia, due to *widely dilated pupils; vision blurred,* due to paralysis of accommodation. Crowding of iris and ciliary muscle into angle of eye chamber may *raise intraocular pressure* by interfering with drainage of aqueous humor. Thus, these drugs are *contraindicated* in patients with *narrow angle glaucoma,* and *caution* is required in all *patients over 40 years old* because of their increased susceptibility to attacks of acute glaucoma.

- *Urinary retention* may occur, owing to loss of bladder tone, especially in elderly males with an enlarged prostate gland. Thus, these drugs are *contraindicated* in patients with *prostatic hypertrophy.* Synthetic

atropinelike drugs with ganglionic blocking component may produce *impotence* in young men.

- *Heart palpitations* and *tachycardia* may occur, owing to loss of vagal control. This may cause coronary insufficiency, chest pain, and cardiac decompensation in patients with a history of heart disease. Thus, *caution* is required in patients with *angina,* etc.

- *Constipation* and possible obstipation, due to reduced tone and motility of G.I. musculature. Thus, *caution* is required in patients with partial *pyloric stenosis,* because of the danger that the narrowed passageway may become completely obstructed.

SUMMARY OF NURSING CONSIDERATIONS WITH ATROPINE AND RELATED DRUGS

- Take special care to make sure that the correct dose is being administered, because the amounts ordered are small and may be written in either the apothecary or the metric system.

- Be alert to recognize the signs and symptoms of atropine poisoning in patients under treatment with this drug. Inform the physician of any marked changes in pulse rate, visual acuity, bladder function, or behavior.

- Do not neglect to tell the patient that certain side effects are likely to occur when he is taking belladonna-type drugs and synthetic cholinergic agents; a brief mention of mouth dryness, blurring of vision, etc., may spare him needless concern. Parents should be in-

formed that flushing is an expected effect of atropine medication in children and not the result of infection and fever.

- Advise patient that he can minimize minor discomforts such as mouth dryness (by sucking on hard candies) and photophobia (by wearing dark glasses).

- Let patients who have had eye drops know when the visual effects will wear off so that they can plan their activities accordingly.

- Caution elderly ambulatory patients to take special care in walking down stairs and in other activities, if they are likely to have visual blurring from these drugs.

SUMMARY OF CLINICAL USES AND ADVERSE REACTIONS OF THE NEUROMUSCULAR BLOCKING AGENTS

- *Clinical Uses*
  Adjuvant in anesthesia
  Adjuvant in electroconvulsive shock therapy
  Intubation procedures (bronchoscopy, esophagoscopy, laryngoscopy, sigmoidoscopy)
  Orthopedic procedures (reduction of dislocations and fractures)
  Neuromuscular spastic disorders (cerebral palsy, hemiplegia, paraplegia, poliomyelitis, athetosis, dystonia, hyperkinesis)

Acute convulsive states (status epilepticus, tetanus, arachnidism)

- *Adverse Reactions*
  Respiratory: Hypoxia and apnea, following respiratory embarrassment and paralysis or bronchial constriction
  Use with caution in patients with asthma or myasthenia gravis; succinylcholine chloride contraindicated

in patients with liver disease, malnutrition, anemia, or plasma cholinesterase deficiency

Circulatory: Hypotension and possible circulatory collapse from partial ganglionic blockade, histamine

release (e.g., tubocurarine); cardiac arrhythmias from hypoxia or vagal blocking actions (e.g., gallamine)

SUMMARY OF NURSING POINTS CONCERNING NEUROMUSCULAR BLOCKING DRUGS

• Make certain that equipment and antidotal drugs (e.g., neostigmine; edrophonium) that may be required for resuscitation are readily available.

• Observe the patient for signs of respiratory embarrassment or apnea and be prepared to assist with such measures as artificial respiration and oxygen administration to sustain the patient until normal breathing

resumes. Note also any signs of asthmatic breathing as a result of tubocurarine-induced release of tissue histamine.

• Watch the patient's pulse and blood pressure carefully; circulatory collapse is a possible effect of tubocurarine administration.

REVIEW QUESTIONS

Antimuscarinic-Type Blocking Agents

1. (a) What is the *exact cellular site* at which atropine and other "antimuscarinic" anticholinergic drugs act?

(b) What is the mechanism by which drugs of this type act to bring about changes in normal physiological function?

2. (a) Name the two most important *natural* anticholinergic alkaloids and list three plants from which they are extracted.

(b) Name two prototype *synthetic* drugs of different types, which were prepared in the search for safer, more effective anticholinergic drugs.

3. (a) Why is it difficult to use atropine for treating gastrointestinal disorders without causing certain side effects?

(b) Give an example of how an action of atropine that is usually considered a side effect may, in other circumstances, be used to produce a desired therapeutic effect.

4. (a) List three clinical situations in which the action of atropinelike drugs on the secretory glands of the mouth and respiratory tract is considered desirable.

(b) What are the undesirable effects of this antisecretory action and in what condition may this drying action constitute a possible danger to the patient?

5. (a) In what condition may the effect of atropine-type drugs on sweat gland function be desirable?

(b) What is the appearance of the skin after atropine overdosage, and what is the possible danger of this action of atropine on the skin?

6. (a) What is the effect of a moderately large dose of atropine on the heart rate, and how is this brought about?

(b) Indicate patients of two types, for whom this cardiac action of atropine is undesirable and its use is contraindicated; list two clinical situations in which atropine may be administered for this cardiac action.

7. (a) Name the two main ocular actions of atropine-like drugs, and indicate some situations in which these actions are considered useful.

(b) What are two ocular side effects which may occur when atropine is administered systemically to produce effects in organs other than the eye; in what type patient are anticholinergic drugs contraindicated?

8. (a) What are several clinical uses of belladonna alkaloids and synthetic anticholinergic drugs based on their action on the smooth muscle of the genitourinary tract?

(b) What is a side effect of this action, and in what type patient is atropine contraindicated because of its effect on the urinary bladder?

9. (a) What are the three main actions of belladonna alkaloids and synthetic anticholinergic drugs on *gastrointestinal* function?

(b) List several clinical conditions in which these actions are utilized.

10. (a) How do dicyclomine (Bentyl) and drugs of its type differ from the belladonna alkaloids in their gastrointestinal actions, and how does this affect their clinical utility?

(b) How do propantheline (Pro-Banthine) and drugs of the same sub-class differ from the natural alkaloids in their G.I. action and what significance, if any, does this have when they are used clinically?

11. (a) What is a possible gastrointestinal side effect of atropine overdosage?

(b) In what type patient may anticholinergic drugs be *contraindicated* because of this G.I. effect?

12. (a) List several clinical conditions and situations in which scopolamine or atropine are administered for their central effects.

(b) What are the C.N.S. signs of atropine overdosage, and what may be the end result of the central action of *toxic* doses of solanaceous alkaloids?

Adrenergic Blocking Agents

1. (a) Explain briefly how adrenergic blocking drugs keep neuroeffectors from responding to sympathetic nervous system stimulation and sympathomimetic amines (i.e., adrenergic drugs).

(b) Explain briefly why adrenergic blocking agents of the *alpha* type fail to keep cardiac receptors from responding to sympathetic stimulation or to sympathomimetic drugs.

2. (a) What is the effect of alpha type adrenergic blocking agents upon the tone of a patient's vascular smooth muscle walls?

(b) What are two effects of such adrenergic blockade upon local blood flow and systemic arterial pressure?

(c) For clinical conditions of what two types should such vascular effects of the alpha adrenergic drugs be useful, at least in theory?

3. (a) What adverse effects of adrenergic blocking drugs such as tolazoline and dibenzyline limit their utility in the treatment of patients with essential hypertension?

(b) In what type patient would such adverse effects be especially dangerous?

(c) With what other drugs may adrenergic blocking agents be combined for reducing such side effects in treating these patients?

4. (a) Explain briefly the manner in which adrenergic blocking drugs such as phentolamine and dibenzyline help to control hypertension caused by pheochromocytoma.

(b) Explain briefly the basis for the use of phentolamine to determine whether a patient's high blood pressure may be due to circulating catecholamines from a pheochromocytoma, rather than from neurogenic sources (as in many cases of essential hypertension).

5. (a) Name several drugs classified as *beta* adrenergic blocking agents and indicate what their predictable effect on heart action should be.

(b) Indicate a couple of clinical conditions which may be improved by treatment with beta receptor blocking drugs and a possible adverse effect of their cardiac action.

6. (a) List drugs of two other types which are capable of reducing hyperactivity of the sympathetic nervous system, and indicate how they differ, in general, from the true adrenergic blocking drugs.

(b) Name some so-called adrenergic nerve blocking drugs, and indicate how their action at the junction between sympathetic postganglionic fibers and neuroeffectors differs from that of the adrenergic blocking agents.

Drugs Acting on Autonomic Neuroeffectors

Ganglionic Stimulants and Blockers

1. (a) What two effects does nicotine have on ganglionic function?

(b) Why cannot nicotine be used clinically as a ganglionic blocking agent?

2. (a) List three cardiovascular effects that may be caused by the small amounts of nicotine inhaled during smoking.

(b) List patients of several types whose conditions may be adversely affected as a result of these pharmacological effects of nicotine.

3. (a) List some gastrointestinal effects from nicotine inhalation during smoking.

(b) Indicate how such actions may prove undesirable for some kinds of patients.

4. (a) Describe the effects of acute nicotine poisoning which are usually the cause of a fatal outcome.

(b) Describe some of the measures taken to prevent death of the patient acutely poisoned by nicotine.

5. (a) Describe the manner in which ganglionic blocking agents interfere with transmission of preganglionic nerve impulses to ganglion cells.

(b) What are the effects of such interference with sympathetic ganglionic transmission upon the blood vessels and upon the systemic circulation in general?

(c) Name two clinical conditions in which these circulatory changes brought about by ganglionic blocking agents are deliberately sought in treatment.

Neuromuscular Blocking Agents

1. Explain briefly the manner in which molecules of tubocurarine and related drugs interfere with impulse transmission from somatic nerve fibers to skeletal muscle fibers.

2. Explain briefly how drugs like succinylcholine and decamethonium act to prevent impulse transmission at the neuromuscular junction.

3. (a) How do the observable effects of neuromuscular blocking drugs of these two types differ, and in what way are they similar?

(b) How do the muscles affected by the competitive and the depolarizing blocking agents differ in their responses to anticholinesterase-type drugs?

4. (a) Indicate the sequence in which different groups of skeletal muscles relax when a neuromuscular blocking agent is slowly infused by vein.

(b) What is the clinical significance of the fact that the amounts of the neuromuscular blocking agents needed to produce block of abdominal muscles are very close to those that will paralyze skeletal muscles?

5. (a) List two pharmacological actions of tubocurarine other than neuromuscular blockade, and indicate the possible clinical significance of such actions.

(b) What properties of succinylcholine are thought to make it somewhat safer than tubocurarine?

(c) In patients of what types may the use of neuro-muscular blocking agents be contraindicated?

6. (a) How does administration of a neuromuscular blocking agent as an adjunct to anesthesia benefit the patient undergoing a surgical procedure that requires muscular relaxation?

(b) What precaution is required in administering tubo-curarine to a patient who is to be anesthetized with ether?

7. (a) List several intubation procedures which may be facilitated by prior curarization.

(b) List some orthopedic, ophthalmological and psy-chiatric situations in which the adjunctive use of neuro-muscular blocking agents may be desirable.

8. (a) What is the main danger in the use of neuro-muscular blocking drugs and what requirements must be met before these agents can be safely employed?

(b) What anticurare drugs are employed as antidotes to overdosage with competitive-type blocking drugs but not with the depolarizing blockers?

(c) What other agents may be used for counteracting toxicity from neuromuscular blocking drugs?

BIBLIOGRAPHY

Antimuscarinic-Type Blocking Agents

Ambache, N.: The use and limitations of atropine for pharmacological studies on autonomic effectors. Pharmacol. Rev., 7:467, 1955.

Craig, F. N.: The effects of atropine, work and heat on heart rate and sweat production in man. J. Appl. Physiol., 4:826, 1952.

Eger, E. I.: Atropine, scopolamine and related compounds. Anesthesiology, 23:365, 1962.

Friend, D.: Gastrointestinal anticholinergic drugs. Clin. Pharmacol. Ther., 4:559, 1963.

Inglefinger, F. J.: The modification of gastrointestinal motility by drugs. New Eng. J. Med., 229:114, 1943.

Longino, F. H., *et al.*: An orally effective quaternary amine, Banthine, capable of reducing gastric motility and secretions. Gastroenterology, 14:301, 1950.

Rodman, M. J.: The anhidrotic action of atropine on human thermoregulatory sweating. J. Am. Pharm. Ass., (Sci. Ed.), 41:484, 1952.

———: The effect of Banthine and Prantal on human thermoregulatory sweating. J. Am. Pharm. Ass. (Sci. Ed.), 42:551, 1953.

———: Drugs in the management of peptic ulcer. R.N., 26:71, 1963 (April).

———: Drugs for G.I. distress. R.N., 28:49, 1965 (June).

Ruffin, J. M., and Cayer, D.: Role of anticholinergic drugs in the treatment of peptic ulcer disease. Ann. N. Y. Acad. Sci., 99:179, 1962.

Smith, V. M.: Newer anticholinergic drugs. Med. Clin. N. Am., 48:399, 1964 (March).

Stoll, H. C.: Pharmacodynamic considerations of atropine and related compounds. Am. J. Med. Sci., 215:577, 1948.

Unna, K. R., *et al.*: Dosage of drugs in infants and children. I. Atropine. Pediatrics, 6:197, 1950.

Adrenergic Blocking Agents

Bradley, E. C., and Weil, M. H.: Vasopressor and vaso-dilator drugs in the treatment of shock. *In* Symposium on Treatment of Shock. Modern Treatment, 4:243, 1967 (March).

Conn, R. D.: Newer drugs in the treatment of cardiac arrhythmia. Med. Clin. N. Am., 51:1223, 1967.

Goldenberg, M., Snyder, C. H., and Aranow, H. Jr.: New test for hypertension due to circulatory epinephrine. J.A.M.A., 135:971, 1947.

Goldfien, A.: Pheochromocytoma: diagnosis and anesthetic and surgical management. Anesthesiology, 24:462, 1963.

Hamer, J., *et al.*: Effect of propranolol (Inderal) in angina pectoris: preliminary report. Brit. Med. J., 2:720, 1964.

Helps, E. P., Robinson, K. C., and Ross, E. J.: Phentola-mine in the diagnosis and management of pheochromo-cytoma. Lancet, 2:267, 1955.

Hillestad, L. K.: Phenoxybenzamine (Dibenzyline) in vascular disease of the hands. Angiology, 13:169, 1962.

Kvale, W. F., *et al.*: Present-day diagnosis and treatment of pheochromocytoma. J.A.M.A., 164:854, 1957.

Rodman, M. J.: Drugs for congestive heart failure and arrhythmias. R.N., 30:51, 1967 (Nov.).

Soffer, A.: Phentolamine (Regitine) and piperoxan (Beno-daine) in the diagnosis of pheochromocytoma. Med. Clin. N. Am., 38:375, 1954.

Turner, J. R. B.: Propranolol in the treatment of digitalis-induced and digitalis-resistant tachycardias. Am. J. Cardiol., 18:450, 1966.

Ganglionic Stimulants and Blockers

Larson, P. S., Haag, H. B., and Silvette, H.: Tobacco Experimental and Clinical Studies. Baltimore, Williams & Wilkins, 1961.

Master, A. M.: Angina pectoris. Guest editorial. J.A.M.A., 162:1542, 1956.

Matousek, W.: Smoking: A basis for advice to the patient. Am. Pract., 8:1226, 1957.

Moyer, J. H.: Treatment of the ambulatory patient with hypertension. G.P., 15:109, 1957.

Piper, D. W., and Raine, J. M.: Effect of smoking on gastric secretion. Lancet, 1:696, 1959.

Report of the Advisory Committee of the Surgeon General: Smoking and Health. Washington, D. C., U. S. Dept. Health, Education and Welfare, 1963.

Rigdon, R. H., and Kirchoff, H.: Smoking and disease. Texas Rep. Biol. Med., *16:*116, 1953.

Roth, G. M., and Shick, R. M.: Effect of smoking on the cardiovascular system of man. Circulation, *17:*443, 1958.

Neuromuscular Blocking Agents

Bennett, A. E.: Preventing traumatic complications in convulsive shock therapy by curare. J.A.M.A., *114:*322, 1940.

Churchill Davidson, H. C.: Neuromuscular block in man. Anesthesiology, *17:*88, 1956.

Foldes, F. F.: The pharmacology of neuromuscular blocking agents in man. Clin. Pharmacol. Ther., *1:*345, 1960.

Friend, D. G.: Pharmacology of muscle relaxants. Clin. Pharmacol. Ther., *5:*871, 1964.

Griffith, H. R., and Johnson, G. E.: The use of curare in general anesthesia. Anesthesiology, *3:*418, 1942.

Levine, I. M.: Muscle relaxants in neurospastic diseases. Med. Clin. N. Am., *45:*1017, 1961.

Rodman, M. J.: Drugs for neuromuscular pain and spasm. R.N., *29:*62, 1966 (May).

———: The muscle relaxants. R.N., *27:*59, 1964 (Aug.).

McIntyre, A. R.: Some physiological effects of curare and their application to clinical medicine. Physiol. Rev., *27:*464, 1947.

Drugs Acting on the Heart and Circulation

Of the patients whom the nurse cares for—whether in the hospital, at home, or in industry—a great many suffer from diseases of the heart and blood vessels. Cardiovascular disease accounts for more disability and more deaths in this country than does any other category of illness. Most people are, of course, aware of these statistics showing the high mortality rate of heart disease and need only see each day's obituary notices to be freshly reminded of the suddeness with which cardiac death can strike. Thus, a diagnosis of heart disease usually hits the patient and his family with a very forceful impact.

Because they associate heart disease with sudden death, people who hear that they have a heart rhythm disorder, a coronary condition, or a failing heart may be overwhelmed by fear and hopelessness at first. Their families often share this despair and are, in addition, alarmed by the thought that, should an emergency arise, the responsibility of obtaining help or even giving the patient emergency care might be theirs alone. They may worry about how helpless they would feel in such a situation, and their uneasiness in the presence of the patient may add to his own anxiety and tension.

The nurse who is called upon to care for a heart patient may also often be troubled by her own responsibilities in what she may view as a life-or-death situation. One way by which she can overcome her apprehension is to gain a fuller understanding of what the risks really are and then prepare herself to deal with them in the most efficient manner. The nurse can, for example, lessen her own doubts by schooling herself thoroughly in the actions and uses of the drugs used in cardiac emergencies.

Actually, the chances are that no sudden emergencies will arise. Many patients with heart disease live with their condition for years and, indeed, die eventually of something else entirely. This has always been so, but it is especially true in this era of rapidly advancing cardiovascular therapy. Some forms of heart disease are now surgically curable, and elec-

tronic pacemakers now keep diseased hearts, that would once have stopped, beating steadily for many years.

These treatments are, of course, quite dramatic. However, most heart patients are still maintained by medical means such as rest, diet and drugs and are able to keep functioning self sufficiently for many years. Contrary to the patient's fears when he hears, for example, that he has "heart failure," this diagnosis is no death sentence. Most patients respond to a regimen of rest and sedation, low sodium intake and other dietary measures, and a combination of a cardiotonic drug of the long established digitalis group with one of the new potent oral diuretic drugs.

In this section, we shall discuss the actions and uses of the most important classes of drugs employed in treating diseases of the heart and blood vessels. Among these drug groups are the following: the digitalis-type plant derivatives which strengthen the beat of the failing heart; the diuretics so effective for removing edema fluids from the tissues of patients with congestive heart failure; the antiarrhythmic agents employed for counteracting irregularities of cardiac rate and rhythm; the anticoagulant chemicals that are used to keep blood from clotting within the vessels of patients who may already be suffering from the effects of a thromboembolic episode (and other drugs that hasten clotting and thus help to stop bleeding); drugs used to dilate the coronary arteries of angina pectoris patients, and medications employed in the management of postcoronary patients with myocardial infarction; drugs for dilating blood vessels outside of the heart—for example, the antihypertensive agents employed to relax the relatively constricted arterioles of the systemic circulation of patients with hypertension (high blood pressure), and the agents used to increase blood flow through the disease-narrowed arterioles of patients with peripheral vascular disease. Finally, we shall study the drugs that affect formation of the blood itself—the vital fluid that the heart pumps through the vessels.

· 18 ·

Review of Cardiovascular Function in Health and Disease

The drugs that are discussed in the various chapters of this section are used to correct or counteract malfunctioning of the circulatory system. In order to gain greater insight into how these drugs bring about their therapeutically useful effects, we must first understand the fundamentals of normal and abnormal cardiovascular functioning. We shall not discuss here in detail the anatomy, the physiology and the pathology of the heart, the blood and the blood vessels; however, we shall review some essential terms and concepts concerning the circulatory system.

THE HEART

The heart is a muscular organ with four hollow chambers (Fig. 18-1). Actually, there are two joined hearts—a right one and a left—and each is divided into two parts, an upper *atrium* and a lower *ventricle*. The right half of the heart, which is separated from the left heart by a partition, or septum, has the task of directing into the lungs the blood brought to it from the body tissues by the veins. The left heart receives the blood after it has been reoxygenated in the lungs and pumps it out into the aorta, from which it flows through the rest of the systemic circulation.

Before we follow the flowing blood to the tissues which it nourishes, let us examine the properties of the muscular pump that propels blood through the 60,000 miles of tubes comprising the rest of the circulatory system.

The heart, which in health beats thousands of millions of times in a lifetime of pumping hundreds of thousands of tons of blood, possesses structural and functional properties different from those of other muscles. The fibers of the myocardium form two intertwining networks, or *syncytia*. This interlacing structure accounts for the fact that first both atria and then

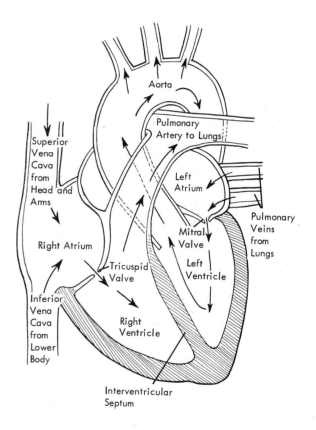

FIG. 18-1. Blood flow, into and out of the heart.

both ventricles contract synchronously when excited by the same rapidly traveling stimulus. Complete simultaneous contraction is a necessary property of a muscle that acts as a pump. A hollow pumping mechanism must also pause long enough to let **its**

275

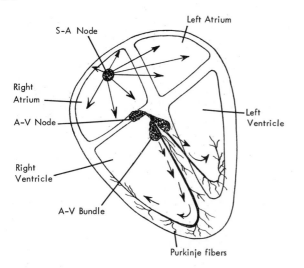

FIG. 18-2. The conducting system of the heart. Impulses originating in the S-A node are transmitted through the atria, into the A-V node to the A-V bundle and by way of the Purkinje fibers through the ventricles.

chambers fill with fluid. Heart muscle does relax long enough to assure adequate filling; and the more fully it fills, the stronger is the contraction that follows as the stretched muscle fibers spring back like elastic bands.

The rhythm of these alternating contractions and relaxations is set by the heart itself. That is, the heart does not need outside stimulation (e.g., by nerve impulses) to make it beat. The stimuli that set off its contractions arise spontaneously in its own tissues. They are believed to arise from the ebb and flow of ions (electrically charged chemical particles) through the membranes of myocardial fiber cells.

This unceasing leakage of sodium and potassium ions through the permeable cell membranes causes changes in electrical potential. Such automatically arising stimuli then spread swiftly through the entire myocardium to set off its contraction. All muscles, of course, possess the property of contractility, and all are excitable—that is, they respond to a stimulus at one point, which is conducted through the whole muscle. However, *self*-excitability, or automatic rhythmicity (*automaticity*), and *conductivity* are especially well developed in cardiac muscle.

Normal Heart-Beat Rhythm

Different tissues within the heart vary in the rate at which they generate electrical impulses. If the various fiber groups all contracted chaotically in response to their own impulses, the muscular walls of the chambers could not contract with the power needed to propel blood out into the vessels. However, the heart has a special system that normally lets the part of the

heart in which impulses arise most rapidly set the pace for the rest of the myocardium.

Ordinarily, the most excitable part of the heart is a knot of tissue on the rear wall of the right atrium. This area—the remains of the sinus-vein-ending seen in the embryo—is located at the point where one of the body's major veins empties into the right atrium and is called the *sino-atrial*, or *S-A, node*. These cells send out their signals at a rate so fast that other cardiac tissues cannot transmit their more slowly generated impulses. Thus, the S-A node is the *pacemaker* that sets off cardiac contractions at a so-called *sinus rhythm*. While the myocardium is contracting it is resistant to impulses arising elsewhere in the heart or impinging upon it from outside by way of its extrinsic nerves. Drugs can sometimes shorten or lengthen this so-called *refractory period* and thus raise or reduce the heart's responsiveness to both normal and abnormal stimuli.

The signal from the S-A node spreads swiftly across both atria and sets off simultaneous contractions in both upper chambers. These beats are followed a fraction of a second later by the coordinated contraction of the ventricles. The speedy response of the ventricles as they become filled with the blood driven into them by the atria is brought about by specialized conducting tissues (Fig. 18-2).

When the wave of impulses crosses the atria it reaches an area of atypical muscle tissue at the junction of the atria and ventricles. This *atrioventricular*, or *A-V, node* picks up the atrial signals and transmits them down into the ventricles. A mass of superconductive tissue located in the septum, or wall, between the two ventricles then speeds the signals along at an accelerated rate. This *A-V bundle*, or *bundle of His*, divides into smaller branches that then pass into the right and left ventricular walls and break up into a network of fine fibers (*Purkinje fibers*), which carry the command to contract to every cardiac muscle fiber group. The coordinated beat of both ventricles occurs only an instant after that of the atria and is delayed just long enough to allow adequate filling.

Nervous Influences

Normally, in response to stimuli originating automatically in the S-A node, the heart beats a bit faster than once every second—about 70 to 80 times a minute. However, the heart's rate is also constantly being adjusted to meet the changing demands of the tissues for oxygenated blood. These adjustments are made as the result of nervous reflexes set off by stimuli from all over the body. The most immediately important stimuli are variations in the pressure of the blood that is pumped out of the heart itself into the first segment of the aorta and into the carotid arteries—the vessels which carry blood to the brain.

The aortic arch and carotid sinuses contain pressure-sensitive receptors which react constantly to slight variations in the pressure of the blood reaching these vessels after cardiac contractions. The sensory signals from these areas to certain brain centers that work constantly to regulate cardiovascular function then stimulate or inhibit their tonic activity. One result of these afferent influences is that these cardioinhibitory and cardioacceleratory centers send out fewer nerve impulses to the heart through the efferent nerves that influence it.

The extrinsic nerves that carry the impulses which alter the heart's automatic sinus rhythm are of two types. The vagus nerves, which are part of the parasympathetic nervous system (Chap. 14), terminate at the S-A and A-V nodes. Impulses arriving at these areas over the vagi slow the heart and weaken its contractions when it is beating too fast and too forcefully. Their activity tends to let the heart rest and conserve its strength. The other nerves that exert an outside influence upon the heart are part of the sympathetic nervous system (Chap. 14). These sympathetic cardioacceleratory nerves speed and strengthen the heartbeat when body tissues require more blood and oxygen for optimal functioning.

This happens naturally during exercise, when the tissues raise their demands for oxygen and the heart responds by beating more rapidly and powerfully to send added blood surging through the arterial circulation. However, heart disease may also set off the same kind of compensatory reflexes for counteracting a lack of adequate tissue oxygenation.

Such tissue hypoxia is one cause of the accelerated heart rate often seen in patients with heart failure. When drugs of the digitalis group (Chap. 19) help the failing heart to beat better, the activity of the cardioacceleratory nerves is reduced and that of the vagus nerves is increased. As a result, the rate of the heart's beating slows as an indirect response to the cardiotonic action of these drugs.

In addition, drugs can slow or speed the heart directly by imitating the actions of autonomic nerve impulses or by blocking such extrinsic impulses. Thus, sympathomimetic drugs accelerate the heart as do vagus blocking drugs like atropine; on the other hand, parasympathomimetic drugs slow the heart rate, as do beta-adrenergic blocking agents.

Cardiac Irregularities

Irregularities in the rhythm of the heart may be caused by many factors besides drugs. The most serious are those that are the result of heart tissue damage. Most often this, in turn, stems from some abnormality in the blood supply to the S-A node or the tissues that make up the pathway from the sinus pacemaker to the terminals of the Purkinje system fibers, including the A-V node, the A-V bundle and its branches. As a result, the atrial and ventricular contractions may become excessively slow (bradycardia) or they may speed up suddenly (paroxysmal tachycardia) or twitch in a wildly irregular manner (fibrillation). These arryhthmias are not all equally serious, but all interfere with cardiac contractile efficiency.

Diseased conducting tissues may, for example, keep impulses originating in the S-A node from being conducted from the atria to the ventricles. In such cases of "heart block," the ventricles beat at a rate which is set by their own slower pacemaker. Sometimes, the decrease in pumping efficiency caused by such bradycardia reduces the blood supply to the person's brain, with resulting dizziness and even "blackouts," or syncopal fainting spells. In addition, these patients have a high incidence of cardiac arrests.

In other cases, impulses arising in diseased tissue (ectopic sites) may trigger contractions at times not set by the sinus pacemaker. Such extrasystoles or premature beats need not be serious, or they may be the prelude to more dangerous arrhythmias, as in digitalis intoxication.

Other cardiac irregularities are atrial flutter, in which these chambers pump almost no blood despite their rapid rate (200–300 beats per minute) and atrial fibrillation. In the latter condition, isolated groups of muscle fibers in the atrial wall contract convulsively but in a completely uncoordinated way. Their chaotic twitching is too weak to drive blood down into the ventricles. This is not immediately dangerous, as the ventricles do still receive and send out blood. However, the doctor may desire to stop the atria from fibrillation, because the churning blood within them may tend to form clots on their inner walls (mural thrombi). Besides, many of the impulses being generated in the atria at a rate of 400 to 600 per minute may be conducted to the ventricles and cause tachycardia. Ventricular tachycardia may, in turn, lead to ventricular fibrillation, a condition which is usually rapidly fatal because the twitching ventricles fail to pump blood out into the aorta and the rest of the systemic circulation. (See Chap. 21 for further details concerning the various kinds of cardiac arrhythmias and their treatment.)

THE CIRCULATION (FIG. 18-3)

The purpose of the heart's unceasing pumping action is to keep blood flowing to and from all the body's tissues. Blood brings the cells the oxygen and nutrients they need for producing energy, and it carries away carbon dioxide and other metabolic waste products. This steady circulation of blood is essential for proper functioning of all the body's organs, including the heart itself. Thus, we should review certain aspects of blood flow through the heart and the pulmonary and systemic circuits. This will help us to understand the various clinical conditions that develop when such

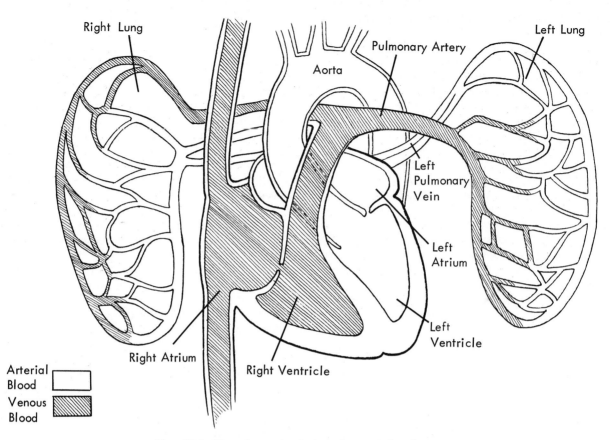

FIG. 18-3. Heart-lung circulation. See text for discussion.

circulation is interfered with, as well as the actions of the drugs used to treat these disorders.

Heart-Lung Circulation

The blood that returns to the right heart by way of the venous portion of the systemic circulation pours first into the right atrium. A contraction of the thin muscular wall of this chamber sends this oxygen-spent blood into the right ventricle which squeezes it, in turn, into the pulmonary artery. This vessel enters the lungs and divides into smaller and smaller channels through which the blood flows until it spreads out in a thin sheet in the pulmonary capillaries. These thin-walled vessels are in direct contact with another wispy membrane lining the alveoli, the terminal cells for air inhaled with each breath. Here oxygen diffuses across these thin walls and is picked up by the blood pigment hemoglobin.

The oxygenated blood is now transferred into vessels that grow from capillary size into venules and, finally, into the pulmonary vein, which carries it into the left atrium. From here the oxygenated blood spills into the left ventricle. The thick muscular wall of this chamber drives the blood out into the aorta, the body's largest artery. Branches of the aorta carry blood to the heart, head, lungs, liver, kidneys and other vital organs.

The Coronary Circulation

The heart muscle itself requires a constant supply of oxygenated blood in order to keep contracting. The myocardium receives its own nourishment through two coronary arteries. These vessels are called "coronary" because they branch off from the aorta just as it leaves the left ventricle and then circle around the upper part of the heart in a pattern resembling a coronet, or crown. The oxygenated blood that is thus immediately fed back into the heart reaches every cardiac fiber, since these main vessels branch, divide, and subdivide throughout the myocardium.

Normally, when the heart's own output of blood is adequate, enough of the flow from the aorta is forced through the coronary vessels to meet the demands of the myocardium for oxygen and nutrients. However, in heart failure (with low cardiac output) and in circulatory collapse (when the arterial blood pressure drops to shock levels) the coronary flow may be reduced, and the myocardium may become hypoxic, thus further reducing its capacity to contract efficiently.

Another cause of inadequate heart muscle circulation may be disease of the coronary arterioles themselves. These vessels are often so narrowed by atherosclerosis that they carry a markedly reduced quantity of blood to the myocardium. If the vessels do not widen when physical exertion or emotional stress make the heart beat more vigorously, the failure to deliver as much oxygen as the myocardium demands may lead to painful attacks of angina pectoris.

If a major branch of a coronary vessel is blocked off by a blood clot or closed down by severe spasm, the prolonged coronary occlusion can result in death of the heart tissue that is deprived of its blood supply. Such a myocardial infarction can then prevent the heart from pumping with enough contractile force to keep the blood circulating properly throughout the body. (See Chap. 22 for a fuller discussion of these pathophysiological processes.)

Systemic Arterial Pressure

The contraction of the left ventricle which sends blood surging out into the aorta creates a pressure that continues to force the blood through all of its divisions. This pressure against the arterial walls is greatest during systole (the contractile phase of the cardiac cycle), and it falls to its lowest level during diastole. Thus, in determining a patient's blood pressure, we measure both the systolic and diastolic pressures.

This head of pressure in the arteries must stay high enough to ensure a sufficient flow of blood to all the body tissues. If it falls too steeply for any reason—for example, through a reduction in cardiac output—tissue function soon fails. A sharp drop of pressure in the carotid arteries is followed by a marked reduction of blood flow to the brain. This leads to loss of consciousness in just a few seconds. Reduced renal arterial pressure interferes with kidney function. This plays an important part in producing edema in congestive heart failure and in keeping patients of other kinds edematous. A very severe fall in pressure following sudden circulatory collapse can kill very quickly, by bringing about a state of irreversible shock that leads to the death of blood-deprived vital organs.

On the other hand, too high a level of arterial blood pressure is also undesirable. Such hypertensive pressure may damage the arterioles and even lead eventually to rupture of a major blood vessel in the brain or other vital organs. Hypertension puts an added burden on the heart which must use up more energy in driving blood out into a relatively resistant circulatory tree.

The cause of most cases of hypertension remains unknown, despite numerous hypotheses. These theories are all based upon the presence of some abnormality in one or another of the complex nervous, hormonal and kidney mechanisms known to play a part in regulating the level of a person's arterial pressure. While high blood pressure is not necessarily caused by excessive vasoconstrictor nerve impulses, many of the drugs employed in treating hypertension (Chap. 23) produce their pressure-reducing effects by lessening the flow of such impulses to the blood vessels; so we should briefly review the ways in which arterial pressure responds to variations in nervous regulation.

Vasomotor Tone. The smooth muscle walls of the blood vessels receive nerve fibers from the sympathetic nervous system. Impulses passing continuously over these fibers to the vascular walls keep the vessels in a constant, or tonic, state of moderate constriction. Any increase in the output of vasoconstrictor impulses by the vasomotor center in the brain stem tends to raise the tone of the vascular musculature and increase the pressure of the blood passing through the narrowed arterioles. A reduction in the number of tonic nerve impulses reaching the smooth muscle walls lets them relax. This dilates the arterioles and results in a lessening of the pressure of the blood on the walls of the vessels.

Although impulses carried by certain nerves may also directly relax vascular smooth muscle, such vasodilator nerves do not play an important role in the control of systemic arterial pressure. Instead, when the blood pressure tends to rise too high, the vasomotor center lessens its output of vasoconstrictor signals. This is accomplished by so-called buffer reflexes which are intensified by pressure rises in the carotid arteries carrying blood to the brain. Many drugs act to lower (or raise) arterial pressure by their effects upon these vasomotor reflex mechanisms.

Venous Pressure

Pressure in the veins may also sometimes rise above normal. This may happen, for example, when the heart cannot adequately cope with all the blood being returned to it by the venous circulation. One sign of the heart's failure to handle this load of blood is a rise in pressure in the right atrium. This, in turn, leads to increased pressure in the veins which empty into this chamber as the venous blood that is attempting to flow into the atrium meets with resistance.

Blood that becomes dammed in the veins behind a weakened heart causes a rise in the venous pressure of many organs, including the lungs, liver, spleen and kidneys. The hydrostatic pressure in the capillaries rises, leading to leakage of fluid into the tissue spaces. This accounts for the pulmonary edema that makes breathing difficult in acute left ventricular failure. It is also a factor in the congestive signs and symptoms of right heart failure—the enlarged liver, fluid-filled abdomen, and pitting edema of the extremities.

However, other mechanisms besides raised venous pressure operate in the production of the congestion of heart failure. Besides the reduction in renal arterial pressure already mentioned, hormonal factors contribute to the kidneys' reduced ability to remove sodium and to the resulting retention of salty fluids in the tissues. For example, the kidney sends out chemical messengers that make the adrenal cortex step up the secretion of the mineralocorticoid hormone, aldosterone. This hormone then stimulates the kidney tubule cells to transport more sodium back into the blood and the fluids bathing the body tissues.

Hypoproteinemia (a reduced amount of plasma proteins) may be a cause of reduced blood volume. This is because these colloid molecules exert an osmotic force (oncotic pressure) which ordinarily helps to retain fluids within the circulatory tree. When the synthesis of plasma proteins is reduced (in liver disease, for example), or when albumin is lost through a leaky glomerular membrane (in nephrosis), fluid tends to move out of the plasma and into the extravascular spaces to form pools of edema. (See Chaps. 19 and 20 for further discussion of the pathophysiologic mechanisms which operate in congestive heart failure, hepatic cirrhosis, nephrosis and other edema states.)

In summary, we have reviewed some aspects of the functioning of the circulatory system. Some of the things that sometimes go wrong with cardiovascular function have been emphasized. An understanding of the importance of the circulation and the necessity to keep this system working as close to normal as possible will lead to a better appreciation of the value of the drugs which we administer to patients with disorders of the heart and blood vessels. Drugs acting upon the cardiovascular system in various ways are discussed in the following chapters of this section.

REVIEW QUESTIONS

1. (a) What structural property of heart muscle fibers accounts for the ability of all the atrial muscle and all the ventricular muscle to contract as a unit with maximal pumping power?

(b) List three physiological properties of heart muscle which help to make it an especially efficient pumping mechanism.

2. (a) List the several parts of the heart's specialized system for generating and conducting the impulses that set off myocardial contractions.

(b) What does the heart gain by having such a specialized pacemaking and conducting system?

3. (a) Name two types of extrinsic nerves that exert influence upon the rate and strength of the heart beat.

(b) How, in general, are such changes set off and brought about?

4. (a) What is the cause of heart block? What are the effects on the patient?

(b) List some cardiac arrhythmias marked by rapid, irregular cardiac muscle fiber contractions.

5. (a) Trace the pathway taken by blood through the heart and lungs and out into the systemic circulation.

(b) How does the heart itself receive nourishment, and what are two conditions which may result from interference with blood flow to the myocardial tissues?

6. (a) What are the two phases of arterial pressure that are measured in taking a patient's blood pressure?

(b) What are some possible results of sharp sustained drops in blood pressure?

(c) What are some possible adverse effects of long-sustained elevation of blood pressure to excessively high levels?

7. (a) What factor largely determines the degree to which blood vessels are kept in a state of partial constriction?

(b) What is the main way by which the extent of tonic vascular constriction is increased or decreased?

8. (a) What may be the result of a rise in venous pressure?

(b) What may be the result of a reduction in plasma protein content?

(c) What are some clinical conditions in which venous pressure may be raised or in which hypoproteinemia may occur?

· 19 ·

Digitalis and Related Heart Drugs

SOURCES OF DIGITALIS PRINCIPLES

Digitalis, a plant that doctors have known and employed for hundreds of years, is more widely used today than ever before. According to one recent survey, close to ten per cent of hospitalized patients receive a digitalis product during their stay. No synthetic drug has yet been discovered that is capable of producing the desirable cardiac actions of this plant and its purified principles.

The British physician William Withering brought this old vegetable drug into modern medicine. In 1775 he singled out the foxglove plant as the active ingredient of an old wives' secret recipe for treating "dropsy," as edema was then called. After studying the effects of the leaf and its watery extracts for ten years, he published his findings in *An Account of the Foxglove*—a classic paper that still makes fascinating reading. Withering, although he thought of the drug as a diuretic rather than a heart stimulant, had obviously learned both the value of digitalis and its dangers.

The most important species employed medicinally in this country is *Digitalis purpurea*, so named for its purplish finger-like flowers. The dried, powdered leaf is official in the U. S. Pharmacopeia and an alcoholic tincture is included in the National Formulary. This plant and another species, *Digitalis lanata*, are also the source of several pure crystalline glycosides of great potency.

Although we shall discuss mainly digitalis in this chapter, other plants also contain principles with digitalis-like action. Some of these botanicals, such as strophanthus, are the source of heart-strengthening drugs that are in use in this country (e.g., ouabain, etc.–Table 19-1). Plants that are used mainly abroad may come to our attention when children occasionally eat parts of flowering ornamental plants, such as the lily of the valley (Convallaria), the Christmas rose (Helleborus), the sea onion bulb (Squill), or the oleander shrub. Substances that have been found in the skin secretions of toads exert the same poisonous yet remarkably useful action that digitalis has upon the pumping action of the heart.

Pharmacological Actions and Clinical Uses

Contractile Action. Digitalis has several actions on the heart, but the most important of these is its ability to increase the strength of the heart beat. This ability to make the myocardium contract more forcefully is demonstrated most clearly in patients with congestive heart failure, a condition that develops when this muscular pump has been weakened by disease.

But what is so special about that? Other drugs such as the sympathomimetic agents epinephrine and isoproterenol (Chap. 16) also strengthen the heart beat. Yet these adrenergic drugs are contraindicated for most cardiac patients, because they force the heart to work too hard, causing it to pound, race, and demand more oxygen than its coronary vessels can deliver. Digitalis, on the other hand, slows the heart beat as it strengthens it. The heart muscle fibers contract more fully and more efficiently, as is indicated by the fact that each systolic contraction drives a greater amount of blood out of the heart without consuming more oxygen while doing the extra work.

Mechanism of Action. Just how digitalis does this is still uncertain, in spite of many studies of its metabolic and electrochemical effects on the heart. All we can say here is that digitalis somehow helps the heart turn more of its chemical (metabolic) energy into mechanical energy. This may be brought about by the drug's action on the contractile protein actomyosin or on an associated enzyme adenosinetriphosphatase—both part of the intracellular energy converting system. On the other hand, digitalis may act on the cell's membrane to affect the transport into and out of the cell of potassium, sodium, calcium and other ions involved in cellular enzyme activity.

Scientists would like to know precisely which phys-

281

TABLE 19-1
CARDIOTONIC DRUGS AND DOSAGE SCHEDULES *

Nonproprietary Name	Proprietary Name or Synonym	Range of Total (Full) Digitalizing Doses	Daily Maintenance Dose
Acetyldigitoxin	Acylanid	1.0–2.0 mg. oral	0.1–0.2 mg.
Acetylstrophanthidin	–	0.6 mg. I.V.	–
Deslanoside, N.F.	Cedilanid D	1.2–1.6 mg. I.V.	0.4 mg. I.V.
Digitalis glycosides, purified	Digalen; Digifolin; Digiglusin	10–15 U.S.P. units oral; 4 units I.V.	0.8–1.6 U.S.P. units
Digitalis, Powdered (dried leaf), U.S.P.	Digifortis; Digitora	1.0–2 Gm. oral	100–200 mg.
Digitalis, Tincture, N.F.	–	10–15 ml. oral	0.75–1.5 ml.
Digitoxin, U.S.P.	Crystodigin; Digisidin; Digitaline Nativelle; Purodigin	1.0–1.5 mg. oral or I.V.	0.05–0.2 mg.
Digoxin, U.S.P.	Lanoxin	2.0–3.0 mg. oral; 1 mg. I.V.	0.25–0.75 mg.
Gitalin (amorphous)	Gitaligin	4.0–8.0 mg. oral	0.25–1.0 mg.
Lanatoside C, N.F.	Cedilanid	5.0–10.0 mg. oral; 1.2–1.6 mg. I.V.	0.5–2.0 mg.
Lanatoside A, B, and C, mixed	Digilanid	3.0–6.0 mg. oral; 0.8–0.16 mg. I.V.	0.33–0.66 mg.
Ouabain, Injection, U.S.P.	G-Strophanthin	0.5 mg.–1 mg. I.V.	–
Squill glycoside, amorphous	Scillaren B	0.5 mg. I.V.	–
Squill glycosides, mixtures A and B	Scillaren	9.6–14.4 mg. oral	0.8–3.2 mg.
Squill glycosides, water insoluble	Urginin	6.0–12.0 mg. oral	0.5–1.0 mg.
Strophanthin	K-Strophanthin	0.5–0.75 mg. I.V.	–

* These doses should be considered as approximations and used as a guide in checking dosage, which is, of course, highly individualized. Full digitalization may be achieved by a series of fractional doses or by a single larger dose (see p. 287).

iochemical functions or chemical steps are affected so favorably by the drug, because such knowledge would give them a deeper insight into the pathological physiology of the failing heart. So far, however, despite much study, the exact mechanism of action of digitalis eludes them.

The Failing Heart. In order to appreciate the benefits of digitalis, we must first picture the patient with congestive heart failure. His signs and symptoms of course vary, depending upon whether his case is mild or severe, acute or chronic. Often, the failing heart is enlarged and its rate is accelerated. Such cardiomegaly and tachycardia are the results of compensatory mechanisms—means by which the handicapped heart has made extra efforts to fulfill its function of keeping all the body's tissues supplied with an adequate flow of blood.

Many kinds of conditions can bring the heart to this state by making it work overtime and use up its reserve energy: In hypertensive vascular disease, the heart has to work harder to overcome the resistance offered by a relatively constricted peripheral circulatory system. Coronary arteriosclerosis gradually reduces the heart's pumping power, and, in cases of acute myocardial infarction, the part of the heart muscle that is deprived of blood and oxygen is too severely injured to force blood out into the circulatory system. The patient whose valves have been scarred and twisted by rheumatic fever, syphilis and other heart-damaging diseases must use up extra energy in repumping part of each previous stroke's output, which keeps flowing back into the chambers by way of the leaky, incompetent valves.

In order to compensate for these defects and the

resulting tissue hypoxia, certain cardiac reflexes set the heart to beating faster. In addition, the larger load of blood that must be pumped by each beat makes the myocardial mass grow greater. Even during diastole, the heart's chambers are dilated by unpumped blood left behind after each systole. Before long, this increased pressure within the ventricles is transmitted back to the great veins that empty blood into the heart, and the relative amount of blood in the arteries, including those of the patient's kidneys, is reduced.

Edema and Congestion. The heart's inability to drive enough blood out of its ventricles to meet the needs of the kidneys and other tissues soon leads to signs and symptoms of circulatory failure. These may

be mild and make their appearance only upon exertion, or they may be severe enough to disable the patient totally and put his life in immediate danger.

The patient's difficulties develop as the pressure in the veins of his lungs and other tissues rises, while the pressure of the blood in the arteries of his kidneys falls, and urine production drops. As a result of the increased hydrostatic pressure of the blood in the engorged veins and the kidneys' failure to remove enough sodium, salty fluids soon begin to ooze out of the venous capillaries and into the extravascular tissue spaces.

The earliest signs of such congestion in right heart failure may be a pitting edema in the ankles, feet or legs. The patient's liver becomes enlarged (hepato-

TABLE 19-2

CARDIAC DECOMPENSATION AND RESPONSE TO DIGITALIS

Signs and Symptoms *	During Decompensation	After Full Digitalization †
Heart Rate, Rhythm, and Size	Heart hypertrophied and dilated; rate often rapid, rhythm irregular (e.g., gallop rhythm, pulse alternation). Patient may complain of awareness of palpitations.	Resting rate slowed to between 70 and 80 beats per minute. Heart size (dilation) reduced, but hypertrophy may still exist.
Lungs	Dyspnea ("breathlessness," or "shortness of breath") on slight effort or when lying flat in bed (orthopnea). Sudden attacks of breath shortness (paroxysmal nocturnal dyspnea or cardiac asthma), and periodic (Cheyne-Stokes) breathing. Pulmonary edema, rales at base of lungs, cough, expectoration, and hemoptysis (bloody sputum).	Breathing improved, but other drugs (e.g., aminophylline and mercurial diuretics) may also be required for relief of bronchospasm and edema, and morphine may be desirable for allaying restlessness, struggling and excitement.
Peripheral Congestion	Pitting edema of dependent parts (i.e., feet, legs, lower abdomen); enlarged liver; accumulation of fluid in abdominal cavity (ascites); veins distended with rise in venous pressure; prolongation of circulation time; cyanosis—dusky blue color of lips, nail beds and elsewhere on the skin surfaces; oliguria and nocturia (increased urine volume at night).	Increased cardiac output and relief of renal anoxia leads to diuresis. Loss of large quantity of salty fluids in urine results in relief of all congestion symptoms and better skin color.
Other	Weakness, fatigue, insomnia; anorexia, nausea, vomiting, abdominal pain.	Strength and appetite return.

* Because the clinical picture in heart failure varies with stage and degree of severity, the signs and symptoms may vary considerably in different patients.

† Digitalis will not overcome similar symptoms when they are caused by conditions other than heart failure. Overdosage may actually cause symptoms similar to those of heart failure (e.g., anorexia, nausea, and vomiting; cardiac arrhythmias; peripheral congestion).

megaly), and fluid leaking out of swollen hepatic venous capillaries accumulates in the abdominal cavity (ascites). The patient's neck veins may be seen to swell and throb, and fluid may also accumulate in subcutaneous tissues throughout his body (anasarca).

Most distressing to the patient is the dyspnea that often develops in left sided heart failure. His discomfort may be especially severe when he lies flat (orthopnea), and it may be relieved only when he sits erect or stands up. These breathing difficulties and pulmonary edema (waterlogging of the lung tissues, with resultant reduction in ventilation) stem primarily from failure of the left ventricle to rid itself of the blood being brought to it by the pulmonary veins by way of the left atrium.

As a result of this left ventricular failure, the pulmonary vein capillaries become distended and fluid is pushed out into the alveolar air sacs of the lungs. In chronic cases, such encroachment upon the air spaces causes cough and the rales which can be heard with the stethoscope. In acute pulmonary edema—a major medical emergency which may develop following a myocardial infarction—symptoms such as cyanosis, blood-tinged frothy sputum and hemoptysis may be further indications of how severely the heart's failure is interfering with the patient's respiratory exchange. Prompt and vigorous action is required both for symptomatic relief and to reverse the fundamental difficulty—heart failure—if the patient's death by drowning in his own fluids is to be prevented.

Treatment of Heart Failure. Measures of many kinds are employed to relieve the various disabling signs and symptoms of cardiac decompensation and circulatory failure. In mild cases, the doctor may merely suggest that the patient take off some weight and that he cut down his physical activity. This, like bed rest, which is ordered for the patient with signs and symptoms of acute congestive heart failure, is intended to reduce the body's demands for blood.

Other measures for control of chronic failure, including reduction of the sodium content of the patient's diet and the use of diuretics (Chap. 20), are intended to remove edema and to keep new fluid from accumulating in the tissues. Patients with acute left ventricular failure usually require administration of oxygen in high concentration. Morphine may be ordered for patients with acute dyspnea in order to lessen their breathing difficulties.

Most important are various medical and even surgical measures for narrowing the gap between the demand for oxygenated blood and the heart's inadequate ability to supply it. Often today, heart surgery can correct a cardiac lesion and overcome congestive failure. New antihypertensive agents (Chap. 23) that bring down the blood pressure of the patient with hypertensive heart disease also often help to ameliorate the pulmonary and other symptoms of congestive failure. Digitalis, however, remains the most important means of increasing the output of the failing heart.

Beneficial Effects of Digitalis. The strengthening action of digitalis on the contractions of the weakened, hypodynamic heart usually produces prompt and, often, dramatic relief of signs and symptoms of congestive heart failure. The improved circulatory competence is apparent, in part, in desirable changes in the rate, rhythm and size of the heart itself. Benefits of better circulatory function are also observed in the kidneys, lungs, and other organs.

Cardiac Improvement. As the ventricles become able to empty themselves more completely, the amount of blood left in these chambers after each systolic contraction is much less than before. This results in a reduction in the diastolic size of the heart—an objective sign of improvement readily visible in chest X-rays. This in itself adds to the heart's pumping power, because a smaller, stronger heart has greater mechanical efficiency than a large, flabby one.

The digitalis-induced increase in stroke volume (the blood pumped by each beat) and cardiac output sets in motion reflex circulatory changes that tend to slow a speeding heart and to increase its efficiency still further. As the tissues begin to get adequate quantities of blood, the stimuli which had set off the cardio-acceleratory compensatory reflexes are removed. The heart rate of patients whose hearts had speeded up (sinus tachycardia) in an effort to meet the needs of the tissues for blood commonly drops by about thirty per cent after adequate digitalization has helped improve the circulation. Other digitalis actions on the rate of the heart (see below) often slow the heart still further.

Circulatory Improvement. Because the ventricles empty more completely, they can cope more readily with the load of blood being brought back to the heart by the veins. At the same time, the kidneys, which now receive a better flow of fresh, oxygenated blood, are better able to perform their filtering function.

This circulatory improvement, which is a hemodynamic consequence of the primary contraction-strengthening action of the heart, permits edema fluid to drain out of the waterlogged tissues. As this fluid is transferred into the arterial portion of the circulation, the pressure in the previously engorged veins falls. This reduction in venous hydrostatic pressure leads, in turn, to relief of lung congestion and of the signs of edema in the skin, limbs, abdomen and elsewhere. Better kidney function is manifested by a marked increase in urine production, which may rise from as little as half a pint or less (oliguria) to as much as several quarts (diuresis).

As fluid leaves the lungs of a patient with pulmonary edema, his dyspnea is usually relieved. With easier breathing, the nurse will note a reduction in the patient's anxiety and restlessness and the restoration of better skin color as cyanosis lessens. In patients with right heart failure, abdominal distention lessens, and pitting no longer occurs when skin of an extremity is pressed.

Diuretic Action. Unlike the drugs discussed in Chapter 20, digitalis is not a true diuretic. It does not (for instance) act upon the cells lining the renal tubules to reduce their capacity for absorbing sodium and water from the glomerular filtrate. In congestive failure digitalis improves kidney function indirectly, by helping the weakened heart to pump a greater amount of blood through the renal arteries. This, of course, raises the reduced glomerular filtration pressure and results in a larger volume of filtrate reaching the tubules.

A smaller proportion than previously of the sodium and water in this filtrate now gets back into the blood. This is because the better blood flow and higher filtration pressure leads to a reversal of the complex nervous and hormonal compensatory mechanisms (see Chap. 20) that had stimulated the renal tubules to absorb excessive amounts of sodium. As a result of decreased renal tubular absorption of sodium, the salty fluid carried to the kidneys is removed from the body as urine, instead of returning to the extracellular spaces.

The nurse should carefully record the patient's urinary output and note the extent of his weight loss, because these signs are a useful index of the drug's desirable action. If improvement of edema is incomplete, the doctor may order addition of a true diuretic to the patient's treatment regimen to bring him down to his "dry weight."

Other Cardiac Actions. We have seen that the main action of digitalis—its ability to strengthen weakened myocardial contractions—can lead to secondary slowing of the heart in patients with sinus tachycardia. In addition to this desirable effect, which stems from the patient's improved circulatory status, digitalis possesses actions that directly and indirectly affect cardiac rate and rhythm. Some of these changes add to the drug's usefulness in heart failure and account for its effectiveness in treating certain cardiac arrhythmias; other cardiac actions of digitalis are the cause of dangerous toxic reactions to overdosage.

Digitalis slows the heart, in part, by raising vagal tone—that is, by increasing the number of impulses that pass down the vagus nerves to exert a braking action on the heart. This ability to slow a speeding heart may be observed not only in patients in heart failure with sinus tachycardia but also in those with other cardiac irregularities. Thus, digitalis is sometimes effective for converting paroxysmal atrial tachycardia to a sinus rhythm after various other drugs and measures have failed. This condition and *A-V nodal tachycardia* are often brought under control by cholinergic drugs such as methacholine (Chap. 15),

which directly stimulate vagal receptors in the cells of the nodal tissues. Emetic drugs and measures such as pressure on the eyeballs or on the carotid sinuses in the neck may also be employed to increase vagal tone indirectly. Addition of digitalis to this regimen further increases reflex vagal stimulation and sensitizes the S-A node to such stimuli. As a result, digitalis often stops an attack of atrial tachycardia which had not responded to parasympathomimetic drugs or to ocular and carotid sinus pressure alone.

Extravagal Effects. Another desirable cardiac action of digitalis is its ability to lessen the number of atrial impulses that reach the ventricles. The drug does this by depressing the ability of the conducting tissues—the A-V node, bundle of His, and Purkinje fibers—to carry the impulses that make the ventricles contract. This extravagal action accounts for a further slowing of the racing heart of the patient in failure—especially desirable for patients who are suffering from atrial fibrillation.

In this arrhythmia, impulses arising in atrial ectopic foci bombard the A-V node at rates of 400 to 600 per minute. The conducting tissues are insensitive to most of these impulses because they arrive during the refractory period. Usually, however, enough impulses can get through to force the ventricles into a rapid, irregular beat. This further reduces the contractile efficiency of the failing heart. Thus, pulse deficit (a difference between the patient's apical pulse and the pulse taken at the wrist) is common in those with this arrhythmia. The ventricles are sometimes stimulated to contract so soon after the start of diastole that little or no blood may be pumped out into the aorta and other peripheral arteries.

The depressant action of digitalis on the conducting tissues helps to lengthen the refractory period and thus ward off most of the impulses that are being showered on the ventricles from such supraventricular sources. Digitalis reduces the ventricular rate, eliminates the pulse deficit and restores the efficiency of the myocardium. Patients with atrial fibrillation who are not in failure also often benefit by digitalis-induced protection against bombardment by excessive impulses from ectopic foci in the atria.

Digitalis is sometimes used to treat another cardiac irregularity—atrial flutter. In part, it is used here, again, to protect the ventricles by producing a partial block of atrioventricular conduction. In addition, the drug may sometimes help convert the flutter to a normal sinus rhythm. Oddly, this often happens only after digitalis has first sent the fluttering atria into fibrillation. If the drug is then discontinued the atria often stop fibrillating spontaneously and begin beating normally. If they fail to do so, atrial fibrillation can usually be overcome by careful administration of the antiarrhythmic drugs quinidine and procainamide or by such new measures as cardioversion (Chap. 21).

The Toxic Effects of Digitalis Overdosage

In the preceding section we have emphasized the desirable effects of digitalis upon the functioning of the failing heart. However, overdosage with this potent drug can actually send a compensated heart patient into failure. Also, as we have seen, digitalis is useful for treating several cardiac arrhythmias—yet extension of the drug's rhythm-altering actions into the toxic range can be the *cause* of almost every kind of cardiac irregularity. Thus, the nurse must be alert and quick to recognize the various types of cardiac toxicity caused by digitalis intoxication, as well as the extracardiac effects which often serve as the first signs of approaching poisoning.

Cardiac Toxicity. Digitalis overdosage tends to cause adverse effects of two different kinds: (1) excessive slowing of the heart, and (2) a variety of cardiac arrhythmias, including ventricular tachycardia, in which the heart beats too rapidly and irregularly. Often the irregular beats begin to develop while the rate of the heart is still generally quite slow. These confusing effects may pose a difficult diagnostic problem for the doctor, who must decide whether the patient needs more digitalis, or has already had too much.

The nurse's observations of signs such as pulse rate, rhythm, and deficit can help the physician in his task of regulating the dosage of digitalis, so that the patient gains the maximum therapeutic benefits of this valuable drug while suffering as little of undesirable drug actions as possible.

A-V Block. We have indicated that the depressant action of digitalis that keeps excessive atrial impulses from reaching the ventricles is a desirable effect. However, as the digitalis accumulates to toxic levels, the number of atrial impulses able to pass through the increasingly refractory conducting tissues may fall too low. As a result, some atrial beats may not be followed by ventricular contractions. Such partial heart block may later become complete, with the atria and the ventricles contracting at entirely different rates. (The doctor can follow these changes on the electrocardiogram, which reflects them first in a lengthening of the P-R interval and later in a dissociation between P waves and QRS complexes on the ECG.)

When heart block is complete, the ventricles continue to beat, but at a rate lower than when the S-A node was setting a pace of about 70 to 80 beats per minute. The ventricular pacemaker sends out its impulses at a rate of 60 or less per minute. Thus, if the nurse, in checking the patient's apical pulse, notes a fall below 60 beats per minute, she should report this to the doctor. (Most physicians try to give just enough digitalis to drop the patient's apical pulse at rest to between 60 to 80 beats per minute. When it falls below 60, they consider this a sign of incipient toxicity.)

If digitalis dosage is continued, the patient's pulse may become so infrequent and irregular (e.g., 35 per min.) that his brain may be periodically deprived of blood. To avoid dizziness, weakness and fainting spells, the doctor discontinues digitalis for a while, until the excess of the drug in the patient's myocardium is eliminated. Sometimes, if syncopal episodes occur so frequently that the doctor fears cardiac arrest, he may administer the adrenergic drug isoproterenol. (See Chap. 21 for a discussion of the use of this agent in treating A-V block in patients with Stokes-Adams disease.)

Increased Cardiac Automaticity. Although isoproterenol may help those patients in whom digitalis has induced heart block, its ventricular stimulating action could be harmful to others. This is because overdoses of digitalis often make the heart excessively responsive to stimuli, including those originating in the ventricle itself. As a result of this increasing rhythmicity or automaticity, impulses may begin to be generated irregularly in various parts of the ventricles other than the normal pacemaker. The impulses arising in such ectopic foci set off extrasystoles.

The ectopic beat most commonly caused by digitalis overdosage is bigeminy, or "coupling," in which the regular beat is followed almost immediately by a weak beat. The nurse should report coupled beats, trigeminy, and other irregularities including the pulse deficits found when extrasystoles felt apically fail to evoke a pulse at the wrist. The doctor then ordinarily orders a temporary halt to digitalis administration. If digitalis is not discontinued, the extrasystoles may become more frequent, the premature beats may take on the rhythm of ventricular tachycardia, and, unless the racing heart is slowed down, fatal ventricular fibrillation may follow.

Other Indications of Overdosage. Often, before any of the cardiac irregularities mentioned appear, the nurse may detect early signs of overdigitalization. These extracardiac effects are often the result of the drug's action on the nervous system and the gastrointestinal tract. Most commonly, the patient may complain of headache and nausea. He may also display a marked aversion to food when his tray is brought to him. Such anorexia should be promptly reported to the doctor, since it is often a sign that the patient is fully digitalized and is entering an early toxic state.

Anorexia and nausea are often followed by salivation, vomiting, abdominal pain and diarrhea. Late vomiting is significant, because it means that digitalis has accumulated in the heart in amounts sufficient to stimulate the central vomiting mechanism. This vomiting is *not* the result of gastrointestinal tract irritation; it can even occur when digitalis glycosides are given by vein rather than orally. It usually indicates that the level of drug in the patient's plasma is high enough to stimulate the chemoreceptor trigger zone (CTZ) in the medulla (Chap. 38), or that its vagal action on the heart is setting off reflexes that indirectly stimulate the vomiting center.

On the other hand, vomiting that occurs soon after administration of the first dose of digitalis does not, of course, indicate overdosage. This is probably caused by the irritating action of the drug. It occurs more frequently with crude drug products such as powdered digitalis leaf and tincture of digitalis, which contain extraneous irritants, than when the pure glycosidal principles are employed. The nurse can help lessen local irritation and the resulting vomiting by giving these preparations shortly after meals.

Other direct effects of digitalis on the nervous system include drowsiness, feelings of fatigue, and, rarely, convulsions. Sometimes, especially in elderly patients with cerebral arteriosclerosis, disorientation, confusion and delirium may occur. Patients may mention that their vision is impaired. They may say that they see flickering yellowish-green lights or note the presence of white dots or "snowflakes," and white borders or frost on various objects. Some patients may show allergic skin reactions or suffer severe facial neuralgia.

All such complaints should be heeded, for they may be early warning signs of digitalis toxicity. In addition, if a parenteral digitalis preparation is employed, the nurse should watch for signs of tissue irritation, which can become severe enough to cause sloughing. Parenteral digitalization is usually reserved for emergencies because of the irritating effects of these drugs, and even then the slow infusion of a dilute solution into a vein is preferred to the more irritating intramuscular and subcutaneous routes.

Prevention and Treatment of Overdosage

It is always better to prevent the full effects of digitalis overdosages from developing in the first place than to subject the patient to the dangerous cardiac toxicity that can occur. If the nurse recognizes the early danger signals, and the doctor promptly orders the digitalis product discontinued, the signs of toxicity may soon disappear. On the other hand, continued administration of the drug, on the false assumption that the return of tachycardia and other signs of heart failure reflects underdosage, may lead to fatal ventricular fibrillation.

The doctor may tell the nurse to terminate the administration of diuretic drugs also at this time, since today's potent diuretic agents may affect electrolyte balance in ways that increase digitalis toxicity. For example, they can cause excessive elimination of the body's stores of potassium. Digitalis is believed to produce its cardiac effects by causing the release of this ion from heart muscle cells. Thus, when a diuretic causes a further fall in plasma potassium levels, the cardiac actions of digitalis are intensified.

Giving potassium salts by mouth may quickly overcome the cardiac toxicity of digitalis. When the cardiac arrhythmias are especially severe, the physician may inject solutions of potassium salts cautiously by vein. To prevent postassium overdosage in such cases, it is important to check the patient's kidney function. The doctor may also monitor the patient's heart action by means of the electrocardiograph during infusion of the antidotal salt solution, in order to detect any effects of excessive potassium before they become serious.

Another electrolyte that plays a part in digitalis toxicity is the calcium which is present in blood and tissues. This ion tends to increase the heart's responsiveness to digitalis. Thus, attempts have been made recently to lower serum calcium levels in order to reduce digitalis-induced arrhythmias. Intravenous infusion of disodium edetate (Endrate), a drug that ties up excess calcium and removes it from the body, has helped counteract the toxic effects of digitalis on the heart.

The antifibrillatory drugs quinidine and procainamide are sometimes employed to reverse the ventricular arrhythmias brought on by digitalis overdosage. The doctor, if he decides to employ these potent cardiac depressants, gives them with great caution, perhaps with electrocardiographic monitoring. For, if these cardiac depressants affect the regular ventricular pacemaker as well as the ectopi foci responsible for the ventricular tachycardia and other arrhythmias, they may cause cardiac arrest of ventricular fibrillation.

The beta adrenergic blocking agent propranolol (Inderal, Chap. 17) has recently been advocated for controlling digitalis-induced ventricular arrhythmias. However, this drug may itself induce heart failure, because it tends to reduce myocardial contractility and cause a decrease in cardiac output in these patients whose stores of myocardial catecholamines are already depleted by their heart disease.

DOSAGE AND ADMINISTRATION OF DIGITALIS

The main aim in administering any digitalis preparation is to give just enough of the drug to reduce heart failure symptoms, causing only minimal minor side effects and avoiding cardiac toxicity entirely. Once effective cardiac concentrations are attained by saturating heart tissues with high initial doses, this "digitalized" state is maintained indefinitely by administering smaller doses of the drug.

Digitalization. The margin between fully effective doses of any available digitalis preparation and amounts that cause side effects is always somewhat narrow. Thus, during digitalization—the initial period of intensive dosage when relatively large doses are given at rather short intervals—the nurse must watch the patient very carefully for signs of improvement and of toxicity, as indicated previously.

The nurse need not be afraid to administer these relatively large doses, but she should always remember that differences of only a fraction of a milligram of the modern potent purified glycoside preparations may determine whether the drug will produce its desired therapeutic effects or an extremely undesirable toxic reaction. Even with the less powerful galenical preparations, such as the tincture of digitalis, the nurse must very carefully measure out the exact number of minims or milliliters that the doctor has ordered.

Some patients who present only mild signs of congestion may be digitalized gradually over a period of several days by administering relatively small fractions of the full oral dose at intervals that allow the drug to accumulate slowly in tissues. More seriously ill patients, such as those with acute left ventricular failure, dyspnea and pulmonary edema, are digitalized more rapidly, sometimes by intravenous injection of fast-acting glycosides in comparatively large doses. In either case, the doctor reduces the amounts administered when the patient shows signs of full digitalization or early toxicity.

Maintenance Dosage. After the patient in failure is adequately digitalized and his congestive symptoms subside, he will probably have to go on taking a digitalis product for the rest of his life. However, he will require much less of the drug each day than was administered during digitalization when the aim was to make the drug accumulate to effective levels as quickly as possible. All that is needed during maintenance therapy is administration of just enough drug to replace the amount eliminated by the body since the last dose.

Even though the daily maintenance dosage of digitalis is smaller, the risk of toxicity remains. For, if the daily dose is just a little higher than the amount eliminated daily, the excess drug will accumulate and cause the insidious development of poisoning. On the other hand, if the daily dose is a bit too low, the patient may slowly slide back into heart failure.

These dosage difficulties indicate the need for teaching the patient and his family the importance of making regular visits to the doctor and of following the doctor's directions for taking the drug carefully and accurately. This puts a special burden on public health and outpatient nurses, whose duties bring them most frequently into contact with such people. To help minimize medication errors, the patient should be supplied with a calibrated (standardized) dropper, teaspoon or vial if he is taking a liquid preparation, such as tincture of digitalis, or a dilution of some other strong digitalis solution. Patients taking tablets of the potent, pure glycosides should understand the importance of never taking two tablets if one is called

for and of never skipping a dose. (Some patients may try to save money by cutting down the number of daily tablets they take.)

The nurse should take extra time to instruct elderly patients. Older people tend to become confused by a barrage of rapid-fire directives; so, after the doctor has finished, the nurse might sit down with the patient and make a written summary of his instructions. She should also give the patient an opportunity to ask questions.

A common query is whether taking digitalis continually will harm the heart. Most patients do not distinguish between the need to take a drug like digitalis indefinitely and the development of dependence or addiction with potent pain-relieving drugs. Thus, if the patient seems uneasy and alarmed when he asks whether he is getting a drug "habit" or if dependence on the drug could make his heart weaker, the nurse can assure him that he will not be harmed physically or emotionally in any way by continuing to take digitalis for prolonged periods.

In language adapted to the level of the patient's intellect and education, the nurse should explain that the drug will help his heart, so that he will feel better and be better able to carry on his daily activities. She can explain at this time, in ways that won't alarm the patient, that though the drug is safe it is important to watch for certain signs and symptoms and to report them to her or to the doctor.

When the patient is seen periodically, the nurse should have *him* explain to *her* how he is taking his medicine. Many older patients may forget the doctor's orders or, because of failing eyesight, not read the instructions on the label of the bottle correctly. They may often forget to take the drug or sometimes take it twice on the same day due to forgetfulness.

All such oversights can best be discovered by asking the patient directly, "How many pills do you take? How often do you take them? Do you have a system for remembering what you took today?" This makes for better instruction than just relying on repetition while the patient says, "Yes" and nods his head without really listening.

The nurse can also show the patient or his family how to keep a record of medicine taken—for example, making a medicine check-off card that can be kept inside the medicine cabinet. Such a card can be made up each week, and patients on daily medication can check off each dose as they take it.

It may seem unrealistic for the nurse in a busy clinic to take the time to teach an elderly man how to take his digitalis and to check each time he returns to see whether he remembers and is following instructions. Yet, if such small measures that show personal concern for the patient are neglected and he is left on his own, we may next hear of him after he has been brought into the emergency room at

2 A.M., unable to breathe, cyanotic, and fearfully struggling for breath. Yet such an illness and the prolonged disability which will probably follow need not happen at all. If someone—and that someone might well be the nurse—had been willing to work with this elderly patient, he could probably have kept a part-time job for another five years. Instead of retaining his independence and taking care of himself, the old person with no one to help him may now never be able to work again—all because no one took the time to go over with him the doctor's recommendations concerning digitalis and diuretic dosage, the importance of staying on his low sodium diet, and the need to pace himself in a program that provided both rest and work.

These general points apply, of course, not only to administration of digitalis, a drug often used for long periods of chronic cardiac illness, but also to the care of patients who are partially or completely disabled by other chronic illnesses. It is sad enough that our society often offers too little emotional or financial support to such people. But it is doubly frustrating that chronically ill elderly patients too often fail to profit fully from available modern treatment measures.

This may be because the need to communicate the little details that make for conscientious care has been too little emphasized. Yet it is just these small points which can add up to success or failure in a chronic cardiac illness requiring long-term digitalis therapy. The nurse working in such a situation—with patients who aren't ever going to be wholly cured and may get gradually worse—should make an extra effort to minimize the adverse effects of the patient's ignorance, carelessness, poverty, or age. She should always function on the basis of a calculated plan of action and yet be willing to alter it in accordance with changes in the patient's condition.

Types of Products. Many different digitalis preparations are available. These fall into three main categories: (1) the powdered leaf of digitalis and galenical preparations made from the crude drug, such as tincture of digitalis; (2) pure glycosides extracted from digitalis species, such as digitoxin, obtained from *Digitalis purpurea*, and digoxin, a glycoside from *Digitalis lanata;* (3) mixtures of all the glycosides of a particular species of digitalis, squill or other plant that contains cardiotonic principles. Such purified mixtures, made up of several active glycosides in the same proportions as found in the plant but free of the inert material in the crude drug, include digalen, digilanid, scillaren, urginin, etc.

Much larger amounts of the powdered digitalis leaf and the tincture made from it must be taken than of a pure glycoside. Thus, for example, a thousand times more digitalis powder must be administered (100 mg.) than the amount of digitoxin (0.1 mg.) that will produce an equivalent effect.

Many doctors now prefer the pure principles, because they are more stable in potency and because the tiny quantities that are required are less likely to cause early vomiting. The crude drug, on the other hand, contains extraneous inactive substances which may irritate the gastrointestinal mucosa and cause nausea and vomiting even early in the digitalizing procedure. (Of course, all digitalis products cause G.I. upset as they build up toward toxic levels.)

Despite frequent claims to the contrary, the different digitalis glycosides do not differ significantly in their relative safety and effectiveness. Biologically equal doses produce essentially the same degree of stimulation of the heart and central nervous system. All the glycosides have about the same safety margin between the therapeutically effective dose for a particular patient and the dose that produces toxic signs and symptoms. In all products, the dose that is required for effective digitalization is said to be about half the dose that causes minor toxicity, and the latter is, in turn, about half the amount that may prove lethal.

Although no one preparation is superior to the others in therapeutic index, differences in the way they are handled by the body may make some products preferable to others in particular clinical situations. For example, the fact that some glycosides are more rapid in onset of action, or that others produce a more prolonged effect are factors that often determine which one the doctor decides to use.

Patients with acute congestive failure and pulmonary edema are best treated with rapidly acting glycosides such as deslanoside, and digoxin, or the ultra-short-acting agents acetyl strophanthidin and ouabain. These drugs begin to act within 10 to 30 minutes after slow intravenous injection. While this route is relatively dangerous, the comparatively rapid rate at which these drugs are eliminated minimizes the chance of severe toxicity. In any case, these drugs are often lifesaving in patients with myocardial infarction who might die before slower-acting glycosides could become effective.

In cases of chronic congestive failure rapid onset of action is less important than a persisting effect. Digitoxin (or the crude leaf and tincture containing this long-lasting glycoside) is often preferred for maintenance therapy because of its slow elimination. Because this drug exerts a long-lasting effect on the myocardium, a patient who happens to miss a day's dosage is in no great danger of slipping back into congestive failure.

A disadvantage of digitoxin's relatively long duration of action is the possibility of prolonged toxicity, in case of overdosage. Because it is so slowly excreted, the toxic effects may not wear off for several days. Similarly, even though its onset of action is relatively slow, digitoxin has a cumulative effect and a small daily overdosage during maintenance therapy can lead to toxic symptoms of gradual and insidious onset.

Two derivatives of *Digitalis lanata*—digoxin and lanatoside C—possess properties that have made them increasingly popular recently. Both act promptly enough to be effective in emergencies, yet, unlike ouabain, they can be given by mouth and cause effects that last long enough to permit their use during maintenance therapy. On the other hand, because they are more easily eliminated than digitoxin, the effects of overdosage by these lanata glycosides are less prolonged and more readily overcome.

Most doctors try to familiarize themselves with only two or three digitalis products which they learn to use with skill. The nurse, on the other hand, may have to administer the varied choices of many doctors. Thus, it is always desirable to check up on the special properties of any relatively unfamiliar preparation that may be ordered.

SUMMARY OF CARDIAC ACTIONS OF DIGITALIS

- **Desirable Actions**

  Increased contractility: each beat of the hypodynamic heart is strengthened, resulting in a larger stroke volume and increased cardiac output, which, in turn, sets into motion desirable circulatory changes.

  Slowing of the heart:

  (1) Secondary to the improved circulation and consequent reduction in cardioacceleratory reflex activity.

  (2) Increased vagal tone sends more parasympathomimetic heart-braking impulses to sensitized S-A and A-V nodes.

  (3) Depressed conduction of impulses in conducting tissues—A-V node, bundle of His, and Purkinje fibers protects ventricles from excessive atrial stimuli.

- **Undesirable (Toxic) Actions**

  Excessive slowing of the heart (60–35 b.p.m.) as a result of partial or complete heart block may lead to dizziness, weakness and fainting spells.

  Increased automaticity leads to various cardiac arrhythmias, including premature beats or extrasystoles, bigeminy or coupling, pulse deficit, ventricular tachycardia, and ventricular fibrillation.

SUMMARY OF POINTS THAT THE NURSE SHOULD REMEMBER DURING DIGITALIS ADMINISTRATION

- Observe the patient for signs of clinical improvement, including the following:

  (1) Gradual slowing of the pulse to between 70 and 80 beats per minute, with reduction in pulse deficit (the difference between the patient's apical pulse and that taken at the wrist). In counting the pulse (for at least a full minute), observe its rhythm as well as its rate.

  (2) Reduction in signs and symptoms of pulmonary congestion such as dyspnea, orthopnea, cyanosis, cough, hemoptysis, and anxiety, restlessness, or other emotional reactions.

  (3) Reduction of generalized edema, as indicated by reduced abdominal size and lessened discomfort or pain upon pressure: absence of pitting when the surfaces of the extremities are pressed; an increase in the patient's daily urinary output and a decrease in his daily weight, both of which should be recorded.

- Before giving each dose of the drug, observe the patient for signs of digitalis overdosage, including:

  (1) An excessive slowing of the heart or the appearance of rhythmic changes such as bigeminy. If the apical pulse rate falls below 60 per minute, the next dose is usually withheld until the doctor has been consulted. (Do not withhold digitalis on the basis of the radial pulse, which may well be below 60, while the apical rate is, for example, 84.)

  (2) Loss of interest in food by a patient who has usually had a good appetite. Ask him whether he feels nauseated and, if so, report this to the doctor to avoid the discomforting vomiting which will probably follow further dosage, and, of course, to prevent cardiac toxicity.

  (3) Listen for complaints of headache, neuralgic facial pain, and unusual visual disturbances.

• Take special care in checking the labels of digitalis products: the names of many of these products are similar and may be readily confused.

• Take particular care to check the accuracy of medication measurements: administration of precisely correct amounts of these extremely potent drugs is essential to the success of treatment and the patient's safety.

• Take time to teach the patient and his family how to follow the doctor's directions for taking these drugs during long-term maintenance therapy. For example:

(1) If possible, write out the doctor's recommendation and go over them with the patient; later, have him tell you how much he is taking and how often.

(2) Show him how to make up a chart on which he can make a check each time a dose is taken, and, in doing so, take the opportunity to emphasize the importance of accuracy in self-administration of this medication.

(3) In answering the patient's questions, try to reassure him of the harmlessness of these drugs when taken as directed and indicate the benefits of faithful adherence to his treatment program.

(4) Help him to understand the importance of reporting to the doctor any symptoms such as loss of appetite and nausea.

(5) Be aware of special problems that may arise with elderly patients whose eyesight and memory may be failing and who may be short of funds and without family or friends.

REVIEW QUESTIONS

1. (a) Name two species of digitalis plants that are the sources of cardiotonic glycosides used in treatment of heart disorders.

(b) Name several plants that are the sources of cardiotonic glycosides with digitalislike activity.

2. (a) What action of digitalis upon the heart is therapeutically most important for patients with congestive heart failure?

(b) In what way does digitalis differ from epinephrine in exerting this action on the heart?

3. (a) Describe the likely condition and action of a hypodynamic heart, i.e., the heart of a patient with chronic failure.

(b) Describe the signs and symptoms of pulmonary and peripheral venous congestion in a patient with congestive heart failure, using some technical terms to picture the patient's condition.

4. (a) What measures besides digitalis treatment may be beneficial to the patients with chronic cardiac decompensation?

(b) What are the earliest signs of digitalis-induced improvement in cardiac function and how are these effects brought about by the drug?

5. (a) Explain how the primary contraction-strengthening action of digitalis brings about improvement of the patient's circulation.

(b) Explain how the digitalis-induced improvement in the patient's circulation leads to removal of salty fluids from the body by diuresis.

6. (a) Explain how the effect of digitalis upon vagal tone can help to convert certain cardiac arrhythmias to a more regular heart beat.

(b) Explain how the extravagal cardiac effects of digitalis may be desirable for patients with heart irregularities of other types.

7. (a) In taking the patient's pulse rates (apical and wrist), what signs indicate improvement under digitalis therapy and which serve as warnings of oncoming drug-induced toxicity?

(b) Indicate two actions of digitalis on the heart that may lead to cardiac toxicity and tend to reduce the heart's efficiency.

8. What are some early extracardiac signs of digitalis toxicity that the nurse should watch for, in

(a) Gastrointestinal system?

(b) Nervous system?

9. (a) What measures may the doctor order to prevent digitalis toxicity from advancing?

(b) What measures may be employed for treating digitalis toxicity?

10. (a) What is meant by *digitalization* and how may digitalis be administered to attain this state?

(b) How does *maintenance* dosage with digitalis differ from initial digitalization?

11. (a) What are some measures the nurse may take to help minimize medication errors by patients taking digitalis?

(b) What are some other suggestions which the nurse may make in teaching patients how to take digitalis correctly over long periods?

12. (a) What property of *digitoxin* makes it desirable for maintenance therapy of chronic congestive failure patients?

(b) What properties of *digoxin* make it desirable in comparison to ouabain or to digitoxin in some situations?

(c) What are some drugs which are preferred for patients with acute failure and pulmonary edema and what property makes them preferable?

CLINICAL PROBLEMS

Mrs. Warren came to the hospital with a diagnosis of congestive heart failure. While in the hospital, she received 0.1 mg. of digitoxin daily and 0.5 Gm. of chlorothiazide b.i.d. Her doctor also prescribed 8 ounces of orange juice daily.

As a result of a regimen of rest, low-sodium diet, and this drug therapy, Mrs. Warren's symptoms improved and she was ready to follow her treatment at home.

Describe:

1. The instructions you would give Mrs. Warren before discharge about taking digitalis and chlorothiazide at home.

2. The observations you, as the public health nurse, would make in regard to the way Mrs. Warren was carrying out her drug therapy.

3. How you would respond to Mr. Warren's uneasy question about whether the drugs his wife was taking were habit-forming.

4. The way you would answer Mrs. Warren's query concerning whether she could substitute prune juice for her daily orange juice.

BIBLIOGRAPHY

Blumgart, H. L., and Zoll, P. M.: The clinical management of congestive heart failure. Circulation, *21:*218, 1960.

Bryfogle, J. W., Santilli, T., Salzman, H. A., and Bellet, S.: Therapeutic and toxic indices of digitalis. New Eng. J. Med., *256:*767, 1957.

Friend, D. W.: Current concepts in therapy (with) cardiac glycosides. New Eng. J. Med., *266:*88–89; 187–189; 300–302; 402–404, 1962.

Frohman, I. P.: Digitalis and its derivatives. Am. J. Nurs., *57:*172, 1957.

Groom, D.: Drugs for cardiac patients. Am. J. Nurs., *56:*1125, 1957.

Harris, A. W.: Management of patients with congestive heart failure *in* Symposium on Treatment of Heart Failure. Modern Treatment, *2:*247, 1965 (March).

Kay, C. F.: Current status of therapy for congestive heart failure. Report to the Council on Drugs. J.A.M.A., *164:*657, 1957.

Krantz, J. C.: The cardiac glycosides in medical practice. Postgrad. Med., *24:*224, 1958.

Lyon, A. F., and DeGraff, A. C.: The neurotoxic effects of digitalis. Am. Heart J., *65:*839, 1963.

Modell, W.: The clinical pharmacology of digitalis materials. Clin. Pharmacol. Ther., *2:*177, 1961.

Pastor, B. H.: The use and abuse of digitalis. G.P., *22:*85, 1960.

Rodensky, P. L., and Wasserman, F.: Observations on digitalis intoxication. Arch. Int. Med., *108:*171, 1961.

Rodman, M. J.: Drugs for heart failure and arrhythmias. R.N., *30:*51, 1957 (Nov.).

———: Drugs for heart failure. R.N., *23:*37, 1960 (Oct.).

———: The manner of action of cardiovascular drugs. R.N., *20:*76, 1957 (Jan.).

Somylo, A. P.: The toxicology of digitalis. Am. J. Cardiol., *5:*523, 1960.

Taylor, R. R., *et al.:* Reversal of digitalis intoxication by beta adrenergic blockade with pronethalol. New Eng. J. Med., *271:*877, 1964.

Diuretics for Edema Management

Diuretics are commonly defined as drugs that cause an increased flow of urine. Actually, most of the clinically useful diuretics do more than merely stimulate the kidneys to produce greater amounts of fluid wastes. By aiding the renal excretion of electrolytes, or dissolved salts, these agents can also alter the chemical composition of the blood and body fluids.

This property is employed clinically for counteracting *edema*. In this state—which occurs, for example, in patients with various disorders of the heart, liver or kidneys—the volume of fluid retained in the spaces between the capillaries and the cells of the tissues is abnormally large. This increase in the percentage of the body's water and dissolved salts that stays outside of both the cells and the blood stream—that is, in the *extracellular compartment*—can have adverse effects on a person's comfort and health.

In heart disease, for example, fluid accumulating in the lungs (i.e., pulmonary edema) and distending the abdomen (i.e., ascites) tends both to make the patient uncomfortable and to increase the burden on his already overworked heart. The edema of congestive heart failure, like edema in other conditions, is the result of a decrease in the excretion of water and electrolytes by the kidneys. Diuretics help the kidneys remove this salty fluid by aiding the renal excretion of the sodium, chloride, bicarbonate and other ions which have helped to keep water trapped in the extracellular fluids that bathe the body tissues.

The value of diuretics for helping edematous patients become more comfortable cannot be overestimated. It is satisfying to see the change in a patient as edema subsides after a few days of treatment. As fluid leaves his abdomen, legs, ankles and face, he loses the bloated look that had distorted his features. This change in appearance alone is a source of great encouragement to the patient and his family. In addition, the patient whose edema fluid has been mobilized and removed usually regains his appetite, feels more energetic, breathes more easily, and moves around more.

During this period, when potent diuretics are exerting their sometimes dramatic effects, the patient often voids copious quantities of urine. The patient should be assured that the often alarming frequency and quantity of his urinary output is a natural reaction to the diuretic drug that he was given. The nurse should see to it that a bedpan or urinal is available to the patient at all times. If the patient is permitted to go to the bathroom, he should still be given these utensils, so that his urine can be measured before being discarded. The doctor may also order daily weighings to check on whether his patient is losing watery weight and to determine when he has arrived at his "dry" weight. If so, the patient should be weighed at the same time each day.

Before discussing in detail how diuretic drugs can affect the chemical equilibrium of the body for better or worse, we should, first, briefly review the role of the kidneys in maintaining *homeostasis*, the internal steady state that is needed for normal body functioning (see also Chap. 45).

REVIEW OF KIDNEY ANATOMY AND PHYSIOLOGY

The kidneys, two bean-shaped, fist-sized organs located on either side of the vertebral column behind the abdominal wall, have been called the body's "master chemists." They do, indeed, play a crucial part in controlling the chemical constancy of the internal environment. By a series of delicately precise physical and chemical mechanisms, they perform the following functions:

1. They rid the body of nitrogenous waste substances of protein metabolism, such as urea and uric acid while, at the same time, conserving the metabolites and minerals necessary for life.

2. They keep the acid-base balance of body fluids in adjustment, mainly by their ability to remove the acid residues of metabolism.

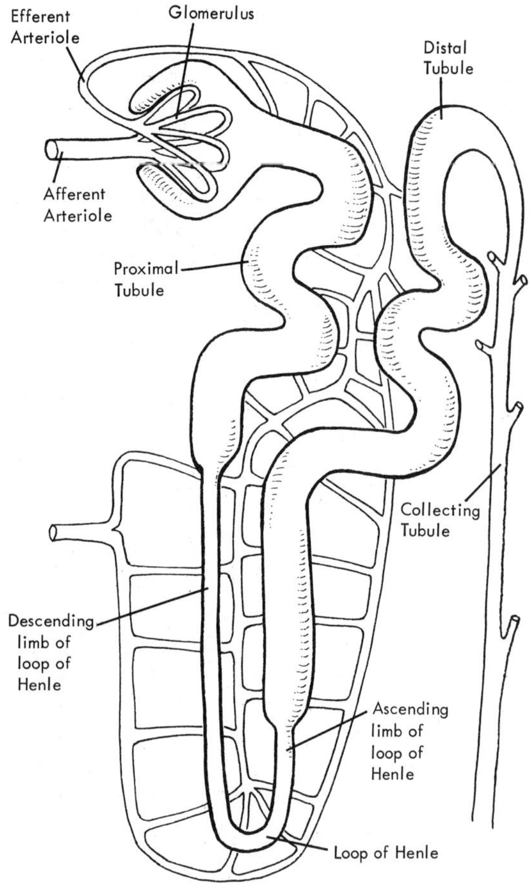

Fig. 20-1. The nephron—the functional unit of the kidney. Secretion and absorption of water, electrolytes and other solutes in the proximal and the distal tubule can be influenced by drugs of many types.

3. They maintain the osmotic balance between the blood and the extravascular fluids that bathe the tissues, mainly by their ability to adjust the concentrations of ions such as sodium, chloride, and bicarbonate in the body's fluid compartments.

The importance of the kidneys in the control of the volume and composition of the body fluids may be seen from the fact that although they make up less than one half of one per cent of body weight, they receive almost one quarter of the blood pumped out of the heart. About 1,700 quarts of blood pass through the kidneys for cleansing daily. From this huge volume of liquid, the kidneys filter out the waste products, foreign materials, and excesses of electrolytes. Most of the fluid is sent back to the blood, along with other essential substances. The

filtered wastes, together with some undesirable substances secreted by the kidneys themselves, are dissolved in a relatively small amount of water and passed out of the body as urine.

These three processes—*filtration, reabsorption,* and *secretion*—are carried out by each of about two million tiny functional units called *nephrons* (Fig. 20-1). Each nephron consists of (1) a *glomerulus,* a microscopic ball of blood vessels enclosed in a membranous capsule (Bowman's capsule), and (2) a hair-thin *tubule,* made up of several segments, which runs a twisted course before it empties into a collecting duct. Each tubule spans a distance of less than two inches, but so serpentine are its windings that the total length of all the renal tubules is estimated to be between 60 and 75 miles!

The *glomerulus* functions as an ultra-fine filter. Normally, its semipermeable membranes keep blood cells, plasma proteins, and lipids inside the capillary vessels, but hydrostatic forces push plasma constituents of smaller molecular size through the tiny membranous pores, along with the water in which they are dissolved. About 125 milliliters of fluid are filtered per minute, or a total of around 180 quarts a day.

Most of this filtered fluid (about 99 out of every 100 milliliters) is returned to the blood as the filtrate makes its way through the tubules. Cells lining the first segment, or the *proximal* portion of the tubules, begin promptly to draw all the essential substances in the filtrate back into the blood vessels closely entwined around the tubules. Sodium, chloride, bicarbonate, and other important cations and anions, and nutrients such as glucose, vitamins, and amino acids are all transported back to the blood by *reabsorptive processes* in the loop of Henle and the distal as well as the proximal portions of the tubule.

Most of the water (about 80 per cent) in which these substances are dissolved, diffuses back *passively,* along with the solutes. The remaining one fifth of the water is pulled out of the tubules and back into the blood by the cells lining the far end, or the *distal* portion, of the *convoluted tubule* and the *collecting duct.* All such mechanisms for *actively* transporting water and solutes require work and the expenditure of energy. This energy is supplied by enzymatically catalyzed chemical reactions. Some of these processes are influenced by hormones of the posterior pituitary gland and the adrenal cortex, and, as we shall see, these cellular enzymes can be affected by drugs in ways that alter the ability of the tubules to reabsorb sodium and other ions.

The epithelial cells that line the renal tubules are capable of carrying certain ions and various foreign substances (e.g., penicillin) in the *reverse* direction also. This process of *tubular secretion* plays an important part in regulating acid-base balance. The tubular cells secrete ammonia, for example, and they transport hydrogen ions into the glomerular filtrate in exchange for sodium ions. This helps to conserve the body's stores of base and results in production of an acid urine. Drugs that interfere with hydrogen-ion formation and secretion cause an increase in the elimination of sodium and bicarbonate. The loss of these ions that combat metabolic acidosis, plus the retention of chloride ions, tends to make the tissues less alkaline than usual, a condition called *hyperchloremic acidosis.*

THE EFFECTS OF DRUGS ON URINE-FORMING PROCESSES

It is important to understand that diuretic drugs are *not* useful for stimulating failing kidneys. In fact, the administration of diuretics is contraindicated when renal function is markedly impaired. Glomeruli and tubules that are severely scarred by disease cannot be whipped into performing their functions more efficiently by administration of diuretics. Uremia and distortions of the internal environment such as acidosis and alkalosis are treated either by removing excess electrolytes and waste materials by physical procedures (e.g., hemodialysis with an artificial kidney), or by replacing missing electrolytes (e.g., potassium) in just the right quantities required to rectify the imbalance caused by kidney failure.

On the other hand, when the kidneys are capable of functioning, diuretic drugs can act to influence the processes of *glomerular filtration, tubular reabsorption,* and *tubular secretion* in ways that produce a copious flow of salty urine. This action is useful primarily for treating the edema that occurs when the extra-vascular salt stores trap water in the spaces between the body cells and the blood vessels. Edema occurs in many different diseases and as a result of derangements of various types. No matter what the underlying cause of the edema may be, it is often possible to relieve the disabling tissue swelling with drugs that increase the renal excretion of sodium ions and water.

Tubular Reabsorption. The most effective diuretic drugs are those that *alter tubular reabsorption.* Agents such as the organic mercurial compounds and the sulfonamide diuretics are believed to act in this way. It is thought that they inhibit the enzymes that produce the energy needed to reabsorb filtered ions from the tubular fluid. The tubular epithelial cells then fail to pull back some of the sodium (for example) in the glomerular filtrate, and these ions pass on to the collecting tubules, carrying with them the water which would otherwise have been reabsorbed into the blood and would have leaked into the tissue spaces. If acid chloride ions are excreted in excess along with sodium, and tissue bicarbonate stores become relatively elevated, a condition called *hypochloremic alkalosis* may develop.

Since 99 per cent of the filtered water is ordinarily reabsorbed and only 1 per cent ends up as urine, it takes only a 1 per cent decrease in tubular reabsorption to double the amount of urine produced. (That is, if the 1% of filtrate not absorbed makes 1 quart of urine, a drug that keeps the tubules from reabsorbing 2% of the filtrate will raise the volume of urine to 2 quarts.) The excretion of this additional amount of urine may spell the difference between chronic invalidism and a state of relative well-being.

Tubular secretion also can be altered by drugs, with a resultant removal of excess sodium and water. For example, drug-induced inhibition of the enzyme carbonic anhydrase results in decreased production and secretion of hydrogen ions by the renal tubular epithelial cells. When fewer hydrogen ions are available to be exchanged for sodium ions, the water-trapping sodium winds up in the urine instead of moving back into the blood and the fluids in the extravascular tissue spaces. The simultaneous loss of bicarbonate ions and retention of chloride causes a relative tissue acidosis.

Glomerular filtration may be increased by drugs that bring an increased amount of blood to the capillary filter beds. Digitalis, as we have seen, often causes a copious diuresis by strengthening the heart beat and increasing the cardiac output. The resulting rise in renal blood flow produces a greater amount of glomerular filtrate containing considerable salt drained from engorged tissues. Sodium and chloride ions, when they are delivered to the tubules in amounts exceeding the reabsorptive capacity of the lining cells, are passed on into the collecting tubules, carrying water along with them in a copious urine flow.

Drugs of the xanthine class, such as aminophylline, are also thought to act, in part, by increasing the amount of blood filtered by the glomeruli. This may be the result of their heart-stimulating action and the consequent circulatory improvement, or it may be due to direct dilatation of renal arterioles. In any case, a somewhat larger volume of filtrate is formed and this, together with some decrease in the tubular reabsorption of filtered sodium and chloride ions, is thought to account for the diuresis produced by these drugs.

THE CLINICAL USES OF DIURETICS

Diuretic drugs are used primarily for providing symptomatic relief of the many conditions in which sodium and water are retained in the tissues. Some are also employed for treating certain disorders in which visible edema does not occur. Before discussing the several different classes of diuretic drugs, we shall first briefly review some of the specific clinical conditions for which diuretic therapy is indicated.

Congestive Heart Failure. We have already seen (Chap. 19) how the stimulating effect of digitalis on the heart and subsequent improvement in renal circulation may lead indirectly to the removal of fluid from the tissues by way of the kidneys. Sometimes, however, digitalis alone may not produce adequate diuresis. This may be because heart failure sets in motion a vicious cycle of *hormonal* events that interferes with kidney function.

For example, the reduced renal blood flow may stimulate secretion of the adrenal cortical hormone *aldosterone*, a substance that acts on certain renal tubular cells to make them reabsorb sodium from the glomerular filtrate more efficiently. Retention of this electrolyte in turn stimulates the release of the *antidiuretic hormone* (ADH) from the posterior pituitary gland. ADH aids the reabsorption of water by the cells lining the distal portion of the convoluted tubule (see Chap. 27).

Administration of a potent diuretic may break this cycle by blocking the tubular reabsorption of sodium and water. The resulting elimination of great quantities of salty fluids both reduces the gross edema and decreases the abnormally large blood volume and the high venous pressure which also had tended to drive fluids out of the blood stream and into the extravascular spaces.

Hepatic Ascites. Several factors contribute to the formation of fluid in the abdomen of patients with cirrhosis and other liver diseases. Rising pressure in the capillaries of the portal vein tends to push fluid out into the peritoneal cavity. On the other hand, the ability of the blood to retain fluid is reduced because of lowered production by the liver of the plasma proteins that normally tend to pull fluid back into the blood by their colloidal osmotic (oncotic) pressure. In addition, the damaged liver has a low detoxifying capacity and does not readily inactivate the fluid-retaining hormones that have been secreted by the adrenal and posterior pituitary glands.

The introduction of potent diuretics in recent years has reduced the need to draw off fluid periodically from the patient's abdomen by paracentesis, or tapping, an operation involving puncture with a trochar, and further loss of protein. These drugs act, of course, not to improve liver function but by reducing the amount of sodium that is reabsorbed into the blood stream by the renal tubules after glomerular filtration.

Renal Edema. Loss of protein is also a factor in the edema of the *nephrotic syndrome*, a condition in which the damaged kidney glomeruli hold back sodium and permit plasma proteins to leak out into the tubules to be lost in the urine. Diuretics of various kinds are used cautiously to remove sodium retained in the tissues because of decreased glomerular filtration and reduced colloid pressure in the blood. Many children with this disease also benefit from treatment with corticotropin (ACTH) and corticosteroids, which sometimes bring the permeability of the glomerular capillaries back to normal.

Drug-Induced Edema. In many chronic conditions, administration of corticosteroids may cause rather than cure edema (Chap. 28). Cortisone and hydrocortisone, for example, tend to stimulate renal tubular reabsorption of sodium. Thus, patients with severe rheumatoid arthritis, asthma, or other conditions that require prolonged steroid treatment may often benefit from daily administration of oral diuretic drugs, to counteract the tendency of corticosteroids to cause fluid retention.

Premenstrual Edema and Tension. During the last days of the menstrual cycle, many women develop edema and varying degrees of increased nervous tension. The new diuretic drugs that can be conveniently taken by mouth have recently been employed for relief of symptoms such as breast fullness and subcutaneous swelling or puffiness. Emotional tension also appears to be reduced when excess fluids are eliminated at this time.

Edema of Pregnancy. Hormonal imbalance may be one of the factors involved in edema of pregnancy. Patients who show signs of fluid retention in early pregnancy are now often maintained on diuretics. When toxemia threatens, diuretics are often prescribed together with antihypertensive agents which are employed to keep the patient's pressure from rising to dangerous levels.

Hypertension. The sulfonamide-type diuretics, such as chlorothiazide, are widely employed, either alone or combined with more specific blood pressure reducing drugs, in the management of hypertension. The exact nature of their action in this non-edematous condition is not fully understood. It has been suggested that these saluretic, or salt-removing, compounds may lower the salt content of the patient's arterial walls, and that this may make the arterioles less responsive to vasoconstrictor hormones and nerve impulses. (See also Chap. 23.)

Other Non-Edematous States. Diuretics of the carbonic-anhydrase-inhibitor type are sometimes used in the treatment of acute glaucoma (Chap. 42) and in selected cases of epilepsy (Chap. 8). Occasionally, diuretics may be employed in the treatment of poisoning to hasten renal elimination of the toxic substance. Bromide intoxication has been successfully treated in this way. It is also common practice to force fluids in order to dilute the concentration of nephrotoxic substances that might damage the kidney during their elimination. Intravenous administration of osmotic diuretics (p. 302) along with hydrating solutions has been advocated to protect the kidneys and prevent acute renal failure in conditions marked by severe reduction in renal blood flow.

CLASSES OF DIURETIC DRUGS

The Organic Mercurial Diuretics

Actions and Use. The mercurial compounds, when administered parenterally, produce a powerful diuretic action in patients with severe edema. This is the result of the inhibiting action of mercury ions on certain enzymes essential to the tubular reabsorption of sodium and chloride ions. The loss of salt and of the water in which it is dissolved is often very large in waterlogged patients. As much as ten quarts of urine may be voided after a single intramuscular injection. The diuretic action may then be maintained by daily administration of oral doses of mercurials or other agents.

Once the diuretic action begins, it may continue for many hours. Thus, mercurials are best administered in the morning to avoid disturbing the patient's rest during the night. The patient should be warned that the injection may cause copious diuresis, so that he will not be alarmed by the frequency and urgency of his need to void all through the day. A bedpan or urinal should be readily available for the patient's convenience during the drug's peak action (about four to eight hours after injection).

Untoward Reactions and Precautions. Despite their potency and reliability, the mercurial diuretics have been largely replaced in recent years by the sulfonamide-type diuretics, which are safer and more convenient to administer. The mercury ion is capable of causing both local irritation and systemic toxicity. The irritating action of mercury on the kidney tubules makes these diuretics unsafe for patients with acute nephritis; also, they should be used only with great caution in patients with chronic renal disease, and the urine should be checked periodically for the presence of albumin, blood cells, and casts.

Patients who are *hypersensitive to mercury* sometimes show signs of stomatitis (mouth irritation), skin eruptions, fever, dizziness and stomach upset. *Chlormerodrin* (Neohydrin; see Drug Digest), which is an orally effective mercurial, causes gastric distress more frequently than do the oral diuretics of the sulfonamide class.

Muscle cramps and weakness sometimes result from excessive loss of electrolytes in copious diuresis—a *low-salt syndrome* similar to that found in heat prostration. Patients who have been on a low salt diet should be most carefully watched for signs of salt depletion during mercurial diuresis.

Excessive salt loss (*hyponatremia* and *hypochloremia*) may make patients unresponsive to further treatment with mercurial diuretics. Paradoxically, the administration of sodium chloride may then get diuresis going once more. Patients are also often primed with *ammonium chloride* for this purpose prior to administration of mercurial diuretics. More

recently, *l*-lysine monohydrochloride and *l*-arginine hydrochloride have been introduced for overcoming resistance to mercurial diuresis in patients with such *hypochloremic alkalosis*. These acidifying chloride compounds are said to be safer than ammonium chloride in patients with liver disease, in whom the ammonium salt may sometimes precipitate hepatic coma.

Intravenously injected mercurials have occasionally caused fatal ventricular arrhythmias. These drugs are now rarely given by vein; however, the occurrence of such arrhythmias indicates the need for caution when diuretics of this class are being given by any route to patients with a history of heart irregularities. Special care must be taken when potent mercurials are administered to patients who are heavily digitalized after a recent myocardial infarction.

Various substances are commonly combined with mercurials to decrease local irritation and pain or to increase their effectiveness. The addition of small amounts of *theophylline* is claimed to increase absorption of the mercurial from intramuscular injection sites and thus reduce local irritation. *Merethoxylline procaine* contains a local anesthetic to deaden the injection site. The nurse can minimize such discomfort by making the injection deep into the muscle, beneath the subcutaneous fat, and then massaging the area vigorously.

In the mercurial compound *mercaptomerin* (Thiomerin; see Drug Digest), mercury is combined with sodium thioglycollate, a sulfur-containing compound that is said to counteract the toxicity of the mercury ions. It is claimed that mercaptomerin is less irritating than other combinations and that it can be injected subcutaneously with greater safety. This drug may be given rectally in the form of a suppository, with less likelihood of causing proctitis than other mercurial compounds. Nonetheless, the nurse should examine the patient's rectum regularly for signs of developing irritation during treatment.

Summary. The organic mercurials are often still preferred for initiating diuresis in severely edematous patients. However, the possibility of their causing many dangerous side effects has led to a decrease in the use of mercurials for the long-range maintenance of patients requiring continued diuretic therapy. It is likely that the use of these drugs will decline further as a result of the recent introduction of the potent nonmercurial diuretic, sodium ethacrynate (p. 299).

The Sulfonamide Diuretics (Benzothiadiazides, etc.)

Actions and Use. The comparatively recent introduction of the sulfonamide diuretic *chlorothiazide* (Diuril; see Drug Digest) in the late 1950's ushered in an era of safer, more convenient treatment for edema. This compound and its many close congeners (called *thiazides*) and certain other chemical relatives of slightly different structure (phthalimidines, etc.) are, when given by mouth, nearly as effective as parenteral mercurials; moreover, they are less likely than the latter to cause severe toxicity. For example, the sulfonamides are safer for patients with some degree of kidney impairment. Even when the mercurials may be preferred for initiating diuresis, the easy-to-take thiazides are useful for keeping the patient edema-free over long periods. Their relative safety also permits the use of these diuretics in premenstrual edema and other minor conditions for which the use of the more dangerous mercurials had not seemed warranted.

The sulfonamides produce a pattern of electrolyte excretion similar to that caused by the mercurials. Like the latter, they tend to remove sodium and chloride ions in close to equal amounts. The exact mechanism of this saluretic action has not been clarified, but it is believed to stem from the ability of these drugs to block reabsorption of electrolytes and water by the renal tubular cells. As a result, salt and water are removed from edematous tissues and excreted in the urine.

Side Effects and Potential Toxicity. Although the sulfonamide diuretics are better tolerated than the mercurials, the changes which they cause in the patient's electrolyte patterns may lead to various ill effects. Excessive loss of salt and water may, of course, cause the *low-salt syndrome*—muscle weakness, leg cramps, mouth dryness, and dizziness, as well as gastrointestinal disturbances. The excessive excretion of chloride, coupled with the compensatory retention of bicarbonate ions, may cause the acid-base imbalance called *hypochloremic alkalosis,* with resulting weakness, lethargy, epigastric distress, nausea and vomiting.

These drugs may also permit the removal of excessive amounts of potassium ions from the plasma, with resultant *hypokalemia.* This is especially dangerous for patients under digitalis treatment, because low potassium levels sensitize the heart muscle to the irritating action of the cardiac glycosides. Thus, these patients should be closely watched for development of cardiac irregularities or other early signs of possible potassium depletion. It is important to correct hypokalemia or to prevent it by administering potassium supplements or giving fruit juices and foods (e.g., bananas) containing this ion routinely to patients under treatment with thiazide diuretics.

Such natural sources of potassium are certainly preferable to enteric-coated tablets containing this ion. A number of patients have suffered severe damage to the small intestine when they were given products containing potassium chloride combined in this manner with a thiazide diuretic. The tablets became stuck at certain points in the bowel, and the salt reached a high local concentration in the delicate tissues of the jejunum and ileum. This led to bleeding and ulceration, with perforation in some patients and scarring and contraction at the site of the gut lesion in others. Such stenosis, or narrowing, of a portion of the intestine has caused serious obstruction.

This is, of course, *not* an adverse reaction to the thiazide diuretic, nor is it the administration of potassium itself that is undesirable. The danger is that a poorly soluble tablet may get caught at a single spot in the gut and release its entire contents in one place. Commercial solutions of soluble potassium salts such as the acetate, chloride, citrate, bicarbonate and gluconate are also available and seem safe enough.

Physicians may prefer to try to minimize thiazide-induced potassium loss through use of a combination of a diuretic of that class with one that tends to *prevent* potassium loss. The *non*-thiazide diuretics triamterene (Dyrenium) and spironolactone (Aldactone), which are discussed later, are examples of diuretics that tend to reduce potassium loss when they are combined with thiazides.

Cautions and Contraindications. Certain patients other than those taking digitalis—notably those with severe kidney and liver disease—require careful observation while receiving thiazide-type diuretics. Others, with a history of diabetes, gout, or hypersensitivity to sulfonamide drugs, occasionally have been affected adversely during treatment with these diuretics.

Patients with hepatic ascites caused by severe liver damage have sometimes been sent into coma when treated with thiazides. The increased excretion of sodium and potassium induced in these patients may somehow raise the level of ammonia in their blood. The nurse should watch the cirrhotic patient for signs of excessive drowsiness, confusion and muscle tremors when thiazide diuretics are being employed for removal of fluids from his distended abdomen. Patients with severe renal disease do not ordinarily receive diuretics—and, when they are used, the nurse should be especially alert for any indication that kidney function is being further impaired rather than helped. If this occurs, it could lead to cumulation of unexcreted drug in the kidneys and other body tissues.

The thiazides occasionally cause a rise in the blood level of uric acid of persons with gout. This results from reduced renal excretion of uric acid by the kidney, and the doctor can readily correct the condition and prevent a possible attack of acute gouty arthritis by prescribing a uricosuric agent (Chap. 41) to speed the excretion of this metabolite. Diabetic patients may experience reduced glucose tolerance and hyperglycemia during prolonged thiazide diuretic therapy. Although this can be readily corrected by increasing insulin dosage, these diuretics are used with caution in patients with diabetes mellitus. (Oddly, these sulfonamide diuretics act to *reduce* urine production in patients with *diabetes insipidus* [Chap. 27].)

Hypersensitivity reactions similar to those sometimes observed with the antibacterial sulfonamides used to treat infections have occurred with these diuretics. These allergic responses include skin rashes, urticarial reactions, and photosensitivity. More serious (and, fortunately, rare) are reports of blood dyscrasias, including leukopenia, agranulocytosis, and aplastic anemia.

Newer Sulfonamides. Each new sulfonamide diuretic that is introduced is claimed to be superior to the earlier agents of this class. Actually, these drugs differ mainly in the dose needed to produce saluresis. Some of these compounds are close to a hundred times as potent, milligram for milligram, as others, in their sodium-excreting capacity. This, in itself, is not an advantage, since their potassium-depleting effect runs more or less parallel. Since these drugs do not differ much in their maximum edema-removing ability, their clinical effects are essentially similar. Some of these sulfonamide diuretics are, however, more slowly eliminated and, consequently, produce a diuresis of longer duration. Chlorthalidone (Hygroton), methyclothiazide (Enduron), polythiazide (Renese), and trichlormethiazide (Metahydrin; Naqua) are among these long-lasting diuretics which need be given only once a day, or even only every other day, for keeping patients edema-free.

New Diuretics of Increased Potency

Recently, two new diuretics have been introduced that are claimed to be more effective than previously available drugs. These agents, *ethacrynic acid* (Edecrin) and *furosemide* (Lasix), are said to remove edema in patients who had proved refractory to treatment with other diuretics. These compounds have in common an unusual property—the capacity to produce continued diuresis even after their action has created hypochloremic alkalosis.

It will be recalled from our discussion of the organic mercurials (p. 297) that patients tend to become unresponsive to further diuretic treatment after elimination of an excess of chloride ions. With the newer drugs, on the other hand, diuresis persists even after hypochloremia and alkalosis or acidosis have developed. Although this continuing action in the presence of diuretic-induced electrolyte imbalances adds to their effectiveness for removing edema fluid, it also makes more likely the possible development of serious fluid-electrolyte disturbances.

For this reason, it is recommended that patients who require these potent diuretics receive them for the first time in the hospital, where laboratory facilities are available for keeping close check on plasma levels of chloride, potassium and sodium ions and upon the state of the patients' acid-base balance. Such studies, together with close clinical observation during the period of initial dosage adjustment, are particularly important for preventing hepatic encephalopathy in cirrhotic patients and cardiac arrhythmias in digitalized heart failure patients.

The nurse should be particularly alert with these drugs for signs and symptoms of the syndromes that can occur as a result of too vigorous diuresis (see summaries, p. 304). The doctor may also have the nurse weigh the patient daily during treatment with ethacrynic acid or furosemide. From her reports, he may be able to determine and then order the smallest dose of these diuretics that will produce the desired gradual loss of weight. Although these drugs can remove as much as 20 pounds of fluid in 24 hours, it is safer to administer them in individualized doses that bring about a weight loss only of one or two pounds a day.

These two potent new diuretics are chemically different from one another. Furosemide is a *non*-thiazide sulfonamide derivative; the other, ethacrynic acid, is an organic acid of unusual structure. Yet both drugs apparently exert a similar effect on sodium ion reabsorption at the same renal tubular site—the ascending limb of the loop of Henle. This action, together with their interference with tubular reabsorption of sodium ions elsewhere in the tubule, may account for their unusual potency and rapid onset. The oral administration of either drug usually produces diuresis in one half to one hour. Injection of the soluble salt of ethacrynic acid, *sodium ethacrynate*, by vein has reportedly doubled urine production within 15 minutes. This has helped to save the lives of some patients suffering from severe pulmonary edema.

Other Diuretics

Various other substances with diuretic properties are employed in special circumstances. Although these drugs do not possess the potency of the organic mercurial agents or the long-term safety and effectiveness of the sulfonamide diuretics, they are sometimes more valuable for a particular patient than the more widely used drugs.

Spironolactone (Aldactone) is a synthetic steroid drug that structurally resembles the adrenal hormone *aldosterone*. It acts by blocking the effects of this hormone on the cells of the kidney tubules. Aldosterone secretion plays a part in perpetuating the edema of cardiac, kidney and liver disease by stimulating the return of sodium to the blood from the filtered fluid that is passing through the renal tubules.

An advantage of spironolactone over most other diuretics is that it does not cause the loss of potassium: in fact, this drug tends to decrease the excretion of potassium. Thus, it is often given in combination with thiazide-type diuretics (e.g., hydrochlorothiazide) in order to counteract their tendency to cause the elimination of too much potassium. This, of course, lessens the likelihood of hypokalemia.

An added advantage claimed for combination of spironolactone with a thiazide diuretic is that the effect of the two drugs on sodium excretion is additive. This may be because the thiazides interfere with the tubular reabsorption of sodium mainly at the *proximal* portion of the renal tubule, whereas spironolactone exerts its retarding effect on sodium reabsorption in the *distal* end of the tubule.

Spironolactone is reserved mainly for patients whose edema has resisted treatment with other diuretics. Such patients are often suffering from hyperaldosteronism, a hormone imbalance that sometimes develops secondary to severe cardiac, hepatic, and kidney disorders. However, this drug is not used for patients with severe renal insufficiency, because its potassium-retaining action could lead to development of *hyper*kalemia in such patients. Excessive plasma potassium loss might then affect cardiac function adversely.

Triamterene (Dyrenium). This relatively new synthetic diuretic possesses properties similar to those of spironolactone and the thiazides, but it also differs from them in various ways. Like the thiazides, this drug has the capacity to increase the excretion of sodium and chloride ions. Unlike the thiazides, it does not eliminate potassium ions. In this respect, it resembles spironolactone. However, the mechanism by which triamterene tends to cause retention of potassium in the tissues differs from that of spironolactone; that is, triamterene is *not* an aldosterone antagonist.

This diuretic is used alone, only when patients have proved resistant to thiazide diuretics or suffer allergic or other adverse effects from them. It is administered mainly in combination with a thiazide (e.g., hydrochlorothiazide). The main advantage of such combinations over a thiazide alone is that the patient is less likely to lose excessive amounts of potassium. As indicated earlier, hypokalemia is especially dangerous in digitalized patients. Thus, triamterene-thiazide combinations are especially suited for patients being treated for chronic congestive heart failure. Triamterene and spironolactone are now also recommended as adjuncts to therapy of cirrhotic patients with the potent new diuretics ethacrynic acid and furosemide.

Triamterene has caused few serious adverse effects. However, *hyper*kalemia may result from potassium retention unless proper precautions are taken. Thus, if a patient who has been taking thiazides has triamterene added to his regimen, the doctor will probably have him discontinue his potassium supplements. This is especially true in patients whose impaired kidneys might be unable to remove the extra potassium.

Triamterene, like the thiazides, has a saluretic action. However, it is not ordinarily employed for treatment of high blood pressure, as are the thiazide diuretics, because it does not have a consistent enough hypotensive action to be therapeutically useful. Triamterene may sometimes potentiate the action of an antihypertensive drug that the patient may be taking, which could lead to an unexpectedly steep drop in the patient's blood pressure.

Carbonic Anhydrase Inhibitors. The enzyme carbonic anhydrase (CA) plays an important role in certain cellular chemical reactions. In the kidney tubule cells, for example, its action helps to produce free hydrogen ions. These are then secreted into the tubular fluid in exchange for sodium ions. This is one of the ways by which the body conserves its stores of base while excreting the acids formed during metabolism.

Certain substances were found to inhibit carbonic anhydrase in renal tubular cells. This block of CA activity leads to reduced hydrogen ion secretion and, in turn, to the loss of sodium and bicarbonate ions in a copious flow of alkaline urine. Drugs of this kind— the CA inhibitors—were among the first orally effective diuretics to be introduced. However, they have largely been replaced in edema treatment by the more dependable and longer-acting thiazide diuretics.

The CA inhibitors—acetazolamide, etc. (Table 20-1)—are still employed for certain specialized purposes. They are effective, for example, as adjuncts to miotic drugs in the treatment of glaucoma (Chap. 42), and they are sometimes administered together with anticonvulsant drugs for the control of epileptic seizures of the petit mal and grand mal types (Chap. 8). Their usefulness in these conditions may be due, in part, to their ability to dehydrate the patient and acidify his tissues. On the other hand, they may act by inhibiting carbonic anhydrase in brain cells and ocular blood vessels or by some other mechanism entirely.

Xanthine-Type Diuretics. Theophylline, theobromine, and caffeine are relatively weak diuretics when given in small oral doses. They have largely been replaced in recent years by more dependable diuretics. The xanthines are, however, still commonly employed for other purposes—for example, as bronchodilators in the management of asthma (Chap. 40). One drug of this class, *aminophylline*, is sometimes especially useful for patients with pulmonary edema following left-sided heart failure (Chap. 19). In such cases of so-called cardiac asthma, this drug, administered intravenously, sometimes produces dramatic relief of dyspnea in patients who had failed to respond to treatment with digitalis and mercurial diuretics. This response to aminophylline probably results not only from its diuretic action but also from its bronchodilator effects and its digitalis-like stimulating action on the heart.

Cytosine-Type Diuretics. These synthetic drugs are distantly related chemically to the xanthines and share some of their properties. *Aminometradine* and *amiso-*

TABLE 20-1
DIURETIC DRUGS

Nonproprietary Name	Trade Name	Usual Daily Dosage Range
Sulfonamide-Type Diuretics		
Bendroflumethiazide	Naturetin; Benuron	2.5 to 5 mg. orally
Benzthiazide	Exna	25 to 100 mg. orally
Chlorothiazide N.F.	Diuril	500 to 1000 mg. orally
Chlorothiazide sodium	Lyovac Diuril	500 mg. to 2 Gm. I.V.
Chlorthalidone	Hygroton	50 to 100 mg. orally at first (100 to 200 mg. 3 times weekly)
Cyclothiazide	Anhydron	2 mg. (1 mg. 2 or 3 times a week)
Flumethiazide	Ademol	500 mg. to 2 Gm. orally
Furosemide	Lasix	40 to 200 mg. orally
Hydroflumethiazide	Saluron	25 to 200 mg. orally
Hydrochlorothiazide U.S.P.	Esidrix; HydroDiuril; Oretic	25 to 200 mg. orally; maintenance, 75 to 100 mg.
Methyclothiazide	Enduron	2.5 to 10 mg. orally
Polythiazide	Renese	1 to 4 mg. orally
Quinethazone	Hydromox	50 to 100 mg. orally
Trichlormethiazide	Metahydrin; Naqua	2 to 8 mg. orally
Carbonic Anhydrase Inhibitors		
Acetazolamide U.S.P.	Diamox	250 to 375 mg. orally
Acetazolamide sodium U.S.P.	Diamox Sodium	275 to 415 mg. I.M.
Dichlorphenamide U.S.P.	Daranide; Oratrol	100 to 200 mg. orally initially; 25 to 150 mg. maintenance
Ethoxzolamide	Cardrase; Ethamide	62.5 to 250 mg. orally (intermittently) (but also up to 750 to 1,000 mg.)
Methazolamide U.S.P.	Neptazane	50 to 200 mg. orally
Organic Mercurial Diuretics		
Chlormerodrin N.F.	Neohydrin	55 to 110 mg. orally
Meralluride U.S.P.	Mercuhydrin Sodium	1 to 2 ml. parenterally
Mercaptomerin sodium U.S.P.	Thiomerin	130 mg. (in 1 ml.) parenterally once or twice a week
Mercumatilin sodium	Cumertilin Sodium	Test dose: 0.5 ml.; maintenance, 2 ml. I.M., or 1 to 2 ml. I.V., at biweekly intervals
Mercurophylline N.F.	Mercuzanthine	200 mg. orally; 1 ml. (135 mg.) I.M., once or twice a week
Merethoxylline procaine	Dicurin Procaine	0.5 to 2 ml. S.C. or I.M.
Mersalyl sodium and theophylline	Salyrgan-Theophylline	Initial dose 0.5 ml.; maintenance, 1 to 2 ml. I.M. or I.V.
Xanthine and Cytosine Diuretics		
Aminometradine	Mincard	200 to 800 mg. orally
Aminophylline U.S.P.	Theophylline-Ethylene-diamine	100 to 200 mg. orally; 250 to 500 mg. rectally; 250 to 500 mg. I.V. slowly
Amisometradine	Rolicton	800 to 1,600 mg. orally
Chlorazanil	Daquin	—
Diphylline	Neothylline	200 to 600 mg. orally
Oxtriphylline	Choledyl	200 to 1,600 mg. orally
Theobromine N.F.	—	500 mg.

TABLE 20-1 (Cont'd)

Nonproprietary Name	Trade Name	Usual Daily Dosage Range
Xanthine and Cytosine Diuretics (*Cont'd*)		
Theobromine sodium acetate N.F.	Thesodate	250 to 750 mg. orally
Theobromine and sodium salicylate	Diuretin	600 to 3,000 mg. orally
Theobromine calcium salicylate	Theocalcin	500 to 1,500 mg. orally
Theophylline N.F.	Theocin	200 to 800 mg. orally
Theophylline Calcium	Phyllicin	500 to 1,000 mg. orally
Miscellaneous Diuretic and Anti-Edema Agents		
Osmotic diuretics (*Nonelectrolytes*)		
Dextrose	Glucose	25 to 50 Gm. I.V.
Mannitol N.F.	Osmitrol	50 to 200 Gm. I.V.
Urea U.S.P.	Carbamide	25 to 60 Gm. orally
Urea in invert sugar or in dextrose solution	Ureaphil; Urevert	100 to 1,000 mg. per Kg. of body weight, infused slowly by vein as a 30 per cent solution
Acid-forming salts and compounds		
Ammonium chloride U.S.P.	—	1 to 8 Gm. divided (e.g., single doses of 300 to 2,000 mg. orally); 100 to 500 ml. of a 2 per cent solution, I.V.
Ammonium nitrate	—	6 to 12 Gm., divided
Calcium chloride	—	4 to 8 Gm., divided
Lysine monohydrochloride	—	—
Aldosterone antagonists		
Spironolactone U.S.P.	Aldactone	25 mg., 2 to 4 times daily
Unclassified		
Ethacrynic acid	Edecrin	25 to 200 mg. orally
Sodium ethacrynate	Lyovac Sodium Edecrin	0.5 to 1 mg. per Kg. body weight, I.V.
Triamterene	Dyrenium	100 to 200 mg. orally; maintenance, 100 mg.
Nondiuretic anti-edema aids		
Albumin, human, salt poor	—	20 to 50 ml. I.V.
Carbacrylamine resin	Carbo-Resin	48 to 100 Gm. orally

metradine, for example, are relatively weak diuretics, and, like the xanthines, they tend to cause some gastrointestinal distress. Thus, they are best given after meals to lessen possible nausea and vomiting. Like the xanthines, these drugs have been largely replaced by the more potent and dependable thiazides.

Osmotic Diuretics. Molecules filtered from the plasma by the glomeruli vary in the extent to which they are reabsorbed into the blood by the renal tubules. Some, such as *glucose,* are normally reabsorbed completely; another sugar, *mannitol,* is not reabsorbed at all and soon appears in the voided urine. *Urea,* another nonelectrolyte, is also classed as a so-called *low-threshold* substance, because only about half of the amount that normally reaches the tubule is reabsorbed; the rest is excreted in the urine.

When such substances are given in large amounts, the portion that is not reabsorbed carries with it extra amounts of water as it leaves the nephron. Although, in theory, urea and glucose can be used to reduce chronic edema, their use for this purpose is not very practical because of the large quantities that have to be injected to remove adequate amounts of sodium. The increase in plasma volume may sometimes make congestive heart failure worse. Hypertonic solutions of urea may cause tissue injury; and glucose has to be given in amounts that cause diabetes-like hyperglycemia—that is, the diuretic action of glucose depends upon its being administered in amounts that exceed the kidney's capacity to reabsorb it. As in actual diabetes mellitus, diuresis results because the excess glucose keeps in the tubules water which would otherwise be reabsorbed into the blood. Despite such polyuria, the amount of sodium excreted is relatively limited.

Nevertheless, the ability of certain of these substances to keep filtered fluid from being reabsorbed from the renal tubules makes them useful in the treatment of certain serious conditions. For example, urea (see Drug Digest) is often useful in cerebral edema. When they are injected intravenously, urea solutions tend to draw fluid from the brain and carry it to the kidneys for excretion. The resulting reduction in intracranial pressure benefits patients with brain injuries requiring neurosurgery. Reduction of cerebrospinal pressure relieves headaches and stops projectile vomiting. Intravenous urea may also be employed to reduce intraocular pressure in glaucoma and prior to eye operations such as surgery for a detached retina.

Mannitol infusions are often employed to prevent oliguria and acute kidney failure. The increased flow of fluid through the kidney reverses renal failure in patients suffering from shock following severe hemorrhage, injuries, and surgical procedures such as open-heart operations. In poisoning by nephrotoxic agents such as mercury bichloride, the increased amount of water in the tubules tends to dilute the poison and limit its toxic effects on the tubular tissues. (For further information on uses and dosage of mannitol see Drug Digest.)

These osmotic diuretics must not, however, be used when kidney function is severely impaired. For, if the kidney cannot eliminate them, the molecules may carry fluid into the blood and tissues, thus overloading the circulation. Mannitol is not administered to patients with congestive heart failure because it may produce pulmonary edema in patients with low cardiac reserve.

Miscellaneous Agents. Certain substances which are only weak diuretics or not diuretics at all are sometimes employed in the management of edema. The acidifying salts such as *ammonium chloride* are used mainly to make the kidneys more responsive to mercurial diuretics. Used alone, their effect is fleeting, largely because the kidney quickly compensates for the drug-induced tissue acidity. Even in enteric-coated form, the large amounts required often cause epigastric distress.

Ion exchange resins such as *carbacrylamine* help to remove dietary sodium from the intestine before it can be absorbed from the gastrointestinal tract. Unfortunately, other important ions such as potassium and calcium also tend to become tied to the resin and leave the body in the feces in excess amounts. This and various other drawbacks have led to these substances' being largely replaced by oral thiazide diuretics.

SUMMARY OF SIDE EFFECTS, TOXICITY, AND CONTRAINDICATIONS OF CERTAIN POTENT DIURETICS

- **Organic Mercurial Compounds**

  Hypersensitivity reactions: Dermatitis, fever, dizziness, stomatitis, nausea and vomiting; intravenous injections have caused fatal ventricular arrhythmias.

  Local irritation: Pain at sites of injection; epigastric distress from tablets; proctitis from suppositories.

  Electrolyte depletion: Excessive salt loss may cause muscle weakness or cramps, lethargy, circulatory collapse, oliguria and azotemia.

  Contraindications: Acute nephritis; repeated injections should not be given to patients who fail to respond. (Hypertonic sodium chloride injections may be required to correct low-salt syndrome, or ammonium chloride to correct hypochloremic alkalosis.)

- **Sulfonamide-Type Compounds** (Benzothiazides, etc.)

  Electrolyte imbalances: Muscle weakness or cramps, thirst, dizziness, paresthesias, nausea, vomiting, diar-

rhea; (if severe and unrecognized) oliguria, hypotension, convulsions, coma. (Administer sodium chloride for hyponatremia and hypochloremia, potassium salts for hypokalemia and alkalosis.)

  Hypersensitivity reactions: Skin eruptions of maculopapular type, photosensitivity, leukopenia, agranulocytosis, thrombocytic purpura.

  Cautions and contraindications: Patients with poor kidney functions may retain blood urea nitrogen (BUN), nonprotein nitrogen (NPN), and creatinine; gout patients may get acute attacks from higher uric acid levels; diabetes patients may need more insulin; heart irregularities may occur in digitalized heart patients.

- **New Potent Diuretics** (Furosemide and Ethacrynic Acid)

  Electrolyte imbalances: Too vigorous diuresis may lead to dehydration and excessive loss of sodium, chloride and potassium ions. Signs of hyponatremia, hypokalemia and hypochloremic alkalosis include muscle cramps, weakness, thirst and paresthesias. (Weigh the patient daily during the period of dosage adjustment to avoid excessive diuresis. Administer supplemental potassium chloride to prevent hypokalemia.)

Other adverse effects: Gastrointestinal complaints include anorexia, nausea and vomiting. Mild diarrhea may occur with both compounds, but the occasional profuse watery diarrhea caused by ethacrynic acid requires discontinuation of drug treatment. Readministration of this diuretic in such cases is contraindicated.

Other cautions and contraindications: These drugs are contraindicated in the presence of anuria and should be withdrawn if increasing oliguria or azotemia is noted during treatment. Particular caution is required with the following patients:

1. Those with advanced liver cirrhosis: diuretic drug-induced electrolyte imbalances may lead to encephalopathy, hepatic coma and death

2. Patients receiving digitalis for cardiac decompensation: diuretic drug-induced hypokalemia can cause fatal arrhythmias

3. Patients taking antihypertensive drugs, who are subject to episodes of postural hypotension

4. Diabetic patients, in whom hyperglycemia may develop

5. Gout patients in whom an acute gout attack may be precipitated by a rise in plasma levels of uric acid

6. Patients who have previously exhibited sensitivity to these drugs resulting in leukopenia or thrombocytopenia

- **Carbonic Anhydrase Inhibitors**

Electrolyte imbalances: Potassium depletion and sodium bicarbonate loss cause hypokalemia and mild metabolic acidosis, leading to gastrointestinal upset (anorexia, nausea, vomiting, mouth dryness), nervous system signs and symptoms (drowsiness, dizziness, headache, tinnitus, tremor, paresthesias—i.e., numbness and tingling of face and extremities, especially lips, fingers and toes).

Hypersensitivity reactions: Skin rashes, fever, bone marrow depression, crystalluria, and renal calculi.

Cautions and contraindications: Patients with renal failure; Addison's disease and adrenocortical insufficiency; respiratory disorders with reduced pulmonary ventilation leading to hyperchloremic acidosis.

- **Aldosterone Antagonists** (Spironolactone)

Electrolyte imbalances: Caution is required in patients with impaired renal function because of the danger of potassium retention, leading to serious *hyperkalemia.* Patients with severe liver disease may lose excessive sodium and suffer the effects of *hyponatremia* and subsequent stupor or transient hepatic coma.

SUMMARY OF POINTS FOR THE NURSE TO REMEMBER DURING DIURETIC THERAPY

- Keep an accurate record of the patient's fluid intake and urinary output.

- Weigh the patient once daily, at the same time each day, to determine whether he is losing watery weight. Patients may lose 10 to 20 pounds in one day of diuretic action.

- Record any visible decrease in edema, such as the absence of pitting when fingers are pressed into the flesh of the extremities, and note any reduction in the protrusion of the abdomen, in ascites.

- Explain to the patient that these drugs may produce a copious flow of urine, so that he will not be alarmed by the frequency and urgency of his need to void

within a few hours after a potent diuretic has been administered.

- See to it that a urinal, bedpan, or other facility for voiding are readily available. Patients may eliminate several quarts of urine in the course of a day after a mercurial diuretic has been administered by injection in the early morning. If the diuretic is one that is given once during the day, administer it in the morning, so that its effects will have diminished by bedtime, and the patient will not have his sleep disturbed by the need to void frequently.

- Know the signs and symptoms of the various syndromes that may result from excessive loss of electrolytes and water and how they may be prevented or counteracted. Gastrointestinal, muscular, and nervous disorders may be the secondary result of dehydration, potassium depletion, low-salt syndrome, hypochloremic alkalosis, or hyperchloremic acidosis.

- Know the signs and symptoms of the hypersensitivity reactions and direct tissue toxicity that sometimes occur with mercurial diuretics.

- Make intramuscular injections or mercurials deep into the muscles, avoiding subcutaneous fat pads and edematous areas. Massage the area vigorously to enhance absorption and reduce local pain and irritation. When mercurial suppositories are employed, examine the patient's rectum for signs of irritation.

- Report any reduction in urine production after repeated diuretic administration. This may alert the doctor to the need for supplementary electrolytes to overcome refractoriness. In the case of mercurials, it may prevent kidney injury, with consequent cumulation of the metal to toxic levels in renal and other tissues.

REVIEW QUESTIONS

1. (a) What are diuretics and what, in general, do they do that helps to overcome edema?

(b) Describe some of the changes in the appearance and attitudes of a patient whose edema has been relieved by treatment with a diuretic.

(c) What are some ways in which the nurse can be of assistance to the patient during diuretic therapy and what changes in his condition should she watch for?

2. (a) List the three main *functions* of the kidneys.

(b) List the three *processes* by which the kidneys carry out these functions.

3. (a) How, in general, do diuretics that alter *tubular reabsorption* aid in removing edema?

(b) How, in general, can a drug that reduces *tubular secretion* of hydrogen ions aid in removing edema?

(c) How, in general, do drugs that increase *glomerular filtration* aid in removing edema?

4. (a) List six clinical conditions in which diuretics may be indicated for treating edema.

(b) Indicate briefly how an excess of two natural hormones may help to cause edema in congestive heart failure, hepatic cirrhosis, and other conditions.

(c) What role does a reduction in plasma proteins play in the mechanism of hepatic and renal edema formation?

5. (a) Under what circumstances are organic mercurial diuretics mainly used today, and how are they usually administered?

(b) What can the nurse do to minimize pain from the parenteral administration of mercurial diuretics?

6. (a) List some substances that are sometimes combined with organic mercurial diuretics to lessen local tissue irritation and pain.

(b) List some substances that are sometimes administered to patients to increase responsiveness to organic mercurial diuretics.

7. (a) List some signs of hypersensitivity to the mercury ion in an organic mercurial diuretic.

(b) Name two fluid and electrolyte disturbances that may result from excessive diuresis induced by organic mercurials, and indicate some signs of electrolyte depletion.

8. (a) What are the main advantages of the thiazides and related sulfonamide diuretics?

(b) What is the meaning of the following sentence concerning the sulfonamide diuretics? "They are employed to produce *saluresis,* but excessive *natriuresis* and *chloruresis* may lead to *hyponatremia* and *hypochloremic alkalosis.* In addition, *kaluresis* commonly leads to *hypokalemia.*"

9. (a) What are some of the ways by which the loss of potassium sometimes caused by sulfonamide diuretics may be counteracted?

(b) What advantage may the newer sulfonamide diuretics such as chlorthalidone, methyclothiazide, and polythiazide have over earlier drugs of this class?

10. (a) List patients of several types who should not receive sulfonamide diuretics or in whom these drugs must be administered with caution.

(b) What adjunctive drugs may need to be administered along with thiazide diuretics when patients with gout or diabetes who require diuretic therapy suffer a drug-induced exacerbation of these chronic conditions?

11. (a) What property of the potent new diuretics, ethacrynic acid and furosemide, appears to account for their increased effectiveness?

(b) What measures may be taken to prevent the occurrence of fluid-electrolyte imbalances as a result of production of too vigorous diuresis by these drugs?

12. (a) How does spironolactone exert its diuretic effects, and what are the results of its action upon the movement of sodium and potassium ions?

(b) What are the advantages of combining spironolactone with a thiazide diuretic?

(c) For what type patient is spironolactone indicated and in whom is it contraindicated?

13. (a) How does the effect of triamterene resemble that of thiazide diuretics and how do they differ in their effects upon the handling of sodium and potassium by the kidney?

(b) For what type patient may this drug be a preferred diuretic and in whom is it contraindicated?

14. (a) How does drug-induced inhibition of the enzyme carbonic anhydrase lead to increased excretion of sodium ions?

(b) List several CA inhibitor drugs and indicate two

clinical conditions besides edema in which they are employed.

15. (a) How do substances such as glucose, mannitol, and urea bring about a more copious flow of urine?

(b) List some clinical conditions in which osmotic diuretics are employed and others in which these drugs are ineffective or even contraindicated.

BIBLIOGRAPHY

Baker, D. R., Schrader, W. H., and Hitchcock, C. R.: Small bowel ulceration apparently associated with thiazide and potassium therapy. J.A.M.A., *190*:586, 1964.

Beyer, K. H., and Baer, J. E.: Physiological basis for the action of newer diuretic agents. Pharmacol. Rev., *13*:517, 1961.

Chinard, F. P.: Current status of therapy in the nephrotic syndrome in adults. J.A.M.A., *178*:312, 1961.

Ford, R. V.: The new diuretics. Med. Clin. N. Am., *45*:961, 1961

Friedberg, C. K.: Treatment of heart failure . . . with diuretics. J.A.M.A., *174*:2129, 1960.

Friend, D. C.: Modern diuretics and diuretic therapy. Clin. Pharmacol. Ther., *1*:5, 1960.

Fries, E. D., and Sappington, R. F.: Long-term effect of probenecid on diuretic-induced hyperuricemia. J.A.M.A., *198*:127, 1966.

Gold, H.: Present status of the management of congestive heart failure and advances in diuretic therapy. J. New Drugs, *1*:160, 1961.

Heath, W. C., and Freis, E. D.: Triamterene with hydrochlorothiazide in the treatment of hypertension. J.A.M.A., *186*:119, 1963.

Javid, M.: Urea—new use of an old agent. Surg. Clin. N. Am., Aug., 1958.

Kessler, R.: Clinical pharmacology of chlorothiazide compounds. Clin. Pharmacol. Ther., *3*:109, 1962.

Leiter, L.: Mechanisms and management of edema. Bull. N. Y. Acad. Med., *40*:432, 1964.

Moyer, J. H.: Diuretics. Ab. J. Nurs., *59*:1119, 1959.

Rodman, M. J.: Diuretics to fight edema. R.N., *22*:33, 1959 (June).

———: Roundup of the diuretics. R.N., *26*:77, 1963 (Nov.).

Rodman, M. J.: Drugs for congestive heart failure and cardiac arrhythmias. R.N., *30*:51, 1967 (Nov.).

Tublin, I. N.: Treatment of edema with an orally administered spirolactone. J.A.M.A., *174*:869, 1960.

Walker, G. W.: The clinical use of furosemide and ethacrynic acid, Med. Clin. N. Am., *51*:1277, 1967.

Warshaw, L. J.: Acute attacks of gout precipitated by chlorothiazide induced diuresis. J.A.M.A., *172*:802, 1960.

Antiarrhythmic Drugs

CARDIAC ARRHYTHMIAS

As we have seen (Chap. 18), the heart contracts and relaxes in response to impulses that arise regularly at the sinoatrial pacemaker and spread swiftly through the atria, the specialized conducting tissues, and the ventricles. Many factors may interfere with the orderly origin of these waves of excitation or with their spread through the heart muscle fibers where normally they induce contraction. The irregular rhythms that then result may markedly reduce the pumping efficiency of the heart and thus interfere with blood flow to vital organs.

Disorders of the heart beat (ectopic rhythms) may develop when a disease-damaged bit of heart muscle tissue outside of the sinoatrial (S-A) node becomes hyperirritable and takes over the pacemaker function. Such ectopic foci are often the source of rapid rhythms—*premature beats, atrial flutter* and *tachycardia,* and *ventricular tachycardia.* According to other theories, many arrhythmias occur when the waves of excitation take abnormal pathways through the heart muscle. As a result, the impulses may—for example—travel in circles (circus movements), continuing to stimulate the same small fiber bundle rings instead of activating the whole atrial or ventricular muscle mass to contract at once. *Atrial* and *ventricular fibrillation* are examples of these arrhythmias, in which isolated groups of fibers contract rapidly but weakly with a resultant loss of coordinated pumping power.

Disturbances in the conduction of impulses from the atria to the ventricles may lead to still another kind of cardiac irregularity—atrioventricular (A-V) *heart block.* This may occur in elderly patients because of a poor blood supply to the conducting tissues as a result of atherosclerosis of coronary arterioles, or the A-V node may be damaged by an acute coronary occlusion. In either case, impulses arising in the atria may be delayed in their passage to the ventricles (partial block), or they may fail to reach the ventricles at all (complete heart block).

In this chapter, we shall deal mainly with two classes of drugs that directly affect the excitability, conductivity, rhythmicity, and other properties of the heart:

1. *Drugs that depress the myocardium* (Quinidine, procainamide, etc.). These reduce its irritability and slow the rate at which the waves that activate contractions are conducted through the heart. These drugs are most useful in heart conditions characterized by very rapid ventricular rates (140 to 180 beats per minute) even though the arrhythmias may sometimes originate in the atria. In many such critical cases, the careful parenteral administration of a cardiac depressant may restore normal sinus rhythm. Even when the supraventricular arrhythmias cannot be abolished, these drugs may succeed in slowing the ventricular rate. Daily oral doses often help to reduce the number and severity of recurrent attacks of atrial tachycardia or atrial fibrillation.

2. *Drugs that increase cardiac rhythmicity* (isoproterenol, ephedrine, epinephrine). These drugs are used to speed up hearts that are beating with excessive slowness, or even sometimes to restart a heart that has stopped (cardiac arrest). In complete heart block, for example, the ventricles take up a slow beat of their own when atrial stimuli fail to reach them through the blocked conducting tissues. However, this idioventricular rhythm may be too slow (below 36 beats per minute) to supply an adequate flow of blood to the brain. Drugs of this class help to increase the rate and output of the slowed heart.

CARDIAC DEPRESSANTS

The cardiac arrhythmias that are caused by abnormal impulses that arise in hyperirritable areas of the heart and take abnormal pathways through its tissues are often treated with cardiac depressant drugs. It may seem undesirable to depress the functions of a heart that is already beating abnormally. However, when properly employed, these antiarrhythmic agents can convert an inefficiently contracting heart back to one with a strong normal sinus rhythm. This, of course, restores alternate contraction and relaxation at a rate that enables the ventricles to work with maximum pumping power.

Mainly, drugs of two chemical classes are commonly employed for counteracting rapid, irregular cardiac rhythms. These drugs are (1) *quinidine,* an alkaloid derived from the bark of the cinchona tree, which is also the source of the antimalarial drug quinine (Chap. 36), and (2) *procainamide HCl,* a close chemical relative of the local anesthetic agent procaine (Chap. 11). In addition, the continuing search for safer and more effective antiarrhythmic drugs has led to the recent trial of several experimental antifibrillatory agents. These include the beta adrenergic blocking agent propranolol (Inderal); the local anesthetic lidocaine; and other drugs that act to stabilize cardiac cell membranes such as antazoline (Antistine) and diphenylhydantoin (Dilantin).

Although the ways in which drugs restore normal rhythm to irregular hearts are not yet fully understood, quinidine and procainamide probably act in essentially the same way. This involves depression of cardiac functions as follows:

1. *They prolong the effective refractory period* of all parts of the heart. (That is, these drugs lengthen the time during which the atria, ventricles and conducting tissues remain unresponsive to stimuli that ordinarily set off contractions.)

2. They *slow* the *conduction* of impulses through the cardiac tissues.

3. They reduce the rate at which areas of heart muscle discharge spontaneously in a rhythmic manner. (Such *suppression* of *automaticity* occurs much more readily in ectopic foci than in the normal cardiac pacemakers, fortunately.)

4. They counteract the activity of the vagus nerve. (Excessive vagal tone, even though it slows the heart, tends to increase its susceptibility to certain arrhythmias.)

Although a combination of these actions probably accounts for the clinical effectiveness of these drugs, it also accounts—together with their capacity for reducing cardiac contractile power—for the toxicity of these drugs when administered to some patients with arrhythmias, particularly when dosage is not most carefully controlled.

Quinidine Salts (See Drug Digest)

Actions and Uses. Quinidine is especially effective for terminating *atrial fibrillation* and restoring a normal sinus rhythm. In this condition, as we have said, atrial impulses are generated at a rapid rate in ectopic foci or sent out as waves of excitation that take abnormal pathways in traveling through the atrial musculature. The overstimulated atrial fibers twitch and quiver chaotically. Moreover, the ventricles also beat rapidly and irregularly, because many of the several hundred impulses generated in the atria each minute bombard the A-V node and break through the conducting tissues to stimulate ventricular contractions. The resulting secondary ventricular tachycardia tends to make the heart vulnerable to ventricular fibrillation, a rapidly fatal arrhythmia.

We have seen (Chap. 19) that digitalis is given to patients with atrial fibrillation to protect the ventricles from stimulation by excessive atrial impulses. However, digitalis does not stop the atria themselves from fibrillating, and their continuing uncontrolled irregularity may further reduce the heart's energy reserves. Quinidine, on the contrary, actually abolishes atrial fibrillations in most cases, especially when the arrhythmia is of recent origin. Both drugs depress the conduction of atrial impulses through the A-V node to the ventricles. However, only quinidine reduces the excitability of the atria themselves and lengthens their refractory period. This often leads to re-establishment of a normal sinus rhythm. (Some doctors prefer to reduce a rapid ventricular rate by digitalization, before administering quinidine to convert the fibrillating atria to normal.)

Despite its effectiveness in *atrial* fibrillation, quinidine cannot be expected to overcome clinical *ventricular* fibrillation. Once this deadly condition develops, no drug—quinidine included—can ordinarily be given quickly enough to stop it and restore the blood flow to vital organs. (The fibrillating ventricles can, however, be stopped electrically and restarted with further electric shocks.) If it is administered in time, *before* the ventricles begin fibrillating, *prophylactic* quinidine can often keep this disastrous condition from occurring in patients whose hearts might otherwise be unable to withstand the strain of persistent ventricular extrasystoles and ventricular tachycardia.

Quinidine is also very useful in various conditions in which the atria are beating rapidly and inefficiently, such as atrial flutter, atrial extrasystoles, and paroxysmal atrial tachycardia. Atrial flutter is characterized by a very rapid but regular beat in contrast to the mere irregular muscular twitching of atrial fibrillation. In both conditions, however, the same danger—overstimulation of the ventricles—exists. Quinidine not only reduces atrioventricular conduction but also often converts the atrial flutter to a normal sinus rhythm by depressing the atrial ectopic foci. The same myocardial depressant action often stops atrial extrasystoles and, by depressing overstimulated nodal tissues, can halt attacks of atrial tachycardia.

Cardiotoxic Effects. Quinidine has certain cardiac actions which are almost never desirable, and, indeed, the useful properties may themselves be a source of danger if the drug's effects are permitted to go too far.

Thus, the depressant action of quinidine on impulse conduction—the very effect sought in order to protect the ventricles—may constitute a hazard. For, when atrioventricular conduction is completely blocked and the ventricular tissues are also depressed, ventricular fibrillation or cardiac arrest can occur. Therefore, the doctor must monitor the patient's electrocardiogram to detect any indication of excessively slowed conduction. The idioventricular pacemaker responsible for running the ventricles may itself be depressed by overdoses of quinidine, and this loss of automatic rhythmicity can result in cardiac standstill.

Quinidine can sometimes make the heart speed up dangerously. This happens when it depresses the vagal nerves which help to keep the heart slowed down. Thus, by removing this vagal brake before conduction is adequately slowed, quinidine can cause a dangerous increase in atrial and ventricular rates. This is one reason why some doctors prefer first to administer digitalis—a drug that stimulates vagal activity and reduces A-V conduction—before trying quinidine for conversion of atrial fibrillation. Another undesirable cardiac effect of quinidine, in addition to the vagal blocking effect, is its depressant action on myocardial contractility. The decreased strength of the heart beat, together with dilation of blood vessels, may lead to serious falls in blood pressure. For these reasons, the doctor may request the nurse to take the patient's pulse and read his blood pressure before administering each dose of quinidine. The rate and quality of the pulse should be noted carefully and recorded. Any sudden slowing, acceleration, or irregularity must be promptly reported.

Other Side Effects. More common than these dangerous depressant actions on the heart are a variety of extracardiac side effects that are sometimes observed when quinidine is employed. Oral doses may cause gastrointestinal irritation that leads to nausea, vomiting, cramps, and diarrhea. The salt quinidine polygalacturonate (Cardioquin) is claimed to cause less gastrointestinal distress than the sulfate or the hydrochloride. However, all quinidine salts are capable of causing certain other central and peripheral signs of overdosage (cinchonism) and various kinds of allergic hypersensitization reactions.

Cinchonism, a syndrome sometimes seen in malaria patients being treated with quinine, is manifested by tinnitus (ringing in the ears), visual disturbances (blurred or double vision), dizziness, headache, confusion, and delirium. Hypersensitivity reactions may be of the histamine-release type—e.g., urticaria, angioneurotic edema, and asthma. Another kind of idiosyncracy occasionally results in destruction of blood platelets by an antigen-antibody reaction. This may lead to bleeding into the mucous membranes of the mouth and petechial hemorrhages in the skin. Thus, quinidine is contraindicated in some patients, especially elderly women with a history of thrombocytic purpura and earlier episodes of severe sensitivity. Of course, this drug should not be administered to patients with complete heart block, severe cardiac failure with hypertrophy, or acute bacterial endocarditis.

Dosage and Administration. Obviously, quinidine administration is something of a two-edged sword. However, the drug is very valuable when it is administered with proper precautions to patients whose serious cardiac status warrants the risk of using this always potentially hazardous agent.

The drug is safest when given by mouth in gradually increasing doses. A single tablet (0.2 Gm.) is often administered initially to test whether the patient is allergic to quinidine. If this dose is well tolerated, the drug is continued on any of several schedules which permit a build-up to blood and tissue levels that are both safe and effective. Once the cardiac rhythm returns to normal, the drug may be stopped or its dosage may be reset at a long-term maintenance level. The nurse should repeatedly impress the patient with the importance of taking all of his prescribed daily doses and the need to take them at the proper intervals (usually every three or four hours, except with certain extended-action tablets that are administered at eight- to twelve-hour intervals).

Parenteral administration is usually reserved for emergencies or for patients unable to take quinidine by mouth. Quinidine gluconate may be injected intramuscularly—for example, in patients who are vomiting or unconscious. When minutes matter, this compound and another soluble salt, quinidine lactate, may be given by slow intravenous infusion. An electrocardiogram is always recorded simultaneously so that the doctor can detect the onset of desirable changes in cardiac rhythm and maintain administration at a rate that avoids excessive reduction of cardiac excitability, conductivity, and contractility. Fortunately, ectopic foci are more sensitive to quinidine than are normal pacemaker tissues. Thus, the doctor's task is to determine the smallest dose that will reduce ectopic activity without interfering with A-V conductivity or the automatic rhythmicity of ventricular muscle tissues.

Procainamide Hydrochloride (See Drug Digest)

Actions and Uses. Of various drugs shown by laboratory procedures to possess antiarrhythmic, or antifibrillatory, activity the only one that has been employed clinically to an extent comparable with quinidine is procainamide. The actions and uses of this agent are essentially similar to those of quinidine. Despite claims to the contrary, it is no safer than quinidine. However, because procainamide is somewhat less potent than the alkaloid, it may afford somewhat more margin for error in the event of accidental overdosage.

Procainamide reduces the excitability of both the atria and the ventricles as well as the atrioventricular conducting tissues. Best results have been obtained in the protection of patients from the cardiac arrhythmias that sometimes develop during anesthesia and surgery. It is often administered prior to intrathoracic surgery, endotracheal intubation procedures, and induction of cyclopropane anesthesia, because occurrence of arrhythmias is not uncommon in these situations, especially in patients with heart disease.

Procainamide can often prevent premature ventricular beats and ventricular tachycardia from progressing to fatal ventricular fibrillation. Thus, in digitalis overdosage, this drug has been used to control ventricular hyperexcitability. However, administration of procainamide for this purpose requires great care, because (as with quinidine) disastrous cardiac standstill may result from depression of ventricular automatic rhythmicity at a time when digitalis has already caused heart block.

Toxicity. Procainamide produces its most dramatic conversion of ventricular arrhythmias to normal when it is administered intravenously. However, the likelihood of dangerous reactions is also greatest when the drug is given by this route. The drug is infused very slowly, with electrocardiographic monitoring, in order to detect early signs of depressed conduction and thus avoid ventricular arrest and fibrillation. Patients are kept lying flat during the infusion, and blood pressure readings are taken continuously to detect any tendency toward hypotension. The infusion can then be halted if such signs are observed, thus avoiding the sudden precipitous drops in blood pressure sometimes observed when this drug is injected by vein.

As with quinidine, the hazard of cardiac toxicity is reduced when procainamide is given by mouth for attacks of atrial fibrillation or flutter. Occasionally, however, conversion to a stronger atrial beat may result in the breaking away of blood clots from the walls of the atria to cause a disastrous embolic episode. Actually, this is not a toxic effect of the drug but a consequence of chronic atrial fibrillation, which often tends to produce mural thrombi. Quinidine sometimes can cause similar clot dislodgement when it succeeds in converting long-standing atrial twitching to a forceful rhythmic beat. Patients are sometimes pretreated with anticoagulant drugs to prevent this.

In addition to gastrointestinal upsets and allergic reactions, procainamide has reportedly produced two much rarer but more dangerous toxic reactions. These are a syndrome resembling the collagen disease lupus erythematosus, and the blood dyscrasia, agranulocytosis. Therefore, patients should be instructed to report symptoms such as sore throat or upper respiratory infections that develop during long-term procainamide maintenance therapy.

Miscellaneous Antifibrillatory Agents

The danger inherent in administering quinidine or procainamide to patients with acute cardiac arrhythmias has stimulated a search for safer drugs. Recently, several agents have been widely employed experimentally in certain clinical situations, including arrhythmias caused by overdosage of digitalis and diuretics. These drugs are not intended to take the place of the traditional drugs in the treatment of chronic arrhythmias. However, their relatively rapid onset and short duration of action make them especially suited for use in emergency situations such as the development of sudden severe arrhythmias during anesthesia and surgery—particularly cardiac surgery—and for postoperative and postcoronary patients.

Propranolol (Inderal; see Chap. 17), the first of the beta adrenergic blocking agents to prove clinically useful, has been found particularly effective in arrhythmias caused by excessive circulating catecholamines and in digitalis overdosage. It has also proved useful in arrhythmias induced by certain anesthetics, in patients with supraventricular arrhythmias refractory to digitalis, and in ventricular arrhythmias not controlled by quinidine and procainamide.

This drug's primary action stems from its ability to occupy cardiac beta adrenergic receptors (Chap. 14) and thus protect the heart against overstimulation by sympathetic cardioacceleratory nerve impulses or by the epinephrine released from the chromaffin cell tumor tissues of patients with pheochromocytoma. The main effect of this action is a decrease in excessively rapid and irregular heartbeats.

Thus, this drug has helped to slow the rapid ventricular rate of patients with atrial fibrillation, especially when the ventricular tachycardia has persisted despite attempts to digitalize the patient. The combined use of propranolol and digitalis is often not only desirable but necessary in heart failure patients. Propranolol alone may precipitate heart failure by slowing the heart and reducing cardiac contractility and output. However, if the patient is first fully digitalized, his heart can continue to beat strongly, since propranolol counteracts digitalis-induced arrhythmias without interfering with the heart-strengthening (inotropic) action of digitalis.

The side effects of propranolol are ordinarily minor and transient. However, certain categories of patients must be carefully observed. Diabetics, for example, must be watched for signs of insulin overdosage, because propranolol tends to mask some of the early warning signs of hypoglycemia (see Chap. 32). Patients receiving reserpine are prone to suffer excessive cardiac slowing following propranolol, as are those who are being anesthetized with ether.

Lidocaine (Xylocaine; see Chap. 11) is a local anesthetic that acts like procainamide and procaine itself in stabilizing the cell membranes of heart muscle as well as those of nerve fibers. This drug's ability to reduce cardiac excitability and conductivity has led to its experimental use in treating acute ventricular arrhythmias. Some authorities claim that this drug is more uniformly effective than the older agents for control of cardiac irregularities following acute myocardial infarction (Chap. 22). It is also indicated for use by coronary care units, in counteracting digitalis-induced arrhythmias, and by anesthesiologists for prevention of cardiac irregularities during induction of anesthesia and during the surgical procedures that follow, particularly when patients have a history of arrhythmias.

Diphenylhydantoin (Dilantin; see Chap. 8) also has a stabilizing effect on the cell membranes of cardiac muscle that protects the myocardium against excessive stimuli arising in ectopic foci. It is reportedly effective in protecting the ventricles against digitalis-induced supraventricular arrhythmias and in the control of various acute and recurrent atrial and ventricular arrhythmias resistant to treatment with the older antifibrillatory agents. Its ultimate utility, like that of the other experimental antiarrhythmic drugs, still remains to be established.

CARDIAC STIMULANTS

In many patients with heart disease, the main symptom may be a marked slowing of the heart. Such slowing usually occurs either because impulses are initiated only sluggishly by the sinoatrial pacemaker, or because the passage of the excitatory impulses through the cardiac tissues is blocked at some point. Conditions of the first type—sinus bradycardia, for example—may cause few circulatory symptoms. However, when the heart rate falls below 35 beats per minute, as it frequently does when complete atrioventricular heart block occurs, serious circulatory impairment may develop.

Thus, some patients with very slow heart rates may show shortness of breath, chest pain, and symptoms of heart failure. Frequently, they complain of dizziness and faintness, and sometimes, during periods of transient cardiac standstill, cerebral hypoxia may result in syncope (fainting) and convulsions. Such seizures are characteristics of the Stokes-Adams syndrome, a condition that is the most common cause of death in patients with complete heart block. Fortunately, Stokes-Adams seizures now can often be counteracted and prevented by the use of certain sympathomimetic (adrenergic) drugs and with various electronic pacemakers.

Adrenergic Drugs (See also Chap. 16)

Drugs of this class increase the speed and strength of the heart beat. Thus, they may be useful for starting up a heart that has gone into standstill during an acute attack and for maintaining an adequate heart beat in the intervals between attacks. At one time, the neurohormone epinephrine (Adrenalin) was widely used for overcoming Stokes-Adams seizures. Sometimes, however, this drug tends to increase cardiac irritability and precipitate fatal ventricular fibrillation. Thus, it has recently been largely replaced for this purpose by isoproterenol (Isuprel, see Drug Digest), a drug that acts more powerfully than epinephrine on the cardiac pacemakers and with fewer irritating effects on ectopic foci.

Isoproterenol is now considered the best drug for the management of Stokes-Adams seizures and for raising the heart rate in other conditions marked by a very slow beat and transient cardiac standstill episodes, such as the carotid sinus syndrome. During actual or impending standstill, the drug is injected intravenously or directly into the heart to increase ventricular contractions and to stimulate S-A and A-V node pacemakers. Later, intramuscular or subcutaneous administration may be substituted, and for long-term therapy the drug is usually taken sublingually. This dosage form is both rapid-acting and long-lasting. Thus, the patient who is taking the drug every four hours or so is often instructed to take an extra dose when he feels signs of an attack coming on.

A long-acting oral form of isoproterenol has been tried out recently, but it is considered to be not entirely dependable. Other sympathomimetic drugs which are better absorbed than orally administered isoproterenol are sometimes taken to prevent attacks. These include ephedrine (see Drug Digest) and hydroxyamphetamine (Paredrine), which are often administered orally about four times a day. Because they tend to cause nervousness and insomnia, these centrally acting adrenergic drugs are usually combined with sedative doses of barbiturates.

Anticholinergic Drugs

In addition to the adrenergic drugs, which stimulate the heart directly, certain agents that block the effects of vagal slowing may be used to speed up slow hearts in some cases. Sinus bradycardia, for example, is a condition caused usually by excessive numbers of vagal nerve impulses impinging upon the sinoatrial pacemaker. Patients with an excessively sensitive carotid sinus mechanism are also subject to attacks of heart slowing caused by overactive vagal tone. Sometimes, when such a patient wears a tight collar or even twists his neck in a way that presses on the carotid sinus, the vagal reflexes that are set off are so strong that the patient's heart rate drops drastically, or the heart may even stop briefly. He may then get giddy and suffer a black-out because of the reduced flow of blood to the brain.

Atropine, methantheline (Banthine), and other anticholinergic drugs (Chap. 17) are often used to counteract arrhythmias marked by too great a vagal action on the S-A and A-V nodes. These drugs act to keep the acetylcholine released by vagal nerve endings from reaching the effector cells in the right atrium and in the nodal conducting tissues. As a result of this blocking action, the braking effect of vagal nerve stimulation on the heart is eliminated, and the heart rate is increased.

Although this blockade of parasympathetic cardiac effects is often beneficial, the drugs have various drawbacks. Their effects are relatively short in duration; side effects such as mouth dryness, blurring of vision, constipation, and bladder difficulties are often troublesome, and these agents do not overcome cardiac slowing that is the result not of vagal overstimulation but of such metabolic changes as hypoxia or acid-base and electrolyte imbalances.

Alkalinizing Agents

When excessive slowing of the heart is secondary to acidosis, excessive plasma potassium levels, and anoxia, the heart rate may sometimes be raised by injec-
tion of alkalinizing solutions. Among the most commonly used of these is sodium lactate, a substance that is broken down to metabolites that raise the pH of the blood and lower its potassium content. When this occurs, the heart speeds up and also becomes more responsive to sympathetic nerve stimulation, circulating catecholamines, and adrenergic drugs.

A one-sixth molar solution of sodium lactate has been used with some success to increase the heart rate in Stokes-Adams seizures. This alkalinizer has even helped to restore the heart beat in cases of cardiac arrest that had not responded to isoproterenol and other adrenergic drugs. Lactate solution works best when it is given within a minute or two after the heart has gone into standstill. In such emergencies, the solution is injected rapidly by vein. Once the heart starts up, the solution is infused very slowly, until the heart's own pacemakers take over.

Electric Pacemakers

Cardiac arrest and ventricular fibrillation are probably best treated by stimulating the heart electrically.

TABLE 21-1
ANTIARRHYTHMIC DRUGS

Nonproprietary Name	Trade Name	Usual Dosage Range
Cardiac Depressant Drugs		
Diphenylhydantoin	Dilantin	5 to 10 mg. per Kg. I.V., in dilute solution, slowly
Lidocaine	Xylocaine	50 to 100 mg. I.V., rapidly, at a rate up to 500 mg. to 750 mg. per hour
Procainamide hydrochloride U.S.P.	Pronestyl	0.5 to 2 Gm. oral or I.M.; 50 to 250 mg. I.V.
Propranolol	Inderal	10 to 30 mg. 3 or 4 times daily, orally; 1 to 3 mg. at a rate of 1 mg. per minute, I.V.
Quinidine gluconate U.S.P.	Quinaglute	0.3 to 0.5 Gm. I.M.
Quinidine hydrochloride	—	0.2 to 0.6 Gm.
Quinidinine lactate	—	0.4 to 0.8 Gm. I.M.
Quinidine polygalacturonate	Cardioquin	0.2 to 0.6 Gm.
Quinidine sulfate U.S.P.	—	0.2 to 0.6 Gm.
Cardiac Stimulant Drugs		
Atropine sulfate U.S.P.	—	0.5 to 2 mg.
Ephedrine sulfate U.S.P.	—	15 to 50 mg.
Epinephrine U.S.P.	Adrenalin	0.25 to 1 ml. of a 1:1,000 sol., intracardiac
Hydroxyamphetamine HBr U.S.P.	Paredrine	20 to 60 mg.
Isoproterenol HCl U.S.P.	Isuprel	10 to 20 mg. sublingual; 0.2 mg. S.C. or I.M.; 0.02 mg. I.V. or intracardiac
Methantheline bromide N.F.	Banthine	50 to 100 mg.
Sodium lactate injection U.S.P.	—	10 to 80 ml. I.V. (⅙ molar sol.)

Normal heart beats can now be restored by external pacemakers and defibrillators—devices that successfully shock the heart through the intact chest. On the other hand, many patients with Stokes-Adams syndrome and complete A-V heart block have recently had cardiac pacemakers implanted internally for long-term steady stimulation of hearts prone to go into standstill. A recent modification eliminates continuous artificial stimulation and the pacemaker goes into action only when the heart fails to beat after a preset interval.

A new electronic device is now being employed to treat conditions marked by excessively rapid ectopic rhythms. The cardioverter, as this instrument is called, is claimed to be more effective than quinidine and procainamide for terminating arrhythmias such as atrial fibrillation and flutter and atrial or ventricular tachycardia. Cardioversion does not, however, do away with the need for antiarrhythmic drugs, which must still be used to maintain the normal rhythm once it is established.

SUMMARY OF TOXIC EFFECTS OF THE ANTIARRHYTHMIC AGENTS QUINIDINE AND PROCAINAMIDE

- **Cardiovascular Toxicity**

  Vagus-blocking effect may cause excessive acceleration of the ventricular rate.

  Excessive slowing of conduction may cause complete A-V block with ventricular extrasystoles and fibrillation, or cardiac arrest (when idioventricular automatic rhythmicity is also depressed).

  Excessive reduction in the contractile force of the heart beat, combined with vasodilation, may cause sharp falls in blood pressure and CV collapse.

  Conversion of chronic atrial fibrillation may cause fresh clots to break loose and lead to thromboembolic complications.

- **Extracardiac Toxicity**

  Quinidine

  Cinchonism: tinnitus, visual disturbances, dizziness, headache, confusion.

  Gastrointestinal: nausea, vomiting, abdominal cramps, and diarrhea.

  Hypersensitivity: fever, skin rashes, angioneurotic edema, asthma, respiratory depression, cyanosis; thrombocytic purpura.

  Procainamide

  Gastrointestinal: nausea, vomiting, diarrhea.

  Allergic reactions: urticaria, skin rash, etc.

  Rare idiosyncracies: agranulocytosis; collagen disease syndrome resembling lupus erythematosus.

SUMMARY OF USEFUL CARDIAC ACTIONS, CLINICAL INDICATIONS AND OBJECTIVES OF THE CARDIAC DEPRESSANT DRUGS

- Drugs act by preferentially depressing ectopic foci and by reducing excitability, conductivity, and automatic rhythmicity of myocardium. The effective refractory period of cardiac tissue is prolonged and the period of latency is lengthened. This protects against reaction to stimuli rapidly arising in ectopic foci.

- Drugs are used in the treatment of both atrial and ventricular arrhythmias, including atrial premature beats, atrial flutter, atrial fibrillation, and paroxysmal atrial tachycardia; ventricular extrasystoles and ventricular

tachycardia. They prevent ventricular fibrillation but cannot ordinarily be given in time to reverse it. (Electrical defibrillation is preferred for this purpose.)

- Drugs may be useful in the following ways:

  To restore normal rhythm in acute tachyarrhythmias caused by digitalis toxicity, certain anesthetics, excessive circulating catecholamines (e.g., pheochromocytoma), and in disorders marked by myocardial ischemia and other organic lesions.

  To produce physiological improvement even when

reversion to normal rhythm does not occur. For example, in patients with atrial flutter or atrial fibrillation, these drugs may protect the ventricles from excessive supraventricular impulses by depressing AV conduction. This reduces the ventricular rate despite the possibly continuing atrial arrhythmia.

To prevent development of acute episodes or their extension (for example, keep ventricular tachycardia from going on to fatal ventricular fibrillation); and, by their *prophylactic effects, to reduce the number and severity of attacks* in conditions such as paroxysmal atrial tachycardia and paroxysmal atrial fibrillation.

SUMMARY OF POINTS FOR NURSES TO REMEMBER WHEN GIVING ANTIARRHYTHMIC DRUGS

• Observe patients receiving quinidine compounds or procainamide carefully for signs of cardiac and extracardiac toxicity and report these promptly to the doctor, if they should occur.

• Count the pulse of patients receiving these drugs for at least one full minute (not for 15 to 30 seconds, as is sometimes done in routinely taking pulse rates). Carefully note and chart not only the rate and the quality of the pulse but also any detectable disturbances in rhythm. If a pulse deficit exists, it is important to note and chart both the apical and the radial pulse rates.

• If the patient is being treated on the ward rather than in the intensive care unit, and no device for continuous cardiac monitoring is available, the patient should be placed where he can be observed frequently. Because of the possibility of sudden and serious changes in the patient's condition, he should preferably be put in a room directly across from the nurses' station, rather than in a room at the far end of the corridor.

• Check the availability of resuscitative adrenergic drugs and the working order of emergency equipment such as the cardiac pacemaker when caring for a patient who is receiving drugs to combat cardiac arrhythmias.

REVIEW QUESTIONS

1. (a) What properties do quinidine and procainamide have in common which account for their usefulness in treating rapid cardiac irregularities?

(b) What property do quinidine and digitalis have in common and in what way are their respective actions different when both are used in treating patients with atrial fibrillation?

2. (a) List several types of atrial arrhythmia for which quinidine is employed and indicate how the drug converts these ectopic rhythms to normal.

(b) Compare the usefulness of quinidine in overcoming ventricular tachycardia with its status in the treatment of ventricular fibrillation.

3. (a) List several potentially dangerous effects that quinidine may have on cardiac rhythm.

(b) Explain how quinidine may both slow and accelerate the heart rate excessively.

4. (a) List some signs and symptoms of cinchonism.

(b) What other extracardiac toxic effects make the use of quinidine undesirable in certain patients?

5. (a) Indicate the manner in which quinidine is ordinarily administered.

(b) Indicate which quinidine compounds are preferred in emergencies and a precaution commonly employed during injection of these soluble salts.

6. (a) List several clinical situations in which procainamide is commonly used to prevent cardiac arrhythmias.

(b) What effects may occur as a result of the combined actions of procainamide (or quinidine) and digitalis (i.e., how may each type of drug counteract the undesirable cardiac effects of the other or add to them)?

7. (a) List several cardiovascular toxic reactions that may occur with procainamide and indicate some measures that are used to prevent them.

(b) List some unusual reactions reported for procainamide.

8. (a) What advantage does procainamide have over procaine, in regard to protection of patients against cardiac arrhythmias?

(b) List another local anesthetic and other agents that have been tried experimentally for treatment of cardiac arrhythmias.

9. (a) Indicate the drug of choice for the treatment of Stokes-Adams seizures and state the reason for its superiority over epinephrine in cases of cardiac standstill.

(b) List several other adrenergic drugs used in the maintenance therapy of Stokes-Adams syndrome and indicate how they differ from the drug of choice in manner of administration.

(c) What are the main extracardiac side effects of these adrenergic drugs and how are these counteracted?

10. (a) List a couple of cardiac arrhythmias which are sometimes treated by atropine and related anticholinergic drugs and indicate the manner in which these drugs overcome certain types of cardiac slowing.

(b) What are some of the drawbacks of atropine-type drugs in treating excessive cardiac slowing?

BIBLIOGRAPHY

Bellet, S.: Clinical pharmacology of antiarrhythmic drugs. Clin. Pharmacol. Ther., 2:345, 1961.

Bernstein, H.: Drug treatment of cardiac arrhythmias. Am. J. Nurs., 64:118, 1964 (July).

Bernstein, H., et al.: Sodium diphenylhydantoin in the treatment of recurrent cardiac arrhythmias. J.A.M.A., 191:695, 1965.

Conn, R. D.: Newer drugs in the treatment of cardiac arrhythmias. Med. Clin. N. Am., 51:1223, 1967 (Sept.).

Dack, S., and Robbin, S. R.: Treatment of heart block and Adams-Stokes syndrome. J.A.M.A., 176:505, 1961.

Freeman, I., and Wexler, J.: Quinidine in chronic atrial fibrillation. Am. J. Med. Sci., 239:181, 1960.

Frieden, J.: Antiarrhythmic drugs. 7. Lidocaine as an antiarrhythmic agent. Am. Heart J., 70:713, 1965.

Gold, H.: Quinidine in Disorders of the Heart. New York, Paul B. Hoeber, 1950.

Hurst, J. W., et al.: Management of patients with atrial fibrillation. Am. J. Med., 37:728, 1964.

Lembert, L., et al.: Pacemaking on demand in A-V block. J.A.M.A., 191:12, 1965.

Lown, B.: "Cardioversion" of arrhythmias, I and II. Mod. Concepts Cardiovasc. Dis., 33:863, 1964 (July and Aug.).

Marriott, H. J. L.: Rational approach to quinidine therapy. Mod. Concepts Cardiovasc. Dis., 31:745, 1962 (Sept.).

Reynolds, E. W., Jr., and Johnston, F. D.: The management of the cardiac arrhythmias. G.P., 18:131, 1958.

Rodman, M. J.: Drugs for the irregular heart. R.N., 25:53, 1962 (Aug.).

————: Drugs for congestive heart failure and arrhythmias. R.N., 30:51, 1967 (Nov.).

Drugs Used in Coronary Artery Disease

CORONARY INSUFFICIENCY

We have seen (Chap. 18) that the heart muscle must get a constant supply of oxygen and nutrients in order to keep up its ceaseless pumping action. The substances that serve as the source of energy for the working myocardium are brought to it by way of blood carried in the coronary arteries, which branch off from the aorta and spread down through the heart muscle. These vessels divide and subdivide, forming fine arterioles and capillaries that feed the heart muscle fibers with a rich supply of blood.

Ordinarily, the myocardium receives an adequate quantity of blood as long as the aortic pressure stays high enough to keep the coronary vessels fully perfused. Sometimes, however, these blood vessels become narrowed by fatty deposits that develop just underneath their inner lining. This condition (coronary atherosclerosis) gradually reduces the flow of blood to some parts of the heart muscle. Often, the person so affected may suffer no symptoms, because his heart has time to compensate for its inadequate blood supply by developing additional vascular channels—a secondary, or collateral, circulation.

In many cases, however, the atherosclerotic process may progress until blood flow is so reduced as to cause episodes of acute coronary insufficiency. These episodes are most severe when the blood flow through a major artery is cut off completely—that is, the blood vessel is occluded. Acute coronary occlusion occurs most often when the blood moving sluggishly through the narrowed vessel suddenly forms a solid clot, called a thrombus, which blocks further flow. As a result of such a coronary thrombus, the cardiac tissues below the blocked part of the arteriole are deprived of the oxygen and nutrients that they need, and they then usually suffer permanent damage. This condition is referred to as myocardial infarction, and it often ends fatally.

On the other hand, a person may suffer many episodes of acute coronary insufficiency without actually having an occlusion. Although hypoxia caused by transient cardiac ischemia is usually painful and alarming, the heart may show no permanent ill effects once an adequate flow of blood is restored to the myocardial tissues which were made temporarily hypoxic. Sometimes, such painful attacks are caused by a sudden spasm in some of the already narrowed coronary vessels. This seems to be brought on by physical exertion or emotional stress, which increase the work load of the heart. If the person's atherosclerotic coronary vessels cannot cope with the demands of the cardiac tissues for extra blood, he may suffer an anginal attack.

An attack of angina pectoris can be extremely painful and frightening. The Latin term means literally, "a choking of the chest," and the patient may, in fact, feel as if he were strangling, as sudden severe pain radiates up into his throat from a point behind his breastbone. Yet, unlike the pangs of a true coronary occlusion, the pain of an anginal attack will usually wear off gradually if the patient heeds its warning and stops all physical exertion for a few minutes. However, recovery is more rapid if the patient takes certain drugs of the coronary vasodilator class.

Coronary Vasodilator Drugs

Drugs that dilate the coronary arterioles are not usually very effective for relieving the pain of an acute coronary occlusion; however, they are often quite useful for helping to overcome anginal attacks. These drugs are thought to act mainly by relaxing spasms of the coronary arterioles. The resulting dilation of these vessels is believed to bring a better flow of blood to the hypoxic myocardial tissues.

Several different classes of chemicals (Table 22-1) are said to have the ability to abort an anginal attack. Some of these agents are also employed on a long-term basis in an attempt to aid the development of a collateral coronary circulation. This, it is hoped, will help the heart to meet the demands of physical and

TABLE 22-1
CORONARY VASODILATOR DRUGS

Nonproprietary Name	Trade Name or Synonym	Usual Dosage
Aminophylline U.S.P.	Theophylline ethylenediamine	200 to 500 mg.
Amyl nitrite N.F.	Aspirols; Vaporols; etc.	0.2 to 0.3 ml. by inhalation
Dioxyline phosphate	Paveril	100 to 300 mg.
Dipyridamole	Persantin	25 to 50 mg.
Erythrityl tetranitrate	Cardilate	5 to 10 mg. sublingually and orally
Ethaverine HCl	Ethquinol, etc.	30 mg.
Nitroglycerin U.S.P.	Glyceryl trinitrate	0.4 to 0.6 mg. sublingually
Inositol hexanitrate	Tolanate	10 mg.
Isosorbide dinitrate	Isordil	5 mg. sublingually or orally
Mannitol hexanitrate	Maxitate, Nitranitol	15 to 60 mg.
Octyl nitrite	Octrite	750 mg. inhaler
Oxtriphylline	Choledyl	100 to 200 mg.
Papaverine HCl N.F.	—	100 mg. orally; 30 mg. I.M.
Pentaerythritol tetranitrate	Peritrate, etc.	10 to 20 mg.
Theophylline N.F.	Theocin	200 mg.
Theophylline sodium acetate N.F.	Theocin soluble	200 mg.
Theophylline sodium glycinate N.F.	Theoglycinate, etc.	300 mg.
Trolnitrate phosphate	Metamine; Nitritamin	8 to 16 mg. daily

mental stress and thus actually prevent or, at least, reduce the frequency of anginal attacks.

We shall first discuss in detail the nitrites and other coronary vasodilators that are used mainly in the management of angina pectoris. Then, we shall summarize the manner in which drugs of this and several other classes are employed in the management of myocardial infarctions. Finally, we shall look briefly at the status of the various measures that are presently being tried for prophylaxis or control of coronary atherosclerosis, the underlying cause of these conditions.

The Nitrites and Nitrates (See Drug Digests)

Actions and Uses. The inorganic and organic chemicals of this class have the ability to relax smooth muscle of all types. These drugs act directly on the muscle fibers themselves rather than by blocking constrictor nerve impulses. As a result, spastic smooth muscles in various viscera relax and the pain produced by such spasms vanishes. Although the nitrites are capable of relaxing the musculature of the biliary, bronchial, urinary, and gastrointestinal tracts, they are rarely used for such purposes, since various other antispasmodic drugs that act more effectively at these visceral sites are available.

The nitrites (the term is employed traditionally for *both* the nitrites and the nitrates) are especially effective for relaxing the smooth muscle walls of the blood vessels. Such relaxation leads to vasodilation, i.e., enlargement of the lumen in arterioles, venules, and capillaries. Generalized vasodilation can, of course, cause a fall in blood pressure, and large doses of nitrites do, indeed, produce acute hypotensive effects. Nitrites have been employed in the treatment of essential hypertension, but they are not used extensively today for this purpose and any sudden drops in blood pressure produced by these drugs are considered undesirable side effects.

A much more important result of nitrite-induced vasodilation is the increased local flow of blood. This is especially desirable for overcoming the coronary constriction and myocardial ischemia which are the causes of the sudden severe pain in attacks of angina pectoris. These drugs are often used to prevent such attacks or, at least, to reduce their frequency and severity.

Glyceryl Trinitrate (Nitroglycerin). This drug is the nitrite most widely used for terminating acute anginal attacks. Its exact mechanism is still not entirely understood, despite its having been employed as a specific for over 80 years. Its effectiveness is most probably the result of a rapid relaxing action on the coronary vessels that have gone into spasm and upon nearby arterioles. By widening these channels, the drug is thought to cause an increase in the flow of blood through the oxygen-starved heart muscle. However, recent evidence indicates that nitroglycerin may also act by reducing the work load of the heart and, possibly, by producing desirable changes in myocardial metabolism.

In any case, patients prone to suffer frequent anginal attacks should carry a vial of fresh nitroglycerin tablets for use in aborting an acute attack or helping to prevent one. Whenever the patient feels an anginal attack coming on, he places a tiny tablet (0.3 to 0.6 mg. usually) under his tongue and sits or lies down. Within a few minutes usually, the strangling chest pain passes off and, even though the drug's action is relatively short, relief may last for quite some time afterward.

Hospitalized patients who need nitroglycerin for quick use when an attack strikes are often allowed to keep a supply at their bedsides. Nurses may have misgivings about a patient's taking a drug without first consulting them, because, in most hospitals, administration of medications is the nurse's responsibility, and there are strict rules against leaving drugs in the hands of the patient for self-administration.

Actually, there is no reason why an anginal patient who has been using nitroglycerin for years to cope with his attacks should not continue to do so while he is in the hospital. Instead of indicating that she disapproves of his taking medication on his own initiative, the nurse should see to it that the patient has an adequate supply of nitroglycerin available at all times for immediate use. Because (as we have said) the pain of an attack can be both excruciating and terrifying, the patient should not be deprived of the security of knowing that he can take care of himself if he has to.

Of course, even though the patient may have received permission to take his own nitroglycerin p.r.n., the nurse is not relieved of her own responsibilities in the matter. She needs to know, for example, how much nitroglycerin the patient requires for relief of an attack and how often he needs to take a dose of the drug. This can best be ascertained in casual conversation with the patient, rather than by brusquely opening his bedside table drawer and counting the number of tablets left in his vial. Such action implies that the patient is somehow not to be trusted and indicates disrespect for his judgment or his motives.

The nurse should also observe how the patient responds to the drug when he takes it. She should note not only whether any side effects occur, but also whether the patient gets complete or only partial relief from nitroglycerin. Such indications of developing tolerance should be promptly reported to the doctor, who may then decide to increase the dose or to switch to a different vasodilator for a time. The physician should also be informed if the patient seems to show signs of impaired judgment or memory. If the patient becomes careless or forgetful enough to make the nurse doubt the wisdom of his continuing to control his own treatment, despite its having been ordered by the doctor, she should talk to the physician about it, giving him a careful report of the patient's behavior.

Communication between nurse, doctor, and patient is important in regard to the concern the patient may feel over the possible long-term dangers of his continuing to take nitroglycerin. The patient may, for example, express alarm over whether this drug may cause the kind of dependence he may have read about in relation to narcotics or corticosteroids. The nurse should avoid answering such questions immediately and try, instead, to arrange for the patient to get this information from the doctor directly. She should, if possible, be present during this discussion, or should check with the doctor later as to what the patient has been told. Then, if the patient asks the nurse a question, her reply will be consistent with the information imparted by the doctor and the patient won't be worried because he has perhaps been told two somewhat different stories.

Thus, the nurse should know exactly what the doctor told the patient about the possibility of his developing tolerance to nitroglycerin. Tolerance to nitrites is a nuisance, which the doctor will try to avoid or delay. It is not, however, accompanied by psychic or physical dependence, as is the case with the opiates and other narcotic analgesics. Thus, the patient should be aware of the likelihood of his requiring larger doses, but the nurse should be careful to say nothing that might differ from what he may have been told by the doctor about this matter and alarm him unnecessarily.

The nurse can also teach the patient hospitalized for the first time with angina how best to take his nitroglycerin. He should know, for example, what side effects to expect and how to minimize them. Thus, for example, she should teach him to sit down before taking the drug, in order to avoid the faintness that some people experience if they are standing upright when the systemic vasodilator effects of this drug come on. With guidance of this kind by the nurse, the hospitalized patient can learn to carry out his own nitroglycerin treatment safely and effectively when he gets home.

Other Rapid-Acting Nitrites. Most other nitrites are too slow in the onset of their action to be of very much value in an actual attack. However, two volatile compounds, octyl nitrite and amyl nitrite, act even faster than nitroglycerin. When inhaled, their effects may begin to come on within seconds, compared to the two to five minutes required with sublingual nitroglycerin. These inhalant forms have not, however, attained much popularity. Amyl nitrite is a liquid that comes in a fabric-covered glass ampule that has to be broken in a handkerchief from which the vapors are inhaled. Patients often consider this cumbersome and find it embarrassing to use the drug in public because of its unpleasant odor. In addition, the very rapid action of amyl nitrite tends to set off some rather unpleasant circulatory side effects.

Prophylactic Use. NITROGLYCERIN is used in two ways to prevent anginal attacks. The patient may slip a tablet under his tongue a few minutes before undertaking a task which, experience has taught him, will produce chest pain. For example, shortly before going out for a walk in cold weather, he may take a sublingual tablet of nitroglycerin. This helps to supply the improved blood flow that his heart will require in order to meet the stress of physical exertion during the next half hour. Nitroglycerin is also available in oral dosage forms, for a longer-lasting preventive effect. However, most of any dose that is swallowed is destroyed in the liver, and some doctors doubt that oral nitroglycerin actually has the more sustained coronary vasodilation action claimed for it.

OTHER NITRITES. A number of nitrites with action that is slower in onset but much longer in duration than that of nitroglycerin are usually preferred for long-term use. The effects of a single dose of pentaerythritol tetranitrate (Peritrate, etc.), erythrityl tetranitrate (Cardilate), isosorbide dinitrate (Isordil), and similar compounds are said to last from three to five hours. Sustained-action dosage forms from which certain of these vasodilator drugs are slowly released may provide therapeutic drug levels for up to twelve hours. Some of these drugs are also taken sublingually for coping with an acute attack, but none seems to act as quickly or to be as effective as nitroglycerin for that purpose.

Long-term nitrite therapy is supposed to keep the heart muscle supplied with more of the oxygen and nutrients it needs, thus reducing the number of anginal attacks and the need for frequent nitroglycerin medication. Use of the long-acting nitrites in this way is claimed to stimulate development of the heart's collateral circulation. This action could, of course, be useful during the convalescence of patients recovering from an acute myocardial infarction, and some of the long-acting agents are recommended for postcoronary patients, once their blood pressure has stabilized.

The actual effectiveness of long-term nitrites for these purposes is a matter of controversy at present. Evidence from animal experiments indicates that these drugs encourage development of an enlarged cardiac collateral circulation; however, some doctors doubt that these agents offer any real help to patients with coronary insufficiency. Although numerous clinical reports that have been published claim that patients have benefited from treatment with pentaerythritol tetranitrate and related long-acting nitrites, many cardiologists look upon these drugs as mere placebos and continue to express skepticism concerning their actual ability to raise the patient's cardiac reserve.

Tolerance to Nitrites. The failure of nitrite-treated patients to maintain early improvement in their ability to work without suffering chest pains may be the result of the rapidity with which tolerance to these agents develops. Nitrites are notorious for the speed with which they lose their initial effectiveness. It is often necessary for the doctor to begin ordering larger doses of nitrites after several days of treatment, and patients often stop responding to them at all after a few weeks of continuous nitrite therapy. For this reason, the doctor may temporarily discontinue the use of nitrites and switch to vasodilator drugs of some other chemical class, until the patient has lost his tolerance to nitrites and his vessels have regained their responsiveness to the vasodilator action of these drugs.

Other Disadvantages. The tendency of nitrites to dilate cranial arterioles may make them dangerous to use in patients with raised intracranial or intraocular pressure. Thus, they must be used cautiously, if at all, for managing angina pectoris in patients who also have a history of glaucoma. Patients with obvious anemia should have their hemoglobin levels brought back to normal before starting long-term nitrite treatment. One reason, of course, is that patients are more prone to anginal attacks when their blood has a relatively low oxygen-carrying capacity. This—in theory, at least—can be accentuated by nitrites, since these drugs are capable of converting part of the hemoglobin of the blood to methemoglobin, which does not have the ability to transport oxygen from the lungs to the tissues.

Side Effects. The most common side effects of all the fast-acting nitrites are the result of the dilation of vessels other than those in the heart. For example, nitroglycerin and its chemical relatives tend to dilate blood vessels in the meningeal coverings of the brain. This is believed to account for the throbbing headache that this drug often causes. More serious is the systemic vasodilation, which occasionally causes a sharp drop in blood pressure and reflex racing of the heart. Patients should be advised to lie down in order to avoid the cardiac palpitations and the feeling of faintness, weakness, and dizziness which may be brought on by such drug-induced postural hypotension and tachycardia. They should also be warned not to drink alcoholic beverages (except as prescribed), because nitrite syncope—a severe shocklike state—occurs most commonly in individuals who take nitrites when they have been drinking excessively. Other side effects sometimes seen with nitrites include nausea and vomiting, drowsiness, and visual disturbances, especially when the drugs of longer duration are being employed in long-term prophylactic therapy.

Toxicity. Actually, serious degrees of methemoglobinemia rarely occur during routine nitrite therapy. Poisoning is usually the result of the accidental ingestion of overdoses of sodium nitrite, a salt used in minute amounts as a meat preservative. Babies who have been fed formulas prepared with well water high in nitrites have become cyanotic as a result of severe methemoglobinemia. Unlike most asphyxial conditions, nitrite poisoning does not respond to inhalation of high concentrations of oxygen. First, a methylene blue solution must be administered by slow intravenous injection. This reducing chemical returns the hemoglobin to normal and restores the blood's ability to pick up oxygen and carry it to the tissues. The skin then quickly loses its bluish cast, and the patient soon recovers.

Other Vasodilator Drugs

Many non-nitrite vasodilator drugs have been tried in the long-term treatment of angina pectoris. Despite frequent claims for the effectiveness of various kinds of old and new drugs, none of these agents seems superior to the nitrites for reducing the frequency of anginal attacks. Those drugs that act at all are usually reserved for use in patients who have become tolerant to nitrites.

Papaverine and Its Synthetic Analogues. Papaverine, a non-narcotic alkaloid obtained from opium, is an excellent smooth muscle antispasmodic. It is sometimes combined with morphine for administration to patients with biliary and renal colic. Papaverine has little analgesic activity; however, it often helps to relieve these painful conditions by relaxing the spastic biliary and ureteral musculature. The drug also relaxes the smooth muscles of various vascular beds to permit increased blood flow through the tissues which receive their blood supply from the constricted or partially blocked vessels. Among the conditions for which papaverine has been employed are pulmonary embolism and various other peripheral, cerebrovascular, and cardiac artery thromboembolic disorders.

Papaverine is most effective for these conditions when given intramuscularly. It is thought to act by relaxing the reflexly constricted arteries adjacent to the ones blocked by a thrombus or embolus. This, of course, increases the collateral circulation and tends to limit the area of tissue damage following blood clots in the brain, ergot poisoning, and even coronary occlusion. Yet, despite its occasional effectiveness in such more serious occlusive conditions, papaverine has not proved very useful in the long-term preventive management of angina pectoris when administered orally, nor is it as reliable as nitroglycerin for terminating acute anginal episodes.

Two related compounds, ethaverine and dioxyline phosphate (Paveril), are claimed to cause fewer side effects than papaverine when employed to relax coronary vessel spasm in angina pectoris. However, these drugs cause gastrointestinal upset, dizziness, and drowsiness. These papaverine relatives appear to produce some antispasmodic effects, but their prophylactic value in the long-term management of angina is

slight. (For further discussion of papaverine, see Drug Digest.)

Theophylline and Related Xanthines. Periodically, various drugs of the xanthine class are claimed to be valuable coronary vasodilators in the routine management of angina pectoris. However, the usefulness of theophylline and its more soluble salts in this condition is actually controversial. For, although these drugs relax smooth muscle spasm, doctors differ in their opinions whether the xanthines really help to dilate the coronary vessels enough to keep anginal symptoms under control during long-term oral administration.

Administered intravenously, aminophylline is sometimes employed for treating patients who show signs of heart failure following an acute coronary occlusion. In such cases, the drug is given primarily for its rapid digitalislike cardiac actions. That is, it increases the contractility of the myocardium and tends to remove edema fluid in congestive failure by its circulatory and diuretic actions. Parenterally administered aminophylline is sometimes especially effective for relief of the pulmonary edema of left-sided heart failure. The drug's relaxing effect on bronchial smooth muscle may also play a part in relieving the dyspnea, or difficult breathing, of what is sometimes called cardiac asthma. However, some doctors believe that aminophylline and its relatives do little to improve the nutrition of the heart muscle because, even if these drugs do dilate the coronary vessels, they may also stimulate the heart to work harder and thus use up any extra oxygen carried to the heart by way of the widened channels.

Because theophylline and its derivatives often tend to cause gastrointestinal irritation, they may be prescribed in doses too low to reach effective levels in the coronary vessels. As a result, attempts have been made to increase the rapidity and completeness of the absorption of theophylline and related xanthines from the G.I. tract. Certain hydroalcoholic solutions of theophylline and theophylline sodium glycinate have recently been found effective for controlling anginal symptoms. Alcohol apparently aids absorption of these drugs, and although it is itself not a coronary vasodilator, some patients may benefit from the prompt pain-relieving and sedative actions of ethyl alcohol (Chap. 12). (See Drug Digest for dosage and administration of theophylline.)

Aminophylline, oxtriphylline (Choledyl), and other solubilized theophylline derivatives are employed most commonly today in the treatment of bronchial asthma. (A detailed discussion of their side effects and toxicity will be found in Chap. 40.)

Dipyridamole (Persantin) is one of the newest of the non-nitrite coronary vasodilators. Despite its effectiveness when given to experimental animals by vein, the oral form of this drug does not seem to be useful for reducing the frequency of painful anginal attacks. However, the drug is sometimes ordered for patients with various clinical conditions caused by reduced coronary blood flow. Its utility in angina, arteriosclerotic heart disease, and postmyocardial infarction is still not well established.

Nonspecific Drug Treatment of Angina

Since emotional stress as well as physical exertion can precipitate anginal pain, the doctor often orders sedatives and tranquilizers (Chaps. 6 and 7) to help protect the patient from the adverse effects of anxiety. The barbiturates—especially phenobarbital, for daytime use, and pentobarbital (Nembutal) and secobarbital (Seconal), at night—are commonly employed for this purpose. The minor tranquilizers meprobamate (Miltown) and hydroxyzine (Atarax) are often combined with pentaerythritol tetranitrate in antianginal products, and chlordiazepoxide (Librium) is also often prescribed with coronary vasodilators for reducing tension in patients with this and other cardiac conditions.

Antidepressant drugs of the monoamine oxidase inhibitor type (Chap. 7) have also been employed for treating angina pectoris. Although these drugs may somehow affect the catecholamine metabolism of the heart favorably, they do not dilate the coronary vessels significantly. Most probably, these drugs, including isocarboxazid (Marplan), nialamide (Niamid), and phenelzine (Nardil), produce their pain-relieving effects in angina by their effects on the central nervous system. That is, these mood-elevating agents seem to reduce the patient's awareness of and concern with his chest pains. Obviously, such patients may then tend to ignore warning signals to slow down. This, and the increased motor activity often induced by these drugs, may lead some patients to put too great a strain on their hearts. In addition, these drugs are capable of producing numerous side effects during long-term use. Doctors, with increased awareness of the potential toxicity of these MAO inhibitors, are now using these drugs in angina less frequently than they did during the period of early enthusiasm.

The fact that all these centrally acting drugs often reduce anginal symptoms (as, indeed, placebos also often do) indicates the importance of keeping these patients calm and relaxed. Thus, it is desirable for the doctor and the nurse to win the patient's confidence. This not only helps to lessen the apprehension that often triggers anginal attacks, but also makes the patient more likely to accept advice about how he can best live with his cardiac disability. Although physical activity should not be too severely restricted, patients with angina must be taught to readjust their way of life in order to protect themselves from environmental stresses that tend to precipitate attacks of chest pain.

We should be aware, however, that even when they follow all the physician's instructions carefully and make the most judicious use of their medication, some anginal patients will continue to have attacks. Thus, we should do what we can to help the patient adjust to the idea that limiting his activities and taking his medication faithfully will not necessarily succeed in wholly controlling his painful symptoms. Accepting this may help to allay the patient's feeling of frustration and his understandable anger, resentment, or despair—emotions that may adversely affect this cardiac condition.

THE MANAGEMENT OF MYOCARDIAL INFARCTION

Block of a major coronary artery by a blood clot or by an unusually prolonged and severe spasm may damage and destroy the heart muscle tissue that receives its oxygen and nutrients by way of the blocked vessel. Oxygen lack causes the death of the muscle fibers located in the center of the ischemic (blood-deprived) area, which is surrounded by a border of injured, but still living, muscle cells. The necrotic myocardial area is filled in by a fibrous connective tissue scar over a period of several weeks of healing.

If this myocardial infarction can be kept small and the bordering muscle fibers restored to full function, the patient's heart may recover most of its former contractile power. This is the basis for the use of long-acting coronary vasodilators during convalescence. However, some authorities say that anoxia itself is actually the most powerful stimulus for increasing the circulation locally in the border area. Thus (they argue) the use of vasodilator drugs for this purpose seems superfluous and may, indeed, prove harmful if it interferes with the heart's own compensatory mechanisms for increasing the collateral circulation.

Coronary vasodilator drugs are also administered to relieve ischemic cardiac pain. These drugs are not nearly as effective for relieving the pain of a coronary occlusion as they may have been against that of the patient's early anginal attacks. In fact, the failure of nitroglycerin to bring the usual relief may be a sign that he has suffered a more serious occlusion. In some cases, large doses of papaverine or theophylline, as well as nitroglycerin, may give some pain relief by dilating reflexly constricted coronary vessels in the surrounding, non-infarcted areas. However, these drugs may, in such large doses, dilate systemic blood vessels also and thus cause a further fall in the blood pressure of a patient already close to circulatory collapse. Consequently, such vasodilator drugs, if they are used at all, may be withheld until the patient's blood pressure has returned to near normal levels.

Actually, the severe chest pain following an acute coronary attack is best relieved not by these vasodilator drugs but by the administration of narcotic analgesics (Chap. 9). Many physicians prefer to give morphine for this purpose, since its tranquilizing properties help to reduce the patient's apprehension, and its somnifacient effects aid in producing periods of restful sleep. Other doctors tend to rely on meperidine (Demerol), which is less constipating than morphine. Because it is less sedating than morphine, meperidine must be combined with a sedative-hypnotic such as phenobarbital if the patient is restless and wakeful. Some patients are started on morphine, which is replaced after a few days by meperidine combined with phenobarbital or promethazine (Phenergan); then, they may be switched to only the sedative or the tranquilizer, and, finally, they may get no nerve-quieting medication at all.

Many other drugs and medical measures are employed to prevent and overcome complications such as cardiac arrhythmias, cardiogenic shock, congestive heart failure, and pulmonary embolism. The various kinds of drugs used for this purpose are discussed in detail elsewhere; however, some major points concerning their employment in the management of a myocardial infarction are summarized briefly here.

Antiarrhythmic Agents (See Chap. 21)

Sudden cardiac arrest (asystole) and ventricular fibrillation are the main causes of death during the first hours after a coronary occlusion. Apparently, differences in the degree of oxygenation of adjacent cardiac tissues set up a state of electrical instability between well oxygenated and hypoxic areas. As a result, the heart of the postcoronary patient may then suffer an electrical failure that is thought to arise in the poorly oxygenated tissues at the margin of the infarcted area.

The patient gets pure oxygen by mask, and, if premature systoles persist or ventricular tachycardia develops, quinidine or procainamide may be administered to dampen possible ectopic foci. The doctor usually monitors the patient's heart action with electrocardiograms during administration of these antiarrhythmic drugs or when potassium salts are being infused to counteract irregular cardiac rhythms. For complete heart block which may be a prelude to sudden cardiac arrest, isoproterenol and molar sodium lactate may be infused intravenously. If the heart actually stops, 0.1 mg. of isoproterenol or 0.5 ml. of a 1:10,000 solution of epinephrine (the official 1:1,000 solution is diluted tenfold) may be injected intracardially. Some authorities advocate use of a smaller quantity (0.25 ml.) of the 1:1,000 solution. This condition and ventricular fibrillation are now often treated with electrical pacemakers and defibrillators.

Adrenergic Vasopressors

The infarcted heart may pump less blood than normal out into the aorta. Since adequate coronary circulation depends upon perfusion from the aorta, this drop in cardiac output may interfere still further with cardiac action, thus setting off a vicious cycle which may cause cardiogenic shock. The drugs most commonly employed for raising the systemic blood pressure and for increasing cardiac efficiency are levarterenol (Levophed) and metaraminol (Aramine; Pressonex). These adrenergic drugs are said to precipitate fewer arrhythmias than other agents of this class. However, they must be administered with great care (see Chap. 16) to avoid both excessive blood pressure rises and the occurrence of cardiac irregularities.

Cardiotonic and Diuretic Drugs

Many patients develop some degree of heart failure following an acute infarction. Mild failure often responds to rest, sedation, and oxygen. Others, in whom left ventricular failure causes fluid to collect in the lungs, require cardiotonic and diuretic drugs to drain away the pulmonary fluid and relieve dyspnea. Such patients are usually digitalized with one of the more rapid acting of the glycosides (see Chap. 19), and they may receive a mercurial diuretic parenterally at the same time. This is often followed by an orally administered thiazide-type diuretic to keep the patient free of edema, and, if necessary, maintenance therapy may be instituted with a long-acting digitalis derivative such as digitoxin.

Anticoagulant Therapy (See Chap. 24)

Most patients with myocardial infarction do not suffer any thromboembolic complications. However, patients whose history makes them seem likely to develop peripheral venous thrombosis and, possibly, pulmonary embolism during prolonged bed rest may require anticoagulant therapy. The frequency of thromboses may also be reduced by measures such as reducing the period of absolute bed rest, getting the patient to move his feet, and slightly elevating the *foot* of his bed but *not* the knee gatch. Such patients usually receive heparin parenterally at once and are started, at the same time, on an orally administered anticoagulant of the prothrombin-reducing type (e.g., Dicoumarol or coumadin).

The heparin may be given by vein or injected subcutaneously in an area, such as the abdominal fat pads, to form a depot from which absorption is relatively slow and steady and the likelihood of hematoma is low. The heparin is discontinued after a few days when the hypoprothrombinemic agents have succeeded in lowering plasma prothrombin levels to therapeutically desirable levels. This is usually accomplished by administering a drug such as Dicoumarol for three days in descending dosage—300 mg.; 200 mg.; 100 mg.

The patient may then be continued on long-term maintenance dosage of anticoagulants, as determined by periodic prothrombin-time tests, if the doctor thinks that he may be subject to future thrombo-embolic episodes of the kind that had caused the infarction. Some authorities, however, do not feel that the prolonged use of anticoagulants routinely is desirable for most postcoronary patients. Similarly, there is disagreement as to the utility of putting the patient on special dietary and drug regimens for reducing plasma levels of cholesterol and other lipids in order to attempt reversal of coronary atherosclerotic processes.

Drug and Dietary Treatment of Atherosclerosis

Atherosclerosis

The underlying cause of coronary artery disease is atherosclerosis, a condition in which lipid deposits are laid down within the intima, the inner layer of the arterial wall. By narrowing the lumen, or channel, of the artery, such cholesterol-containing masses interfere with blood flow. In addition, blood is more likely to clot as it passes over the roughened inner surface of atherosclerotic vessels. Because this pathogenic process predisposes people to strokes and peripheral vascular obstructions as well as coronary occlusions, it is a very common cause of death and disability.

The exact cause of what has been called "medical public enemy number one" in the United States and Europe is still obscure. However, authorities agree that these fatty thickenings of the arterial walls occur most commonly in people with abnormalities in their serum lipid patterns. For example, people with a history of familial hypercholesterolemia (high blood cholesterol levels) are known to have a higher incidence of atheromata (atherosclerotic plaques) and to suffer myocardial infarctions more frequently than those with normal amounts of this lipid in their plasma.

Although not all the relationships between atheroma formation and high lipid levels are understood, many authorities believe that it is desirable for some patients to have their high cholesterol levels lowered. People considered candidates for dietary measures and drug therapy to accomplish this reduction include: (1) those who have already had one or more coronary attacks or strokes and who seem prone to recurrences, and (2) those with a family history of atherosclerotic disease, who show elevated blood cholesterol, high blood pressure, and overweight, even though they may not yet have suffered any attacks.

Dietary Measures. Most of the body's cholesterol is synthesized from other substances, including metabolites derived from protein and carbohydrates as well as from fat. Thus, it does little good merely to eliminate cholesterol-containing foods from the patient's diet. It is necessary for the patient to reduce his total caloric intake and also to alter the amount and type of fat ingested. It has been found, for ex-

ample, that serum cholesterol is somehow lowered when certain vegetable and fish oils rich in unsaturated fatty acids are substituted for foods high in saturated fats. ("Saturation" refers to the extent to which certain links between carbon atoms are occupied by hydrogen; most saturated fats are of animal origin.)

Patients are now sometimes put on diets relatively low in all fats, and the proportion of polyunsaturated fatty acids in their dietary intake is raised. Among the fats high in these fatty acids that contain several hydrogen-free double bonds are vegetable oils such as corn, cottonseed, peanut, soybean, olive and safflower. The patient may simply take an ounce of corn oil with each meal, or a product may be prescribed containing emulsified safflower oil plus a supplementary amount of pyridoxine (Vitamin B_6). If these oils replace an equal amount of fat from foods such as whole milk, cream, cheese, butter, eggs, and meat, the patient's lipid levels are likely to fall. However, there is still no proof that products containing corn oil, safflower oil, etc., have any ability to reduce the atherosclerotic lesions or to increase the patient's life expectancy.

Hypocholesterolemic and Antilipemic Agents. A number of new drugs have been introduced in recent years for the reduction of plasma levels of cholesterol and other lipids. When employed steadily as adjuncts to a diet low in saturated fats and total calories, some of these drugs seem able to turn abnormal plasma lipid patterns back toward normal for a time. However, these hypocholesterolemic agents have not been shown to improve the condition of disease-damaged blood vessels.

The exact manner in which most of these drugs act is not entirely clear. They are thought mainly to alter cholesterol metabolism in one way or another. That is, they may interfere with the absorption of dietary cholesterol, inhibit its biosynthesis by the liver, or speed its breakdown to bile acids which are then excreted, instead of being built up to cholesterol again. All of these mechanisms play a part in the cholesterol-lowering actions of various drugs. Often, however, after an initial drop, plasma cholesterol levels tend to rebound to the original abnormally high planes.

This may be, in part, the result of bodily compensatory mechanisms. For example, when drugs increase the rate of cholesterol degradation, the liver may simply speed up its rate of synthesis of the lipid. On the other hand, the real reason may be the patient's failure to continue taking his medication regularly. This is understandable, since these drugs do nothing to make the patient feel that he is improving and their side effects may even make him feel worse. However, despite a lack of any clear-cut evidence of their usefulness, the use of some of these hypocholesterolemic agents is considered justified in "poor-risk" patients whose high lipid levels do not drop significantly with dietary measures alone.

Some of the individual drugs that are being employed clinically or experimentally are discussed briefly below. The bibliography should be consulted for more detailed information.

Nicotinic Acid (niacin). This B-complex vitamin, when given in massive doses (up to 50 times the daily requirements), often causes a decrease in serum cholesterol and various other plasma lipids. The most common side effects include flushing and itching of the face and neck, and anorexia, nausea, and vomiting. These reactions are claimed to occur less frequently with aluminum nicotinate (Nicalex), a salt that releases nicotinic acid slowly as it hydrolyzes in the gastrointestinal tract.

Dextrothyroxine Sodium (Choloxin). Thyroid hormones have long been known to reduce plasma cholesterol levels when administered to hypothyroid patients. However, this cholesterol-lowering effect is usually accompanied by other metabolic effects typical of thyroid hormones, including an increase in cardiac work (see Chap. 31). This drug is one of several thyroid derivatives that are said to be less stimulating to the heart and to possess hypocholesterolemic activity. However, all these analogues are capable of causing anginal attacks when administered to patients with a tendency toward coronary insufficiency. Thus, their use obviously requires caution in patients whose high cholesterol levels have to be lowered because they have had a coronary attack or are considered candidates for one.

Sitosterols (Cytellin). These plant sterols are thought to interfere with the absorption of dietary cholesterol and increase its fecal excretion. Large daily doses must be ingested, and these occasionally cause anorexia, cramps, and diarrhea. Serum cholesterol may still remain high because of the synthesis of this substance from other sources. Thus, the dietary measures mentioned previously must be employed simultaneously, if these drugs are to have any significant effect on cholesterol levels.

Estrogens. The use of female sex hormones for heart patients was suggested because of the observation that the incidence of coronary atherosclerosis was relatively low in premenopausal women. The doses of estrogens which are required in order to lower elevated serum lipid levels have had undesirable feminizing effects in men and caused uterine bleeding in postmenopausal women. Recently, however, it has been claimed that doses of certain estrogens too small to reduce lipid levels have nevertheless increased the survival rates of patients with a history of recurrent myocardial infarction. This "protective action" is said to be achieved with doses of conjugated estrogens that have few feminizing side effects. Large-scale studies are in progress to determine the validity of these observations.

Other Agents. Many other agents have reportedly produced beneficial effects.

Heparin (Chap. 24) is known to clear up plasma made cloudy by fats absorbed during a meal. This occurs when the drug is given intravenously as an anticoagulant. However, this antilipemic effect is not observed when heparin is given by the more convenient oral route. A sublingual preparation for reducing lipemia has been marketed, but its usefulness has not been established.

Cholestyramine (Cuemid; Questran), introduced for relief of itching in biliary disease, is said to be capable of lowering serum cholesterol levels. It is a resin which binds bile acids in the gastrointestinal tract and removes them in the feces. This prevents their reabsorption into the blood and return to the liver. As a result, the liver produces more of the bile acids needed for digestion by breaking down part of its cholesterol stores. Often, this results in a decrease in serum cholesterol. However, in many cases cholesterol eventually rises once more to the original abnormally high plasma levels. Thus, the true utility of this agent in hypercholesterolemia still remains to be established.

Clofibrate (Atromid S) is a recently introduced antihyperlipidemic agent claimed to be capable of reducing elevated serum triglycerides as well as cholesterol. The drug is also said to bring about a desirable reduction in the coagulability of the blood. The manner in which it brings about these effects is not fully understood. Some evidence suggests that the drug in part acts indirectly to interfere with cholesterol synthesis by the liver. Since *Triparanol*, an agent that also interferes with hepatic biosynthesis, had to be withdrawn when long-term toxic effects developed, doctors are now cautious in their use of drugs known to act in this way and hope that this new agent functions in some other manner.

Clofibrate, however, has caused no impairment of liver or adrenal gland function in humans, and the side effects so far reported seem minor. These include nausea, flatulence, loose stools and abdominal distress. Patients who are taking anticoagulants of the hypoprothrombinemic type (see Chap. 24) may require reduction in the dosage of these drugs when clofibrate is added to the regimen, lest additive effects result in hemorrhagic complications.

This drug may be ordered for patients with ischemic heart disease, and cerebral or peripheral vascular diseases when it seems desirable to lower the patient's elevated lipid levels. It is also sometimes administered to patients with xanthomatosis in order to bring about regression of the fatty skin lesions by reducing circulating triglyceride levels.

The search for drugs to treat atherosclerosis goes on. At present, however, no agent has established itself as outstandingly useful even for lowering plasma cholesterol and keeping it low indefinitely. And, if a drug did succeed in doing so, there is, as yet, no proof that this would reverse atherosclerotic lesions or increase the life expectancy of patients with a history of myocardial infarction.

SUMMARY OF POINTS FOR THE NURSE TO REMEMBER CONCERNING CORONARY VASODILATOR DRUGS

- Nitroglycerin tablets should be available to the anginal patient at all times, including his stay in the hospital, and he should be allowed to assume responsibility for administering the drug to himself when he decides that he requires it.

- Nitroglycerin is almost always administered sublingually. The ordinary tablets should *not* be swallowed, because the patient will experience little relief from oral administration of nitroglycerin unless it is given in much larger doses.

- If the patient's chest pain is not relieved 15 or 20 minutes after he has taken his nitroglycerin sublingually, the doctor should be notified at once and the patient kept at complete rest until the physician comes. (The patient may have suffered a coronary occlusion rather than an anginal attack.)

- Patients should be told how to minimize the side effects of nitroglycerin. By sitting down before taking the drug, for example, the patient may spare himself the feelings of faintness and weakness that often occur when he is standing.

- Watch how the patient reacts to the nitroglycerin that he takes, in order to be able to tell the doctor whether tolerance is developing or unusual side effects occur.

- Be especially aware of the coronary patient's emotional state, since his general condition and his response to drug therapy is frequently affected by environmental stress and personal relationships. If the patient has confidence in those caring for him, he is more likely to accept advice and follow instructions that will help him to live with his disability.

REVIEW QUESTIONS

1. (a) Explain the manner in which the rapid-acting nitrites are believed to act to overcome the pain of an angina pectoris attack.

   (b) What is the rationale for long-term therapy with the nitrites of longer action?

2. (a) How is nitroglycerin usually taken to abort an anginal attack or to prevent one prior to physical exertion?

   (b) What other dosage forms are available and for what purposes are these employed?

3. What are some points that the nurse should remember in caring for the hospitalized patient who is taking nitroglycerin for angina?

4. (a) List some common side effects of nitrite therapy of angina pectoris.

   (b) In what patients are nitrites given only with caution if at all?

5. (a) How does the doctor try to deal with tolerance to nitrites when it develops in anginal patients?

   (b) What is a toxic effect of nitrite overdosage and how may the doctor try to deal with it?

6. (a) What is the manner in which papaverine is thought to act when administered to patients who have suffered an arterial occlusion?

   (b) What are some of the clinical conditions for which papaverine is sometimes employed?

7. (a) List several pharmacological effects of theophylline and related xanthine compounds.

   (b) How is aminophylline thought to benefit some patients with left-sided heart failure?

8. (a) What is the role of sedatives and tranquilizers in the management of angina pectoris?

   (b) What are some possible dangers in the use of monoamine-oxidase-inhibitor-type antidepressants in the management of angina pectoris?

9. List six kinds of drugs employed in the management of a myocardial infarction and its complications, and indicate briefly the basis for the use of each type.

10. List six kinds of drugs used in the management of hypercholesterolemia in patients with atherosclerosis, and indicate the general and the specific limitations of such treatment.

BIBLIOGRAPHY

Drugs for Coronary Artery Disease

Bruce, T. A., and Bing, R. J.: Clinical management of myocardial infarction. J.A.M.A., *191*:124, 1965.

Ellis, L. B., and Hancock, E. W.: Current status of therapy in coronary artery disease. J.A.M.A., *163*:445, 1957.

Friend, D. G.: Angina pectoris therapy. Clin. Pharmacol. Ther., *5*:385, 1964.

Lown, B., *et al.:* The coronary care unit. J.A.M.A., *199*:188, 1967.

Modell, W.: Clinical pharmacology of antianginal drugs. Clin. Pharmacol. Ther., *3*:97, 1962.

Riseman, J. E. F.: The treatment of angina pectoris. New Eng. J. Med., *261*:1126, 1959.

Rodman, M. J.: Drugs for coronary disease. R.N., *23*:43, 1960 (Nov.).

————: Drugs used in heart disease, Part I. R.N., *27*:37, 1964 (May).

————: Drugs used in coronary and cerebral vascular diseases. R.N., *29*:63, 1966 (Sept.)

Russek, H. I.: Glyceryl trinitrate in angina pectoris. J.A.M.A., *189*:108, 1964.

Silber, E. N.: Medical management of angina pectoris. Am. J. Nurs., *55*:168, 1955.

Drugs and Diet in Atherosclerosis

Ahrens, E. H., *et al.:* Symposium on significance of lowered cholesterol levels. J.A.M.A., *170*:2198, 1959.

Altschul, R.: Nicotinic acid and cholesterol metabolism. G.P., *21*:115, 1960.

Best, M. M., and Duncan, C. H.: Comparative effects of thyroxin analogues as hypocholesteremic agents. Circulation, *24*:58, 1961.

Brown, D. F., *et al.:* Dextro-triiodothyronine, effects on serum lipid levels of patients with ischemic heart disease. J.A.M.A., *180*:643, 1962.

Danowski, T. S., *et al.:* Hypolipidemic effect of chlorphenoxyisobutyrate (clofibrate). Clin. Pharmacol. Ther., *7*:631, 1966.

Frederickson, D. S.: Current attitudes about atherosclerosis. G.P., *28*:102, 1958.

Goldsmith, G. A.: Highlights on the cholesterol fats, diets and atherosclerosis problem. J.A.M.A., *176*:783, 1961.

Hashim, S. A.: The relation of diet to atherosclerosis and infarction. Am. J. Nurs., *60*:348, 1960.

Marmoston, J., *et al.:* Estrogen therapy in men with myocardial infarction. J.A.M.A., *174*:241, 1960.

Moses, C.: Pharmacology of drugs used in the control of hypercholesterolemia. Angiology, *13*:59, 1962.

Stamler, J., *et al.:* Effectiveness of estrogens for therapy of myocardial infarction in middle-age men. J.A.M.A., *183*:632, 1963.

Van Itallie, T. B., and Hashim, S. A.: Clinical and experimental aspects of bile acid metabolism. Med. Clin. N. Am., *47*:629, 1963 (May).

Drugs Used in Hypertension

HYPERTENSION

Hypertension, or high blood pressure, has been defined as a condition in which a person's systolic pressure stays consistently above 160 mm. of Hg., or his diastolic pressure taken at rest reads 95 mm. of Hg. or more during several different examinations. Since pressure normally stays under 140 mm. systolic and 90 mm. diastolic, these arbitrary criteria are set well beyond the bounds of borderline cases.

The words *consistently, at rest,* and *several different examinations* in the above definition are especially significant. Blood pressure can, of course, rise far above normal for brief periods in many situations. Fear—even the uneasiness many patients feel during a medical examination—and exercise, including climbing stairs to the doctor's office, may cause a temporary rise to high levels. However, when a nurse takes a patient's pressure at intervals while he is at ease, she can usually tell whether abnormally high readings are the result of environmental factors or are indicative of a true hypertensive state.

The doctor, of course, makes his diagnosis on the basis of additional tests. He may, for example, look at the patient's eye-grounds with an ophthalmoscope to see if the arterioles in the fundus of the eye are excessively constricted or whether the optic disc is edematous (papilledema). He may take chest roentgenograms and take an electrocardiogram to see whether the heart is enlarged or shows signs of strain from overloading. These tests may indicate that the heart has been working too hard in its efforts to force blood through narrowed arterioles—that is, against high peripheral resistance.

Hypertension is commonly classified, on the basis of the extent of any complications present, as being of *mild, moderate,* or *severe* degree. Most early cases are mild and free of symptoms or complications. People with this type condition—so-called *labile* hypertension—often react to stressful situations with a rise in blood pressure, but their pressure returns readily to normal when the emotional strain is removed.

Later in life, however, the pressure of people with such *labile* hypertension may stabilize at an abnormally high level. Persistent elevation of arterial pressure leads to damage of blood vessel walls. It may also speed up atherosclerotic processes in the arteries of the heart, brain, and kidneys. Depending on how high the pressure stays and the degree of vascular damage, this condition is classed as moderate or severe hypertension.

Severe hypertension, including the rapidly progressive malignant form and the sudden acute crises observed in the toxemias of pregnancy, may cause fatal complications. Strokes due to cerebral thrombosis or hemorrhage are common in older patients, and dangerous eclamptic convulsions may occur in pregnant women who are predisposed to toxemic hypertension. In other patients, severe hypertension may end in heart failure or in renal insufficiency and fatal uremia.

The specific causes of hypertension are known in only a small minority of cases. Some of these cases that are *secondary* to a definite organic cause—for example, pheochromocytoma, the chromaffin cell tumors, which were discussed in Chapter 17—are curable by surgery.

In most cases of hypertension, however, the cause of the patient's arterial pressure is unknown, and there are, at present, no surgical or pharmacological means by which the still undiscovered basic defect of the *primary,* or *essential,* type hypertension can be overcome.

Nonetheless, many of the milder cases of primary hypertension can now be kept from getting worse or may even be reversed, and the dangerous late complications can often be prevented. Sometimes, all that is needed is a regimen of rest, reassurance, moderate exercise, and reduced intake of sodium. In other patients the addition of relatively safe sedative and diuretic drugs may be required to halt the advance of the disease.

For patients with moderate to severe hypertension, several new kinds of antihypertensive drugs have become available in the past fifteen years or so, and have already helped to lengthen thousands of lives. These potent drugs are not, however, a true cure for the condition, nor do they help all patients. Many people with moderate hypertension who might benefit from these more powerful antihypertensive agents are unwilling or unable to withstand the discomforts which these drugs often cause. Thus, these agents are sometimes reserved for patients with malignant and other severe forms of hypertension.

DRUG TREATMENT OF HYPERTENSION

Indications. Doctors used to think that it was not wise to try to bring the blood pressure of a hypertensive patient down by means of drugs. They reasoned that the rise in arterial pressure was the body's way of keeping enough blood flowing through the vessels feeding the heart, brain, and kidneys. Restoring pressure to normal with drugs, they felt, might dangerously reduce the perfusion of these vital organs with blood.

Today, however, it is generally held that it is more dangerous to let a patient's pressure stay high, because of the progressive blood vessel damage that tends to develop. Early treatment with drugs is aimed at preventing mild cases from progressing to the more severe forms. Drug treatment of the more serious grades of hypertension has as its goal a reduction in the vascular complications of high blood pressure, including hypertensive encephalopathy, heart muscle damage, and renal insufficiency.

Fortunately, several classes of drugs have been developed in recent years that now make it possible to achieve these goals of keeping mild disease from getting worse and severe hypertension from leading to deadly complications. None of the presently available drugs actually counteract the causes of high blood pressure. Rather, they act to relax constricted arterioles and thus reduce the high peripheral resistance of the narrowed arterial system.

These new antihypertensive agents are by no means ideal. All are capable of causing side effects some of which are severe. These can, however, be minimized by tailoring the patient's treatment to fit his disease. Since the severity of the side effects is often related to the potency of the drug, the doctor uses the weakest drug that will keep a patient's pressure down to near normal levels. He reserves the more toxic drugs for patients with severe, sustained hypertension. Even in such cases, he tries to minimize toxicity by the use of adjunctive drugs and other measures.

Treatment Programs. Although hypertension regimens vary in detail from doctor to doctor and clinic to clinic, we may make some generalizations in regard to how this condition is treated today. The available drugs can be classified broadly on the basis of the grades of hypertension for which each type seems best suited.

The least severe cases of hypertension are often handled with no drug treatment at all except, occasionally, a sedative. *Barbiturates* have been used traditionally for this purpose. Recently, certain tranquilizers have been employed to dampen the patient's reaction to emotional stress. The minor tranquilizers chlordiazepoxide (Librium) and meprobamate (Equanil, Miltown) sometimes help to keep the blood pressure of patients with labile hypertension from rising when they become upset by difficulties in their daily lives. A phenothiazine derivative, acetophenazine (Tindal), has been recommended as a calmative for patients with hypertensive heart disease.

Certain agents that possess a sedative component are thought to act in other ways to lower blood pressure. A derivative of meprobamate called mebutamate (Capla) is claimed to reduce the sensitivity of the brain's vasomotor center to incoming nerve impulses. As a result, the nerve cells of this center send out fewer vasoconstrictor impulses to the smooth muscle walls of the blood vessels. Thus, some patients with mild degrees of hypertension are said to show a gradual moderate lowering of pressure.

The rauwolfia alkaloids (another tranquilizer group) are the agents most widely used for control of the less serious forms of hypertension. Used alone or in combination with one of the sulfonamide type diuretic drugs (Chap. 20) these rauwolfia plant derivatives are capable of controlling most of the milder cases of hypertension by a combination of central and peripheral effects that reduce sympathetic nerve impulses to the heart and blood vessels.

Combinations of rauwolfia alkaloids and sulfonamide diuretics usually are not effective alone for treating moderate to severe grades of hypertension. However, these drugs do tend to increase the effectiveness and reduce the toxicity of more potent drugs such as hydralazine (Apresoline), the veratrum alkaloids, and the ganglionic blocking agents. Thus, when patients receive rauwolfia-diuretic combinations concurrently, the previously required dosage of these potent hypotensive drugs and of newer ones such as guanethidine (Ismelin), pargyline (Eutonyl), and methyldopa (Aldomet) can be cut in half. This, in turn, leads to reduction of some of the side effects caused by full therapeutic doses of the more powerful drugs.

These potent drugs and certain others, including sodium nitroprusside, are sometimes employed parenterally in malignant hypertension and in emergency situations to counteract sudden steep rises in blood pressure. Such acute hypertensive reactions require the parenteral administration of large doses to prevent the very high blood pressure from causing brain damage or heart failure.

In toxemias of pregnancy, for example, the intravenous administration of a ganglionic blocking agent such as trimethaphan (Arfonad) may relieve severe headache and prevent convulsions. Similarly, infusion of nitroprusside solution or of protoveratrines A and B (Veralba) (which is done only by intensive-care teams trained in the use of these drugs) can often rouse stuporous or comatose patients in hypertensive crisis by bringing about a rapid drop in blood pressure and intracranial tension.

THE SEVERAL CLASSES OF ANTIHYPERTENSIVE AGENTS

The drugs used for hypertension act either on the nervous system or directly upon the heart and blood vessels to lower blood pressure. Although, as we have said, these drugs do not correct the underlying conditions responsible for the rise in the patient's pressure, they do counteract the rise itself in most cases. The manner of action of some of these agents is well understood, but the way in which others act is still somewhat obscure.

In general, as the following discussions of the several classes of drugs will reveal, these agents act:

1. To reduce the number of nerve impulses passing out of the central nervous system and over sympathetic efferent pathways to the circulatory system. (Some act directly on the vasomotor center; others act indirectly as a result of their primary peripheral effects.)

2. To relax blood vessels and bring about vasodilation by a depressant effect directly on the vascular smooth muscle walls.

In the following discussions of the various kinds of antihypertensive drugs we shall take up, among other things, (1) the manner in which they are thought to act, (2) their side effects, potential toxicity and other limitations, and (3) their current status in the management of the various types of hypertension.

The Rauwolfia Alkaloids (See Drug Digests)

History. The powdered root of the shrub *Rauwolfia serpentina* has been used in India for centuries in the treatment of many medical conditions. It was introduced in this country in the early 1950's for the treatment of hypertension and was later widely used as a tranquilizer for mentally ill patients (see Chap. 7).

Later, chemists succeeded in extracting the several alkaloids responsible for the pharmacological effects of the whole plant. They have also synthesized hundreds of derivatives, some in which the central seda-

TABLE 23-1
RAUWOLFIA-TYPE PRODUCTS

Nonproprietary Name	Trade Name	Usual Daily Dosage
Alseroxylon	Rauwiloid, Rautensin, etc.	2 to 4 mg.
Deserpidine	Harmonyl	0.1 to 0.5 mg.
Rescinnamine	Moderil	0.1 to 0.5 mg.
Reserpine U.S.P.	Serpasil, Sandril, etc.	0.1 to 0.25 mg.
Syrosingopine N.F.	Singoserp	0.5 to 3 mg.

tive effect predominates, and others that act mainly peripherally (i.e., in the tissues of the heart and blood vessels).

Manner of Action. Despite great scientific interest in the subject, the exact mode of action of the natural and semisynthetic rauwolfia alkaloids is still not entirely clear. The natural alkaloids reserpine, rescinnamine, and deserpidine (see Table 23-1 for trade names and doses) act, in part, by suppressing the sympathetic outflow from the vasomotor center in the brain.

Recently, reserpine and its relatives have been shown to act peripherally, also, to reduce sympathetic stimulation of the heart and arterioles. In some manner, these drugs deplete the catecholamines, including norepinephrine, that are stored in these tissues. (See Chap. 14 for a review of catecholamine metabolism in sympathetic nervous system transmission.)

Syrosingopine (Singoserp) is said to cause less central depression than reserpine and others, presumably because the drug acts mainly peripherally to release norepinephrine bound in the tissues. The neurohormone is then destroyed in enzymatically catalyzed chemical reactions. Then, sympathetic nerve impulses arriving at nerve endings fail to release the usual quantities of norepinephrine and, as a result, the heart is slowed, blood vessels dilate, and the blood pressure falls gradually.

Current Status. The rauwolfia alkaloids are recommended mainly for treating the mild, labile forms of hypertension. Administered orally in small doses (e.g., 0.25 mg. a day for reserpine), either alone or in combination with a sulfonamide diuretic, the rauwolfia alkaloids are often the antihypertensive agents to be administered in initiating treatment.

These drugs are also used as a foundation upon which the doctor sometimes builds a structure for treating more severe degrees of hypertension. That is, the doctor may add more potent drugs to the initial regimen of rauwolfia alkaloids and diuretics, if he finds that the first-administered drugs alone fail to lower the patient's pressure adequately. Simultaneous administration of the reserpine-type drugs and the diuretic tends to increase the effectiveness of the more potent drugs, and, because this permits their dosage to be lowered, the toxicity of these potent drugs is consequently reduced.

Reserpine and related drugs are occasionally administered intramuscularly in large doses in acute hypertensive crises. However, because large amounts of these depressant drugs may make the patient very drowsy or even stuporous for several days, other agents are usually preferred for managing hypertensive emergencies.

Side Effects, Toxicity, and Cautions. The rauwolfia alkaloids cause many minor side effects, but these are not usually severe enough to require that the drugs be discontinued. Some of these adverse effects are the result of reduced sympathetic nervous system transmission and a relative increase in parasympathetic predominance. Thus, local vasodilation in the nasal-sinus mucosa often leads to nasal congestion and obstruction and occasionally to nosebleed. The increased gastrointestinal secretion and motility which often occur with these drugs can cause cramps and diarrhea or even make a healed peptic ulcer become active again.

In addition to these and other effects of autonomic imbalance, the rauwolfia alkaloids cause various central effects. Least serious is the drowsiness that often develops during the early days of treatment. Most dangerous is mental depression, at times so serious that the patient may try to commit suicide. Thus, the nurse should watch all patients, and especially those with a history of depression, for any signs of personality change while they are taking rauwolfia alkaloids for hypertension. Patients who have been taking these drugs may suffer severe convulsions and prolonged apnea if subjected to electroshock therapy for depression.

The Sulfonamide Diuretics (*See Drug Digests*)

These drugs, including chlorothiazide (Diuril) and its many congeners, are most commonly employed in the management of edema (see Chap. 20 for a more detailed discussion). However, they are now widely used in hypertension, even when the patient is not edematous.

Manner of Action. These drugs act by removing excess sodium from the body. Just how this helps to reduce high blood pressure is still somewhat obscure. One view is that the loss of sodium and the water in which it is dissolved reduces the volume of blood in the vascular tree. Another suggestion is that reduction of the sodium content of the blood vessel walls makes them less sensitive to the constricting action of nor-

epinephrine released by sympathetic vasomotor nerve impulses.

Current Status. These drugs, which are used both alone and combined with other antihypertensive agents, are now commonly employed more than any other single group of drugs used for high blood pressure. The use of these saluretic, or salt removing, drugs has made rigid sodium restriction less important than it used to be. Availability of these diuretics has not, however, done away with the need for patients to keep their sodium intake at low levels, and, in fact, some doctors still prefer to put patients on a low sodium regimen rather than run the risk of potassium loss and the other side effects that may occur even with these relatively safe drugs.

By combining these diuretics with the ganglionic blocking agents and other potent antihypertensive agents smaller, less toxic doses of the powerful hypotensives can be used. This often helps to lower the stubbornly high blood pressure of patients with moderate to severe hypertension without subjecting them to disabling side effects.

The Ganglionic Blocking Agents (*See Drug Digests*)

Manner of Action. As has been indicated in Chap. 17, drugs that block transmission of nerve impulses through sympathetic ganglia are able to reduce high blood pressure even in severe cases of hypertension. Interruption of vasoconstrictor impulses results in a relaxation of vascular walls. The resulting vasodilation tends to let blood pool in the vessels of the lower limbs, especially when the patient is standing. This, in turn, leads to a reduction in the return of blood to the heart by way of the veins, and the diminished cardiac output causes a fall in systolic blood pressure.

Ordinarily, a reduction of the amount of blood being pumped out of the heart sets off reflex nervous mechanisms that increase the number of nervous impulses passing out of the brain's circulatory control centers. These usually speed up the heart rate and constrict the blood vessels—a combination of effects that quickly brings the pressure back up to normal.

After administration of ganglionic blocking agents, however, such compensatory circulatory effects fail to occur. The reason is that the nerve impulses which must pass over sympathetic nervous pathways are interrupted when they reach the sympathetic ganglia. Thus, the patient's pressure remains down. This same ganglioplegic (ganglion-paralyzing) effect also keeps the patient's blood pressure from reflexly stabilizing itself when he stands up suddenly. As a result, most people taking these drugs suffer from so-called *postural hypotension* to a small or a great degree (see Side Effects).

Side Effects. Although these drugs are usually effective for producing a drop in blood pressure, their actions cause many annoying and even dangerous side effects. Some of these are the result of too great a degree of sympathetic ganglion blockade; other distressing symptoms are caused by blockade of parasympathetic ganglia.

Side Effects of Sympathetic Blockade. The side effect of the ganglionic blocking agents that occurs most commonly is *postural*, or *orthostatic*, *hypotension*, an excessive and uncompensated fall in blood pressure when the patient rises from a recumbent position. The reflex nervous responses that usually act promptly, when we stand up suddenly, to pump more blood out of the heart and into the head fail in such cases because of the ganglionic blockade. As a result, the patient feels giddy, faint, and lightheaded. The dizziness of fainting may make the patient fall. Thus, serious injury is an ever-present hazard against which the patient must be taught to guard himself.

This side effect—which is, after all, merely an extension of the drugs' desired action—may be minimized by very careful adjustment of dosage of the ganglionic blocking agents. Thus, the doctor may specifically state that the next dose of the drug is to be given only after checking the patient's blood pressure. He may even leave specific instructions as to *when* the patient's blood pressure should be taken and in *what position* the patient must be. The nurse should then note on the chart whether the patient was sitting, standing, or lying down when his pressure was taken.

Teaching the patient or a member of his family to take blood pressure readings at home may also be part of the nurse's responsibility in preventing overdosage and hypotension. Of course, the doctor may not want some patients to be preoccupied with their blood pressure at all. Thus, the nurse should always talk to the physician to find out what he has taught the patient and how much he feels the patient should be told in discussing his condition with him.

The patient should also be warned about getting out of bed too fast, lest he faint, fall, and injure himself. He should, for instance, let the telephone ring, rather than bound out of bed to answer it. He may have to sit on the edge of the bed for a couple of minutes before getting up. If he gets weak while walking to the toilet, he should lie horizontal on the floor or sit down promptly with his head down between his knees rather than risk a fall against a fixture upon reaching the bathroom.

The patient may also be told—if the doctor wants him to have such information—about the need to adjust dosage downward in warm weather because of the greater degree of natural vasodilation during the summer. Patients going south in midwinter, for instance, may need to lower the dosage of ganglionic blocking drugs and other antihypertensive medications, since what had previously been safe doses may cause postural hypotension.

Ordinarily, the patient's blood pressure stabilizes at the desired lower level after the dosage is adjusted to his needs over a period of days or weeks. This is best accomplished by beginning at a very low dosage level and building up gradually to fully effective amounts.

However, some kinds of patients are poor candidates for treatment with ganglionic blockers, no matter how carefully these potent drugs are given. Patients with marked cerebral atherosclerosis or a history of a recent cerebral or myocardial infarction, for example, may be endangered by these and other potent pressure reducers. Blood flow through the narrowed vessels of their vital organs may be reduced too much, and the resulting ischemia could cause coronary insufficiency or precipitate an episode of cerebral thrombosis.

Side Effects from Parasympathetic Blockade. One of the great disadvantages of the ganglionic blocking agents is that doses that effectively lower blood pressure block the parasympathetic as well as the sympathetic ganglia. Normal nerve impulses are kept from passing down the postganglionic fibers to many structures that usually receive strong parasympathetic stimulation. This results in widespread side effects resembling those of atropine overdosage.

The side effects include constipation, blurring of vision, difficulty in urinating (especially in elderly men), and sexual impotence in younger men. Laxatives to counteract constipation are commonly prescribed as an adjunct to ganglioplegic drug therapy. Certain cholinergic drugs such as neostigmine and bethanechol may be administered to prevent bowel paralysis and urinary retention. Pilocarpine eye drops tend to relieve some of the visual difficulties, and oral administration of this cholinergic stimulant sometimes reduces dryness of the skin and mouth caused by parasympathetic ganglion blockade.

The measure most effective for lessening such discomforts is the concurrent administration of a sulfonamide diuretic. This permits a marked reduction in the amount of the ganglionic blocking agent needed to lower blood pressure. As a result of the smaller dose employed, parasympathetic ganglion blockade and the side effects stemming from this action are diminished.

Current Status. The ganglionic blocking agents are effective for treating even severe cases of hypertension; however, their many side effects and the need to regulate dosage with extreme care are distinct drawbacks. These drugs are presently being replaced in the treatment of moderate to severe hypertension by other potent agents that cause fewer side effects because of greater specificity for the sympathetic nervous pathways. With methyldopa (Aldomet) and guanethidine (Ismelin), for example, patients do not suffer the disabling atropinelike side effects of parasympathetic blockade observed with these ganglioplegics.

Newer Potent Antihypertensive Agents

Several potent pressure-reducing drugs that do not interfere with parasympathetic nervous system function have been replacing the ganglionic blockers in the treatment of patients with moderate to severe hypertension. It is claimed that these drugs tend to reduce pressure, to some extent, while the patient is lying down as well as while he is in the standing position. Side effects are somewhat less frequent and severe than with the ganglionic blocking agents.

Guanethidine (Ismelin). This drug acts at sympathetic postganglionic fibers to reduce the number of nerve impulses that reach the muscular walls of the arterioles. Unlike the adrenergic blocking agents (Chap. 17), guanethidine does not set up a barrier to the neurohormone norepinephrine. It is thought to act, instead, to alter the rate of synthesis and release of the neurotransmitter.

The chief advantage of guanethidine over the ganglionic blockers lies in its relatively selective action in suppressing sympathetic nervous transmission without affecting parasympathetic function. Thus, it does not cause ocular or urinary bladder dysfunctions or constipation. On the contrary, diarrhea is a common side effect of suppression of sympathetic inhibitory impulses to the gut and the resulting relative increase in parasympathetic stimulation of peristalsis.

Guanethidine must be used with caution when patients have a history of peptic ulcer or spastic colitis, because these conditions may be aggravated by increased parasympathetic secretory and motor activity. Similarly, the vagal slowing of the heart may be undesirable for patients with certain kinds of cardiac difficulties. The reduction in cardiac output and, consequently, in glomerular filtration may lead to edema and congestive heart failure. Patients should be watched for signs of weight gain from fluid which can then usually be eliminated by administration of a sulfonamide diuretic.

Patients should be warned about postural hypotension with this drug, just as with the ganglionic blockers. Dosage must be carefully regulated, since too great a fall in blood pressure may be especially harmful to patients with a history of hypertensive encephalopathy or a recent myocardial infarction, or with severe coronary or renal insufficiency—in all of whom blood flow to the brain, heart, and kidneys may be dangerously reduced. (See also Drug Digest.)

Pargyline (Eutonyl). This drug is related in its actions to some of the antidepressant drugs that are discussed in Chapter 7. Like them, it inhibits the enzyme monoamine oxidase (MAO), which plays a part in the catalytic destruction of catecholamines. The resulting rise in norepinephrine would be expected to cause a rise in blood pressure, but, paradoxically, this drug causes a drop, instead.

Pargyline, whatever its mechanism, seems to be useful for reducing the blood pressure of selected patients with moderate to severe cases of hypertension. It is *not* used in mild cases or in very severe ones such as malignant hypertension, or in pheochromocytoma. It is often administered with a sulfonamide diuretic to reduce edema. This lowers the patient's weight if the gain was the result of fluid retention, but it does not, of course, prevent the weight gain that often follows the increase in appetite sometimes caused by pargyline.

Patients should be warned of the possibility of postural hypotension, so that they can take measures similar to those described for the ganglionic blocking agents. Special care is, of course, required to avoid sharp falls in blood pressure in patients with coronary, cerebrovascular, or renal insufficiency. Since MAO inhibitors sometimes make patients with angina pectoris feel better without really increasing their coronary blood flow, patients should be warned against becoming overactive on the false assumption that their underlying cardiac condition is really improved.

Pargyline, like other potent drugs for treating hypertension, is potentiated by sulfonamide diuretics. Simultaneous administration of a saluretic is especially useful in patients who develop edema while taking pargyline. The drug, however, is usually not given together with reserpine, because it has been found that rauwolfia alkaloids (and the other catecholamine-releasing drug, guanethidine) may cause a *rise* in blood pressure when injected in animals pretreated with the MAO-inhibitor drug.

The potentiating effect of pargyline on a wide variety of drugs that depress and stimulate the central nervous system must also be considered if unexpected reactions are to be avoided. Thus, if patients who are on a pargyline regimen take antihistamine drugs for a cold, they may be made excessively sleepy. If they take barbiturates or alcohol, or are given a narcotic analgesic drug such as meperidine (Demerol), they may become deeply depressed. On the other hand, if they use nose drops containing adrenergic drugs, they may become excessively excited. Even the stimulating effects of caffeine in coffee may be potentiated by pargyline. Thus, all the precautions outlined in Chapter 7 for the MAO-type antidepressant drugs should be followed when pargyline is being employed for treating hypertensive patients. (See Drug Digest for dosage and administration.)

Methyldopa (Aldomet). This synthetic drug, a close chemical relative of the catecholamines, was prepared in a deliberate attempt to develop a drug that would interfere with one of the steps by which the body builds norepinephrine. A reduction in the rate of biosynthesis of this sympathetic neurotransmitter should, of course, lead to a lowering of the arterial blood pressure.

Methyldopa does indeed inhibit dopa decarboxylase, an enzyme that is important in norepinephrine biosynthesis, and the drug causes a reduction in peripheral resistance which leads to drops in blood pressure of patients with moderate to severe hypertension. However, it is now thought that this drug does more than merely inhibit the catecholamine-synthesizing enzyme. Instead, methyldopa may, itself, be metabolized in the terminals of adrenergic nerves to form, not norepinephrine, but a false neurotransmitter. When this substance, alpha methylnorepinephrine, is released by nerve impulses in place of the transmitter, norepinephrine, that is normally stored in nerve endings, it fails to carry vasoconstrictor signals to the vascular smooth muscles.

The drug has benefited some patients who had not been responsive to earlier agents, and it seems to cause fewer side effects than do most other potent antihypertensive agents. Postural hypotension is said to occur less frequently with methyldopa than with other potent drugs. Although the patient's blood pressure tends to fall more when he is standing, a significant drop in pressure is found also while he is lying down. On the other hand, some patients fail to show a sustained drop in pressure, and others tend to become tolerant during treatment with this drug. (See the Drug Digest for further details on dosage, side effects, etc.)

Older Potent Antihypertensive Agents

Among the potent drugs for reducing blood pressure are the chemicals hydralazine and sodium nitroprusside, and the alkaloids of the hellebore plants, *Veratrum album* and *V. viride*. These drugs are all occasionally used in hypertensive emergencies to bring blood pressure down rapidly. However, their routine use in oral forms for maintenance therapy of moderate hypertension has diminished considerably in recent years, with the development of drugs less likely to cause severe side effects.

Veratrum Alkaloids. These natural substances reflexly stimulate the vasomotor center to send out nerve impulses that slow the heart and dilate the blood vessels. As a result, blood pressure drops—often dramatically when the purified alkaloids are infused by vein in acute hypertensive crises.

Unfortunately, these drugs also stimulate the central emetic mechanism. Thus, it is difficult to produce the desired reduction in blood pressure on a regular basis without at the same time causing some nausea and vomiting. The various alkaloids are still sometimes combined in low doses with other antihypertensive agents in attempts to minimize vomiting and other side effects, but the routine use of veratrum products has diminished in recent years. (See Drug Digest (protoveratrines A and B) for typical administrative procedures.)

Hydralazine (Apresoline). This synthetic chemical has complex central and peripheral effects that account for its antihypertensive activity. It acts both at the vasomotor center and directly on the smooth muscles of the blood vessels to produce a reduction in peripheral resistance. This vasodilator action is often accompanied by an increase in cardiac output.

This cardiac effect is unusual and may be desirable for maintaining a good flow of blood to the kidneys; however, the stimulating effect on the heart can be harmful for patients with cardiac damage and coronary insufficiency. The combination of hydralazine with drugs such as Rauwolfia and Veratrum alkaloids, which tend to slow the heart, is intended to prevent tachycardia and cardiac palpitations.

The many minor side effects which accompany the

TABLE 23-2
GANGLIONIC BLOCKING AGENTS

Nonproprietary Name	Trade Name	Usual Daily Dosage Range *
Chlorisondamine chloride	Ecolid	12.5 (initial) to 200 mg.
Hexamethonium chloride	Bistrium, Methium, etc.	125 (initial) to 1500 mg.
Mecamylamine HCl U.S.P.	Inversine	5 (initial) to 25 mg.
Pentolinium tartrate	Ansolysen	60 to 600 mg.
Tetraethylammonium chloride	Etamon	200 to 500 mg. I.V. or 1000 to 1200 mg. I.M.
Trimethaphan camsylate	Arfonad	1 to 4 mg. per minute, I.V. as needed.
Trimethidinium methosulfate	Ostensin	40 to 300 mg.

* The wide range of doses reflects the need for adjusting the dosage to the requirements and the tolerance of each individual patient.

use of this drug (e.g., headache, fever, general malaise, loss of appetite, and gastrointestinal irritation) and the need for painstaking adjustment of dosage have led doctors recently to abandon this sometimes useful drug in favor of newer agents such as methyldopa in the management of moderate degrees of hypertension. Hydralazine is now given alone only rarely, in hypertensive crises. For a long-range therapy, it is usually prescribed in combination with hydrochlorothiazide and reserpine (see Drug Digest).

Sodium Nitroprusside. This powerful direct depressant of the blood vessel walls is now rarely used. How-

ever, in the hands of an emergency team whose members are familiar with its dangers, nitroprusside sometimes produces rapid restoration of normal blood pressure in patients who are having an acute hypertensive episode.

Infused intravenously in a dextrose solution, nitroprusside helps to prevent hypertensive encephalopathy, an adverse effect of sudden rises in blood pressure on the brain. Severe hypertensive headaches may be relieved and convulsive seizures prevented by prompt employment of this drug in such situations.

TABLE 23-3
MISCELLANEOUS ANTIHYPERTENSIVE AGENTS

Nonproprietary Name	Trade Name	Usual Daily Dosage Range
Alkavervir	Veriloid	9 to 15 mg.
Cryptenamine acetates	Unitensin Acetates	0.05 mg./ml. I.V. or I.M. as needed.
Cryptenamine tannates	Unitensin Tannates	2 to 6 mg.
Guanethidine sulfate U.S.P.	Ismelin	10 to 50 mg.
Hydralazine HCl N.F.	Apresoline	40 to 400 mg.
Methyldopa	Aldomet	375 to 750 mg.
Methyldopate HCl	Aldomet Ester	1000 to 3000 mg. I.V.
Pargyline	Eutonyl	25 to 50 mg.
Protoveratrine A	Protalba	0.2 to 0.4 mg.
Protoveratrines A and B	Veralba	2 mg. orally, I.V. or I.M. as needed.
Protoveratrines A and B, maleate	Provell	1 to 2.5 mg.
Sodium nitroprusside		I.V. as needed.

SUMMARY OF SIDE EFFECTS AND CAUTIONS: RAUWOLFIA ALKALOIDS

• *Mild Side Effects and Measures for Counteracting Them*

Nasal stuffiness	Use vasoconstrictor-decongestant nose drops.
Intestinal cramps, diarrhea	Use belladonna-type antispasmodic drugs.
Increased gastric acidity	Use antacids and antisecretory-anticholinergic agents; drug contraindicated in patients with peptic ulcer.
Drowsiness	Use mild cerebral stimulants that do not affect blood pressure.
Increased appetite and weight gain	Watch diet.

• *More Serious Toxicity*

Mental depression	Watch patient for early signs of personality change.
Severe sinusitis	Watch for early signs of nasal obstruction.
Severe intestinal irritation	Watch for cramps and diarrhea; drug contraindicated in patients with spastic colitis.
Tremor, rigidity and other signs of Parkinsonism	These signs of overdosage, which are sometimes seen in psychiatric patients taking high doses, are rare in hypertension; they disappear when the drug is withdrawn.
Sudden severe falls in blood pressure and possible cardiac arrest during general anesthesia	Surgical operations should be postponed until several weeks after the drug is withdrawn.

SUMMARY OF SIDE EFFECTS AND CAUTIONS: GANGLIONIC BLOCKING AGENTS

• **Sympathetic Ganglionic Blockade**

Postural (orthostatic) hypotension may cause dizziness, weakness, fainting, and falls.

Reduced blood flow to *brain, heart,* and *kidneys* may be dangerous for patients with a recent history of a *heart attack, cerebrovascular accident,* or *renal insufficiency.*

• **Parasympathetic Ganglionic Blockade**

Blurring of vision	Counteract with cholinergic eye drops.
Mouth dryness	Counteract by sucking candy or taking pilocarpine.
Constipation	Counteract with laxatives.
Urinary retention	Counteract with cholinergic drugs
Impotence in the male	Reduce dosage by combining G B A with a sulfonamide diuretic.

• **Contraindications** include: glaucoma; enlarged prostate gland in elderly male patients; or a tendency toward constipation, which could develop into paralytic ileus.

SUMMARY OF SIDE EFFECTS, CAUTIONS, AND CONTRAINDICATIONS: MISCELLANEOUS ANTIHYPERTENSIVE DRUGS

• **Guanethidine** (Ismelin)
Side Effects: Postural hypotension, bradycardia, nasal congestion, diarrhea, etc.
Caution: in patients with history of peptic ulcer, spastic colitis, recent myocardial infarction, coronary insufficiency, cerebrovascular and renal disease.
Contraindicated: in patients with pheochromocytoma.

• **Pargyline** (Eutonyl)
Side Effects: Postural hypotension, weakness, headache, dizziness, fainting; mouth dryness, constipation, impotence; weight gain.
Caution: May potentiate actions of other drugs.
Contraindicated: in patients with pheochromocytoma, hyperthyroidism, advanced renal disease, and paranoid schizophrenia.

• **Methyldopa** (Aldomet)
Side Effects: Drowsiness, dizziness, lightheadedness; nausea, vomiting, epigastric distress, constipation; fever, malaise, jaundice, and edema.
Caution: Liver function and blood tests are performed, and drug is discontinued if tests indicate reactions.
Contraindicated: in patients with active liver disease, or with pheochromocytoma.

• **Veratrum Alkaloids**
Side Effects: Nausea, vomiting, hiccough, substernal oppression, flushing, bradycardia and extrasystoles.

• **Hydralazine** (Apresoline)
Side Effects: Tachycardia, palpitations, dizziness, faintness, flushing, nausea and vomiting, paresthesias, and general malaise.

```
┌─────────────────────────────────────────────────────┐
│   SUMMARY OF POINTS TO REMEMBER ABOUT                │
│   DRUGS USED IN TREATING HYPERTENSION                │
└─────────────────────────────────────────────────────┘
```

- Instruct the patient in measures that will help him avoid postural hypotension (e.g., never to rise suddenly but to get up slowly after sitting on the edge of the bed for a couple of minutes).
- Take the patient's blood pressure as frequently as ordered and in accordance with the conditions directed (i.e., sitting, standing, etc.).

- Observe the patient carefully for any early signs and symptoms of drug toxicity and report these promptly to the physician.
- Follow the doctor's instructions for dosage regulation very carefully, because timing of the intervals between doses properly is essential for smooth maintenance of blood pressure at a safe level.

REVIEW QUESTIONS

1. (a) List some non-pharmacological measures which are often adequate for the control of high blood pressure of the early, mild, labile type.

(b) What kinds of drugs are sometimes added to the regimen of patients whose pressure cannot be kept at normal levels by such measures alone?

(c) For what type cases are the more recently introduced potent and potentially toxic antihypertensive drugs reserved?

2. (a) List several drugs with predominantly *central* effects which are used as adjuncts to other measure for controlling high blood pressure.

(b) List several drugs sometimes injected to reduce blood pressure rapidly in acute hypertensive crises.

(c) By what two broad mechanisms can the antihypertensive drugs be said generally to act in bringing blood pressure down?

3. (a) Indicate two ways in which drugs such as reserpine and syrosingopine are thought to cause their cardiovascular effects.

(b) Indicate two ways in which reserpine and other rauwolfia-type drugs are employed in treating cases of hypertension more severe than the mild cases for which small oral doses of these drugs are usually given.

4. (a) List several common side effects of the rauwolfia alkaloids and indicate how they may be counteracted.

(b) List several possible dangers from the rauwolfia alkaloids and indicate the precautions required to avoid these untoward reactions and the kinds of cases in which these drugs may be contraindicated.

5. (a) Indicate two ways in which the sulfonamide diuretics (e.g., hydrochlorothiazide) may act in helping to reduce high blood pressure.

(b) List some of the potent drugs with which these diuretics are often combined and explain the advantage of such combinations.

(c) List several side effects resulting from diuretic-induced fluid and electrolyte imbalance and indicate a common supplemental measure for preventing excessive loss of one important ion.

6. (a) Explain briefly the manner in which the ganglionic blocking agents produce their effects on blood pressure.

(b) Explain briefly how excessive sympathetic ganglionic blockade causes postural hypotension.

7. (a) What are some measures by which the doctor, the patient, and the nurse may all help to minimize the danger of overdosage of ganglionic blockers and the resulting hypotension?

(b) List several conditions that make patients poor candidates for treatment with ganglionic blocking agents, in whom the drugs must be used very cautiously, if at all.

8. (a) List several common side effects which can occur as a result of excessive blockade of parasympathetic ganglia.

(b) List several drugs which may be administered as adjuncts to the ganglioplegic drugs in order to reduce specific side effects of the blockade of various parasympathetic ganglia, or to reduce parasympathetic effects in general.

9. (a) Explain briefly the manner in which guanethidine acts to produce vasodilation and a fall in blood pressure.

(b) What advantage does such a mechanism of action offer over the ganglionic blocking agents?

(c) What side effects can be expected from the sympathetic suppressant action of this drug?

10. (a) Name the enzyme that is *inhibited* by the antihypertensive agent pargyline and the one that is *blocked* by *methyldopa*.

(b) For what type hypertensive patients are both these drugs indicated?

11. (a) List some of the side effects sometimes observed during treatment with pargyline.

(b) List some of the side effects caused by treatment with methyldopa.

12. (a) List some difficulties that limit the utility of the veratrum alkaloids and hydralazine in the routine management of moderate hypertension.

(b) What measures are sometimes taken to minimize these difficulties?

(c) In what circumstances are these drugs and sodium nitroprusside still employed by parenteral administration?

BIBLIOGRAPHY

Brest, A. N., and Moyer, J. H.: Enzyme inhibitors—in the treatment of hypertension. Am. J. Med. Sci., *240:*729, 1961.

————: Newer approaches to antihypertensive therapy. J.A.M.A., *172:*1041, 1960.

Cranston, W. I.: Treatment of benign hypertension. Modern Treatment, *3:*21, 1966 (Jan.).

Dollery, C. T.: Alpha-methyldopa (Aldomet) in the treatment of hypertension. Med. Clin. N. Am., *48:*335, 1964 (March).

————: Treatment of malignant hypertension. Modern Treatment, *3:*39, 1966 (Jan.).

Dupler, D. A., Greenwood, R. J., and Connell, J. T.: Present status of the treatment of hypertension. J.A.M.A., *174:*123, 1960.

Finnerty, F. A., Jr.: Newer antihypertensive drugs. Med. Clin. N. Am., *48:*329, 1964 (March).

Ford, R. V.: Pharmacology and clinical use of ganglionic blocking agents in the treatment of hypertension. Am. J. Cardiol., *9:*860, 1962 (June).

Friend, D.: Antihypertensive drugs. Clin. Pharmacol. Ther., *3:*269, 1962.

Fries, E. D., *et al.:* Chlorothiazide in hypertensive and normotensive patients. Ann. N. Y. Acad. Sci., *71:*450, 1958.

Fries, E. D., and Lodge, M. P.: Treatment and nursing care of hypertension. Am. J. Nurs., *54:*1336, 1954.

Grollman, A.: Clinical pharmacology of antihypertensive agents. Clin. Pharmacol. Ther., *1:*735, 1960.

Hoobler, S. W.: Practical plan for long-term treatment of hypertension. J.A.M.A., *165:*2143, 1957.

New Drugs and Development in Therapeutics: Pargyline Hydrochloride (Eutonyl), Statement of the Council on Drugs, A.M.A. J.A.M.A., *184:*887, 1963.

Page, I. H., Hurley, R. E., and Dustan, H. P.: The prolonged treatment of hypertension with guanethidine. J.A.M.A., *175:*543, 1961.

Rodman, M. J.: New drugs for high blood pressure. R.N., *22:*57, 1959 (Feb.).

————: Drugs for treating high blood pressure. R.N., *25:*75, 1962 (Feb.).

Schroeder, H. A., and Perry, H. M., Jr.: Current status of therapy in hypertension. J.A.M.A., *175:*543, 1961.

Wilkins, R. W.: New drugs for hypertension. Ann. Int. Med., *50:*1, 1959.

Wilson, W. R.: Treatment of hypertensive encephalopathy and crisis. Modern Treatment, *3:*50, 1966 (Jan.).

· 24 ·

Drugs Affecting Blood Coagulation

BLOOD COAGULATION

Blood circulating within the vascular tree ordinarily stays in the liquid state as long as the vessels remain intact. When a blood vessel breaks or is torn, and hemorrhage results, part of the blood escaping at the point of injury turns solid. This clotted blood quickly plugs the opening and stops the bleeding. The ability of the blood to flow freely within the vessels and to solidify when necessary to prevent hemorrhage is the result of the continual functioning of certain complicated mechanisms for controlling the physicochemical state of the blood.

In order to understand how drugs affect the clotting of blood, we must first have some idea of how these mechanisms operate to regulate the formation and resolution of blood clots. Recent research has revealed how very complex are those reactions that keep the blood in the vessels always liquid, yet always ready to clot when necessary to help close a wound. These reactions can best be understood by dividing them into four broad phases and considering each separately in terms of those aspects of each stage that can later be related to the actions of the important drugs affecting blood coagulation. The four main steps or stages are, in brief, as follows:

1. The formation of activated *thromboplastin* from inactive blood and tissue precursors.

2. The formation of *thrombin* from prothrombin under the influence of thromboplastin, etc.

3. The formation of *fibrin* from fibrinogen under the influence of thrombin.

4. The *breakdown* of fibrin under the influence of *fibrinolysin (plasmin)*.

This series of reactions can be influenced by the intervention of drugs that alter the delicate balance between various of the factors that must be present in adequate amounts for each step to proceed. Thus, in order better to understand how the several classes of drugs act, we should first consider more closely how

some of these factors are formed and how they interact with one another. Figure 24-1 offers a simplified outline of the complex series of biochemical steps by which inactive proenzymes are converted to active enzymes that in turn activate other proenzymes, until coagulation occurs and, finally, the clot so formed is resolved.

Stage I. Formation of Activated Thromboplastin

The clotting sequence is started when injury to tissues and to blood platelets (thrombocytes) results in formation of thromboplastin from an inactive precursor. People with a platelet deficiency or lacking the accessory factors antihemophilic globulin (AHG) and plasma thromboplastin component (PTC) may suffer from certain hemorrhagic disorders such as thrombocytic purpura and hemophilia.

Stage II. Conversion of Prothrombin to Thrombin

The thromboplastin generated in the first stage quickly converts the plasma protein, prothrombin, to the proteolytic enzyme *thrombin*. Prothrombin and certain other plasma proteins essential to this reaction, such as accelerin and factor VII, or proconvertin, are synthesized in the liver. Thus, patients with serious liver disease may be subject to bleeding episodes. Similarly, a lack of Vitamin K can cause bleeding, because the vitamin normally plays a part in the biosynthesis by the liver of these plasma proteins. Calcium ions are also needed in this reaction, but blood calcium never gets low enough to cause bleeding.

Stage III. Conversion of Fibrinogen to Fibrin

The *thrombin* formed from prothrombin then acts as an enzyme that helps to split two peptide links from the soluble plasma protein *fibrinogen*. This change in the structure of the molecule converts it to an insoluble protein called *fibrin*, which precipitates out in the form of fine needles and threads. These

338

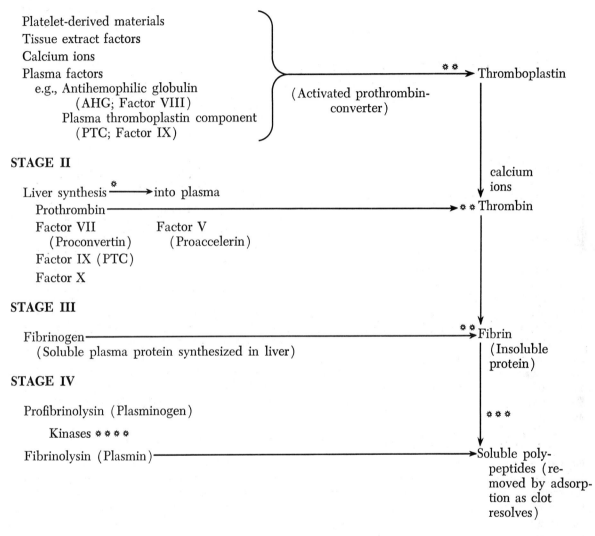

STAGE I

Platelet-derived materials
Tissue extract factors
Calcium ions
Plasma factors
    e.g., Antihemophilic globulin
        (AHG; Factor VIII)
        Plasma thromboplastin component
          (PTC; Factor IX)

(Activated prothrombin-converter)   ✲ ✲ → Thromboplastin

STAGE II

Liver synthesis ✲⟶ into plasma

Prothrombin ⟶ ✲ ✲ Thrombin

calcium ions

Factor VII   Factor V
  (Proconvertin)   (Proaccelerin)

Factor IX (PTC)

Factor X

STAGE III

Fibrinogen ⟶ ✲ ✲ Fibrin
  (Soluble plasma protein synthesized in liver)   (Insoluble protein)

STAGE IV

Profibrinolysin (Plasminogen)

✲ ✲ ✲

Kinases ✲ ✲ ✲ ✲

Fibrinolysin (Plasmin) ⟶ Soluble polypeptides (removed by adsorption as clot resolves)

Fig. 24-1. Simplified schematic outline of the interactions that result in blood coagulation and blood clot resolution.

✲—Site of action of vitamin K and of coumarin and indanedione drugs.
✲ ✲ —Sites of action of heparin.
✲ ✲ ✲—Site of action of fibrinolytic agents.
✲ ✲ ✲ ✲—Site of action of aminocaproic acid.

threads become woven together into a mesh that traps red cells, white cells and platelets, thus forming the gelatinous clot.

Stage IV. Resolution of the Blood Clot

The fibrin framework of the clot is sooner or later broken up by another enzymatically catalyzed reaction. The enzyme responsible for the breakdown of fibrin is *fibrinolysin,* or *plasmin.* It is itself formed from an inactive precursor, the plasma protein *profibrinolysin,* or *plasminogen.* Here, certain enzymes called *kinases* are required to split off the amino acids lysine and arginine from the inactive precursor in order to generate enough fibrinolysin to shift the balance of continuous biochemical reactions in favor of clot destruction. Finally, as the fibrin matrix of the clot is cut into smaller and smaller fragments of soluble protein, the clot breaks up and disappears.

In this chapter we shall deal with drugs that act in one way or another to retard or to speed up one or more of these steps. Such drugs can be used (1) to prevent clots from forming or enlarging within the patient's blood vessels (*anticoagulants*), (2) to increase the rate at which blood clots resolve (*thrombolytic agents*), and (3) to correct internal bleeding tendencies or to stop bleeding by helping clots to form locally at the bleeding point (*hemostatics*). Drugs that affect bleeding and coagulation in other ways (e.g., vascular actions) will be discussed briefly.

ANTICOAGULANTS

The complex reactions that cause both bleeding and clotting are going on unceasingly and simultaneously within our vascular systems. Yet so delicate is the balance maintained between the remarkable chemical processes outlined above, that, in normal health, hemorrhage or thrombosis only rarely becomes a threat to a person's life. Abnormal bleeding is always a cause for concern and often calls for quick action; however, the risk of disability and death from blood clots is far greater than it is from hemorrhage.

Thromboembolic disorders strike down more than a million Americans annually. These conditions cause more deaths in people over fifty years old than any other disease processes including cancer. Such fatalities are most commonly the result of the blocking off of blood flow in a major blood vessel of a vital organ. This frequently happens where a thrombus (blood clot) forms at the site of an atherosclerotic lesion on the inner lining of an artery that has been damaged and narrowed by disease. Also, arterial occlusion can occur when a blood clot that is only partially blocking a vein or artery breaks loose, goes whirling through the circulation as an embolus, and finally lodges in a major artery of the lungs, brain, or heart. Such an obstruction in a vital organ can cause death in a mat-

ter of minutes, and an acute arterial occlusion in an extremity may lead to loss of the limb.

The anticoagulant drugs are often used in treating patients with pulmonary embolism, coronary artery occlusion, and with conditions that make the patient seem especially susceptible to thromboembolic complications. These drugs do *not* dissolve blood clots: doctors use them cautiously to keep an existing clot from extending, or to prevent new clots from forming, when the patient's present condition or past history indicates the possibility of such recurrences. Even then, physicians are often unwilling to prescribe these potentially dangerous drugs for long periods unless the patient can be closely observed to detect any early tendency toward bleeding.

Clinical Indications. Although anticoagulant therapy has been advocated in the management of many conditions, these drugs are not equally effective in all thromboembolic disorders. Considerable controversy exists even among authorities as to whether the long-term employment of anticoagulants is justified in various clinical situations. Without entering into these currently unresolved areas of argument, we can agree with the view of those who feel that the potential toxicity of these agents makes it mandatory to keep patients who are taking them under close observation. Thus, prolonged employment of anticoagulants is generally reserved for selected cases in which the doctor thinks the risks are warranted and can be minimized.

Most doctors agree that the anticoagulants have proved most beneficial for patients with *venous thrombosis*—clots formed in the veins (of the legs usually) as a result of sluggish circulation in the limbs and minor injury to the inner walls of these vessels. Such clots are always painful and sometimes crippling, but the real danger of thrombophlebitis and phlebothrombosis is that bits of the clot may break off or be dislodged to become dangerous emboli.

Pulmonary embolism is a condition that occurs when emboli reach the lungs, where they block the flow of blood through the vessels. Pressure rises in the pulmonary arteries, but there is often a sharp drop in systemic blood pressure and cardiac output. The condition causes an estimated 35,000 deaths each year in this country. Anticoagulants have reduced the death rate somewhat by keeping further clots from forming during the patient's recovery. The drugs are also often given prophylactically to patients known to be especially susceptible to embolism. These include patients with rheumatic heart disease and atrial fibrillation; patients who have suffered injuries that have damaged blood vessels, and patients undergoing vascular surgery and major operations in the abdominal, thoracic, and pelvic regions.

Coronary Occlusion. Anticoagulant therapy has a definite place in the treatment of patients with *acute coronary occlusion with myocardial infarction.* It is said to have helped cut the death rate in half during the first weeks after an episode of coronary thrombosis. On the basis of this success in preventing enlargement of coronary vessel clots and formation of new thrombi or emboli during the early recovery period, these drugs have been employed on a long-term basis for preventing recurrent occlusions. Despite several extensive studies, the status of this sort of prolonged anticoagulant therapy is still unsettled. Some authorities advocate the use of these drugs indefinitely in selected postcoronary cases; others claim that the continued use of anticoagulants does not benefit most patients with coronary atherosclerosis and that the drugs may often do harm.

Strokes. Anticoagulants are used in the prevention and treatment of strokes caused by *emboli* and *cerebral thrombi.* Doctors agree that the occurrence of cerebral infarction can be reduced in patients who are having transient attacks of cerebral ischemia or other signs of an impending stroke by administering anticoagulants to reduce the sludging of their blood. The desirability of employing anticoagulants in the management of patients who have had a stroke is controversial. Some authorities fear that the anticoagulants may cause bleeding in the damaged brain areas; others argue that, by keeping cerebral arterial clots from growing and blocking larger brain vessels, the anticoagulants reduce the chances of complications to an extent that more than makes up for any risk of hemorrhage. Once the patient has recovered from the stroke, some authorities suggest the long-term use of anticoagulants to help prevent recurrences in selected patients; others argue that the usefulness of such prophylaxis is too limited to warrant the risks. All agree that they must first make certain that the stroke was caused by a clot, and not by intracranial bleeding, before employing anticoagulant drugs as an adjunct to other management measures.

Contraindications. The main danger in the use of anticoagulant drugs is that they may set off spontaneous bleeding. Such hemorrhaging is most likely to occur in patients whose conditions make them susceptible to bleeding episodes. Thus, the drugs are not used when there is evidence of weakened blood vessel walls or of possible defects in the patient's clotting mechanisms.

Patients with peptic ulcer and other chronic ulcerative diseases of the gastrointestinal tract are considered poor risks for anticoagulant therapy. Use of such drugs is generally avoided after neurosurgery because of the danger that they may induce bleeding in the brain and spinal cord. Patients with liver disease should not be given those anticoagulants that act by interfering with liver biosynthesis of plasma protein clotting factors, because such patients may already be suffering from deficiencies that make them prone to bleed. In addition, patients with hepatic and renal insufficiency may have difficulty in metabolizing and eliminating these drugs, with resultant cumulative toxicity which would not readily respond to treatment with the antidotal drug.

The most important contraindication to long-term anticoagulant therapy is lack of facilities for conducting the tests needed to determine proper dosage for each patient individually. If adequate tests cannot be performed regularly, the continued use of these drugs is undesirable, since overdosage may lead to bleeding, or underdosage to possible clot formation. The patient must be made to understand the need to report regularly for these blood tests and to follow all oral and written directions explicitly. Doctors often withhold anticoagulant drugs from patients who fail to keep their clinic appointments faithfully or do not follow instructions correctly for any reason. Use of these drugs usually is avoided in the treatment of alcoholics, mentally defective or mentally depressed patients, and others with emotional problems that keep them from cooperating fully.

We shall now consider the two major kinds of anticoagulants: (1) *heparin,* the rapid-acting agent preferred in emergencies, and (2) the *coumarin* derivatives and the *coumarinlike* indanedione derivatives often employed in long-term thromboembolic therapy.

Heparin

Heparin is a mixture of natural chemicals usually obtained from the lungs of animals. (It was first found in liver and named from *hepar,* the Greek word for that organ.)

Heparin is produced by human mast cells, which are concentrated around capillaries. Some scientists think that the substance is secreted locally, after an injury, to keep clots from enlarging too much and spreading too far; others doubt that heparin actually plays any important part in preventing blood from clotting within the vessels. In any case, when injected from an outside source, heparin reacts with a plasma protein cofactor to form a complex that acts in several ways to interfere with the clotting mechanisms of the blood.

Mechanism of Action. Heparin is a highly acidic substance and carries a strong electronegative charge. This may account for its ability to block the chain of clotting reactions at several points. First, the heparin-protein complex inactivates thromboplastin, the first-phase substance needed to start the series of clotting steps. This, in turn, interferes with the second step—conversion of prothrombin to thrombin. In addition, heparin appears to have a direct antithrombin action—that is, it inactivates any molecules of thrombin which manage to form. As a result, fibrinogen retains its original structure and stays in the liquid state instead of precipitating out as fibrin. There is even some evidence that heparin promotes the breakdown of newly formed clots and that it keeps blood platelets from sticking together in the way that ordinarily helps to set off new clotting.

Heparin thus has many properties that amply account for its quick and dependable anticoagulant effect on blood, both in and out of blood vessels. Heparin can be used, for example, to keep blood drawn for transfusion from clotting, and it is now routinely added to blood that is routed out of the body and into a heart-lung machine (the extracorporeal shunt employed in open-heart surgery and other operations) in order to keep the blood fluid while it is outside the body.

Advantages. The main advantage of heparin is its immediate action. Its ability to begin acting at once makes it more useful in emergencies than are the coumarin compounds, which take many hours or several days to develop their full anticlotting effects. Thus, heparin is preferred for initiating treatment of patients with pulmonary embolism, acute coronary occlusion, and other conditions in which it is imperative to prevent extension of an already massive clot or to halt further embolization.

When administered by vein, heparin produces more or less predictable effects, which the doctor can usually control readily. For example, he can perform a simple bedside test (the Lee-White test) to determine the drug's effect on clotting time. If the coagulation time is lengthened from the normal 5 to 8 minutes to less than the 30 to 60 minutes usually considered desirable, the next dose of heparin may be given sooner or the rate of infusion may be increased. On the other hand, when the test reveals too long a clotting time, the doctor may order that the next dose be delayed or even omitted. Even if bleeding does develop, it can be readily counteracted, usually, by blood transfusions that supply clotting factors or by injection of the specific chemical antidote protamine sulfate. Injected intravenously, this and certain other heparin antagonists can promptly neutralize the circulating anticoagulant by reacting with it chemically. This keeps heparin from reacting with the circulating clotting factors. Thus, coagulation time quickly returns to normal and drug-induced bleeding is halted.

Disadvantages. The greatest drawback of heparin is that it has to be given parenterally. The fact that it cannot be taken by mouth, coupled with its short duration of action, makes the drug unsuitable for long-term maintenance therapy of ambulatory patients. In order to keep heparin at effective anticlotting levels, it usually has to be administered by frequent intravenous injection or even by continuous infusion. Obviously, this requires hospitalization, which adds further to the expense of administering a drug which is itself relatively costly.

The duration of action can be lengthened by injecting the drug subcutaneously or intramuscularly in the form of a slowly absorbed suspension that need be injected only once daily. However, the absorption of heparin from such tissue depots is somewhat irregular, and repeated injections may cause painful hematomas and sloughing of tissues. Bleeding that may occur is, of course, less readily controlled while heparin continues to be absorbed from such repository forms than when it is given by vein in the short-acting aqueous solution. However, absorption from the injection site may be slowed by application of an ice bag. Protamine injections may have to be given repeatedly to counteract overdosage by heparin in repository form, and several transfusions of whole fresh blood may be required.

Side Effects and Contraindications. Spontaneous bleeding from mucous membranes is the only truly toxic effect of heparin. The doctor can usually prevent or counteract this by employing the measures described in the preceding section and by withholding the drug from patients who are poor risks. These include, in addition to those already mentioned, patients who have lost large areas of skin, those requiring continuous tube drainage of the stomach or small intestine, and patients with conditions that increase capillary fragility or cause clotting-factor deficiencies. Thus, the drug may be dangerous for patients with subacute bacterial endocarditis or mesenteric thrombosis, or after operations on the biliary tract. Allergic reactions to heparin may occur in patients sensitive to substances of animal origin. This may be manifested by redness and itching of the skin and sometimes by urticarial wheals. Breathing difficulties and anaphylactoid reactions are rare.

Coumarin and Indanedione Derivatives

The second class of anticoagulants includes drugs with chemical structures of two somewhat different types. Both kinds act, however, in essentially the same manner to lengthen the clotting time of the blood some time after they have been taken by mouth. The first of these drugs was discovered as a result of research into the cause of a bleeding disorder that occurred in cattle that had fed on sweet clover spoiled by improper storage. Hemorrhaging in the animals was found to be the result of a reduction in plasma prothrombin brought about by a coumarin derivative formed in the fodder. This substance was isolated and was identified as bishydroxycoumarin; it is now prepared synthetically and marketed as Dicumarol.

Mechanism of Action. Bishydroxycoumarin and all the other coumarin derivatives (Table 24-1), as well as the indanediones (compounds of a somewhat different structure), all act in essentially the same way: they keep vitamin K from entering into the biosynthetic reactions by which the liver synthesizes the proteins that take part in the second step of the clotting series. Because of their structural similarity to

TABLE 24-1

ANTICOAGULANT DRUGS

Nonproprietary or Official Name	Trade Name or Synonym	Recommended Ranges of Total Daily Dosage *
Hypoprothrombinemic Agents (Coumarins and Indanediones)		
Acenocoumarol	Sintrom	20–12–8 mg. days 1 to 3. 2–10 mg. maintenance
Anisindione	Miradon	300 mg. initially; 50–100 mg. maintenance
Bishydroxycoumarin U.S.P.	Dicumarol	200 mg. initially; up to 300 mg. thereafter
Cyclocoumarol	Cumopyran, etc.	150 mg. initially; 10–50 mg. for maintenance
Diphenadione N.F.	Dipaxin	20–30 mg. initially; 3–30 mg. maintenance
Ethyl biscoumacetate N.F.	Tromexan	1.2–1.8 Gm. initially; 300–900 maintenance
Phenindione	Danilone; Hedulin, etc.	200–300 mg. initially; 50–100 mg. maintenance
Phenprocoumon	Liquamar; Marcoumar	21–9–3 mg., days 1 to 3. 1–4 mg. maintenance
Sodium Warfarin U.S.P.	Coumadin; Panwarfin; Prothromadin, etc.	25–75 mg. initially; 5–10 mg. maintenance oral or I.V.
Other Anticoagulant and Fibrinolytic Agents		
Sodium Heparin Injection U.S.P.		5000 U.S.P. units every 4 to 6 hours I.V.; 20,000–40,000 units of repository form I.M. in accordance with coagulation times
Fibrinolysin (Human)	Actase; purified plasmin; Thrombolysin	variable
Streptokinase		variable
Urokinase		variable

* Maintenance dosage is in accordance with prothrombin time determinations.

vitamin K, these substances compete with this essential metabolite for a place on the surface of an enzyme required for the synthesis of prothrombin and related clotting factors, including, especially, proconvertin (factor VII). As a result of this competitive inhibition by these antimetabolites, the plasma levels of the blood coagulation proteins drop gradually—a condition commonly called hypoprothrombinemia, although failure of factor VII is now known to be the primary deficiency leading to prolonged clotting time of the blood.

Prothrombin Time Testing. These drugs do not keep drawn blood from coagulating. This is because, unlike heparin, they have no effect on clotting factors already in the circulation. However, once this plasma prothrombin has been used up, and the drugs have prevented it from being fully replaced by newly synthesized proteins, the signs of clotting factor deficiency can be measured. The fall in prothrombin activity is best measured by so-called prothrombin time tests, which compare the time required for the patient's normal plasma to clot (when mixed with thromboplastin and calcium under standard conditions) with the clotting time during treatment by hypoprothrombinemic drugs.

Normal prothrombin time usually ranges between 11 and 13 seconds. Doctors have learned by experience that, when the time it takes for the patient's plasma to clot is kept at between 2 and 2.5 times normal (about 24 to 30 seconds in many tests), the coagulability of his blood is lowered enough to lessen the likelihood of thrombosis without serious danger of spontaneous bleeding developing. Lengthening of the prothrombin time to this degree indicates that prothrombin activity is between 10 and 30 per cent of normal for that particular patient.

During long-term maintenance therapy the doctor tries to adjust the daily dosage to an amount that will keep the patient's prothrombin activity at about 20 per cent of normal. This is not always easy to accomplish. For one thing, patients vary so greatly in their responses that the standard dose does not mean much. In fact, the same patient may differ from time to time in his responsiveness to a set dosage schedule. And, just as it is the doctor's responsibility to determine dosage on the basis of the patient's prothrombin time and general status, the nurse is responsible for administering these drugs safely.

Precautions. During the first few days of treatment, patients often receive both heparin and a hypoprothrombinemic agent simultaneously. Heparin is discontinued as the effects of the coumarin-type drugs become apparent—*which can be determined only by daily prothrombin time tests.* Thus, the nurse should not administer each day's dosage order until the doctor has had a chance to check the patient's prothrombin time and evaluate its significance. Certainly she should not go on giving these drugs repeatedly in any setting that does not include regularly scheduled testing and evaluation. Instead, she should make use of whatever channels exist in the particular hospital for discussing the matter with the doctor or with her supervisor, since she bears responsibility for any harm that might come to the patient from anticoagulant drug overdosage.

Even minor bleeding that would be unimportant in other patients is significant when it occurs in a patient receiving anticoagulants. Thus, the patient's bed pan should be carefully scrutinized for signs of hematuria and tarry stools. The patient's emesis basin and tooth brush should also be unobtrusively observed for bleeding. Auxiliary personnel must be instructed (not, of course, in the patient's presence) to look for such signs in the containers that they empty in the utility room, and they should also be told to save the contents for the nurse's inspection if they are in any doubt as to whether blood is present. In these ways the nurse, without arousing the patient's apprehension, can keep him protected from the main danger of these drugs—serious and possibly fatal hemorrhage. By promptly reporting any signs of bleeding, however slight, the nurse gives the doctor an opportunity to make an immediate adjustment in the dosage of the anticoagulant.

Once the patient's prothrombin time has been stabilized, the interval between tests is gradually increased to about once a week. Often, patients on long-term therapy need be tested only once a month after their blood prothrombin levels are well stabilized. Such patients often need, nevertheless, to be urged to keep reporting for their tests. Nurses—especially industrial and public health nurses—are in an excellent position to encourage patients to continue with their medication and periodic prothrombin time tests.

Also, nurses can instruct patients in regard to procedures that enhance the safety of anticoagulant drug treatment. Of course, any information the nurse offers should conform to the doctor's previous instructions to the patient. The most effective way to accomplish this is to ask the doctor directly to tell you exactly what the patient has been told about his treatment. If the doctor has supplied the patient with a printed booklet or procedural manual, the nurse should be aware of what rules and suggestions it contains. In this way, when the patient seeks information from the nurse, she can help him to interpret the doctor's instructions rather than run the risk of giving conflicting suggestions.

It takes tact and judgment to convey the importance of the patient's following the doctor's instructions without frightening him into thinking that he is about to bleed to death. The patient's family also should be made aware of what to look for, and they, too, must be taught to be observant without alarming the patient. The wife who peers, frets, wrings her hands and calls the doctor whenever she finds a drop of blood on her husband's towel after he has shaved will only keep everyone in a state of needless alarm. If a patient and his family react with unusually marked anxiety and cannot learn to live with the risks of anticoagulant therapy, the doctor may have to discontinue such treatment and, thus, deprive the patient with thromboembolic disease of the benefits of these drugs.

The patient should be alerted to the need to watch for warning signs of approaching toxicity. These include the presence of slight discolorations or "bruises" on the skin of the arms and thighs; continued oozing from slight skin abrasions; nosebleeds, blood in the urine, and "black" stools. If any of these appear, he is to discontinue the drug and get in touch with his doctor, who may suggest that he take a vitamin K capsule and come in for a prothrombin time test. Patients should be made aware that diarrhea may diminish the effectiveness of anticoagulant therapy, and infections—especially if they require antibiotic drug therapy—may increase their anticoagulant requirements; thus, they should call their doctor to report any illness. Patients must be warned to avoid taking aspirin and other salicylates without consulting the physician, since these substances can themselves interfere with the same clotting mechanisms that the coumarin-type anticoagulants act on. They should not drink alcoholic beverages to excess, nor should they make any drastic dietary changes that may affect the absorption of the anticoagulant drugs or of vitamin K from the intestine.

Antidotal Measures. If recognized in time, the effects of anticoagulant drug overdosage usually can be readily reversed by administration of phytonadione (vitamin K_1) by vein. This substance begins to bring blood prothrombin levels back to safe levels within a few hours. It acts by displacing the competing anticoagulant drugs that have blocked the liver enzyme systems required for the biosynthesis of prothrombin and related clotting factors. During the time required for enough prothrombin to be synthesized and to enter the blood stream in amounts adequate to stop the bleeding, this clotting factor can be supplied ready-made in the form of fresh whole blood. This is often done when patients taking anticoagulants have been injured or require emergency surgery; in other cases the doctor often prefers to avoid transfusions, if the patient's condition warrants waiting the four to twelve hours required for vitamin K_1 to act.

The nurse should see to it that vitamin K_1, and the heparin antidote protamine sulfate, as well, are on hand in the ward medicine cabinet when any patient on her hospital floor is receiving anticoagulant therapy. The fact that these are emergency drugs is sometimes forgotten by hospital administrators. This can lead to the delay often involved in trying to pry these drugs loose from the pharmacy—a procedure sometimes requiring reams of requisitions and the waiting for slow moving elevators to take you from floor to floor. Thus, it is the nurse's responsibility to work out these problems in advance through discussion with the doctor and supervisor, lest any patient be deprived of an immediately required antidote.

Individual Drugs. The various drugs that reduce plasma prothrombin levels are listed in Table 24-1, and the two most widely employed drugs, bishydroxycoumarin (Dicumarol) and warfarin sodium (Coumadin, etc.), are discussed in more detail in the Drug Digests. All of these drugs have the advantage over heparin of being effective when administered by mouth. Warfarin is the only one that is also available for parenteral injection. This dosage form offers an advantage not only because it reduces to as little as twelve hours the time required for onset of anticoagulant action, but also because it permits use of the drug in patients who may be unconscious, vomiting or unable to swallow.

An advantage of both bishydroxycoumarin and warfarin is their relatively long duration of action, which makes it easier to maintain low prothrombin levels for long periods. Thus, if a patient fails to take his medicine for a day or two he still stays protected against a sudden thromboembolic episode. Other

drugs, such as ethyl biscoumacetate (Tromexan) and phenindione (Hedulin, etc.), are more rapid in action but are also rather rapidly eliminated. This may be desirable in case of overdosage but, otherwise, it may make it more difficult to maintain stable anticoagulant effects. Some of the newer drugs have greater milligram potency, but this is not necessarily an advantage. As in the case of the many digitalis products available, most doctors try to learn how best to use only one or two of the many available anticoagulant hypoprothrombinemic drugs.

THROMBOLYTIC AGENTS

As we have noted, the anticoagulant drugs do not dissolve blood clots; they only keep them from enlarging. Recently, attempts have been made to break down freshly formed thrombi by injecting certain fibrinolytic (fibrin-dissolving) agents directly into the circulatory tree. This therapeutic approach to thromboembolic disease appears to possess great potential utility. At present, however, the available agents have only limited utility, and various problems have to be solved before they can be considered useful in most clotting conditions.

Manner of Action. Three fibrinolytic agents have been employed, all of which act in the fourth phase of the clotting cycle.

1. *Streptokinase* is a bacterial enzyme, which may be injected intravenously to activate the patient's own plasminogen and convert it to plasmin.

2. *Urokinase* is an enzyme found in traces in human liver. This plasminogen-activating kinase, which is sometimes the cause of hematuria, has recently been purified and used clinically in the treatment of patients suffering from pulmonary embolism. These clinical trials also indicate its potential usefulness following coronary thrombosis.

3. *Fibrinolysin* (Actase; Thrombolysin) is a product prepared by activating human plasma with purified streptokinase outside of the body. This results in a mixture of direct-acting human plasmin, or fibrinolysin, together with residual activator capable of converting still more plasminogen into plasmin.

These products should, in theory, be able to push the patient's clotting-anticlotting balance in favor of fibrin breakdown. As a result of the increase in plasma thrombolytic activity, vascular blood clots should be broken down more readily.

Indications. In actual practice, these thrombolytic agents have only limited utility at present. Injected intravenously along with heparin, human fibrinolysin has apparently helped to speed destruction of clots in the leg, in some patients with acute, uncomplicated thrombophlebitis. However, its use is often accompanied by adverse reactions. Fibrinolysin (purified plasmin) is also sometimes injected directly into a blocked peripheral artery, while the patient is being prepared for arterial surgery. Occasionally, the drug has succeeded in opening a channel wide enough to permit blood flow and save the limb. More often, surgery is still required, but, even in this case, the prior treatment with plasmin is said to help reduce postoperative thromboembolic complications. Unfortunately, fibrinolysin, or plasmin, has not proved useful against coronary and cerebrovascular clots. In fact, its use in these conditions is contraindicated, at present, because the large doses required to restore blood flow rapidly enough to save heart and brain tissue are likely to set off severe toxic reactions in these seriously ill patients.

Adverse Reactions. Toxic reactions are mainly of two types: (1) febrile and allergic reactions, and (2) hemorrhage (a dose-related risk). Reactions of the first type are thought to be due mainly to the residual streptokinase activator, which acts as an antigen. These are marked by a rise in body temperature, and headache, chest, back and epigastric pain, and nausea, vomiting, and dizziness. These ill effects may be partly counteracted by administration of analgesic-antipyretic and antihistaminic drugs, and sedatives.

The possibility of generalized bleeding limits the utility of the thrombolytic agents in some patients. However, the availability of the antiplasmin substance aminocaproic acid (see p. 347), recently introduced, may help to overcome this drawback. In case of hemorrhage, the doctor can now administer aminocaproic acid as an antidote to fibrinolysin, just as he gives protamine sulfate to counteract heparin overdosage.

DRUGS TO CONTROL BLEEDING

Most commonly, bleeding occurs as a result of injury to blood vessels. Normally, bleeding caused by accidental trauma or by surgical and dental procedures soon stops spontaneously as a clot quickly forms and plugs the opening in the vascular wall. Various mechanical measures that help accelerate clotting—ligatures, sutures and gentle pressure, for example—help to hasten control of hemorrhage from major vessels.

Ordinarily, drugs are not an important means of dealing with bleeding. For, if a person's own clotting mechanisms are functioning normally, no drug is likely to improve their efficiency. There are, however, two situations in which the use of substances from outside sources may speed the formation of clots at the site of a wound or at other bleeding points within the body: (1) when patients have a definite defect in one of the steps in the hemostatic mechanism, and (2) when blood oozes persistently from tiny capil-

laries that cannot be readily tied off or from vessels in tissues too soft for holding instruments in place.

Systemically Active Agents for Blood Coagulation

Most people with a history of nose bleeds, skin bruise marks and slightly delayed laboratory bleeding times have minor vascular weaknesses rather than any serious clotting defects. However, in some patients, especially children, episodes of unusual bleeding sometimes occur that can be traced by tests and through the patient's history to a congenital or acquired deficiency in one of the essential clotting elements. Once the doctor determines which factor specifically is lacking, he can order the plasma fractions or drugs needed to correct the deficiency that is the cause of the bleeding. To furnish the missing elements and prevent circulatory collapse, there is, of course, nothing better than transfusions of *fresh* whole blood and normal human plasma. However, in many hemorrhagic disorders, it is desirable to counteract the specific deficiency by replacing the missing clotting factor directly or by administering drugs that aid the body's own efforts to restore its hemostatic mechanisms to normal.

Clinical Applications

We shall not discuss the total management of all bleeding disorders; however, we shall look briefly at some of the more common conditions seen clinically and at the agents employed in their control.

Thrombocytic Purpura and Hemophilia. These hemorrhagic disorders are the result of a lack of factors required in the first stage of clotting. As indicated previously, blood clotting begins with the breakdown of platelets or thrombocytes. This releases a substance that works along with other factors, such as the antihemophilic globulin (AHG), plasma thromboplastin component (PTC), and other reactants to form active thromboplastin. Thus, when there is a deficiency of platelets or when any of the many factors involved in the complex first stage of clotting is missing, bleeding is likely to occur.

Drugs ordinarily are not effective for counteracting bleeding in thrombocytic purpura or in hemophilia. However, administration of *adrenocorticosteroids* (Chap. 28) is often helpful in the former condition for reducing petechial bleeding and even for bringing about a rise in platelets. In the acute stage, concentrated packed platelets may have to be transfused, along with fresh whole blood, for control of massive hemorrhaging.

Hemophilia is a common cause of serious chronic bleeding in children. Its management involves many measures, including orthopedic care to reduce crippling deformities from chronic bleeding into joints (hemarthrosis). Fresh frozen plasma transfusions are the chief source of the deficient antihemophilic globulin (AHG). Injected intravenously, *Antihemophilic Human Plasma U.S.P.* usually halts the bleeding episode. However, the amounts sometimes needed may tend to overload the circulation, and, therefore, fractions of human and animal blood containing AHG in more concentrated form are sometimes employed, despite various drawbacks that limit their use. The locally applied hemostatic agents (discussed later in this chapter and in the Drug Digests) are sometimes applied at certain accessible bleeding points.

Hypoprothrombinemia. When adequate amounts of thromboplastin are being produced in stage I, the prothrombin in the blood of most people is quickly converted to sufficient thrombin (in Stage II) to permit normal clotting. However, although hereditary defects of prothrombin and related proteins such as factor VII are very rare, deficiencies of these substances occur commonly secondary to other conditions. In acute emergencies, whole blood or plasma administration is the best way to replace these missing factors rapidly. However, since vitamin K is so safe and so effective for correcting the coagulation defects responsible for bleeding of this type (provided that liver function is adequate), it is usually administered simultaneously.

VITAMIN K. The importance of this substance in the biosynthesis of prothrombin, proconvertin (Factor VII) and other clotting factors and its use to counteract toxicity caused by overdoses of certain anticoagulant drugs has already been discussed. Several forms of natural and synthetic vitamin K are effective for treating hypoprothrombinemic bleeding in other medical and surgical situations also.

The medical disorders most commonly requiring vitamin K therapy are caused by defects—of the intestinal tract, the bile ducts or the liver—that interfere with the synthesis, absorption and utilization of natural vitamin K. Normally, this fat-soluble vitamin is readily available from many foods, and, in addition, it is manufactured by bacteria in the intestinal tract. It is then absorbed with bile-emulsified fat by way of the lymph channels and carried to the liver where it participates in the synthesis of prothrombin by the liver cells.

Bile duct blockage tends to reduce absorption of vitamin K, and this deficiency leads in turn to a lack of prothrombin. Patients requiring biliary-tract surgery were thus especially likely to suffer from postoperative bleeding before this vitamin became medically available. Today, such patients may receive one of the water-soluble forms of *menadione*, a synthetic vitamin K, which is absorbed even in the absence of bile. If *phytonadione* (the natural fat-soluble form) is used, bile salts must be administered simultaneously to assure its absorption. Both types of vitamin K are effective when the intestinal tract is bypassed by parenteral administration of the product, before and after biliary-tract surgery.

Patients with celiac disease, cystic fibrosis or sprue may require oral or parenteral vitamin K, because (as in patients with ulcerative colitis) the normally available vitamin may be absorbed in inadequate amounts from their defective intestinal tracts. Patients who have had large parts of the intestine removed or are under prolonged treatment with anti-infective drugs that eliminate the intestinal bacteria that synthesize this vitamin may be subject to hypoprothrombinemic bleeding. Injections of vitamin K are effective for returning their plasma prothrombin levels to normal and this can quickly control bleeding in such cases.

Newborn infants have naturally low plasma levels of prothrombin until bacteria become established in the intestine and begin to biosynthesize vitamin K in the amounts needed to step up liver production of the essential blood clotting factors. Because hemorrhagic disease of the newborn may lead to dangerous intracranial bleeding, many authorities now suggest that vitamin K be administered routinely to the newborn infant or to the mother shortly before the birth of her child.

Vitamin-K products are less effective for treating bleeding in severe liver disease, because the damaged hepatic cells may be unable to use the vitamin in the manufacture of the clotting factors. Thus, patients with cirrhosis of the liver or with hepatitis of toxic or infectious origin may require transfusions of fresh whole blood or plasma to obtain enough prothrombin to counteract bleeding when vitamin K alone cannot stimulate adequate biosynthesis.

Hypofibrinogenemia. A congenital lack of the clotting factor fibrinogen is not often a cause of serious bleeding. However, hypofibrinogenemia may occur in certain medical and surgical situations in which the fibrin-destroying mechanism becomes abnormally hyperactive. Such an increase in activity of the fourth stage in the clotting-anticlotting reaction series can so reduce the amount of fibrinogen available for conversion to fibrin by thrombin (in Stage III) that lifethreatening hemorrhage may result.

Again, whole blood and plasma transfusions are the best means of replacing the missing fibrinogen factor and restoring the lost blood volume. A concentrated fibrinogen blood fraction is also available for intravenous administration. Recently, certain other substances have been claimed to be effective for counteracting excessive fibrinolytic activity. These include female sex hormones and a potent synthetic antifibrinolytic agent called aminocaproic acid (Amicar).

Aminocaproic acid has proved useful for stopping the bleeding in several medical and surgical conditions marked by hypofibrinogenemic hemorrhaging. In all such situations, the body's stores of plasminogen are somehow activated. This results in the formation of an excess of plasmin, the fibrin-destroying enzyme. (Purified plasmin, or fibrinolysin (see p. 345), is employed as a thrombolytic agent for dissolving intravascular clots in certain thromboembolic conditions.) Abnormally high plasma levels of the enzyme tend to reduce the blood's fibrinogen content too much, and the resulting deficiency of the clotting factor can cause spontaneous hemorrhaging.

As indicated on page 346, aminocaproic acid can serve as an antidote to overdosage with thrombolytic agents such as plasmin and streptokinase. It also counteracts bleeding that occurs in various obstetrical complications including abruptio placentae, amniotic fluid embolism, and after death of the fetus in utero. Certain surgical procedures also are followed by fibrinolytic bleeding—heart, chest, liver or prostate operations, for example—and medical conditions marked by hemorrhaging of this type include leukemia, hepatic cirrhosis, and metastatic carcinoma of the prostate.

Aminocaproic acid is effective in these conditions because it blocks the biochemical reaction that converts the inactive precursor plasminogen to active, fibrin-dissolving plasmin. In this reaction, it will be recalled, certain enzymes called kinases split off the amino acids lysine and arginine from plasminogen, thus forming plasmin. Aminocaproic acid, which is very similar in chemical structure to these amino acids, acts as a competitive antagonist of the kinase enzymes. Thus, it keeps the enzymes from converting inactive plasminogen into excessive quantities of fibrinolytic plasmin.

Estrogens, which are sometimes employed for treating men with carcinoma of the prostate (Chap. 29), have reportedly helped to control fibrinolytic bleeding in this condition. Conjugated equine estrogens (Premarin), a female hormone product, is claimed to be effective against bleeding in other conditions also. Thus, its intravenous administration is advocated for control of capillary bleeding following various surgical procedures, including tonsillectomies.

These estrogens are said to act not only by inhibiting the activation of plasminogen but also by several other mechanisms, including an action on the blood vessel walls rather than on plasma clotting factors. Most hematologists are not convinced that this and various other hemostatics claimed to have vascular actions are actually effective when administered orally or parenterally for reducing postoperative and posttraumatic bleeding.

Other Agents for Vascular Effects. Various substances besides the conjugated estrogens of equine origin are claimed to counteract capillary bleeding by decreasing the permeability of the walls of these vessels. Among them is ascorbic acid (vitamin C), which may overcome the bleeding from the gums seen in scurvy by its effects on the so-called capillary cement

substances. However, ascorbic acid is ineffective against bleeding that is not caused by a deficiency of this vitamin.

Other substances obtained from citrus fruits and other sources and called collectively vitamin P (for permeability), or flavonoids, have been advocated for treating capillary bleeding. Despite clinical reports claiming that agents such as rutin, quercetin, hesperidin and similar substances have reduced capillary blood leakage in many medical conditions, proof that these substances are truly effective seems to be lacking. The same may be said for a host of other substances marketed for oral and parenteral use to control capillary bleeding in a wide variety of conditions.

LOCALLY ACTIVE HEMOSTATIC AGENTS

In contrast to the systemically administered substances, a number of materials that are applied locally to bleeding surfaces definitely do speed clotting in one way or another. Some of these hemostatics are natural clotting factors—thromboplastin, thrombin and fibrin, for example—which have been made available in purified form. Others, such as absorbable gelatin sponge, and oxidized cellulose, do not enter directly into the natural hemostatic reactions of the blood and body tissue components. These also are useful in various surgical and medical conditions marked by difficult-to-control capillary bleeding.

All these substances (see Drug Digests) are used mainly to control continued oozing from abraded and denuded surfaces. Applied to organs such as the brain, liver and kidney, these materials do what cannot be done readily with ligatures; they form a real or artificial clot or a mechanical barrier to blood flow. If left in place within the wound, in most anatomical sites both the natural clots and the other organic materials (i.e., the specially treated gelatin or cotton gauze) are gradually digested, or absorbed from the tissues without interfering in any way with natural healing processes. (Substances such as oxidized cellulose—see also Drug Digest—should not, however, be packed permanently into fractures.) In addition to being used in neurological surgery, skin grafts and other operations, some of these substances are taken internally by stomach tube to control gastroduodenal bleeding in peptic ulcer.

Summary: This chapter has dealt mainly with drugs that keep blood from clotting and with agents which accelerate blood coagulation. Major emphasis was placed upon the anticoagulants, because these drugs are so widely used in the prevention and treatment of the thromboembolic disorders—a major cause of death and disability. However, hemostatics also are important, especially to the operating room nurse. Both classes of drugs are employed most efficiently by those who understand how blood clots naturally and how these agents affect clotting.

TABLE 24-2
ANTIHEMORRHAGIC AGENTS

NONPROPRIETARY OR OFFICIAL NAME	SYNONYM OR TRADE NAME	DOSAGE
Systematically Active Agents		
Prothrombogenic Substances		
Menadiol sodium phosphate U.S.P.	Synkayvite; Kappadione	4 to 8 mg. parenteral
Menadiol sodium phosphate tablets N.F.		5 mg. oral
Menadione U.S.P.	Vitamin K$_3$ (synthetic); Kappaxin; Kayquinone, etc.	1–5 mg. oral
Menadione capsules N.F.		2 mg. oral
Menadione injection N.F.		1–2 mg.
Menadione sodium bisulfite N.F.	Hykinone	2 mg. I.V. and S.C.
Phytonadione U.S.P.	Vitamin K$_1$; Konakion; Mephyton	20 mg. oral; 5 mg. I.V. or I.M.
Anti-Heparin Substances		
Hexadimethrine bromide	Polybrene	1 mg. per mg. of heparin
Protamine sulfate injection U.S.P.		50 mg. I.V. repeated as necessary
Tolonium chloride	Blutene	200–300 mg.
Miscellaneous		
Aminocaproic acid	Amicar	5 Gm. oral or by slow I.V., initial, then 1 Gm./hour
Carbazochrome salicylate	Adrenosem	1–5 mg. oral; 5 mg. I.M.
Conjugated estrogens (equine)	Premarin I.V.	20 mg. I.V.
Fibrinogen, Human U.S.P.	Parenogen	2 Gm. I.V.
Plasma, Antihemophilic, Human U.S.P.		250 ml. I.V.
Rutin	Quercetin glucoside	20–50 mg.
Topically Active Agents (Local Hemostatics)		
Absorbable Gelatin Sponge U.S.P.	Gelfoam	
Fibrin Foam		
Oxidized Cellulose U.S.P.	Hemo-Pak; Oxycel	
Thrombin N.F.		
Thromboplastin U.S.P.	Thrombokinase	

SUMMARY OF THROMBOEMBOLIC DISORDERS AND OTHER CLINICAL SITUATIONS IN WHICH THE ANTICOAGULANTS ARE EMPLOYED

- Thrombophlebitis

- Phlebothrombosis

- Occlusion due to embolism or thrombosis of peripheral, pulmonary, or coronary arteries (e.g., pulmonary embolism; coronary thrombosis; arteriosclerosis obliterans; thromboangiitis obliterans); management of gangrene of the extremities secondary to trauma or diabetes; and prophylaxis against thrombosis after blood vessel injury or surgery

- Cerebral ischemia (i.e., transient attacks that may herald an impending stroke)

- Progressing, or evolving, stroke (but *not* immediately after the end of a stroke)

- Prophylaxis against recurring strokes in selected patients

SUMMARY OF CONDITIONS IN WHICH ANTICOAGULANT THERAPY IS CONTRAINDICATED OR USED ONLY WITH EXTREME CAUTION

- Ulcerative and other diseases of the gastrointestinal tract (e.g., peptic ulcer; ulcerative colitis; bleeding hemorrhoids).

- Neurosurgical patients (e.g., following brain and spinal cord operations and recent trauma to the central nervous system).

- Severe liver and kidney disease (e.g., hepatitis; renal calculus, raised blood urea nitrogen).

- Blood dyscrasias (e.g., thrombocytopenic purpura); a vitamin K deficiency state and conditions which may lead to it such as biliary disease, steatorrhea, and gastrointestinal malabsorption.

- Uncontrolled cardiac failure, subacute bacterial endocarditis, malignant hypertension, especially when retinopathy is present.

- Patients who have lost large areas of skin; those requiring continuous tube drainage of the upper gastrointestinal tract and those with mesenteric thrombosis.

- Patients who have shown previous hypersensitivity to heparin, coumarin, or phenindione compounds.

- Patients lacking in the intelligence required for cooperation in long-term therapy or those whose personality difficulties make them unreliable (e.g., alcoholics) in keeping appointments for prothrombin time tests and in following medication schedules.

- Patients requiring intensive salicylate therapy.

- Pregnancy.

SUMMARY OF POINTS THE NURSE SHOULD REMEMBER WHEN CARING FOR PATIENTS RECEIVING ANTICOAGULANTS

- Carefully observe the patient for any bleeding, and report it promptly to the physician if it occurs.

- If the patient is to receive anticoagulants at home, help him to understand the need to notice and report bleeding, and the importance of returning to his physician's office or to the clinic for tests of his prothrombin time. The family also should be given this information. Teaching should be carried out in a way which emphasizes the importance of these measures but does not cause the patient and family alarm.

- Make certain that antidotes for these drugs (vitamin K_1, and protamine sulfate, for example) are readily available if any patient on the ward is receiving anticoagulants.

- Remember that dicoumarol and related drugs are safely given only when the prothrombin time is periodically checked and evaluated by the physician. In acute illness, such testing and evaluation usually occurs daily; in long-term therapy, it is done regularly but at less frequent intervals. If such safeguards are not being employed, discuss the matter with your supervisor or with the physician before administering the medication.

- In emergency situations, the physician often orders immediate administration of both heparin and dicoumarol. This does not constitute a "double dose," because heparin takes effect quickly, whereas dicoumarol is slow to begin its action.

CLINICAL PROBLEMS

Mr. Johnson suffered an acute myocardial infarction. In addition to bed rest and a soft diet, his physician prescribed 15 mg. of morphine q.4 h. p.r.n., and an initial dose of 300 mg. of Dicumarol.

1. What observations should the nurse make in relation to Mr. Johnson's Dicumarol therapy?

2. Why is each dose of Dicumarol ordered individually, rather than having a standing order for daily administration?

3. What side effects of morphine therapy are especially important to watch for in Mr. Johnson's situation?

REVIEW QUESTIONS

1. (a) List, in brief, the four main steps of blood clot formation and breakdown.

(b) Indicate, in more detail, the main factor formed in each phase and some of the necessary accessory factors or substances.

2. (a) For what general purpose do doctors administer the anticoagulant drugs?

(b) List several clinical conditions in which the anticoagulant drugs are routinely employed.

3. (a) List patients of several types in whom anticoagulant therapy is usually contraindicated.

(b) Indicate two clinical conditions or situations in which the desirability of employing anticoagulants is presently a subject of controversy.

4. (a) How does heparin exert its anticlotting action?

(b) How do the site and mechanism of heparin's action influence the speed of its onset and the ease with which it can be counteracted by an injectable antidote?

5. (a) In what circumstances is heparin preferred to other anticoagulant drugs?

(b) What are two disadvantages of heparin?

6. (a) What are the site and the mechanism of action of the coumarin- and indanedione-type anticoagulants?

(b) What is the significance of this in terms of the onset of action of these drugs and the time required for antidotal therapy to take effect?

7. (a) What is the significance of the prothrombin time test in determining the dosage of anticoagulant drugs of the coumarin class?

(b) List some precautions that the nurse can take to help ensure the safety of patients receiving anticoagulants and some points that she should be sure the patient remembers from the list of instructions given him by the doctor.

8. (a) What are some of the advantages of warfarin sodium?

(b) What type toxicity has sometimes been observed with certain indanedione derivatives?

9. Explain how human fibrinolysin and streptokinase act when injected into the vascular system of a patient with a blood clot.

10. (a) In what conditions is the administration of human fibrinolysin indicated?

(b) In what conditions is this product considered relatively useless or even contraindicated?

11. Indicate the two types of toxic reactions caused by injection of human fibrinolysin and explain how each of these can be counteracted.

12. (a) What step in the clotting sequence is inadequate in cases of thrombocytic purpura and hemophilia?

(b) What substances are employed to make up for the specific deficiencies in each of these bleeding disorders?

13. (a) Why are patients with bile duct obstructions or fistulas especially susceptible to postsurgical bleeding unless special measures are taken?

(b) Which vitamin K preparation is preferred for oral administration in cases of obstructive jaundice and what other means of overcoming deficiency of this vitamin are available?

(c) Which form of vitamin K is preferred as an antidote for overdosage by coumarin- and indanedione-type anticoagulants and for preventing hemorrhagic episodes in newborn infants?

(d) Name some other clinical conditions in which vitamin K may be employed to counteract hypoprothrombinemic bleeding.

14. (a) What blood clotting defect accounts for the bleeding that sometimes occurs in patients with certain obstetrical complications?

(b) What concentrated blood fraction may be transfused for best results in such cases and in other medical and surgical situations in which the same clotting deficiency is the cause of the patient's bleeding?

(c) Explain in your own words why the synthetic drug *aminocaproic acid* (Amicar) is sometimes effective for speeding blood coagulation in such cases.

15. (a) List some types of surgical procedures in which locally acting hemostatics are employed.

(b) In what medical condition are certain of these agents (e.g., absorbable gelatin) used and what precaution is taken to prevent them from being made ineffective for this purpose?

(c) Compare the manner of action of thrombin with the way in which oxidized cellulose exerts its hemostatic effect.

(d) How must thrombin *never* be administered?

(e) In what tissues should oxidized cellulose *never* be left as an implant or dressing?

BIBLIOGRAPHY

Alexander, B.: Anticoagulant therapy with coumarin congeners. Am. J. Med., *33*:679, 1962.

Conley, C. L.: Management of hemorrhagic diseases. J.A.M.A., *181*:985, 1962.

Fletcher, A. P., *et al.*: Evaluation of human fibrinolysin. J.A.M.A., *172*:912, 1960.

Friedberg, C. K.: Should we abandon anticoagulant therapy in acute myocardial infarction? J.A.M.A., *180*:307, 1962.

Gaston, L. W.: The blood clotting factors. New Eng. J. Med., *270*:236, 290, 1964.

Griffith, G. C., *et al.*: Conservative anticoagulant therapy of acute myocardial infarction. Ann. Intern. Med., *57*:254, 1962.

Hartman, J. R., and Bolduc, R. A.: Hemophilia. Am. J. Nurs., *56*:169, 1956.

Hartman, J. R., *et al.*: Bleeding disorders in children. G.P., *32*:145, 1965.

Howard, F. A.: The anticoagulants. Clin. Pharmacol. Ther., *2*:423, 1961.

Jorpes, J. E.: Heparin: its chemistry, pharmacology and clinical use. Am. J. Med., *33*:692, 1962.

Lewis, J. H., and Doyle, A. P.: Effects of aminocaproic acid on coagulation and fibrinolytic mechanisms. J.A.M.A., *188*:56, 1964.

McDowell, F. H.: Initial treatment of cerebrovascular disease. *In* Treatment of Stroke. Modern Treatment, *2*:15, 1965 (Jan.).

Moser, K. M.: Current status of clot dissolution therapy. G.P., *26*:95, 1962.

Owren, P. A.: Indications for anticoagulant therapy. New Eng. J. Med., *268*:1173, 1963.

Rodman, M. J.: Drugs to treat blood clots. R.N., *22*:37, 1959 (April).

———: The anticoagulant and thrombolytic drugs. R.N., *25*:43, 1962 (Oct.).

———: Drugs for the control of bleeding. R.N., *28*:45, 1965 (May).

Sawyer, W. D., *et al.*: Thrombolytic therapy. Arch. Int. Med., *107*:274, 1961.

Sherry, S., and Fletcher, A. P.: Proteolytic enzymes, a therapeutic evaluation. Clin. Pharmacol. Ther., *1*:202, 1960.

Whisnant, J. P.: Anticoagulant treatment of transient ischemic attacks and progressing strokes. *In* Treatment of Stroke. Modern Treatment, *2*:25, 1965 (Jan.).

Wietti, T. J., *et al.*: Vitamin K, prophylaxis in the newborn. J.A.M.A., *176*:791, 1961.

Wright, I. S.: Treatment of thromboembolic diseases. J.A.M.A., *174*:1921, 1960.

· 25 ·

Drugs Used for Treating the Anemias (Antianemic Drugs)

THE BLOOD

The previous chapters of this section have dealt mainly with drugs that improve the functioning of the circulatory system. Yet the heart, arteries, veins and capillaries are important only because of the vital fluid which they handle—*the blood*—for it is this life-giving liquid that brings to the brain and all other organs and tissues the oxygen and nutrients without which they could not survive. In this chapter, we shall study some of the substances that are administered when it becomes necessary to improve the *quality* of a patient's blood supply.

Composition of the Blood

Blood is a fluid tissue that serves many important protective and regulatory functions. These depend upon the properties of its two component parts: (1) the plasma, a light yellowish liquid, in which (2) the formed elements of the blood—red blood cells, white blood cells, and platelets—are suspended. The platelets, or thrombocytes, play an important part in setting off the series of reactions that results in blood clotting (Chap. 24). The white cells, or leukocytes, make up one of the body's major defense mechanisms against invading microorganisms. Our main concern here, however, will be with the red cells, or erythrocytes, which are responsible for the respiratory functions of the blood, including its ability to transport oxygen to the tissues.

Erythrocyte Production

The bone marrow elements that become red cells pass through successive stages of development. Beginning as *megaloblasts*, large immature cells containing a nucleus but no hemoglobin, at each stage the cells become gradually smaller and more pigmented. Ordi-

narily, the form that is finally discharged into the blood stream is the small non-nucleated *reticulocyte*. These cells soon turn into fully formed erythrocytes.

The erythrocytes are produced by the bone marrow in enormous numbers. The red cells that are synthesized there are constantly being poured out into the blood stream to replace the millions of erythrocytes that wear out and disintegrate every second. The circulating blood contains many trillions of red cells, each of which lasts about four months on the average before it wears out and is destroyed. Ordinarily, the bone marrow factory can keep the number of erythrocytes at normal levels by reusing most of the chemical elements of the disintegrated red cells along with added raw materials obtained from foodstuffs.

Supplied with certain essential nutrients, the healthy marrow in the long bones, ribs, vertebrae, and skull carries out the complicated process of red cell formation, or erythropoiesis, without ever faltering. This involves the synthesis of substances of two types:

1. *Hemoglobin,* a bright red respiratory pigment. Each molecule is made up of globin, a large protein portion, to which is attached an iron-containing non-protein chemical called heme.

2. The *stroma*—a thin membranous supporting structure which serves merely as a container for the many millions of hemoglobin molecules in a single red cell.

To make hemoglobin the marrow requires protein, certain vitamins, iron and traces of other metals. Ordinarily, the diet contains adequate amounts of all these substances. Sometimes, however, iron may be drained from the body at a rate greater than the rate at which it can readily be replaced from foods alone. Similarly, the nutrients that are needed to bring the red cells to maturity and form an erythrocyte with a stromal structure strong enough to resist early destruction are abundantly available in a normal diet. However, some people are unable to absorb enough of the substances—cyanocobalamin (vitamin B$_{12}$) and folic acid, mainly—that are required for proper red cell maturation. As a result, the weak-walled red cells cannot long withstand the buffeting that erythrocytes must take as they are hurled about in the larger vessels and squeezed through the narrow capillaries. When they are destroyed at too rapid a rate, the bone marrow becomes unable to keep up with the demand for fresh, fully formed erythrocytes, and their number in the blood stream becomes markedly reduced.

THE ANEMIAS

The condition that develops when the bone marrow cannot obtain sufficient iron for adequate hemoglobin synthesis or enough of the factors needed for red cell maturation is called anemia. This term, which means literally "no blood," describes states in which either the number of erythrocytes or the amount of hemoglobin (or both) in the circulating blood is reduced significantly below normal. Lack of red cells and their respiratory pigment reduces the blood's ability to pick up oxygen in the pulmonary capillaries and transport it to the tissues. Thus, the many discomforting or even disabling signs and symptoms of anemia are essentially the result of oxygen deficiency.

Clinically, the nutritional anemias are mainly of two types: (1) those that are due primarily to a deficiency of iron, and (2) those that are the result of a lack of the B-complex vitamins cyanocobalamin and folic acid. Except in cases of extreme starvation, anemia rarely results from a deficiency of protein or of the other vitamins and trace metals needed for red cell synthesis.

The red cells produced during a period of iron deficiency contain less than normal amounts of hemoglobin, and they look relatively pale under the microscope. They are, in addition, smaller than normal red cells, because they were retained in the bone marrow overlong. Because of these red cell characteristics, iron-deficiency anemia is often called the *hypochromic microcytic* type.

The anemias that result from a lack of erythrocyte maturation factors are frequently referred to as *hyperchromic* and *macrocytic,* because the blood contains an abnormally high proportion of large cells (*macrocytes*). Although each of these cells is crammed with more hemoglobin than is contained in normal erythrocytes, the total number of cells (and thus the total amount of hemoglobin) is abnormally low. Also, the circulating blood sometimes contains an unusual number of megaloblasts, which have left the bone marrow prematurely. This is characteristic of the condition called pernicious anemia.

Treatment of the Anemias

Once the doctor determines which type anemia his patient has, he can quickly correct the blood picture by supplying adequate amounts of the missing hematopoietic (blood-cell-producing) substances. Thus, the hyperchromic macrocytic, or megaloblastic, anemias usually respond readily to replacement therapy with folic acid and vitamin B$_{12}$ when these *hematinics* (blood-formers) are administered in a form that can be assimilated. Similarly, treatment with hematinic iron salts supplied in medicinal doses that permit adequate amounts to be absorbed soon corrects anemia of the hypochromic microcytic type.

Iron-Deficiency Anemia

When a person takes in less iron from his diet than he is losing through normal elimination or by abnormal means such as bleeding, the body's stores of that element become gradually depleted. Even before any appreciable fall in erythrocytes or in hemoglobin levels can be detected, the iron-deficient person may often suffer a variety of vague complaints. These include feelings of weakness and fatigue, loss of appetite, headaches and dizziness.

Early symptoms of this sort sometimes disappear quite dramatically in a day or two when the person begins to take iron. Doctors still argue as to whether this is merely a placebo response or the result of re-activation of iron-containing cellular enzyme systems needed for producing energy. (Trace amounts of iron are present in *all* cells and play an important role in cellular respiration.) In any case, the treatment of a true hypochromic microcytic anemia requires not days but, usually, many months of treatment. After the patient's blood picture has returned to normal and symptoms of hypoxia, such as skin pallor and dyspnea, have been relieved, it may take months to restore the patient's iron reserve to normal.

Iron Metabolism. In order to understand what happens during the development of iron deficiency anemia and during its treatment with medicinal iron, we must first recall how this element is absorbed, transported, stored, used and excreted by the body. New knowledge of iron metabolism, acquired recently by the use of radioactive isotopes to trace the pathways taken by this metal in the body, has helped to put the treatment of this type anemia on a more rational basis.

Absorption. The iron in foods is tied up in forms from which it is not readily released. Normally, only about 5 to 10 per cent of it is absorbed into the blood stream from the gastrointestinal tract. However, people who have an iron deficiency may manage to assimilate as much as 30 per cent of the available iron. This may be because, during an iron deficiency, the biochemical mechanism that normally limits the absorption of iron by the cells lining the G.I. tract is partially suppressed. When this mucosal barrier is lowered, larger amounts of iron can pass through these cells and enter the blood.

The presence of stomach acids in the duodenum aids iron absorption by converting some of it to soluble inorganic salts. Ascorbic acid (vitamin C) also increases the amount absorbed by favoring the formation of the ferrous form of iron which is more easily assimilated than ferric iron. At best, however, the amount of iron that people can get from food is limited. Thus, patients with iron-deficiency anemia require large quantities of medicinal ferrous salts. When these salts are given in amounts as high as the patient can tolerate, enough iron gets by the mucosal block in the duodenum to increase the blood level of hemoglobin by 1 per cent or more each day.

Transport and Storage. Once it enters the blood, iron is bound to a plasma protein that is called *transferrin* because it transports the metal to its storage sites in the bone marrow, liver and spleen. Transferrin is capable of carrying much more iron than it ordinarily does. This is why the doctor sometimes orders the iron to be injected when he desires to build up the patient's iron reserves very rapidly. By thus by-passing the G.I. barrier and saturating the patient's plasma transferrin, the parenterally administered iron speeds hemoglobin synthesis.

Utilization and Excretion. When iron is needed for red cell synthesis, it is mobilized from its storage sites. Along with iron derived from food, medicines and disintegrating erythrocytes, the freed element is transported to the immature bone marrow cells. There, the iron atoms are built into heme, the iron-containing part of the hemoglobin molecule. Very little iron is lost by the body ordinarily. Most of the amount excreted daily is contained in cells that slough off from the intestinal lining. The rest is lost with flaking skin, falling hair and in body fluids such as urine, sweat and bile. The total loss of iron by these routes is only about 0.5 to 1 mg. daily. However, menstruating women may, in a few days, lose an amount of iron that is at least equal to that excreted by all other routes during the rest of the month.

Iron Requirements. Because of its ability to conserve its stores of iron, the body ordinarily needs to take in very little of the element in order to meet the demands of the bone marrow and all other cells. Since the same stores are used over and over again, only the 1 mg. or less lost daily by excretion has to be made up from dietary sources. Although only a small percentage of the iron contained in even the best diet is absorbed, this is usually enough to keep most people in positive iron balance indefinitely.

Indications for Medicinal Iron. Drugstores stock scores of iron-containing tonics. Iron alone or in combination with many other minerals, as well as with multiple vitamins, is an ingredient of many products widely advertised to the public for self-treatment. How necessary are such sources of extra iron and under what circumstances should they be taken?

We have seen that the body conserves its stores of iron tenaciously and that an ordinary diet usually offers enough iron to replace the small daily loss. This means that—among adult men and in women past the menopause, at least—iron deficiency is much less common than the television commercials for hematinic products for self-medication would lead people to believe. People suffering from the vague symptoms so graphically described in the "tired-blood"-type advertisement are very often doing themselves a disservice when they diagnose their condition as an iron-deficiency anemia and buy a pharmaceutical liquid or capsule for self-treatment.

Why is this so, and why should the nurse urge such people to see their doctors instead? First, because their signs and symptoms may be those of some serious condition other than anemia. In that case, the patient's weakness, dizziness and dyspnea will not, of course, be helped by his taking many bottles of a costly iron tonic. More serious than the unnecessary expense is the possible delay in diagnosing a progressing cardiac or pulmonary condition or other dangerous disorder with early symptoms similar to those of iron-deficiency anemia. (Few who watch a TV commercial heed the announcer's quickly mumbled "check with your doctor," before they go to the drugstore to buy the advertised product.)

A second reason for advising people to see their physician is that if a person is, indeed, suffering from an iron-deficiency anemia, it is vitally important that a doctor discover its *cause* and take steps to correct the underlying condition as well as the anemia itself—because the most common cause of iron deficiency in men and in women past the child-bearing age is undetected bleeding!

Thus, when the laboratory notifies the doctor that one of his patients has an abnormally low hemoglobin and other signs of hypochromic microcytic anemia, his first concern is with whether the patient is losing blood internally. To the alert doctor, an iron-deficiency anemia is not a disease in itself but a *symptom* that serves as a warning signal. This leads him to look for occult bleeding or other signs of disease, especially in the gastrointestinal tract.

The following facts are important in understanding the treatment of iron-deficiency anemia: (1) Inadequate dietary intake of iron is rarely the cause of iron-deficiency anemia in healthy American men of any age or in women over fifty. (2) Failure to absorb enough iron from an ordinary diet is relatively rare today. People with pathological malabsorption problems usually have a history of prior G.I. tract disease that makes the reason for their deficiency readily detectable. (3) The most common cause of an unusual increase in a person's iron requirements is *loss of blood by hemorrhage.*

Is it not essential, then, to send such a patient to a doctor who will seek the source of such bleeding? It may be something as readily correctible as bleeding hemorrhoids or a hidden gastroduodenal ulcer. Or it could be an early carcinoma of the stomach or colon.

In such cases, an iron tonic could well clear up the patient's anemia, while the undetected cancer continues to grow until it reaches an inoperable stage!

Other Indications. In addition to patients with pathologic states that lead to anemia, there are persons whose naturally higher-than-normal iron requirements may cause them to develop a hemoglobin deficiency. These individuals, in whom special circumstances cause an increased demand for iron, include infants, adolescent girls, and women with excessive menstrual bleeding or frequent pregnancies (especially if they breast-feed their babies). Medicinal iron is by no means indicated in *all* such cases. However, negative iron balance (a state in which tissue stores become gradually depleted because more iron is being utilized than is being supplied) is more likely during such periods of life.

Premenopausal women tend to lose between 14 and 28 mg. of iron in the blood shed during even a normal menstrual period. This means that their added daily iron loss is about equal to the amount normally excreted by the usual routes—i.e., 0.5 to 1 mg. Often, the extra iron is readily absorbed and assimilated from foods such as meats and dairy products eaten as part of a diet that also contains cereal grains, green and yellow vegetables, and citrus fruits or tomatoes.

However, if (as is often true with teen-age girls) they neglect to eat an adequate diet, young women may readily suffer an iron deficiency. Obviously, if a girl had barely been in positive iron balance on a diet that supplied the 0.5 to 1 mg. she needed as a pre-pubescent child, she will lose that precarious equilibrium when she both begins to menstruate regularly and enters a time of rapid growth and development. Even if she eats well and increases her food iron intake, she may not get quite enough dietary iron to meet her new needs.

Women with menorrhagia (an unusually heavy menstrual flow) are especially likely to become iron deficient, as are those with metrorrhagia (bleeding at times in the menstrual month other than the regular period). Often, such women may fail to consult a physician about their condition, because they think that it is normal for them. Thus, the nurse who gains such information in casual conversation with a woman may do well to suggest that she see a doctor and have her hemoglobin level and red cell count checked. The character of the menstrual flow should be noted in taking the medical histories of all premenopausal women.

During pregnancy, of course, no loss of menstrual blood iron occurs. However, the growing fetus may take an even greater quantity of iron out of the mother's reserves. Thus, a multipara whose pregnancies have come within a relatively few years may suffer from an iron-deficiency anemia that requires treatment with hematinics. Such iron tonics are probably best taken during the third trimester of pregnancy when the demands of the rapidly growing fetus are greatest. It is probably best to avoid this kind of medication, *and all others,* during the early weeks and months of pregnancy when the embryo and fetus are most susceptible to drug-induced damage which could lead to developmental abnormalities.

The newborn baby does not ordinarily need extra iron. Although his diet is largely milk—a food deficient in iron—the stores he has obtained transplacentally usually last for several months. However, between the ages of 6 months and 2 years, when his body size and blood volume are increasing so greatly, the infant's demands for iron with which to synthesize new hemoglobin-containing red cells may become greater than his diet can supply. In such cases, the very young child may require pediatric iron drops or even parenterally administered iron.

Iron-Containing Pharmaceuticals. Ordinarily, patients with iron-deficiency anemia cannot build up their hemoglobin levels by diet alone. To absorb enough of the element for rapid erythropoiesis, patients need to take large amounts of medicinal iron. Most of the extra iron given by mouth never gets into the blood stream at all but leaves the body in the feces. However, enough of the metal is absorbed to begin producing objective improvement within a week or two. Often, after a month or more of treatment, the patient's hemoglobin level has returned to normal.

However, it may be many more months or even years before the patient's depleted tissue reserves of iron can be raised to optimal levels, even after the cause of blood loss has been discovered and corrected. This means that the patient on long-term hematinic therapy may be put to considerable expense, if the doctor has prescribed a costly product. The nurse cannot, of course, do anything about this. However, because many people whom she meets may be medicating themselves with *non*-prescription iron products, the nurse *can* offer information that will help save them money and yet assure adequate hematinic therapy.

The point is—despite the persuasive claims of drug manufacturers aimed at both the public and members of the health professions—*the most effective iron products available are also the least expensive ones.* Specifically, the simple inorganic iron salts ferrous sulfate, ferrous gluconate, and ferrous fumarate—all official in the U.S.P.—produce as rapid and complete a response as more complex iron compounds which cost the patient four to six times as much for a day's treatment.

Criteria for Oral Iron Products. Besides being cheap, an iron product must meet two tests: (1) The elemental iron in it must be readily absorbable, and (2) it should not cause excessive gastrointestinal upset when taken by mouth. Pharmaceutical companies currently market about two hundred hematinic products, and the manufacturer of each one claims that the form of iron offered in his product is both the most absorbable and the best tolerated.

Actually, no single iron compound can be *both* the most readily absorbed and the least irritating. The reason is this: Any iron salt is absorbed only in proportion to the degree that it can be converted to soluble elemental iron in the patient's G.I. tract. Furthermore, the extent of local mucosal irritation produced by any particular product also depends on the amount of free (ionic or elemental) iron that the molecule releases. In practice, this means that the inexpensive iron salts such as ferrous sulfate are both the best absorbed and the most likely to cause G.I. irritation, whereas the compounds that contain iron bound up into a complex molecule from which it is only slowly released will be both least well absorbed and less irritating. If the doctor believes that the newer iron complexes cause fewer side effects, he may prescribe them despite their greater cost to the patient. On the other hand, he may order the relatively inexpensive simple salts and suggest ways by which the patient may minimize G.I. difficulties.

Administration of Oral Iron. Iron salts are absorbed best when taken on an empty stomach, because foods contain proteins, phosphates and other substances that tend to tie the iron up into insoluble unabsorbable complexes. Since the erythropoietic response is most rapid when the absorption of elemental iron is most complete, some doctors now order between-meal administration of iron. They may also suggest that it be given with a glass of orange juice, because ascorbic acid (vitamin C) is said to aid iron absorption.

Some patients may complain, on the basis of previous experience, that they can't take iron. They mean that the drug's irritating action on the upper G.I. tract gives them an "upset stomach"—cramping pain, epigastric burning, nausea and even vomiting. The action of iron in the lower tract may cause diarrhea, or (because it has astringent properties) a particular product may prove constipating. In such cases, the doctor may start the patient off on small doses taken right after meals and then gradually raise the dose of iron while lowering food intake to a couple of crackers and a little liquid.

Sometimes the doctor may want the patient to be warned that gastrointestinal upset may occur early in treatment with an iron product. However, the nurse should not volunteer such a warning, because, with some patients, directing the attention to the possibility of ill effects of drugs makes it all the more likely that they will indeed complain of them. The nurse should, however, let the patient know that his stool may be colored dark red or black by an iron prepara-

tion and that this is not an indication of gastrointestinal bleeding.

Patients taking liquid products containing soluble iron salts should be protected against staining of the dental enamel. They should be told to place iron drops well back on the tongue. When such a product is diluted with juice, it should be sipped through a straw or drinking tube.

Parenterally Administered Iron. Most anemic patients respond quite readily to treatment with orally administered iron. Sometimes, however, it becomes necessary to administer the metal by injection. Because this route is relatively painful, expensive, and occasionally dangerous, repeated courses of parenteral iron are rarely given and are usually tried only after oral therapy has failed.

Among the patients who may require an injectable iron preparation are:

1. Persons who are unable to absorb oral iron because of gastrointestinal malabsorptive diseases or after the surgical removal of extensive sections of the G.I. tract.

2. Patients with inflammatory gastrointestinal diseases who would find the irritating action of oral iron intolerable (e.g., ulcerative colitis and regional enteritis patients).

3. Persons, including children, who may be unwilling to withstand even minor discomforts caused by the local irritating effects of iron when taken by mouth; also some elderly and psychiatric patients who cannot be depended upon to remember to take their daily oral doses.

4. Persons in whom it becomes necessary to build up depleted iron stores rather rapidly, especially when they continue to bleed and lose iron faster than it can be replaced by oral therapy.

Parenteral Preparations. The earlier parenteral iron preparations were too irritating to be injected into soft tissues and had to be given by vein. Often, this resulted in inflammatory reactions within the vein (thrombophlebitis) and in damage to extravascular tissues into which they accidentally leaked. Another dangerous drawback was the fairly frequent occurrence of systemic reactions to intravenously administered iron.

Fortunately, less toxic parenteral iron preparations are now available. One of these, *iron dextran* (see Drug Digest), can be injected intramuscularly with little local pain or inflammation. Thus, it does not have to be given by the more dangerous intravenous route. Another, *dextriferron*, is less irritating locally and less likely than the earlier parenteral products to cause systemic reactions when it is injected by vein.

Parenteral Toxicity. The systemic toxic reactions that may occur after iron injections may be acute or chronic.

Chronic Toxicity. Overdosage can result in the body's storage sites being chronically overloaded with iron. Injection of more of the metal than the plasma protein transferrin can carry causes the metal to pile up in tissues such as the liver, pancreas, skin and bone marrow (*hemosiderosis*), which, in turn, can result in damage to these tissues (*hemochromatosis*). This condition, which sometimes also occurs in patients who have had too many blood transfusions, may cause hepatic cirrhosis, diabetes or other illnesses—all the result of damage to tissues by excess iron. Thus, the doctor takes care to calculate the patient's parenteral dose carefully on the basis of the iron deficit indicated by his hemoglobin level.

Acute reactions to injected iron are no longer common when the newer parenteral products are employed. However, reactions of the allergic type are always possible and should be looked for. Some occur within a few minutes of an injection; others are delayed for a day or so. Less severe reactions are marked by dizziness, headache, and muscle and joint pains, with chills and fever. Reactions of the more dangerous anaphylactoid type are marked by breathing difficulties, anginal-type chest pains and blood pressure falls. Very rarely, fatal circulatory collapse may occur.

Accidental Iron Poisoning. Young children have often fallen victim to acute iron toxicity. Attracted by tablets that often resemble brightly colored candies, the child may swallow several. Although 1 to 3 grams of iron may be relatively harmless to an adult, this amount of the soluble iron salts can do severe damage to a child's delicate G.I. tract. (Ferrous sulfate, which gives up its elemental iron most readily, seems to be the most dangerous of the salts when accidentally ingested.)

Manufacturers of products that contain iron in organic complexes, from which the metal is only slowly released, claim that these preparations are less likely to cause serious toxicity. Animal experiments seem to indicate that this is true. However, *all* iron products are potentially toxic, and parents should be warned that hematinic tonics are *not* simply harmless mixtures of the same vitamins and minerals found in food. They should be advised to keep iron products—and, indeed, all medicines—where children cannot get at them.

Toxicity and Treatment. Overdosage with iron salts causes both local and systemic toxicity. The nausea, vomiting and abdominal pain produced by the corrosive action of iron may be followed by a shocklike state. Death may occur from cardiovascular collapse within a few hours or after a delay of a day or so, during which the child may appear to be recovering.

In addition to symptomatic treatment with pressure-raising drugs, oxygen, systemic alkalinizers and anticonvulsants, efforts are made to tie the iron up into insoluble complexes and to remove it from both the gastrointestinal tract and the systemic circulation. If the child is seen soon after taking iron tablets, it may be desirable to induce vomiting or to wash out the stomach with sodium bicarbonate solution. Later, tissue erosion may make these measures too dangerous.

Recently, chelating agents have been employed to bind and remove the iron both from the G.I. tract (by gavage) and from the plasma and tissues (after parenteral administration). The most successful compound for removing excess iron seems to be *deferoxamine* (*Desferal*). This drug, which converts both free and tissue-bound iron to a harmless complex and carries it to the kidneys for excretion, has also been employed in chronic iron storage disease (hemochromatosis).

Megaloblastic Anemias

We have seen that, in order to develop properly in the bone marrow, the precursors of the red cells of the blood require certain essential dietary substances. When the blood-building B-complex vitamins cyanocobalamin and folic acid are unavailable, the megaloblasts stay large and immature. The bone marrow becomes loaded with these cells, which, in turn, produce many macrocytes—abnormally large hemoglobin-loaded red cells that have only a relatively short life span in the circulating blood. Because they are destroyed in 45 days (on the average) instead of the 125 days that is normal for erythrocytes, both the red cell count and total hemoglobin become markedly lowered.

This hematological picture is characteristic of a number of clinical conditions. These disorders, in which the blood abnormalities are the result of failure to take in or, more often, to absorb vitamin B_{12} or folic acid include pernicious anemia, the megaloblastic anemias of pregnancy and of infancy, sprue, celiac disease and other conditions such as fish tapeworm infestation and gastric carcinoma.

Pernicious anemia is a disease that was once considered incurable. The megaloblastic anemia that develops is only one sign of a widespread metabolic disorder that affects all the cells of the body including those of the nervous system and the lining of the gastrointestinal tract. Patients lose their appetites, have difficulty in walking, weaken progressively to the point of prostration, and—before the discovery of its cause and treatment—they invariably died.

This disease was shown in the 1920's to be the result of a gastric disorder which prevented absorption of an essential substance present in the diet. It was found that feeding large amounts of liver, which is rich in this dietary "extrinsic factor," often helped pernicious anemia patients despite their lack of the gastric "intrinsic factor."

At first, it was thought that these two factors combined to form a third—the *erythrocyte maturation factor* (*EMF*) or *anti-pernicious-anemia* (*APA*) *principle.* Later, it was learned that liver cures pernicious anemia because it contains large amounts of vitamin B_{12} and that the latter substance was *both* the extrinsic factor and the erythrocyte maturation factor. That is, once the vitamin breaks away in the stomach from the dietary protein to which it is bound and makes its way through the intestinal wall (with the aid of the intrinsic factor), it acts on the bone marrow precursors, converting them to mature erythrocytes.

During the search for the APA principle in liver extracts, another substance was discovered that also counteracted the megaloblastic anemia, although it failed to reverse the neurological lesions of pernicious anemia. This substance, which was named *folic acid* because of its presence in leafy vegetables and other foliage, is also found in brewer's yeast and in various other foods (see p. 360). Like vitamin B_{12}, folic acid plays a vital role in the metabolism of rapidly growing cells. The two vitamins have some metabolic functions in common. For example, both participate in some of the steps by which rapidly reproducing cells synthesize the nucleoproteins needed for cell division. When the bone marrow cells, for example, fail to get enough of either of these substances, their nuclei do not make enough DNA. As a result, the cells grow to giant size without dividing.

Vitamin B_{12}

Deficiency States. The dark red crystals finally isolated from liver extract concentrates in 1948 proved to be the most potent vitamin ever found. Only one *micro*gram—a millionth of a gram—must be absorbed from dietary sources to meet the body's daily need for vitamin B_{12}. Amounts much larger than that are available in liver, muscle meats, seafood, eggs and milk. Thus, vitamin-B_{12} deficiency is rarely the result—in this country, at least—of a lack of B_{12} in the diet. However, because B_{12} is absent in plants, vegetarians—especially those who eat no eggs, milk or cheese as well as meat—may occasionally become deficient. Even then, it takes several years for the body's stores of the vitamin to drop enough for signs of deficiency to appear.

The main cause of vitamin-B_{12} deficiency is the failure to absorb the minute amount needed to replace the tiny quantity lost each day. As we have already noted, a so-called *intrinsic factor* secreted by stomach cells is needed to aid the intestinal absorption of dietary B_{12}. When this factor is lacking (not only in pernicious anemia patients but also in those who have had large parts, or even all, of their stomach removed), the vitamin taken in when animal protein foods are eaten cannot get through the mucosal wall of the ileum and into the blood stream. Some patients with intestinal disease, as well as those with gastric carcinoma or perforating peptic ulcer, who require subtotal gastrectomy or other massive surgical resec-

tions of the upper G.I. tract, may develop a gradual deficiency of vitamin B_{12}.

Parenteral Administration. Once the patient's symptoms have been diagnosed as definitely due to a deficiency of vitamin B_{12}, the body's depleted reserves can be rapidly built up by administering the pure crystalline substance. There is now no need to use liver extract injections and run the risk of causing allergic reactions. The pure vitamin, prepared by microbial synthesis, is inexpensive, completely free of toxicity, and painless when injected.

The preferred preparation is the *Cyanocobalamin Injection* official in the U.S.P. (this name indicates the presence of a cobalt atom linked to a cyanide radical within the extremely complex molecule). Injected intramuscularly or deep into subcutaneous tissues, the aqueous solution of the vitamin promptly enters the blood and is carried to the liver and other storage sites, which periodically release the small amounts required by the bone marrow for red cell synthesis and maturation.

At first, the B_{12}-deficient patient receives *daily doses* of between 30 and 100 micrograms—or, on another common schedule, 200 micrograms 3 times a week. The purpose of high initial doses is rapid replenishment of the patient's low stores. Later, the same doses may be injected at somewhat longer intervals, such as once weekly. Finally, after about four to six weeks, when the patient has attained maximum benefits, B_{12}-administration is required only once a month. An injection of 100 micrograms at monthly intervals is considered adequate for making up for the daily loss of the vitamin over a period of several weeks.

It is important to make it clear to the patient and his family that he must continue to receive injections for the rest of his life at the intervals specified by his physician. They should be made to understand that in most cases the underlying cause that led to the B_{12}-deficiency cannot be corrected. Thus, if the patient neglects to keep getting his treatment because he "feels fine," his stores of B_{12} will inevitably slide to subnormal levels. Then, if he does not heed the early warning signs of deficiency—weariness and malaise—the patient may suffer insidious damage to his nervous system without being aware that the disease is progressing.

Response to Treatment. As long as he continues to get adequate B_{12} dosage periodically, the patient maintains the remarkable improvement seen soon after treatment is undertaken. Within a day or two after a person with pernicious anemia begins to get daily injections, he feels stronger and his appetite returns. Soon, showers of reticulocytes appear in his blood stream, and then the count of normal erythrocytes increases daily while the number of macrocytes and other abnormally shaped blood cells drops. Although the color index of the blood decreases, total hemoglobin rises to normal.

In addition to this favorable hematological response, the patient's digestive complaints—glossitis and diarrhea, for example—are largely eliminated. His sore tongue heals, and symptoms of intestinal irritation are lessened, as the mucosal epithelial cells lining the G.I. tract are restored. Of course, the atrophied stomach cells do not recover their ability to secrete gastric acid and intrinsic factor. Similarly, although the milder symptoms of nervous system damage (numbness and tingling of the extremities, for example) may be relieved with continued treatment, little improvement can be expected in functions controlled by parts of the brain and spinal cord in which the neurons have already degenerated. However, further neurological damage is arrested by B_{12} treatment.

Oral Preparations. Vitamin B_{12} can, of course, be given by mouth in combination with a concentrated intrinsic factor prepared from the dried stomach and duodenum of food animals. Supplying the substance missing in the stomach of the pernicious-anemia patient permits adequate intestinal absorption of the vitamin. However, this route is ordinarily not recommended, because it is not as reliable as the injections, which bypass the G.I. tract entirely. Besides, this oral product is much more expensive than the injectable B_{12} solution—a situation different from what is true ordinarily.

Patients can be further spared expense if someone in the family can be taught to administer their B_{12} injections. However, since such patients are often elderly and victims of a chronic and incurable illness, they should be urged not to neglect periodic visits to the physician for routine examination. This will still be true even if a cheap and completely dependable oral preparation is developed, or if one of the longer-acting depot forms of vitamin B_{12} being currently tested lengthens considerably the time between injections. *Hydroxocobalamin*, another member of the cobalamin family, is claimed to reach higher plasma levels and last longer in the blood and body tissues than cyanocobalamin. However, neither this nor other suggested B_{12} substitutes have yet been proved superior to the official compound for maintaining pernicious anemia patients in remission.

Other Indications. Vitamin B_{12} is often prescribed for treating conditions that are not the result of a deficiency of this vitamin. People with symptoms similar to those observed in pernicious anemia patients and others with a definite B_{12} deficiency sometimes receive massive doses of the vitamin. It is highly unlikely that cyanocobalamin has any pharmacological effects which would make it useful for patients who do not suffer from a B_{12} deficiency.

Although favorable reports have frequently appeared concerning the efficacy of B_{12} in nervous and mental disorders, there is no real proof of its value in these conditions. That is, the fact that B_{12} injections often clear up the numbness and tingling that pernicious-anemia patients feel in their fingers and toes does not mean that this vitamin will help patients with paresthesias of the hands and feet which are not caused by a lack of dietary B_{12}. The same can be said of claims that B_{12} injections are sometimes of value in trigeminal neuralgia, multiple sclerosis, and some psychiatric conditions marked by mental defects and emotional upsets of the kind that occur in pernicious-anemia patients as a result of their B_{12} deficiency.

The best that can be said for the use of B_{12} in these conditions is that the drug seems to be completely free of toxicity. Thus, it may act as a harmless placebo while the doctor is trying to determine the real cause and the cure of the patient's condition. Administration of the drug itself to elderly patients and children in poor nutritional states because of lack of appetite, probably does little good. However, the better general care these patients get while in the doctor's hands may help them gain weight and strength.

Folic Acid

Folic acid is needed by the body because it is converted to a coenzyme that plays an important part in some of the metabolic reactions by which cells reproduce themselves. Deficiencies of folic acid show up first in those tissues that grow at the most rapid rates, including cancerous tissues, the bone marrow blood cell precursors, and the epithelial cells that line the gastrointestinal tract. That is why the *anti*folic drugs—chemicals that keep rapidly reproducing cells from utilizing dietary folic acid—are useful in treating leukemia and other neoplastic disorders. It is also the cause of the toxic hematological and G.I.-tract effects of these anticancer drugs, which are discussed in Chapter 44.

Deficiency States. Ordinarily, people have no difficulty in meeting their need for folic acid. It is found in most foods and is highest in green vegetables such as spinach, lettuce and asparagus as well as in liver, eggs and milk. Sometimes, however, people in tropical lands and others who may be suffering from general malnutrition do not get an adequate dietary supply of folic acid. People eating diets on the borderline of adequacy may be thrown into negative balance when their requirements for folic acid become abnormally increased—late in pregnancy, for instance, when the rapidly growing fetus drains off much of the mother's stores of this vitamin. Megaloblastic anemia of pregnancy is seen most commonly in women who have given birth to twins, especially after several earlier births.

In addition to these and other anemias due to malnutrition, anemia may result from failure to absorb enough folic acid from a diet that is entirely adequate.

Such malabsorptive conditions include tropical and nontropical sprue, celiac disease and severe organic diseases of the small intestine.

Patients deficient in folic acid develop a megaloblastic anemia that does not differ from that found in pernicious anemia. As in the latter disorder, gastrointestinal symptoms such as glossitis and diarrhea may occur. However, a lack of folic acid does not lead to the neurological damage that results from a deficiency of vitamin B_{12}. This is probably because nerve cells do not reproduce themselves. (Vitamin B_{12} is probably needed for a metabolic step in the synthesis of nerve cell lipids such as myelin; folic acid is not needed in the synthesis of the myelin sheath lipids of neurons.)

Response to Treatment. Once the doctor has definitely diagnosed the patient's anemia as the result of a folic acid deficiency, he can readily remedy the condition by administering this vitamin by mouth or by injection. Patients who are not severely ill with a malabsorptive syndrome respond to oral doses of as little as 0.5 mg. daily; however, many hematologists prefer to start the patient on much higher doses (10 to 30 mg., or more), and, even after hematologic remission has occurred, the patient continues to receive 5 to 10 mg. daily. This drug is *never* used alone when there is a possibility that the patient may be suffering from pernicious anemia. For folic acid will return the blood picture to normal and even correct the G.I. symptoms of pernicious anemia, but the nerve cell damage would not be checked at all!

Panhematinic Preparations. Because of the possibility—and the danger—of obscuring the diagnosis of pernicous anemia, all hematologists deplore the presence of folic acid in many antianemia products. These so-called panhematinics are claimed to contain all the

TABLE 25-1
DRUGS FOR TREATING THE ANEMIAS

Nonproprietary Name	Synonym or Trade Name	Total Daily Dosage
Iron Compounds		
Dextriferron	Astrafer: Iron-dextrin	1.5–5 ml. I.V. (30–100 mg. Fe)
Ferrocholinate	Chel-Iron; Ferrolip	1–2 Gm.
Ferrous fumarate U.S.P.	Ircon; Toleron, etc.	600–800 mg.
Ferrous gluconate N.F.	Fergon, etc.	900 mg.
Ferrous sulfate U.S.P.	Iron sulfate, hydrated	900 mg.
Dried ferrous sulfate U.S.P.	Feosol, etc.	600–800 mg.
Iron dextran injection U.S.P.	Imferon	1–5 ml. I.M. (50–250 mg. Fe)
Iron sorbitex (iron–sorbitol–citric acid complex)	Jectofer	2–4 ml. I.M. (100–200 mg. Fe)
Polyferose	Iron carbohydrate chelate; Jefron	600–800 mg.
Hematopoietic Vitamins and Related Substances		
Cyanocobalamin injection U.S.P.	Vitamin B_{12}, etc.	1–100 mcg. (10–100 mcg. at weekly or monthly intervals)
Folic acid U.S.P. (injection and tablets)	Folvite	10 mg.
Hydroxocobalamin	Vitamin B_{12a}, etc.	50 mcg. every other week
Intrinsic factor concentrate		300 mg.
Liver injection N.F.		equiv. of 1 mcg. B_{12} (10–15 mcg. at intervals of 10–15 days)
Vitamin B_{12} with intrinsic factor concentrate		10 mcg. B_{12} and 300 mg. I.F.

vitamins and minerals required for red cell synthesis. At best, such mixtures are unnecessarily expensive, because the vast majority of anemic patients respond promptly to *iron* alone and do not profit from inclusion of vitamin B_{12}, intrinsic factor, folic acid or minerals such as copper, cobalt, zinc, manganese and molybdenum (substances that are rarely, if ever, lacking in the diet).

Much more serious, however, is this: A patient with undiagnosed pernicious anemia may get enough folic acid to return his blood picture to normal if he takes a "shotgun" type antianemia product that is aimed at correcting anemias of every type, regardless of cause. The danger is that, even when the product also contains vitamin B_{12}, that anti-pernicious anemia principle may be present in too small an amount to meet the needs of the patient's nervous tissues. As a result of this lack of absorbable B_{12}, the patient's nervous system may continue to degenerate to a point beyond repair, despite the normal appearance of his blood.

Thus, the nurse should always urge patients not to treat themselves for anemia with multivitamin-multimineral panhematinic products but to get a definite diagnosis of the specific deficiency responsible for the anemia from a hematologist. If it is found that they require iron, this is what the doctor will usually prescribe *alone*. If all they need is folic acid *or* cyanocobalamin, that is *all* they should get.

The Food and Drug Administration no longer permits the presence of intrinsic factor in *non*-prescription products, because it cannot be counted on to aid the absorption of enough vitamin B_{12} to clear up all symptoms of pernicious anemia. Similarly, over-the-counter hematinics may now contain only enough folic acid to make up for a deficiency of that vitamin; the amount of folic acid is kept at a level below that which would overcome the megaloblastic picture in pernicious anemia and thus mask the diagnosis of that condition until it would be too late to treat the neurological damage.

Citrovorum factor (folinic acid; leucovorin) is the coenzyme to which folic acid is converted in the tissues. Administering it directly has no advantage over folic acid itself, except in one important situation—overdosage of the *anti*folic drugs used in the treatment of neoplastic diseases. These folic acid antagonists (Chap. 44) act by keeping folic acid from being enzymatically changed to folinic acid, the form that all cells need. Thus, in cases of toxic reactions resulting from antifol drugs such as amethopterin, folinic acid may be injected to counteract the intoxication directly.

SUMMARY OF POINTS FOR THE NURSE TO REMEMBER ABOUT DRUGS USED FOR TREATING ANEMIA

- The nurse should advise people to have a doctor diagnose their problem instead of buying advertised hematinic products for self-medication. Taking such products is not only often an unnecessary expense but also potentially dangerous. If the patient is actually anemic, the *cause*, which is often *loss of blood*, should be sought. Besides, certain products may mask the presence of pernicious anemia without counteracting the most dangerous effects of this disease.

- If a patient complains that he "can't take iron" because it causes gastrointestinal upset, she should advise him to consult his physician as to whether a change in the dosage or method of administration of the drug might be possible, or even as to whether a less irritating product might not be prescribed.

- Do not suggest the likelihood of nausea, vomiting, cramps, diarrhea or constipation unless the doctor specifically wants the patient warned beforehand that such side effects are possible. Do let the patient know that a darkening of the stool is to be expected and that this does not mean that he is bleeding but is quite harmless. (The nurse, too, should check on whether *any patient* with a dark stool is taking iron before deciding that this is a sign of bleeding.)

- For most rapid and complete absorption, soluble iron salts are sometimes taken in orange juice. Remember that liquid iron sometimes stains the teeth and have the patient take it through a straw or a drinking tube. Drops should be placed well back on the patient's tongue.

- Remember that iron-containing products are potentially toxic when taken in large quantity, and alert parents to the need for storing such substances out of the reach of young children.

- Patients should be urged not to forget to visit their physician for B_{12} injections when the symptoms of pernicious anemia and similar deficiency disorders are in remission. If the doctor desires, they can be taught to administer B_{12} injections periodically at home, in order to reduce the high cost of long-term treatment of this lifelong illness.

CLINICAL PROBLEM

Miss Swenson, age 52, has just learned that she has pernicious anemia. Her doctor has prescribed vitamin B_{12} 1 cc. I.M. weekly, indicating that later it may be possible to decrease the frequency of injections to 1 cc. every other week. He explained to Miss Swenson, however, that she would continue to require vitamin B_{12} injections for the rest of her life. The public health nurse visits weekly to give the injections.

One day, while the nurse is preparing the injection, Miss Swenson says, "I know that you are giving me a vitamin. The doctor explained to me why I need it, but I've forgotten a lot of what he said. I've always eaten a good diet. Why is it that I'm not getting the vitamin from my food?"

Later, she says, "I have to keep taking this medicine all my life. Could it have harmful effects on me after a while?"

How would you reply to Miss Swenson's questions?

REVIEW QUESTIONS

1. (a) Substances of what two types are synthesized by the bone marrow during erythropoiesis?

(b) List some dietary substances that are needed for the formation of adequate numbers of healthy red blood cells.

2. (a) What is the appearance of red blood cells produced during a period of iron deficiency? What terms describe such cells?

(b) What is the appearance of the red cells when substances such as cyanocobalamin and folic acid are lacking? What terms describe such cells?

3. (a) List some symptoms of early iron deficiency and some signs typical of the anemia that develops in such states.

(b) What are some circumstances in which the amount of iron absorbed from the G.I. tract tends to increase?

4. (a) How is iron carried to and from its storage sites in the body? Where are these iron reserves largely located?

(b) How is iron ordinarily excreted by the body and about how much is lost daily by these routes?

5. (a) What are two important reasons for urging people to see a doctor before trying to treat themselves with an iron-containing hematinic product?

(b) What are three possible ways in which people may develop an iron-deficiency anemia, and which of these is most likely to be the cause of a definitely diagnosed anemia in an American male and in women past the child-bearing age in this country?

6. (a) List the kinds of people who are most likely to become so deficient in their iron stores as to require medicinal iron.

(b) Explain some of the circumstances that make such people susceptible to development of iron deficiency anemia.

7. (a) List three characteristics considered desirable in an iron-containing hematinic product.

(b) What must happen to iron-containing chemical complexes before they can be absorbed from the G.I. tract,

and how does this affect their local action on the G.I. mucosa?

8. (a) Which of the available oral iron compounds is considered least expensive and yet as completely effective as any of the more costly iron complexes?

(b) What is the main adverse effect of this and similar iron salts and what suggestions may be made to a patient in order to minimize this problem?

9. (a) What measures may be taken to assure the most complete absorption of oral iron by patients who have no complaints of discomfort from products that are taken by mouth?

(b) What should be done for the patient to prevent staining of his teeth by liquid iron preparations?

10. (a) List several types of patients for whom parenterally administered iron may be indicated.

(b) What are some advantages of iron dextran injection over earlier forms of injectable iron?

11. (a) What adverse effects may result from chronic iron overload?

(b) What are some possible reactions to intravenous iron?

12. (a) What advice would you give to a young mother who has received a prescription for an iron tonic?

(b) What are some general measures employed in treating iron toxicity and what is one specific chemical antidote for iron poisoning?

13. (a) List several clinical conditions in which the blood picture is characterized by a markedly reduced erythrocyte count and an unusually high percentage of large cells (macrocytes) and some bone marrow elements (megaloblasts).

(b) What defect in pernicious-anemia patients leads to the deficiency that results in megaloblastic anemia and other signs and symptoms?

14. (a) What other type patient may suffer from absorptive defects that can result eventually in a deficiency of vitamin B_{12}?

(b) How are all such patients best treated for rapid and sustained remission of their symptoms?

15. (a) What advice can the nurse give to pernicious anemia patients in remission, or to their families?

(b) Describe the response of a pernicious-anemia patient to cyanocobalamin injections.

16. (a) Give some examples of situations in which people may become deficient in folic acid and indicate the main symptoms of the lack of this essential nutrient.

(b) What difference in the metabolic functions of vitamin B_{12} and folic acid results in the latter's not being adequate treatment for patients with pernicious anemia?

BIBLIOGRAPHY

Amerman, E. E., *et al.:* Ferrous sulfate poisoning. J. Pediat., *53:*476, 1958.

Bethell, F., *et al.:* Present status of treatment of pernicious anemia. J.A.M.A., *171:*2092, 1959.

Block, M.: The clinical pharmacology of trace metals and iron. Clin. Pharmacol. Ther., *1:*748, 1960.

Castle, W. B.: Nutritional megaloblastic anemias: etiological considerations. Med. Clin. N. Am., *50:*1245, 1966.

Committee on Toxicology: Accidental iron poisoning in children. J.A.M.A., *170:*676, 1959.

Ellison, A. B. C.: Pernicious anemia masked by multivitamins containing folic acid. J.A.M.A., *173:*240, 1960.

Franklin, M., *et al.:* Chelate iron therapy. J.A.M.A., *166:*1685, 1958.

Friend, D. G.: Iron therapy. Clin. Pharmacol. Ther., *4:*419, 1963.

Henderson, F., *et al.:* The use of desferrioxamine in the treatment of acute iron toxicity due to ferrous gluconate. J.A.M.A., *186:*1139, 1963.

Herbert, V.: The diagnosis and treatment of folic acid deficiency. Med. Clin. N. Am., *46:*1365, 1962.

————: Current concepts of therapy. Megaloblastic anemia. New Eng. J. Med., *268:*201; 368, 1963.

Herbert, V., and Castle, W. B.: Intrinsic factor. New Eng. J. Med., *270:*1181, 1964.

Lichtman, H. C.: Current status of therapy in anemias. J.A.M.A., *167:*735, 1958.

McKenna, P. J., and Erslev, A. J.: Treatment of anemias. Med. Clin. N. Am., *49:*1371, 1965.

Moore, C. V., and Dubach, R.: Metabolism and requirements of iron in the human. J.A.M.A., *162:*197, 1956.

Rodman, M. J.: Blood-building B-vitamins and how they work. R.N., *22:*33, 1959 (Nov.).

Unglaub, W. G., and Goldsmith, G. A.: Folic acid and vitamin B_{12} in medical practice. J.A.M.A., *161:*623, 1956.

Vilter, R. W.: Vitamins, minerals, and anemia. J.A.M.A., *175:*1000, 1961.

· 26 ·

Drugs Used in Peripheral Vascular Disease

PERIPHERAL VASCULAR DISEASE

We have previously discussed various drugs that are used in treating coronary and cerebral vascular diseases (Chaps. 22 and 23). The results of the sudden block or rupture of an artery carrying blood to the heart or brain are so serious that we tend to forget that similar circulatory disturbances often occur elsewhere in the body, including the limbs. Yet, although the effects of a reduction in the blood supply of *the extremities* are usually less dramatic and not as immediately deadly as a heart attack or stroke, these disorders—the *peripheral vascular diseases*—can have very serious consequences.

A severe reduction of the blood supply to a limb—which may come on gradually when the lumen of a major vessel is progressively narrowed by atherosclerosis, or with dramatic suddenness when a blood clot blocks the main channel completely—can cause so much injury to tissues that amputation becomes necessary. Diminished blood supply of less severe degree, such as occurs with excessive vasoconstriction, can have painful and, finally, disabling consequences for the patient. As the chronic forms of arterial or venous insufficiency advance, the patient may become too crippled to walk or to work with his hands. Often ugly skin ulcers or gangrene of deeper tissues develop and require eventual surgical intervention.

The management of peripheral vascular diseases calls for many medical and surgical measures, as well as physical therapy. There are, in addition, numerous details of nursing care that can help to foster better circulation and prevent the more dangerous complications of peripheral vascular disorders. The nurse is also often in a position to instruct the patient in the proper home care of his skin and feet, the desirable and appropriate clothing, and other aspects of personal hygiene—all of which will help to prevent the injuries and infections that so commonly lead to ulcers and even gangrene in persons with poor peripheral circulation.

Pathological Physiology. The flow of blood to the fingers or toes may be slowed or stopped by various mechanisms. Sometimes, the patient's arteries are narrowed by an excessive number of nerve impulses arriving at the vascular walls by way of sympathetic vasoconstrictor nerve fibers. Adrenergic drugs (Chap. 16) or other smooth muscle contracting agents, such as the ergot alkaloids (Chap. 41), may cause vasospasm and reduced blood flow to local tissues.

More difficult to deal with are conditions caused by structural rather than functional abnormalities. Hardening of the arterial walls, for example, or damage to the inner lining of the vessels, with subsequent development of atherosclerotic plaques (Chap. 22) may gradually impair peripheral circulation. Clots that suddenly form or lodge in such narrowed channels may then cut off blood flow completely to the parts below the block. Sometimes, certain diseases that do not damage the artery itself may lessen peripheral circulation by pressing upon the vessel (e.g., in scleroderma), or inadequate local circulation may stem from a systemic disease (e.g., anemia; hyperthyroidism).

DRUG TREATMENT OF ARTERIAL DISEASES

Drugs of several classes discussed elsewhere in this book are often used to treat disorders of the outlying arteries and veins and to counteract the complications of these peripheral vascular diseases. These include the *anticoagulant agents,* employed to prevent the extension of thrombi and emboli in the vessels; the *thrombolytic agents* that sometimes hasten the breakdown of venous blood clots; *antibiotics,* for controlling infections in ischemic tissues; *analgesics* and *anti-inflammatory* agents, to reduce pain and local edema; and *dermatological agents* for relief of skin rashes and itching. However, we shall limit our discussion here mainly to the *peripheral vasodilator drugs*—agents

365

given in an effort to widen the channels of narrowed arterioles and thus increase the local circulation to ischemic tissues in the extremities.

Vasodilatation. Drugs act in various ways to enlarge the caliber of constricted arterioles and bring a flow of fresh blood to tissues deprived of oxygen and nutrients. However, before discussing the several classes of chemicals which exert their vasodilator actions at various sites, we should note that the value of any drug therapy of vascular diseases is relatively limited. This is especially true in those peripheral vascular diseases that are marked by degenerative changes in the blood vessel walls. Vessels made rigid by arteriosclerosis, for example, are relatively resistant to the action of drugs intended to relax vascular smooth muscle walls and thus to enlarge the lumen.

These drugs are most likely to be of some benefit in conditions caused by *vasospasm*, especially when the reflexly constricted vessels are not also partially occluded by atherosclerotic plaques or blocked by blood clots. Even in these relatively responsive disorders, vasodilatation is limited, occurring largely in the patient's skin rather than the vessels located deep within the muscles. At best, despite claims to the contrary, a drug-induced increase in blood flow is usually of short duration, so that frequent administration is required to produce sustained vasodilatation in these chronic conditions.

Adrenergic Blocking Agents

Drugs of this class are often effective for reduction of vasospasm caused by the action of the sympathetic neurohormone norepinephrine upon alpha type adrenergic neuroeffectors in vascular smooth muscle. As indicated in Chapter 17, molecules of these drugs occupy the alpha adrenergic receptors and thus tend to keep the chemical transmitter released from sympathetic nerve endings from exerting its tonic vasoconstrictor effects.

Partial blockade of sympathetic nerve impulses in this manner proves most beneficial in conditions caused by excessive vasoconstrictor tone. *Raynaud's disease,* a vasospastic condition in which peripheral vessels tend to become reflexly constricted, especially upon exposure of the body to cold or as a result of emotional upset, is an example of a functional arteriolar disorder that often responds to treatment with drugs of this class. It occurs mainly in young women and may, if uncontrolled, lead to painful ulcers on the fingertips and elsewhere. Unless delayed by vasodilator drug therapy, so-called trophic changes occur in the skin which is often stretched tightly over the fingers. Such skin damage is relatively rare in a related condition called *acrocyanosis,* in which the skin turns blue and cold but without pain or permanent disability.

Phenoxybenzamine (Dibenzyline) is considered one of the best of the alpha adrenergic blockers for reducing vasoconstriction because of the relatively long duration of its blocking action upon the sympathetically innervated excitatory neuroeffectors in vascular smooth muscle. This reduction in vasoconstrictor tone lessens the likelihood of attacks in Raynaud's disease upon exposure to cold. Increased circulation in the fingertips and toes, as well as the skin of the ears, nose and cheeks, may reduce the rate of progress of this disorder and help to prevent infection, blisters, indolent ulcers or local gangrene. If the patient appears to respond well, even temporarily, to drug treatment of this type (which has been called a *chemical* sympathectomy), he may be a good candidate for surgical sympathectomy, the treatment of choice for progressive peripheral vascular disorders of this type.

The vasodilator action of adrenergic blocking drugs is not, however, entirely limited to reduction in sympathetic nervous system impulse transmission. *Tolazoline* and *azapetine* (see Drug Digests) have a histaminelike ability to relax vascular smooth muscle directly, as well. Their actions at other sites cause side effects such as gastrointestinal upset. With all the adrenergic blockers, dosage must be carefully adjusted to avoid precipitating undesirable cardiovascular side effects.

Side Effects and Contraindications. Too high dosage of these drugs tend to cause systemic as well as local vasodilatation. The resulting fall in blood pressure can, of course, cause headache, dizziness, weakness and feelings of faintness and fatigue. Such episodes of postural hypotension and the reflex tachycardia it evokes are best avoided by raising the dosage of adrenergic blocking agents only gradually, or by injecting the drugs intra-arterially. Such injection directly into the major channel carrying blood to the involved peripheral part is often more effective and produces fewer circulatory side effects than intravenous administration.

The cardiac effects of these drugs make them especially undesirable for patients with coronary atherosclerosis. *Alpha* adrenergic blocking drugs of this type do not prevent reflex cardioacceleration caused by stimulation of *beta* receptors in the myocardium (see Chap. 17). Thus, if overdosage of these drugs tends to cause a fall in blood pressure and sets off compensatory tachycardia in such a patient, his hardened coronary arteries may be unable to dilate enough to meet the demands of the racing heart for more blood. Such cardiac effects can be especially severe with systemically administered tolazoline, a drug that tends to stimulate the heart directly as well as reflexly. Its administration in excessive doses can cause attacks of angina pectoris or even precipitate a patient with compensated congestive heart failure into frank failure.

Ganglionic Blocking Agents

These drugs (as indicated in Chaps. 17 and 23) reduce excessive transmission of vasoconstrictor impulses at the sympathetic ganglionic relay stations between the brain and the blood vessels (see Fig. 14-1). Because of their ability to counteract vasospasm resulting from overactive sympathetic reflexes, agents such as *chlorisondamine, mecamylamine, pentolinium,* and *trimethaphan* (see Drug Digests) are all capable of producing increased local blood flow to ischemic limbs in some circumstances by producing a partial and temporary chemical sympathectomy.

Like the adrenergic blockers, these agents are most useful when a vasospastic component is the predominant feature of the patient's peripheral vascular disease. Thus, they may be effective for counteracting the after-effects of local *frostbite* by eliminating excessive reflex vasoconstriction and allowing a flow of fresh blood to warm the skin, especially in the lower limbs. Similarly, in *causalgia*—an extremely painful condition resulting from trauma to sympathetic nerve fibers—sympathetic blockers of both types sometimes relieve the burning pain in the patient's hand or foot by their "sympatholytic" vasodilator effects.

Unfortunately, ganglionic blockade is not very useful when the patient's circulatory insufficiency stems from chronic occlusive vascular diseases such as *atherosclerosis obliterans* and *thromboangiitis obliterans* (*Buerger's disease*). In these conditions, in which the channels of the blood vessels are progressively obliterated by organic obstructions, drug-induced vasodilatation does little to aid local blood flow to the ischemic tissues and prevent the damage that often requires amputation of parts of the limbs.

Occasionally, in these chronic conditions and after acute occlusion of a major artery by a thrombus or embolus, these sympathetic blockers may help to increase the flow of blood through unblocked adjacent arterioles. In such situations, the reflex vasospasm that often develops in the neighboring arteries can be counteracted by chemical blockade of the sympathetic ganglia. This tends to relieve the severe pain and limits the extent of ischemic tissue damage. However, despite this drug-induced increase in collateral circulation, the blood clot in the blocked vessel itself is not likely to be dislodged. Embolectomy or other kinds of vascular surgery are required if the limb is to be saved.

Cautions and Contraindications. Ganglionic blockade of sympathetic vasoconstrictor impulses does not affect all vascular beds equally. Thus, the skin may become flushed and warm, but, often, blood flow to the brain and to the legs may not be increased significantly and may, in fact, be reduced in some circumstances.

The effects of systemically administered ganglionic blocking agents are not usually limited to the local area that the doctor desires to treat. Thus, generalized vasodilatation and a marked fall in blood pressure may follow the administration of excessive doses of these drugs. The resulting reduction in overall perfusion pressure may then lead to an actual *diminution* of the local flow of blood. This is especially likely to happen in those organs in which the blood vessels are arteriosclerotic and thus cannot benefit from the vasodilator action of these drugs.

For this reason, the ganglionic blocking agents may be especially undesirable for treating those patients with peripheral vascular disease who suffer from cerebrovascular atherosclerosis also. A marked fall in systemic pressure in such cases may lessen blood flow not only to the ischemic limb but also to the brain, thus precipitating an episode of cerebral vascular insufficiency or even causing a stroke. Similarly, these drugs are contraindicated for patients with a history of coronary or renal circulatory difficulties, since reduced blood flow to the heart and kidneys could cause infarctions in these organs also.

Sympathomimetic Amines

Certain synthetic substances with a structural resemblance to epinephrine are sometimes used to increase blood flow to ischemic vessels in the skeletal muscles of the limbs. These vascular beds, unlike those of the skin, contain mainly *beta*-type, or inhibitory, adrenergic receptors. Consequently, these vascular walls respond to natural catecholamines and to synthetic sympathomimetic drugs by relaxing. The resulting dilatation of the arterioles in the skeletal muscles is claimed to be desirable in *intermittent claudication*. This is a condition marked by cramping pain in the patient's calves which develops when he walks a little way. It is the result of reduced blood flow, which leads to an imbalance between the metabolic requirements of the patient's muscles and the quantity of blood the vessels can deliver.

Most authorities doubt that these, or any other vasodilator drugs, actually dilate the atherosclerotic vessels in the patient's legs. An increase in the collateral circulation to the limbs may account for the ability to walk greater distances and the reduction in ischemic night cramps in calves and thighs sometimes reported by patients taking *nylidrin* (see Drug Digest) or *isoxsuprine,* two drugs of this class.

Both of these agents, although they are adrenergic compounds, appear to be relatively free of the side effects typical of most sympathomimetic drugs. For example, they do not tend ordinarily to produce a rise in blood pressure, tachycardia, or excessive central excitement. Nylidrin and isoxsuprine should, however, be employed only with caution for aiding circulation in the extremities of patients who have a history of coronary artery disease or other conditions in which adrenergic drugs are contraindicated.

Parasympathomimetic (Cholinergic) Agents

Certain blood vessels respond to release of *acetylcholine,* the cholinergic neurohormone, by dilating. The effects of acetylcholine itself are too fleeting for clinical utility; however, the longer-lasting choline ester, *methacholine* (Chap. 15), has been employed to produce peripheral vasodilatation in the skin of patients with Raynaud's disease, phlebitis and chronic varicose ulcers.

Large oral doses of this cholinergic agent sometimes help skin ulcers to heal by relaxing vasospastic vessels, but the improved local blood flow is often bought at the expense of undesirable muscarinic side effects such as diarrhea. To avoid the systemic actions of methacholine, it is sometimes administered by iontophoresis, a procedure in which the drug is introduced directly into the skin by means of an electric current. The expense and technical skill required limit the utility of this method of localizing the action of methacholine.

Direct-Acting Vasodilator Drugs

The side effects that often accompany the use of autonomic blocking and stimulating drugs has led to a search for drugs that would act more specifically upon the peripheral blood vessels themselves. Drugs do not, of course, have to block or imitate autonomic nerve impulses to produce vascular dilatation. We have seen (Chap. 22) that the nitrites and papaverine relax spastic coronary vessels and thus increase local blood flow in the myocardium. Recently, drugs have been introduced that act directly on the vascular smooth muscles of peripheral vascular beds.

Cyclandelate (see Drug Digest) is an example of a drug with a direct relaxant effect on the smooth muscles of blood vessels and other organs. The resulting increase in local circulation of the skin has reportedly helped to heal ulcerated areas, and increased blood flow to the muscles is said to relieve the pain of intermittent claudication. The drug has been reported to be beneficial in Buerger's disease and for diabetic vascular difficulties, but its usefulness in patients with such degenerative and obstructive blood vessel disorders is not yet truly established.

Cyclandelate seems to produce fewer and less severe circulatory system side effects than the vasodilators that act through their effects on autonomic nervous transmission. Overdosage sometimes causes headaches and dizziness, as with nitrites, and flushing, tingling and itching of the skin, as with *nicotinic acid* (p. 324). A derivative of the latter drug, *nicotinyl tartrate,* is another direct-acting vasodilator. It is available alone in a long-acting form, and combined with *aminophylline,* for relief of vascular spasm and to increase local circulation in patients with varicose and decubital ulcers and chilblains. Transient flushing, and occasional skin rashes and stomach upset are side effects.

Drugs Acting on the Heart and Circulation

DRUG TREATMENT OF VENOUS DISEASES

Various conditions often interfere with the flow of blood back to the heart by way of the veins. This need not be serious, since there are so very many venous pathways that the blood can readily bypass most minor obstructions. On the other hand, *chronic* venous insufficiency and varicose veins can cause considerable discomfort and disability. *Acute* inflammation of veins with blood-clot formation in the deep channels of the legs can cause a long period of disability or result in fatal pulmonary embolism.

Phlebitis. The main groups of drugs used in the treatment of phlebitis and venous thrombosis are the anticoagulant and thrombolytic agents discussed in Chapter 24. Prompt treatment with heparin injections followed by the oral anticoagulants has helped to reduce the death rate from pulmonary embolism in patients with thrombophlebitis. The use of salicylates and anti-inflammatory agents such as phenylbutazone also tends to relieve local tenderness and edema in phlebitis when combined with watchful nursing care.

Many *locally acting* medications are used for control of the complications of phlebitis, including the deep ulcers that sometimes develop around the patient's ankles. The treatment of such stasis ulcers often involves soaks with astringent solutions, the use of local and systemic antibiotics to control infection, and application of gelatin boot bandages impregnated with anti-inflammatory and antipruritic agents to speed healing and control itching. The locally acting dermatological agents and the antibiotics, as well as the diuretic and corticosteroid drugs often employed to control postphlebitic complications, are discussed elsewhere in this book (see Index).

Varicose Veins. In contrast to the many kinds of medications used for phlebitis, drugs are of only limited usefulness for varicose, or dilated, veins, and surgery is today's treatment of choice for varicosities. Of course, prevention of varicose veins by minimizing the factors that lead to this common condition is the best procedure of all, but even this is not always successful, since many people have a hereditary predisposition toward venous disorders.

Physiology. Our veins contain a built-in pumping system that helps to propel blood back toward the heart. As we walk, for example, contractions of the calf muscles drive the venous blood forward. When these muscles relax, one-way valves within the veins keep the blood from flowing backward. When these valves are stretched and become incompetent, the blood in the veins tends to be pulled downward by the force of gravity. This increasing pressure makes the walls of the veins bulge outward.

Pregnancy is a common cause of aggravation of previously existing weaknesses, as the distending uterus puts increasing pressure on the engorged veins of the woman's lower limbs. Obesity also aggravates lower-limb vascular weaknesses. People who must stand for long periods at their jobs are prone to develop varicose veins, as are those who have to lift heavy loads in their work.

Sclerosing Agents for Varicose Veins

The only drugs that are used specifically for venous disorders are the so-called *sclerosing agents*. These are irritating chemicals that are sometimes injected into small superficial varicose veins in order to close them off. These substances act by damaging the inner lining of the vein, causing an injury that leads to formation of blood clots in the isolated segment of the vessel. The clot is then gradually converted into fibrous connective tissue which permanently occludes the overly dilated vein.

Not all varicosities require or benefit from injection therapy with sclerosing solutions. Most small varicose veins cause no discomfort; larger varicosities are best treated surgically, because they tend to reopen shortly after sclerosing treatment. However, small superficial leg veins that become dilated during pregnancy, for example, and continue to cause aching, cramping, itching, and feelings of fullness and burning in the limbs may often be permanently obliterated with these chemicals.

TABLE 26-1
DRUGS USED IN TREATING PERIPHERAL VASCULAR DISEASES

Nonproprietary Name	Proprietary Name	Usual Oral Single Dose
Vasodilators for Arterial Disease		
Adrenergic Blocking Agents		
Azapetine phosphate	Ilidar	50–75 mg.
Phenoxybenzamine HCl	Dibenzyline	20–60 mg.
Phentolamine HCl	Regitine	50–100 mg.
Tolazoline HCl	Priscoline	50–75 mg.
Ganglionic Blocking Agents		
Chlorisondamine chloride	Ecolid	10–50 mg.
Mecamylamine HCl U.S.P.	Inversine	2.5–25 mg.
Pentolinium tartrate	Ansolysen	20–60 mg.
Trimethidinium methosulfate	Ostensin	20–40 mg.
Sympathomimetic Amines		
Isoxsuprine HCl	Vasodilan	10–20 mg.
Nylidrin HCl N.F.	Arlidin	6 mg.
Parasympathetic (cholinergic) Agents		
Methacholine bromide N.F.	Mecholyl Br	200 mg.
Methacholine chloride N.F.	Mecholyl Cl	20 mg. S.C. and 0.2–0.5% sol. for iontophoresis
Direct-Acting Vascular Antispasmodics		
Cyclandelate	Cyclospasmol	200 mg.
Nicotinyl tartrate	Roniacol	50–150 mg.
Sclerosing Solutions for Varicose Veins		
Ethylamine oleate	Etalate	
Monoethanolamine oleate	Etholate; Monolate	
Quinine and urea HCl injection U.S.P.		
Sodium morrhuate injection	in Morusul	
Sodium psylliate	Sylnasol	
Sodium ricinoleate	Soricin	
Sodium tetradecyl sulfate	Sotradecol	

Among the substances employed for this purpose are the sodium salts of certain natural fatty acids. *Sodium morrhuate* injection, for example, comes from cod liver oil; *sodium psylliate* is obtained from psyllium seed oil. These and similar natural chemicals sometimes cause sensitization and allergic reactions. This is why the doctor often injects only a small test dose and waits a few minutes before following with further injections. *Sodium tetradecyl sulfate*, a synthetic sclerosing chemical, is claimed less likely to cause allergic reactions than the substances of animal and vegetable origin. However, patients should still receive a test dose for detecting allergic susceptibility to the drug prior to completion of the course of injections with it. It is recommended that such courses of treatment be completed within a few days to avoid development of sensitization which would preclude future use of the sclerosing agent.

The injection of these irritant chemicals is often followed by local pain, but this may be reduced by the addition of agents with local anesthetic properties. The doctor takes special care to avoid letting the sclerosing agent leak into tissues outside of the vein. Such extravascular spillage may cause necrotic abscesses and sloughing off of subcutaneous tissues. The injected area is kept clamped with compression bandages to keep the veins collapsed, and the patient is instructed to wear elastic stockings over the bandages day and night for several weeks so that the "glued" together inner surfaces will "set."

Other Measures for Patient Care

It is important to remember always that drugs do not ordinarily cure peripheral arterial and venous disorders. Other measures must be employed simultaneously to relieve symptoms, slow the progress of these vascular diseases, and prevent their often disabling complications. Since most patients with chronic conditions are treated at home, it is essential to teach the patient not only to take his prescribed medication but also to care for himself by adhering to a program of

personal hygiene to aid local circulation and avoid stagnation and infection.

Among the practical points often suggested to patients with peripheral vascular diseases are these:

Keep the entire body warm at all times. Chilling tends to cause reflex constriction of blood vessels. (*Local* heat should, of course, be used only very judiciously.)

Avoid wearing clothing that constricts the thighs or legs. Round garters and tight girdles are especially undesirable for patients with circulatory difficulty: they tend to cause excessive congestion of superficial veins and reduce arterial flow.

Walk (within the limits recommended by the doctor). *Light exercise* of this kind is desirable even in patients with intermittent claudication or severe varicosities in order to maintain muscle tone, develop collateral circulatory pathways, and prevent obesity which aggravates peripheral vascular difficulties.

Rest is desirable. *It is important* to sit or lie in positions that aid blood flow to and from the limbs. Patients with *venous* difficulties should have their limbs elevated to reduce local tenderness and edema in the legs. Those with *arterial* disease must keep their legs lowered—for example, the head of the bed should be raised on shock blocks, in order to keep the patient's legs low.

Avoid smoking and the use of vasoconstrictive drugs such as amphetamine, ephedrine and ergotamine, as well as external preparations that may irritate the skin, which should be kept clean and supple.

In summary, the nurse's willingness to work with patients with peripheral vascular diseases may, in the last analysis, be the most important factor in determining whether pain will lessen, an ulcer will heal, or a limb will be lost or saved. This kind of patient-care can thus be rewarding even though the peripheral vascular diseases, which are becoming increasingly common as the number of elderly people increases, tend to improve only very slowly or not at all.

SUMMARY OF POINTS FOR NURSES TO REMEMBER CONCERNING DRUG TREATMENT OF PERIPHERAL VASCULAR DISEASES

• Treatment for many patients consists of careful attention to details; one of these important details involves administration of the prescribed drug and careful observation of its effects. Is the patient able to walk farther without pain? Is his foot warmer?

• Instruction of the patient and his family in measures that promote improved circulation and lessen the possibility of complications is essential. Nurses can carry out such instructions in the hospital, home, and industry. Particular nursing vigilance is required in settings where there are many elderly people, such as in nursing homes. For example, the nurse should promptly report any tiny ulcer, or any change in the temperature of an extremity, to the doctor.

- Relief of pain is an important problem. Ideally, pain is relieved by improving the blood supply. Actually, analgesics may be required if blood supply cannot be sufficiently improved. Since pain tends to be chronic, be especially vigilant in noting it and in using pre-scribed measures to relieve it. If these measures are not effective, be sure to discuss this with the physician. Opiates are avoided, not because the pain is trivial, but because of the danger of addiction.

- When applying any medicine locally to an ulcer, use careful aseptic technique. Owing to impaired blood supply, the patient is particularly hampered in fight-ing infection which can then lead to gangrene and necessitate amputation.

REVIEW QUESTIONS

1. (a) List several peripheral vascular diseases with a vasospastic component, which may be benefited by vaso-dilator drug treatment.

(b) List several peripheral vascular diseases with or-ganic occlusive vascular lesions, which do *not* respond very well to vasodilator drug treatment.

2. (a) By what mechanism do the adrenergic blocking agents aid the peripheral circulation of patients with Raynaud's syndrome and related vasospastic conditions?

(b) What undesirable cardiovascular effects can result from administration of excessive doses of adrenergic block-ing agents to such patients?

(c) In patients of what types may overdosage of the adrenergic blocker *tolazoline* be especially undesirable?

3. (a) Under what circumstances may the administra-tion of a ganglionic blocking agent bring an increased flow of blood to a limb in which a major vessel has been oc-cluded by a blood clot lodged in a channel narrowed by organic obstructive disease?

(b) Under what circumstances may the administration of a ganglionic blocking agent lead to an actual lessening of blood flow to the limbs of a patient with atherosclerosis obliterans or with Buerger's disease?

(c) In patients of what types may the use of ganglionic blocking agents for treating peripheral vascular diseases be contraindicated?

4. (a) In what manner may an adrenergic agent such as nylidrin aid blood flow in intermittent claudication?

(b) In patients of what types may the use of vasodilator drugs of the sympathomimetic type be undesirable?

(c) What special method of administration is some-times employed to lessen systemic side effects when the parasympathomimetic drug methacholine is employed for increasing cutaneous blood flow in peripheral vascular dis-eases?

5. (a) What is the manner of action of the vasodilator drugs cyclandelate and nicotinyl tartrate, and what are some conditions in which they are claimed effective?

(b) What are some side effects of agents of this type?

6. (a) List several classes of drugs employed in the management of thrombophlebitis and postphlebitic com-plications.

(b) List several sclerosing agents and indicate the pur-pose for which they are employed.

7. (a) What precautions does the doctor take in mak-ing injections of sclerosing solutions?

(b) What measures may be suggested to patients with peripheral vascular diseases to aid local circulation and prevent complications from their conditions?

BIBLIOGRAPHY

Beck, L., and Brody, M. J.: The physiology of vasodilation. Angiology, *12:*202, 1961.

Friend, D.: Drugs for peripheral vascular disease. Clin. Pharmacol. Ther., *5:*666, 1964.

Le Fevre, F.: Management of occlusive arterial diseases of the extremities. J.A.M.A., *147:*1401, 1951.

Lippman, H. L.: Intra-arterial Priscoline (tolazoline) ther-apy for peripheral vascular disturbances. Angiology, *3:* 69, 1952.

Moser, M., *et al.*: Clinical experience with sympathetic blocking agents in peripheral vascular disease. Ann. Int. Med., *38:*1245, 1953.

Rodman, M. J.: Vasodilator drugs in peripheral vascular disease. R.N., *26:*39, 1963 (March).

———: Drug management in peripheral vascular disease. R.N., *29:*61, 1966 (Aug.).

Spittell, J. A., Jr. (ed.): Symposium on treatment of venous disorders. Modern Treatment, *2:*1061, 1965 (Nov.).

Wright, I. S.: Treatment of occlusive arterial disease. J.A.M.A., *183:*186, 1963.

Drugs That
Affect Metabolism

· 27 ·

Pituitary Gland Hormones

ANATOMICAL ASPECTS
OF THE PITUITARY BODY

The pituitary gland is a tiny organ, hardly larger than a fingertip. It is located deep in the head just below the brain, to which it is connected by a stalk containing nerve fibers and blood vessels. Its true importance went unrecognized until this century, and, in fact, the name *pituitary*, derived from the Latin word for mucus, indicates the fact that for a long time its function was thought to be merely to supply moisture for the mucous membranes of the nose. (Another name for this body is *"hypophysis,"* which comes from the Greek for "undergrowth" and, at least, describes its anatomical relation to the brain accurately.)

It is now known that the pituitary gland exerts a profound influence over many vital metabolic processes. The forward, or anterior, portion of the pituitary body is the master gland of the entire *endocrine system*. In addition, through its vascular connections with the brain, the anterior pituitary gland is influenced by *nervous system* activity. Thus, it is now known that the body's two chief systems for controlling and integrating the activities of all the body's countless cells for the good of the whole organism are linked together at this point.

Actually, the pituitary body consists of two separate parts pushed together by an anatomical accident rather than by any shared function. Its anterior and posterior lobes have their origins in different parts of the embryo and then move toward one another to meet midway. The anterior lobe, or *adenohypophysis* (Gr. *adeno = gland*), which starts out in the embryo as part of the mouth, is made up of true glandular secretory tissue; the posterior portion develops from the floor of the brain, to which it remains connected, and it is made up largely of nerve fibers. Thus, this so-called *neural lobe*, or *neurohypophysis*, does not make its own secretions at all but only stores and releases hormones, which are made in the hypothalamic portion of the brain and transported to the posterior pituitary for storage.

The pituitary hormones, which play a vital physiological role by their influence on many metabolic functions, have had relatively few uses in medical treatment up to this time. However, as purified hormones become available and chemists learn to synthesize their active portions, these secretions may become much more important as therapeutic agents than they have been thus far.

In any case, we should have some familiarity with the actions of these hormones. This is so, not merely because of their occasional use as replacement therapy in certain relatively rare conditions in which patients with pituitary disease lack the natural secretions. A more important reason for understanding the actions of the pituitary hormones is that this will give us deeper insight into the functioning of other endocrine glands, such as the ovaries, thyroid, and adrenals, and into some ways by which various important metabolic functions—such as growth and water balance, for instance—are regulated.

THE POSTERIOR PITUITARY GLAND
AND ITS HORMONES

The neural lobe of the pituitary body, together with tissue that rises midway between it and the brain (the median eminence of the hypothalamus), makes up the neurohypophysis. It contains cells called *pituicytes*, which were once thought to synthesize the posterior pituitary hormones. This is now known not to be the case. Instead, these cells serve only as a storage depot for secretions that are made by certain nerve cells in the hypothalamus. The granules of these neurosecretions then travel down the nerve cell fibers (axons) that pass down the pituitary stalk to end in the neural lobe. When these hormones, which accumulate at the nerve fiber terminals, are required by body tissues, they are released from these storage sites by signals sent down to the posterior pituitary by way of these same hypothalamic nerve tracts.

This secretory material is made up of two substances: (1) the *oxytocic hormone* (oxy*tocin*), and (2) the *antidiuretic hormone* (ADH; vasopressin). Structurally, these substances are small peptide molecules made up of linked amino acids. These chains can now be built synthetically, and the pure synthetic hormones are, in fact, now available for clinical use. However, their most common source is still the dried, powdered glands of certain domestic animals and glandular extracts, from which each of the two hormones may be separated in purified form.

Oxytocin is thought to play a part in parturition, or childbirth, and in releasing the flow of milk from the mother's breast. Thus, this hormone is believed to initiate labor when it is released from the pituitary lobe as the result of a reflex set off by distention of the uterus and dilatation of the cervix.

Similarly, the suckling infant causes afferent nerve impulses to pass from the breast to the hypothalamus. Certain nerve cells in this portion of the brain then both secrete oxytocin and send down the nerve impulses that release the previously synthesized hormone from its storage sites in the posterior pituitary neural lobe. The hormone then drains into the blood stream which carries it to target tissues in the breast. This results in the ejection of milk from the alveoli of the mammary gland into the large ducts and sinuses that direct it into the baby's mouth. (The clinical use of oxytocin for this purpose is discussed in Chap. 39, together with the use of the purified natural and synthetic hormone in obstetrics.)

Vasopressin, or ADH, has a physiological regulatory function that is even more important, because it operates continuously rather than only occasionally. It acts constantly to keep the body from becoming excessively dehydrated, by acting on the kidneys in a manner that helps to conserve water that might otherwise be lost in the urine. Released from the posterior pituitary as required, this antidiuretic hormone is carried by the blood to its primary target tissues—certain portions of the renal tubular epithelium. Here, the hormone's action helps to increase the permeability of this tissue to the filtered water still contained in the tubules. Thus, this water re-enters the blood stream, instead of staying in the tubules and collecting ducts of the kidneys to be carried out of the body in the urine.

The Therapeutic Uses of Vasopressin

Diabetes insipidus, a condition marked by the excretion of copious quantities of sugar-free urine, is caused by a deficiency of the antidiuretic hormone. The lack of this secretion is, in turn, usually the result of a brain tumor or trauma affecting the hypothalamic neuro-

secretory cells and their nerve fiber tracts running in the pituitary stalk.

Sometimes, after surgical removal of the whole pituitary body (*hypophysectomy*), the patient may suffer a temporary episode of diabetes insipidus. However, if the hypothalamus and most of the nerve fibers in the stalk were not damaged during the operation, the patient quickly recovers his water-conserving ability. (Since the source of ADH is in these nerve cells, the mere removal of the posterior pituitary gland storage site does not keep more of the hormone from being produced and released directly into the blood stream as required.)

On the other hand, injury to the hypothalamo-hypophyseal tract or removal of tissue with a tumor at the base of the brain may result in varying degrees of permanent polyuria. As long as the patient can make up for his water loss by drinking equally large quantities of water (*polydipsia*, or excessive thirst), he is in little danger of severe dehydration. Nevertheless, when a patient is inconvenienced by the need to pass more than three or four liters of urine daily, replacement therapy with posterior pituitary extracts or with the purified hormone vasopressin is indicated. For the few patients who suffer from the distress and danger of having to void as much as 20 to 30 liters of urine each day, control of their condition by administration of the hormone from an outside source is essential and life-saving.

Properly administered, posterior pituitary extracts or vasopressin itself can help to conserve about 90 per cent of the water which would otherwise be lost by way of the kidneys of the diabetes insipidus patient. Administered by injection or by application to the mucous membranes of the nose, the exogenous hormone is absorbed and transported to the kidney tubular tissues that require it for adequate reabsorption of water from the glomerular filtrate. As a result, the patient with diabetes insipidus, who would otherwise lose large quantities of hypotonic urine, produces instead a scanty flow of highly concentrated fluid.

Administered in much larger doses, vasopressin causes contractions of the smooth muscles of the blood vessels and the gastrointestinal tract. These pharmacological actions are occasionally utilized clinically, but, because they also lead to adverse effects, other agents are usually preferred. For example, for patients in shock the adrenergic vasopressor drugs (Chap. 16) are considered more desirable than vasopressin because this hormone may constrict coronary vessels as well as peripheral arterioles. This could, of course, cause anginal pain, and it would be especially dangerous for patients who were in shock following a myocardial infarction.

Other uses of vasopressin injection are based upon its ability to increase the propulsive motility of the gastrointestinal tract of patients with postoperative abdominal distention. Here, however, cholinergic stimulants such as neostigmine are usually preferred. Similarly, vasopressin has been used for hastening elimination of gas from the intestine prior to X-ray of the gallbladder or other abdominal organs; however, most physicians prefer to order a cathartic such as castor oil for this purpose.

The relatively small replacement doses of vasopressin employed for diabetes insipidus cause few, if any, ill effects. However, administration of excessive amounts may cause abdominal cramps, nausea, and facial pallor. A more serious result of over-treatment with the antidiuretic hormone may be development of water intoxication. That is, the patient who has received an overdose of a long-acting hormone preparation such as vasopressin tannate in oil might be unable to rid his body of water that he had drunk. The reabsorbed fluid from this water load might then waterlog his tissues, with potentially dangerous results.

Preparations. For many patients application of dry powdered posterior pituitary extract to the nasal mucosa produces an adequate antidiuretic action, lasting about four to eight hours. When the patient's urinary volume is greater than seven or eight liters daily, he may require injections of vasopressin. A watery solution of this hormone controls such moderately severe cases when injected subcutaneously or intramuscularly. A suspension of vasopressin tannate in peanut oil provides very much longer-lasting symptomatic relief when absorbed slowly from an intramuscular depot injection site.

The Anterior Pituitary Gland and Its Hormones

The anterior pituitary gland contains cells of several different types, each capable of secreting a specific hormone. So far, six hormones have been obtained from this portion of the pituitary body. They are the *growth hormone somatotropin* (STH), which directly influences metabolic processes in many types of body tissues, and several so-called *tropic* (or *trophic*) hormones, which indirectly affect many body functions by their stimulating effects upon various other endocrine glands. The adenohypophyseal hormones of this kind include two *gonadotropic hormones,* which affect the functioning of the male and female sex glands; the *adrenocorticotropic hormone* (corticotropin; ACTH), which exerts its stimulating action on the cortex of the adrenal glands; the *thyrotropic hormone* (TSH), which activates the thyroid gland; and *prolactin* (luteotropin; LTH), which in humans acts mainly on the mammary glands but may also stimulate the corpus luteum of the ovaries of various animal species (Fig. 27-1).

Like the posterior pituitary, the anterior pituitary gland is under the regulatory control of the hypothalamus. Here, however, the glandular cells are made to secrete not by nerve impulses but by chemicals released by the brain cells. These neurosecretions, or neurohormones, of the hypothalamus are picked up by the blood in the capillary network between the brain and pituitary and are channeled directly to the gland cells without entering the general circulation.

Apparently, each type of anterior pituitary secretory cell is stimulated by a different peptide produced by the cells in the base of the brain. When each of these neurohormones arrives in the adenohypophysis by way of the special portal veins between the brain and the master gland, it stimulates secretion of a specific tropic hormone. Each of these, in turn, enters the systemic circulation and is carried to the endocrine target gland that it specifically stimulates. Thus, a so-called corticotropin-releasing factor from the brain (CRF) initiates the release of corticotropin from the anterior pituitary into the blood stream. This hormone then stimulates adrenal-gland synthesis of the steroid hormones that affect body tissue metabolism in many complex ways.

The secretion of the various tropic hormones of the anterior pituitary gland is itself regulated by the hormones of the endocrine glands that they stimulate. That is, there seems to be a mutual or reciprocal regulation between these hormones. Thus, when the level of thyroid hormones in the blood is low, the hypothalamus signals the pituitary gland to step up its secretion of thyrotropin, the thyroid-stimulating hormone (TSH). The resulting rise in the amount of thyroid hormone poured out into the blood leads to suppression of pituitary production of TSH and this, in turn, leads to a drop in thyroid-gland hormone production. Such *negative feedback* mechanisms assume considerable importance clinically when patients are being treated with pharmacological doses of adrenal cortex and sex gland hormones also.

Therapeutic Uses. Disease of the anterior pituitary gland leads to the partial failure of the intermediate or end-organ glands that depend upon the pituitary hormones for tropic stimulation. Although patients suffering from pituitary gland failure could be treated by replacement therapy with tropic pituitary hormones, their use is not considered clinically practicable at present.

Patients who show deficiencies of the target endocrine glands are treated with the hormones of those glands. Thus, thyroid hormone, sex steroids, etc., from an outside source are administered, because the pituitary hormones that might be given to make the person's own glands produce these secretions are more expensive, less reliable, and more difficult to administer. Because the pituitary hormones are proteins or polypeptides which would be digested if taken by mouth, they must be given by injection; also, as foreign proteins, they stimulate production of antibodies that may lead to allergic reactions as well as, eventually, to a lessening of their effectiveness.

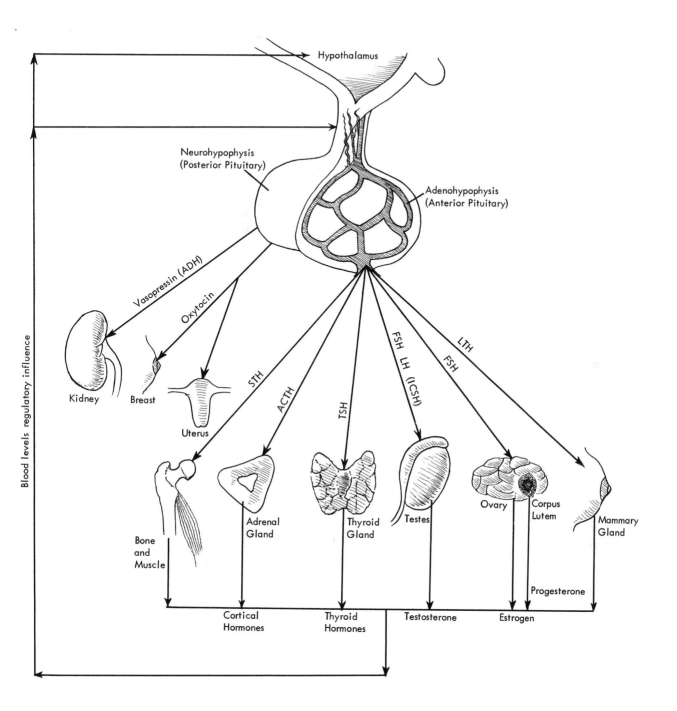

Hypothalamus

Neurohypophysis
(Posterior Pituitary)

Adenohypophysis
(Anterior Pituitary)

Blood levels regulatory influence

Vasopressin (ADH)

Oxytocin

STH

ACTH

TSH

FSH LH (ICSH)

FSH

LTH

Kidney

Breast

Uterus

Bone
and
Muscle

Adrenal
Gland

Thyroid
Gland

Testes

Ovary   Corpus
Lutem

Mammary
Gland

Cortical
Hormones

Thyroid
Hormones

Testosterone

Estrogen

Progesterone

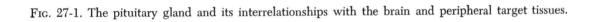

Fig. 27-1. The pituitary gland and its interrelationships with the brain and peripheral target tissues.

Nevertheless, there are some circumstances in which certain of the anterior pituitary hormones are employed. Their use may well increase in the future, as purified human pituitary hormones or their synthetic or semisynthetic modifications become more readily available. Thus, it seems desirable to discuss the current clinical status of several anterior pituitary hormones.

Human Growth Hormone

Children born with defective pituitary glands may remain midgets. This condition—hypopituitary dwarfism—results mainly from lack of growth hormone (somatotropin; STH). This substance, unlike the tropic hormones, acts not on other endocrine glands but upon all body tissues directly. Lack of this hormone leads to reduced protein formation and failure of bone growth, among other abnormalities. Replacement therapy overcomes the retarded growth of children with this condition.

Unfortunately, unlike most glandular extracts of pigs and cattle, the growth hormone obtained from these animals is ineffective in children. Apparently, people respond only to the secretion from the glands of monkeys and man. Human growth hormone (HGH) extracted from human pituitary glands removed at autopsy is now available, but it is, of course, in short supply and likely to remain so. According to one authority, only about 400 of an estimated 10,000 children with growth problems were being treated with HGH in 1968. Scientists hope, however, that they will be able to determine which part of the hormone molecule is responsible for its activity and, then, to synthesize the active fragment.

Meanwhile, human growth hormone has been used successfully to increase the height of several hundred youngsters. Small doses, injected 3 times weekly for several years, have helped these dwarfed adolescents develop to the height of small but normal adults. The hormone seems safe except for those with diabetic tendencies, in whom its anti-insulin action may bring about full-blown diabetes. All patients must have their blood sugar and glucose tolerance checked frequently to detect the presence of any diabetogenic effects from the growth hormone. (This action might be found to be therapeutically useful for patients with *hypogly-cemia*, if more of the hormone were available for trial in conditions other than pituitary dwarfism.)

The Adrenocorticotropic Hormone (ACTH)

The adrenocorticotropic hormone is produced by certain cells of the anterior pituitary gland and is released into the systemic circulation when that gland receives stimuli from the brain. The hypothalamus secretes a neurohormone, the corticotropin-releasing factor, CRF, which signals the pituitary cells to secrete the previously synthesized hormone. Carried by the blood stream to the adrenal glands, corticotropin then stimulates the outer coat, or cortex, to increase production of hormones—the several kinds of adrenocortical steroids (glucocorticoids, mineralocorticoids, and sex hormones).

Clinical Uses of Corticotropin (ACTH). In theory, corticotropin, or ACTH, should be therapeutically useful in most of the clinical conditions that are responsive to treatment with the adrenocorticosteroid drugs (Chap. 28). In practice, however, most such conditions are today treated with the *synthetic* corticosteroids rather than by attempting to stimulate increased secretion of the patient's own adrenal steroids by administering ACTH. For one thing, the patient's response to the synthetic steroids from an outside source is more predictable than the response of the patient's own adrenals to prodding by ACTH. In addition, the steroids can often be given in relatively convenient and less costly tablet form, whereas corticotropin must always be injected because it is a polypeptide that would be digested if taken by mouth. Also, such injections of ACTH, which is obtained from animal pituitary glands, sometimes cause allergic reactions. For these reasons, ACTH is being used less frequently today than it once was.

Some physicians, however, still prefer ACTH to the synthetic adrenal steroid hormones for some patients, because ACTH stimulates the adrenal cortex to release *all* the natural steroid hormones, including the male sex hormone. The latter hormone has *anabolic*, or protein-building, effects (Chap. 30). These are thought to be beneficial for patients with neuromuscular conditions which might be made worse by the muscle-wasting effects of therapy with synthetic glucosteroids alone.

Other doctors disagree with this view and prefer the corticosteroids to ACTH even in such cases. They argue that an anabolic agent can be added to the corticosteroid regimen, if desirable for a particular patient, and the disadvantages of ACTH therapy could thus be avoided. One of the most serious is this hormone's tendency to stimulate adrenal gland secretion of mineralocorticoids, the hormones responsible for retention of sodium and water and loss of potassium ions from the body (as indicated in Chap. 28, the new synthetic corticosteroids ordinarily do not do this).

Actually, ACTH is being used today mainly for diagnostic purposes in pituitary and adrenal diseases and for stimulating the adrenal glands of patients from whom corticosteroid drugs are being withdrawn after long-term treatment. To understand the theoretical basis for such therapy, we should briefly review the manner in which the pituitary and adrenal glands interact.

Regulation of Corticotropin Secretion. The rate of adrenal cortex secretion is, as we have seen, controlled by corticotropin released by the pituitary gland. The reverse is also true: when the circulating adrenal steroids reach the brain, they tend to suppress secretion of the hypothalamic nerve cell substances (i.e., CRF) responsible for the release of ACTH by the pituitary. This negative feedback mechanism serves to reduce further production of corticosteroids by the adrenal glands (Fig. 27-2).

In times of physical and emotional stress, the hypothalamic-pituitary secretion mechanism is released from inhibition by circulating steroids. The pituitary gland continues to pump out ACTH, and this, in turn, stimulates the adrenal glands to keep pouring out greater amounts of its hormones to help the body meet the stressful situation.

Use of ACTH in Steroid Withdrawal. In patients who have been taking steroid drugs the high levels of circulating *exogenous* steroids (i.e., from an outside source) suppress natural pituitary secretion of ACTH and this, in turn, leads to at least partial atrophy of the adrenal glands. Thus, these patients are deprived of a natural defense mechanism and, when the corticosteroid dosage is reduced or withdrawn, may be endangered by the body's inability to cope with sudden stressful emergencies (Chap. 28).

For this reason, some physicians try to reactivate the patient's adrenal glands by injecting ACTH during the time when corticosteroid drug therapy is gradually being withdrawn. Courses of ACTH given at this time are said to help stimulate the secretion of *endogenous* corticosteroids (i.e., by the patient's own adrenal glands). This also reduces the tendency to deterioration of the patient's condition when the drugs are withdrawn.

A disadvantage of corticotropin is its short duration of action. Thus, when given by vein, the drip must usually be continued for about eight hours; intramuscular injections of aqueous ACTH solutions must be repeated every six hours or so. To overcome this, repository forms have been developed which are slowly absorbed from intramuscular depot sites, so that the effects of a single injection upon the patient's adrenal glands will last up to 24 hours.

Metyrapone Test of Pituitary Function

Patients with severe pituitary deficiency (i.e., panhypopituitarism) are readily recognized: the clinical picture typically presents hypothyroidism, hypoadren-

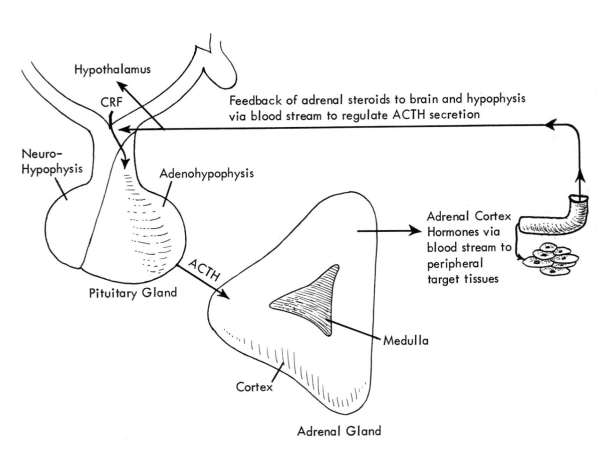

FIG. 27-2. Interrelationships between corticotropin secretion and adrenal cortical function.

ocorticism and hypogonadism—the result of hypofunctioning of target endocrine glands that are unstimulated by pituitary tropic hormones. However, borderline hypopituitarism is not so simple to detect. For example, the patient's pituitary gland may secrete adequate amounts of corticotropin (ACTH) under ordinary circumstances, and, consequently, his adrenal function may seem normal or only slightly abnormal.

However, when a patient with partial hypopituitarism is subjected to stress, the pituitary gland may be unable to respond with added corticotropin production. This, in turn, may send the patient into severe adrenal insufficiency. To prevent such an episode, in suspicious cases the doctor sometimes tries to evaluate the patient's pituitary reserve by subjecting him to a test to determine the gland's ability to step up corticotropin production under stress.

This is done by administering an agent called *metyrapone* or *methopyrapone* (Metopirone). This drug acts on the adrenal glands to block the biosynthesis of adrenal steroids. In people with normally functioning pituitary and adrenal glands, the resulting drop in plasma steroid levels releases the hypothalamus and pituitary from negative feedback inhibition by circulating steroids. This leads to intense stimulation of these areas; the pituitary gland then pours out increased corticotropin secretions in order to stimulate the adrenals and compensate for the low level of plasma corticosteroids.

The increase in corticotropin itself is not detectable by presently employed chemical tests of the blood and urine. However, the effects of adrenocorticotropic stimulation may be measured by the outpouring of adrenal steroid *precursors* into the patient's blood. The adrenals cannot produce the steroids themselves because the metyrapone previously administered prevents completion of their biosynthesis. Thus, only the precursors and their metabolites appear in the patient's urine.

Contrary to the case in people with normal pituitary function, patients with *impaired* pituitary function do not react to the stress of metyrapone administration with stepped-up production of adrenal steroid precursors. That is, the low plasma levels of corticosteroids brought about by this diagnostic drug fail to stimulate the patient's inadequate hypothalamic-pituitary mechanism to increase its output of corticotropin. Thus, measurement of the patient's blood and urine reveals abnormally low levels of adrenal gland products. Obviously, in order for this test to be meaningful, the patient's adrenal glands must be responsive to increased corticotropin secretion. This is determined by administering exogenous ACTH prior to performing the metyrapone test.

The Gonadotropic Hormones

As previously indicated, the anterior pituitary gland produces two gonad-stimulating hormones of different types. (1) the follicle-stimulating hormone (FSH), and (2) the luteinizing or interstitial-cell-stimulating hormone (LH or ICSH). A third pituitary hormone, prolactin, also has gonadotropic activity in some species.

Neither these pituitary secretions nor the gonad stimulating substances obtained from *non*-pituitary sources have ever had more than limited clinical utility. However, their physiological functioning is well worth discussing for two reasons: first, because some knowledge of the ebb and flow and the regulatory functions of pituitary gonadotropins is needed in order to understand the actions and clinical uses of the natural and synthetic gonadal hormones (the *estrogens, progestins,* and *androgens* discussed in Chaps. 29 and 30); second, because the results of recent studies in which human pituitary gonadotropin preparations have been employed for overcoming infertility indicate that their use for this important purpose may soon become practicable.

The Follicle-Stimulating Hormone. FSH is a glycoprotein first secreted by the anterior pituitary gland in large amounts at puberty. At that time of life, a preset "biological clock" within the brain apparently sets off changes in hypothalamic-hypophyseal function which lead to increased pituitary production of this hormone. In the female, FSH stimulates the ovaries to step up their secretion of the estrogens. These sex hormones then act to turn an immature girl into a woman capable of bearing children. The testes of the male are also prepared for their role in reproduction by the action of FSH.

Actions of FSH on the Ovary. After puberty, FSH continues to affect ovarian function cyclically all through the reproductive years of a woman's life. Early in each cycle, FSH released by the pituitary stimulates several primordial follicles in the ovary to grow. As they enlarge and develop under the influence of FSH (together, probably, with small amounts of LH), these follicles secrete *estrogens*. These ovarian sex hormones then act on the woman's reproductive system, including the inner lining of the uterus, or *endometrium*, which gradually grows in thickness (Fig. 27-3) during this so-called *proliferative phase* of the ovulatory cycle.

At the same time, the rising level of estrogens affects the production of pituitary gonadotropins. Through a negative feedback mechanism, the estrogens suppress the production and secretion of FSH. In addition, the female sex hormones trigger increased pituitary production of the second, or luteinizing, gonadotropin, LH (see below). Midway in the average 28-day menstrual cycle, the combined action of a sudden spurt of LH and the small amount of FSH still being released by the pituitary brings the ovarian follicle to maturity and causes the ripened egg sac to release an ovum, in the process called *ovulation* (Fig. 27-3).

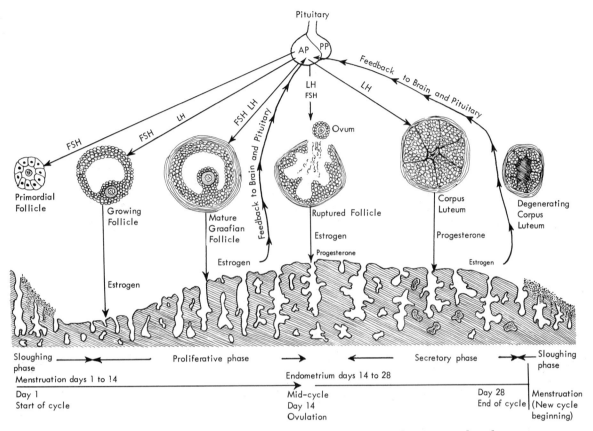

Fig. 27-3. Changes in the endometrium and ovary during the menstrual cycle.

Action of FSH on the Testis. In the male, FSH has only one function. It does *not* stimulate secretion of androgens, or male sex hormone, but it does have an effect on sperm production analogous to its role in helping to produce ova in females. Specifically, FSH produces this gametogenic effect in the male by stimulating the development of the seminiferous tubules of the testes. Such stimulation of testicular germinal epithelium influences *spermatogenesis,* the complex series of steps by which spermatozoa are produced and brought to maturity.

The Luteinizing Hormone. LH, or ICSH, the second gonadotropin produced by the anterior pituitary gland of both males and females, serves to stimulate hormone production by the gonads of both sexes.

Action of LH on the Ovary. As we have seen, LH plays an important part in causing ovulation to occur. Under its influence, the wall of the ripening follicle becomes thinner and thinner, until the tissue finally ruptures and the mature ovum is flushed out by the pressure of follicular fluid, which then floats it away from the ovary and into the opening of the oviduct or fallopian tube.

After the follicle breaks, LH continues to act upon the collapsed capsule. Under its influence, this thin epithelial membrane is converted into a thick, folded,

firm, glandular body, bright orange in color—the corpus luteum (Fig. 27-3). The luteal cells of this ovarian gland secrete a second kind of steroid in addition to estrogens. This substance, *progesterone,* acts upon the uterus which had been previously primed by estrogens. It converts the proliferative endometrium into the *secretory* type which is especially suited for receiving, implanting and nourishing a fertilized ovum.

In humans, this luteinizing hormone probably possesses *luteotropic* activity also. That is, it not only produces the corpus luteum but continues to sustain it and to stimulate its production of progesterone. Finally, however, if the ovum has not been fertilized, the rising level of ovarian hormones exerts its negative feedback effect on gonadotropin production by the pituitary. Apparently, the sex steroids signal certain hypothalamic nerve cells to suppress pituitary secretion of LH. Deprived of its hormonal support, the corpus luteum then shrivels and dies. This, in turn, leads to deterioration of the endometrium and to the onset of menstruation (Fig. 27-3).

If, however, the ovum is fertilized and forms a blastocyst that sinks roots (i.e., its outer layer of cells) down into the endometrium, the corpus luteum continues to produce progesterone. This occurs even though secretion of the *pituitary* gonadotropin, LH, has been inhibited, because the trophoblastic cells that will eventually help to form the placenta begin immediately to produce a gonadotropin with luteinizing and luteotropic activity (that is, the ability to continue to stimulate secretion of progesterone by the corpus luteum).

This *non*-pituitary hormone is *human chorionic gonadotropin* (HCG), which begins to appear in a woman's urine within a week or so after she becomes pregnant—a fact that forms the basis for several pregnancy tests. HCG obtained from pregnancy urine has been the gonadotropin chiefly employed clinically in the treatment of both males and females deficient in the pituitary luteinizing hormone, LH (see Therapeutic Uses).

Action of LH on the Testis. In the male, LH is known as the interstitial cell stimulating hormone (ICSH), because it stimulates the Leydig cells located in the interstices, or spaces, between the seminiferous tubules. These cells then secrete *androgens* (male sex hormones)—mainly testosterone, the growth hormone of the male accessory sex organs (Chap. 30). Thus, in theory at least, this gonadotropin might be expected to stimulate sluggish male gonads to secrete more testosterone when administered from an outside source.

The Luteotropic (LTH) or Lactogenic Hormone (Prolactin). In humans, this hormone—which, in some species, acts to keep the corpus luteum functioning— is believed to be responsible for initiating milk secretion by mammary glands previously prepared by the actions of female sex hormones. Such prior priming of the breasts by estrogens and progestins must precede the action of the lactogenic hormone (prolactin), yet these same hormones also suppress secretion of prolactin by the pituitary.

Therapeutic Uses. From the foregoing, one would expect that purified gonadotropic extracts should be useful in various clinical conditions caused by a lack of stimulation of a person's gonads by his own pituitary hormones. Such hypogonadism should respond to treatment with gonadotropins, in ways that would lead to maturity in cases of sexual infantilism and to ovulation and sperm production respectively in previously infertile females and males.

In practice, gonadotropins obtained from animal pituitary glands and other non-human sources (e.g., the serum of pregnant mares) have not proved to be very effective as therapeutic agents, partly because the patients quickly react to the foreign protein by forming antibodies that tend to destroy the animal-derived hormones. Hormones from human pituitary glands do not induce such antihormone production; however, such extracts have been in short supply, owing to the same conditions that have limited the availability of human growth hormone (p. 376).

Anovulation. Recently, purified gonadotropic hormones obtained from human pituitaries post mortem and from the urine of postmenopausal women have proved clinically effective. (Postmenopausal urine is rich in gonadotropins, because of their increased production by the pituitary when that gland is released from feedback inhibition by estrogens, secondary to gradual ovarian failure.) Startling results have reportedly been obtained when one of these purified products called *menotropins* (Pergonal) which is high in FSH activity, has been used in conjunction with human chorionic gonadotropin (high in LH) in the treatment of infertile women whose problem had been an inability to produce mature ova (only 5 to 10% of infertility cases).

These hormonal combinations have been employed successfully for stimulating ovulation. First, the FSH preparations from human pituitaries or from postmenopausal urine are injected daily usually for about ten days. When follicular stimulation has reached its peak, the doctor orders injection of human chorionic gonadotropin (HCG) daily, for one to four days. The luteinizing activity of this pregnancy urine extract causes the ripened follicle of the ovary to rupture and release its ovum, which may then be fertilized during its passage down the oviduct.

This treatment is said to have resulted in pregnancies in more than half the previously infertile women so treated. Undesirable effects seem to result mainly from overstimulation. For example, an unusual number of such pregnancies have resulted in *multiple* births, including quadruplets, quintuplets, and even miscarried septuplets! Another common complication has been a tendency for the ovaries of treated women to become excessively enlarged and hemorrhagic. Obviously, considerable study will be required before the use of human pituitary gonadotropins for this purpose and for treating infertility in males can be considered safe and effective.

Cryptorchidism. Human chorionic gonadotropin (HCG) has, up to now, been employed mainly for treating males rather than females, although its LH activity should, in theory, make it useful for helping to sustain the corpus luteum of women with amenorrhea resulting from failure of progesterone secretion. In practice, the new synthetic progestins, which can be conveniently taken by mouth, are preferred to injectable HCG for this purpose and for others requiring progestational activity, such as functional uterine bleeding (see Chap. 29).

HCG is, however, the preparation of choice in cryptorchidism, or undescended testicle. This is a condition in which the testes of young boys fail to descend from their fetal position in the abdomen. If uncorrected, this can lead to sterility as a result of damage to the germinal epithelium, with subsequent failure of sperm production. In such cases, provided that there is no mechanical obstruction requiring surgery, a course of HCG injections can often bring the testes down into the boy's scrotal sac.

Apparently, the interstitial-cell-stimulating (ICSH) activity of this extract leads to production of the male hormone, the action of which brings about descent of the testis. Failure of HCG to accomplish this or to elicit any other androgenic responses means that the patient's testes are either absent or atrophied and that he will require treatment with testosterone itself, preferably at puberty, in order to develop his accessory sex organs and secondary sex characteristics (see Chap. 30). On the other hand, youngsters being treated with HCG must be watched for signs of sexual precocity—the result of stimulation of excessive testosterone secretion at too early an age. The occurrence of frequent penile erections in such children serves as a warning that HCG dosage should be reduced or that the hormone should be administered less frequently.

Non-Gonadotropic (Indirect) Ovulation Induction

Some subfertile women have recently been treated successfully with *clomiphene citrate* (Clomid), a synthetic ovulation-inducing drug. This orally effective agent, which is itself neither a steroid nor a gonadotropic hormone, is thought to act by somehow triggering the release of the patient's own pituitary gonadotropins, particularly the luteinizing hormone. Thus, it is indicated for treating carefully selected anovulatory patients who wish to become pregnant.

Patients are selected for clomiphene therapy on the basis of laboratory and physical findings and a detailed history. The presence of tubal obstructions and neoplasms must be ruled out, and the patient must be free of such endocrine disorders as diabetes, thyroid or adrenal disease, and primary pituitary or ovarian failure. Since a functional pituitary gland and responsive ovaries are essential for success, the secretory status of these organs is first evaluated by a battery of tests.

The husband's fertility is, of course, also tested before his wife undertakes a course of clomiphene treatment, and the couple is advised concerning the importance of proper timing of coitus in relation to the days of drug therapy. (Courses of clomiphene are started on the fifth day following the beginning of progestin-induced or spontaneous menstrual bleeding and the patient then checks her basal body temperature pattern as a guide to the time of occurrence of ovulation and maximum fertility.)

Patients should be made aware that the incidence of multiple pregnancy is as much as ten times higher than normal in patients who conceive during a cycle in which they have received clomiphene. Patients are also advised as to possible adverse reactions that may be encountered during therapy, including side effects such as hot flashes, abdominal distention and discomfort, and abnormal ovarian enlargement and pain.

Patients are instructed to report visual symptoms, such as blurring of vision, as this requires discontinuation of treatment and ophthalmological examination. The significance of these visual difficulties is not understood, but patients should be warned not to drive until blurring, spots, and flashes disappear, usually within a few days.

REVIEW QUESTIONS

1. (a) Name the two parts of the pituitary gland and indicate the kind of tissue of which each is made up.

(b) What part of the brain influences pituitary gland function, and how does the mechanism by which posterior pituitary hormones are released differ from the way in which the brain brings about the release of anterior pituitary secretions?

2. (a) Name the two types of posterior pituitary hormone and indicate the target tissues for each secretion.

(b) What are some therapeutic uses of posterior pituitary hormones of each type?

3. (a) Explain briefly how patients who lack the antidiuretic hormone are helped by the action of vasopressin or of posterior pituitary extract administered as replacement therapy.

(b) At what other tissues do pharmacological doses of vasopressin act to produce effects that both have some therapeutic usefulness and also result in adverse reactions that limit the drug's usefulness?

4. (a) List the names of the six main hormones synthesized and secreted by the anterior pituitary gland.

(b) Explain briefly how a tropic hormone of the pituitary (such as TSH, for example) affects the function of another endocrine gland and how that gland, in turn, exerts a negative feedback effect upon pituitary secretion of that particular tropic hormone.

5. (a) For what purpose is somatotropin employed clinically?

(b) What precautions are required during the long-term use of this hormone?

6. (a) What is the site of action of corticotropin (ACTH) and what is the result of such an action?

(b) What is the effect of high levels of circulating adrenal corticosteroid hormones upon the secretion of ACTH by the pituitary gland?

7. (a) What are some of the disadvantages of ACTH therapy in comparison to corticosteroid therapy in the conditions for which either may be employed?

(b) For what patients is ACTH sometimes preferred to corticosteroid drug therapy?

8. (a) What action of ACTH may be dangerous for patients with cardiovascular diseases?

(b) What other reaction sometimes follows a course of ACTH injections?

9. (a) What is one of the main uses of ACTH therapy in conjunction with corticosteroid drugs?

(b) What is the theoretical basis for such treatment?

10. (a) What property of ACTH makes its administration inconvenient?

(b) What form of ACTH preparation has been developed to overcome this disadvantage?

11. (a) What drug is used in the diagnosis of partial hypopituitarism, and where does it act to produce its primary effects?

(b) How is the difference in normal and abnormal pituitary gland function detected after administration of this diagnostic drug?

12. (a) What is the result of increased pituitary production of FSH at puberty in girls?

(b) What is the result of increased secretion of FSH during the first half of the menstrual month?

13. (a) What is the effect of increasing plasma levels of estrogens upon the production of FSH by the anterior pituitary?

(b) What is the effect of a rise in FSH production upon the testes of the male?

14. (a) What hormones are produced by the ovaries and by the testes under the influence of the pituitary gonadotropin, LH?

(b) What is the effect of a rising level of ovarian hormones upon pituitary production in an ovarian cycle in which a released ovum has not been fertilized; what happens when an ovum is fertilized?

15. (a) What are two present sources of gonadotropins with high FSH activity and one source of gonadotropins high in LH activity?

(b) For what clinical purpose and in what manner are these two gonadotropins being presently employed in women?

(c) Name a *non*-gonadotropic synthetic drug used for this same purpose.

16. (a) For what purpose is clomiphene citrate employed, and what is the manner in which it is thought to bring about its therapeutic action?

(b) What are some points about which couples should be counseled when the wife undertakes clomiphene therapy?

17. (a) For what other general purpose should a preparation with the activity of the pituitary hormone, LH, be useful in treating women?

(b) For what purpose is such a preparation employed in treating young males?

BIBLIOGRAPHY

Vasopressin (ADH)

Cannon, J. F.: Diabetes insipidus. Arch. Int. Med., *96:* 215, 1955.

Randall, R. V.: Treatment of diabetes insipidus. Modern Treatment, 3:180, 1966 (Jan.).

Wagner, H. N., Jr., and Braunwald, E.: The pressor effect of the antidiuretic principle of the posterior pituitary in orthostatic hypotension. J. Clin. Invest., 35:1412, 1956.

Corticotropin (ACTH), etc.

Hench, P. S.: Cortisone and ACTH in clinical medicine. Proc. Mayo Clin., 25:474, 1950.

Liddle, G. W., Duncan, L. E., Jr., and Morley, E. H.: Dual mechanism regulating adrenocortical function in man. Am. J. Med., 21:380, 1956.

Thorn, G. W., *et al.:* Clinical usefulness of ACTH and cortisone. New Eng. J. Med., 242:783; 824; 865, 1950.

Gonadotropins, etc.

Beck, P., *et al.:* Induction of ovulation with clomiphene . . . including comparison with intravenous estrogen and human chorionic gonadotropin. Obstet. Gynec., 27:54, 1966.

Gemzell, C. A.: Induction of ovulation with human pituitary gonadotropins. Fertil. Steril., *13:*153, 1962.

Greenblatt, R. B., *et al.:* Induction of ovulation with MRL/41. J.A.M.A., *178:*101, 1961.

Kistner, R. W.: Further observations on the effects of clomiphene citrate in anovulatory females. Am. J. Obstet. Gynec., *92:*380, 1965.

Growth Hormone

Raben, M. S.: Growth hormone. 1. Physiological aspects. 2. Clinical uses of human growth hormone. New Eng. J. Med., *266:*21; 82, 1962.

Rosenbloom, A. L.: Growth hormone replacement therapy. J.A.M.A., *198:*364, 1966.

The Adrenocorticosteroid Drugs

HISTORICAL ASPECTS

The substances known as adrenocorticosteroids are among the most important therapeutic agents employed in modern medicine. The discovery, in 1948, of the potent anti-inflammatory activity of *cortisone,* an adrenal gland hormone, marked the opening of a new era in medical treatment. Following the announcement by Hench, Kendall and other Mayo Clinic doctors of the dramatic improvement that cortisone had brought about in patients suffering from severe rheumatoid arthritis, this steroid and the even more potent related hormone, *hydrocortisone,* were tried in the treatment of many other acute and chronic clinical conditions.

These natural, gland-produced chemicals and another—*corticotropin* (ACTH), the anterior pituitary hormone that controls their biosynthesis by the adrenal cortex (Chap. 27)—proved strikingly successful for relieving painful and disabling symptoms in dozens of diseases. However, increasing clinical experiences with these so-called miracle drugs revealed that they had many drawbacks and dangers. This set off an intensive search for synthetic corticosteroids which, it was hoped, would be free of the disadvantages of the natural adrenal gland hormones.

Research in this area did, indeed, prove successful in many respects. Small structural changes made at a few key points in the complex corticosteroid molecule resulted in compounds of markedly increased potency and fewer side effects. However, the presently available synthetic adrenocorticosteroids continue to be a two-edged sword capable of doing both great good and much harm. Indeed, their development has been compared with that of atomic energy in terms of the potential of both scientific advances for constructive and destructive activity.

Before discussing the current status of these drugs in modern therapy, we must first review some of the physiological functions of the hormones naturally secreted by the human adrenal cortex.

THE HORMONES OF THE ADRENAL CORTEX

The two adrenal glands are flattened bodies that fit like a cap over the top of each kidney. Each gland is made up of an inner core, the medulla, and an outer shell or bark, the cortex. The adrenal medulla is composed of dark brown chromaffin cells which secrete catecholamines such as *epinephrine.* The physiological functions of this hormone and of *norepinephrine* are discussed in Chapter 16, which deals with the actions of autonomic nervous system neurohormonal substances.

The adrenal cortex, which surrounds the medulla, is made up of three layers of cells, which produce several different kinds of chemicals. These substances, which differ both in their chemical structures and physiological functions, include:

1. The *glucocorticoids*—substances such as *hydrocortisone (cortisol)* and *cortisone,* which, as the name implies, have potent effects upon glucose or carbohydrate metabolism;

2. The *mineralocorticoids,* such as *aldosterone* and *desoxycorticosterone* which influence salt and water metabolism;

3. Certain *sex hormones,* such as the relatively weak androgen or male hormone, *dehydroepiandrosterone,* and smaller amounts of *testosterone* and of the female hormones, such as *progesterone* and *estradiol.*

The adrenal sex steroids are of clinical importance only when secreted in excess in pathological states or when their production, even in ordinary amounts, stimulates the growth of certain sex tissue cancers. The glucocorticoids and mineralocorticoids, on the other hand, are necessary for life, and death occurs

383

rapidly when the adrenal cortex fails to produce these hormones.

THE PHYSIOLOGICAL FUNCTIONS OF ADRENAL CORTEX HORMONES

The adrenocortical steroid hormones have various biological properties that help higher animal organisms—including humans—to cope with the changes constantly taking place in their environment. When these hormones are absent, as a result of disease of the adrenal glands or their surgical removal, profound metabolic imbalances develop. These changes in *electrolyte and water balance*, and in *carbohydrate, protein and fat metabolism* interfere with the individual's ability to keep his internal environment constant (i.e., homeostasis).

Among the hormones most important for survival are those with high *mineralocorticoid* activity. When *aldosterone*, for example, is deficient, the kidney tubules lose their ability to return to the blood some of the sodium that was filtered through the glomeruli. As a result of the steady drain of sodium that then develops, the volume of the blood and extracellular fluid declines steadily. If this condition is unchecked, blood pressure falls to shock levels and the patient dies of circulatory collapse.

The metabolic effects of those adrenal cortex hormones that are classified as *glucocorticoids* are extremely complex. In ways that are still not at all well understood, these steroid substances have widespread direct and indirect effects on many enzymes and on metabolic processes of all types. In this way, the glucocorticoids influence the functioning of various vital organs and systems. In their absence, the individual shows not only marked weakness of the skeletal muscles but a reduction in his capacity to cope with stress. Thus, the glucocorticoids play a vital role in aiding the organism to meet emergencies set off by trauma, infection, and other stressful situations.

ADRENAL INSUFFICIENCY AND ITS TREATMENT

Adrenal Insufficiency. People whose adrenal glands fail to synthesize adequate amounts of corticosteroids sooner or later develop symptoms of adrenal deficiency. Such symptoms may be mild or severe, depending on the extent of the patient's hormonal lack. In some cases, the patient may get along well enough ordinarily and show symptoms only when he is subjected to unusual stress. Other patients may have a complete lack of cortical hormones such that they are in continuous danger of going into acute adrenal crisis unless they receive substitution therapy with adrenal hormones from an outside source.

In the past, the most common cause of adrenal insufficiency was *Addison's disease*. In this condition, the adrenal cortices may be destroyed by tuberculosis or become atrophied owing to various other factors. Today, with the introduction of *adrenalectomy* and *hypophysectomy* (Chap. 44) for the treatment of cancers of certain types, severe diabetes, and other serious disorders, many more patients require replacement of selected adrenal cortical hormones from an outside source, in order to avoid death as a result of their complete and permanent lack of adrenal mineralocorticoids and glucocorticoids.

Another modern cause of adrenal insufficiency is adrenal atrophy resulting from the prolonged use of large doses of glucocorticoids in the treatment of various chronic diseases. As indicated in the previous chapter, such exogenously administered corticosteroids inhibit anterior pituitary release of corticotropin (ACTH), and this, in turn, both reduces adrenal production of hydrocortisone and leads, in time, to a withering of the glands themselves. Then, when the steroid hormone therapy is discontinued, the patient's own atrophied adrenal glands may be incapable of producing enough of these hormones to meet his needs.

Replacement Therapy. Patients who have been tided over an acute adrenal crisis may often be maintained on only small physiological doses of *hydrocortisone* taken together with ample amounts of sodium chloride. Many patients with chronic adrenal insufficiency following adrenalectomy or from addisonian atrophic lesions require only 15 to 30 mg. of hydrocortisone daily to replace the amount of the natural hormone which would ordinarily be secreted. Patients whose adrenal insufficiency stems from a lack of corticotropin following hypophysectomy or from disease of the anterior pituitary gland need even less hydrocortisone—usually only about 5 mg. after each meal.

Most patients, however, must have a steroid with mineralocortical activity higher than that of hydrocortisone. The natural mineralocorticoid *desoxycorticosterone acetate* (see Drug Digest) is often given daily by intramuscular injection to aid the kidney in retaining sodium and thus prevent dehydration and hypotension. Later, the patient may be switched to a longer-acting ester, *desoxycorticosterone trimethyl acetate*, which has salt-retaining effects that last several weeks after a single injection. A synthetic steroid with both glucocorticoid and quite potent mineralocorticoid activity is *fludrocortisone acetate*, which has the advantage of being effective when taken by mouth in a dose as small as 0.1 mg. daily. Thus, patients who once would not have survived are now kept well indefinitely on corticosteroid substitution therapy combined with dietary salt supplements.

PHARMACOLOGICAL EFFECTS OF CORTICOSTEROIDS

Replacement of the missing hormones of patients suffering from adrenal insufficiency often has dramatic and lifesaving effects. However, the use of small, physiological amounts of corticosteroids for such substitution therapy is relatively rare. Very much more often, these substances are administered clinically in amounts much greater than those secreted each day by the adrenal glands. Such *supra*physiologic, or pharmacological, doses are sometimes employed for supporting body functions during severe stress and, most often, for their anti-inflammatory activity in very many conditions in which the patient's own adrenal glands are perfectly capable of producing ordinary amounts of their hormones.

Anti-inflammatory Action. The pharmacological effects of the natural and synthetic corticosteroids that are most commonly sought for in the treatment of many conditions are brought about by their so-called *anti-inflammatory action.* The way in which larger-than-ordinary amounts of these steroids suppress the usual response of body tissues to injury or abnormal stimulation is still very much of a mystery. Yet it is their remarkable ability to inhibit tissue reactions to trauma, irritants, infectious agents and the biologically active chemicals released when cells are injured in an antigen-antibody reaction that accounts for the clinical utility of the corticosteroids in so many and varied conditions.

Inflammation is a complex mechanism that often serves to protect the body from further damage by bacteria, viruses, physical injury, chemical irritants and toxins. Yet, an inflammatory response—which may serve, for example, to wall off and localize invading microorganisms, destroy and remove injurious material, and initiate healing and repair processes—is also the source of some of the most painful and disabling manifestations of disease.

Corticosteroids, administered in adequate doses, suppress the main signs of inflammation—the characteristic local redness, heat and swelling, and the pain that usually accompanies them. This occurs because of the ability of these drugs somehow to affect both the blood vessels and the tissues adjacent to the point of injury. As a result, the increase in capillary permeability that ordinarily leads to leakage of fluid into the tissues, with resulting local edema, fails to occur. Blood vessels do not become dilated and congested, and the phagocytes usually brought to the area by the blood in large numbers no longer make their way out through the vessel walls into the tissues. Under the influence of the natural hormones and the synthetic compounds of this class, the late destructive effects of inflammation also often fail to develop. That

is, the proliferation of capillaries and of tissue cells such as fibroblasts is inhibited, and late scarring by fibrous tissue growth is prevented.

Although the corticosteroids relieve pain and prevent disability, they do not get at the cause of the inflammatory reaction. This means that the steroids *do not cure any of the diseases* for which they are given and, if they are used unwisely, may even make some conditions worse. Obviously, for example, suppression of a local inflammatory response set off by tuberculosis bacteria or other microorganisms may lead to their spread throughout an organ (e.g., the lungs) or even the entire body.

Other Actions. The administration of inflammation-suppressing amounts of the natural adrenal hormones has proved to have other drawbacks also. For example, when hydrocortisone is given for more than a short time in doses much greater than the amounts normally secreted by a person's glands, it can cause potentially dangerous changes of many kinds in metabolic processes and endocrine function.

These adverse effects of supraphysiologic amounts of this hormone include:

1. An alteration in mineral (electrolyte) metabolism that may result in excessive retention of sodium and water and in the loss of potassium.

2. Effects on *carbohydrate, fat* and *protein* metabolism, which may cause signs and symptoms similar to those of *Cushing's syndrome,* a relatively rare endocrine disorder which is caused ordinarily by pituitary or adrenal gland hyperactivity.

3. Suppression of the secretion of *corticotropin* (ACTH) by the anterior pituitary gland, which leads, in turn, to a decrease in production of the patient's own adrenal hormones.

Under continued high doses of hydrocortisone from an outside (*exogenous*) source, *endogenous* secretion of this hormone by the patient's adrenals may cease completely, and the adrenal cortices may become progressively atrophied.

Synthetic Corticosteroids. Organic chemists have tried to alter the naturally occurring steroid molecules in ways that would intensify their desirable anti-inflammatory action while eliminating the other pharmacological effects, which are considered clinically undesirable. Although they have succeeded in developing new synthetic steroid molecules of much greater potency than those built by the body, the molecule-manipulating chemists have been only partially successful in separating the therapeutically useful actions of these synthetic steroids from the adverse effects that limit their utility.

The most important difference between the natural glucocorticoids, such as cortisone and hydrocortisone, and the newer synthetic steroids (Table 28-1) is that most of the latter are relatively free of sodium-retain-

TABLE 28-1

ADRENOCORTICOSTEROID DRUGS *

Nonproprietary or Official Name	Synonym or Proprietary Name	Usual Doses † and Dosage Ranges
Betamethasone N.F.	Celestone	600 mcg. to 4.8 mg. daily, oral
Cortisone acetate N.F.	Cortogen; Cortone	Oral 25 mg. q.i.d.; I.M. 100 mg. daily
Dexamethasone N.F.	Decadron; Deronil; Decameth; Gammacorten; Hexadrol	500 mcg. to 6 mg. daily; 750 mcg. 2 to 4 times daily
Dexamethasone sodium phosphate N.F.	Decadron phosphate	0.4 to 6 mg. per local injection
Hydrocortisone U.S.P.	Cortisol; Cortef; Cortifan; Cortril; Hydrocortone, etc.	10 to 300 mg. daily; oral 10 mg. up to 4 times a day
Hydrocortisone acetate U.S.P.	Cortef acetate, etc.	10 to 50 mg. intra-articular
Hydrocortisone cypionate	Cortef fluid	Initially 20 to 500 mg.; maintenance 10 to 260 mg.
Hydrocortisone sodium succinate U.S.P.	Solucortef	50 to 300 mg. daily I.V. or I.M.
Methylprednisolone sodium succinate N.F.	—	10 to 40 mg. daily I.V. or I.M.
Methylprednisolone N.F.	Medrol	Oral 4 mg. q.i.d. or 2 to 60 mg. daily
Paramethasone acetate	Haldrone	Oral 6 to 12 mg. initially; 1 to 8 mg. maintenance
Prednisolone U.S.P.	Delta Cortef; Hydeltra; Meticortelone; Metiderm; Paracortol; Sterane; Sterolone	Oral 5 mg. 1 to 4 times daily for 2 to 7 days; then 5 mg. one or more times a day. Range: 5 to 80 mg. daily
Prednisolone acetate U.S.P.	Sterane	5 to 50 mg. intra-articular; 5 to 80 mg. daily I.M.
Prednisolone sodium phosphate U.S.P.	Hydeltrasol	10 to 100 mg. I.M. or IV.
Prednisone U.S.P.	Deltasone; Deltra; Meticorten; Paracort	Initially 5 mg. 2 to 4 times a day for 2 to 7 days; maintenance, up to 5 mg. one or more times a day. Range: 5 to 80 mg. daily
Triamcinolone	Aristocort; Kenacort	Initially 8 to 30 mg. daily orally for adults; 4 to 16 mg. daily for children; reduce for maintenance

* These drugs are administered orally or parenterally for systemic or intra-articular actions of an anti-inflammatory or anti-stress type. Other steroids and dosage forms are available for topical application and for mineralocorticoid activity.

† Doses vary very widely, depending on the nature and severity of the condition that is being treated. Equivalent milligram dosages of the glucocorticoids are given in Table 28-2.

ing activity. That is, the natural steroid molecules have been modified in ways that markedly increase their anti-inflammatory potency without a corresponding increase in mineralocorticoid activity.

Actually, the first attempt to alter the biological actions of hydrocortisone by treating it chemically so that a fluorine atom was inserted into one of the rings in the complex steroid molecule (Fig. 28-1) resulted in formation of compounds in which both glucocorticoid and mineralocorticoid activity were markedly increased. *Fludrocortisone*, which is an example of such a synthetic steroid, has so prohibitively high a mineralocorticoid activity that it is never taken internally (except by patients with adrenal insufficiency). Its high glucocorticoid activity is utilized usually only in *topical* administration against inflammatory skin reactions, because of the dangerous edema that may develop, upon systemic administration, as a result of its strong sodium-retaining effect.

The first truly useful fruit of research on the chemical structure–biological activity relationships of adrenocorticosteroid molecules came with the synthesis of *prednisone* and *prednisolone*. These synthetic steroid compounds, which differ from cortisone and hydrocortisone chemically only by the presence of a single double bond in one of the steroid rings, differ from the two natural hormones biologically by being four or five times more powerful in their anti-inflammatory and other glucocorticoid activity while possessing no added salt-retaining potency.

Further research resulted in the discovery of other new families of steroid compounds in which the anti-inflammatory action was selectively increased and the electrolyte-water-retaining effect was entirely eliminated. In practice, this means not only that less than 1 mg. of potent synthetic steroids such as *dexamethasone* and *betamethasone* will do the work of 25 mg. of cortisone (Table 28-2), but that they will do so without causing the tissues to become waterlogged, as equivalent anti-inflammatory doses of cortisone and hydrocortisone do. This property makes them especially useful for patients with heart disease, high blood pressure, and other conditions that would be affected adversely by a drug-induced accumulation of salty fluids in the tissues.

Unfortunately, despite their relative freedom from undesirable edema-producing effects, the synthetic steroids still retain all the rest of the undesirable pharmacological actions of high doses of the natural adrenal hormones. That is, the continued use of even small supraphysiologic doses may depress the patient's own adrenal gland activity; more important, they may bring about a state of hypercorticism marked by Cushingoid signs and symptoms (see Adverse Effects) and expose some patients to other dangers such as diabetes, osteoporosis and peptic ulcer. Thus, the doctor always tries to keep patients taking corticosteroid drugs under close observation and urges the patient to stay in touch with him. The nurse should also make clear to the patient that it is important to visit the clinic for frequent checks while he is taking corticosteroids.

Scientists are still searching for synthetic steroids which will have a *selective anti-inflammatory action* without any of the associated adverse actions of present-day steroid therapy that will be discussed in a later section. Some doctors doubt that this will ever be possible. They reason that the corticosteroids suppress inflammatory reactions by their ability to exert a basic inhibitory effect upon protein metabolism, which, in turn, produces related changes in the way the body handles carbohydrates and fats. Thus, they argue, the prolonged administration of anti-inflammatory doses of any corticosteroid must result inevitably in metabolic signs of steroid activity such as muscle weakness (the result of protein wastage), hyperglycemia such as that found in diabetes (because of conversion of amino acids from proteins into glucose), and a peculiar redistribution of the body's fat deposits, as well as many other undesirable results of corticosteroid-induced changes in metabolism and in mental and endocrine gland functioning.

The practical significance of the failure, thus far, to dissociate the desirable from the undesirable effects of the corticosteroids is this: The *prolonged* use of any corticosteroid for treating chronic conditions is always likely to cause potentially disabling side effects. No matter which drug is employed, pharmacological doses of equivalent anti-inflammatory activity will produce adverse effects when used for more than a few days or weeks. Thus, the doctor has to decide whether the risk of embarking on long-term steroid treatment of a chronic condition is really worth taking. If he decides to do so, the doctor often discusses the risks with the patient and tries to make clear to him the need to return for regular examinations to detect signs of drug toxicity.

THE THERAPEUTIC USES OF THE ADRENOCORTICOSTEROID DRUGS

The adrenocorticosteroids have been used to relieve the symptoms and signs of countless conditions. The remarkable ability of these drugs to inhibit inflammatory reactions and thus to reduce pain and disability accounts for their use in many disorders involving tissues and organs of every type. In addition, however, both the natural hormones and their synthetic analogues possess a capacity for carrying critically ill patients past periods of very severe stress. Thus, although these steroids do not, as we have noted, constitute a cure for any disease, their combined *anti-inflammatory* and *antistress* actions sometimes help to save patients whose lives are threatened by acute illnesses. These drugs also aid in prolonging the lives of patients suf-

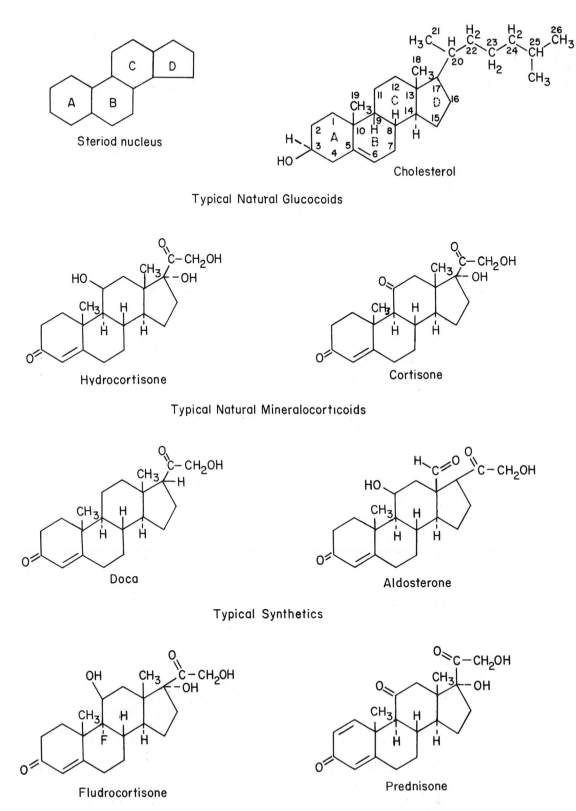

FIG. 28-1. Examples of typical corticosteroids. The action of the compound is related to the structural variations in the molecule. (See text, pp. 385 and 387, for discussion.)

fering from diseases that are presently considered incurable.

How the doctor uses these drugs—or, indeed, whether he decides to use them at all—depends upon many factors. From the following discussion of their therapeutic uses, certain *general principles* in regard to appropriate and effective employment of these drugs in various conditions should become clear. More detailed discussion of the use of specific kinds of corticosteroid preparations in particular clinical conditions is reserved for various chapters in Section 7.

Pathological States

The corticosteroids are used in conditions so varied in etiology and so numerous that any attempt to classify the diseases that have been reported to be responsive to treatment is doomed to failure. However, because even a broad and overlapping classification may make it easier for the student to remember the bewildering array of disorders for which steroid therapy has been advocated, the following grouping of steroid-responsive diseases, which is based primarily on resemblances in their underlying pathology, is offered as an aid to study:

Collagen Diseases. These are conditions in which certain characteristic changes occur in the connective tissue of various organs (*collagen* is a connective tissue protein found in the deeper layers of the skin, in the joints and elsewhere). Although the diseases of this tissue are grouped together, they probably do not have a common cause and they vary considerably in their end results. All are serious: some are disabling rather than deadly; others are invariably fatal. Among these conditions, which have in common a responsiveness to treatment with corticosteroids, which often afford temporary relief, are: rheumatoid arthritis, rheumatic fever, disseminated lupus erythematosus, dermatomyositis, scleroderma, periarteritis nodosa, and pemphigus.

Allergic and Infectious Diseases of the Skin and the Mucous Membranes. This is a very broad grouping of conditions, based only on the fact that corticosteroids often suppress the nonspecific inflammatory response of the epithelial tissues to both antigen-antibody reactions and invasion by infectious bacteria. It includes allergic dermatoses; allergic rhinitis and pollinosis; allergic and bacterial conjunctivitis, and inflammation of many other eye structures; bronchial asthma and status asthmaticus.

Hematological and Neoplastic Conditions. In these serious conditions, including the leukemias and most especially the kinds of leukemia that involve the lymphoid tissues, such as acute and chronic lymphocytic leukemia, the corticosteroids often produce remarkable although temporary remissions. In other kinds of leukemia (e.g., the acute granulocytic type), in *non-neoplastic* blood dyscrasias (e.g., aplastic anemia,

agranulocytosis), and in patients with solid tumors (e.g., carcinoma of the breast), steroid drugs are often beneficial in that they make the patient feel better, even when they do little to produce a remission of physical symptoms.

Miscellaneous Acute Emergencies. In many conditions besides adrenal insufficiency, large doses of corticosteroids often help to overcome states of shock or otherwise to tide the patient over in a life-threatening situation. Among these are conditions involving the central nervous system (e.g., encephalitis; meningitis) or the heart (e.g., acute heart block in myocarditis), and various fulminating bacterial infections caused by gram negative or tuberculosis microorganisms (e.g., endotoxic shock, bacteremia, tuberculous meningitis).

Miscellaneous Chronic Conditions. Examples of serious conditions which may be controlled by long-term steroid therapy (and by steroids during acute flare-ups as well) are ulcerative colitis and idiopathic nephrosis. In the former condition, corticosteroids are best given by retention enema if the intestinal inflammation can be reached by topically applied steroids and as long as it remains responsive to them. In more severe and widespread colitis and in the chronic kidney disease large doses may have to be administered intermittently for long periods, despite the risk of steroid toxicity.

DOSAGE AND ADMINISTRATION OF CORTICOSTEROIDS

Once the doctor decides to employ steroid drugs, he must try to determine the dose that will give the particular patient good symptomatic relief without causing disabling drug-induced side effects. The amount of adrenocorticoids that the doctor orders varies very widely, depending upon the severity of the illness and the patient's response to these drugs and the other medications with which he is being treated. The following sampling of several kinds of conditions that are sometimes treated with steroids is intended to indicate some of the different ways in which steroid drugs are administered.

Chronic Nonfatal Conditions

Patients with chronic diseases that almost never pose direct threat to life are kept off steroid drug treatment as long as possible. Thus, in *rheumatoid arthritis* the patient is always managed first by more conservative treatment measures. As indicated in Chapter 41, these include a regimen of rest, physical therapy, corrective exercises and salicylates. Most doctors prefer to try other antirheumatic drugs such as phenylbutazone, indomethacin, and even courses of gold salts or the so-called antimalarial drugs (e.g., chloroquine) before turning to corticosteroid therapy. The reason for this is that once arthritic patients have gained the remarkable relief that corticosteroids can bring they are often unwilling to give these drugs up despite their dangers.

The same is true of patients with another chronic condition, *bronchial asthma,* who also often tend to become psychologically and physically dependent upon corticosteroids. The steroid drugs often affect the patient's mood; they may have a euphoric effect—i.e., conferring a sense of well-being that stems from C.N.S. stimulation rather than from relief of pain and discomfort alone. This action, as well as the tendency of these chronic conditions to flare up into acute episodes, makes withdrawal of steroids from patients with chronic arthritis or asthma often very difficult. (See p. 393 for a further discussion of how steroids are best withdrawn.)

In some circumstances, however, the continued use of corticosteroids for such patients is considered justified. When none of the more conservative measures serves to control the progress of the patient's chronic disorder and he is threatened with permanent disability and possible loss of his livelihood, the doctor may reluctantly turn to corticosteroids. For example, if chronic intractable asthma threatens to produce deformity of the patient's rib cage or seems likely to lead to severe emphysema, the patient may justifiably be placed on steroid drug therapy.

The doctor starts out in such cases by adding to the patient's present regimen a relatively small daily dose of a steroid drug—for example, about 10 mg. of prednisone or equivalent dosage of one of the newer synthetic steroids (Table 28-2). Such small initial amounts are then raised very slowly to levels that will keep the patient comfortable and able to work at his job. The doctor does not, however, aim at eliminating *all* of the arthritic or asthmatic patient's symptoms, and, in fact, he tries to cut back on corticosteroid dosage periodically, even if this increases the patient's complaints somewhat. The reason for keeping steroid dosage at the minimum that will give adequate relief is that doses of prednisone much above 5 mg.—or any other steroid in the amount that will give equivalent anti-inflammatory effects (Table 28-2)—must sooner or later produce signs and symptoms of mild and, later, of moderate or severe hypercorticism (see Adverse Effects, p. 391).

The clinic nurse, or the nurse in the doctor's office, can often help explain to the patient the need for reducing his steroid dosage. The patient must be made to understand the importance of following the physician's orders for gradually decreasing his dose of these drugs, even if this seems to make his symptoms worse. If the patient does not understand the reason for reducing steroid dosage to avoid toxicity, he may not retain the self-control required to keep from taking more of the drug than has been ordered. The nurse can, by providing encouragement and support, help

patients deal with this difficult aspect of their total treatment plan.

Some patients may have their systemic steroid dosage kept at a minimum by the periodic employment of topical preparations that are poorly absorbed. For example, some asthmatic patients may inhale a steroid vapor several times daily for symptomatic relief. This acts locally in the lungs with minimal systemic absorption, as do isoproterenol, epinephrine, and the other adrenergic bronchodilators (Chaps. 16 and 40) that are often administered in aerosol mists for relief of asthma.

Similarly, in osteoarthritis and in cases of rheumatoid arthritis involving only a few joints, certain steroid compounds are injected directly into the joints to produce a prolonged local effect, with little likelihood of systemic absorption in amounts that would cause hypercorticism. The acetate esters of various steroids, which are only slightly soluble and absorbable, seem best suited to such intra-articular or intrasynovial administration (see Chap. 41).

Acute Episodes and Crises

Patients who suffer acute exacerbations of *arthritic* or *asthmatic* disease are treated on an entirely different dosage schedule. Instead of initiating therapy with the small doses employed in chronic cases, the doctor starts the acutely ill patient off with large doses —for example, 40 to 60 mg. of prednisone or an equivalent amount of one of the newer synthetic steroids. This high dosage level is gradually lowered as the acute episode is brought under control. Later the steroid dosage is discontinued entirely, but only very slowly (1 or 2 mg. every week or two), in order not to set off steroid withdrawal symptoms.

This method of administering short courses of steroids in relatively high doses is used both in acute flare-ups of disabling diseases, such as rheumatoid arthritis, that do not endanger life, and in cases of rheumatic fever with myocarditis or of severe status asthmaticus, both of which often threaten to cause the patient's death. (See Chaps. 40 and 41 for discussion of the water-soluble succinate esters of certain steroids (e.g., hydrocortisone sodium succinate Drug Digest) in these life-threatening conditions.)

Patients in the *acute stages of fatal diseases* or at the *crisis* of an explosive, overwhelming infection or other life-endangering disorder often receive massive steroid dosage without any regard to the possible hypercortical side effects. Very large doses of steroids (60 to 120 mg. of prednisone daily, or its equivalent) sometimes produce remissions lasting several months in systemic lupus and in pemphigus, for example, and relatively high doses are then continued for long periods in these chronic and eventually fatal diseases. Doctors reason that the hypercorticism that inevitably results from such suppressive doses of steroids is less disabling than the uncontrolled diseases themselves. Sometimes, however, these patients die of corticosteroid complications such as hemorrhage from a perforated peptic ulcer.

There is, of course, little or no danger of such steroid complications when massive doses are employed for only brief periods, as, for example, at the height of a fulminating infection or during endotoxic shock, or in acute adrenal insufficiency crises. Here, such large doses, given for only a few days, are harmless and often life-saving.

Acute Self-Limiting Conditions

Patients with acute, self-limiting conditions that do not require prolonged treatment are the ones most likely to benefit from steroid therapy. This is true especially in skin and mucous membrane inflammations, which can be treated with topically applied corticosteroids. Thus, steroids have proved particularly useful in dermatology where they have largely replaced earlier remedies for various conditions. Applied to the skin in the form of creams, lotions, ointments, emulsions and aerosol sprays, certain steroids are often remarkably effective for relief of itching, burning and pain in acute contact dermatoses such as poison ivy, in severe sunburn and in eruptions of other types (see Chap. 43).

Various eye disorders can now be controlled by topical application of steroids in ophthalmic solutions and ointments. By their ability to suppress edema formation and scarring of the delicate ocular tissues, steroids have saved the sight of many patients whose eyes might once have been damaged beyond repair by inflammatory reactions accompanying infection and other conditions (see Chap. 42). Of course, systemic therapy also is often necessary for treating ocular conditions originating deep in the eye, in structures behind the iris. Similarly, in the acute spreading phase of severe psoriasis and in the fatal collagen diseases with characteristic skin symptoms—pemphigus, for example, with its periodic eruptions of blisters all over the body—systemic rather than topical corticosteroid therapy is usually required for relief.

THE ADVERSE EFFECTS OF CORTICOSTEROID THERAPY

The administration of small, physiological doses of corticosteroids as replacement therapy is rarely attended by adverse effects. Even very high dosage need not be harmful when given for only a few days. For example, patients in shock and critically ill from a severe bacteremic or nervous system infection suffer no ill effects from intravenous infusion of massive steroid doses, provided that they simultaneously receive treatment with antibiotics or other anti-infective agents that strike specifically at the pathogenic microorganisms.

On the other hand, long-continued use of steroids in doses only slightly above the amounts normally secreted will lead eventually to toxicity, and, of course, higher doses will produce dangerous toxic reactions in a relatively short time—i.e., two weeks, or so. Some patients are especially susceptible to certain severe complications from steroids because of the presence either of the underlying disease for which these drugs are being used or of certain other physical and mental states that are adversely affected by steroids. If the doctor decides to employ extended steroid therapy in such patients at all, he keeps them under especially close observation and uses every means of minimizing drug-induced adverse reactions.

Cushing's Syndrome. Most patients who have to be maintained for any length of time on steroid dose levels about three or four times the amounts naturally secreted by the person's adrenals show signs and symptoms similar to those seen with certain adrenal and pituitary gland tumors. The patient with such Cushingoid features first shows a characteristic fullness or rounding of the face. On his face, neck and shoulders the skin may become flushed, and growth of excess hair and an acnelike eruption may occur. The patient's trunk may also show the effects of the corticosteroids on fat distribution, as the abdomen becomes heavy and humps of fat appear behind the shoulders and above the collarbones—so-called buffalo hump and supraclavicular fat pads.

In contrast, the patient's arms and legs often look thin. This is no mere illusion but the result of an actual wasting away of muscle tissue. The patient may complain of weakness in his leg muscles and of pains in his back. These signs and symptoms stem from the effects of high steroid dosage on protein metabolism—the result of actions which are characterized as both *catabolic* and *anti-anabolic*. That is, the corticosteroids both speed the breakdown of tissue protein to amino acids and prevent these building blocks from being readily reutilized in the synthesis of new muscle, skin, and bone.

Despite this, most patients on steroids tend to put on weight, often to the point of obesity. This may be due, in part, to the patient's increased appetite when he is relieved of pain and discomfort and becomes high-spirited. However, it may also be metabolic in origin. Even while protein is wasting away and the patient goes into negative nitrogen balance, his body is producing increased amounts of glucose—an effect on carbohydrate metabolism that sometimes manifests itself in the hyperglycemia and glycosuria of a newly developing diabetes.

All of the synthetic steroids share these metabolic effects, which, as we have already indicated, are probably the basis of their desirable anti-inflammatory effects as well as of these undesired changes in the patient's appearance and physical condition. Because of this, doses of *all* these drugs that produce equal degrees of anti-inflammatory activity can be expected to cause essentially the same toxic signs and symptoms. One synthetic steroid, *triamcinolone,* seems less likely to cause the characteristic voracious increase in appetite and gain in weight, but it is also the one with which tissue wasting and muscle weakness are probably most likely to occur.

Required Precautions. In order to prevent muscle weakness and wasting (*myopathy*), steroid-treated patients are kept on a diet rich in protein and potassium. Those who require surgery may sometimes also receive *anabolic agents* (Chap. 30) to stimulate protein synthesis. This may help both to build them up and to speed the healing of suture wounds, which tends to be slowed in patients with steroid-induced negative nitrogen balance.

Reduction of synthesis of skin components as a result of the effect of the corticosteroids on protein metabolism may increase susceptibility to bed sores. A similar reduction in synthesis of the elements that make up mucous membranes may be one factor in the increased occurrence of *peptic ulcer*—one of the more common of the potentially serious reactions to steroids. Rheumatic patients seem especially susceptible to development of such gastrointestinal lesions. Ulcer can be especially dangerous, because the steroid drugs may suppress gastric pain and other warning symptoms until the ulcer finally perforates, or the patient begins to bleed internally. For this reason, the G.I. tract is often X-rayed before steroid therapy is started, and roentgenography is repeated periodically during treatment. The drugs are usually taken after meals and with antacids to minimize gastric irritation, and some patients—especially those with a previous history of peptic ulcer—are placed on a special ulcer diet and receive antisecretory-antispasmodic drugs as adjuncts to steroid therapy.

Another danger that must be watched for is the development of *osteoporosis*, with possible fractures of the vertebrae, ribs and femur. This complication of prolonged steroid therapy is most common in elderly, debilitated patients and especially in postmenopausal women or in women with low estrogen levels following surgical removal of the ovaries. Bedridden rheumatoid arthritis patients are also especially susceptible to this difficulty which may result from steroid-induced negative nitrogen and calcium balances. When warned by signs of mineral depletion in such patients, the doctor often orders a protein-rich diet, calcium salt supplements, and anabolic agents (Chaps. 30 and 45) to counteract the adverse effects of corticosteroids. In patients with osteoporosis, it may be necessary to discontinue steroid therapy (if the patient's condition

permits) or to gradually reduce the dosage of these drugs.

The possibility of development of *diabetes* during steroid therapy in susceptible patients requires periodic tests for sugar in the blood and urine, especially when others in the family are diabetic. However, corticosteroids are not necessarily contraindicated for diabetics, provided that the hyperglycemia and glycosuria can be kept under control by added insulin and a dietary regimen richer than previously in protein.

Steroid-Spread Infections. The cellular effects of steroids that reduce inflammation also tend to inhibit the body's mechanisms for defending itself against invasion by microorganisms. Such reduction in resistance to infection often poses a problem in patients being treated with steroids, especially when they are already weakened by disease. Not only do steroids lower the patient's capacity to localize and control the invaders, but they often tend also to mask the presence of the infection until it is far advanced, by suppressing the usual rise in body temperature and by keeping leukocyte levels low.

Once the infection is diagnosed and the microorganism causing it is identified, the doctor tries to hit it with high doses of the most effective antibiotic available. He does *not* discontinue steroids in such cases but may even increase their dosage. This is necessary because, during prolonged steroid medication, the patient's own adrenal glands have probably lost much of their own hormone-producing capacity. This adrenal insufficiency may keep him from coping adequately with the stress of a severe infection.

Massive doses of steroids are sometimes employed in overwhelming infections for their anti-stress effects, despite their admitted tendency to spread infection. For example, patients in shock from severe blood poisoning or meningitis, who have not been responding adequately to vasopressor drugs and antibiotics, have sometimes been aided remarkably and helped to survive by such steroid medication. Among patients reportedly saved by the timely addition of steroids to their regimen have been some with severe bacteremias, bacterial endocarditis, viral hepatitis, encephalitis from measles, mumps or mononucleosis, and pneumococcal and tuberculous meningitis.

Despite their lifesaving effects in such fulminating tubercular infections, steroid drugs are ordinarily *contraindicated* for patients with a history of tuberculosis. Because of the danger that they may reactivate healed lesions, the use of these drugs by patients with arrested tuberculosis is generally considered undesirable. If steroid treatment of another serious disorder becomes necessary for such patients, the doctor often orders preventive antituberculosis medication (Chap. 35) and checks the patient periodically by means of chest X-rays and sputum studies in order to detect any steroid-induced escape of tubercle bacilli that had been previously walled off in supposedly healed lesions.

Corticosteroid therapy is also contraindicated in the presence of viral and fungal infections for which no effective anti-infective therapy is yet available. Thus, topical and systemic steroid therapy, which is often helpful in bacterial infections of the eye when combined with appropriate antibacterial agents (e.g., neomycin), is considered contraindicated in fungal infections of various eye structures and in herpes simplex virus invasions of the cornea. The viruses of chickenpox and other exanthematous diseases may be disseminated during administration of steroid medication. This is one reason why some doctors avoid long-term administration of steroids to children, who are especially susceptible to such virus infections (another reason is the fact that long-term treatment with corticosteroids tends to suppress the growth of children).

Mental Effects. Early in the use of steroids in the treatment of rheumatoid arthritis, doctors noted that many patients became unusually happy and talkative. At first, this change of mood was attributed to their natural joy at the dramatic relief of the painfully disabling condition. Often, however, this euphoria progressed to a hypomanic state, in which the patient became increasingly restless and overactive. Sometimes, the patient's mood swung to one of agitated depression, which increased in severity upon withdrawal of steroid therapy.

The accumulated experience of many years now indicates that corticosteroids are capable of producing abnormal behavior in many patients. Some actually become psychotic as a result of the mental effects of these drugs. Such psychoses are most often of the manic-depressive type, but schizophrenic reactions also sometimes occur. Thus, the nurse should watch for changes in the mood and behavior of patients taking steroids and report these to the doctor. The physician will then try to lower the daily dosage of these drugs.

The causes of such psychological changes brought about by steroids are obscure; however, these difficulties are most likely to occur in patients who have a history of emotional instability. Thus, the doctor tries to avoid administering these drugs to patients with such tendencies, and the drugs are definitely contraindicated for people who are already overtly psychotic. Steroid therapy is also considered undesirable for patients with epilepsy, because their convulsive seizure activity is often increased by these drugs.

Steroid Withdrawal. It often becomes desirable to reduce or discontinue steroid dosage, either because the patient's condition goes into remission or because of the appearance of severe side effects. In such instances, doctors have learned that reduction of steroid dosage must proceed very gradually. It has been found that the underlying disease tends to increase in severity if steroids are withdrawn too suddenly. For

TABLE 28-2

	Equivalent Milligram Doses	Relative Anti-inflammatory Potency
Cortisone	25 mg.	0.8
Hydrocortisone	20 mg.	1.0
Prednisone	5 mg.	4.0
Prednisolone	5 mg.	4.0
Methylprednisolone	4 mg.	5.0
Triamcinolone	4 mg.	5.0
Paramethasone	2 mg.	10.0
Dexamethasone	0.75 mg. (750 mcg.)	25.0
Betamethasone	0.60 mg (600 mcg.)	30.0

example, in rheumatoid arthritis, joint symptoms sometimes return with increased severity when steroids are withdrawn, and asthmatic patients often suffer a flareup of breathing difficulties when taken off steroids.

In addition, patients who have been weaned away from long-continued steroid therapy may suffer from latent adrenal insufficiency for some time afterward. The effects of suppression of their own adrenal secretions during prolonged dosage with steroids may not be readily seen. If, however, within the next few months, they are suddenly subjected to unusual stress of some sort—a severe illness, accidental trauma or a surgical operation, for example—the reduced pituitary-adrenal responsiveness sometimes becomes apparent in their sudden severe collapse.

Thus, it is very important for the doctor to know whether a patient has been under steroid therapy during the previous year. If so, the physician may order administration of high doses of hydrocortisone or a similar steroid to help tide the patient over the emergency. Patients taking steroids may be advised to carry a card indicating that fact, so that if they should be injured and unconscious, they will not be deprived of these drugs just when they need their support more than ever to meet the stressful situation.

Patients who are being withdrawn from steroids should get all possible medical and emotional support. Thus, rheumatic and asthmatic patients who have been taking steroids during an acute attack are not abruptly deprived of medication when the emergency is over. The steroid dosage is reduced only gradually, often with supplemental injections of corticotropin (ACTH) to help tide the patient over the period during which his own adrenals are not functioning adequately (Chap. 27). Also, other medications must be substituted for the steroids in order to reduce the return of discomforting symptoms.

It is essential that the patient receive a careful explanation of the reasons for taking him off the medicine that may have been giving him gratifying relief. If the drugs are withdrawn without adequate discussion of why this is necessary, the patient who is left with little to sustain him may go from doctor to doctor, trying to find one who will prescribe the continued use of steroids. The patient is likely to do better physically if he gets both personal reassurance and continued treatment with other medications, than if he feels deprived both of his drugs and of the physician's concern for his well-being.

SOME CLINICAL CONDITIONS RESPONSIVE TO CORTICOSTEROID THERAPY

- **Collagen Diseases and Nonarticular Musculoskeletal Disorders**
  Rheumatoid arthritis (and related disorders, such as rheumatoid spondylitis, Still's disease, psoriatic arthritis, acute and chronic gout and gouty arthritis).
  Acute rheumatic fever
  Bursitis, fibrositis, synovitis, myositis, tendinitis
  Disseminated lupus erythematosus
  Pemphigus
  Scleroderma
  Periarteritis nodosa
  Dermatomyositis

- **Allergic, Infectious, and Other Inflammatory Disorders of the Skin and Ocular and Respiratory Mucous Membranes**
  Bronchial asthma, including status asthmaticus
  Pulmonary fibrosis and emphysema
  Pollinosis (hay fever)
  Rhinitis (perennial vasomotor; allergic)
  Skin disorders such as atopic dermatitis (eczema), contact dermatitis, poison ivy dermatitis, neurodermatitis, exfoliative dermatitis, angioneurotic edema, urticara, seborrheic dermatitis, pruritus vulvi or ani, dermatitis herpetiformis.
  Eye disorders such as allergic conjunctivitis, iritis, iridocyclitis, choroiditis, chorioretinitis, keratitis, uveitis, corneal ulcers, secondary glaucoma.

  Severe allergic reactions including anaphylactic shock, transfusion reactions, Stevens-Johnson syndrome.

- **Hematological and Neoplastic Conditions**
  Acute leukemia; chronic lymphocytic leukemia
  Autoimmune hemolytic anemia
  Acquired hemolytic anemia
  Idiopathic thrombocytic purpura
  Blood dyscrasias such as agranulocytosis and aplastic anemia
  Breast cancer (advanced metastatic mammary carcinoma)
  Hodgkin's disease and other lymphomatous neoplasms
  Pulmonary granulomatosis

- **Miscellaneous**
  Nephrotic syndrome
  Adrenogenital syndrome
  Ulcerative colitis
  Thyroiditis
  Sarcoidosis
  Hepatitis and cirrhosis
  Parotitis (mumps)
  Neuritis
  Bell's palsy
  Myocarditis and other cardiac conditions, including heart block and congestive heart failure.
  Shock—hemorrhagic, endotoxic, bacteremic, postoperative, etc.
  Adrenocortical insufficiency

SUMMARY OF SIDE EFFECTS AND TOXICITY OF ADRENOCORTICOSTEROID DRUGS

- Cushingoid signs such as:
  Rounding of the face (moon face), with flushing, sweating, acne, and hirsutism; thinning of hair on the scalp, supraclavicular fat pads, buffalo hump, abdominal distention and striae; weight gain.

- Protein depletion, with osteoporosis and spontaneous fractures; myopathy, with weakness of muscles, thighs, pelvis, and lower back; aseptic necrosis of the hip and humerus.

- Thrombophlebitis, thromboembolism, petechiae, purpura, necrotizing angiitis.

- Peptic ulcer, gastrointestinal hemorrhage, ulcerative esophagitis, acute pancreatitis.

- Headache, vertigo, increased intracranial pressure, increased intraocular pressure, posterior subcapsular cataracts requiring extraction.

- Psychic disturbances, marked mainly by euphoria but sometimes by depression; insomnia, fatigue; convulsions.

- Suppression of growth in children

- Aggravation of infection

- Aggravation of diabetes mellitus

- Increase in blood pressure

- Amenorrhea and other menstrual irregularities

SUMMARY OF CONTRAINDICATIONS AND PRECAUTIONS WITH CORTICOSTEROID DRUGS

- **Contraindications (Absolute and Relative)**
  Infections, including active, questionably healed, or latent tuberculosis; herpes simplex keratitis; and sometimes fungal or exanthematous diseases, such as chickenpox
  Osteoporosis; myasthenia gravis
  Peptic ulcer, diverticulitis, fresh intestinal anastomoses; thrombophlebitis
  Diabetes mellitus; hyperthyroidism
  Psychic or marked emotional disturbances
  Hypertension; acute coronary disease; acute glomerular nephritis and renal insufficiency
  Pregnancy, especially in first trimester

- **Precautions**
  Patients with a history of peptic ulcer are placed on an antiulcer regimen including antacid and anticholinergic drugs, diet, and rest. If they complain of abdominal pain, they are X-rayed (steroids may mask symptoms of perforation).
  Patients with a history of tuberculosis should receive prophylactic doses of antituberculosis drugs. If infection develops in these or other patients, high dosage of appropriate anti-infective drugs is required. Steroids should *not* be withdrawn abruptly in acute infections (or other severe stress, such as surgery or trauma); dosage may actually be increased.
  Patients with a history of well controlled diabetes are closely watched and their insulin dosage increased if glycosuria or hyperglycemia develops.
  Patients should be closely watched for signs of possible adrenocortical insufficiency, periarteritis nodosa and ocular changes. Children on prolonged steroid therapy are observed for signs of growth retardation.

SUMMARY OF NURSING POINTS TO REMEMBER IN CORTICOSTEROID THERAPY

- Observe the patient carefully for signs of hypercorticism (Cushingoid signs) or others typical of toxicity, and report these to the physician.

- Encourage the patient on long-term corticosteroid therapy to keep his appointments with the clinic or his private physician, so that all observations and tests for adverse effects can be made and gradual withdrawal of the steroid drugs can be begun promptly if toxicity is detected.

- Reinforce the doctor's explanations to the patient of why dosage reduction or even withdrawal of the steroid drugs may be necessary. Such measures may be facilitated if the patient understands from the beginning that he will not be able to depend indefinitely on these drugs, and if other measures are taken to ease his symptoms during withdrawal. Psychological and emotional support should be offered the patient who continues to have symptoms of his illness while dosage is being reduced on account of side effects.

CLINICAL PROBLEMS

Miss Washington suffers from severe rheumatoid arthritis. Her pain is no longer relieved by salicylates, and the physician has ordered 5 mg. of prednisone t.i.d. Miss Washington's symptoms were markedly relieved, and the physician advised decreasing the dose gradually to 5 mg. b.i.d., and finally to 5 mg. q.d. Miss Washington confided to the clinic nurse that because she had recurrence of symptoms when the amount of medication was decreased, she has continued taking three tablets daily, despite the physician's recommendation.

How would you, as the clinic nurse, deal with this problem in your interaction with Miss Washington and her physician?

REVIEW QUESTIONS

1. (a) What three kinds of hormones are produced naturally by the adrenal cortex?

(b) Give an example of a steroid of each type and indicate, in a general way, the physiological functions of the two types that are essential for life.

2. (a) What are several situations that may result in chronic or acute adrenal insufficiency?

(b) Name several corticosteroids that are employed in small physiological doses as replacement therapy in adrenal insufficiency.

3. (a) Of what two general types are the pharmacological effects that are sought with pharmacological doses of corticosteroid drugs?

(b) Of what three general types are the adverse effects that may result from prolonged administration of *supraphysiologic* doses of corticosteroid drugs?

4. (a) What is the most important practical difference between the natural adrenal glucocorticoids (e.g., hydrocortisone) and the newer synthetic corticosteroids?

(b) What are the two most potent synthetic corticosteroids and how does their anti-inflammatory potency compare with that of the natural hormone, cortisone?

5. (a) List several collagen diseases commonly treated with corticosteroid drugs.

(b) List several allergic disorders so treated.

6. (a) What drugs and other measures does the doctor employ for relief of rheumatoid arthritis before deciding to add a steroid drug to the patient's regimen?

(b) What dosage procedure does the doctor usually employ in such chronic conditions, and how may the nurse help him and the patient attain the therapeutic objective?

7. (a) List several disorders in which it is desirable to start patients off on large doses of corticosteroid drugs.

(b) List several situations in which corticosteroid drugs may be applied topically or injected for their local action.

8. (a) What are some characteristic (Cushingoid) signs of corticosteroid overdosage?

(b) What are several clinical conditions which may develop as the result of the adverse effects of prolonged corticosteroid therapy and what measures may be taken to detect and counteract such toxic reactions?

9. (a) List some severe infections in which massive doses of steroids may sometimes prove lifesaving?

(b) List some situations in which corticosteroid drugs are contraindicated because of the presence of active or latent infection.

10. (a) Which patients typically must be kept under close observation during corticosteroid therapy, because of their special susceptibility to adverse central or peripheral effects?

(b) What measures does the doctor take in withdrawing corticosteroid medication, and how may the nurse help make this procedure easier for the patient?

BIBLIOGRAPHY

Bollet, A. J., *et al.*: Major undesirable effects from prednisolone and prednisone. J.A.M.A., *158*:459, 1955.

Bunim, J. J., *et al.*: Studies on dexamethasone, a new synthetic steroid in rheumatoid arthritis. Arthritis Rheum., *1*:313, 1958.

Dameshek, W.: Use of corticosteroids in hematological therapy. Ann. N. Y. Acad. Sci., *82*:924, 1959.

Dubois, E. L.: Current therapy of systemic lupus erythematosus. J.A.M.A., *173*:1633, 1960.

Ensign, D. C., Sigler, J. W., and Wilson, G. M.: Steroids

in rheumatoid arthritis. Arch. Int. Med., *104:*949, 1959.

Frohman, I. P.: The steroids. Am. J. Nurs., *59:*518, 1959.

Harter, J. G., Reddy, W. J., and Thorn, G. W.: Studies on an intermittent corticosteroid dosage regimen. New Eng. J. Med., *269:*591, 1963.

Leopold, I. H.: Steroid therapy in ophthalmic lesions. J.A.M.A., *170:*1547, 1959.

Liddle, G. W.: Clinical pharmacology of the anti-inflammatory steroids. Clin. Pharmacol. Ther., *2:*615, 1961.

Nelson, D. H.: Relative merits of the corticosteroids. Ann. Rev. Med., *13:*241, 1962.

Neustadt, D. H.: Corticosteroid therapy in rheumatoid arthritis. J.A.M.A., *170:*1253, 1959.

Quarton, G. C., *et al.:* Mental disturbances associated with ACTH and cortisone. Medicine, *34:*13, 1955.

Rodman, M. J.: The use of the corticosteroids. R.N., *23:*39, 1960 (March).

———: The corticosteroids, a progress report. R.N., *21:*50, 1958 (Oct.).

Romansky, M. J.: Steroid therapy in systemic infections. J.A.M.A., *170:*1179, 1959.

Thorn, G. W., *et al.:* Clinical usefulness of ACTH and cortisone. New Eng. J. Med., *242:*783; 824; 865, 1950.

Thorn, G. W.: Clinical considerations in the use of corticosteroids. New Eng. J. Med., *274:*775, 1966.

The Female Sex Hormones

ESTROGENS AND PROGESTINS

The female sex glands, or ovaries, synthesize and secrete hormones mainly of two types: (1) The *estrogens* and (2) the *progestins*. These sex steroids, which are first produced in significant amounts at puberty, can be said to control the continuation of the human species. The estrogens bring about the changes that turn immature girls into women and, together with the progestins, they set the stage for pregnancy and childbearing. In addition to their direct effects on the reproductive system, these steroids affect the functioning of other body tissues and they even possess subtle psychological actions.

These hormones and certain synthetic substances now available that share many of their properties are widely used in gynecology and other areas of medicine. In order to understand their many clinical uses, it is essential that we know what effects the natural ovarian secretions have on the various tissues that serve as their targets. Once we have seen how the hormones produced by the gonads of women influence the reproductive system and the metabolism of other body tissues, we may better comprehend the reasons for their administration as medications in the management of various clinical conditions.

We shall discuss first the physiological functions of the *estrogens*, since these are the first female hormones produced at puberty and the ones secreted during the earliest part of each monthly ovulatory cycle. Then, after we have related various of the natural actions of the estrogens to their therapeutic uses, we shall examine in the same manner the *progestational steroids* that are produced in the latter half of the ovulatory cycle and during pregnancy.

ESTROGENS

Physiological Effects

The compounds called estrogens are biosynthesized by the ovary from cholesterol in a series of compli-

cated chemical steps. The principal product secreted by the ovaries is *estradiol,* which circulates in the blood along with such related steroids as *estrone* and *estriol.* Before being excreted in the urine in the free form or after conjugation with glucuronic and sulfuric acids, these estrogenic substances influence the functioning of genital as well as other tissues.

Reproductive Tissues

Estrogens can be considered the *growth hormone* of all the tissues involved in reproductive processes, including the uterus, oviducts, vagina and breasts. The effects of estrogens on these organs are most noticeable at puberty. At that time these accessory sex organs are brought to maturity, as the ovaries step up their secretion of female hormones when stimulated by pituitary gonadotropins that are themselves released in increased quantities upon signals from certain hypothalamic areas of the brain (Chap. 27). Thereafter, these sexual tissues continue to respond to fluctuations in the amounts of estrogens secreted during each monthly ovulatory cycle, until they finally undergo gradual atrophic changes in the years following the menopause when estrogenic secretion by the ovaries falls to lower and lower levels.

The Uterus. Estrogens influence the growth and development of both the muscular and mucosal elements of the uterus and the oviducts, or fallopian tubes.

The myometrium attains adult size under pubertal estrogen stimulation, and part of its great growth during pregnancy is the result of the response of this smooth muscle to the estrogens poured out by the placenta. Estrogens also tend to stimulate the thickening uterine muscle to contract, but this is counteracted by the presence of progestins in the latter half of each menstrual month and during pregnancy.

The Endometrium. The most marked effects of estrogens upon the endometrium occur during the first half of the menstrual cycle. During this so-called *proliferative phase,* this inner lining of the uterus, which had been destroyed and sloughed off during the previous menstrual period, is rebuilt under the influence of follicular estrogenic hormones. The endometrial epithelium increases tenfold in thickness at this time and its initially short glands grow into long narrow tubes. The glands in the inner lining of the *cervix*—the endocervical glands—are also stimulated to secrete a thin watery fluid, which is most profuse at the midcyclic estrogen peak.

The vaginal tract mucosa is kept thick by the action of ovarian estrogens upon its epithelium, and a reduction in the glandular secretion of these hormones at the menopause is accompanied by a thinning of these epithelial layers and an increased susceptibility to vaginal infections.

The breast tissues are affected by estrogens both at puberty and during pregnancy, as well as in each ovulatory cycle. Through the complicated interactions between these and other hormones, the mammary gland ducts and alveoli (the secreting sacs) grow and develop to full functional maturity. Yet, when actual lactation occurs after childbirth, estrogens are at relatively low levels, and estrogens tend to suppress milk production by their direct and indirect actions on the lactating breasts.

Effects on Other Tissues

The estrogens influence the metabolism of *non*-sexual tissues in ways that account for their utility in certain clinical conditions and for some undesired reactions. Among these *metabolic actions* are some that are believed to account for the weight gain seen in some women at times during the menstrual month when estrogen levels are high. This is, in part, the result of tissue retention of sodium and water. In addition, estrogens often exert an *anabolic action,* in which dietary nitrogen and other elements are more readily turned into body protein.

Estrogens may also help to prevent negative calcium balance and to aid the deposition of this mineral in the protein matrix of the bones. These female hormones seem to increase the number of elastic elements in the skin. They also tend to keep plasma cholesterol at relatively low levels and may, in this way, delay the development of atherosclerotic processes in the walls of blood vessels.

Pituitary Actions of Estrogens

As has already been indicated, estrogens have the ability to suppress the secretion of the follicle-stimulating hormone (FSH) by the anterior pituitary gland while increasing its production of the luteinizing hormone (LH). These effects help to bring about midcyclic ovulation, and they are thus sometimes sought in the estrogen treatment of infertile women who lack natural estrogens. However, potent synthetic estrogens

are employed more commonly today to *inhibit* FSH production and, in this way, prevent ovulation and pregnancy from occurring (see the discussion of oral contraceptives, p. 409).

Estrogens are also thought to exert an inhibitory control over the secretion of the luteotropic or lactogenic hormone. Some authorities believe that it is the lowering of estrogen levels at childbirth that leads to pituitary release of prolactin and resultant lactation. Similarly, some think that administration of estrogens at this time stops postpartum lactation by suppressing pituitary secretion of this lactogenic hormone.

Therapeutic Uses of the Estrogens

Estrogens are employed in many clinical conditions. Most often these hormones are used in small doses for *replacement* purposes in girls or women who complain of various disturbances of menstrual flow arising from partial or complete lack of natural ovarian steroid secretions. On the other hand, natural and synthetic estrogens are sometimes administered in pharmacological, rather than physiological, doses in order to produce various other effects, not only on female genital tissues but also elsewhere in the body. Indeed, doses of these female hormones are sometimes administered to men as well as women.

The Menopause or Female Climacteric

This syndrome, which women often call "the change of life," is a physiological process that occurs most often during a woman's middle to late forties. It is set in motion by a gradual reduction in ovarian function. The resulting deficiency in estrogen secretion is accompanied by menstrual irregularities and by a variety of other more or less discomforting physical complaints and emotional symptoms.

Most menopausal complaints can be readily controlled through the use of estrogens in doses individualized to meet each patient's need for replacement therapy. The amount of estrogens required to remedy this deficiency state is now often determined by vaginal cytology. That is, the doctor studies vaginal smears, using the percentage of mature epithelial cells as a guide to estrogen dosage. Proper dosage provides prompt relief of hot flushes, night sweats, heart palpitations, headaches, dizziness and other cardiovascular and nervous system symptoms. Cyclic therapy with progestational steroids (which is discussed later) also can control the menstrual irregularities of the menopause.

Nurses who hear women complain of what are obviously menopausal symptoms should advise them to see a physician. Some women seem reluctant to visit a doctor despite their distress—perhaps because they are loath to acknowledge that the "change" is occurring, or because of a mistaken belief that estrogen therapy can cause cancer. The nurse can help the patient by offering factual information to counteract old wives' tales of various kinds.

Some women go through the menopause with relatively few symptoms, whereas others show many signs of emotional and mental imbalance, including sleeplessness, spells of crying, intense uneasiness and anxiety or agitated depression. For this reason, some doctors have tended to look upon menopausal symptoms as psychogenic and related to factors in a woman's life situation other than ovarian failure. Thus, they have advocated that these women be treated by psychotherapy and with sedative, tranquilizer and antidepressant drugs rather than with estrogens.

This conservative attitude appears to be changing at present. Most gynecological authorities now appear to agree that, in view of the relative lack of toxicity of estrogens compared to their possible benefits, a trial of hormone therapy is usually worthwhile. This seems especially true when a woman takes only small doses of estrogens under a doctor's supervision for the few months—or at most a year or two—during which her physical and emotional menopausal discomforts are at their peak. The prompt return to a stable state with estrogen replacement is generally thought to be well worth the minor and readily controllable side effects that sometimes occur.

Postmenopausal Disorders

In addition to the temporary employment of estrogens to help women adjust to menopausal changes, which has gained general acceptance, a few physicians have suggested that most women would benefit by continuing to take these hormones well beyond the transitional period. They argue that older women may postpone or prevent many of the ills that accompany aging by continuing to take estrogens indefinitely during their postmenopausal years. The reasoning behind this advocacy of prolonged postmenopausal estrogens is that these hormones exert *non*-sexual metabolic effects that play an important part in protecting the well-being of practically every tissue, organ and system in the body. Thus, the doctors claim that continued estrogenic therapy not only will help to keep breasts firm and skin supple, but may help to avoid serious disorders such as osteoporosis and coronary atherosclerosis.

Osteoporosis. This skeletal disorder, which sometimes thins the bones of elderly men as well as women, is often treated with either estrogens or androgens, or sometimes with combinations of sex steroids of both types. It is believed that the anabolic effects of the two kinds of hormones are helpful for providing the protein framework into which calcium is laid down by bone cells. (When given together, the anabolic effects of estrogens and androgens are additive, whereas their actions on sexual tissues tend to cancel one another out.) Patients are also often put on a diet high in protein and milk, with supplementary calcium salts and perhaps Vitamin D and fluorides.

Estrogens seem to relieve back pain caused by weakened vertebrae, even though there seems to be no clear-cut X-ray evidence that these bones are thickened or that compression fractures are less likely to occur. Nevertheless, the continued use of these hormones for preventive purposes during the postmenopausal period has been recommended as a means of keeping the bones strong and hard and less liable to fracture. Prophylactic therapy with estrogens or other anabolic steroids is considered especially desirable during treatment of menopausal or postmenopausal patients with corticosteroids.

Coronary Atherosclerosis. The prophylactic use of estrogens for preventing heart attacks in both men and women has been advocated recently. The theoretical basis for this therapy, which is also discussed in Chapter 22, is the fact that *pre*menopausal women are relatively free of coronary artery disease, whereas women who have had their ovaries removed show a sharp rise in atherosclerosis. Similarly, postmenopausal women have about the same rate of myocardial infarctions as men in the same age range.

The effectiveness of such prophylaxis has not yet been established. Large doses of the potent synthetic estrogen, *ethinyl estradiol,* appeared to lower cholesterol levels and the cholesterol-phospholipid ratio of the plasma. However, although the development of feminizing effects such as gynecomastia (mammary gland growth in the male) and a lessening of the libido was observed, the survival rate of men treated in this manner was *not* increased. On the other hand, for reasons not readily explainable, the survival rate among men who had suffered several infarctions is claimed to have been significantly improved by treatment with doses of *natural conjugated estrogens* so small that they caused none of the physical changes mentioned above.

Despite the uncertain status of this treatment, some doctors now prescribe estrogens for postmenopausal women not only to maintain physical and mental well-being but with the thought that replacement of these hormones will lessen their chances of suffering from coronary vascular disease as well. Estrogens employed for this purpose are probably harmless to women; however, such hormone therapy may create problems for some male patients. A man who can detect no obvious benefits insofar as his cardiac condition is concerned but who clearly sees undesirable physical changes in himself will often want to stop taking prescribed estrogens. The nurse can help support such a patient's will to continue treatment by making it clear that she recognizes his manliness and respects him as a man, despite some superficial changes in his secondary sex characteristics.

Vaginal Mucous Membranes and Skin

Changes in the thickness of the vaginal epithelium are among the earliest signs of deficient ovarian estrogen production. Atrophic changes in the vaginal lining tend to increase a woman's susceptibility to vaginitis. Estrogens have long been administered orally and by local application to help thicken these epithelial layers in women with *senile vaginitis*. In the treatment of vaginitis in immature girls (and in conjunction with antibiotics) the hormones have been used to convert the vaginal mucosa into the mature, more infection-resistant type.

The nurse can help make the use of local estrogenic medications more convenient by suggesting measures for proper use of vaginal creams and suppositories. For example, it should not be assumed that patients will be aware of how to use suppositories. The nurse should suggest that this medication be refrigerated to avoid its melting in warm weather. She should instruct the patient to wash her hands before and after inserting the suppository and explain that the foil must be peeled off prior to insertion.

Similarly, when creams are to be applied intravaginally, or on the external genitalia for relief of itching in *pruritus vulvae* and *kraurosis vulvae*, the patient should be told how to use a perineal pad to avoid soiling clothing. Patients treated in the doctor's office should be provided with a pad before they get dressed. Such attention to the patient's comfort and esthetic sensibilities will make it easier for her to follow through with a treatment that might otherwise seem tedious and messy.

Children are usually treated with *locally acting* estrogens, in order to alter the vaginal mucosa without producing other premature pubertal changes. However, if the sex hormones are given systemically to produce vaginal changes or for any other purposes (e.g., sexual infantilism), the child's parents should be carefully instructed concerning the possible effects of hormone therapy upon her secondary sex characteristics (e.g., changes in the breasts, body contours and behavior). They should be given an opportunity to discuss their concern about the child's future ability to have children and also receive answers to any other questions that may be troubling them.

Administration of estrogens to postmenopausal women has recently been claimed to produce *regenerative changes* in *aging skin*. This is part of the widely publicized and emotionally appealing claim that estrogen replacement therapy can keep women young and attractive indefinitely. Women who ask questions about such still unestablished assertions are best advised to consult their physicians concerning the desirability of long-term estrogens *for them.*

They should be made to understand that the doctor has to decide whether such therapy is desirable on an individual basis, following a complete physical examination and in the light of each patient's medical history. It should be explained that once she starts such treatment, the woman must not neglect to return for examinations at the intervals specified by her physician. He will, of course, be concerned with much more than the state of her skin during such regular follow-up visits and will probably perform breast and pelvic examinations, as well as a "Pap" smear and vaginal cell count.

Female Hypogonadism

We have seen that estrogen replacement therapy is desirable during the menopause and probably all through the *post*menopausal period. The indefinitely continued use of these hormones is also desirable for maintaining the femininity and general health and well-being of young women whose ovaries have had to be removed for medical reasons.

Even more dramatic than their effects in such ovariectomized (i.e., castrated) women is the response to estrogen administration in girls of adolescent age or older who have failed to develop sexually. This condition may be the result either of congenital absence of the ovaries or of the failure of the ovaries to respond to pituitary gonadotropin secretion at the time for normal onset of puberty. In either case, patients with such *sexual infantilism* are best treated with estrogens. Hormone administration induces growth and development of the accessory sex organs and development of the female secondary sex characteristics.

Such girls cannot, of course, bear children if ovaries are absent from birth, or if a normal ovulatory cycle cannot occur. They can, however, marry and have normal sexual relationships. Their *primary amenorrhea* can best be overcome by adding progestational steroids to the estrogens for a few days each month and then withdrawing both hormones for a brief period (see p. 407).

Other Uses of Estrogens

In addition to their use as replacement therapy in the conditions discussed in the preceding paragraphs and in menstrual disturbances such as uterine bleeding, the estrogens are often employed for their *pharmacological effects* in certain other situations. Synthetic estrogens, such as *diethylstilbestrol*, for example, are commonly used to overcome painful postpartum engorgement of the breasts with milk. Once the woman's breasts have been freed of milk by pumping or by the use of the posterior pituitary hormone oxytocin, high doses of estrogens are administered for several days. This is thought to suppress production of prolactin by the pituitary and thus to inhibit further lactation.

High doses of estrogens are sometimes used to stop the growth of girls who are becoming excessively tall because of ovarian failure. One of the effects of *both* male and female sex hormones is to close *the epiphyses* after the final spurt of growth at puberty. The ephiphyses are the cartilage-coated ends of the youthful long-bone shafts. During childhood and early adolescence the expanding connective tissue layer just beneath the ephiphyses forces these bone ends forward ahead of the growing shaft. This keeps the ephiphyses separated from the bone that is being continually laid down beneath the cartilage. Finally, at puberty, bone cells invade the cartilage from below and close the gap between the shafts of the long bones and their knobby ends. Closure of this epiphyseal "expansion joint" brings growth in height to an end. Thus, it is easily understood that, just as a lack of such hormones may lead to excessive height unless counteracted by hormone treatment, administration of hormones prior to puberty may result in shortened stature. To avoid this, as well as the danger of setting off precocious pubertal changes, estrogens are administered to children topically, when required at all, rather than systemically.

Men with carcinoma of the prostate gland are frequently treated with high doses of a synthetic estrogen such as diethylstilbestrol, as discussed in Chapter 44. Although estrogens are contraindicated for women with a history of breast cancer, these hormones are sometimes administered to patients with mammary carcinoma who are at least five years *past* the menopause.

Adverse Effects of Estrogens

Among the reasons for withholding treatment with products containing estrogens (and progestins) is the fear that these hormones might cause cancer of the genital tissues and breasts. This attitude appears to be *totally unwarranted* by the evidence, and there seems to be no reason to believe that the female sex hormones have ever caused the development of genital or mammary malignancies. In fact, recent studies indicate that administration of female sex steroids may actually have a protective action in patients with abnormal (precancerous) cervival tissue.

Nevertheless, because the growth of sexual tissue tumors is dependent upon such hormones, the use of estrogens is *contraindicated* in women who have such cancers or even show evidence of precancerous lesions. Caution is suggested in women whose family history indicates a possible tendency toward malignancies of these types, and the hormones should be withheld from women with uterine bleeding until the presence of genital carcinoma has been ruled out by pelvic examinations and other diagnostic procedures.

Patients taking estrogens occasionally have episodes of *"breakthrough" bleeding*. This usually stems from the breakdown of portions of the proliferative endometrium that has been built up under the influence of the estrogens. Such bleeding, which occurs when the patient's endometrium grows too thick to be maintained by its own blood supply, can be counteracted either by lowering or by raising estrogen dosage, but it is probably best avoided by periodically *withdrawing* the drug for a week or so. Such rest periods prevent overstimulation of the endometrium and result in *cyclic bleeding* at a predictable time. When withdrawal of estrogen is preceded by a few days of progestational steroid therapy, an even more normal menstrual period ensues.

Postmenopausal women who are placed on cyclic estrogen therapy should understand that they will have a menstrual period when the hormones are withdrawn every few weeks. It should be explained that this is actually *pseudo*menstruation and that they have not been made fertile once more and likely to become pregnant. They should, of course, be cautioned to report any bleeding that occurs while the drug is being administered.

The most common complaint of women taking large doses of estrogens (especially the synthetic type such as diethylstilbestrol) is a tendency toward loss of appetite, nausea and even vomiting and diarrhea. Such symptoms are similar to those of early pregnancy, and, like the latter, they tend to disappear as the patient becomes tolerant of the gastrointestinal side effects of the female hormones. These symptoms or the headaches and dizziness of which a few patients sometimes complain rarely require permanent withdrawal of estrogen therapy.

Available Estrogenic Products

Substances with estrogenic activity can be broadly classified as: (1) *the natural steroids* (and their esters and semisynthetic derivatives) and (2) certain *nonsteroidal synthetic chemicals* capable of eliciting essentially similar effects. Compounds of both types are available in oral and parenteral preparations. The products that can be given by mouth are preferred for most purposes because of their convenience and the fact that their effects are more predictable and more readily controlled.

In addition to the natural hormones themselves (*estradiol, estrone* and *estriol*), a commonly employed mixture of natural estrogens is *conjugated estrogenic substances* (Premarin, etc.), which is claimed to have certain special properties (see Drug Digest). These substances are effective when administered orally, as are *ethinyl estradiol* and *mestranol,* two semisynthetic derivatives which are especially potent, in part because their chemical side-chain structures protect the natural estrogenic nucleus from rapid inactivation in the liver and other tissues. The injectable esters of estradiol (e.g., the *dibenzoate, dipropionate, cypionate* and *valerate*) are also long acting, primarily because they are absorbed very slowly from intramuscular injection sites. These esters may exert effects for as long as a month or more after a single injection. They are used ordinarily only in certain special situations, because the orally administered products bring about menstruation in a more natural manner when discontinued (see Drug Digest).

The prototype of the *non-steroidal estrogenic substances* is *diethylstilbestrol* (see Drug Digest), which is cheap in comparison to the natural hormones and is capable of producing all their physiological effects. The various other synthetic estrogens listed in Table 29-1 are similar in their actions but are claimed to be less likely to cause nausea and vomiting than is diethylstilbestrol. This may be only because they are less rapidly and completely absorbed from the intestinal tract than the latter (when diethylstilbestrol is made available in more slowly absorbed forms, gastrointestinal upset is minimized).

PROGESTERONE AND THE SYNTHETIC PROGESTINS

Progesterone is a steroid hormone synthesized by the ovaries and the adrenal glands, and—during pregnancy—by the placenta. Ordinarily, it is produced mainly during the latter half of the menstrual month by the corpus luteum under the influence of luteinizing and luteotrophic hormones (Chap. 27). When the corpus luteum regresses, progesterone production drops and menstruation soon follows. On the other hand, if the ovum becomes fertilized, the corpus luteum continues to function for several months under the influence of chorionic gonadotropins and progesterone levels remain high. Later, after the final failure of the corpus luteum, the placenta continues to pour out progesterone, which reaches peak plasma levels late in pregnancy.

Because of the importance of progesterone in pro-

TABLE 29-1
NATURAL AND SYNTHETIC ESTROGENS

Nonproprietary or Official Name	Proprietary Name	Usual Dosage
Natural Steroid Estrogens and Derivatives		
Estradiol N.F.	Aquadiol; Diogyn; Ovocyclin; Progynon, etc.	250 mcg.
Estradiol benzoate N.F.	Diogyn B; Progynon B; etc.	1 mg. I.M.
Estradiol cypionate N.F.	Depo-Estradiol	1–5 mg. I.M., every 4 weeks
Estradiol dipropionate N.F.	Dimenformon dipropionate, etc.	1 mg. I.M.
Estradiol valerate U.S.P.	Delestrogen	10–40 mg.
Estriol	Theelol	240 mcg.
Estrone N.F.	Theelin, etc.	1 mg. I.M.
Estrogenic substances, conjugated, U.S.P.	Premarin, etc.	0.3–2.5 mg.
Ethinyl estradiol U.S.P.	Estinyl, etc.	0.01–0.5 mg.
Mestranol	Ethinyl estradiol-3-methyl ether	100 mcg.
Piperazine estrone sulfate	Sulestrex	1.5 mg.
Non-Steroid Synthetic Estrogens		
Benzestrol N.F.	Chemestrogen	2.5 mg.
Chlortrianisene N.F.	Tace	24 mg.
Dienestrol N.F.	Synestrol, etc.	0.5 mg.
Diethylstilbestrol U.S.P.	Stilbestrol; Stilbetin	0.1–25 mg.
Diethylstilbestrol dipropionate N.F.	Stilbestrol D.P.	0.5–5 mg.
Hexestrol	Esta-Plex, etc.	0.2–3 mg.
Methallenestril	Vallestril	3–20 mg.
Promethestrol dipropionate	Meprane	1 mg.

ducing normal menstrual bleeding and for maintaining pregnancy, doctors eagerly seized upon this substance when it was isolated from the corpora lutea of pigs and later purified and synthesized. Unfortunately, the natural ovarian hormone had several drawbacks that has limited its clinical usefulness. For one thing, its low potency when taken orally made injections necessary. These were painful and had to be repeated frequently because of the rapid breakdown of progesterone by the liver to the inactive metabolite pregnanediol, which is then excreted by the kidneys. In addition, the repeated administration of progesterone as substitution therapy all through a pregnancy was prohibitively expensive.

The clinical inadequacy of the natural hormone stimulated a search for synthetic steroids with progestational activity. This culminated, in the 1950's, in the introduction of several families of synthetic compounds derived from progesterone and from testosterone. These newly prepared progestational steroids differ from progesterone and from one another in some of their properties, but all are many times more effective than the natural hormone in evoking certain clinically important effects when administered by mouth, and some have a markedly prolonged duration of action when given by injection.

Gynecologists quickly began to employ these synthetic progestins, alone or in combination with estrogens, in the management of many clinical conditions.

Before discussing their therapeutic application in treating various menstrual disturbances and for dealing with problems related to female fertility, we shall first briefly review the physiological effects of progesterone. Some knowledge of the main natural actions of this hormone during the ovarian cycle is essential if we are truly to understand the reasoning behind the use of the new synthetic progestational steroids in the medical management of certain gynecological disorders which once usually required surgery (e.g., dysfunctional uterine bleeding; endometriosis). Similarly, a review of the physiological role of progesterone in pregnancy will help to clarify the rationale for the use of the progestins both to aid infertile women to conceive and in the temporary prevention of conception.

Physiological Actions

Actions on the Uterus

Progesterone acts upon both the thick muscle mass of the uterus and on its inner mucous lining in ways that are significant for the survival of the fertilized ovum and the embryo. The endometrial actions of progesterone prepare the uterine mucosa for reception and implantation of the egg, and the quieting effect of this luteal secretion on the myometrium keeps the embryo from being dislodged by muscular contractions of the uterus.

The endometrium, which has been previously primed by the proliferative effects of the estrogens, undergoes so-called *secretory* changes under the influence of progesterone. Its glands multiply rapidly and secrete large amounts of glycogen, a carbohydrate that will serve as the first source of energy for the rapidly dividing fertilized ovum. The accumulating secretions fill the glands and make them swell and twist into corkscrew shapes that give the pregravid endometrium a characteristic lacelike appearance in microscopic cross-section (Fig. 29-1).

During pregnancy, however, under the continued influence of progesterone, the dilated glands become narrow and their spirals straighten out as a result of secretory exhaustion (Fig. 29-1). These atrophic changes in the glands and in their underlying framework, or stroma, are also seen during long-term treatment with progesterone or synthetic progestins. This pregnancy-type endometrium offers an *un*favorable environment to the ovum that might be released from the ovary and fertilized. The glands in the inner lining of the cervix—the endocervical glands—produce a secretion under the influence of progesterone that is quite different from that induced by estrogens (p. 397). This pregnancy-type secretion is thick and viscid. It tends to form a cervical plug which acts as a barrier to sperm cells during pregnancy and progestin administration.

The myometrium tends to relax under the influence of progesterone. Such suppression of rhythmic uterine contractions favors implantation of the fertilized egg and, later, protects the placenta from being dislodged and, with the embryo, expelled prematurely. Throughout fetal development progesterone continues to counteract uterine spasms that could lead to spontaneous abortion. Finally, a falling off in progesterone production late in pregnancy is thought to play a part in initiating labor, since lack of this hormone may sensitize the myometrium to the contractile effects of oxytocin (Chap. 39).

Pituitary Actions of Progesterone

Like the estrogens, progesterone acts to suppress the secretion of pituitary gonadotropins. Late in the menstrual month, the progesterone produced by the corpus luteum reaches levels that inhibit the hypothalamic cells which control pituitary secretion of the luteinizing hormone (Chap. 27). This, in turn, causes regression of the corpus luteum, a fall in further production of progesterone and, finally, the failure of the secretory endometrium, which leads to its desquamation during menstruation.

During pregnancy, the continued production of progesterone by the corpus luteum and placenta keeps pituitary secretion of gonadotropins suppressed. This negative feedback effect of progesterone on hypothalamic-hypophyseal function stops the ovaries from

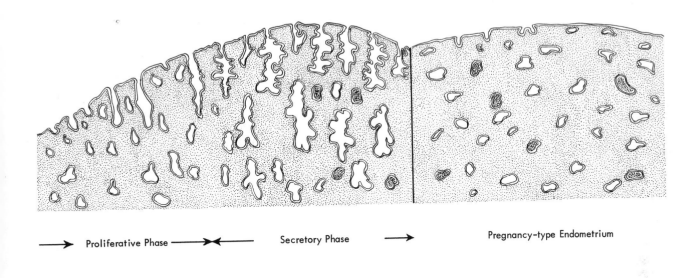

Fig. 29-1. The endometrium. (*Left*) Alterations during normal ovulatory cycle. (*Right*) During pregnancy or treatment with exogenous estrogens and progestins the endometrium shows signs of secretory exhaustion.

producing ova during pregnancy. Knowledge of this physiological suppression of ovulation by progesterone during the luteal phase of the ovulatory cycle and in pregnancy led researchers to study the possible use of this "pregnancy-supporting" hormone for *contraceptive* purposes.

Other Actions of Progesterone

Like estrogen, progesterone has effects on the breasts, vaginal mucosa and other body tissues. Its action on the breasts helps to bring about development of their alveolar secretory sacs during pregnancy. However, although these grapelike clusters within the mammary gland grow and fill with fluid in late pregnancy, lactation occurs only *after* the levels of progesterone and estrogen *fall* at the time of the baby's birth. Apparently, this helps to release from the mother's pituitary gland the milk-producing hormone, prolactin, which then stimulates the steroid-prepared secretory cells in the breasts. *Increasing the progestational activity by administering progestins can suppress the lactogenic hormone, inhibit lactation and relieve postpartum engorgement of the breasts* in a manner presumably similar to that of the

estrogens which are commonly employed for this purpose.

Progesterone, like estrogen, has various metabolic effects, but these differ from those of the other ovarian hormones in various ways. Its effects on the kidneys, for example, are of a kind that tend to increase salt and water excretion, whereas the estrogens seem to support electrolyte and fluid retention. Apparently, progesterone antagonizes the effects of the adrenal mineralocorticoid aldosterone upon the renal tubules. This anti-aldosterone (and anti-estrogen) action has led to trial of progestins in the treatment of premenstrual edema and tension. Still other metabolic effects of progesterone may account for the rise in body temperature that occurs midway in the menstrual cycle when progesterone production rises at the time of ovulation. This increase in temperature has been used to determine whether a woman is capable of ovulating, and, if so, to chart her times of maximum fertility.

Therapeutic Uses of Progesterone and the Progestins

When progesterone first became available, gynecologists tried to employ it in the treatment of menstrual and reproductive difficulties that stemmed from a lack of the natural hormone. They reasoned that many women failed to menstruate, or bled excessively, because a deficiency of endogenous progesterone led to endometrial abnormalities. Similarly, many women with no organic defects of the reproductive tract remained childless as a result of deficient production of this hormone.

It was thought that replacement of the lacking luteal hormone which prepares the endometrium to embed a fertilized egg (nidation) would correct infertility in some women. Giving progesterone and then withdrawing it should help other women to menstruate more normally. Administration of the hormone, isolated from animal ovaries and purified, was expected to be useful for preventing some miscarriages that may occur in the early months of pregnancy if the placenta fails to produce enough progesterone to keep the uterine musculature quiet.

In practice, progesterone proved disappointing. Although the hormone seemed useful in some menstrual disorders and in certain selected cases of endocrine infertility and habitual or threatened abortion, the need to administer either massive oral doses or frequent painful injections put severe practical limitations upon the use of the natural hormone. Many of these difficulties seem to have been eliminated with the advent of the synthetic progestins.

Some of these progestins are preferred to others for various clinical uses, because they possess properties that make them superior for particular purposes. Thus, few of the synthetic progestins are purely progesta-tional. Some have, in addition, slight estrogenic or androgenic (male hormone) actions, which affect their suitability for treating various conditions. However, all these compounds are sufficiently similar to permit certain generalizations about their utility in the clinical situations we shall discuss here.

Infertility

Infertility, of course, may have many causes, including, not infrequently, the husband's inability to produce adequate numbers of lively, motile sperm. The usefulness of progestins is limited, even in theory, to those cases in which these hormones may work to correct some abnormality in a woman's menstrual rhythm and thus help her ovaries to release an ovum, or prepare the endometrium for implantation of a fertilized egg.

The new synthetic steroids seem to have proved most effective in those women whose infertility can be traced back to a poorly functioning corpus luteum that fails to produce enough progesterone to maintain an adequate secretory endometrium. The administration of small daily oral doses of synthetic progestins (combined with estrogens) during the *post*ovulatory phase of the menstrual cycle is claimed to have helped some women with luteal phase defects to conceive and bear children.

In such cases of infertility, the progestins serve as substitutional therapy. That is, when administered daily from the time when a rise in the woman's body temperature indicates that ovulation has occurred, these synthetic hormones supplement the patient's

TABLE 29-2

PROGESTATIONAL STEROIDS *

Nonproprietary Name	Proprietary Name or Synonym	Dosage Range
Chlormadinone acetate	Lormin	2–20 mg.
Dydrogesterone	Duphaston	5–30 mg.
Ethisterone N.F.	Ethinyl testosterone; Pranone; Progesterol, etc.	25–100 mg.
Ethynodiol diacetate	in Ovulen	1 mg.
Hydroxyprogesterone acetate	Prodox	25–50 mg.
Hydroxyprogesterone caproate	Delalutin	250 mg. I.M.
Medroxyprogesterone acetate U.S.P.	Provera	2.5–40 mg.
Norethindrone	Norethisterone; Norlutin	5–30 mg.
Norethindrone acetate	Norlutate	2.5–15 mg.
Norethynodrel	in Enovid	2.5–30 mg.
Progesterone N.F.	Colprosterone; Lipo-Lutin; Lucorteum; Lutocylin, etc.	10–25 mg.

* See also Table 29-3.

own inadequate progesterone production. Under their influence, the woman's proliferative endometrium is converted into the secretory type that is capable of receiving and nourishing a fertilized egg. Repetition of such steroid replacement therapy during several menstrual cycles eventually leads to pregnancy, provided that the woman with luteal phase deficiency is capable of producing an ovum, and viable sperm reach it during its descent through the oviduct.

The progestins have apparently proved useful even in some women whose infertility stemmed from failure to ovulate. The manner in which the progestins stimulate ovulation in such cases is still uncertain. Unlike treatment with gonadotropins or clomiphene (Chap. 29), progestins do not stimulate either the ovaries or the pituitary gland directly. On the contrary, the progestins act, at first, to produce a *pseudo-pregnancy* situation, in which pituitary gonadotropin secretion is suppressed and ovulation is, of course, impossible.

Reportedly, when progestin-estrogen therapy was stopped after several such cycles, the ovaries of some women whose infertility stemmed from failure to ovulate were indirectly stimulated to produce ova, and the women soon became pregnant. This so-called rebound-effect, which may result from the rest afforded a sluggish pituitary gland, is said to account for the seeming *increase* in fertility of women who stop taking oral steroid contraceptives when they wish to become pregnant.

Spontaneous Abortion

Spontaneous abortion occurs in about 10 per cent of all pregnancies and thus accounts for the termination of very many desired pregnancies. Some women abort repeatedly, and those who have had three or more consecutive miscarriages are termed "habitual" or "recurrent" aborters. Progesterone has been employed in such cases for many years, on the assumption that at least some abortions result from a failure of the placenta to secrete enough of the hormone to keep the uterus quiet. Administered in large and frequent doses all through pregnancy, progesterone is claimed to counteract the contractile effects of estrogens on the myometrium and thus to prevent premature expulsion of the embryo or fetus from the uterus.

Some of the synthetic progestins are claimed to be even more effective than progesterone itself for maintaining pregnancies in patients who have aborted habitually and for other women when staining and uterine cramps indicate that abortion is a threat. For example, daily administration of oral doses of medroxyprogesterone acetate (see Drug Digest) during pregnancy is claimed to have helped to salvage fetuses. A long-acting ester derivative, *hydroxyprogesterone acetate* (see Drug Digest), which requires less frequent injection than the natural luteal hormone, is also claimed to be helpful for maintenance of pregnancies. Thus, although there is still some controversy as to whether treatment with progesterone and its derivatives is truly more effective in threatened abortion than bed rest and sedation alone, many doctors now feel that the use of the new synthetic progestins is worth a trial when a woman who badly wants her baby seems in danger of losing it.

These drugs cannot, of course, prevent spontaneous abortions that are due to defects in the embryo. Many miscarriages are inevitable because of some fundamental defect in the germ plasm. In some cases, the embryo has died even before signs such as vaginal staining and colicky pains in the lower abdomen appear. In such circumstances, the progestins are, of course, ineffective, since they are given too late to do any good.

Certain of the synthetic progestins are considered undesirable for use in the long-term treatment of threatened abortion. These include the testosterone derivatives, *ethisterone* and *norethindrone* (see Drug Digest), which possess a slight androgenic action. This has occasionally led to clitoral enlargement and other masculinizing effects on the external genitalia of female fetuses. Such virilizing effects have, in rare instances, occurred after treatment with progesterone itself as well as after use of norethynodrel—a progestin which, if anything, has slight estrogenic rather than androgenic activity.

Menstrual Disorders

The menstrual cycle depends upon a delicately balanced sequence of steps involving interactions between the pituitary gland and the ovaries. Failure of any link in this pituitary-ovary-uterus axis can lead to a lack or excess of the ovarian hormones that affect the functioning of the uterus. Such disruption of uterine function may be marked by any of a variety of menstruation disturbances. These include (1) *amenorrhea* (the absence of menstruation), (2) *hypermenorrhea* (excessive menstrual bleeding, and other kinds of dysfunctional uterine bleeding), and (3) *dysmenorrhea* (painful menstruation).

In all of these conditions, and in others such as *endometriosis* and *premenstrual tension*, the introduction of convenient, orally effective synthetic progestins has led to better control. Combined with estrogens, or administered alternately with them in accordance with the principles of menstrual cycle physiology, the progestins seem to help correct many of the hormonal imbalances responsible for menstrual abnormalities.

Amenorrhea may have many causes. Failure to menstruate can be entirely physiological—in pregnancy, for example, or following the menopause; absence of menstruation may, on the other hand, be secondary to many systemic diseases and endocrine malfunctions. Once the cause has been determined by a variety of diagnostic tests, treatment to establish normal menstrual bleeding can be undertaken. The new and potent synthetic progestins are often useful for both the diagnosis and treatment of amenorrhea.

Primary Amenorrhea. In a normal menstrual cycle, female sex hormones of both types must be secreted in adequate amounts and exert their sequential proliferative and secretory effects upon the endometrium. Then, when ovarian secretion drops off late in the menstrual month, the mucous membrane breaks down and menstruation occurs. Thus, in the hypogonadal girl menarche (i.e., the beginning of menstrual function) never does occur (*primary* amenorrhea), because she lacks ovarian estrogens. Successful treatment of the hypo-ovarianism by gonadotropic stimulation or by estrogen replacement therapy helps to produce the proliferative endometrium upon which progestational compounds can then act. Withdrawal of these hormones then leads to breakdown of the secretory endometrium and menstrual bleeding. (In girls and women without functioning ovaries, this is, of course, *pseudo*menstruation.)

Secondary Amenorrhea. In secondary amenorrhea—i.e., the kind that develops in women who have previously menstruated—the administration of estrogen-progestin combinations in a way that imitates normal cyclic production can, of course, also be used to bring about menstruation upon periodic withdrawal. Therapy of this kind often results, after several such artificial cycles, in spontaneous menstruation presumably because this treatment stimulates pituitary hormone production, and the gonadotropins in turn stimulate natural ovarian hormone secretion in proper amounts and timing.

Progestins administered during the latter half of the menstrual cycle will produce a secretory endometrium and withdrawal bleeding only if ovarian estrogens have first built up a proliferative endometrium. Thus, continued amenorrhea following administration of progestins alone indicates a lack of prior estrogenic priming. This may serve as a diagnostic test of whether a patient's ovaries are producing adequate amounts of endogenous estrogens.

On the other hand, when bleeding fails to occur within several days of withdrawal of combined estrogens and progestins, such amenorrhea is indicative of pregnancy. This hormonal pregnancy test is based upon the assumption that the patient's amenorrhea is caused by the continued secretion of endogenous progesterone, which is being produced by the developing chorionic membranes. If the patient were not pregnant, the endometrium would deteriorate and menstruation would follow within a few days after withdrawal of the hormonal support from an outside source.

Uterine bleeding that is of endocrine origin and not due to organic disease—that is, "functional," or (perhaps better put) "*dysfunctional*," bleeding—can now be rather readily controlled by hormonal treatment and recurrence prevented by continued cyclic administration of estrogen-progestin drug combinations. Abnormal bleeding occurs most commonly at puberty —when the ovulatory cycle is not yet well established— and at the climacteric, when ovarian function is failing. (Doctors distinguish between two types of uterine hemorrhage: *menorrhagia*, which is marked by excessive blood loss during a normal menstrual period, and *metrorrhagia*, a term which refers to bleeding at irregular intervals at times other than menstrual periods.)

Such bleeding episodes are the end-result of either too little estrogen production or too long continued estrogen secretion in the absence of a source of progesterone.

The latter situation may occur as the result of ovulatory failure. In such an anovulatory cycle, no corpus luteum is formed; as a result, a progesterone deficiency occurs and the proliferative endometrium is not converted to the secretory type. Since it is then being stimulated solely by estrogens, it continues to proliferate and grows quite thick. Finally, however, this proliferative endometrium outgrows its blood supply and begins to break down at various weak spots. This leads to bleeding that is irregular and often prolonged and excessive, because the hyperplastic endometrial tissue does not slough off completely and all at one time.

Acute uterine hemorrhaging can be *halted* by injections of estrogens or progesterone, or even by the male hormone, testosterone. On the other hand, the synthetic progestin *norethindrone*, which also has some slight estrogenic and androgenic activity, effectively *controls* bleeding. When given *by mouth* several times a day for a week or two, this drug (and other progestins) repairs the necrotic endometrial areas. Then, the withdrawal of the progestational steroids at the end of that time is followed by shedding of the endometrium, with what appears to be essentially normal bleeding. Such a hormone-induced removal of the uterine mucous membrane frequently does away with the need for dilatation and curettage, a procedure considered undesirable in young unmarried women. Often after several such intermittent "medical curettage" treatments with a progestin or with combined estrogens and progestins, the woman's normal cycles are re-established and excessive bleeding episodes no longer occur.

Dysmenorrhea. Many women with no evidence of organic pelvic disease suffer disabling uterine cramps during their menstrual periods. Numerous drugs, including analgesics, sedatives and antispasmodics are employed for symptomatic relief, and a variety of hormones including thyroid, insulin and even the male hormone have been tried. However, all drug treatments and even the ovarian uterus-relaxing hormones, lututrin (Chap. 39) and progesterone, have offered only inconsistent relief.

Progesterone injections just prior to the menstrual period were first employed as replacement therapy on the assumption that the uterine contractions in this condition are the result of a lack of this myometrium-quieting hormone. However, this treatment did not help many patients. Although this *premenstrual* progesterone treatment did not help many patients, the oral administration of either synthetic progestins or estrogens, or a combination of the two steroids, *early in the menstrual month*, has recently been reported to be followed by painless menstruation after withdrawal.

Such treatment, which suppresses pituitary gonadotropin secretion, prevents ovulation from occurring. It is now thought that inhibition of ovulation is somehow responsible for the resulting relative freedom from menstrual cramps. Thus, the same steroid combinations which are employed as oral contraceptives are now being used to treat women with dysmenorrhea. When the combined oral estrogens and progestins are withdrawn at the end of each cycle, painless menstrual bleeding usually occurs. If such cyclic steroid therapy is continued indefinitely, it will, of course, interfere with fertility.

Endometriosis

In this condition, according to one theory, pieces of endometrial tissue, which have been carried (by retrograde menstrual flow) from the uterus through the oviducts up into the abdominal cavity, become implanted upon pelvic organs. These vagrant bits of uterine mucosa form masses on organs such as the ovaries, fallopian tubes, ureters, urinary bladder and colon. Periodic bleeding then causes surface swellings that may be painful and may interfere with the proper functioning of these organs. By blocking the tubes, for example, such masses may cause infertility, and the rupture of blood-filled ovarian cysts may result in sterility.

Until recently, severe endometriosis was treated mainly by surgical removal of the ovaries and uterus. Such hysterectomy and castration, of course, halted the disease but also ended the woman's childbearing years and brought about a premature menopause. Today, this serious condition is being successfully treated by the continuous administration of progestins, alone or combined with estrogens, for many months. Such a regimen not only prevents the painful menstruation of this condition but also often leads to regression of the growths within the abdomen.

The *pseudo*pregnancy brought about by such progestin therapy is effective for several reasons. By suppressing pituitary function, ovulation, and menstrua-

tion such steroid treatment prevents the pathological extrauterine bleeding which otherwise occurs in this condition at the time of each menstrual period. Even more important than the drug-induced amenorrhea is the fact that the bits of displaced endometrial tissue often become fibrotic and reduced in size during prolonged progestin therapy. When the drug is withdrawn after six to nine months, normal ovulation and menstruation soon resume but, in most cases, the ectopic endometrial implants do not become reactivated. As a result, many women with endometriosis-induced infertility have been able to conceive and bear children.

Other Uses of Uninterrupted Progestational Therapy. The drug-induced amenorrhea that results when progestin-estrogen combinations are administered and *not* withdrawn periodically is being put to various other uses. Gynecologists agree that there is no harm in postponing menstruation and that many women may benefit from the longer than monthly cycles which can be brought about and regulated by these drugs. For example, since menstrual bleeding leads to significant iron loss (Chap. 25), steroid-induced amenorrhea may often be a desirable adjunct to the standard treatment of iron-deficiency anemia and may also be applicable in the prevention of anemia in women who are being prepared for surgery.

Premenstrual Edema and Tension

Many women tend to retain fluid as their menstrual periods approach. Weight gain, painful breast fullness, backache and headache are some of the physical complaints in this premenstrual condition. In addition, some women suffer from emotional upsets of varying intensity. Although its cause is uncertain, some physicians have suggested that this syndrome results from inadequate production of progesterone by the corpus luteum and a resulting relative excess of fluid-retaining estrogens.

The new oral progestins have been administered as replacement therapy, alone or combined with oral diuretics and sedatives, during the latter half of the menstrual month. This regimen has been claimed to be effective for relief of premenstrual crankiness and irritability as well as for removal of retained fluid. The administration of progestin-estrogen combinations to suppress ovulation and thus eliminate the inadequate luteal phase thought to be responsible for the emotional upsets and physical symptoms is also said to have proved effective for counteracting premenstrual distress.

Oral Contraception

In addition to all their other and varied gynecological uses, combinations of progestins and estrogens have been widely employed recently to prevent conception. The nurse, regardless of her personal religious convictions in regard to contraception, must be informed concerning the use of sex steroids for this purpose, in order to participate intelligently in the care of these patients. Thus, the current status of the presently available steroid combinations employed as oral contraceptives (Table 29-3) will be briefly discussed here.

Administration. Generally, products of two types, which are administered on somewhat different dosage schedules, are in use today. Both kinds of contraceptive preparations contain a progestin in combination with one or another of several potent estrogens. Most of these combinations are prepared as a single tablet which is taken orally for 20 days, beginning on the fifth day after the onset of menstruation and ending on the twenty-fourth day. In a few products, *two* tablets, one containing only estrogen and the other a combination of progestin and estrogen, are employed in a so-called sequential regimen. The estrogen tablet is taken for about 15 days and followed for 5 days with the combined steroids. In both schedules, withdrawal of the combination tablet therapy is fol-

lowed by breakdown of the secretory endometrium that had been induced by the presence of the progestational steroid in the combination. Thus menstruation usually occurs within a few days.

Manner of Action. Products of both types produce their contraceptive effect primarily by their ability to suppress ovulation through the reduction of gonadotropic hormone secretion by the anterior pituitary gland. In addition, steroid combinations may have *extra*ovulatory effects that would probably prevent pregnancy even if an ovum were released. For example, the effects of synthetic progestins upon the endometrium and the endocervical glandular secretions (see Fig. 29-1 and discussion on p. 404) would probably prevent a sperm from reaching the egg and would keep a fertilized ovum from becoming implanted.

Effectiveness and Acceptability. All authorities agree that, when a woman takes her daily steroid tablet faithfully, either regimen is virtually 100 per cent effective for preventing conception. The efficacy and convenience of this contraceptive method has led

TABLE 29-3
STEROID COMBINATIONS USED AS ORAL CONTRACEPTIVES, ETC.

SYNTHETIC PROGESTIN	SYNTHETIC ESTROGEN	PRODUCT NAME
Chlormadinone, 2 mg.	Mestranol, 0.08 mg. + Mestranol, 0.08 mg.	C-Quens (S)
Dimethisterone, 25 mg.	Ethinyl estradiol, 0.1 mg. + Ethinyl estradiol, 0.1 mg.	Oracon (S)
Ethinylestrenol (Lynestrenol), 5 mg.	Mestranol, 0.15 mg.	Lyndiol
Ethynodiol diacetate, 1 mg.	Mestranol, 0.1 mg.	Ovulen Ovulen 21
Medroxyprogesterone acetate (Provera), 10 mg.	Ethinyl estradiol, 0.05 mg.	Provest
Megestrol acetate, 4 mg.	Ethinyl estradiol, 0.05 mg.	Volidan
Norethindrone, 2 mg.	Mestranol, 0.1 mg.	Norinyl; Ortho-Novum
Norethindrone, 2 mg.	Mestranol, 0.08 mg. + Mestranol, 0.08 mg.	Norquen; Ortho-Novum SQ (S)
Norethindrone acetate (Norlutate), 2.5 mg.	Ethinyl estradiol, 0.05 mg.	Norlestrin
Norethynodrel, 2.5 mg.	Mestranol, 0.1 mg.	Enovid E

(S) = Sequential

to its wide acceptance by married couples who had previously depended upon the use of mechanical barriers to conception in their family planning efforts. However, a number of women have tried and then discontinued oral contraceptives, because they were unwilling to put up with various unpleasant reactions resulting from the systemic actions of these steroids.

The most common undesirable effects resemble those of early pregnancy, and, like the latter, they tend to diminish or disappear after several monthly cycles. These include nausea and vomiting, headache and dizziness, weight gain, breast fullness and discomfort and, occasionally, acne and chloasma (an increase in skin pigmentation). Another reaction that some women find frightening and confusing is the occurrence of breakthrough bleeding, or spotting, during their cycle, or, on the other hand, failure to menstruate upon withdrawal of the drugs at the end of the cycle.

Despite these distressing symptoms, most women seem willing to continue taking oral contraceptives through the first few cycles, after which—as in pregnancy—nausea and other discomforts lessen. Most side effects are, in any case, controllable. Nausea, for example, can be reduced by taking the tablet at bedtime with a glass of milk. Breakthrough bleeding can be overcome by *increasing* the steroid dosage to prevent premature endometrial breakdown.

Actually, most women with prior menstrual irregularities find that these steroid combinations exert a regularizing effect upon their menstrual cycles. This has helped some women to employ the so-called rhythm method of birth control with a greater degree of security. (Thus, the *temporary* use of these products for this purpose is acceptable to the Catholic Church, which does not, of course, disapprove of family planning for medical, economic or social reasons, but recognizes only the rhythm method as a licit means of limiting the size of the family.)

These drugs are simple to use and are usually available in special calendar packages that are intended to help the patient keep track of tablet taking. However, women with emotional problems may be unable to cope with the responsibility of remembering the required dosage schedule. Similarly, some women, especially uneducated ones, tend to worry needlessly that taking these drugs may be dangerous or that their use will prevent future desired pregnancy. In all such cases, the nurse can help by providing an opportunity for the woman and her husband to discuss their doubts and fears with their doctor, who can then instruct them in how best to use these drugs and what to expect of them.

Long-term Safety. Although no truly toxic effects have been traced to these steroid combinations, serious concern has often been expressed as to the possible adverse results of prolonged administration of these drugs. Doctors are still studying the long-range effects

of these medications on glandular function and reproductive capacity, and on the blood vessels, among other organs. In certain situations, it is felt that the risk of using these substances for contraceptive purposes is not warranted.

Women with a history of *thromboembolic disease*, for example, are warned to avoid the use of oral contraceptives, until it is known for certain whether taking these steroids might make them more prone to develop blood clotting disorders. Some doctors have reported cases in which young women suffered from thrombophlebitis, pulmonary embolism and clot-caused eye damage while using this contraceptive method. Even though no link has so far been found between administration of these drugs and the occurrence of these dangerous conditions, caution seems indicated until any causal relationship can be definitely disproved.

Another question that has disturbed some doctors is whether these synthetic sex hormone combinations might cause cancer when taken for long periods as contraceptives. Careful studies of thousands of patients have revealed no evidence of genital tract cancer, and there is instead some indication that these drugs may have some protective action against uterine carcinoma. However, the presence of estrogens tends to increase the growth of uterine fibroid tumors, and these hormones might also stimulate growth of an undetected mammary or genital carcinoma. Thus, the use of oral contraceptives is contraindicated in patients with a previous history of such cancers, and the steroids are discontinued if enlargement of fibromas is detected.

Caution is also required in patients with a history of liver disease, mental depression, and various disorders that might be adversely affected by steroid-induced fluid retention—e.g., epilepsy, migraine headaches, asthma, or cardiovascular disease. Patients with thyroid disease, diabetes, and other endocrine disorders must be closely watched for signs of worsening of their conditions while taking these drugs.

On the other hand, fears that these drugs might adversely affect a woman's future fertility seem unfounded. Most women who want to conceive have no difficulty in doing so shortly after discontinuing the contraceptive drugs. Babies born to former users of steroid contraceptive seem normal in every way. Studies of the long-term effects on the patient's pituitary gland and ovaries are still continuing, but there is no indication thus far that these drugs might delay a woman's menopause or lengthen her child-bearing years.

In summary, it seems that the synthetic sex steroids, although they cause frequent minor side effects (that tend to decrease with continued use), have proved safe in terms of capacity to cause true toxicity. Most women who wish to avoid conception for a time are willing to bear the occasional disagreeable effects, and some women apparently gain bonus benefits such as improvement in menstrual regularity, with reduced cramps and blood flow. New contraceptive drugs now being tested may prove somewhat more convenient to take—for example, *one-a-month* administration or

tablets that are effective when taken *after* intercourse; however, the agents of the future will probably be no safer or more effective than the drugs presently available.

SUMMARY OF POINTS FOR THE NURSE TO REMEMBER CONCERNING THE FEMALE SEX HORMONE

- Be alert for comments and complaints that indicate distress over normal physiological processes (such as the menopause) and encourage the women to seek medical advice.

- Help male patients who require estrogen therapy for coronary atherosclerosis or cancer to cope with their emotional reactions to feminizing side effects. Show that you recognize the patient's essential manliness despite such changes as gynecomastia induced by these female sex hormones.

- Instruct women carefully in how to insert suppositories and apply creams containing estrogens. Suggest ways to store suppositories and to avoid soiling clothing after use of such medications.

- Make certain that all girls—or the parents in the case of children—who are being treated with female sex hormones in doses high enough to bring about changes in secondary sex characteristics know in advance what to expect from the physiological actions of these substances. See that their fears are allayed and that they are given an opportunity to ask questions about the significance of such changes.

- If a woman raises questions concerning the possibility of estrogens causing cancer, suggest that she discuss her fears with her physician. He will assure her of the safety of these hormones for women who first

have a full physical examination and continue to take the drug under medical supervision.

- Indicate the desirability of regular visits to the physician during prolonged estrogen therapy, since the only established hazard in such therapy is failure to follow treatment with regular examinations.

- Women should be told that the occurrence of bleeding when estrogens are withdrawn is natural. It should be carefully explained that such bleeding in *post*menopausal women is *pseudo*menstruation and does not, of course, mean that they have regained fertility and are capable of becoming pregnant. Bleeding at other times is *not* natural and should be reported to the doctor so that he can rule out any organic causes.

- Encourage the woman who is taking oral contraceptives to report any discomforting side effects to her physician, so that he can seek their cause and deal with them.

- Recognize that the same sex steroids can be used for widely different purposes. Thus, estrogen-progestin combinations can be used both to promote fertility and to prevent conception.

- Remember that it is essential to respect the decision of the patient in regard to the desirability of employing contraceptive drugs, regardless of one's personal religious views.

CLINICAL PROBLEMS

Mrs. Johansen, who is 46 years old, visited the gynecologic clinic because of nervousness, sweating, and a feeling of depression. Her menstrual periods have become irregular, and Mrs. Johansen told the clinic doctor that she thought her symptoms were due to "change of life." After talking with her and examining her, the doctor stated

that he, too, believed her symptoms were due to menopause. He prescribed Premarin 2.5 mg. t.i.d. As Mrs. Johansen was leaving the clinic, she said to the nurse, "The doctor says I must take female hormones. I've heard that they cause cancer—is that true?"

How would you reply to Mrs. Johansen?

SUMMARY OF SIDE EFFECTS, CAUTIONS, AND CONTRAINDICATIONS OF THE FEMALE SEX HORMONES

- **Estrogens**

    Anorexia, nausea and vomiting; sometimes diarrhea also.

    Headache, dizziness, fatigue.

    Vaginal bleeding from a hyperplastic proliferative endometrium (i.e., "breakthrough bleeding," etc.).

    Contraindicated in *pre*menopausal women with mammary carcinoma and in all women with genital-tissue cancers; also possibly contraindicated in women with a personal or family history of breast or genital malignancy.

    Gynecomastia or breast soreness (in *men*).

    Hypercalcemia (in cancer treatment).

    Loss of libido; testicular atrophy (in the male).

    Precocious puberty, premature closure of the epiphysis, if administered systemically in overdoses to prepubertal children.

- **Progestins**

    Masculinization of female fetuses.

    Presence of malignancy should be ruled out before using for control of uterine bleeding.

    Acne, hirsutism and chloasma occasionally.

    Increase in size of uterine fibroids.

    Reduced menstrual flow.

    Caution in patients with a history of thromboembolic disease (when used for long-term contraception in combination with estrogens).

    Caution in similar use for patients with a history of hepatic, renal, or cardiovascular disease, including hypertension; also in asthma, epilepsy, or migraine.

REVIEW QUESTIONS

1. Indicate briefly the *physiological* effects of estrogens upon the following tissues: (a) the *endometrium*, (b) the *vaginal mucosa*, (c) *pituitary* (gonadotropin-producing cells), (d) skin, bone, and other *non*-reproductive tissues.

2. What are some menopausal symptoms of which women may complain, and what seems to be the current status of estrogen-replacement therapy for treating the menopause? (i.e., What advice might a nurse offer concerning the safety and efficacy of estrogen prescribed for this purpose?)

3. (a) What is the rationale for the use of estrogens *post*menopausally in osteoporosis?

(b) Why are these hormones sometimes used for men as well as postmenopausal women, and what may be the side effects of their use in males?

4. List several conditions in which estrogens are administered topically and indicate some suggestions that might be made to women receiving such dosage forms.

5. (a) What is the rationale for the use of estrogens in sexual infantilism?

(b) What attitude should the nurse assume toward patients (and their parents) when they are to receive hormones in doses high enough to bring about sexual changes?

6. (a) At what site are estrogens thought to act to suppress postpartum lactation?

(b) At what site do estrogens act to stop growth in a girl's height?

7. (a) What is the most common side effect of estrogen therapy?

(b) What is the cause of occasional "breakthrough bleeding" during estrogen therapy, and how is it best avoided?

8. (a) What advice can be given to a patient who expresses fear of developing genital or breast cancer during estrogen therapy?

(b) What advice can be given to women who are confused and disturbed by withdrawal bleeding during prolonged postmenopausal cyclic estrogen therapy?

9. (a) List three estrogens from natural sources.

(b) List two potent semisynthetic estrogens.

(c) List two synthetic non-steroid drugs with estrogenic activity.

10. (a) What are the usual sources of the female sex hormone, progesterone, during a normal menstrual (ovarian) cycle and during pregnancy?

(b) What are some drawbacks limiting the use of progesterone clinically, and what are the advantages of the new synthetic progestational steroids?

11. (a) What is the ordinary effect of progesterone upon the endometrium?

(b) Indicate why continued action of progesterone upon the endometrium and upon the endocervical glands might make fertilization and implantation of an ovum more *difficult* rather than easier.

12. (a) What is the effect of progesterone and its derivatives upon the myometrium?

(b) What is the effect of excessive progesterone upon the production of pituitary gonadotropins?

13. (a) Explain how administration of progestins as substitution therapy may help some women who are infertile (even though they ovulate) to become pregnant.

(b) Explain how cyclic progestin treatment may sometimes help to overcome infertility in women with anovulatory cycles.

14. (a) Name two progesterone derivatives employed for treating habitual and threatened abortion and indicate the rationale for their use.

(b) Name two synthetic progestins considered undesirable for this purpose and indicate the type of difficulty that has followed their use.

15. (a) How does the administration of estrogens and progestins act to produce menstrual bleeding in amenorrhea?

(b) What does failure to bleed after withdrawal of combined estrogens and progestins probably indicate, and why is this so?

16. (a) What is the reason for excessive uterine bleeding in women who fail to ovulate?

(b) How does administration and then withdrawal of a progestin control such abnormal bleeding?

17. (a) How are orally administered progestin-estrogen combinations believed to act to relieve dysmenorrhea?

(b) How does administration of progestins benefit patients with endometriosis?

18. (a) How do the two presently available types of oral contraceptives differ in their administration schedules?

(b) What is the primary manner of action of oral contraceptive products of both types?

19. (a) List some of the most common side effects of contraceptive therapy.

(b) How may adverse gastrointestinal and uterine effects be reduced?

20. (a) List several conditions in which oral contraceptive products are employed with caution or actually contraindicated.

(b) What advice can be offered women who express fear of cancer or of future inability to conceive after taking prescribed oral contraceptive medication for some time?

BIBLIOGRAPHY

Estrogens

Davis, M. E.: Long-term estrogen substitution after the menopause. Clin. Obstet. Gynec., 7:558, 1964.

Davis, M. E., Strandjford, N. M., and Lanzl, L. H.: Estrogens and the aging process. J.A.M.A., *196*:219, 1966.

Lammert, A.: The menopause: a physiologic process. Am. J. Nurs., *62*:56, 1962.

Marmoston, J., *et al.*: Effect of Premarin on survival in men with myocardial infarctions. Proc. Soc. Exp. Biol. Med., *105*:618, 1960.

Progestins (and Estrogens)

Berczeller, P. H., Young, I. S., and Kupperman, H. S.: The therapeutic use of progestational steroids. Clin. Pharmacol. Ther., 5:216, 1964.

Cole, M.: Strokes in young women using oral contraceptives. Arch. Int. Med., *120*:551, 1967 (Nov.).

Control of Fertility. Report of Committee on Human Reproduction. J.A.M.A., *194*:462, 1965.

de Alvarez, R. R., and Smith, E. K.: Physiological basis for hormone therapy in the female. J.A.M.A., *168*:489, 1958.

Epstein, J. A., and Kupperman, H. S.: Oral antifertility measures. Clin. Pharmacol. Ther., 3:216, 1962.

Gold, J. J., Scommegna, A., and Borushek, S.: The clinical use of ovulation suppressants. Med. Clin. N. Am., 47: 131, 1963.

Oliver, M. F., and Boyd, G. S.: The influence of reduction of serum lipids on prognosis of coronary heart disease, a five year study using estrogens. Lancet, 2:499, 1961.

Rodman, M. J.: Drugs in gynecology (I). R.N., *24*:45, 1961 (July).

Rogers, J.: Current status of therapy of the menopause. J.A.M.A., *175*:1167, 1961.

Wallach, S., and Henneman, P. H.: Prolonged estrogen therapy in postmenopausal women. J.A.M.A., *171*:1637, 1959.

Goldzieher, J. W.: Newer drugs in oral contraception. Med. Clin. N. Am., *48*:529, 1964.

Kupperman, H. S.: Functional uterine bleeding. G.P., *25*: 100, 1962.

Kister, R. W.: The use of steroidal substances in endometriosis. Clin. Pharmacol. Ther., *1*:525, 1960.

Rodman, M. J.: Drugs in gynecology (II). R.N., *24*:29, 1961 (August).

———: The oral contraceptives. R.N., *29*:51, 1966 (March).

———: The female sex hormones. R.N., *31*:41, 1968 (May).

Tyler, E. T.: Current status of oral contraception. J.A.M.A., *187*:562, 1964.

Wilkins, L.: Masculinization of female fetus due to use of orally given progestins. J.A.M.A., *172*:1028, 1960.

· 30 ·

The Male Sex Hormones
and Anabolic Agents

THE MALE SEX HORMONE

Even primitive peoples were well aware of the relationship between the testes and maleness. The practice of castrating young men to make eunuch caretakers of harems has persisted in the Orient from remote antiquity to modern times. Fortunately, the male soprano, or "castrato," voice so prized in early Italian opera is no longer developed by training the voices of young men castrated for this purpose prior to puberty. (The high-pitched countertenor voice occasionally heard today is presumably a natural attribute of its male possessor, obtained without sacrifice of his masculinity.)

Isolation and purification of the testicular secretion responsible for male physical and mental characteristics became possible as a result of chemical advances in the first quarter of this century. Only in this generation has this hormone, *testosterone*, been employed in medicine for treating male endocrine dysfunctions. Indeed, testosterone and its derivatives are being used today not only to replace hormones missing in men because of testicular loss or deficiency diseases, but also in treating women and children with various *nonendocrine* disorders.

Before we discuss the therapeutic uses of testosterone and the compounds derived by altering its molecular structure in various ways, we shall review briefly the physiology of the male hormone. This will enable us better to understand the actions that the doctor is seeking when he orders these drugs, as well as the adverse effects which he wishes to avoid.

Physiology of the Male Hormone

As indicated in Chapter 27, the functions of the testes are under the control of anterior pituitary gonadotropins. The pituitary hormone FSH, which, in women, stimulates the ovarian follicles to bring their ova to maturity, has an analogous function in the male —i.e., it influences sperm development (spermatogenesis) by its stimulating action on the seminiferous tubular tissues of the testes. FSH does *not*, however, simultaneously stimulate testicular secretion of the male hormone, in the way in which it prods the ovaries to produce estrogens.

Testosterone production is, instead, under the influence of another anterior pituitary gonadotropin. This hormone, known in the female as the luteinizing hormone (LH), acts upon the cells of Leydig, located in the spaces or interstices between the seminiferous tubules of the testes. Thus, in the male, it is called the interstitial-cell stimulating hormone (ICSH). The testosterone secreted by these cells, in turn, plays a part in regulating pituitary gonadotropin production. That is, high levels of androgens (male hormones) in the blood tend to suppress the secretion of FSH and ICSH. This negative feedback mechanism is, however, probably not the only way in which gonadotropic production, release, and secretion is inhibited.

Functions of Testosterone

The functions of testosterone may be broadly classified as: (1) *sexual* and (2) *metabolic*. These actions become dramatically evident at puberty when previously suppressed gonadotropic hormones are released in large amounts upon a signal from the hypothalamus. The outpouring of testosterone that follows such gonadotropic stimulation of the boy's testes produces effects of the two types (sexual and metabolic) upon all the tissues of the body. That is, the testicular secretions act as a growth hormone not only to the boy's sex organs but also to such structures as the skeletal muscles and the bones. The skin and hair are also affected, and protein metabolism in general is

415

stimulated, so that dietary nitrogen is retained in the tissues in larger amounts (an *anabolic* action).

Sexual Function. The accessory sex organs—the penis, prostate gland, seminal vesicles and vas deferens—grow in size and functional capacity under the influence of pubertal testosterone. The testes themselves grow in size as does the scrotal sac in which they are contained. The seminiferous tubules of the testes share in this growth, and, under the combined influence of testosterone and FSH, spermatogenesis begins. Sperm production is maintained throughout the man's reproductive life by the balanced effects of these testicular and pituitary hormones. Oddly, oligospermia, or low sperm counts, can result from either too little or too much testosterone. In the latter case, too much testosterone shuts off pituitary secretion of the FSH needed to maintain seminiferous tubule function.

The secondary sex characteristics of the male also make their appearance at puberty under the influence of testosterone. At this time, the boy's high-pitched voice deepens as his vocal cords thicken under the influence of this hormone. Hair begins to grow, not only in the axillary and pubic areas but also on his arms, legs and trunk. Interestingly, some young people predisposed to baldness by heredity begin to show the first signs of future loss of hair at this time. Apparently, testosterone plays a part in producing so-called male pattern baldness. Facial hair makes its first appearance at this time, and the beard continues to come in gradually over the next few years. Testosterone also stimulates the skin's sebaceous glands to grow in size and secretory capacity. As indicated in Chapter 43, this plays a part in the pathogenesis of acne, a condition very common in adolescence.

Metabolic Function. The greater growth of the male's skeletal structures is also attributable to testosterone. This hormone somehow stimulates tissue-building processes by aiding retention of the dietary protein nitrogen needed for formation of the amino

TABLE 30-1

ANDROGENIC AND ANABOLIC AGENTS

NONPROPRIETARY OR OFFICIAL NAME	TRADE NAMES	USUAL DOSE
Preparations Used Mainly for Their Androgenic Effects		
Fluoxymesterone	Halotestin; Ora-Testryl; Ultandren	2 to 20 mg.
Methyltestosterone N.F.	Metandren; Neo-Hombreol M; Oreton Methyl	buccal, 5 mg.
Testosterone N.F.	Androlin; Neo-Hombreol F; Oreton; Testryl	buccal, 10 mg. I.M. 25 mg. Pellet implantation, 300 mg.
Testosterone cypionate U.S.P.	Depo-Testosterone cypionate	I.M. 50 to 100 mg. every 7 to 14 days
Testosterone enanthate N.F.	Delatestryl	I.M. 200 mg. every 2 to 4 weeks
Testosterone phenylacetate	Perandren phenylacetate	I.M. 50 mg.
Testosterone propionate U.S.P.	Neo-Hombreol; Oreton propionate; Perandren	I.M. 25 mg. daily or 3 times a week
Preparations Used Mainly for Their Anabolic Effects		
Dromstanolone propionate	Drolban; Masterone	100 mg. 3 times weekly
Ethylestrenol	Maxibolin	8 to 16 mg. oral
Methandrostenolone	Dianabol	5 mg. oral
Nandrolone decanoate	Deca-Durabolin	I.M. 50 to 100 mg. every 3 or 4 weeks
Nandrolone phenpropionate	Durabolin	I.M. 25 mg. once a week
Norethandrolone	Nilevar	10 to 30 mg. I.M. or oral
Oxandrolone	Anavar	5 to 20 mg. oral
Oxymetholone	Androyd; Anadrol	5 to 10 mg. oral
Stanozolol	Winstrol	2 mg. oral 3 times a day

acids from which new muscle is built. At the same time, less nitrogen is lost from the pool of chemical fragments formed in the constant breakdown of body tissues. This hormone-regulated combination of increased anabolism and decreased catabolism of protein helps to produce the larger, more powerful muscles of the male.

The boy's bones also begin to grow in thickness and in length. This stems from testosterone's stimulating action at two sites: (1) the protein-tissue bed in which bone is laid down by the osteoblasts, and (2) the epiphyses, the ends of the long bones, which are separated from the shafts by a layer of cartilage. However, after stimulating a sudden spurt of growth at puberty, the hormone also finally puts an end to any further growth in height. It does so by hastening the conversion of the cartilaginous tissues to bone, thus permanently closing off these "expansion joints."

PREPARATIONS AND ROUTES OF ADMINISTRATION

Preparations of *testosterone* include aqueous suspensions and oily solutions for intramuscular injection, solid pellets for implantation under the skin, and tablets for absorption through the sublingual and buccal mucosa—*not* for oral ingestion, because the hormone is largely destroyed in the liver after absorption from the upper gastrointestinal tract. Because injected esters of testosterone are absorbed more slowly from tissue depots and thus have a more prolonged duration of action, they are usually preferred for the long-term replacement therapy that ordinarily is necessary.

The propionic acid ester, testosterone propionate (see Drug Digest), is administered in an oily solution which is absorbed at a moderately slow, steady rate that produces hormonal effects for a period of two or three days. Testosterone cypionate (Drug Digest) and testosterone enanthate (Table 30-1) are much longer-lasting in their hormonal activity, and the oily solutions of these esters need be given only once every one to four weeks for replacement therapy and other purposes. Of the esters, only testosterone phenylacetate is available in an aqueous suspension. Methyltestosterone (also administered sublingually) and fluoxymesterone (Halotestin), a synthetic halogenated steroid, produce androgenic effects when administered orally.

THE THERAPEUTIC USES OF THE ANDROGENS

Androgen Therapy in Men

Testosterone and its derivatives are used in medicine mainly as replacement therapy in males who lack the hormone. Such hypogonadism may become apparent at puberty when the boy fails to develop normally, or it may occur in men at some time after the masculinizing changes of adolescence have taken place. Eunuchism, as a result of castration, or eunuchoidism from testicular hypofunction or failure, can also be successfully treated with testosterone preparations of various kinds.

Eunuchism and eunuchoidism may both be treated with testosterone preparations. However, when the extent to which the patient's testes may be capable of producing hormones is uncertain, doctors may first administer gonadotropins to see whether the gonads may be stimulated to secrete endogenous testosterone. The preparation used for this purpose is human chorionic gonadotropin (HCG), an extract of pregnancy urine rich in ICSH and thus—in theory—capable of stimulating the patient's testes to produce and secrete the hormone. If this treatment fails to bring about pubertal changes, however, the patient's hypogonadism is diagnosed as primary—that is, the result of lack of responsive testicular tissue—rather than secondary to a lack of pituitary gonadotropins. Treatment, preferably with a long-acting testosterone preparation, is then undertaken.

The effects of such male hormone replacement therapy upon the young patient's physical and psychic development are often truly dramatic. Administered in doses and intervals intended to imitate the natural rate of testicular hormone secretion, these preparations almost literally make a man of the boy. Some of these changes—in height, depth of voice, size of sex organs, and pattern of hair distribution, for example—are permanent. However, hypogonadal patients must continue to receive hormone replacement therapy indefinitely in order to maintain muscular strength, physical vigor and libido, or sex drive.

Men who develop a hormone deficiency after sexual development has occurred naturally at puberty do not need as intensive treatment as does the young eunuch or eunuchoid. Thus, treatment may begin with injections of testosterone esters, and then these patients may often be maintained with oral therapy, using methyltestosterone or its synthetic derivative, fluoxymesterone. The latter agent is somewhat more potent and is claimed unlikely to cause the jaundice that sometimes occurs with methyltestosterone.

The male climacteric is a condition analogous to the menopause in women. The symptoms also—hot flashes, heart palpitations, nervous irritability or fretting over minor matters, failure of concentration and memory and insomnia—are somewhat similar. They are often so vague and subjective that some doctors tend to feel that the condition is psychogenic and a mental depressive state rather than the result of an endocrine imbalance stemming from testicular failure. Differential diagnosis is important, since symptoms resulting from a true hormone deficiency will respond readily to replacement therapy, whereas a depressive neurosis or psychosis may require psychotherapy, antidepressant drugs, or even electroshock if—as sometimes happens—the patient develops suicidal tendencies.

The doctor may order laboratory studies of the hormone levels in the patient's blood and urine to help determine whether the patient actually is suffering from the relatively rare male climacteric. If these tests indicate that the patient's urine is low in testosterone metabolites and that his blood is correspondingly high in pituitary gonadotropins, the doctor may start the patient on testosterone propionate injections for a trial period. Often dramatic improvement follows one or two weeks of treatment. Not only do the patient's cardiovascular and mental symptoms clear up, but he often gains in physical vigor, sense of well being, and restoration of lost libido and potency.

If the patient's subjective response is too rapid and dramatic, the doctor may suspect that his condition is indeed psychogenic. He may then substitute a placebo—the oily solvent *without* the hormone—to see whether the patient's improvement continues or whether his symptoms return. If the results of this test are positive—that is, if relapse occurs during the placebo period—the doctor may decide to put the patient on long-term therapy with one of the testosterone esters with a longer duration of action.

Before proceeding with such maintenance treatment with exogenous male hormone, the doctor tries to rule out the presence of prostate-gland growths, which are not uncommon in men of late middle age and might be stimulated into more rapid activity by hormone treatment. Similarly, such men are examined frequently during treatment to detect any signs of possible prostatic carcinoma, since such a hormone-dependent neoplasm might grow rapidly and spread to other sites in the body.

Other adverse effects of excessive amounts of testosterone which must be guarded against are: (1) a steroid-induced retention of salty fluids, that may tend to raise the patient's blood pressure or send a person with previous cardiovascular difficulties into congestive heart failure; and (2) psychological and physical changes, including an unseemly increase in libido that might prove socially embarrassing to a middle-aged man. Both of these reactions, including increased sex drive, are unlikely with carefully regulated replacement therapy, but they may occur in *women* receiving pharmacological doses of the male hormone.

Cryptorchidism, or undescended testicle, is a condition caused either by an obstruction of the inguinal canal or a lack of testosterone. In the latter case, as indicated in Chapter 29, it is customary to treat the boy with a course of human chorionic gonadotropin (HCG) injections. Even if this ICSH-containing substance fails to stimulate enough secretion of endogenous testosterone to let the testes descend from the abdomen into the scrotum, it helps to facilitate the surgery that may be required later. If the doctor decides to try testosterone from an outside source, he must regulate the dosage very carefully to avoid precipitating premature puberty in the youngster. For, as when HCG is used in such patients, the sex hormone may cause too-early development of accessory sex structures and secondary sex characteristics.

Oligospermia, a lack of viable, motile sperm in the semen, is commonly a cause of male infertility. It is unlikely to be corrected by testosterone treatment alone, because high doses of the hormone are likely to suppress pituitary secretion of FSH, the gonadotropin that ordinarily stimulates the seminiferous tubules. Occasionally, however, such temporary suppression of the pituitary by testosterone may sometimes be followed by a rebound in secretion of FSH when testosterone therapy is withdrawn. This, and the resulting rise in sperm counts, is analogous to the increased gonadotropin production and the increased chances of ovulation and pregnancy when oral contraceptive therapy with estrogen-progestins is withdrawn from women (see p. 406).

Another treatment that has been tried for male infertility has involved administration of methyltestosterone together with injections of pregnant mare's serum, a product containing FSH. The two together are said to stimulate sperm production in previously infertile men sometimes.

Androgen Therapy in Women

Testosterone therapy is not limited to men and boys. Women also are often treated with the male hormone. The main reason for this is that androgens antagonize the effects of excessive amounts of estrogens on the endometrium of the uterus and on the breasts. Of course, testosterone is capable of suppressing the secretion of certain anterior pituitary gland hormones in the woman as well as in the man. In addition, testosterone or one of its derivatives may sometimes be administered for its anabolic, or tissue-building, effects in debilitated women.

Since the recent introduction of potent synthetic female sex hormones capable of suppressing pituitary gonadotropins and of producing various endometrial changes with few side effects, testosterone is not widely used in treating the menstrual disorders briefly described below. Most doctors prefer to use the synthetic estrogens and progestins discussed in Chapter 29, and only a minority still employ androgens for these purposes. Sometimes androgens and estrogens are administered in combination in the management of menopausal symptoms and in postmenopausal years. In such combinations, it is the anabolic effect of the male hormone rather than its sexual effects that is desired.

Menorrhagia and metrorrhagia—conditions marked by excessive uterine bleeding—are usually treated today with the new synthetic estrogen-progestin combinations mentioned above. However, in episodes of acute hemorrhaging unresponsive to these agents, testosterone propionate injections sometimes have an excellent hemostatic effect. This has sometimes helped young women avoid the surgical curettage that might otherwise be required for control of endometrial bleeding. Androgens, like estrogens, are sometimes combined with progestins for this purpose. Then, when the endometrium has been repaired and converted to the secretory state, the progestin is discontinued. This is followed in a few days by a more or less normal menstrual period.

Dysmenorrhea and premenstrual tension also are now mainly treated with oral estrogens and progestins (Chap. 29). However, some doctors prefer to employ methyltestosterone tablets or androgen-estrogen combinations for control of the symptoms of these conditions. Administered during the latter half of the cycle in doses adequate for influencing pituitary, ovarian, and uterine function without producing masculinizing effects, androgens often help to control premenstrual mental and physical distress. That is, their use sometimes prevents the annoying nervousness and fluid retention, including painful premenstrual mastalgia. The painful uterine contractions also are sometimes suppressed by such androgenic therapy.

Suppression of lactation is sometimes accomplished by androgen administration during or immediately after childbirth. Like the estrogens now more commonly employed for this purpose, testosterone esters inhibit release of the pituitary hormone responsible for initiating lactation. This prevents postpartum breast engorgement in women who do not intend to nurse their babies.

Metastatic carcinoma of the breast that has spread beyond the reach of surgery or radiation therapy is a condition in which large doses of androgens are administered to women. The symptomatic relief sometimes obtained in such cases (see Chap. 44) is occasionally accompanied by masculinizing effects. Thus, these patients are watched for early signs such as growth of facial hair and development of acne. Withdrawal of hormone treatment results in clearing of these skin symptoms and prevents permanent signs of virilization such as deepening of the voice and clitoral enlargement. The patient is often willing to endure such virilizing effects in order to obtain the feeling of well being and the relief of pain that hormone treatment often offers.

The nurse should, of course, be sensitive to the woman's emotional responses to the physical and psychological effects of hormone therapy. For example, the woman may discuss such matters as her hormone-induced increase in libido with the nurse rather than the doctor, and the nurse can then bring such subjective responses to the doctor's attention. Such patients must then be watched for sudden development of signs and symptoms of more serious toxicity. A marked rise in plasma calcium levels, for example, calls for prompt withdrawal of androgen therapy and administration of fluids to avoid formation of renal calculi. The short-acting ester, testosterone propionate, is preferred over the long-acting cypionate and enanthate esters, the effects of which would tend to continue and contribute to persistent hypercalcemia. A new synthetic derivative, dromstanolone (Drolban, etc.) is said to be safer than the testosterone preparations. It is claimed less likely to precipitate hypercalcemic reactions in advanced breast cancer patients with progressive osteolytic metastases. Masculinizing effects, jaundice, and edema are also said to be rare with this derivative.

THE ACTIONS AND THERAPEUTIC USES OF ANABOLIC AGENTS

Doctors often want to stimulate the flagging appetites of debilitated patients and to reverse the processes responsible for protein wastage and subsequent weight loss. When it was found that testosterone possessed anabolic activity that could produce positive nitrogen balance in patients who were in negative balance, physicians tried administering the hormone in such cases. Although it often brought a return of appetite and a feeling of well being, the hormone's sexual effects limited its usefulness for women and children and caused mental and physical changes undesirable even in male patients.

Chemists have tried to modify the testosterone molecule in attempts to devise compounds free of sexual effects, yet capable of stimulating muscle growth and strength in the manner of the hormone. Several synthetic anabolic steroids which are now available (Table 30-1) are capable of increasing protein anabolism when administered in doses that are less likely to cause undesired masculinizing activity than are doses of testosterone that cause comparable anabolic activity. However, a complete separation of the sexual effects from the anabolic effects has not yet been achieved. Thus, patients taking any of these drugs must be watched for possible development of virilizing and other toxic effects of testosterone.

Clinical Uses

The clinical uses of these anabolic steroids with reduced androgenic activity are potentially very varied. These substances might prove useful in any of many conditions marked by inadequate protein bio-synthesis or excessive protein breakdown. However, it has been hard to prove that patients actually do better on these drugs, which tend to stimulate the appetite, than they would by simply eating a diet adequate in proteins and other food factors. This difficulty, as well as the possibility of causing un-desired side effects, particularly in women and children, has limited the acceptance of these agents.

Patients being treated with corticosteroid drugs (Chap. 28) sometimes receive adjunctive anabolic steroids. The catabolic, or protein-breakdown, effects of the corticosteroids are especially dangerous for patients with arthritis who are confined to bed or inactive. These patients are subject to *osteoporosis* resulting from disease of their limbs. Like elderly patients with senile osteoporosis, they may suffer bone fractures as a result of calcium loss from the protein matrix of osseous structures. Administration of ana-bolic steroids in such cases is said to help prevent osteoporosis. These drugs often relieve the patient's pain; however, there is still some doubt as to whether the disabling disease process is actually reversed. One view is that these drugs do help to stop the loss of calcium from the bones, especially when taken to-gether with a calcium and fluoride supplement and a high protein diet. Other studies have failed to demonstrate any improvement in the patient's bone density in X-ray pictures.

Convalescent patients sometimes receive a course of treatment with an anabolic agent. Patients who have suffered the stress of surgery or other trauma are often in negative nitrogen balance. Administration of anabolic agents in such cases or in patients who have suffered fractures, deep extensive burns, or weakening virus infections such as influenza some-times helps to retain nitrogenous compounds that would otherwise be lost to the body, and to convert them into the amino acids from which new tissues are built. Here too, however, it has been hard to prove that patients actually recover more rapidly than they would with good nursing care and an adequate diet only.

Some patients with severe anemias or wasting dis-eases such as tuberculosis and carcinosis are claimed to benefit from the protein-building action of these drugs. (They cannot, of course, be used in patients with prostatic carcinoma, because the retained andro-genic component, though less potent than that of testosterone, may be sufficient to stimulate growth and spread of the hormone-dependent cancer.) In other neoplastic diseases, patients who are anemic may make more hemoglobin under the protein-pro-ducing effects of these drugs. In aplastic anemia and other anemias unresponsive to ordinary measures, treatment with testosterone or with one of the less androgenic anabolic steroids may stimulate production of showers of new reticulocytes and erythrocytes.

Children whose growth is retarded or who eat poorly and are weak and anemic may sometimes re-spond to small doses of these drugs. However, most doctors do not lightly undertake such therapy, since children may be especially sensitive to the androgenic component in all these drugs. This could, of course, have adverse effects on the child's ability to achieve his full height. That is, an initial increase in weight and a spurt in growth might be bought at the expense of early closure of the epiphyses. To avoid this, the doctor may consult an authority on growth and de-velopment before beginning treatment with anabolic drugs. Then, in the intervals between courses, the ends of the long bones are examined by X-ray to detect any early changes which might indicate the start of premature ossification that could keep the child from further growth. The child is also watched for signs of premature puberty, which would require withdrawal of the anabolic agents.

Perhaps further research in this field will succeed in entirely separating the sexual from the metabolic effects of these compounds. Such drugs could then be used with greater safety in children, women with senile or disuse type osteoporosis, and men debilitated by metastatic prostate cancer.

REVIEW QUESTIONS

1. What is the nature of the interrelationships between the anterior pituitary gland hormones ICSH and FSH and the male gonads?

2. Describe the changes that take place at puberty in a boy, under the influence of the male sex hormone secreted by the testes, or in a eunuchoid individual receiving testos-terone from an outside source as replacement therapy.

3. Compare testosterone propionate with testosterone cypionate in terms of duration of action and the advan-tages of each over the other in particular clinical situations.

4. What is the doctor's purpose in first administering a course of human chorionic gonadotropin to a eunuchoid male before proceeding with testosterone replacement therapy?

5. (a) What are some complaints typical of patients who may be suffering from the male climacteric?

(b) Laboratory tests of what type are required to con-firm a diagnosis of male climacteric, thus warranting a trial of testosterone therapy?

6. (a) What condition must be ruled out before an older man receives extended courses of testosterone therapy (i.e., what is a contraindication to testosterone therapy?)?

(b) What kinds of side effects must be watched for in men receiving testosterone injections?

7. (a) What hormone other than testosterone from an outside source is preferred for treating cryptorchidism?

(b) What should be carefully watched for, when either this hormone or testosterone is being employed in treating cryptorchidism in prepubertal boys?

8. (a) What is the rationale for employing testosterone in the treatment of oligospermia?

(b) What other combination of hormones has been tried for treating this condition?

9. (a) What is the effect of administering testosterone injections to a young woman with menorrhagia or metrorrhagia?

(b) What is the effect of administering testosterone ester injections to women in the postpartum period?

10. (a) What physical and psychological side effects can be anticipated in women receiving testosterone treatment of advanced mammary carcinoma?

(b) What toxic effect may sometimes develop suddenly in women being treated for this condition with testosterone derivatives?

11. (a) What is the main advantage of the testosterone-related compounds called *anabolic agents* over the male hormone itself?

(b) What kinds of side effects must nonetheless be watched for in patients being treated with anabolic agents?

12. (a) What are some kinds of clinical conditions in which anabolic agents may be beneficial when combined with dietary therapy?

(b) What special precautions are required when anabolic agents are being employed in the treatment of children?

BIBLIOGRAPHY

Berczeller, P. H., and Kupperman, H. S.: The anabolic steroids. Clin. Pharmacol. Ther., *1:*464, 1960.

Bishop, P. M. F.: The male sex hormones. Brit. M. J., *167:* 184, 1960.

Frohman, I. P.: The steroids. Am. J. Nurs., 59:518, 1959.

Fruehan, A. E., and Frawley, T. H.: Current status of anabolic steroids. J.A.M.A., *184:*527, 1963.

Heller, C. G., and Myers, G. B.: Male climacteric, its symptomatology, diagnosis, and treatment. J.A.M.A., *126:*472, 1944.

McGavack, T. H.: The male climacterium. J. Am. Geriat. Soc., 3:639, 1955.

Rodman, M. J.: The male sex hormone and anabolic steroids. R.N., *30:*41, 1967 (May).

Werner, A. A.: Male climacteric. J.A.M.A., *132:*188, 1946.

The Thyroid Hormones
and Antithyroid Drugs

THE THYROID GLAND

The thyroid gland is located in the neck, where it surrounds the trachea and seems to protect the windpipe like a shield. (It gets its name from the Greek word for one kind of shield.) The large size and prominence of the thyroid was the subject of some quaint speculation by the early anatomists. Some, noting that the thyroid was larger in women, suggested that the gland served to filter a woman's blood before it passed to the brain, in a vain attempt to reduce the effects of elements in that fluid which contribute to the flighty female emotional state. Kinder, but no more scientific, observers suggested that the gland was there to give a comely shape to a girl's neck.

Late in the last century, however, these and similarly worthless theories of the thyroid's function were swept away by the work of the pioneering endocrinologists. First they noted what happened when they removed this gland from the necks of experimental animals; then they prepared and injected thyroid extracts capable of overcoming most of the signs and symptoms produced by the prior surgical ablation of the gland. Later, physicians found that they could counteract the low metabolic rate of hypothyroid patients by simply giving them powdered thyroid gland by mouth.

We now know that the thyroid gland regulates the rate of metabolism in almost all body cells. That is, the thyroid gland secretes hormones that control the speed of the combustion processes by which body tissues burn food to derive the energy needed for normal function and for growth and development. The exact chemical nature of the secretions synthesized by the thyroid is also known. The glandular follicles are filled with a colloidal fluid containing a protein called *thyroglobulin.* This serves as a storage

site for two iodinated amino acids: (1) *thyroxine,* or *tetraiodothyronine,* and (2) *triiodothyronine,* or *liothyronine.* These are the chemicals that are secreted into the circulation to seek out their metabolic targets in the body's tissues.

We still do not know precisely how these two thyroid hormones control the rate of cellular metabolic processes. However, we are very much aware of what happens to a person when his thyroid gland fails to function properly. In this chapter, we shall discuss the drugs that are used to treat clinical conditions caused by the underfunctioning and the overactivity of the thyroid gland.

THYROID DISORDERS

Thyroid gland disorders may be broadly classified as (1) *hypothyroidism*—conditions marked by a decrease in the production and secretion of thyroid hormones, and (2) *hyperthyroidism*—conditions in which the thyroid gland produces and secretes excessive amounts of its hormones into the systemic circulation. In hypothyroid conditions, body metabolism slows down to subnormal levels, rates of growth and development are reduced, and the effects of sluggish metabolism are apparent in many body systems including the central nervous system. In hyperthyroidism, on the other hand, the metabolic rate is abnormally elevated, with far-reaching effects on many systems, including the cardiovascular system particularly. (The signs and symptoms accompanying full-blown hypo- and hyperthyroidism are summarized in Table 31-1.)

Simple non-toxic goiter is a thyroid disorder of another type. The thyroid gland is enlarged but the secretion of its hormones may be more or less normal. This so-called *euthyroid,* or essentially normal, state

TABLE 31-1
SIGNS AND SYMPTOMS OF THYROID DYSFUNCTION

	HYPOTHYROIDISM	HYPERTHYROIDISM
Central Nervous System	*Functions depressed:* hypoactive reflexes (hyporeflexia), lethargy, emotional dullness, sleepiness, slow speech, stupid appearance.	*Functions stimulated:* hyperactive reflexes, anxiety, nervousness, restlessness, insomnia, tremors.
Cardiovascular-Renal	*Functions depressed:* bradycardia, hypotension, increased circulation time, oliguria, anemia, decreased secretion of catecholamines and decreased sensitivity to catecholamines and to adrenergic drugs.	*Functions stimulated:* tachycardia, palpitations, decreased circulation time, increased pulse pressure, systolic hypertension, increased secretion of catecholamines and increased sensitivity to catecholamines and to adrenergic drugs.
Skin and Other Epithelial Structures	Skin pale, coarse, dry, thickened, especially on hands and face which is puffy about the eyelids, cheeks and elsewhere; hair coarse and thinned on scalp and in eyebrows; nails thick and hard.	Skin flushed, thin, warm, moist due to vasodilation and sweating; hair fine and soft; nails soft and thin.
Metabolism Rate	*Decreased,* with body temperature reduced, intolerance of cold, decreased appetite, with more of food intake converted to fat, including cholesterol (i.e., tendency toward weight gain and definite hypercholesterolemia).	*Increased,* with body temperature raised (low-grade fever), intolerance of heat, increased appetite, but with tendency toward weight loss, which may be severe sometimes and accompanied by muscle wasting and weakness (thyrotoxic myopathy).
Generalized Myxedema	Including accumulation of mucopolysaccharides in heart (cardiomegaly), tongue and vocal cords (hoarseness and thickened speech), periorbital areas.	*Localized,* with accumulations of mucopolysaccharides in the orbits, eyeballs and ocular muscles; periorbital edema, puffiness of eyelids, lid lag, and exophthalmos; occasional pretibial edema.
Ovarian Function	Decreased, with tendency toward menorrhagia, possible habitual abortion or sterility.	Altered, with tendency toward oligomenorrhea or amenorrhea.
Goiter	Relatively rare and of simple, nontoxic type.	Diffuse, highly vascular and murmurous (bruit), is very frequent.

occurs because the gland has grown enough to compensate for conditions which would otherwise result in deficient secretion. The most common cause of simple goiter is a lack of dietary iodine which tends to reduce thyroid hormone production. However, the compensatory increase in the size of the gland and its greater blood supply helps the thyroid to extract maximal amounts of iodine from the circulation. As a result, enough thyroid hormones are usually produced to maintain normal metabolism. Nonetheless, such thyroid enlargement indicates an abnormal functional state which requires correction.

BIOSYNTHESIS AND RELEASE OF THYROID HORMONES

Before undertaking our discussion of the treatment of hypothyroidism, hyperthyroidism and simple goiter, it is desirable that we review the way in which the production and secretion of thyroid hormones are controlled and carried out. The reason for this is that nearly every kind of thyroid function disorder stems fundamentally from some defect that alters the normal rate of thyroid hormone synthesis and release.

Thyroid-Pituitary Relationships

The rate of thyroid activity is regulated by the anterior pituitary gland. Among the tropic hormones secreted by that structure is one that specifically increases the activities of thyroid gland cells. This substance, *thyrotropin,* or *thyroid stimulating hormone* (TSH), causes a prompt increase in the secretion of stored thyroid hormones into the blood stream, which then carries them to the body tissues that are their ultimate targets. In addition, TSH causes an increase in the total mass of thyroid tissue and in the number and size of the blood vessels that run through it. These changes result in both an increased capacity to extract iodine from the blood and a greater ability to build this element into the molecules of thyroid hormones, which are then released into the circulation in increased quantities.

These thyroid hormones, in turn, exert a *negative feedback* effect upon pituitary production and secretion. Thus, ordinarily, there is a delicate balance between the reciprocally acting hormones of these two glands. If the amount of thyroid hormone in the blood rises even slightly above normal, pituitary secretion of TSH is suppressed, and this of course leads to a reduction in thyroid hormone production. The reverse is also true: if the level of thyroxine in the blood reaching the pituitary is reduced, that gland steps up its secretion of TSH, which then causes the thyroid to grow and secrete more of its hormones. This accounts for the glandular enlargement in goiters.

Biosynthetic Steps

The production of the two thyroid hormones thyroxine and triiodothyronine takes place in three stages: (1) iodine trapping; (2) attachment of iodine atoms to the amino acid tyrosine; and (3) coupling of iodotyrosine molecules to form the final hormones. If we study these steps in a bit more detail at this time, we shall be better able to understand how certain hypothyroid states develop and how certain of the drugs used in treating hyperthyroidism act to bring about reduction of excessive thyroid gland activity.

Iodine is present in small but adequate amounts in the diets of most people. It is found in seafood and in the drinking water and the soil in which leafy vegetables are grown in most coastal areas. In certain parts of the world, including Switzerland and parts of the midwestern United States, the latter sources of dietary iodine are inadequate, and goiter once occurred endemically in these regions. Now, however, it is cus-tomary to add tiny supplements of iodine salts (iodides) to table salt in order to avoid iodine-deficiency diseases.

The thyroid gland possesses a powerful mechanism for rapidly removing iodine from the blood passing through it and for concentrating the element within the gland in amounts much greater than the plasma iodine content. This so-called *iodide trap* may occasionally fail to operate as a result of a congenital enzymatic defect. The glandular device for capturing iodide may also be blocked by certain chemicals (p. 430). In either case, the result is similar to what occurs when there is a persistent dietary deficiency of iodine —i.e., the lack of this vital element prevents the synthesis of thyroid hormones, and the person may suffer the signs and symptoms of hypothyroidism.

Once iodide is taken up by thyroid tissue it is enzymatically oxidized to active iodine atoms which are then attached to the amino acid tyrosine. The iodinated tyrosine molecules made in this way are of two types—*mono*iodotyrosine and *di*iodotyrosine. A congenital lack of the enzymes needed to oxidize iodide to atomic iodine and then bind the element to tyrosine may lead to hypothyroidism—the condition that is the result of failure to manufacture enough thyroid hormones. Some of the drugs that are used in the treatment of hyperthyroidism inhibit enzymatic oxidation of the iodide trapped by the overactive thyroid gland; in this and other ways, these agents succeed in slowing down the production and outpouring of hormones in the excessive amounts responsible for the signs and symptoms of *thyrotoxicosis* (Table 31-1).

In the final biosynthetic step, two molecules of *di*iodotyrosine are coupled (again, by specific oxidative enzymes that may occasionally be missing as a result of a genetic defect) to form *tetra*iodothyronine, which is the hormone *thyroxine.* In much smaller amounts (about 10% of the total hormonal output), *triiodothyronine* is produced by the condensation of one molecule of *mono*iodotyrosine with one molecule of *di*iodotyrosine. Both thyroid hormones are stored in the glandular follicles as part of the mucoprotein molecule called *thyroglobulin,* which is too large to leak out of the cell membranes. However, when the tissues demand more thyroid hormones, the smaller active molecules are split off from the protein storage form and secreted into the blood stream.

HYPOTHYROIDISM

A lack of thyroid hormone leads to two clear-cut deficiency syndromes:

1. *Cretinism,* which is the result of glandular failure in infancy

2. *Myxedema,* which is a condition that sometimes develops in adults and older children (juvenile myxedema).

In addition to these obvious deficiency states, some patients apparently suffer from a *partial* or *borderline* type hypothyroidism. These patients, who often seem to have more or less normal thyroid activity, complain of various vague symptoms, which are often dramatically improved by the administration of thyroid.

Cretinism

Cretinism, or congenital hypothyroidism, may result (as we have indicated above) from an inborn enzymatic defect that interferes with iodine uptake and utilization. More commonly, the child is born without a thyroid gland (athyreosis) or with one that has failed to develop properly. The routine use of iodized salt has largely eliminated endemic goiter in this country, but a lack of iodine in the mother's diet may still account for cases of cretinism in certain isolated mountainous regions elsewhere in the world.

Growth and development of the nervous and skeletal systems are retarded in congenitally hypothyroid infants. If the pediatrician recognizes the condition early and treats it with adequate doses of thyroid hormones, the child may develop normally. However, in those who are hypothyroid during fetal development and in infants whose condition goes unrecognized and untreated for more than a few months, the likelihood of permanent mental retardation is very high.

Once the cretinous condition is recognized from the baby's failure to grow normally and by other clinical signs and laboratory tests, thyroid replacement therapy is promptly instituted. Doctors may differ in regard to the particular thyroid product that they prefer, but all agree that it is desirable to administer full doses of any preparation from the start. Infants apparently require relatively large doses and are able to tolerate them. After thyroid treatment has been begun, the doctor determines the maintenance dose which will be required, through frequent checks of the levels of protein-bound iodine (PBI; see Summary of Tests for Thyroid Function) and by periodic X-ray films intended to follow the baby's bone development.

Myxedema

Myxedema may be the result of a primary failure of the thyroid gland, or it may be secondary to failure of the pituitary to produce adequate amounts of the thyroid stimulating hormone (TSH). In myxedema of pituitary origin, the patient usually shows signs of sex hormone deficiency and lack of adrenal cortex hormones as well as the classic signs and symptoms of adult hypothyroidism (Table 31-1) of which the following are most characteristic: the face is puffy, with pale, dry skin; the look is dull and lethargic, and the speech slow and thickened.

Primary myxedema most often develops slowly as the person's thyroid gland becomes fibrous or atrophies for reasons not well understood. Occasionally, this condition follows acute inflammatory destruction of the gland (thyroiditis), or is a result of a gradually progressive glandular degeneration which is thought to stem from an autoimmune reaction (Hashimoto's thyroiditis, or struma). Hypothyroidism that is secondary to pituitary failure most often follows postpartum hemorrhagic destruction of the hypophysis or is caused by growth of a pituitary gland tumor.

Treatment of Myxedema

The administration of adequate doses of thyroid hormones has a remarkable effect upon the mental and physical condition of the myxedematous patient. Even small amounts of thyroid quickly make a great difference in the patient's appearance and behavior. The puffiness disappears as most of the retained fluids are removed from the tissues by way of the kidneys. The dull, expressionless look is replaced by an alert, interested appearance, and physical sluggishness gives way to normal activity. Once the patient achieves normal hormonal balance, he can be kept in such functional equilibrium indefinitely by maintenance thyroid therapy.

The aim of treatment in primary myxedema is to bring about the greatest possible improvement with the lowest dosage of thyroid. That is, the patient is returned to as close to normal a state as possible without pushing him into a *hyper*thyroid state. Ordinarily this is done by administering relatively small doses which are raised gradually to exert a cumulative effect over a period of several weeks. Special care is taken to avoid overdosage in elderly patients and in those with a history of cardiac complications of myxedema.

In myxedema that arises secondary to pituitary gland damage—as in hemorrhagic postpartum necrosis —thyroid treatment is helpful. Here, however, and in the case of hypophysectomized patients, the doctor may also order sex hormones and adrenal corticosteroids to make up for the lack of these secretions following the loss of the gonadotropic and adrenocorticotropic hormones of the pituitary. Replacement of corticosteroids is especially important when thyroid hormones are being administered, because the increased tissue metabolism brought about by the latter may send the patient into a state of adrenal insufficiency. (Pituitary myxedema may be differentiated from primary myxedema by the administration of thyrotropin (Thytropar), which, of course, produces changes in the results obtained with standard laboratory tests for hypothyroidism in the former but not in the latter condition.)

Borderline Hypothyroidism

Hypometabolism is a term sometimes used to describe the state of a group of patients who do *not* show the multiple symptoms of full-blown myxedema but who nonetheless complain of various vague symptoms which are traceable to a thyroid gland that is functioning at only a low normal level. When symptoms such as muscle weakness and pain, fatigue, lethargy, headaches and emotional upsets are recognized to be the result of a *mild*, or *borderline*, hypothyroidism and thyroid therapy is administered, the patient may respond with a remarkable improvement.

Ordinarily, such patients have a history of some sort of thyroid disorder such as simple goiter (see p. 422) or thyroiditis, and their condition can be confirmed by laboratory tests which, taken together, offer some suggestion of a low thyroid reserve. Sometimes, however, neither the history nor laboratory and clinical findings—other than the excellent response to thyroid therapy—indicate the true cause of the patient's varied and vague discomforts.

Non-Thyroid-Deficiency Conditions

Thyroid medication has long been advocated for treating many *non*-myxedematous conditions which are marked by the presence of one or more signs and symptoms found in hypothyroidism. Obviously, since inadequate thyroid secretion can affect the functioning of nearly every body tissue, there are a great number of signs and symptoms that might in theory respond to thyroid replacement therapy. There is no reason to believe, however, that thyroid treatment will be effective for these conditions in the *absence of hypothyroidism*. Nonetheless, the fact that patients with seemingly normal thyroid gland activity sometimes respond well to thyroid administration, has encouraged the *misuse* of thyroid drugs as a panacea.

Obesity. Thyroid medication has often played a part in weight reduction regimens. Its use for this purpose seems unjustified and potentially dangerous. Although thyroid replacement therapy often reduces the flabbiness and puffiness of a myxedematous patient, it will speed neither fat metabolism nor removal of fluids from the tissues of a patient whose thyroid function is normal. Of course, the administration of thyroid from an outside source tends to suppress pituitary production of TSH (p. 424), and this in turn lowers the secretion of endogenous thyroid hormones by the patient's own thyroid gland.

If the dosage of thyroid drugs is pushed very high, the exogenous thyroid product may produce the *pharmacological effects* of the hormone on the patient's metabolic processes. The accelerated rate of tissue metabolism that may then result, with a more rapid burning of stored fat and carbohydrates, may also stimulate the patient's appetite. This, of course, makes it all the harder for him to carry out the only truly effective weight reduction measure—*reduction of his caloric intake*. In addition, an obese patient with some underlying cardiovascular difficulty may be endangered by the adverse metabolic effects of thyroid

drugs on cardiac function (see Summary of Adverse Effects).

The nurse can explain to women who ask whether thyroid would help them to lose weight that this hormone medication is prescribed by the doctor for those whose own glandular secretion is inadequate. She can help them understand that the overweight individual should consult her doctor for proper diagnosis and for whatever treatment he may order, including thyroid if he decides that replacement therapy is needed. The same advice applies in female reproductive disorders, in relation to which women sometimes inquire about thyroid therapy.

OB-GYN Disorders. The reproductive system tissues are adversely affected by a lack of thyroid secretion. Frequently, hypothyroid women may suffer (for example) from a secondary deficiency of ovarian hormones. This lack of estrogens or progesterone often leads to menstrual irregularities, including menorrhagia. The fact that the administration of thyroid hormones sometimes helps to regularize the menstrual cycle of such *hypothyroid* patients does *not* mean that thyroid drug administration will be useful for treating abnormal menses in *euthyroid* women. Yet thyroid has often been administered routinely in *unselected* cases of amenorrhea, dysmenorrhea, premenstrual tension and other gynecological disorders.

Similarly, some cases of sterility and habitual abortion have also been treated with thyroid, even when no clear-cut indication of hypothyroidism could be detected. It has been suggested that the hormone may speed up ovarian and uterine metabolism in a manner that favors conception and the ability to carry a fetus to term. This view is based upon the idea that a seemingly normal thyroid gland may be unable to meet the increased demands made upon it by pregnancy. Although this is purely speculative, some authorities feel that a trial of thyroid therapy is justified in women whose infertility or tendency to abort cannot be explained in terms of other causes.

Other Conditions. The use of thyroid seems much less justified—even in theory—in dermatological, musculoskeletal, and other conditions marked by signs and symptoms similar to some found in hypothyroidism. Thus, although the myxedematous patient's skin may be dry and scaly, thyroid is no panacea for such symptoms when they occur in *euthyroid* individuals. Similarly, thyroid often relieves muscular cramps and joint pains in overt hypothyroidism, but it is no cure-all in arthritis and myositis; nor does the reversal of anemia by thyroid treatment of hypothyroidism mean that thyroid is ever a substitute for the adequate diagnosis and specific treatment of anemia with iron salts or other hematinics (Chap. 25). Finally, thyroid is no substitute for psychotherapy in neurasthenia, even though its administration in myxedema relieves fatigue, irritability, emotional instability, and mental sluggishness.

Simple goiter is a more logical indication for the administration of thyroid drugs. As we have already indicated, the enlargement of the thyroid gland in non-toxic goiter is most often the result of an attempt to compensate for a dietary iodine deficiency. That is, the low plasma level of thyroid hormones causes the anterior pituitary gland to secrete the thyroid-stimulating hormone (TSH). The compensatory action of extra thyrotropin often helps to keep the patient in a euthyroid state, but the thyroid gland of such a person often tends to grow abnormally large. This is especially likely to occur during adolescence and pregnancy, when the iodine-deficient gland is called upon to manufacture more than normal amounts of thyroid hormones.

Although this condition can be prevented by supplementing the diet with iodides in endemic areas, the administration of iodine in this way is effective only in the early stages of simple goiter. The hormone imbalance in this condition is best corrected—even in the absence of overt hypothyroidism—by having the patient take full doses of a thyroid product. The thyroid administered in this way inhibits pituitary production of TSH, thus eliminating the source of continued stimulation of glandular growth. Of course, the hyperplastic gland may sometimes have already undergone permanent changes which require surgical, rather than medical, treatment especially if there is discomfort from pressure upon the patient's windpipe or even danger that his oxygen supply may be cut off.

THYROID PREPARATIONS

Thyroid products of several types are available for oral administration. These are:

1. The *dried defatted powder* prepared from the whole glands of animals; also, thyroglobulin, the purified protein extracted from the glands and standardized so that its dosage is comparable to that of ordinary thyroid;

2. *Sodium levothyroxine,* the levo isomer of the most abundant thyroid hormone, which is about 600 times as potent as the whole gland from which it is extracted;

3. *Sodium dextrothyroxine,* the recently introduced dextro isomer, which is less likely to overstimulate the heart than is the levo isomer; and

4. *Sodium liothyronine* (triiodothyronine), which is the most potent and most rapid acting of the thyroid derivatives. It is about three or four times as active as levothyroxine and its effects begin to come on in hours instead of days; its duration of action also is relatively short.

Opinions differ as to which type thyroid product is preferable, and each has its advocates. Actually, all have the same kinds of actions and differ only in ways which are ordinarily of relatively minor significance. Thus, even though it would appear that administration of the much more potent purified hormonal principles should offer advantages over treatment with the powdered whole gland, this is rarely the case. That is, little is gained by giving sodium levothyroxine, even though 100 micrograms (0.1 mg.) of this hormone has the effectiveness of about six hundred times that amount of the thyroid powder; further, sodium liothyronine, even though it is about three to four times as active as sodium levothyroxine, also has relatively few clinical advantages over the powdered whole gland.

Sodium liothyronine (see Drug Digest) does have an advantage in clinical situations requiring relatively rapid thyroid action, such as *myxedema coma.* However, this is an uncommon complication, and, in the much more commonly encountered myxedematous states, too rapid an onset of action may have adverse cardiac and nervous system effects. It may be argued that the short duration of action of sodium liothyronine following withdrawal offers a safety factor in the event of overdosage. However, the longer duration of the whole gland product seems preferable for maintenance therapy, since the patient who forgets or neglects to take his medication for a few days is less likely to slide down into myxedema.

Sodium dextrothyroxine is said to be safer than the levo isomer for patients with cardiac complications. It is claimed to lower blood cholesterol levels when administered in doses that do not significantly increase tissue metabolism and increase the load on the heart. All thyroid products are capable of reducing hypercholesterolemia in hypothyroid patients by raising the rate of cholesterol breakdown and excretion. They may, however, have adverse cardiac effects, especially in those patients who are most likely to require plasma cholesterol reduction because of a history of atherosclerotic disease of the heart. Sodium dextrothyroxine —the newest of the thyroid derivatives—may prove useful for treating such patients. However, patients must still be closely watched for signs of angina, and the drug is used only with caution in patients with a history of cardiovascular disease. (See also Chapter 22.)

Overdosage with thyroid products results in the appearance of adverse cardiac effects and other signs and symptoms similar to those of hyperthyroidism or thyrotoxicosis (Table 31-1). The heart muscle is forced to work harder to meet the demands of the rapidly metabolizing peripheral tissues for blood. As a result, the rapidly beating heart may tend to outrun the capacity of its own coronary vessels to supply the myocardium with oxygenated blood. Anginal chest pains then occur as a result of such myocardial ischemia. Older patients with some prior degree of coronary insufficiency may be precipitated into congestive heart failure if they receive too high a dose of a thyroid preparation. Patients taking thyroid should not be treated with catecholamines or other adrenergic drugs, because of the possible adverse cardiac effects of the combination.

HYPERTHYROIDISM

This condition is characterized by the excessive secretion of thyroid hormones, which increase the rate of oxidative metabolism in almost all the tissues of the body. This results in signs and symptoms (Table 31-1) which are distressing and dangerous. Although the underlying cause of Graves' disease—the most common of the conditions marked by hyperactive thyroid

function—is not known, the gland of such patients seems to have escaped from the mechanisms which normally regulate its activity (p. 424). Thus, not only is the thyroid gland's ability to take up iodine from the blood and convert it into hormones enormously increased, but the circulating hormones do not succeed in shutting off further iodine uptake and hormone synthesis in the manner previously described.

This is demonstrated in the so-called *thyroid-suppression* test for hyperthyroidism, which consists in administration of sodium liothyronine, the rapid-acting form of the hormone, followed some time later by a tracer dose of sodium radioiodide I 131 (see Drug Digest). In euthyroid individuals, prior administration of the thyroid hormone suppresses pituitary thyrotropin secretion, and the resulting reduction of TSH

TABLE 31-2
DRUGS USED IN TREATMENT AND DIAGNOSIS OF THYROID DISORDERS

OFFICIAL, GENERIC, OR USAN NAME	PROPRIETARY NAME	DAILY DOSAGE
Drugs Used in Hypothyroidism		
Sodium dextrothyroxine	Choloxin	Initially 1 to 2 mg. daily; maintenance 4 to 8 mg.
Sodium levothyroxine U.S.P.	Synthroid; Letter	Initially 100 mcg. daily; maintenance 150 mcg. to 400 mcg.
Sodium liothyronine U.S.P.	Cytomel; triiodothyronine	Initially 5 mcg. daily; maintenance 5 to 100 mcg.
Thyroglobulin	Proloid	60 to 180 mg.
Thyroid U.S.P.	desiccated thyroid	15 to 180 mg.
Drugs Used in Hyperthyroidism		
Antithyroid Drugs (Thiocarbamides)		
Iothiouracil sodium	Itrumil	150 to 300 mg.
Methimazole U.S.P.	Tapazole	5 to 20 mg.
Methylthiouracil N.F.	Methiacil; Thimecil	50 to 200 mg.
Propylthiouracil U.S.P.		50 to 500 mg.
Iodides and Iodine		
Sodium iodide U.S.P.		300 mg. to 1 Gm.
Sodium iodide I 131 U.S.P.	Iodotope; Oriodide; Radiocaps; Theriodide; Tracervial	Oral or I.V. *Diagnostic:* the equivalent of 1 to 100 *micro-*curies. *Therapeutic:* the equivalent of 1 to 100 *milli*curies
Strong iodine solution U.S.P.	Lugol's solution	0.1 to 1 ml.
Iodine Uptake Inhibitors		
Potassium perchlorate		200 to 400 mg. every 6 to 8 hours
Potassium thiocyanate		1 Gm. daily
Anterior Pituitary Hormone (for Diagnosis and Treatment)		
Thyrotropin	Thyroid-stimulating hormone; TSH; Thytropar	10 international units

stimulation of the thyroid reduces the gland's uptake of radioactive iodide. In the hyperthyroid patient, the gland continues to concentrate large quantities of the iodide isotope and turn it into hormones *despite TSH suppression* by the previously administered dose of liothyronine. This suggests that in thyrotoxicosis, the gland is functioning autonomously or that it is being continuously stimulated by some still unknown thyroid-stimulating substance.

Treatment of Hyperthyroidism

Even though its exact cause is not known, the symptoms of hyperthyroidism can now be readily controlled, and, in many cases, the condition can actually be cured. The main forms of treatment are: (1) The administration of one or more of the so-called *antithyroid drugs;* (2) *radiation therapy* employing the radioactive iodine isotope, I 131; (3) subtotal surgical excision of the gland (*thyroidectomy*). Radiation or surgery permanently reduces the functioning mass of the gland. On the other hand, antithyroid drugs do not damage the thyroid irreparably as do the other treatments; however, these agents also often succeed in bringing about permanent remissions of hyperthyroidism. At the very least, they relieve the patient's signs and symptoms and help to prepare him for safer surgery.

Antithyroid Drugs

Drugs of several different kinds act in one way or another to interfere with the biosynthesis of hormones by the thyroid gland. The most widely used are the thiouracil derivatives such as *methimazole* (see Drug Digest) and the other thiocarbamides listed in Table 31-2. These chemicals inhibit the oxidative enzymes that catalyze the iodination and coupling steps in the synthesis of thyroxine and liothyronine. As a result, the gland soon stops secreting the excessive amounts of hormones responsible for the signs and symptoms of hyperthyroidism. Even though the thyroid then undergoes compensatory enlargement, the patient's condition improves over a period of weeks. (These drugs are sometimes called goitrogens, because their ability to reduce glandular secretion sets in motion the same sort of compensatory increase in the size of the thyroid gland that occurs in simple, non-toxic goiter.)

Of hyperthyroid patients who take one of these drugs faithfully for a year or more, more than half may never again have a recurrence of hyperthyroidism. It is important to encourage patients to take the drug regularly and exactly as directed, since, if they neglect to continue taking the drugs daily for many months and at the proper times of day until control is established, the condition may recur. They should also be urged to report any symptoms of illness immediately: sore throat, fever, rash, or jaundice may be signs of drug reactions calling for prompt withdrawal of these drugs. Only a small minority of patients develop adverse reactions, which, however, may include serious disorders such as agranulocytosis and hepatitis.

Preparation for Surgery. Although a third or more of hyperthyroid patients cannot be cured with drugs alone, the administration of *propylthiouracil* or one of its relatives is useful in preparing patients for subtotal thyroidectomy. After taking daily doses of an antithyroid drug for several weeks, the patient's metabolism is brought back closer to normal and his cardiovascular system is stabilized. The only difficulty with such drug therapy is that the patient's gland tends to grow larger and is more likely to bleed excessively during the operation. To prevent this, the surgeon has the patient take a few drops of an iodide solution such as Lugol's solution (Table 31-2) daily for a week or ten days before the surgical procedure is to be done.

Iodides. Until the introduction of the thiouracil derivatives, the only medical treatment for hyperthyroidism was the administration of iodine salts in amounts much larger than those employed in preventing simple goiter. Just how such iodides work to control this condition is still not well understood. However, they often have a rapid effect in reducing hyperactive thyroid function and in returning the patient to a euthyroid condition for a while. This action lasts only for weeks or, at most, months and is thus not suited to the long-range control of hyperthyroidism. It is, nonetheless, very useful for reducing the size and vascularity of the spongy goitrous gland, thus lessening the likelihood of heavy bleeding during surgery. The small amounts of Lugol's solution or of saturated solution of potassium iodide that are ordered for this purpose must be accurately measured, and the drops should be added to fruit juice or milk to disguise the unpleasant taste.

One of the antithyroid drugs, *iothiouracil* (Table 31-2), has iodine already incorporated in the thiouracil molecule. The presence of the iodine is said to keep the gland from enlarging (as it does when other drugs of this class are given to reduce formation of hormone). Instead, in response to the iodine content of this drug the patient's thyroid becomes smaller and firmer and is less likely to bleed. At the same time, of course, hormonal synthesis is suppressed, so that the hyperthyroid patient's symptoms are relieved. The main disadvantage of this drug is that the presence of organically bound iodine interferes with the protein bound iodine (PBI) test and the radioactive iodine uptake test (see Summary) of thyroid function for as long as several months.

Radioactive Iodine. The iodine isotope ^{131}I is trapped by the thyroid gland in the same manner as ordinary iodides. Reaching very high concentrations there, it gives off beta and gamma radiations in amounts that are useful for both the diagnosis of thyroid disorders and the treatment of some cases of hyperthyroidism. Tiny tracer doses are administered to determine the thyroid gland's capacity to store iodine; much larger amounts are administered deliberately to destroy thyroid tissue—for example, in patients for whom surgery does not seem safe and whose hyperthyroidism has not responded to drugs.

THE DIAGNOSTIC USE of sodium radioiodide solution is based on the measurable differences in retention and excretion of iodine. In myxedema only a small proportion of any administered dose is taken up by the patient's thyroid gland, and the rest is excreted in the urine. In the hyperthyroid patient, on the other hand, the thyroid retains a high percentage of the amount administered, and relatively little radioactivity is detected in the urine. The small doses of radioiodide give off enough gamma rays so that such determinations may readily be made; the beta rays are so few that there is little danger of damage to the patient's thyroid or other tissues.

THE THERAPEUTIC USE of sodium iodide 131 involves the administration of perhaps a thousand times as high a dose of the radioisotope. The drug is given either as a single large dose or in a series of smaller cumulative doses. In either case, the iodine isotope accumulates in the patient's thyroid in amounts as much as 10,000 times as high as that in other body tissues. The very short range beta rays that are then given off thus destroy thyroid tissue without harming other cells. As a result of the gradual reduction in hormone secretion, the symptoms of hyperthyroidism are gradually reduced, and the patient's metabolic rate may become normal in about twelve weeks.

Sometimes, if the first dose fails to bring about a remission, the patient receives a second, somewhat larger dose of radioiodide. On the other hand, even a single dose may destroy too much thyroid tissue. Therefore, the patient is examined periodically for signs of *hypo*thyroidism, and, if any tendency toward myxedema is noted, thyroid therapy is instituted. Just as in hypothyroidism caused by surgical removal of too much thyroid tissue, the patient who is made myxedematous by too great a destructive action of radioactive iodine may require replacement thyroid therapy for the rest of his life.

An even more serious concern has been the possibility that the beta radiations might cause thyroid cancer. However, this has not occurred, and fears of this kind have abated. Nevertheless, radioactive iodine

is ordinarily not administered to children (who are thought to be especially susceptible to cancer) or to young adults or pregnant women (because of the possibility of genetic changes and fetal damage). This form of treatment of hyperthyroidism is considered especially desirable for elderly patients with cardiac or kidney diseases that make them poor surgical risks.

In caring for patients who are taking radioactive iodide, the nurse should check on what precautions are necessary. The doses employed for diagnostic purposes are so small that special care is not required, but therapeutic doses can result in potential dangers. Thus, the nurse should read the product literature and other references in regard to current practices in radiation therapy, so that she can then work more closely with personnel in the hospital's radiation therapy department.

Other Goitrogenic Chemicals. Numerous natural and synthetic substances stop the synthesis of thyroid hormones and thus induce compensatory glandular enlargement. The seeds and leaves of certain plants, including cabbage, contain such goitrogens. Aminotriazole, a weed-killing chemical that was used to control weeds in cranberry bogs, was shown to cause goiters in rats. When traces of this compound were found in the fruit one year recently, the F.D.A. ordered much of the crop kept off the market. Certain sulfonamides and the blood-pressure-reducing drug, potassium thiocyanate, have been shown to cause thyroid enlargement at times during therapy.

One goitrogen, *potassium perchlorate*, has found a place in the treatment of hyperthyroidism. Administered in several small daily doses with food to reduce gastric irritation, this drug quickly reduces the signs and symptoms of thyrotoxicosis. Like the thiocarbamide-type goitrogens, this chemical has sometimes caused blood dyscrasias. Unlike the latter group of antithyroid drugs, perchlorate can*not* be used preoperatively along with iodides to prepare the person for thyroid gland surgery. The reason for this lies in this drug's manner of action: the perchlorate ion competes with the iodide ion and keeps it from being taken up from the blood by the patient's thyroid gland. This, of course, accounts for its clinical utility in reducing the synthesis of excessive amounts of hormones in hyperthyroid individuals, but it also keeps these patients from profiting from the ability of iodides to shrink a hyperplastic, brittle thyroid gland before thyroidectomy.

SUMMARY OF TESTS FOR THYROID FUNCTION *

- *The Basal Metabolic Rate (B.M.R.)*

    This test is intended to measure the extent to which the patient's tissues are using up oxygen in carrying out combustion processes when the patient is in the resting state. When properly performed, it not only helps to differentiate euthyroid from hyperthyroid and hypothyroid individuals but also aids the doctor in following his patient's response to circulating thyroid hormones administered as replacement therapy, or the drop in tissue response to such hormones under the influence of antithyroid drugs.

- *Radioactive Iodine Uptake (R.A.I 131)*

    This test is intended to measure the thyroid gland's capacity for trapping and concentrating radioiodide. The

* All of these laboratory diagnostic tests are often useful when evaluated simultaneously. However, all are subject to error and serve best when the doctor uses the results to supplement his clinical judgment as based upon the patient's history and physical examination.

gland of hypothyroid patients takes up only a small fraction of the orally administered tracer dose of the isotope, whereas hyperthyroid patients show accumulation of a large percentage of the amount of I 131 that was taken 24 hours before. (The iodine uptake of a normal gland is suppressed by prior administration of the hormone sodium liothyronine; in Graves' disease, the patient's hyperplastic gland continues to concentrate radioactive iodide even after thyroid suppression of pituitary TSH production.)

- *Protein Bound Iodine (P.B.I.)*

    This test is intended to determine the amount of thyroid hormone circulating in loose combination with plasma carrier proteins. The P.B.I. is high in hyperthyroidism and low in hypothyroidism. A more accurate modification, the *Butanol-Extractable Iodine (B.E.I.)* test, measures only the thyroxine content of the plasma and *not* other circulating iodine-containing compounds that may also be present in addition to the hormone.

SUMMARY OF POINTS FOR THE NURSE TO REMEMBER

- Thyroid preparations sometimes cause unpleasant side effects. Observe the patient for signs and symptoms such as nervousness and insomnia; report the symptoms to the physician if they should occur, and teach the patient to do so.

- Misconceptions concerning the appropriate use of thyroid preparations are widespread. The nurse can help to clarify the legitimate use of thyroid preparations and encourage patients to seek medical advice for conditions such as fatigue and weight gain.

- Regular and persistent drug therapy are especially important in the treatment of patients with hyperthyroidism. Because many of these patients continue drug treatment at home for extended periods, it is particu-

larly important to instruct them in the importance of regular and continued drug therapy as prescribed by the physician.

- Particular care should be taken in accurate measurement of the small amounts of liquid iodide preparations ordinarily prescribed. The disagreeable taste of these drugs can be disguised by placing them in milk or fruit juice.

- Special precautions are ordinarily not required when radioactive iodide is administered for diagnostic purposes. However, the nurse should confer with personnel of the radiation therapy department of the hospital in regard to necessary precautions when using any radioactive isotope.

SUMMARY OF THE CLINICAL USES OF THYROID PREPARATIONS AS REPLACEMENT THERAPY IN *HYPOTHYROIDISM* OR *ATHYREOSIS*

- Myxedema (adult and juvenile)

- Cretinism (after very early diagnosis)

- Gynecological disorders (amenorrhea, dysmenorrhea, habitual abortion, etc., when these are the result of thyroid hormone deficiency)

- Male infertility (as a result of oligospermia stemming from reduced thyroid function)

- Goiter, simple, non-toxic type

- Hypometabolism as a result of borderline hypothyroid deficiency with signs and symptoms such as dry skin and hair, loss of scalp hair, brittle nails, intolerance to cold, feelings of fatigue and sluggishness, and obesity.

SUMMARY OF ADVERSE EFFECTS, PRECAUTIONS AND CONTRAINDICATIONS WITH THYROID PRODUCTS

- *Signs and Symptoms of Overdosage*

    Tachycardia, cardiac arrhythmias, elevated pulse pressure, anginal-type chest pains, dyspnea, possible precipitation of congestive failure; excessive sweating, intolerance to heat, fever, flushing; nervousness, irritability, insomnia, headache; increased gastrointestinal motility, abdominal cramps, diarrhea, nausea, increased appetite.

- *Cautions and Contraindications*

    Caution in patients with a history of angina pectoris, recent myocardial infarction or congestive heart failure, and hypertension.

    Contraindicated in adrenal insufficiency, or in hypopituitarism, unless adrenal deficiency is first corrected by administration of adequate doses of cortisone or hydrocortisone.

REVIEW QUESTIONS

1. (a) What is the main function of the thyroid gland?
(b) What are the two active hormones of the thyroid gland, and what is the storage form of the thyroid secretion called?
2. (a) What are some of the characteristic signs and symptoms of full-blown *hypo*thyroidism?
(b) What are some of the characteristic signs and symptoms of a similar degree of hyperthyroidism?
3. (a) Describe briefly the way in which the rate of thyroid secretion is regulated.
(b) What accounts for the glandular enlargement which occurs in simple, non-toxic goiter?
4. (a) Describe briefly the three steps by which the thyroid gland biosynthesizes the thyroid hormones.
(b) In what ways may the gland be kept from synthesizing either normal or excessive amounts of these hormones?

5. (a) What are the two major deficiency syndromes which are treated by replacement therapy with thyroid products?
6. (a) What is the chief complication of thyroid overdosage and in patients with what conditions must thyroid therapy be undertaken with great caution if at all?
(b) Why must special measures be employed when thyroid is administered to an individual whose adrenal function may also be subnormal?
7. (a) In what respects does sodium liothyronine differ from other available thyroid products?
(b) In what respects do these properties make this thyroid hormone more or less useful or safe in various clinical situations?
8. (a) In what respect does sodium dextrothyroxine differ from sodium levothyroxine and other available thyroid products?

(b) For what patients is this form of thyroid hormone especially advocated? What manifestation of toxicity must be closely watched for when it is used for treating these patients?

9. (a) What is meant by the term hypometabolism, or borderline hypothyroidism, and what may be the response of such a patient's symptoms to thyroid therapy?

(b) What are some clinical conditions in which thyroid therapy has often been undertaken even when there was no evidence of the existence of a hypothyroid state?

(c) What explanation may the nurse give to a patient who thinks that thyroid preparations are a cure-all for a variety of complaints such as fatigue, dry skin and hair, and weight gain?

10. (a) What measure is commonly employed to prevent development of endemic goiters of the simple, nontoxic type?

(b) What is the manner in which the administration of a thyroid product to such patients prevents further growth of the enlarged thyroid gland in this condition?

(c) What explanation can the nurse give in regard to the practice of adding small amounts of iodides to table salt?

11. (a) What is the manner in which methimazole and similar drugs produce their desirable effect on thyroid gland function in the treatment of hyperthyroidism?

(b) What effect do drugs such as methimazole and propylthiouracil have upon the size and physical character of the thyroid glands of patients to whom they are administered?

12. (a) What adverse reactions have been reported in patients taking antithyroid drugs of the thiouracil derivative type?

(b) What signs and symptoms should patients taking these drugs be warned to report to their doctor?

13. (a) What action of iodides accounts for their use in patients in the period prior to their undergoing subtotal thyroidectomy?

(b) In what manner does the administration of relatively large doses of radioactive sodium iodide produce effects that are useful for treating hyperthyroidism?

(c) In what ways may the unpleasant taste of iodides be disguised?

14. (a) For which hyperthyroid patients is sodium iodide I 131 indicated, and for which patients is its use considered least desirable?

(b) What can be learned about the functional state of a patient's thyroid gland by the administration of tracer doses of sodium iodide I 131?

(c) From what sources may the nurse obtain information concerning the precautions required when giving I 131?

BIBLIOGRAPHY

Asper, S. P.: Physiological approach to correction of hypothyroidism. Arch. Int. Med., *107*:112, 1961.

Astwood, E. B.: Management of thyroid disorders. J.A.M.A., *186*:585, 1963.

Clark, D., and Rule, J. H.: Radioactive iodine or surgery in treatment of hyperthyroidism. J.A.M.A., *159*:995, 1955.

De Groot, L. J.: Therapy of thyrotoxicosis. Mod. Treatm., *1*:176, 1964.

Greer, M. A.: The treatment of myxedema. G.P., *22*:123, 1960.

Lerman, J.: Treatment of hypothyroidism. Mod. Treatm., *1*:146, 1964.

McGirr, E. M.: Sporadic goitrous cretinism. Brit. Med. Bull., *16*:113, 1960.

Rodman, M. J.: Drugs used in thyroid diseases. R.N., *25*: 61, 1962 (March).

————: The thyroid and antithyroid drugs. R.N., *31*:55, 1968 (Feb.).

Selenkow, H. A., and Collaco, F. M.: Clinical pharmacology of antithyroid compounds. Clin. Pharmacol. Ther., *2*:191, 1961.

Drugs Used in Diabetes

DIABETES MELLITUS

Diabetes is the most common of all the metabolic diseases. About two million people in this country are known diabetics, and an estimated million more have not yet come to medical attention. The number of diabetics is expected to increase as more people live to middle and old age—the age at which four out of five cases are first recognized.

Actually, because predisposition to development of diabetes is hereditary, the disease can, in one sense, be said to begin at birth or even earlier. That is, the authorities now believe that long before sugar begins to appear in the blood in excessive quantities and starts to spill over into the urine, the unknown genetic defect is already doing its damage. The diabetic person's pancreas fights to keep his carbohydrate metabolism within normal limits and succeeds in doing so for variable periods of time. Finally, however, the body's compensatory mechanisms fail, and overt clinical symptoms of diabetes become detectable.

Diabetes first manifests itself as *hyperglycemia* (fasting sugar levels of over 110 mg. per 100 ml. of venous blood) and *glycosuria* (the presence of *any* sugar in the urine). However, despite this focusing of attention on sugar (the term "mellitus" means "honeyed"), diabetes is a disease not only of carbohydrate metabolism but also of protein and fat metabolism. In fact, even though screening tests and diagnostic techniques for detecting diabetes are based upon finding evidence of defects in carbohydrate metabolism, the most dangerous of both the acute and the chronic complications of diabetes are the result of abnormalities in fat and protein chemistry.

The metabolic abnormalities of diabetes stem from a lack of effective insulin activity. Insulin is a hormone secreted into the blood stream by the endocrine portions of the pancreas. These are the so-called *beta cells* located in tiny islets of tissue scattered through the rest of the pancreas, an organ which also produces exocrine digestive juices. (The Latin word *insula* means *island.*)

In diabetes, the patient's metabolism seems to function as though he were fasting, even when he is actually eating and absorbing the products of digestion. This occurs either because his pancreas fails to produce adequate amounts of insulin or because the hormone which is produced does not carry out its metabolic functions effectively.

Why this should be so is still not well understood. For, although the pancreatic beta cells of many diabetics secrete little or no insulin, this may be a *result* rather than the *cause* of the disease. That is, the beta cells may have become exhausted after years of producing abnormally large amounts of insulin in a futile effort to keep up with unusual demands brought on by a non-pancreatic difficulty. Thus, the primary genetic defect may affect the peripheral tissues rather than the pancreas in a manner that leads to an eventual lack of metabolically effective insulin.

Insulin secreted in adequate quantities may, for example, be inactivated by enzymes or antibodies that destroy it; or the hormone may be bound to blood proteins in a form that prevents it from acting effectively on its target tissues. On the other hand, abnormalities in pituitary, adrenal, or thyroid gland function may also affect carbohydrate metabolism in ways that put a strain on the insulin-producing capacity of the pancreatic islets. Excessive production of corticotropin, corticosteroids, or growth hormone could, for example, cause a very slight but persistent tendency toward hyperglycemia which would keep the pancreas in a state of constant activity. In any case, the beta cells sooner or later lose their ability to synthesize, store and secrete insulin. When these endocrine tissues can no longer respond adequately to demands for more insulin, the signs and symptoms typical of overt diabetes begin to appear.

THE ROLE OF INSULIN
IN REGULATING METABOLISM

The relationship between the pancreas and carbohydrate metabolism was first recognized late in the last century, when dogs whose pancreases had been surgically removed developed diabeteslike signs. In 1922, the Canadian scientists Banting and Best gave an extract of pancreatic islet tissue to a boy dying of diabetes. His dramatic recovery demonstrated the ability of insulin to correct the metabolic abnormality responsible for his severe illness.

Later, insulin was prepared in pure crystalline form from extracts of the pancreatic tissues of animals. This led to its use as replacement therapy in patients with diabetes mellitus whose own pancreatic beta cells failed to secrete enough active insulin. Before discussing the use of insulin in diabetes, we must first review the physiological functions of this hormone.

The Action of Insulin

Body cells burn fragments of digested foodstuffs to produce energy. The products of the digestion of carbohydrates, fats, and proteins must first be absorbed into the blood from the intestine. They are then transported to the tissues and released into the extracellular fluids and, finally, they make their way through the membranes of the cells of all the various tissues. Only after it gets inside the cell can a molecule of a substance such as glucose enter the metabolic mill—the series of enzymatically catalyzed intracellular oxidation-reduction reactions—and be converted into energy.

Some cells, including those of muscle and fat, do not let sugars simply diffuse into their metabolic machinery from the surrounding fluids. Instead, they seem to set up a barrier to free passage of these final fragments of carbohydrate digestion. One of the main actions of insulin is its capacity to act on the cell membrane in such a way as to carry glucose molecules through it and into the cell. Nerve cells and liver cells (among others) can carry sugars across their membranes without the help of insulin, but the transport systems of muscle and fat cells require activation by this hormone. Thus, without insulin to spring the trap door in their outer membranes, glucose cannot readily enter these cells.

Muscle Cells. The glucose that is taken out of the circulation by muscle cells under the influence of insulin may be used immediately or incorporated into glycogen. This storage form of carbohydrate can be quickly converted into glucose again, whenever the cells need more energy. The glucose that enters the cell or that is released from the glycogen molecule is then burnt by way of the Krebs tricarboxylic acid cycle.

In this process of *oxidative phosphorylation,* which is carried out in the mitochondria—the tiny structures within the cells that contain the necessary enzymatic assembly line—the energy of glucose is transferred to the cellular storage battery *adenosine triphosphate* (ATP), and carbon dioxide and water are produced as by-products. (When oxygen is in short supply, glucose can still be converted into energy, but the process—*anaerobic glycolysis*—is relatively inefficient.)

Fat Cells. The glucose that insulin lets get into the cells of fatty tissue is also stored for future use. The carbon, hydrogen, and oxygen atoms from this carbohydrate are used to form fatty acids, which (like the free dietary fatty acids absorbed from the gut) are then combined with phosphoglycerol to form triglyceride molecules. This so-called neutral fat—a highly concentrated fuel—is stored in adipose tissue until it is needed—as, for example, when intracellular glucose falls to a low level.

The burning of free fatty acids in various body tissues produces large amounts of energy rapidly, but the waste products of fat metabolism in the liver are not as readily removed as those produced when glucose alone is being metabolized. Instead of carbon dioxide and water, the keto-acid *aceto-acetic acid* and its by-products beta-hydroxybutyric acid and acetone are formed. Some of these ketone bodies are metabolized in the muscle tissue; the accumulation of excess ketones in the patient's blood that occurs when insulin is lacking leads to development of acidosis (see p. 436).

Protein metabolism is also affected by the presence or absence of insulin, among other hormones. For one thing, insulin speeds the passage of dietary amino acids into muscle cells, where they are then built into tissue protein. On the other hand, when insulin is lacking and glucose therefore cannot enter the muscle cell in adequate amounts, its proteins break down and their amino acids move back into the blood. (This muscle-wasting effect leads to a loss of strength; also, the diabetic patient's negative nitrogen balance slows the healing of skin wounds.)

Certain of the hormones secreted by the adrenal cortex tend, in such circumstances, to accelerate tissue wastage. These glucocorticoids aid the movement of amino acids from the muscles to the liver by way of the blood stream. In that organ, the amino acids are deaminated and—when the tissue cells are low in glucose and demand other sources of energy—some of these metabolic fragments, or carbon residues, are converted to glucose, while others form fatty acids and ketone bodies. (This is probably one reason why the continued administration of high doses of corticosteroids causes hyperglycemia, obesity, and muscular weakness in patients who are being treated with these drugs—see Chap. 28.)

Liver cells, unlike muscle and fat cells, do not need insulin to ease the entry of glucose. However, insulin helps the liver to keep glucose in storage in the form of glycogen. When insulin is lacking, this glycogen is reconverted to glucose which then enters the blood. However, this glucose cannot now make its way into muscle cells and adipose tissues because of the low levels of insulin, and hyperglycemia results. Another substance that stimulates the breakdown of liver glycogen to glucose is *glucagon,* a secretion produced by the *alpha* cells of the pancreas. The adrenal medullary hormone epinephrine causes the conversion of glycogen to glucose in muscle cells as well as in the liver.

METABOLIC ABNORMALITIES
IN INSULIN DEFICIENCY

Normal Regulation. Insulin plays the most important part of all the hormones involved in regulating the concentration of glucose in the blood and tissues. Normally, when glucose begins to enter the blood from the gut during the digestion of food, the beta cells of the pancreas are somehow immediately stimulated to step up their secretion of insulin. As the hormone has its effects on the cell membranes of the muscle cells and adipose tissues and on the liver, the excess glucose is promptly removed from the blood. When the level of blood sugar returns to normal, the beta cells of the pancreas stop secreting insulin; biosynthesis of the hormone continues there, but, instead of being released, the insulin granules are stored in little intracellular capsules.

On the other hand, when a person is fasting, rather than feeding, all insulin activity ceases. As a result, the tissues do not take up glucose from the blood as readily as before. Not only is blood sugar spared by this means, but the lack of insulin brings about changes in protein and fat metabolism that also help to conserve blood glucose. Muscle protein breaks down to amino acids that the liver can convert to glucose, and to ketone bodies. Most of these and the fatty acids freed from the adipose tissues are metabolized in the muscles to meet the body's energy needs. Any excess of keto-acids is combined with alkali and excreted by the kidney.

Signs and Symptoms of Deficiency. The onset of acute diabetes in a person who had previously shown no overt signs may be slow and insidious, or it may occur with dramatic suddenness. At one extreme, the patient may complain only of being chronically tired; at the other, the first sign may be a swift slide into diabetic coma. In general, however, acute diabetes of moderate severity is marked by a classic clinical picture.

In addition to feelings of fatigue and complaints of pruritus (itching of the skin and genital area) the patient may become aware of being excessively thirsty and hungry. These symptoms persist even when he drinks large amounts of fluid and eats heavily. Weight loss is common in young patients; obesity frequently occurs in older ones. The patient produces large amounts of urine, which tests reveal to be loaded with sugar and, often, with acetone or other ketones. Blood tests also show the presence of high glucose and ketone levels.

All of these features of this phase of diabetes can be explained in terms of the underlying metabolic defect. The hyperglycemia, as we have indicated, stems from the lack of effective insulin for shunting blood glucose into muscle cells, adipose tissues and liver glycogen. The patient's polyuria and glycosuria develop when the amount of sugar filtered by the glomeruli of the kidneys is greater than the renal tubules can reabsorb. Because the sugar dissolved in the tubular fluid drags water along with it by osmotic action as it drains out into the ureters, the diabetic patient tends to become dehydrated.

Diabetic Ketoacidosis and Coma. This acute complication resulting from a lack of insulin is most dangerous. It occurs most frequently in youngsters with *juvenile-onset* diabetes—i.e., diabetes diagnosed between birth and about age twenty. However, older people, in whom so-called *maturity-onset* diabetes usually manifests itself after age forty in a relatively mild form, sometimes go suddenly from an asymptomatic state into severe acidosis and coma. This condition, which is a medical emergency requiring prompt diagnosis and vigorous treatment, is the result of a vicious cycle of events set in motion by the absence of insulin. Patients whose condition had previously been controlled by insulin from an outside source may be precipitated into acidosis and coma when they develop an acute infection.

The process that finally results in uncontrolled diabetes is initiated when the patient's insulin lack and consequent failure to utilize glucose leads to the breakdown of tissue proteins and fats for use as fuel. The fatty acids formed in this way flood the liver with metabolic fragments that are converted to ketones. When these pile up to levels higher than the tissues can handle by burning for energy, they accumulate in the blood (ketonemia) and are carried to the kidneys for excretion in the urine (ketonuria). Some are also carried to the lungs for elimination and account for the fruity odor on the patient's breath.

For a time the patient's kidneys and lungs can compensate for ketoacidosis. The lungs remove large quantities of carbon dioxide; and the kidneys secrete ammonia for binding and eliminating the strong organic acids. However, the continued accumulation of ketones and hydrogen ions begins also to use up the body's bicarbonate buffer system, and sodium and potassium ions are then excreted in combination with the keto-acids. As the body's alkaline reserves drop and more fluids and electrolytes are lost through vomiting and osmotic diuresis, the dehydrated patient may go into shock.

The fall in renal blood flow and glomerular filtration, and the oliguria that follows, then lead to an accelerated accumulation of ketones in the central nervous system. At first, this stimulates the respiratory center of the patient with decompensated acidosis. This accounts for the characteristic Kussmaul-type hyperpnea. Finally, however, the higher brain centers are depressed and the comatose patient expires, unless adequate insulin dosage is administered and other supportive measures are taken.

INSULIN IN THE TREATMENT OF DIABETES

Some diabetics can be controlled by diet alone; others may now be managed by diet together with one of the new orally administered synthetic hypoglycemic agents (Table 32-1). However, the injection of insulin remains the single most important measure for managing every type of diabetic patient. Insulin has now been prepared synthetically, but all of the commercially available insulins are purified extracts of animal pancreatic tissues.

The main advances in insulin therapy in recent years have been in the development of a variety of preparations with different durations of action (Table 32-1). The doctor tries to select the preparation best suited to each patient. He schedules its administration in relation to the times of the patient's meals and supplements the patient's ordinary insulin dosage when an infection develops or other stresses occur. The patient—or the nurse—must never substitute insulin of one type for another but always use the particular preparation that was ordered. All the various insulins should be stored in the refrigerator. Insulin that is turbid, or in which separation of the suspension has occurred, should be rotated gently rather than shaken vigorously, to avoid formation of bubbles and foam.

Dosage of insulin products and duration of action vary from patient to patient. Thus, adjustment of dosage is made only under the doctor's direction, and the patient should be carefully instructed in administration of insulin. He should also be urged to make himself completely conversant with the portions of the product's package insert that offer directions for administration and additional information.

Initial Therapy

Most authorities believe that all newly diagnosed diabetic patients should be hospitalized in order to have their needs for insulin determined. At the same time, the patient receives his first instructions concerning the nature of his disease, the manner of calculating his dietary needs, and the relationship of exercise and acute illness to his daily insulin requirements. The nurse, of course, has an important responsibility in this initial orientation and in the subsequent instruction of the diabetic patient.

During this period of evaluation, most internists start the patient on injections of the *unmodified*, or regular, *insulin* (see Drug Digest), beginning with doses of about 10 units before breakfast and, then, adding further doses before other meals and at bedtime. Depending upon the patient's response pattern as determined by tests of his blood and urine, the doctor decides whether he can be managed by dietary therapy alone; by diet and one of the synthetic oral hypoglycemic agents; or by one of the modified forms of insulin, in which the hormone is reacted with another protein· such as protamine or precipitated as large zinc-containing crystals.

If tests show that insulin is required, the patient now usually receives one of the intermediate-acting preparations of insulin. A single dose of a product such as the *insulin zinc suspension* (see Drug Digest) is injected each morning before breakfast in an amount calculated on the basis of the total daily dose of regular insulin that had been found necessary. Many patients with mild to moderate diabetes of the maturity-onset type can get along on a single daily dose of fewer units of one of these longer-acting preparations, thus avoiding the need for frequent injections of the more rapidly eliminated regular insulin.

Other patients with less reserves of metabolically effective insulin of their own may prove more difficult to stabilize in this way. Even when their food intake is carefully calculated and distributed throughout the day, they often show periods of rising blood sugar after meals. In such cases of postprandial hyperglycemia, it is sometimes necessary for the doctor to order supplementary injections of regular insulin.

Sometimes, when blood sugar rises above normal only after breakfast, a single dose of the more rapid-acting regular insulin is added to the early morning intermediate-acting insulin preparation and injected by means of the same syringe after mixing just prior to use. Patients whose blood sugar tends to rise during the night may do best on a long-acting insulin, such as protamine zinc insulin (see Drug Digest), which continues to dissolve slowly from the depot injection site into the blood stream all through the night. Unfortunately, those patients who are most likely to suffer nocturnal hyperglycemia are also the ones whose unstable, or brittle, disease makes them prone to suffer hypoglycemic reactions also.

Insulin in Ketoacidosis

Various kinds of stressful conditions may increase a diabetic patient's need for insulin. Most commonly the occurrence of an acute infection and fever raises the patient's insulin requirements. However, the patient may think that he does not need insulin because he has not eaten on account of nausea and vomiting.

TABLE 32-1

DRUGS USED IN THE TREATMENT OF DIABETES

	PROPRIETARY NAME OR SYNONYM	DOSAGE **	ONSET AND DURATION OF ACTION **
Insulin Preparations			
Rapid-Acting			
Insulin Injection U.S.P.	Regular insulin; regular Iletin	5–100 U.S.P. units S.C. as needed	1–1½ hours onset; 6–8 hours duration
Prompt Insulin Zinc Suspension U.S.P.	Semilente Insulin; Semilente Iletin	10–80 U.S.P. units S.C.	1½–2 hours onset; 12–18 hours duration
Intermediate-Acting			
Isophane Insulin Suspension U.S.P.	NPH Insulin	10–80 U.S.P. units S.C.	1–2 hours onset; 20–32 hours duration
Insulin Zinc Suspension U.S.P.	Lente Insulin; Lente Iletin	10–80 U.S.P. units	1–2 hours onset; 26–30 hours duration
Globin Zinc Insulin		10–80 U.S.P. units	2 to 4 hours onset; 10–22 hours duration
Long-Acting			
Extended Insulin Zinc Suspension U.S.P.	Ultralente Insulin; Ultralente Iletin	10–80 units S.C.	5–8 hours onset; 34–36 hours duration
Protamine Zinc Insulin Suspension U.S.P.	Protamine Zinc Iletin	10–80 U.S.P. units S.C.	7 hours onset; 24–36 hours duration

	PROPRIETARY NAME	USUAL DAILY DOSAGE RANGE	
Oral Hypoglycemic Agents *			
Sulfonylureas †			
Acetohexamide	Dymelor	250 mg.–1.5 Gm.	
Chlorpropamide U.S.P.	Diabinese	100 mg.–250 mg.	
Tolazamide	Tolinase	100 mg.–1.0 Gm.	
Tolbutamide U.S.P.	Orinase	500 mg.–2 Gm.	
Biguanides ‡			
Phenformin tablets	DBI	50–200 mg.	
Phenformin capsules §	DBI-TD	50–100 mg.	

* These drugs are indicated in patients with stable, maturity-onset diabetes of mild to moderate degree who cannot be controlled with diet alone. They are never given alone to unstable, ketotic patients or to patients with the juvenile-onset type diabetes.

† The drugs of this class are almost never given together with insulin after the initial period of conversion from hormone therapy; their main advantage is that their use spares the patient the need to make injections.

‡ These drugs are sometimes used with insulin, to stabilize a "brittle" case and reduce the required dosage of the hormone as well as the peaks and valleys of *hyper-* and *hypo*glycemia. They are also often combined with one of the sulfonylureas for synergistic effects. Used alone, they are sometimes preferred for obese patients.

§ This long-acting form often permits once or twice daily dosage. (Duration of action of capsules 8 to 12 hours, compared with 4 to 6 hours for tablets.)

** Dosage of insulin products and duration of action vary from patient to patient.

Patients are instructed not to neglect taking their insulin in such circumstances. They should, in fact, administer an additional dose of rapid-acting regular insulin if their tests of urine specimens reveal a rising glucose content or persistent ketonuria. It is desirable that a member of the family be instructed to call the doctor and handle the testing of the patient's urine and the necessary adjustments in insulin dosage, since the acutely ill patient may become too drowsy or confused to do so.

Once a definite diagnosis of ketoacidosis or of diabetic coma is made, the patient requires prompt and vigorous treatment with fluids, electrolytes and regular insulin. Delay in diagnosis and treatment still accounts for the loss of a large percentage of very young diabetic children, and the mortality rate in older patients who are comatose when first seen is still about 10 per cent. The nurse must see to it that the supplies that will be needed—insulin, intravenous fluids, etc.—are available and that the prescribed treatment is carried out with meticulous care. Such measures as collection of urine specimens as ordered and careful observation of the patient are also part of the nurse's responsibility, as is seeing that he is protected from injury (by side-rails, for example).

A rapid-acting insulin preparation is injected in relatively large doses to reverse the patient's ketoacidosis as quickly as possible, in order to avoid irreversible damage to the brain. If the patient is in shock, the entire dose is given by vein; otherwise half is sometimes administered subcutaneously and the remainder intravenously. The nurse's responsibilities include taking and recording data such as the patient's pulse, blood pressure, body temperature, fluid intake, and urinary output.

If the first doses of fast-acting insulin succeed in bringing the patient's blood sugar down substantially, the succeeding doses must, of course, be much smaller. On the other hand, some patients with diabetic ketoacidosis and coma may prove unusually resistant to ordinary doses of insulin (20 to 50 units). Patients who fail to respond to the initial insulin injections with a reduction in blood glucose often require repeated large doses of the hormone, along with fluids, electrolytes, and antibiotics or other drugs for treating the illness that set off the episode of acidosis. Rarely, a patient who has developed antibodies to the foreign protein that insulin from beef and pork pancreas represents may show amazing resistance and require thousands of units daily; a concentrated preparation containing 500 units of regular insulin per ml. is available for administration in such cases.

Hypoglycemic Reactions to Insulin

Too much insulin may also cause coma, which must be differentiated from diabetic coma by determination of the patient's blood sugar and ketone levels. It is better, however, to prevent such dangerous reactions by carefully observing the patient for signs of hypoglycemia and administering some food containing readily absorbed glucose. The nurse can help here also, by teaching the patient to recognize the symptoms of hyperinsulinism and take appropriate actions when he detects hypoglycemic symptoms typical of his own pattern.

The symptoms and signs (see Summary, p. 443) vary considerably from patient to patient, and—since the severity of hypoglycemic reactions depends upon how rapidly as well as on how far blood sugar falls—the type of preparation employed also affects the nature of the patient's response to insulin overdosage. Thus, some of the early signs of autonomic nervous system stimulation, which are observed with regular insulin when it reaches its peak of action (only a couple of hours after injection), are largely absent with the more slowly absorbed insulins which lower blood sugar gradually as successive increments slowly enter the blood from the depot site.

Most patients first show the effects of falling blood sugar in the brain, which largely burns glucose alone as its source of energy. Drowsiness and irritability or confusion are often the first signs that the patient and his family should be alerted to look for. If the patient realizes what is happening when he finds it suddenly difficult to concentrate or think clearly, he can often clear up the condition at this stage by taking some candy, orange juice, or other quick source of carbohydrate that he carries with him.

The patient may also know that hypoglycemia threatens when he begins to suffer a sudden series of cardiovascular and gastrointestinal difficulties. These are primarily the result of sympatho-adrenal discharge leading to the release of epinephrine and acetylcholine. The discharge of epinephrine serves the purpose of breaking down liver and muscle glycogen to glucose; it also releases free fatty acids for use as fuel in place of sugar. However, this compensatory mechanism against hypoglycemia often results in cardiac palpitations, anxiety, tremors and profuse sweating. Reflex parasympathetic reactions to such sympathetic stimulation may add to the patient's cardiovascular instability. Parasympathetic hyperactivity often causes G.I. contractions that feel like hunger pangs and increased acid-peptic secretions that cause epigastric distress and nausea.

Severe reactions are most likely in patients who fail to recognize hypoglycemic symptoms or who do nothing to counteract them. This sometimes happens with long-acting insulin preparations, not only because the changes in the patient's personality and mental efficiency may come on more slowly and subtly, but also because these products often reach their peak action during the night while the patient is asleep. As a result, the patient may feel no muscular weakness and fatigue before the sudden onset of motor symptoms such as twitching, athetoid (twisting) movements, clonic spasms and, finally, full-blown tonic seizures. Repeated episodes of continuing convulsions followed —as they often are—by coma may result in permanent cerebral cortical damage.

Treatment of even severe hypoglycemic reactions is simple enough, once the condition is recognized by the finding of a blood sugar level below 50 mg. per 100 ml.: it involves, mainly, giving glucose by vein if the patient is unable to swallow. Often simply the injection of an ounce or two of a concentrated (50%) solution of glucose will produce dramatic recovery. Occasionally, when it is difficult to find a good vein or the patient is thrashing about in delirium, drugs such as epinephrine, hydrocortisone, or glucagon may be administered subcutaneously.

Glucagon (see Drug Digest) is the purified polypeptide extracted from pancreatic alpha cells and acts to speed conversion of the liver's glycogen stores to glucose. It may be useful when no one capable of injecting glucose intravenously is available. Members of the family can readily be taught to give glucagon subcutaneously or I.M. while awaiting the arrival of the doctor, thus avoiding the danger to the patient of delayed awakening. Ordinarily, the patient responds in five to twenty minutes, provided that his liver glycogen had not been previously depleted.

Once the patient recovers consciousness, he should take more carbohydrate by mouth to avoid lapsing into unconsciousness as the effects of the glucagon injections wear off. If the patient's hypoglycemia was caused by a long-acting agent that continues to enter the blood, sources of rapidly available sugar, such as corn syrup or Coca-Cola syrup, should be supplemented by a more slowly digestible form of carbohydrate such as bread and honey. The doctor should always be informed of any hypoglycemic reaction, so that he can examine and question the patient and take measures to prevent future episodes of the same kind.

Prevention of hypoglycemic reactions requires careful adjustment of insulin dosage. The doctor, of course, works out a schedule of injections suited to the needs of each individual. In addition, however, it is necessary to teach the patient how to keep his insulin dosage and food intake in proper balance. The nurse can help to reinforce the physician's instructions for control of hyperglycemia and prevention of hypoglycemic reactions.

Thus, the nurse can help the patient remember the need for adjusting the times of his main meals to the peak activity of the type insulin preparation that he is taking. He is told to replace any meals not eaten with amounts of food containing the missing carbohydrates, fats, and protein. Snacks between meals and at bedtime may also be suggested as a means of neutralizing the amounts of insulin being absorbed at certain hours.

The nurse can also help make the patient aware of the effect of exercise on his insulin requirements. She can point out that sudden strenuous exercise of an unusual nature is undesirable for diabetics taking insulin (regular moderate exercise is, of course, considered desirable). The importance of compensating for the carbohydrate that is burned up in unaccustomed physical activity must be made clear to the patient. He is told that this can be done by taking extra sugary snacks up to a point and that it may also be necessary to reduce his next insulin dose after unusually prolonged exercise.

Children with diabetes—and their parents—require special instruction. When youngsters are told to carry candy or some other source of quick carbohydrates, they are likely to consume these sweets and then not have them when needed for combating a hypoglycemic reaction. They should be warned against this practice and be taught the importance of not missing meals and of not changing their exercise patterns suddenly from day to day, if sudden drops in blood sugar are to be avoided.

Patients with diabetes of long duration sometimes require re-education if their condition becomes unstable. Patients with juvenile-onset type diabetes who have grown older may suddenly become "brittle" in their responses to insulin. They may suffer sudden episodes of severe hypoglycemia that seem to come on with little warning. This calls not only for re-evaluation of their therapeutic program by the physician but also for reminders that they be constantly on the alert for any unusual feelings that may signal the onset of a reaction that requires quick carbohydrate ingestion.

THE ORAL HYPOGLYCEMIC DRUGS

Although the introduction of insulin for control of diabetes mellitus was a landmark in medical history, the need to administer it by injection is a drawback that limits its usefulness in various ways. Many patients balk at taking daily injections for the rest of their days and neglect to do so. Others are prone to painful sensitivity reactions from injections of the foreign protein, even when they follow instructions to change the site of injection frequently and employ antihistamine drug therapy. Some children and women suffer unsightly atrophic or hypertrophic skin changes at local points of parenteral administration.

Despite frequent rumors of the imminent development of oral preparations of insulin ever since the time of discovery of the hormone, no such product has ever actually proved practical. However, during the 1950's two new classes of synthetic chemicals were introduced which were effective for bringing down the high blood sugar levels of many diabetics when taken by mouth. These chemicals—the *sulfonylureas* and the *biguanides*—are *not* "oral insulins" nor are they truly "insulin substitutes." Nevertheless, these oral hypoglycemic agents have proved very valuable for many patients with relatively mild or moderate diabetes who are now spared the nuisance of frequent insulin injections.

The Sulfonylureas (Table 31-1)

This group of drugs was developed as the result of a chance observation in the 1940's that an antibacterial sulfonamide drug caused hypoglycemia in some patients who were being treated for infections. This set off a search for other sulfonamide derivatives that might have an even greater degree of hypoglycemic activity. The introduction of the sulfonylurea compound *tolbutamide* (see Drug Digest) in the mid 1950's marked the successful end of the long search for a drug that would both safely and effectively cause a fall in blood sugar when given orally. Since that time three other drugs of this chemical class have come into use in this country.

Clinical Status

None of these drugs is considered suitable for administration to patients who are likely to develop ketoacidosis or whose diabetes was first diagnosed during childhood or adolescence. This lack of effectiveness in juvenile-onset type diabetes results from the principal manner of action of the sulfonylurea compounds. These drugs act primarily by stimulating the beta cells of the pancreas to release their insulin granules into the patient's blood stream. The hormone secreted in this way is carried, by way of the portal vein, to the liver, where it acts to inhibit the breakdown of glycogen to glucose.

Patients with relatively severe diabetes have few functioning pancreatic islets, or none, and the sulfonylurea drugs cannot, of course, stimulate the secretion of endogenous insulin in such patients. Thus, insulin injections are still indispensable for treating the juvenile-onset patient and the patient who is likely to develop ketoacidosis and coma when an infection, a surgical procedure, or other stressful situation puts too great a demand upon the very limited ability of his pancreas to produce insulin.

Treatment with the sulfonylurea agents is most likely to be effective in patients whose diabetes become apparent relatively late in life—that is, in diabetes of the *maturity-onset* or adult type. Such patients often have more or less adequate amounts of circulating insulin, because their beta pancreatic cells are still functional and may, in fact, be responding excessively to glucose loads. However, in these patients the pancreatic response to high blood sugar levels comes on *too slowly*. As a result, the sluggishly responding secretory cells are continuously being called upon to work overtime. Eventually, just as happens

much earlier in life in the case of patients with the more severe juvenile-onset type diabetes, the beta cells of these over-age-forty patients may become totally exhausted and unable any longer to keep sugar levels normal.

The administration of sulfonylurea-type hypoglycemic agents to these patients often helps their overworked secretory cells to respond more rapidly when blood sugar first begins to rise. By keeping the pancreas from ever falling behind in its efforts to maintain normal blood sugar levels, such drug-induced stimulation of secretion gives the cells a chance to rest and recover. This protective effect of sulfonylurea drug therapy usually tends to bring the patient's diabetes under control and keeps his condition from getting any worse.

Many so-called *prediabetics*—individuals who have not yet developed diabetes but who are known to have a hereditary predisposition to the disease—are receiving sulfonylurea drugs in experimental studies designed to see whether the appearance of overt symptoms can be postponed or prevented entirely.

Secondary failure or relapse sometimes occurs after the condition had been for a while successfully controlled with a sulfonylurea drug such as tolbutamide. This may occur because the patient was not a good candidate for oral drug treatment to begin with and should have been given insulin. On the other hand, relapse may be the result of the patient's own carelessness, particularly in regard to his prescribed diet. One of the drawbacks of oral drug therapy is that it is *too* convenient. Thus, many patients are not as impressed with the seriousness of their condition as they are when they must inject insulin daily. Often, they tend to become careless and are then more likely to suffer various complications (see p. 442).

Choice of Sulfonylurea Compounds

Patients whose diabetes cannot be controlled by diet alone but who can be successfully transferred from insulin to oral drugs are most often started on tolbutamide or chlorpropamide (see Drug Digests)—the two agents with which doctors are most experienced. Tolbutamide seems the safer of the two, mainly because the much longer duration of chlorpropamide's action makes the hypoglycemic reactions that occasionally occur more difficult to deal with. Drug-induced liver disorders and blood dyscrasias occur infrequently with both drugs but must be watched for; therefore the doctor will order liver function and blood tests periodically, especially during the early trials with hypoglycemic drugs.

In most patients taking either of these two drugs, diabetes is satisfactorily controlled. However, some, who tend to suffer secondary failure, or relapse, may do better on one of the two new sulfonylurea compounds, acetohexamide (Dymelor) or tolazamide

(Tolinase). These agents, which have shown a relatively low incidence of adverse reactions, are occasionally effective in patients who failed to respond at all to the older drugs, as well as in those who have relapsed after initial control. Patients who fail to respond to any of the sulfonylureas sometimes can be controlled when they are given one of these drugs in combination with phenformin, especially if they can be kept on proper dietary therapy at the same time.

The Biguanides

The drugs of this group, of which only *phenformin* (see Drug Digest) is currently in use in this country, differ from the sulfonylureas in the way by which they lower the blood sugar of diabetic patients. Their action is *extra*-pancreatic and does not depend upon the production of additional endogenous insulin. In a manner that is still not well understood, phenformin seems to affect the peripheral tissue cells in a way that forces them to pull in and burn up more glucose.

Phenformin is used for essentially the same kinds of patients who are candidates for the sulfonylurea-type oral hypoglycemics; also, as with the others, the use of this drug *alone* is contraindicated in patients whose diabetes can be controlled by diet alone or in those with a tendency toward acute complications such as ketoacidosis. However, its different manner of action sometimes permits the use of phenformin in clinical situations in which the sulfonylureas are not ordinarily employed.

For example, phenformin may be combined with insulin, with benefit to some patients whose blood sugar fluctuates markedly when they take insulin alone. Occasionally, a single daily dose of phenformin in timed-disintegration capsule form helps to stabilize the blood sugar of a patient with labile diabetes, in whom insulin alone tends to cause frequent *hypo*glycemic reactions when it is given in the doses needed to avoid equally frequent episodes of *hyper*glycemia and ketosis. Apparently, the two substances act synergistically in a way that helps to flatten out the peaks and valleys in the patient's blood sugar response patterns.

Similarly, the addition of phenformin to the regimen of some patients who are not being adequately controlled with a sulfonylurea drug alone will sometimes produce satisfactory responses. This may be because of the complementary actions exerted by the two different drugs. The insulin secreted by the pancreatic beta cells under the influence of the sulfonylureas is said to "push" glucose through the membranes of muscle cells, while phenformin "pulls" this sugar into the cell by an action upon anaerobic glycolysis which creates a "space" in the cellular oxidative phosphorylation reactions for the handling of more of the glucose that enters the cells from the surrounding fluids.

Phenformin can, of course, be used by itself, and some patients receiving combination therapy can be gradually weaned away from insulin or from sulfonylureas, after their condition has come under stable control. Some physicians, in fact, claim that phenformin alone is superior to insulin or the sulfonylureas for middle-aged overweight patients, because this drug, unlike endogenous or exogenous insulin, does not tend to encourage fat formation but, instead, decreases lipogenesis. (The presence of close to normal, or even above normal, insulin in the blood of patients with maturity-onset type diabetes may account both for their tendency toward obesity and their relative resistance to ketoacidosis, because the hormone tends to shunt glucose into pathways that favor fat formation, and it counteracts the breakdown of body fats to ketones. See pp. 435 and 436.)

Phenformin may help some patients lose weight in a less desirable way: The drug often produces an unpleasant persistent metallic taste which may sometimes help to reduce the patient's appetite so that he sticks to his prescribed diet more faithfully than do most other diabetics of this age group. If nausea, vomiting, and diarrhea develop, in addition to the bitter, brassy taste and anorexia, the daily dose of this drug should be reduced. It may be adjusted upward once more after a few days, or the timed-disintegration capsule form of phenformin, which is said to be better tolerated than the tablets, may be prescribed.

COMPLICATIONS OF DIABETES

Complications of long-standing diabetes include arteriosclerosis, resulting in retinopathy and blindness, nephropathy, coronary and cerebral vascular disease, and neuropathy. Diabetic patients are also prone to infections of the skin and deeper tissues, which may become gangrenous, particularly in the extremities, and consequent amputation of the foot or the leg may be required.

It is not yet known whether such long-term vascular complications can really be prevented; however, it seems reasonable to assume that patients who make every effort to keep their diabetic condition under control have a better chance of avoiding such late complications. Thus, part of the nurse's responsibility is to teach the patient to take care of himself in every way that may help to minimize such complications. This, of course, includes advising him in proper drug and dietary therapy, as well as in matters of personal hygiene such as skin care and protection of the feet from injury.

SUMMARY

In many patients, diabetes can today be controlled with convenient, orally administered drugs to keep their blood glucose normal and their urine free of sugar. However, the availability of these drugs in no way does away with the traditional therapeutic measures.

Instruction of the patient is intended to help him play his own part—and an important one—in the control of his illness. Without unduly alarming the patient, it must be made clear to him that diabetes is a serious disease and that he must follow the doctor's instructions carefully, so that the possible complications of his condition can be kept to a minimum. Among the points that must always be emphasized are the following:

1. *The need for the patient to store his insulin properly, measure the required amount accurately, and inject it correctly:* The patient should not only be taught what to do; he should also be observed to see how he actually carries out the instructions given him. (One nurse explained that insulin must be injected rather than swallowed. She then proceeded to demonstrate the technique of giving oneself an injection by making an injection through the skin of an orange. Later that day, when she asked the patient to show her how he would go about taking his insulin, he injected the insulin into an orange, which he then began to eat!)

2. *The need for the patient to know the early signs and symptoms of hypoglycemia, hyperglycemia and acidosis and the measures to take to counteract these potentially dangerous conditions:* The patient must be taught to test his own urine routinely and to realize the significance of abnormalities about which the doctor must be notified.

3. *The need for the patient to pay attention to personal hygiene, diet, and exercise:* The patient should know that what he eats, how he eats, and the hour at which he eats, as well as the type and amount of physical activity in which he indulges help to determine his response to the insulin he injects. He should know how to minimize chances of acquiring infections of the skin or other tissues that can lead to serious complications for diabetics.

SIGNS AND SYMPTOMS OF INSULIN-INDUCED HYPOGLYCEMIA

- *Sympathetic and parasympathetic nervous system reactions*

    Profuse sweating; facial pallor; paresthesias.

    Cardiac palpitations; tachycardia (occasionally, bradycardia); rise in blood pressure (occasionally, fall).

    Nausea; hunger pangs; hyperventilation.

- *Central nervous system mental, motor, and other reactions*

    Headache; blurring of vision and diplopia.

    Drowsiness; yawning; difficulty in concentrating; feelings of fatigue and weakness.

    Muscle spasms, twitching; choreiform movements; athetosis; ataxia; clonic or tonic convulsive seizures.

    Nervous irritability; delirium; occasionally, psychotic reactions and late mental retardation.

    Unconsciousness, stupor, and coma.

- *Note: Cause and contributing factors in "insulin shock" are:*

    Overdosage, resulting from
        Error in calculation of dose
        Unpredictable response in patient with labile, or "brittle" diabetes
        Failure to eat
        Unusually vigorous exercise
        Stress due to infection or surgery

SUMMARY OF SIGNS AND SYMPTOMS, AND PRECAUTIONS AND CONTRAINDICATIONS WITH ORAL HYPOGLYCEMIC AGENTS OF THE SULFONYLUREA CLASS

- *Hypoglycemic reactions* are relatively rare but can sometimes be severe in cases of overdosage, or unexpectedly high sensitivity during the period of conversion from insulin (i.e., while the latter is still being given).

- *Gastrointestinal upset*—Anorexia, nausea, vomiting, epigastric distress, diarrhea.

- *Nervous system side effects*—Headache, tinnitus, paresthesias (tingling), weakness, alcohol-like intoxication. (**Note:** an *intolerance to alcohol* similar to that seen with disulfiram has been noted.)

- *Allergic dermatological reactions*—Itching, redness, wheals, measleslike and maculopapular eruptions have been reported.

- *Blood dyscrasias*—Leukopenia, agranulocytosis, thrombocytopenia, and pancytopenia are rare occurrences.

- *Liver disorders* of both the hepatocellular and the cholestatic jaundice types have occurred; tests of liver function are made upon initiation of therapy and periodically during treatment. *These drugs are contraindicated* in patients with liver disease.

- *Contraindicated* in diabetic acidosis, coma, gangrene, pregnancy, infection with fever, and other conditions for which insulin is required.

- *Contraindicated* in patients with renal glycosuria.

- *Caution* in patients taking *thiazide*-type diuretics, sulfonamide antibacterial drugs, phenylbutazone, barbiturates, probenecid, alcohol, and adrenocorticosteroid drugs.

SUMMARY OF POINTS FOR THE NURSE TO REMEMBER CONCERNING DIABETES DRUG TREATMENT

- Carefully observe the patient for signs of hypoglycemia—for example, nervousness, pallor, tremors, and sweating. If you observe such symptoms, administer some readily absorbed food which serves as a quick source of glucose, such as lump sugar, candy, or orange juice. Teach the patient and family to be alert to symptoms of hypoglycemia and how to relieve the symptoms.

- Watch for signs of hyperglycemia and ketoacidosis. For example, the patient may become thirsty, drink a great deal, void copiously, become drowsy, and dehydrated. Instruct the patient and family concerning the significance of such symptoms and the need to continue taking prescribed insulin and to notify the physician immediately, should they occur.

- Insulin should be properly cared for (and the patient should be instructed in these measures) in the following manner:
  1. It should be refrigerated.
  2. Solutions containing particles in suspension should be gently rotated just before the medication is drawn into the syringe, to make certain that an even suspension has been attained.
  3. Care must be taken to use the correct scale on the syringe for measuring insulin. U-40 insulin, for example, should be measured using the U-40 scale on the syringe.

  4. The patient should be taught never to switch from insulin of one type to another except on orders from his doctor.

- When injecting insulin, be certain to rotate the injection sites and teach the patient to do so, in order to minimize trauma to tissues, and to facilitate absorption. Demonstrate the technique of injection, and supervise the patient as he commences giving his own injections.

- Recognize the relationship between duration of the action of the type insulin the patient is receiving, and the timing of his meals, and teach the patient to do so. Be alert to any changes in the timing of the patient's meals—which may be necessitated, for example, by diagnostic tests—and adjust the timing of insulin administration as necessary. For instance, if your patient is fasting for a determination of blood sugar, do not give him regular insulin until you are certain that he may have his breakfast within 10 or 15 minutes.

- Include the family in your teaching. However, whenever feasible, the patient should be encouraged to assume responsibility of his own care, rather than delegate it to a member of the family.

CLINICAL PROBLEM

Miss Jordan, age 22, has newly diagnosed diabetes mellitus. She takes 20 units of N.P.H. Insulin daily. One week after discharge from the hospital, Miss Jordan experienced anorexia and nausea. She was unable to eat, but she took her insulin as usual in the morning. That afternoon, Miss Jordan experienced profuse sweating and was tremulous and apprehensive, and she went to the hospital emergency room. The physician's diagnosis was insulin reaction, brought about when Miss Jordan omitted her usual food intake, owing to her gastrointestinal upset. Miss Jordan was treated at the emergency room with intravenous glucose to relieve hypoglycemia, and chlorpromazine to relieve nausea. After she had rested for an hour, Miss Jordan was ready to return home.

What instructions would you, as the emergency room nurse, give Miss Jordan before she leaves the hospital?

REVIEW QUESTIONS

1. (a) In what way does the action of insulin on muscle cells help to lower hyperglycemia?

(b) What is the effect of insulin upon carbohydrate metabolism in the liver?

2. (a) What terms best describe the character of the blood and urine when a diabetic patient lacks insulin?

(b) What metabolic events lead finally to diabetic coma when insulin is lacking?

3. (a) Which type insulin is ordinarily employed when a newly diagnosed patient's requirements are being determined?

(b) What advantage does insulin zinc suspension possess over regular insulin, and at what time of day is it ordinarily administered?

4. (a) What type insulin would you make available on the ward, if you were advised that a patient in diabetic ketoacidosis was being admitted?

(b) What observations does the nurse have to make during insulin treatment of the patient with diabetic ketoacidosis?

5. (a) What are some signs of hypoglycemia that the nurse should watch for and some symptoms that the patient should be taught to report?

(b) What measures may be taken to counteract hypoglycemia in a diabetic patient, and what instructions may be given to the patient about self-treatment of these symptoms?

6. (a) What are some of the more severe results of hyperinsulinism, and what is the surest way to counteract severe overdosage rapidly in unconscious patients?

(b) What is the main advantage in the use of glucagon in some cases of this kind, and what additional measures should be employed after this substance has produced its early desired effects?

(c) In addition to avoiding dosage miscalculations and taking prompt countermeasures, what should the patient be told about some general aspects of daily living that may help him avoid hypoglycemic reactions to insulin?

7. (a) What is the main advantage of the synthetic hypoglycemic chemicals now available for treating diabetes?

(b) Patients of what types are most likely to respond favorably to transfer from insulin to a sulfonylurea type drug?

(c) Patients with what types of diabetes should never be treated with oral hypoglycemic products alone because of the inability of these agents to control their condition?

8. (a) What is the primary manner of action of a combination of insulin and phenformin, or of phenformin and a sulfonylurea drug, which may account for their synergistic activity in the management of some patients whose diabetes is difficult to control?

(b) Why are insulin and sulfonylurea drugs not ordinarily administered at the same time?

(c) Under what circumstances are newer drugs such as acetohexamide or tolazamide most commonly employed?

9. (a) What is the most characteristic complaint of patients taking phenformin in somewhat excessive amounts?

(b) Name conditions of several types in which the use of oral hypoglycemic agents for control of the patient's diabetes is contraindicated.

10. (a) How might you reply to a query raised by a diabetic patient as to whether complications such as gangrene or blindness can be avoided by following all the doctor's instructions concerning drugs, diet, exercise, etc.?

(b) How would you explain to a diabetic patient the reason for his having to inject insulin instead of swallowing it?

BIBLIOGRAPHY

Barclay, P. L.: Clinical evaluation of phenformin (DBI) in office practice. J.A.M.A., *174:*474, 1960.

Boshell, B. S., and Barrett, J. C.: Oral hypoglycemic agents. Clin. Pharmacol. Ther., *3:*705, 1962.

Bradley, R. F.: Treatment of ketoacidosis and coma. Med. Clin. N. Am., *49:*961, 1965.

Council on Drugs: An oral hypoglycemic agent, acetohexamide (Dymelor). J.A.M.A., *191:*127, 1965.

DiPalma, J. R.: Drugs for diabetes mellitus. R.N., *30:*71, 1967 (Oct.).

Gorman, C. K.: Hypoglycemia, a brief review. Med. Clin. N. Am., *49:*947, 1965.

Marble, A.: Critique of the therapeutic usefulness of the oral agents in diabetes. Am. J. Med., *31:*919, 1961.

Martin, M. M.: The unconscious diabetic patient. Am. J. Nursing, *61:*92, 1961.

Moss, J. M., and De Lawter, D. E.: Oral agents in the management of diabetes mellitus. Am. J. Nursing, *60:*1610, 1960.

Peck, F. B.: Insulin types. *In* Diabetes Mellitus, Diagnosis and Treatment. New York, Am. Diabetes A., 1964.

Rodman, M. J.: Drugs for diabetes treatment. R.N., *24:*51, 1961 (June).

———: Oral drugs for diabetes. R.N., *26:*35, 1963 (Dec.).

Root, H. F., *et al.:* Diabetic coma. Am. J. Nursing, *55:*1196, 1955.

Schulman, J. L., and Greben, S. E.: The effect of glucagon on blood glucose level and the clinical state in the presence of marked insulin hypoglycemia. J. Clin. Invest., *36:*74, 1957.

Shuman, C. R. (ed.): Symposium on treatment of complications of diabetes. Mod. Treatment, *4:*13–119, 1967 (Jan.).

Anti-infective Drugs

General Principles of Anti-infective Therapy

All through the ages medical men have hoped to find drugs capable of controlling infectious diseases. Long before microbes were known to be the cause of infection, doctors tried to treat infected patients with chemicals of natural origin. However, rational attempts at chemotherapy became possible only after the major concepts of microbiology emerged during the last century. Scientific research on drugs for treating systemic infection has finally borne fruit in clinically useful products only in the past fifty years or so.

In this section, we shall take up the drugs in use today in the treatment of infections caused by bacteria, fungi and animal parasites such as protozoa and worms—with a few comments in regard to antiviral drugs, the area in which the next great advance in anti-infective therapy is expected to occur. Our discussion will deal with drugs of two major types: (1) the *antibiotics*, and (2) anti-infective *chemotherapeutic agents*.

Antibiotics are, by definition, chemical compounds produced by living microorganisms which are capable of inhibiting the growth of other microorganisms or even of killing them.

Chemotherapy is a broader term which means something more than merely the treatment of disease with chemicals. In the case of anti-infective drugs, the term embodies the concept of *selective toxicity* (p. 32). That is, a chemotherapeutic agent is a chemical—one *not* produced by living organisms and, ordinarily, synthetic—that strikes selectively at invading pathogenic organisms in the body without doing significant harm to the cells of the host.

In this chapter we shall present some aspects of the historical development of chemotherapy and of antibiotic treatment. Also, we shall indicate some of the major concepts of drug treatment of infectious disease, which have emerged as a result of the experience of the past quarter of a century or so—an era characterized as a "golden age" of anti-infective therapy.

History. Chemicals have been used to treat infectious diseases for many centuries, and the occasional curative properties of soils, plants and other materials containing living molds and bacteria also were recognized by primitive peoples. For example, mercury was used in syphilis from the time of the first recorded outbreak of that disease in Europe about 1500; and ancient Chinese medical manuscripts recommend application of moldy soybean curds to boils, carbuncles and infected wounds.

However, anti-infective drug treatment of systemic infections was put on a rational, scientific basis only with the work of Paul Ehrlich early in this century. Before his pioneer researches, many chemicals were known which eliminated pathogenic organisms when applied topically as antiseptics and disinfectants (Chap. 43). However, such substances were too toxic for internal administration aimed at eliminating microorganisms that had established themselves deep within the tissues of the host.

Ehrlich reasoned that it might be possible to prepare synthetic chemicals that would act selectively on parasitic cells without injuring the person being treated. He felt that drugs might be devised which would have a specific affinity for chemicals present in the microbial cells but absent from human tissues. When injected just once into the infected patient, such a drug would seek out the bacterial invaders and kill them all without harming their host.

In pursuit of his goal of a "Therapia Sterilisans Magna"—a single curative injection which would wipe out all the pathogens while doing no damage to the patient—Ehrlich synthesized hundreds of chemicals and tested them on laboratory animals infected with protozoal and other organisms. In order to compare the potential utility of the various compounds, he introduced the concept of a *chemotherapeutic index*. This is a figure derived by comparing the maximum dose of a drug that the animals could tolerate with the minimum dose needed to cure their infections. The wider the ratio between these two figures, the greater was the efficiency of the anti-infective drug.

In the course of his work, Ehrlich developed drugs with increasingly favorable chemotherapeutic indices, first against mouse trypanosomiasis and later for treating human syphilis. Thus, starting with arsenical compounds with a chemotherapeutic index of only 1—a figure indicating that the chemical was as toxic to the tissues of the animal as it was to the syphilis spirochete—he continued to synthesize organic arsenical molecules with higher indices. His 606th drug, arsphenamine, had the favorable index of 37 and was considered safe enough for use in human syphilitic patients.

Ehrlich never did find his Therapia Sterilisans Magna (or "magic bullet"—as the movies later romanticized it), but his work laid the foundation for later signal successes in the fight against infection. During the decades that followed his death, other scientists employed his concepts and methods to develop chemotherapeutic agents that proved effective against various pathogenic protozoal and spirochetal organisms. Thus, drugs were introduced for treating malaria, amebiasis and various tropical diseases caused by protozoa, as well as syphilis.

For a quarter of a century after Ehrlich's death there were, however, no comparable successes in the treatment of *bacterial* infections. During those years doctors depended upon biologicals—vaccines, to confer active immunity, and antitoxins, to help to tide patients over certain acute infections. These were, however, applicable only to a minority of severe infections and patients continued to die of many common bacterial diseases. Then, in the 1930's, the first *sulfonamide* drug was introduced for treating systemic infections by staphylococci, streptococci, pneumococci, meningococci and other pathogenic bacteria. The success of *sulfanilamide* and its successors (Chap. 35) in curing these and other bacterial infections led scientists to study the antibacterial effectiveness of other new chemical families, including the nitrofurans and others (see also Chap. 35).

Other scientists were stimulated to study crude extracts of the metabolic products secreted by soil microorganisms. Starting with the successful reinvestigation of the antibiotic properties of Penicillium mold culture filtrates (penicillin) by a group of Oxford scientists in the late 1930's (Chap. 34), such studies led to the discovery of dozens of new antibacterial substances of natural origin. Waksman and his group at Rutgers, for example, working in a well-planned way on soil organisms of the Actinomycetes class, discovered streptomycin, neomycin and many other natural antibiotics.

In the course of the development of these anti-infective drugs, various problems arose which had to be dealt with both by the laboratory scientists of various disciplines and by the doctors who put these agents to clinical use. For example, some organisms that were originally quite sensitive to the first antibiotic and chemotherapeutic agents later acquired the ability to withstand these anti-infective agents. On the other hand, microorganisms that never had been susceptible to the early antibiotic agents now sometimes tended to run rampant when released from the inhibitory control of their natural enemies when the latter were eliminated by antibiotic therapy. In addition, doctors had to learn to use these drugs discriminately and with proper respect for their capacity to harm the patient. In general, however, most of these problems have been handled successfully, and today's agents for treating infection can, indeed, be considered among the major "miracle drugs" of modern medicine.

Concepts and Terms. Before studying the various groups of anti-infective agents, we need to have some understanding of the concepts of chemotherapy and antibiotic treatment which have evolved in recent years.

ANTIMICROBIAL SPECTRUM. The presently available anti-infective drugs vary in their degree of effectiveness against different microorganisms. Some are so selective in their inhibitory effects on specialized metabolic processes that their effectiveness is limited to a relatively few microorganisms. Thus, the antifungal antibiotics are said to possess a *narrow spectrum* of activity. At the other extreme are the *broad spectrum* antibiotics—agents that interfere with a biochemical reaction common to many microorganisms, including not only bacteria of the gram positive and gram negative types, but also *non*-bacterial microbes such as rickettsiae and even large viruses.

DEGREES OF ACTIVITY. Anti-infective agents vary considerably in their potency. Some are so active that they exert a *bactericidal* action against sensitive organisms when present in the environment in extremely low concentrations. *Penicillin*, for instance, kills actively multiplying streptococci when as little as 1 microgram of the antibiotic comes in contact with a couple of ounces of culture medium. Other substances are, at best, only *bacteriostatic*. That is, they merely inhibit the growth of previously multiplying microorganisms without actually killing them. However, provided that the patient's own defenses are operating efficiently, bacteriostatic drugs, such as the *tetracyclines* and others, can be very useful for helping the body cope successfully with the microbial invaders. Knowledge of the comparative sensitivity of the infecting pathogen to various agents is of considerable practical importance to the doctor. He often bases his selection of a therapeutic agent upon the results of laboratory tests that determine the degree of the organism's sensitivity to antibiotics and chemotherapeutic drugs of several different types.

MICROBIAL RESISTANCE. Some microorganisms are congenitally resistant to drug actions; other organisms acquire the ability to withstand drugs that once controlled them. Some organisms owe their resistance to their ability to release chemical substances that destroy the antibiotic. Many strains of staphylococci, for example, produce an enzyme that inactivates penicillin. Other organisms become resistant by developing new metabolic pathways for producing energy, so that they are unaffected by drugs that block a biochemical reaction no longer essential.

Acquired resistance, which has led to therapeutic failures, is, of course, a serious practical problem. For example, rapid development of resistance to *streptomycin* often reduces the utility of that antibiotic in the treatment of tuberculosis, and the *sulfonamides* are no longer as effective for treating gonorrhea as they once were. Scientists have done a great deal of work on how organisms become resistant, in order to learn how best to reduce the rate of emergence of resistant strains in the clinical circumstances in which these drugs are employed.

One widely held view is that the drugs themselves serve as a selective force for production of new and resistant microbial strains. That is, as the drugs tend to eliminate the bacteria that are sensitive to them, resistant mutants or variants, which were only a tiny minority of the bacterial population in the beginning, multiply and gradually become the dominant group. This happens because the handful of genetically different organisms have enzyme systems that also are different. As a result, they are unaffected from the start by the anti-infective chemicals that interfere with metabolism, growth, development and reproduction in most organisms of that variety. Another possibility is that the drugs themselves induce the enzymatic changes that make some strains resistant. Recent evidence indicates that resistance of this type may even be transmitted to unrelated organisms.

In either case, it is apparent that resistant strains are more likely to emerge when anti-infective drugs are used widely and unnecessarily for treating conditions in which they either are not needed or are actually ineffective. This is especially true when these drugs are used in less than adequate doses, for the more organisms left alive after inadequate treatment, the greater the likelihood that resistant strains will develop.

Authorities believe resistance can be reduced, first by limiting the use of antibiotics to the treatment of serious conditions caused by organisms known to be specifically sensitive to a given drug. Second, the effective drug should be given in large enough amounts and over a long enough period to eradicate the infection. The addition of antibiotics to animal feeds, or their use for preserving fish or for other commercial purposes are, on the other hand, examples of the misuse of these drugs which some authorities feel has helped to produce resistant bacterial strains.

Reactions to Antibiotics. One difficulty from the widespread indiscriminate use of antibiotics is that the drugs may induce dangerous changes in the patient's own bacterial flora. That is, by eliminating susceptible organisms in the patient's intestinal, respiratory, or genitourinary tract, the drug permits pathogens in these areas, which were previously kept under control by the natural antibiotic activity of their competitors, to grow rapidly and without restraint. As a result of the overgrowth of resistant staphylococci, yeasts and fungi, or strains of Proteus and Pseudomonas, the patient may suffer a *superinfection* more serious by far than the infection that the drug was intended to treat.

Another troublesome result of the too-casual use of anti-infective drugs has been a gerat increase in the number of people who have become *hypersensitive* to them. This means, in practice, that many patients who require antibiotic or sulfonamide therapy cannot be treated with these drugs because of the danger that they may suffer a severe allergic reaction, as a result of prior administration.

Other adverse reactions can result from a drug's *direct toxicity*. Various anti-infective agents can cause kidney or liver damage, deafness, or blood dyscrasias. Thus, although most antibiotic and chemotherapeutic agents are reasonably safe when taken under medical supervision, self-medication may cause a drug-induced illness that may not be detected until too late.

The points made above about how *bacteria* become *resistant* to anti-infective agents and how people become *sensitized* to these drugs are of considerable practical importance from the viewpoint of both personal health and public health. The nurse who understands the significance of these phenomena will be able to explain to people why they should not treat themselves with antibiotics for trivial infections that they may have acquired in one way or another—that is,

1. Such misuse may lead to the unsuspected development of strains of organisms in the community which are not controllable by presently effective drugs. Resistance that microbes acquire against presently effective anti-infective drugs can be disastrous to the person who becomes infected by an organism that was formerly susceptible and no longer responds to treatment.

2. Similarly, when a person takes a drug that he

does not truly need and develops hypersensitivity to it, he may later be unable to tolerate the drug when he needs it to help fight a really severe infection that could have been readily overcome by the antibiotic to which he has become allergic.

Still another difficulty that followed the advent of potent anti-infective agents was a relaxation of concern with strict adherence to the traditional procedures that had been developed for minimizing the spread of infection in hospitals and elsewhere. For a time some doctors and nurses seemed to feel that, since infections could now be readily cured by drug therapy, the danger was not as great as it had formerly been, and so, it was permissible to cut corners in various ways. Fortunately, there appears recently to be a return of emphasis on the need for complete cleanliness and for strict adherence to aseptic technique.

Also, it has become quite clear that these drugs should not be used routinely for prophylaxis of infection, and that, when their use is indicated for prevention, they should be employed only judiciously and in a carefully individualized manner. Thus, it is now known that the routine administration of antibiotics following surgical incisions actually increases rather than reduces the chance of postoperative infection. Similarly, the routine use of these drugs in obstetrics and for prevention of secondary bacterial invasion during respiratory viral infections is considered undesirable. There are some specific situations in which the prophylactic use of anti-infective drugs appears warranted; however, the administration of these agents to prevent infection by any pathogens that may be lurking about the patient's environment is never a substitute for safer physical measures for controlling the growth and transmission of microorganisms.

REVIEW QUESTIONS

1. How do antibiotics and anti-infective chemotherapeutic agents differ from one another?

2. How does the concept of a chemotherapeutic index help to determine the relative usefulness of new anti-infective drugs?

3. What kinds of pathogenic organisms were the first to be controlled by systemically active chemotherapeutic agents?

4. What was the first effective antibacterial chemotherapeutic agent? The first clinically useful antibiotic?

5. What is meant when we speak of a drug's antimicrobial spectrum?

6. What is the difference between bacteriostatic and bactericidal activity?

7. What properties of some microorganisms may make them resistant to the actions of anti-infective drugs?

8. What is one way in which anti-infective drugs may help to bring forth bacterial strains that have acquired the ability to resist drug treatment?

9. What is meant by a superinfection and how may it be brought about by antibiotic treatment?

10. What are two kinds of toxicity that may develop during treatment with anti-infective drugs?

11. What two reasons for not using anti-infective drugs can the nurse give to people who may be misusing these agents?

12. What should be the nurse's attitude toward the control of microbial colonization and transmission in this era of potent anti-infective drugs?

BIBLIOGRAPHY

Bryson, V., and Demerec, M.: Bacterial resistance. Am. J. Med., *18:*723, 1955.

Feingold, D. S.: Antimicrobial chemotherapeutic agents: the nature of their action and selective toxicity. New Eng. J. Med., *206:*900, 957, 1963.

Finland, M.: The new antibiotic era: for better or worse? Antibiotic Med. Clin. Ther., *4:*17, 1957.

Hall, J. W.: Drug therapy in infectious diseases. Am. J. Nursing, *61:*56, 1961.

Jager, B. V.: Untoward reactions to antibiotics. Am. J. Nursing, *54:*966, 1954.

Rodman, M. J.: The status of the antibiotics. R.N., *23:*51, 1960 (Aug.); *23:*51, 1960 (Sept.).

Spink, W. W.: Clinical problems related to the management of infections with antibiotics. J.A.M.A., *152:*585, 1953.

Weinstein, L.: Superinfection, a complication of antimicrobial therapy and prophylaxis. Am. J. Surg., *107:*704, 1964.

Antibiotic Drugs

PENICILLIN

Penicillin, the first of the antibiotics to come into common clinical use, is still considered one of the most important of all available anti-infective agents. Although its spectrum of antibacterial activity is narrow compared to that of some other antibiotics, penicillin is effective against the organisms that cause the most common bacterial infections. Combined with its killing power against these bacteria is a remarkable lack of direct toxicity to the tissues of the patient who is being treated with penicillin.

Manner of Action. This *selective toxicity* seems to be the result of the affinity of penicillin for a biochemical substance required by bacteria but not needed by human cells. Apparently, the presence of penicillin keeps bacteria from picking up and incorporating a component of their cell walls. Deprived of this substance, the bacteria are unable to biosynthesize the outer coat which protects them from osmotic forces in their environment. As a result, the rapidly growing cells swell, become abnormally enlarged, and take on oddly distorted shapes. With further accumulation of fluid, these grossly expanded and misshaped cells finally burst or dissolve. Human cells, on the other hand, are not hurt by penicillin. Because they do not possess cell walls, they are not injured by the penicillin-induced blockade of the vital biochemical substance that bacteria need for synthesis of parts of these outer coats.

Disadvantages. Although penicillin remains superior to other antibiotics in overall clinical value, it falls short of being the ideal antibiotic in several respects. For one thing, penicillin possesses an unfortunate tendency to induce sensitization in a sizable percentage of patients exposed to it. As a result allergic reactions of varying degrees of severity are fairly common.

In addition, certain strains of staphylococci and other bacteria have acquired resistance to natural penicillin. Other microorganisms are, of course, congenitally resistant to this narrow-spectrum antibiotic. Other difficulties encountered in the clinical use of the first natural penicillin products stemmed from the instability of these products in the gastrointestinal tract and the relatively rapid rate at which penicillin is eliminated by the kidneys.

Fortunately, however, research scientists have had considerable success in coping with the various problems that tended to limit the usefulness of this very valuable antibiotic. The continued clinical utility of penicillin is the result of research that has led to the development of new pharmaceutical and chemical forms of penicillin that are relatively free of some of the drawbacks of the first penicillin G products. Penicillins are now available, for example, that are stable in gastric acid, long-lasting in their antibacterial activity, and effective against bacteria that had acquired resistance to penicillin G.

History and Sources of Penicillin. The antibacterial activity of biosynthetic products obtained from certain strains of Penicillium molds was first noted by Sir Alexander Fleming in 1928. Although he tried to use filtrates from these fungi for treating infected wounds, these first penicillin broths proved too weak to affect the pathogens. Fleming's discovery remained a laboratory curiosity until 1939, when a group working at Oxford under the direction of Florey succeeded in making crude but potent extracts from broth cultures of *Penicillium notatum*.

The potential importance of this material, which proved potent but non-toxic in infected experimental animals, was quickly appreciated. In 1940, efforts to prepare penicillin in clinically usable quantities were intensified because of the obvious value of such a systemically safe and effective anti-infective agent for treating the wounded of World War II. By 1943, as the result of government-supported research in the United States, penicillin was being employed for treating infections in American military personnel.

The development of deep-fermentation procedures led to the production of penicillin in enormous quantities, with a consequent drop in its cost. Various types of natural penicillin, all containing the same nucleus but with different side chains, were prepared. Penicillin G, or benzylpenicillin, is the cheapest and most widely used of these. Penicillin V (p. 457), which contains a phenoxymethyl group in place of the benzyl radical, is a specially prepared product of fermentation, as is penicillin O or allylmercaptomethyl penicillin. Penicillins V and O are still used clinically, but other natural penicillins such as X, F, and K are no longer used at all in this country.

Many pharmaceutical forms of these natural penicillins and their salts have been prepared in attempts to alter the metabolism of the antibiotic in the human body. *Benzathine* penicillin G and *procaine* penicillin G suspensions, for example, are preparations of poorly soluble penicillin salts designed to prolong the duration of penicillin's action. In addition, many *chemical* modifications of natural penicillin have been made in further efforts to alter its properties in ways that would enhance the clinical utility of this antibiotic.

Such new chemical congeners are called *semisynthetic* penicillins, because their basic nucleus is obtained by fermentation processes but the chemical groupings that account for their more favorable properties are attached to this natural core by chemical synthesis. Over a thousand of these compounds have been made, mainly by isolating the 6-aminopenicillanic acid portion of the molecule from the medium in which natural fermentation is taking place and then adding all sorts of chemical groupings to this basic intermediate.

Only a handful of these semisynthetic penicillins have come into clinical use (Table 34-1), and none

TABLE 34-1
PENICILLIN PREPARATIONS

Nonproprietary or Official Name	Trade Name or Synonym	Dosage and Administration
Natural Penicillin Derivatives		
Benzathine penicillin G U.S.P.	Bicillin, etc.	500,000 u. orally, or 600,000 u. I.M., at various intervals.
Potassium penicillin G U.S.P.	Pentids, etc.	400,000 u. orally or I.M. q. 6 hours, or I.V. 10 million u. daily.
Potassium phenoxymethyl penicillin U.S.P.	Penicillin V; Pen-Vee K; V-Cillin K, etc.	250 mg. (400,000 u.) q. 6 hours.
Phenoxymethyl penicillin N.F.	Pen-Vee; V-Cillin	125 mg. (200,000 u.) q.i.d.
Procaine penicillin G U.S.P.	Duracillin, etc.	I.M. 300,000 u. q. 12 to 24 hours.
Sodium penicillin G N.F.		400,000 u. orally or I.M. q.i.d. I.V. 10 million units daily.
Sodium penicillin O	Cer-O-Cillin Sodium	300,000 to 600,000 u. I.M., or I.V. daily in divided doses.
Semisynthetic Penicillins		
Ampicillin	Omnipen; Penbritin; Polycillin	250 to 500 mg. orally q. 6 hours.
Cloxacillin sodium monohydrate	Tegopen	500 to 1,000 mg. orally q. 4–6 hrs.
Sodium methicillin U.S.P.	Dimocillin RT; Staphcillin	1 to 1.5 Gm. I.M. q. 4 to 6 hrs.
Nafcillin sodium	Unipen	250 to 1,000 mg. orally q. 4 to 6 hrs.
Oxacillin sodium U.S.P.	Prostaphlin; Resistopen	500 mg. q. 4 to 6 hrs. for 5 or more days.
Phenethicillin potassium N.F.	Phenoxyethyl penicillin; Chemipen; Maxipen; Rocillin; Syncillin, etc.	125 or 250 mg. t.i.d.

of these has replaced penicillin G as the most widely useful form of this antibiotic. However, each of the available derivatives has properties that make it the preferred form of penicillin in certain specific situations (see the following section). Scientists hope to develop synthetic derivatives that will be free of the remaining shortcomings of all the presently available penicillins.

Antimicrobial Spectrum and Therapeutic Uses

The natural penicillins possess a relatively narrow spectrum of antimicrobial activity compared to the tetracyclines and certain other antibiotics. Although the synthetic penicillins—and especially ampicillin—differ somewhat in range and degree of activity, such differences are not great. Thus we shall do well to examine in detail the activity of penicillin G, the prototype of these antibiotics, and then briefly note the similarities and differences in the antimicrobial activity of its semisynthetic relatives.

Penicillin G

Penicillin G (see Drug Digest) is generally effective against most *gram-positive* * cocci and ineffective against most gram-*negative bacilli.* Among the sensitive gram-positive pathogens are those responsible for the most common infections that afflict man. These include the beta hemolytic streptococcus—*Streptococcus pyogenes* (group A)—the cause of the vast majority of cases of bacterial pharyngitis and its frequent follower rheumatic fever. Since this organism is killed by low concentrations of penicillin, penicillin G, certain salts of penicillin G are often administered indefinitely in doses that keep low but effective levels of the antibiotic in the tissues of patients susceptible to rheumatic fever. Such penicillin prophylaxis is credited with having reduced recurrent attacks of rheumatic fever and the incidence of complications from residual cardiac damage. The present practice of promptly administering penicillin to patients with streptococcal pharyngitis also accounts for the relative rarity today of once-common complications such as otitis media, mastoiditis, scarlet fever and streptococcal pneumonia.

The *pneumococcus* remains highly sensitive to penicillin G, which is highly effective both against pneumococcal pneumonia and in the once almost 100-percent fatal meningitis caused by this organism. *Meningococcal* meningitis also usually responds to treatment with penicillin, which, in such cases, is best combined with a sulfonamide such as sulfadiazine (Chap. 35).

The *gonococcus* is less sensitive to penicillin than it

* Bacteria may be broadly differentiated on the basis of their response to treatment with a series of chemical solutions including gentian violet. "Gram-positive" bacteria stain deep violet when treated in the manner described by the Danish bacteriologist Hans Gram. Bacteria that take on a contrasting stain after decolorization are called gram negative.

once was, but adequately high single doses still cure most cases of acute gonococcal urethritis. More prolonged treatment clears up once-common crippling complications such as gonorrheal arthritis and endocarditis. The other major venereal disease, *syphilis*, yields readily to penicillin therapy. The causative spirochete, *Treponema pallidum,* is very sensitive to the antibiotic. Adequate doses of procaine penicillin G, injected intramuscularly within 24 hours of exposure, will protect against syphilis infections. Much smaller amounts of oral penicillin are said to serve as prophylaxis against gonorrhea.

Staphylococcus aureus (*Micrococcus pyogenes* var. *aureus*), the organism most commonly involved in skin and soft tissue infections, was once readily susceptible to treatment with penicillin G. Today, fewer than 5 to 10 per cent of patients who acquire a staph infection in a hospital respond to therapy with natural penicillins. This serious problem is the result of the emergence of resistant strains of staphylococci (see Chap. 33).

These organisms are able to withstand the action of the antibiotic because they have the ability to secrete *penicillinase,* an enzyme that destroys the penicillin molecule by breaking open the chemical ring structure that is essential for its antibacterial activity. The enzyme catalyzes the hydrolytic cleavage of the betalactam ring of penicillin, thus forming inactive penicilloic acid.

Physicians are often faced with the need to treat serious infections caused by resistant staph organisms. Staphylococcal pneumonia, bacteremia and endocarditis—infections with a high mortality rate—have actually increased in incidence after an initial dramatic drop in deaths when penicillin G was first introduced. Failure of a lung infection (for example) to respond to penicillin G may prove fatal, since staphylococci can cause the rapid development of focal abscesses followed by widespread necrosis of pulmonary tissues.

For a time, in the 1950's, this created a very serious situation. Although penicillin G is the preferred antibiotic for pneumonias caused by *susceptible* staphylococci, doctors turned to the tetracyclines and chloramphenicol, to which fewer strains had become resistant. However, results were not as good as they had been with penicillin G, because these antibiotics, although broader in spectrum, are only bacterio*static* and, consequently, not as effective as bacteri*cidal* penicillin in patients whose own natural defenses are low. Two other bactericidal antibiotics, *ristocetin* (Spontin) and *vancomycin* (see Drug Digest), also came into use for treating resistant staphylococcal infections of a serious nature. However, these useful antibiotics are themselves often toxic.

Synthetic Penicillinase-Resistant Penicillins

Fortunately, among the new semisynthetic penicillins introduced in the early 1960's are several which can resist enzymatic cleavage of their molecules by bacterial penicillinase. Although these new synthetic penicillins are not as active as the natural penicillins against most other pathogens, including streptococci, pneumococci and *non*-penicillinase-producing staphylococci, they are often remarkably effective against infections that resist treatment by penicillins G, V, O, and others.

Methicillin (see Drug Digest) is the antibiotic with which most physicians now prefer to initiate treatment of a severe staph infection suspected to be resistant to penicillin G. This drug is administered parenterally, either alone or combined with penicillin G. If laboratory tests prove that the organism is actually sensitive to penicillin G, methicillin is withdrawn and treatment is continued with high parenteral doses of penicillin G alone. On the other hand, if the organism turns out to be, indeed, resistant to penicillin G and responsive to methicillin, injections of the latter are continued every 4 to 6 hours until the infection is brought under control. Many cases of staphylococcal bacteremia, endocarditis and pneumonia require prolonged treatment with methicillin even after their symptoms subside.

Repeated intramuscular injections of methicillin may be painful and may produce sterile abscesses, and intravenous injections are sometimes followed by phlebitis. Thus physicians sometimes prefer to substitute an orally effective penicillin for the parenteral preparation. Several semisynthetic penicillins that resist both bacterial penicillinase and gastric acid are now available for this purpose. One of these, *cloxacillin* (Tegopen) is administered only by mouth in capsule and solution form. Two others, sodium *nafcillin* (Unipen) and sodium *oxacillin* (see Drug Digest), may be given orally or parenterally.

All of these drugs appear to be about equally effective against resistant staph infections in the doses recommended for routine clinical employment. The parenteral preparations are used to start treatment of severe infections. However, the oral forms may be ordered, not only after the severe phase has been controlled but also to initiate treatment of mild to moderate infections of the skin, soft tissues or respiratory tract. When taken by mouth, these drugs are best absorbed from an empty stomach and, consequently, are administered an hour or two before meals.

Among the bacteria that have always been considered relatively insensitive to penicillin are gram-negative organisms such as *E. coli* and *Salmonella, Shigella* and *Proteus* species. However, penicillin products have recently been employed with occasional success in the treatment of infections resistant to treatment by the antibiotics which are more commonly employed against these gram-negative bacilli. Very large doses of penicillin G (for example)—up to 60 million units a day—have recently been employed for this purpose.

Ampicillin (Omnipen; Penbritin; Polycillin), a synthetic penicillin, is more effective than all other penicillins against such gram-negative organisms. Taken by mouth, this drug has sometimes helped to clear up stubborn urinary tract infections caused by strains of *Proteus mirabilis, E. coli,* and others, which had resisted treatment with tetracycline, chloromycetin and streptomycin. Similarly, ampicillin has occasionally proved effective in respiratory infections caused by *Hemophilus influenzae,* an organism usually resistant to penicillin. This drug has occasionally helped patients with enteritis of bacillary origin.

Ampicillin is not effective against all strains of these gram-negative organisms. Its use is preferred mainly when laboratory tests on bacterial cultures taken from the infected patient show the particular strain to be more sensitive to ampicillin than to the standard drugs ordinarily used against such gram-negative bacilli (Table 34-6). Also, the relative safety of this form of penicillin may sometimes make it preferable to tetracyclines, chloramphenicol, streptomycin, etc., for a particular patient.

Ampicillin, despite its uniquely broader spectrum of antibacterial activity, is not effective against resistant staphylococci. It is *not* a substitute for penicillin G against most gram-positive organisms. It may be preferred in certain mixed infections in which it may strike both gram-negative and gram-positive organisms, whereas penicillin G would be ineffective against the gram-negative invader and thus administration in combination with streptomycin would be required.

Penicillin Metabolism and Administration

Scientists have long been concerned with the development of penicillin preparations which would make possible the most efficient use of this valuable antibiotic. To accomplish this, they have carefully studied how the body handles penicillin. From what they have learned of how this antibiotic, as administered by various routes, is absorbed, distributed to different tissues and finally eliminated, they have been able to devise products suited for use in various clinical situations. The doctor picks the type penicillin that seems most effective against the infecting organism and then has to determine the best way to administer it for full effectiveness.

Ordinarily, penicillin is administered parenterally in serious infections or the management of patients who would probably fail to follow instructions concerning its oral use. Penicillin is taken by mouth only after the patient's infection has been brought under control, or when it is not a severe infection to begin with but one mild enough to respond to the relatively low tissue levels attained by the oral route. Oral administration is often preferred during long-term prophylaxis intended to reduce the risk of recurrent streptococcal infections and possible endocarditis, although repository injections (see p. 458) are often used for this purpose.

No matter how it is administered, penicillin must reach a level in the blood and tissues which will inhibit the pathogenic bacteria. This level varies considerably, depending upon the sensitivity of the organism to penicillin and the nature of the infection. A blood level of less than 0.1 unit (0.06 *micro*gram) per milliliter is enough to control certain penicillin-sensitive bacteria. This low level can often be attained with relatively low oral doses or sustained for long periods with repository preparations which permit absorption of small amounts of penicillin into the blood throughout each day.

Some authorities claim that it may not even be necessary to maintain minimal antibacterial levels of penicillin around the clock, as is required with the *sulfonamides* (Chap. 35). They suggest that if penicillin is kept at bactericidal levels for even only a few hours during several periods of the day, it is often able to kill off each new burst of growth in the bacterial population and, in this way, produce both bacteriological and clinical cure.

Nonetheless, control of serious infections by less susceptible organisms may require blood and tissue levels very much higher than those mentioned above. These can be reached and sustained only by the administration of massive doses of penicillin at frequent intervals. For example, in subacute bacterial endocarditis, doses of 100 million units or more of penicillin may be needed every day.

Obviously, the nurse sees to it that all patients for whom penicillin orders have been left receive the antibiotic on time and that no doses are omitted. Since it may be necessary to wake the patient, it is best to take the opportunity to carry out a number of routine tasks at the same time. That is, the patient's temperature, pulse, and respiration may be taken and other aspects of patient care such as giving fluids, etc., can be attended to at that time. It helps, too, to let the patient know why it is necessary to disturb his sleep.

Oral Absorption of Penicillin

With penicillin, as with other drugs, the most convenient and least expensive way to introduce it into the body in therapeutic amounts is by the oral route. An additional advantage of giving penicillin by mouth is that allergic reactions are least likely when the drug is administered by this route. However, because oral administration is at best rather unreliable, parenteral penicillin therapy is preferred for severe infections in which the doctor wants to be absolutely certain of attaining adequate blood and tissue levels.

Most of any orally administered dose of penicillin G never gets into the blood stream. Much of it is destroyed by acid gastric juice or carried down into the large intestine on undigested food particles. There the unabsorbed penicillin is inactivated by penicillinase-producing bacteria.

Despite these difficulties, oral administration of penicillin G is entirely practical today because of the relative inexpensiveness of the antibiotic. The drug is simply administered in several times the dose that would be needed to attain a similar blood level by injection—a procedure that may seem rather wasteful. However, it permits enough penicillin to be absorbed from the duodenum to attain tissue levels adequate for control of most infections caused by penicillin-sensitive pathogens.

Some products contain antacid buffers which are claimed to help retard destruction of penicillin G by gastric acid and thus to favor the absorption of a larger proportion of the ingested penicillin. However, such antacid adjuvants play a smaller part in aiding absorption of penicillin than does following a simple rule for administering the antibiotic: Take penicillin G products between meals, preferably 1 or 2 hours before the next meal or 2 or 3 hours after the last one.

This seems to be true even of new semisynthetic penicillins such as oxacillin, cloxacillin and nafcillin. For, even though these substances are said to resist destruction by stomach acids as well as by intestinal and tissue penicillinase, they are absorbed from an empty stomach more rapidly and completely than in the presence of retarding food particles. It has been claimed, however, that the other acid-stable penicillins, phenoxymethyl penicillin (penicillin V, etc.) and phenoxyethyl penicillin (phenethicillin; Syncillin, etc.) are actually *better* absorbed when taken with a meal than on an empty stomach.

In view of these differences, it may be best for the nurse, when in doubt, to check with the physician to find out when he wants the medication administered (e.g., after meals, or with them) so as to yield the highest blood levels and best results for his patient.

Parenteral Absorption

The absorption of *aqueous* solutions of penicillin that are injected *intramuscularly* is very rapid. The antibiotic reaches very high blood levels in less than half an hour. However, such peaks cannot be maintained, because, once it gets into the blood stream, penicillin is very rapidly removed, through renal excretion (see p. 458). Thus, when a very severe infection makes it necessary to sustain high penicillin levels for long periods, the antibiotic is best given by the continuous intravenous infusion of massive amounts in an aqueous solution to avoid the need for repeated, painful intramuscular injections of the soluble potassium or sodium salts of penicillin.

Much more commonly, however, sustained therapeutic concentrations are achieved in less severe infections by the intramuscular injection of *repository forms* of penicillin. These are preparations containing poorly soluble salts of penicillin, which are sometimes suspended or dissolved in special vehicles that further retard absorption of the antibiotic from the muscle tissue that is the depot site of injection. The penicillin G is then released so slowly that only small amounts of the antibiotic appear in the blood stream at any one time, but these barely therapeutic levels last for relatively long periods.

The most long-lasting of these repository preparations is *benzathine penicillin G* (see Drug Digest). Injected intramuscularly, a single injection of a suspension of this salt is said to offer protection for about one month against streptococcal infections, although twice monthly injections of half that dose are more commonly employed in prophylaxis against recurrences of streptococcal infections in patients with a history of rheumatic fever.

The nurse should make it clear to the patient receiving repository penicillin, or to his family, that he must return on schedule for each injection. The importance of not missing a visit must be emphasized, and the patient should be made to realize the seriousness of letting his protection against infection lapse. Then, if the patient should find it impossible to come on the day of the scheduled visit, he may remember the nurse's warning and call for an alternate appointment instead of skipping the monthly or bimonthly dose of penicillin entirely.

Procaine penicillin G is a salt that is slowly absorbed but its duration of action is not as long as that of benzathine penicillin G. However, an injection of this repository form gives somewhat higher blood levels, which are effective against a greater number of organisms and for more serious infections. It is used, for example, in treating neurosyphilis in a course of treatment requiring moderately high blood levels for 2 or 3 weeks. Administration of single daily doses of 600,000 units of procaine penicillin G in aqueous suspension intramuscularly on each day of the course spares the patient the pain of the several daily injections, which would be required if an aqueous injection of penicillin G itself were employed. This suspension of procaine penicillin G is also preferred for prophylaxis against infection in patients with a history of heart disease who have a tonsillectomy, dental extraction or other surgery. This salt is also available as an oily suspension with aluminum monostearate. When this longer-lasting form is used, only 2 or 3 injections a week are needed.

Excretion of Penicillin

The kidneys clear penicillin from the plasma with amazing efficiency. They not only filter part of it from the blood by way of the glomeruli but also act through tubular secretion. That is, most of the penicillin mole-

cules that escape filtration in passing through the kidneys are promptly secreted into the urine-forming filtrate by the cells lining the renal tubules. This procedure—which would be very useful if penicillin were a poison—posed a difficult problem for doctors trying to keep the drug at effective levels in the days when penicillin was in very short supply. Sometimes, the scientists even tried to recover penicillin from the patient's own urine for re-use!

Later, they worked at developing drugs which would delay the rapid renal excretion of penicillin when administered together with the antibiotic. Among the drugs that do this is *probenecid* (Chap. 41). Its molecules compete with those of penicillin for the tubular transport system that transfers the antibiotic from the blood to the tubular fluid. To the extent that the probenecid molecules occupy this mechanism, the penicillin molecules are blocked from these sites of excretory activity. As a result, the penicillin remains in the blood and tissues at higher levels for longer periods. This kind of combined probenecid-penicillin therapy has sometimes proved useful for potentiating the activity of penicillin in treating patients with subacute bacterial endocarditis or others who require long exposure to large amounts of penicillin. However, the same effect is much more commonly achieved with the repository forms of penicillin discussed earlier, which delay the excretion of the antibiotic by slowing its absorption.

Distribution of Penicillin

Once penicillin is absorbed into the blood stream, it is combined with plasma proteins and carried all over the body. However, passage of penicillin into the fluids bathing different body tissues varies very considerably. Thus, infections of the skin and soft tissues are responsive to systemically administered penicillin, which readily reaches these tissues. (Surgical drainage is, of course, also necessary in many cases.) On the other hand, penicillin penetrates only poorly into the aqueous fluids of the eye. Thus, the antibiotic may have to be injected directly under the conjunctiva to get at a penicillin-susceptible intraocular infection.

Although penicillin is sometimes administered by inhalation as an aerosol mist or dust, this is seldom necessary, since the drug ordinarily penetrates into pulmonary tissues in adequate amounts. Such contact with mucosal surfaces may even sensitize the patient or set off allergic reactions more readily than when the drug is administered systemically. This is also true of topical application of penicillin to the skin. Because of the increased likelihood of sensitization, penicillin is rarely applied directly to skin infections, and less sensitizing antibiotics such as *bacitracin, neomycin, polymyxin,* etc., are preferred for such purposes.

Penicillin does not enter the fluids of the brain and spinal cord readily. Even when massive doses are administered, only a small fraction of the antibiotic ordinarily crosses the blood-brain barrier and the meningeal membranes. Fortunately for patients with meningitis caused by penicillin-susceptible pathogens, the inflamed membranes become more permeable to penicillin, so that enough of the antibiotic enters the subarachnoid space to exert its antibacterial effect. Sometimes, however, massive intravenous doses must be supplemented by *intrathecal* injections to produce adequate antibacterial levels of the antibiotic in the spinal fluid.

The Adverse Effects of Penicillin

Penicillin is a drug of remarkably low direct toxicity. Even massive doses fail to elicit any pharmacological effects, except for some occasional local irritation. In fact, when potassium penicillin G is administered in very large daily doses, there may be more danger from its potassium content than from the penicillin part of the molecule. That is, if the patient is suffering from renal insufficiency, which interferes with potassium elimination, the retained ion may cause hyperkalemia and its ill-effects, though the penicillin which accumulates in his tissues is harmless. This lack of activity on human cells is probably related to the way in which penicillin exerts its antibacterial effect upon rapidly growing microbes (p. 453).

Despite this lack of direct toxicity, penicillin is capable of causing adverse reactions. These are of three types: (1) irritative responses, (2) superinfections by *non*susceptible microbes, and (3) allergic reactions.

Irritative Reactions. Minor manifestations of tissue irritation by concentrated penicillin solutions include pain and discomfort occasionally caused by injections. In muscles this irritation may lead to sterile abscesses, and in veins to phlebitis. More serious is the effect of concentrated penicillin upon nervous tissue when injected intrathecally. The irritation caused by excessively concentrated solutions has sometimes set off convulsive spasms. Thus, when employed for treating meningitis, as mentioned previously, penicillin is injected into the subarachnoid space only in small amounts and well diluted. A concentration of only 1,000 to 2,000 units per ml. and a total of only 20 to 30 ml. is the most that can be safely injected in such cases.

Superinfections. Prolonged penicillin therapy may alter the microbial flora of various parts of the body and thus favor the emergence of fungi and gram-negative pathogens. Such superinfections are less likely to occur with penicillin G, with its narrow spectrum of antibacterial activity, than with the tetracyclines or chloramphenicol. However, monilial infestations, resistant staph overgrowth, and an oral condition called blacktongue have occasionally been reported. It is likely that the incidence of such superinfections may increase with the use of ampicillin, the so-called broad-spectrum penicillin.

Hypersensitivity Reactions. Penicillin does not cause bone marrow depression, though such blood dyscrasias have occasionally been reported recently following the administration of *methicillin*. Very much more common is the occurrence of a variety of reactions of the histamine-release type (Chap. 40).

Allergic reactions to penicillin occur in probably 1 per cent of patients receiving this antibiotic. Although most symptoms are mild and transient, deaths from fatal anaphylaxis are not infrequently reported. The more severe reactions tend to follow intramuscular injections of salts such as procaine penicillin G. However, anaphylactic shock has also occurred in sensitized patients after taking a single penicillin tablet (e.g., for self-treatment of a cold).

Such indiscriminate use of penicillin for trivial infections—for which it is, in any case, ineffective—has made this antibiotic the major cause of drug hypersensitivity. An estimated 15 per cent of people in this country are sensitive to penicillin to some extent. Patients who have previously been exposed to penicillin and had some sort of reaction to it are the most likely candidates for severe reactions upon further exposure to the antibiotic. However, deaths from penicillin anaphylaxis have occurred without warning in people with no prior history of allergy to it.

Nonetheless, it is important to ask each patient if he has ever had a reaction to penicillin and whether he has a history of allergy to other substances. If the doctor is convinced that the patient has truly reacted badly to penicillin before, his best course of action is to order some other antibiotic with a spectrum similar to that of penicillin. Ordinarily, drugs such as erythromycin or triacetyloleandomycin will control most mild penicillin-sensitive infections, and cephalothin will prove effective in the more severe illnesses.

Allergy Tests. When penicillin is obviously the best antibiotic for a particular patient (a patient with subacute bacterial endocarditis, for example), the doctor may feel compelled to try it despite a history suggestive of hypersensitivity. In such cases, he will wish to rule out or confirm the presence of allergy by the use of some objective test. The screening method most commonly used at present is a skin test in which a small amount of penicillin is scratched into the cutaneous surface or introduced intradermally. The rapid development of a red flare and a hive locally is considered a positive indication of sensitivity to penicillin and a sign that the drug should be withheld.

Unfortunately, such skin tests have only limited usefulness. Many patients with negative responses to skin and conjunctival tests nevertheless suffer allergic reactions to injection of a full therapeutic dose of penicillin. A more serious difficulty is that the highly sensitive person who does develop a positive reaction may have one which is generalized rather than local. That is, intradermal injection of penicillin G for screening purposes has sometimes caused severe and even fatal reactions!

Recently, there has been considerable concern in regard to the development of safer and more reliable tests for penicillin sensitivity. One recently suggested test—the *basophil degranulation* procedure—is certainly safe, since it is carried out outside the patient's body. In this test, which can also be used to detect sensitivity to other substances, a drop of the patient's serum is mixed with a drop of penicillin solution in the presence of rabbit basophils. In a positive test, the basophils become degranulated (that is, they swell slowly or suddenly and give up their histamine-containing granules) in the presence of penicillin antigen and antibodies. Unfortunately, this test is difficult to control and has not been widely applied in clinical practice.

A skin test developed recently employs not penicillin but a synthetic penicillin antigen, *penicilloylpolylysine* (PPL). This is a hapten (Chap. 3) prepared by coupling the penicillin catabolite penicilloyl with a polymer of the amino acid lysine. It is said to produce a flare-and-wheal skin reaction in a high percentage of penicillin-allergic people without being itself sensitizing. Patients who develop a strongly positive reaction to PPL are considered much more likely than others to suffer a systemic reaction to administration of penicillin. The PPL test may prove valuable for screening out such patients; on the other hand, it is often positive for patients who are perfectly able to have a therapeutic dose of penicillin without harm. People with a negative reaction to PPL rarely are likely to have a reaction to penicillin; many who respond positively, however, may be unnecessarily deprived of this valuable antibiotic during an illness in which it would be more useful than any other anti-infective measure.

Management of Penicillin Allergy. Penicillin is capable of producing hypersensitivity reactions of all the varied types described in Chapter 3. The severity and number of these reactions can be reduced by use of the measures previously described. However, a few points especially pertinent to the prevention and treatment of reactions to penicillin may be noted here.

First, despite claims to the contrary, patients who are allergic to one type of penicillin are likely to be sensitive to *all* penicillin products. Thus, there is no real proof for the claim that penicillin O is "hypoallergenic." Similarly, patients allergic to penicillin G can be expected to show cross-sensitivity to the new semisynthetic penicillins. This does not mean that reactions will always occur. Patients who have reacted to penicillin G with mild to moderate skin symptoms sometimes take the same drug later without suffering any reaction at all. For example, some may take an oral synthetic penicillin such as phenethicillin, oxacil-

lin, etc. with impunity, despite a history of hives following penicillin G administration on a previous occasion.

Products are available containing penicillin in combination with an antihistaminic agent. The presence of chlorpheniramine, for example, may lessen the incidence of minor reactions such as skin rashes, pruritus, and urticaria, but it is not adequate for fending off anaphylactic reactions in patients highly sensitive to penicillin. Similarly, in the management of an actual reaction, such drugs as diphenhydramine and tripelennamine (Chap. 40) may be expected to control only minor reactions. In treating more severe reactions, the doctor gives relatively low priority to the parenteral employment of these and other antihistamines.

More severe penicillin reactions require treatment with epinephrine (Chap. 16), corticosteroids (Chap. 28) and supplemental oxygen inhalation. These measures are designed to raise blood pressure, dilate bronchioles and counteract the cerebral edema and anoxia which may lead to brain damage that might prove fatal or leave the patient with permanent motor or psychic disability.

A rather interesting, though not widely used, measure for the management of reactions to penicillin involves the use of a highly purified preparation of the enzyme *penicillinase* (Neutrapen). It will be recalled that this is the enzyme secreted by bacteria resistant to penicillin. Apparently, in catalyzing the hydrolysis of a key ring in the penicillin molecule, penicillinase not only inactivates the antibacterial activity of the antibiotic but also stops it from acting as an antigen.

Injected intramuscularly in a patient suffering an allergic reaction, penicillinase seeks out penicillin molecules and destroys them. This, of course, lessens the likelihood of reactions between the antibiotic and circulating penicillin antibodies. The resulting reduction in free histamine release tends to prevent skin rashes, urticaria, bronchial constriction and other symptoms by counteracting their cause.

Penicillinase alone is never used in place of the measures mentioned previously. It seems most useful for treating the delayed serum-sickness type reactions resulting from injection of the long-acting forms of penicillin—procaine penicillin G and benzathine penicillin G. In such cases, the best response is obtained when the purified enzyme is administered immediately after a reaction is seen to begin. Although the action of the enzyme is said to begin quickly and last for as long as four days, additional doses may be required to counteract the long-lasting antigenic action of benzathine penicillin.

Little is known about the usefulness of penicillinase for treating allergic reactions to the newer semisynthetic penicillins methicillin, cloxacillin, oxacillin, and nafcillin. In theory, however, this enzyme should be less useful in such cases, since these drugs are relatively resistant to destruction by bacterial penicillinase. It should also be noted that, since penicillinase is a protein, in theory it could itself act as an antigen. This has, indeed, happened occasionally during a course of treatment with the drug. Thus, the use of penicillinase in a person with demonstrated sensitivity is contraindicated, since the drug itself—administered to treat an allergic reaction to penicillin preparation—may cause a similar reaction.

The nurse plays a most important role, not only in detection of penicillin allergy in its earliest stages and in reduction of the severity of reactions but in regard to prevention also. For example, when the doctor takes a history before ordering penicillin, the patient sometimes neglects to tell him about a reaction to previous exposure. Yet, when the nurse appears with her syringe, he may suddenly say, "Oh, by the way, if that's penicillin, I'm allergic to it!" In such a situation, never proceed without consulting the doctor.

Similarly, should the nurse note a rash on the skin of a patient who has been given penicillin, she should withhold further dosage until she has checked with the doctor. Of course, such consultation should be carried out promptly, so that the patient is not deprived of the anti-infective medication that he requires.

The nurse always tries to teach people about the hazards of using medications left over from the treatment of a previous infection (especially medication prescribed for some other member of the family). In addition, she warns them of the importance of taking *all* the doses of the prescribed medication (people sometimes tend to stop after only three or four doses because they "feel better," which can result in a sudden hard-to-control flare-up of the infection).

THE TETRACYCLINES AND CHLORAMPHENICOL

The impact of the success of penicillin (and of streptomycin) upon the clinical control of serious infections sent scientists back to the soil in a search for other natural substances with antibiotic activity. A systematic screening of soil samples from all over the world turned up two especially useful substances—*chloramphenicol* and *chlortetracycline*—which were introduced in 1948. Despite the similarity of the prefix, these drugs are not related, chemically or otherwise. Chlortetracycline, however, is one of an important family of antibiotics that includes *oxytetracycline* and *tetracycline* among others which have since been discovered (see Table 34-2).

TABLE 34-2

Nonproprietary or Official Name	Trade Name or Synonym	Dosage and Administration
Tetracycline and Chloramphenicol Compounds		
Chloramphenicol U.S.P.	Chloromycetin	50 to 100 mg./Kg. oral or I.V.
Chloramphenicol palmitate U.S.P.	—	86 to 172 mg./Kg. oral
Chloramphenicol sodium succinate U.S.P.	—	70 to 140 mg./Kg. I.M., I.V., or S.C. q. 6 hrs.
Chlortetracycline HCl N.F.	Aureomycin	250 mg. q.i.d. oral or parenteral
Demethylchlortetracycline N.F.; Demeclocycline	Declomycin	150 mg. q.i.d. or 300 mg. b.i.d.
Doxycycline (hyclate and monohydrate)	Vibramycin	Oral 100 mg. q. 12 hrs. on 1st day; maintenance 100 mg. daily, either as single dose or 50 mg. q. 12 hrs.
Oxytetracycline N.F.	Terramycin	250 mg. q.i.d.
Oxytetracycline HCl N.F.	Terramycin	Oral 250 mg. q.i.d., I.V. 500 mg. daily
Rolitetracycline	Syntetrin; Velacycline	I.M. 150 mg. q. 8 hrs., I.V. 350 to 700 mg. q. 8 to 12 hrs.
Tetracycline U.S.P.	Achromycin; Panmycin; Polycycline; Steclin; Tetracyn	Oral 500 mg. q.i.d.
Tetracycline HCl U.S.P.		Oral 500 mg. q.i.d., I.V. 500 mg. b.i.d.
Methacycline	Rondomycin	Oral 600 mg. daily, either 150 mg. q.i.d. or 300 mg. b.i.d.

All these antibiotics have in common an unusually wide antimicrobial spectrum and a considerable degree of safety in most circumstances. As indicated in Table 34-6, the tetracyclines and chloramphenicol are effective against many organisms that resist other anti-infective agents, including the rickettsiae and the so-called large viruses. They are also often selected for treating infections by gram-negative bacilli unresponsive to penicillin. Although such infections respond to streptomycin and certain other antibiotics (Table 34-6), the doctor often prefers to employ a tetracycline because of its comparative safety. On the other hand, penicillin is still usually preferred to these broad-spectrum drugs for treating gram-positive coccal infections, syphilis and gonorrhea.

Therapeutic Uses of the Tetracyclines

All of the tetracyclines are essentially similar in their antimicrobial spectrum and therapeutic uses. They are thought to act by keeping susceptible microbes from synthesizing the protein that they require for growth and reproduction. As a result, these antibiotics exert a bacterio*static* effect that allows the body's own defenses to eliminate the *non*multiplying microbes. Because of this manner of action, it is important to continue treatment with these antibiotics well beyond the disappearance of symptoms, in order to prevent relapses caused by multiplication of unkilled bacteria. Penicillin and other bacteri*cidal* antibiotics are preferred for patients whose defenses against infection are too weak to control organisms whose growth has been only arrested.

Although the tetracyclines are certainly effective in the common respiratory tract infections such as tonsillitis, bronchitis, pneumonia and their complications (otitis media, sinusitis, etc.), these drugs are ordinarily the doctor's second or third choice after penicillin and even erythromycin. This is because relapses are not uncommon after treatment of streptococcal infections is stopped, and because of the emergence of many strains of staphylococci, and some pneumococci, that are resistant to tetracycline therapy. Long-term prophylaxis against recurrences of acute attacks has been employed in patients with chronic bronchitis. However, the continued use of these antibiotics favors the emergence of resistant microorganisms capable of causing dangerous superinfections (see p. 463).

The status of the tetracyclines in the treatment of the common venereal diseases is somewhat similar—that is, penicillin is always preferred for gonorrhea and syphilis, except when the patient is allergic to it. On the other hand, tetracycline is the antibiotic of choice in venereal infections such as lymphogranuloma venereum and granuloma inguinale and it is of value in chancroid.

The tetracyclines are often useful in the management of many *non*venereal infections of the genito-urinary tract. Certain of the gram-negative invaders of this system are still responsive to tetracyclines. Unfortunately, emergence of tetracycline-resistant bacilli such as strains of Proteus and *Pseudomonas aeruginosa* (see pp. 469, 474) has been increasing. For this reason, doctors now tend to order tetracyclines only when the organism proves sensitive to it in laboratory tests, rather than routinely as they once did. (See Chap. 35 for a further discussion of the place of these and other drugs in the management of urinary tract infections.)

The tetracyclines also have a place in the prophylaxis and treatment of *gastrointestinal tract* infections by organisms such as shigella, the cause of bacillary dysentery. Here too, however, the emergence of resistant strains of bacilli has lessened the value of the tetracyclines. Thus, for typhoid fever and other salmonella infections, chloramphenicol is now the drug usually preferred, and for prophylaxis prior to bowel surgery the sulfonamides or neomycin, etc. are employed more commonly than the tetracyclines.

On the other hand, there are certain infections in which the tetracyclines are almost uniquely valuable. *Rickettsial diseases* such as Rocky Mountain spotted fever and the dreaded typhus group often respond dramatically to such medication. Administered in large doses, these antibiotics quickly bring down the patient's high fever, after which continued use of smaller doses during recovery prevents relapses. Other ordinarily difficult-to-treat diseases that still respond very well to the tetracyclines administered alone or in combination with streptomycin include brucellosis, tularemia and relapsing fever.

The condition sometimes called "virus" pneumonia, or primary atypical pneumonia, often responds dramatically to tetracycline therapy, just as do pneumonias caused by a variety of organisms—e.g., the gram-positive pneumococci, strep, and staph, and the gram-negative agents *Klebsiella pneumoniae* (the cause of Friedlander's pneumonia), *Hemophilus influenzae*, and others. The patient's fever often quickly falls and his cough and pulmonary congestion gradually clear with continued tetracycline administration.

Other dangerous diseases responsive to the tetracyclines include psittacosis, or so-called parrot fever, and the blinding eye infection, trachoma. These conditions, like lymphogranuloma venereum, are caused by so-called large viruses, which are untouched by other antibiotics except for chloramphenicol. Like the agent that causes "virus" pneumonia (a PPLO, or pleuro-pneumonialike organism) these large viruses are *not* true viruses.

The last observation may seem exceedingly academic in view of the value of the tetracyclines against this group of agents so far out on the fringes of the microbial spectrum. However, it is important for us to remember that neither the tetracyclines nor any other antibiotics now available are active against the true viruses. Thus, tetracycline therapy is ineffective in measles, mumps, chickenpox, infectious mononucleosis, and the various viral respiratory diseases including influenza and the common cold.

In view of their lack of effectiveness against respiratory viruses, it is interesting to note how very many "cold" and "flu" products contain tetracyclines or some other antibiotic. The pharmaceutical company's rationale for combining an antibiotic with several antihistaminics, analgesics, decongestants, etc. is that the antibiotic will protect the patient against complicating *bacterial* infections. Such employment of antibiotics in products for the symptomatic treatment of trivial conditions, for which they are in any case useless, seems most unwise. It is the indiscriminate use of antibiotics in this manner that has helped produce (1) the large number of patients now allergic to antibiotics, and (2) the emergence of new strains of once-sensitive and now resistant microorganisms.

Adverse Effects of the Tetracyclines

The low incidence of adverse reactions to tetracyclines—less than 3 per cent, reportedly—has contributed to their popularity. However, patients must be carefully watched for signs of untoward effects that may make it necessary for the doctor to order withdrawal of the drug. For, in addition to minor side effects due to local irritation, the tetracyclines can cause (1) severe superinfections, (2) allergic reactions similar to those seen with penicillins, and (3) certain toxic reactions that are a result of the drugs' direct action on body tissues.

Side Effects. The early difficulty most commonly observed in patients taking tetracyclines by mouth is gastrointestinal upset. This is less common with the latest drugs of this class such as *demethylchlortetracycline*, which is taken in smaller amounts, than with the earlier agents such as *chlortetracycline*. It is sometimes suggested that the discomfort caused by gastrointestinal irritation can be lessened by giving the drug with some milk or a small amount of other food. However, it is best to check with the doctor about this, because it is now known that the calcium in milk may interfere with tetracycline absorption. The doctor may not mind the small loss of antibiotic in this way, since it is certainly preferable to loss of the whole dose through vomiting. On the other hand, some pediatricians specify that the tetracyclines *not* be given with an infant's milk formula or other foods and order that the antibiotic be administered at least an hour before the feeding.

Superinfections. The early irritative nausea and vomiting sometimes subsides only to return again with increased severity and accompanied by diarrhea. Such delayed gastrointestinal distress may, however, signal the onset of a much more serious condition, such as staphylococcal gastroenteritis. This infection, caused by the emergence and overgrowth of tetracycline-resistant strains of staph, can lead to a severely dehydrating diarrhea unless promptly treated (see Chap. 38) with fluids and electrolytes, opiate antiperistaltics and, perhaps, with locally acting intestinal adsorbent-demulcents. In most cases, such measures and withdrawal of the drug are enough to cure the condition. Sometimes, however, the doctor may have to determine the sensitivity of the superinfecting strain and then order administration of the antistaphylococcal drug that seems most likely to prove effective.

Overgrowths of the yeastlike fungal organism, *Candida albicans*, may occur not only in the intestine but also on the skin and on the mucous surfaces of the mouth and vagina. Some tetracycline products contain small amounts of antifungal antibiotics such as amphotericin and nystatin for prophylaxis against the development of intestinal moniliasis. It is doubtful, however, that these drugs prevent vulvovaginal or mucocutaneous fungal infections when administered orally, since they are not absorbed in sufficient quantity to attain antifungal concentrations in these areas. The local application of these agents in the form of topical preparations may help to clear up these conditions. Washing the patient's perineal area several times daily is said to reduce drug-induced pruritus.

Allergic Reactions. The tetracyclines sometimes cause skin rashes, urticaria and angioedema in sensitized individuals, but such reactions and anaphylaxis are less common than with penicillin. Some patients taking *demethylchlortetracycline* or other tetracyclines during the summer months have suffered sunburn and other severe skin reactions upon exposure to sunlight. Thus patients with a history of photosensitivity should be told to keep covered when outdoors to avoid development of such photodynamic reactions.

Dental Difficulties. Tetracyclines tend to be tied up with calcium in the bones and teeth. This in itself is not harmful. However, the calcium-tetracycline complex is believed to be responsible for discoloration of children's teeth. This yellow, brown or gray stain occurs most commonly when babies have been given tetracycline during development of the first teeth. Women treated with tetracyclines during pregnancy may bear children whose teeth grow in discolored. Ordinarily, only the deciduous teeth are affected, but long-term treatment with large doses during early childhood may lead to discoloration of the permanent teeth too.

Toxic Effects. The tetracyclines are capable of causing fatty degeneration of the liver when administered in large doses, especially in patients whose kidneys are not functioning properly. Fatalities have been reported in pregnant women who received 3 to 6 grams parenterally for severe infections. Failure to excrete repeated doses of the antibiotic led to its accumulation in the liver in hepatotoxic quantities. It is now suggested that patients with renal impairment receive only a fraction of the full therapeutic dose and that the levels of tetracycline in the plasma of patients on prolonged high doses be determined periodically.

An unusual reaction resembling Fanconi's syndrome but, fortunately, reversible has been reported recently. The signs and symptoms, which stem mainly from impairment of kidney tubule function, include acidosis, aminoaciduria, proteinuria and glycosuria. The patient's illness has been traced to tetracycline products which were outdated or degraded as a result of improper storage. Ordinarily, the nurse checks all drugs for evidence of deterioration which might make the drug ineffective. With tetracyclines, such checks would appear to be doubly necessary because of the possibility of this dangerous reaction. It is important upon receiving tetracycline products from the pharmacy both to be sure that the package expiration date has not passed and to store the container where its contents will not be subjected to excessively high heat and humidity.

Tetracycline Metabolism and Administration

Ordinarily, the tetracyclines are given orally because they are absorbed from the intestine in amounts adequate for treatment of all but the most severe infections. These antibiotics then pass from the plasma into other body fluids and tissues where they reach levels that inhibit bacterial growth. Penetration of these drugs into the cerebrospinal fluid is slow. Thus, in meningitis, they are preferably injected intravenously or intramuscularly—but *not* intrathecally. Also, because not much tetracycline makes its way into the ocular fluids, ophthalmic ointments or freshly prepared solutions for topical application are the preferred products for tetracycline-susceptible eye infections.

Much was made at one time of the purported advantages of one or another type of oral tetracycline product in terms of rapidity and completeness of intestinal absorption. However, all of the available products seem to be absorbed at about the same fairly rapid rate. Effective levels are attained in an hour or two and last for at least six hours. This long-lasting effect is the result of a combination of relatively slow renal clearance and a recycling of part of the absorbed tetracycline between the bile, the intestine and the circulation.

Demethylchlortetracycline (Declomycin) is said to produce somewhat higher and longer-lasting blood levels. This is the result not of better absorption but of a reduced rate of elimination by way of the kidneys. Actually, doctors do not attempt to achieve higher blood levels with oral doses of this drug. Instead, its main advantage is that it can be given in smaller doses than other tetracyclines. An added advantage is the

fact that it stays in the blood in effective levels for a day or two after the last dose. This is desirable for reducing the risk of a flare-up of a streptococcal or other infection in patients who tend to stop taking medication once their symptoms subside.

Methacycline (Rondomycin) and *doxycycline* (Vibramycin), the latest drugs of this class of semisynthetic tetracyclines, possess similar properties and advantages. Doxycycline, for example, is so slowly excreted that administration of a single daily dose is usually enough to maintain effective antibacterial levels once these have been attained with prior priming doses. The low dose is claimed to account for a reduced incidence of such tetracycline-type G.I. side effects as nausea, vomiting and diarrhea.

Parenteral Tetracycline Preparations. Occasionally, the tetracyclines have to be given by injection to assure that therapeutic levels are attained. In severe infections such as meningitis, the drug may have to be placed directly into the blood stream if enough is to penetrate into the infected area. Patients who may be unable to take tetracyclines by mouth or absorb them from the G.I. tract include those who are vomiting or unconscious, as well as others suffering from pathological states that prevent adequate absorption of these drugs from the gut.

Unfortunately, the tetracycline products available for parenteral use are rather unsatisfactory in various respects. Intramuscular injections are often followed by pain and tenderness even when the antibiotic is combined with a local anesthetic to counteract the immediate effects of the irritating tetracycline. Thus, the intravenous route is often preferred when parenteral therapy appears necessary.

Rolitetracycline (Syntetrin; Velacycline), a tetracycline derivative, is said to have certain advantages. Since it is very much more soluble than the parent antibiotic, this substance is more readily absorbed from intramuscular depot sites and is said to reach higher plasma levels and produce longer-lasting effects. It is available in combination with lidocaine for deep, relatively pain-free intramuscular injection. An intravenous form that does not contain the local anesthetic is also available. It must be infused carefully to avoid leakage and subsequent painful tissue and venous inflammation. The risk of liver damage is probably greatest when tetracyclines of any kind are given by the intravenous route. Thus, the doctor tries to transfer the patient to oral tetracycline therapy as soon as high blood levels have been attained with initial parenteral administration.

Chloramphenicol—Current Status

Chloramphenicol has a microbial spectrum as broad as that of the tetracyclines (Table 34-6). When it was first introduced, doctors tended to use it routinely to initiate treatment of infections in which they were uncertain of the causative organisms. Thus, the physician faced with the need to treat a severe respiratory infection of uncertain origin might administer this drug with a good deal of confidence that it would prove effective, even before the reports of laboratory tests were returned. Chloramphenicol was known to inhibit not only the common gram-positive cocci—strep, staph, and pneumococci—but also other respiratory tract invaders such as *Klebsiella pneumoniae, Hemophilus influenzae,* the PPLO *Mycoplasma pneumoniae,* and even the large viruses responsible for ornithosis and psittacosis.

Unfortunately, reports of very serious and sometimes fatal blood dyscrasias in patients treated with chloramphenicol soon began to appear. Although the proportion of such cases was statistically small compared to the number of people treated, this antibiotic became, before long, the leading cause of drug-induced *pancytopenia* (p. 41). The risk of this and other hematological disorders made it apparent that this antibiotic should not be ordered routinely for trivial infections such as colds or for influenza or other common upper respiratory infections, for such use of antibiotic therapy—undesirable at best—is especially dangerous with this drug. Thus, chloramphenicol is at present recommended for use in comparatively limited clinical circumstances.

This antibiotic should be used only after sensitivity tests have shown it to be highly active against the organism causing the patient's infection. Even then, it should not be used when safer antibiotics are effective against the particular pathogen. Thus, although chloramphenicol was used for a while for treating staphylococcal pneumonias caused by organisms resistant to penicillin G, physicians now prefer to initiate treatment of such cases with methicillin or cephalothin. Of course, if the patient is allergic to these drugs or otherwise not able to tolerate them, the doctor can still turn to chloramphenicol.

In such situations and in cases of typhoid fever, *Hemophilus influenzae* meningitis and other severe infections, the doctor may decide that the risk of using chloramphenicol is warranted by the seriousness of his patient's condition. Most authorities believe that the physician is then obligated to have blood studies done frequently during the treatment period. Such studies sometimes detect drug-induced reductions in one or another of the formed elements of the circulating blood—for example, leukopenia—early enough for the drug to be withdrawn before the blood disorder becomes irreversible.

On the other hand, a recent analysis of hundreds of chloramphenicol-associated blood dyscrasias indicates that manifestations of bone marrow depression did not usually appear in most patients until weeks or even months after the course of drug treatment had been completed. Thus, some hematologists now suggest that blood count studies made during treatment with this antibiotic are only rarely useful in preventing illness and death from drug-induced aplastic anemia. They conclude that there is no substitute for good judgment on the part of the doctor in deciding when this drug should or should not be used.

In recent years, direct toxicity of another type has been observed in premature infants and other newborn babies who required chloramphenicol treatment for severe infections developing shortly after birth. This condition has been called the "gray syndrome," because the babies often became cyanotic and ashengray in color. This drug-induced syndrome is characterized by abdominal distention, diarrhea, respiratory irregularities, and peripheral vascular collapse.

This severe illness, which has a high mortality rate, is believed to result from the newborn infant's inability to detoxify and eliminate chloramphenicol. That is, newborn infants, and particularly those born prematurely, do not possess the liver enzyme mechanisms for converting chloramphenicol to an inactive compound that can be readily excreted by the kidneys. As a result, if infants are given ordinary doses calculated on a weight basis, the drug accumulates in the tissues and reaches toxic levels. Thus, all premature babies and full-term infants under two weeks old should receive only half the usual dose (see Drug Digest) and should be observed very closely during all treatment with chloramphenicol so that the drug may be withdrawn in favor of another active antibiotic at the first sign of drug-induced toxicity. The drug must also be discontinued if superinfections of the kind described in relation to the other broad-spectrum antibiotics (the tetracyclines) develop as the result of overgrowth of nonsusceptible microbes.

MISCELLANEOUS ANTIBIOTICS

The search for antibiotics that was set off by the success of penicillin resulted in the introduction of many new anti-infective agents. Some of these are very useful and even life-saving in certain specific situations. However, none can compare with penicillin for combined safety and bactericidal activity or with tetracycline and chloramphenicol for breadth of bacteriostatic antimicrobial spectrum.

Because of their comparatively limited usefulness we need not discuss each of these secondary antibiotics in detail. Despite their sometimes marked individual differences, it is probably better to group them for study purposes into several broad categories based upon certain outstanding characteristics that they seem to have in common. Then we can point out briefly a few of the properties of each agent which seem most pertinent to its current status.

Penicillin Substitutes

A number of antibiotics may be grouped together because of the similarity of their antibacterial spectrum to that of penicillin (Table 34-3). That is, these agents are (with some exceptions) mainly effective against the most important *gram-positive cocci* (e.g., streptococci, pneumococci, staphylococci). Some also hit a few gram-negative cocci (e.g., gonococci, meningococci). Only occasionally do the drugs of this group succeed in controlling some strains of gram-negative bacilli.

These antibiotics have been used mainly in two situations:

1. Most commonly, they are ordered for treatment of patients who ordinarily would have received penicillin but have to be denied that valuable antibiotic because they have become allergic to it.

2. One or another of these antibiotics may sometimes be selected for use against strains of organisms that are not sensitive to penicillin. That is, the doctor may choose one of these drugs when sensitivity tests on bacterial cultures taken from the patient indicate that the organism is more susceptible to that antibiotic than to any other.

Until recently, these second-line antibiotics were most commonly selected to treat infections caused by strains of staphylococci resistant to penicillin and the broad-spectrum agents. However, the success of the new semisynthetic penicillins against penicillinase-producing staphylococci has led to a reduction in the use of these somewhat more toxic antibiotics. In addition, an increasing number of organisms have emerged which are resistant to the older drugs of this group, such as *erythromycin*. Resistance is not yet a problem with newer agents of this group such as *lincomycin*; however, their usefulness, compared to penicillin and the tetracyclines, cannot yet be considered established, and they are employed mainly for patients who cannot tolerate the first-line antibiotics.

Individual Agents

Each of the drugs listed in Table 34-3 will now be discussed briefly to indicate its current clinical status.

Erythromycin (see also Drug Digest). This antibiotic is similar to penicillin in its spectrum. Physicians occasionally prefer it to penicillin in some circumstances. Generally, like the other drugs of this group, it is employed when allergy does not permit the use of penicillin in a particular patient. Numerous derivatives are available for oral and parenteral use. Such salts and esters were devised in efforts to overcome various drawbacks of the erythromycin base.

Erythromycin estolate (Ilosone), for example, is said to be much better absorbed than the base, which is destroyed in the stomach unless administered in specially coated capsules. However, unlike erythromycin itself, which rarely causes any adverse effects except stomach upset, this derivative has reportedly caused allergic liver reactions.

Such hepatic hypersensitivity to erythromycin estolate has been manifested by development of the cholestatic type of jaundice. This distressing condition has its onset after a couple of weeks or so of treatment, with symptoms similar to those of a gallbladder attack. Such early symptoms as abdominal cramps, nausea and vomiting, which precede the development of jaundice, should be promptly reported to the doctor. The

TABLE 34-3
ANTIBIOTICS SIMILAR TO PENICILLINS IN SPECTRUM

Nonproprietary or Official Name	Trade Name or Synonym	Dosage and Administration
Cephalothin	Keflin	0.5 to 1 Gm. I.M. or I.V. 4 to 6 times daily.
Erythromycin U.S.P.	Erythrocin; Ilotycin	Oral or I.V., 1 to 2 Gm. daily.
Lincomycin	Lincocin	500 mg. oral, 600 mg. parenteral.
Novobiocin calcium N.F. Novobiocin sodium N.F.	Albamycin; Cathomycin	250 to 500 mg. oral or I.V.
Oleandomycin phosphate N.F.	Matromycin	250 to 500 mg. oral or parenteral.
Ristocetin U.S.P.	Spontin	25 to 50 mg./Kg. by slow I.V. infusion.
Triacetyloleandomycin N.F.	Cyclamycin; TAO	250 to 500 mg. oral or parenteral.
Vancomycin U.S.P.	Vancocin	500 mg. q. 6 hrs. by slow I.V. infusion.

sooner this drug is discontinued, the more rapidly is the condition likely to clear.

Occasionally, when sensitivity tests on a culture taken from a seriously ill patient show the infecting organism to be highly responsive to this antibiotic, it is administered parenterally. Erythromycin gluceptate is often administered by vein in such circumstances, because intramuscular injections of the lactobionate salt are rather painful. The ethylsuccinate and stearate derivatives are available in palatable forms suitable for pediatric patients.

Triacetyloleandomycin. This ester of oleandomycin is said to be better absorbed than the parent antibiotic and thus to reach higher blood levels. It is similar to erythromycin in bacterial spectrum and, like the latter, it is best reserved for treating serious infections by strains of organisms definitely shown by sensitivity testing to be especially susceptible. Ordinarily, however, penicillin or other less toxic antibiotics are preferred.

Actually, this drug does not often cause adverse reactions. Unfortunately, like erythromycin, this antibiotic occasionally causes cholestatic jaundice in sensitive patients. To reduce the risk of such rare but serious hepatotoxic reactions, a time limit has been set for the continued use of this antibiotic. Present recommendations are that triacetyloleandomycin *not* be used for prophylaxis or in conditions that require more than 10 days of treatment in doses of 1 Gm. or more. If the patient's condition makes use of this drug for longer periods imperative, the patient is closely observed for evidence of liver dysfunction. At the first sign of any abnormality in liver function tests, the drug is discontinued—after which the patient's signs and symptoms soon clear up.

Novobiocin. This antibiotic is sometimes administered by mouth, either alone or combined with tetracycline. It is best reserved for the treatment of severe infections caused by organisms shown by testing to be sensitive to novobiocin but resistant to tetracycline, penicillin and other less toxic antibiotics. In such cases, the drug is administered parenterally, preferably by intravenous injection rather than by the more painful intramuscular route.

Although novobiocin is sometimes used in patients allergic to penicillin, it is itself a strong sensitizing agent. Patients should be carefully observed for the appearance of a rash on the trunk, face, arms or legs. Although such dermal reactions are not dangerous and disappear when the drug is withdrawn, their presence serves as a warning that the patient may be subject to more serious hypersensitivity reactions. Occasional blood dyscrasias and liver damage, for example, have been reported. Thus, blood cell counts are made routinely, and liver function tests are employed if a yellow pigment appears in the patient's plasma.

Lincomycin. This new antibiotic is similar to penicillin and erythromycin in its antibacterial spectrum and is employed mainly for patients who do not tolerate the older drugs on account of allergy or other adverse reactions. Few adverse effects other than gastrointestinal upset have thus far been reported, and the development of resistant strains of bacteria does not yet seem to be a problem. The drug may be administered by the oral, intramuscular, or intravenous routes. Routine blood cell counts are recommended, as is liver function testing in patients taking the drug for longer than two weeks.

Ristocetin. This drug, like *vancomycin* (see Drug Digest), has been employed mainly for treating patients seriously ill with severe staphylococcal infections or subacute bacterial endocarditis that are unresponsive to penicillin and other safer antibiotics. In such cases, this antibiotic is administered only by vein, since it is not absorbed from the gastrointestinal tract and is too irritating for intramuscular injection. Thrombophlebitis not infrequently follows its intravenous injection. The effects of ristocetin upon the blood are among the more serious drawbacks to the use of this drug. Thrombocytopenia, for example, is a potentially toxic hematological effect that makes repeated studies of the blood mandatory. Leukopenia must also be watched for.

The potential toxicity of this drug and of vancomycin severely limits their usefulness. Fortunately, the introduction of semisynthetic penicillins such as *methicillin* and of the related antibiotic *cephalothin* has made the use of these relatively toxic drugs less often necessary.

Cephalothin (Keflin). This antibiotic closely resembles penicillin in its chemical structure and mechanism of action. Like penicillin, it seems to interfere with the synthesis of the cell wall of streptococci, pneumococci and staphylococci. Unlike penicillin G, however, it resists inactivation by bacterial penicillinase, and, unlike the semisynthetic penicillins (which are, of course, also active against penicillinase-producing bacteria), cephalothin does not cause allergic reactions in patients with a history of sensitivity to penicillin.

This antibiotic is presently recommended only for treating relatively serious infections, especially those in which penicillin seems indicated but cannot be tolerated. It has been employed for bacteremia, soft-tissue and respiratory tract infections. In addition, because it is more active than most penicillins—except ampicillin—against certain *gram-negative* invaders of the genitourinary tract, it has been used in infections by strains of such organisms that have been proved sensitive to it by prior laboratory testing.

Few severe adverse effects from cephalothin have been reported up to now, but blood, liver and kidney studies are recommended for patients receiving this new drug. Parenteral administration of this drug seems more irritating than injections of methicillin or oxacillin. Injections should be made deep into the muscle to reduce pain and local soft-tissue damage and sloughing.

Antibiotics Used Mainly Locally

A number of other antibiotics (Table 34-4) may be taken up together because of certain clinical characteristics that they have in common, even though some differ from others chemically and in the nature of their bacterial spectra. In general, the following statements are applicable to most of these drugs:

1. They are *never used routinely* for treating *systemic* infections and are employed only after tests have established that the pathogen is more sensitive to one of these antibiotics than it is to the penicillins, the tetracyclines or other safer agents.

2. In the relatively rare cases in which one of these drugs is chosen for parenteral administration, the patient is observed very closely for *signs of toxicity.* These are most commonly changes in the quantity and content of the urine, since these antibiotics tend to affect *kidney function* adversely. Patients who already suffer from some degree of renal insufficiency are likely to show signs of *neurotoxicity,* including auditory nerve damage that may result in deafness or vertigo. This and other manifestations of direct tox-

icity follow accumulation of the unexcreted antibiotic in body tissues.

3. These drugs are *poorly absorbed* from the gastrointestinal tract. Thus when *oral* administration is ordered, the purpose is not to produce systemically effective blood and tissue levels but to bring about high antibiotic concentrations within the bowel for *treatment* or *prophylaxis* of *intestinal infections.* Systemic toxicity does not ordinarily develop when these drugs are taken by mouth unless the patient's kidney function is so poor that he fails to eliminate the relatively small amounts absorbed through the gut into the blood.

4. These antibiotics are most commonly administered by *topical application* to the skin and mucous membranes. Combinations of these drugs are considered more desirable than ointments, solutions or sprays of penicillin or tetracycline for the treatment of cutaneous infections, for the following reasons: First, strains resistant to these antibiotics have only rarely emerged. Also, allergic hypersensitization, which develops so readily after penicillin and other antibiotics are applied to the skin, rarely occurs with these agents.

Even if sensitization were to occur with these drugs, it would be of much less practical importance than development of allergy to penicillin or the tetracy-

TABLE 34-4
ANTIBIOTICS USED MAINLY ON SKIN AND IN G.I. TRACT

NONPROPRIETARY OR OFFICIAL NAME	TRADE NAME OR SYNONYM	DOSAGE AND ADMINISTRATION
Bacitracin U.S.P.	Baciguent, etc.	I.M. 30,000 to 100,000 u. daily; topically, as ointment containing 500 u. per Gm.
Colistimethate sodium U.S.P.	Coly-Mycin M Injectable	I.M. 2.5 to 5 mg./Kg.
Colistin sulfate	Coly-Mycin S Pediatric	Topically as ointment or solution; orally 3 to 5 mg./Kg.
Gentamicin	Garamycin	Topically as ointment; orally 50 to 100 mg.; I.M. 0.4 mg./Kg.
Kanamycin sulfate U.S.P.	Kantrex	Oral 1 Gm.; I.M. 7.5 mg./Kg.
Neomycin sulfate U.S.P.	Mycifradin; Myciquent, etc.	Topically as ointment, etc.; oral 4 to 12 Gm. daily; I.M. 0.25 Gm.
Polymyxin B sulfate U.S.P.	Aerosporin	Topically as ointment, etc.; I.M. 10,000 to 20,000 u. per Kg. daily
Streptomycin sulfate U.S.P.		I.M. 1 Gm. daily; orally 0.5 to 1 Gm.; topically as ointment, etc.
Tyrothricin N.F.	Soluthricin	Topically in various forms
Zinc Bacitracin U.S.P.		Topically as an ointment containing 500 u. per Gm.

clines through use of an ointment for a minor infection. This is because the antibiotics of this group are rarely required for treating serious systemic infections, in contrast to the frequency with which penicillin and the broad-spectrum drugs must be so employed.

The above generalizations in regard to the bacterial spectrum, clinical uses and potential toxicity of this group may be illustrated by briefly examining some of the characteristics of various individual antibiotics and subclasses of these anti-infective agents.

Individual Agents

Neomycin (see Drug Digest), **kanamycin** and **streptomycin** share many properties. All are effective against the tubercle bacillus—and, indeed, streptomycin is still so important in the treatment of tuberculosis that we shall defer our discussion of that antibiotic until Chapter 35. In addition, all are effective against some of the gram-negative bacilli often responsible for acute and chronic infections of the urinary tract (e.g., *E. coli, Aerobacter aerogenes,* Klebsiella, and some strains of Proteus).

However, the usefulness of these three antibiotics in the treatment of systemic infections is limited by their potential for doing harm. This is especially true in elderly patients and in others whose renal efficiency is impaired. *Nephrotoxic reactions* from neomycin and kanamycin are common in such patients, as is evidenced by frequent albuminuria, cylindruria and hematuria. Such signs sometimes indicate the need to withdraw these drugs, lest they accumulate in the body and damage other tissues. Possible ototoxicity, involving both the cochlear and the vestibular portions of the eighth cranial (auditory) nerve is a constant concern in patients receiving streptomycin and its relatives parenterally. The doctor often orders audiometric testing for early detection of hearing loss, in order to avoid the danger of permanent deafness following treatment.

Polymyxin B sulfate and its close chemical relative **colistin** are limited in their spectrum of activity mainly to gram-negative bacilli. However, along with the new and less well established antibiotic *gentamicin* they are uniquely effective against *Pseudomonas aeruginosa,* an organism which is often quite resistant to other antibiotics. A peculiarity of the antibiotic era is the fact that deaths from pseudomonas infections have increased several fold. Such fatalities from this organism stem from superinfections resulting from overgrowths of these bacteria after their natural microbial competitors have been eliminated by treatment with tetracyclines or other agents to which this organism is resistant.

In serious pseudomonas infections, these antibiotics have often proved life-saving. Pseudomonal meningitis, for example, responds to polymyxin and to colistin injected intrathecally in low doses. The intramuscular route is employed for administration of polymyxin in pseudomonal and other gram-negative urinary tract infections. Because this drug often causes prolonged pain upon injection, some physicians prefer to use a special parenteral form of colistin, sodium colistimethate (Coly-Mycin M Injectable), for this purpose. With both drugs, considerable caution is required to avoid renal toxicity and signs of neurotoxicity ranging from paresthesias to deafness.

Bacitracin and **tyrothricin** (an antibiotic made up of two substances, *gramicidin* and *tyrocidine*) differ from the others of this group in their antibacterial spectrum, since their activity is limited largely to *gram-positive* organisms. They are similar to the others, however, in their systemic toxicity. In the case of tyrothricin, this is so severe that it is *never* administered parenterally. Bacitracin is occasionally injected in the treatment of severe resistant staphylococcal infections. However, its use for this purpose has declined since the introduction of safer antibiotics, such as the new semisynthetic penicillins and cephalothin, to combat infections by penicillinase-producing staphylococci.

These antibiotics are employed mainly by topical application to the skin and the mucous membranes of the throat and eye. Ointments containing these drugs alone or combined with neomycin and polymyxin are very numerous. They are widely employed for treating skin infections such as impetigo, furunculosis (boils) and carbuncles and other pyodermas and for application to wounds, ulcers and other open surface-infections. These antibiotics have been common constituents of eye, ear and nose drops and of troches intended to treat sore throats. However, the Food and Drug Administration recently ordered the removal from the market of self-medication lozenges containing amounts of these antibiotics too small to be effective.

Oral Administration

Gastrointestinal Infections. Almost all of the antibiotics of this group are sometimes administered orally. Taken singly, or sometimes combined with one another or with one of the poorly absorbable sulfonamides (Chap. 35), these antibiotics tend to reach high local concentrations within the bowel, where they exert their inhibitory activity upon susceptible intestinal microorganisms.

Oral administration of neomycin and the other antibiotics of this group is employed for the following purposes:

Treatment and Prevention of Infectious Diarrhea. These antibiotics are available in combination with adsorbents and demulcents such as kaolin, pectin and attapulgite (Chap. 38) for specific therapy of *bacterial diarrhea* and for prophylaxis while traveling abroad.

Actually, the use of products containing neomycin, dihydrostreptomycin, colistin or polymyxin is largely limited to a few days of treatment of relatively mild diarrheas. More severe cases are treated with these antibiotics only when the organism has been specifically identified and shown to be more susceptible to one of these agents than to other anti-infective agents. Ordinarily, the pathogens that are responsible for the most severe types of gastroenteritis are responsive to treatment with the broad-spectrum antibiotics and the sulfonamides. Chloromycetin, for example, is preferred for salmonella infections, especially typhoid fever, the tetracyclines are required in cholera, and both these antibiotics and the sulfonamides are the drugs of choice for bacillary dysentery or shigellosis. (The use of *bacitracin* and other antibiotics including *paromomycin* (see Table 34-5) in the treatment of *amebic* dysentery is discussed in Chap. 38.)

Preoperative Preparation of the Bowel. These antibiotics are often administered for several days prior to abdominal or perineal surgery. It is thought that by their ability to minimize the number of microorganisms in the intestinal tract, these antibiotics tend to reduce the risk of peritonitis from bacterial contamination during surgery.

Some authorities see little value in such so-called sterilization of the bowel by these antibiotics and the sulfonamides. They claim that postoperative infections can be prevented by careful surgical technique and prefer not to run the risks of employing chemical prophylaxis, which, of course, include possible superinfections by overgrowths of resistant organisms.

In any case, when used for this purpose, the antibiotic or chembiotic preparation is begun 24 to 72 hours prior to the time of the planned elective surgery, after the bowel is first emptied through use of a saline cathartic and enema, and the patient has been placed on a low-residue diet.

Occasionally, neomycin solutions have been instilled intraperitoneally to prevent peritonitis when contamination has occurred during surgery. A dangerous reaction that may occur with this procedure is respiratory failure. This effect is believed to be due to the fact that drugs of the neomycin-kanamycin-streptomycin group have a curarelike action on skeletal muscle in high concentrations. Treatment of apnea of this type requires measures similar to those employed in curare overdosage (Chap. 17), including the possible injection of neostigmine.

Adjunct to Hepatic Coma Therapy. These antibiotics are sometimes administered to patients with liver damage who seem likely to pass into hepatic coma. It is thought that these drugs help to lessen production of ammonia and other possible toxins by eliminating the microorganisms that break down nitrogenous materials in the intestine. At the same time, protein is temporarily withdrawn from the patient's diet, and other supportive measures are, of course, employed, if the patient becomes comatose.

Patients must be watched for signs of systemic anti-

biotic toxicity. Ordinarily, as previously indicated, the small amounts of these drugs that may happen to be absorbed are readily excreted by the kidneys. However, patients in hepatic coma may also suffer from renal insufficiency, and, in such cases, an antibiotic such as neomycin may accumulate in the kidneys and other tissues. Drug-induced nephrotoxicity of this type may so interfere with excretion that the antibiotic reaches plasma levels similar to those attained by injection. The patient may then suffer permanent deafness as a result of irreversible damage to the auditory nerve by drugs of the neomycin-kanamycin-streptomycin subgroup.

Antifungal Antibiotics

The antibiotics which we have discussed up to this time have been mainly antibacterial in action. These drugs not only have no effect on fungi but also often tend to bring about overgrowths of yeastlike organisms. Recently, however, a few substances produced by certain soil organisms have been shown to possess antifungal activity. All are being employed in purified form for treating various local fungal infections, and one of these antibiotics is being employed in the treatment of certain systemic fungal infections, for which, previously, no good drug treatment was available.

Amphotericin B (see Drug Digest) is the first truly effective and dependable drug for treating the so-called disseminated mycoses. These are diseases in which certain fungi enter the body by way of the mouth, lungs, or skin and spread to various internal organs including the brain, bones and heart. *Histoplasmosis* is one such condition that is seen with increasing frequency in this country. Inhaled in the dust from pigeon or chicken dung, the fungal organism often causes a pulmonary infection resembling tuberculosis. Other fungi—the causes of *blastomycosis*, *coccidiomycosis*, and *cryptococcosis*, for instance—are even more dangerous because of their rapid spread to the meninges and elsewhere as a generalized infection.

Administered with great care to hospitalized patients, amphotericin B has changed the previously poor prognosis for patients with such systemic fungal infections. Although amphotericin B is a potentially toxic drug, it is less toxic and very much more effective than the chemotherapeutic agents previously employed in these cases. The adverse effects of this life-saving drug can be minimized by close attention to the technical details of its administration by intravenous infusion (see Drug Digest).

Amphotericin B is also used in the treatment and prevention of infections of the skin and mucous membranes by the yeastlike organism, *Candida* (*Monilia*) *albicans*. Although candida occasionally produce septicemia, meningitis and endocarditis—conditions that require intravenous amphotericin B—these organisms are much more commonly the cause of candidiasis

TABLE 34-5
SPECIAL SPECTRUM ANTIBIOTICS (ANTIFUNGAL AND ANTIAMEBIC)

NONPROPRIETARY OR OFFICIAL NAME	TRADE NAME OR SYNONYM	DOSAGE AND ADMINISTRATION
Amphotericin B	Fungizone	I.V. 0.1 to 1.0 mg./Kg.; intrathecal 25 mcg. to 500 mcg. Topical application as ointment, cream, etc.
Candicidin	Candeptin	Topical ointment and vaginal tablets
Fumagillin	Fumidil	10 mg. orally q.i.d.
Griseofulvin U.S.P.	Fulvicin U/F; Grifulvin V; Grisactin	500 mg. to 2 Gm. daily by mouth
Nystatin U.S.P.	Mycostatin	1 to 3 million u. daily by mouth; also, topically and intravaginally
Paromomycin	Humatin	25 to 75 mg./Kg. daily in divided doses, orally

(or moniliasis) of the mouth, vagina, and skin, which can be safely treated by topical application of this antibiotic or with a chemically related antibiotic, *nystatin* (see Drug Digest).

Both these antibiotics are usually effective when applied to the mouth in thrush, administered intravaginally in monilial vaginitis, or spread as a cream between folds of infected skin in intertriginous fungal dermatoses. They are, in addition, often taken orally combined with tetracyclines for prophylactic purposes. Addition of these antifungal agents is thought to prevent superinfections by explosive overgrowth of intestinal candidal organisms when the natural balance of the microbial flora is altered by the broad-spectrum antibiotic. Although the usefulness of such routine administration of amphotericin B or nystatin to all patients has been questioned, it may be desirable for patients with conditions which make them especially susceptible to candida infections.

Griseofulvin (see Drug Digest) is an antifungal antibiotic which is used for purposes entirely different from the other two agents. It is not effective against candida or the other fungi that cause localized or systemic infections. It acts, instead, against various *dermatophytes,* fungi of the genera Microsporum, Trichophyton and Epidermophyton, which cause the most common fungal infections of the skin, hair and nails such as athlete's foot, ringworm and barber's itch, etc.

Although such superficial infections are seldom serious, they sometimes cause intolerable itching and are often disfiguring. They are ordinarily controlled by topical application of creams, ointments and other preparations containing combinations of antifungal and keratolytic chemicals (see Chap. 43).

Such products, although they work reasonably well

in the early stages of acute skin infections, are generally ineffective when the fungi are well established deep in the skin. This is because the tiny parasitic plants burrow down to the base of the keratin layer where some survive an attack from above by topically applied medications. Thus, even when the keratolytic drugs dissolve the dead keratin cells, the newly forming skin, hair and nails carry bits of fungi which begin to grow again.

Griseofulvin has offered dermatologists an entirely new approach to the treatment of such chronic fungal infections. The drug is rarely applied topically, as it apparently penetrates the skin poorly from above. It is instead taken by mouth in tablet form or as an oral suspension. After its absorption into the blood from the intestine, the antibiotic is deposited in the living cells, which are converted to keratin when they die. The drug's continued presence in the keratin layer acts as a barrier to the further growth of fungi already established there. Then, as new cells grow out, they push the fungus-infected tissues before them until they are naturally shed or can be clipped.

The time required for treatment with griseofulvin varies, depending upon various factors, including the location and severity of the fungal infection. Tinea capitis (ringworm of the scalp) and tinea pedis (athlete's foot) require only about four weeks for complete eradication of the fungal invader; tinea unguium (onychomycosis; ringworm of the nails) may need six months to a year of treatment.

Fortunately for patients on long-term therapy, griseofulvin has given little indication of toxicity. Although minor side effects, including headache and gastrointestinal irritation, are the cause of occasional complaints, more serious toxicity has not been reported. Patients taking the drug over a period of many months may be given blood and liver function tests periodically and should be instructed to report the occurrence of sore throat, fever or other unusual symptoms. They should also, of course, be instructed in the measures required to prevent their becoming reinfected (Chap. 43).

Antiviral Therapy

Antibiotic drugs are now available for treating infections caused by pathogenic invaders of every type except viruses. This, then, is the area in which scientists hope to make their next big breakthrough in antibiotic therapy. They have already discovered several *non*-antibiotic agents effective in virus infections. These include idoxuridine (Chap. 42) for herpes simplex eye infections; and amantadine (Chap. 35), which seems effective for preventing influenza caused by one strain of virus. In addition, new vaccines continue to be developed—Mumps Vaccine, for example—for use in conferring active immunity.

TABLE 34-6
ANTIBIOTIC DRUGS OF CHOICE

Organism	Infection	Antibiotics (in Approximate Order of Effectiveness)
Gram-Positive Cocci		
Staphylococcus aureus		
Non-Penicillinase producers	Skin, subcutaneous tissues, eyes, ears, lungs, G.I. tract, bones, joints, blood and meninges	Penicillin G Erythromycin Cephalothin Chloramphenicol Lincomycin Tetracyclines
Penicillinase-producing strains		Cloxacillin Oxacillin Methicillin Nafcillin Cephalothin Lincomycin Erythromycin Novobiocin Vancomycin Ristocetin Chloramphenicol Terramycin
Streptococcus pyogenes; Group A, beta hemolytic, etc.	Upper respiratory infections, including pharyngitis, tonsillitis, sinusitis, otitis media, pneumonia	Penicillin G Ampicillin Cloxacillin Oxacillin Nafcillin Erythromycin Lincomycin Novobiocin Cephalothin Tetracyclines Chloramphenicol
Streptococcus viridans; Enterococcus	Endocarditis, meningitis, urinary tract infections, etc.	Penicillin G, and other penicillins, alone or combined with Streptomycin Cephalothin Erythromycin, etc.

TABLE 34-6 (Continued)

ORGANISM	INFECTION	ANTIBIOTICS (IN APPROXIMATE ORDER OF EFFECTIVENESS)
Gram-Positive Cocci (*Continued*)		
Pneumococcus	Pneumonia, meningitis, endocarditis, etc.	Penicillin G Erythromycin Nafcillin Oxacillin Cloxacillin Cephalothin Lincomycin Tetracyclines
Gram-Negative Cocci		

Meningococcus	Meningococcal meningitis, septicemia	Penicillin G, alone or with
		    Sulfonamides
		    Ampicillin
		    Cephalothin
		    Erythromycin

Gonococcus	Gonorrheal urethritis, salpingitis, vaginitis, arthritis, etc.	Penicillin G Erythromycin Tetracyclines Ampicillin Cloxacillin Oxacillin Nafcillin Lincomycin Cephalothin
Gram-Positive Bacilli		
Bacillus anthracis	Anthrax ("malignant pustule")	Penicillin G Erythromycin Tetracyclines
Listeria species	Meningitis, endocarditis, etc.	Penicillin G Erythromycin Tetracyclines
Corynebacterium diphtheriae	Pharyngitis, laryngitis, tracheitis, pneumonia, etc.	Penicillin G Erythromycin Cephalothin Tetracyclines Lincomycin, etc.
Clostridium tetani	Tetanus	Penicillin G Tetracyclines
Clostridium welchii	Gas gangrene	Penicillin G Tetracyclines, with or without Streptomycin
Gram-Negative Bacilli		
Escherichia coli	Urinary tract infections	Ampicillin Chloramphenicol Tetracyclines Cephalothin

TABLE 34-6 (Continued)

Organism	Infection	Antibiotics (in Approximate Order of Effectiveness)
Gram-Negative Bacilli (*Continued*)		
Escherichia coli (*Continued*)	G.I. tract infections	Oral neomycin Kanamycin
	Septicemia	Chloramphenicol Tetracyclines Kanamycin Neomycin

Klebsiella;
Aerobacter *aerogenes;*
Aerobacter faecalis
	Urinary tract infections; pneumonia, etc.	Chloramphenicol
		Tetracyclines, with or without
		  Streptomycin
		  Kanamycin
		  Neomycin

Proteus mirabilis	Urinary tract, etc.	Ampicillin Penicillin G, etc.

Proteus (other species)	Urinary tract, etc.	Chloramphenicol
		Tetracyclines, with or without
		  Streptomycin
		  Kanamycin
		  Neomycin, etc.

Pseudomonas aeruginosa	Urinary tract, skin and subcutaneous tissues (e.g., burns, wounds), external and middle ear, meningitis, G.I. tract enterocolitis	Polymyxin Colistin Gentamycin
Shigella species	Acute gastroenteritis; bacillary dysentery; shigellosis	Ampicillin Tetracyclines Chloramphenicol Cephalothin Neomycin (oral) Kanamycin (oral)
Salmonella species	Salmonellosis gastroenteritis, typhoid and paratyphoid fevers, septicemia	Ampicillin (milder cases) Chloramphenicol (more severe cases) Tetracyclines Cephalothin
Vibrio comma	Cholera	Tetracyclines Chloramphenicol Streptomycin
Pasteurella pestis	Bubonic plague	Streptomycin Tetracyclines Chloramphenicol
Pasteurella tularensis	Tularemia	Streptomycin Tetracyclines Chloramphenicol
Hemophilus influenzae	Respiratory tract infections, including pneumonia; meningitis	Chloramphenicol Tetracyclines Streptomycin Ampicillin

TABLE 34-6 (Continued)

Organism	Infection	Antibiotics (in Approximate Order of Effectiveness)
Gram-Negative Bacilli (*Continued*)		
Hemophilus ducreyi	Chancroid	Tetracyclines Chloramphenicol Streptomycin
Brucella species	Brucellosis (undulant fever)	Tetracyclines Chloramphenicol, with or without Streptomycin
Acid-Fast Bacilli		
Mycobacterium tuberculosis	Infections of lungs, bones, kidneys, meninges, and all body surfaces (miliary)	Streptomycin Cycloserine Viomycin Kanamycin Neomycin (with such chemotherapeutic agents as Isoniazid Para-amino salicylic acid Pyrazinamide Ethionamide)
Spirochetes		
Treponema pallidum	Syphilis	Penicillin G Tetracyclines Erythromycin
Treponema pertenue	Yaws	Penicillin G Tetracyclines
Borellia recurrentis	Relapsing fever	Tetracyclines Chloramphenicol Penicillin G
Leptospira	Weil's disease	Penicillin G Tetracyclines
Spirillum minus	Ratbite fever	Penicillin G Erythromycin Streptomycin
Rickettsia		
	Typhus fever, Murine typhus, Brill's disease, Q fever, Rocky Mountain spotted fever, etc.	Tetracyclines Chloramphenicol
"Large Viruses"		
Mycoplasma pneumoniae	Atypical viral pneumonia	Tetracyclines Chloramphenicol
Psittacosis agent Ornithosis agent	Parrot fever pneumonia	Tetracyclines Chloramphenicol

TABLE 34-6 (Continued)

Organism	Infection	Antibiotics (in Approximate Order of Effectiveness)
"Large Viruses" (*Continued*)		
Lymphogranuloma venereum agent	Venereal disease	Tetracyclines Chloramphenicol
Trachoma agent	Blinding eye disease	Tetracyclines Chloramphenicol, orally or topically (with sulfonamides)
Fungi		
Aspergillus Blastomyces Cryptococcus Coccidioides Histoplasma Mucor *Candida albicans*	Disseminated (systemic) mycoses in skin, lungs, bones, brain, etc.	Amphotericin B
Candida albicans	Skin and mucous membranes	Nystatin Candicidin Amphotericin B
Dermatophytes	Ringworm of skin, scalp, nails	Griseofulvin
Actinomyces israelii	Granulomas of jaw, brain, lungs, etc.	Penicillin G Tetracyclines
Nocardia asteroides	Nocardiosis of lungs, brain, etc.	Tetracyclines Chloramphenicol Streptomycin Cephalothin Cycloserine (with sulfonamides)

CLINICAL PROBLEM

Miss Jones was admitted to the hospital for treatment of pneumonia. A few minutes after she was given an injection of 300,000 units of penicillin intramuscularly, the patient became restless, developed urticaria, and then fainted. Her roommate observed these symptoms and called the nurse.

• What is the probable reason for Miss Jones's symptoms?

• What actions could you take in this situation? Indicate the order in which you would carry out each task. What equipment and supplies would you prepare for the physician's use?

• What nursing actions are indicated for Miss Jones's roommate?

REVIEW QUESTIONS

1. (a) What two properties of penicillin give it such importance as an anti-infective agent?

(b) Indicate how the manner of penicillin's action on bacterial cells is thought to account, in part, for these desirable properties.

2. (a) List some disadvantages of penicillin G.

(b) By what general means have scientists helped to lessen these drawbacks of natural penicillin?

(c) List some specific penicillin products that were developed as a result of such efforts.

3. (a) List several common pathogens that are still highly sensitive to penicillin.

(b) List infectious diseases of several types which can be controlled or prevented by penicillin.

4. (a) What property of certain strains of staphylococci accounts for their ability to resist treatment with penicillin G?

(b) List several semisynthetic penicillins that are unaffected by this bacterial action and, consequently, kill bacteria unaffected by penicillin G.

5. (a) In what practical respect do methicillin and cloxacillin differ and how does this influence the circumstances under which each of these semisynthetic penicillins is employed?

(b) How does ampicillin differ from other penicillins in its bacterial spectrum?

(c) In what circumstances may ampicillin be preferred to penicillin G or to oxacillin and others, and when would penicillins of the latter kind be more desirable?

6. (a) Under what circumstances is oral administration of penicillin considered adequate and when is parenteral administration of massive amounts of penicillin preferred?

(b) What should be the nurse's attitude toward the orders left with her for administration of penicillin?

7. (a) At what times are most oral penicillin products administered?

(b) Which of the oral penicillins are resistant to gastric acids?

(c) Which of the oral penicillins are claimed to be better absorbed when taken with meals?

8. (a) By what means are the highest blood and tissue levels of penicillin attained and sustained?

(b) By what means are penicillin levels maintained at low but therapeutically effective levels for the longest periods?

9. (a) What should the nurse tell patients who require periodic administration of repository penicillin preparations such as benzathine penicillin G for prophylactic purposes?

(b) For what purposes is procaine penicillin G suspension sometimes employed?

10. (a) By what two processes do the kidneys rapidly remove penicillin from the blood?

(b) How does an adjuvant, such as probenecid, act to keep penicillin levels at higher levels for longer periods?

11. (a) How does the manner in which penicillin is distributed influence the manner in which it may have to be administered in treating meningitis?

(b) What precaution is taken in administering penicillin intrathecally?

12. (a) What should the nurse try to ascertain from the patient before administering a dose of penicillin?

(b) What other measure may the nurse take to help detect the presence of allergic sensitivity to penicillin?

13. (a) Describe briefly a couple of tests for penicillin allergy that the doctor may wish to have done.

(b) List drugs of several types used in the management of reactions to penicillin and indicate in each case what each drug is designed to do.

14. (a) List several organisms and diseases against which broad-spectrum antibiotics such as the tetracyclines and chloramphenicol are uniquely valuable.

(b) List some other clinical conditions in which the tetracyclines are sometimes employed when the patient cannot tolerate penicillin or other more effective antibiotics.

(c) What is the status of the tetracyclines in the treatment of the common cold and other infections caused by true viruses?

15. (a) What side effect is sometimes seen early in treatment with tetracyclines and how may the likelihood of its occurrence be lessened?

(b) Superinfections of what kinds sometimes occur during tetracycline therapy and what measures may be taken to counteract these reactions?

16. (a) What unusual skin reaction has been reported in patients taking tetracyclines?

(b) What dental defect sometimes appears?

(c) What unusual toxic reactions have recently been reported in patients taking tetracyclines?

17. (a) What advantages are claimed for demeclocycline and the recently introduced semisynthetic tetracyclines methacycline and doxycycline over other orally administered tetracycline products?

(b) What advantages is rolitetracycline said to have for patients who require parenteral administration of tetracyclines?

18. (a) List the various organisms responsible for respiratory tract infections that respond to treatment with chloramphenicol.

(b) In what infection is chloramphenicol considered the drug of choice?

19. (a) Dangerous reactions of what types have been reported in patients taking chloramphenicol?

(b) What precautions are taken to detect early signs of these reactions?

20. (a) Under what circumstances are the antibiotics of the group that includes erythromycin and lincomycin mainly employed?

(b) What toxicity has been reported in patients receiving erythromycin estolate and triacetyloleandomycin?

21. (a) What precautions are routinely taken to detect toxic reactions in patients taking novobiocin and in those being treated for long periods with lincomycin?

(b) What are some potential and severe reactions that may limit the utility of ristocetin and of vancomycin?

(c) What newer and seemingly safer antibiotic is now often employed in severe infections that were once treated with ristocetin or vancomycin?

22. (a) What kinds of toxicity are possible when antibiotics of the neomycin, kanamycin, streptomycin subgroup are administered by injection?

(b) In infections of what types may the use of these drugs in this manner sometimes be required?

23. (a) Against what organism are antibiotics of the polymyxin-colistin-gentamycin subgroup especially useful?

(b) How do bacitracin and tyrothricin differ in their antibacterial spectrum from other antibiotics such as polymyxin and neomycin, with which they are often combined?

24. (a) For what purpose are combinations of bacitracin, tyrothricin, neomycin, polymyxin most commonly employed?

(b) What advantages do such combinations have over the topical application of penicillin, or of tetracyclines and other antibiotics?

25. (a) For what three purposes are neomycin and similar antibiotics administered orally?

(b) What danger is present in administering these drugs in this manner to patients with liver and kidney disease?

26. (a) List some disseminated mycoses which have been successfully treated with amphotericin B.

(b) What precautions must be taken to avoid serious toxic reactions to amphotericin?

27. (a) For what purposes are amphotericin and nystatin often applied topically?

(b) For what purposes is griseofulvin taken internally?

BIBLIOGRAPHY

Penicillins and Penicillin-Substitute Type Antibiotics

Dineen, P.: Clinical pharmacology of the semisynthetic penicillins. Clin. Pharmacol. Ther., 3:224, 1962.

Friend, D.: Penicillin G. Clin. Pharmacol. Ther., 7:421, 1966.

Geraci, J. E., Nichols, D. R., and Wellman, W. E.: Vancomycin in serious staphylococcal infections. Arch. Int. Med., 199:507, 1962.

Gilbert, F. L., Jr.: Cholestatic hepatitis caused by esters of erythromycin and oleandomycin. J.A.M.A., 182:1048, 1962.

Griffith, R. S., and Black, H.: Cephalothin, a new antibiotic. J.A.M.A., 189:823, 1964.

Hewitt, W. L.: The penicillins. J.A.M.A., 185:264, 1963.

Klein, J., and Finland, M.: The new penicillins. New Eng. J. Med., 269:1019, 1963.

Koenig, M. G.: The treatment of staphylococcal infections. Med. Clin. N. Am., 47:1231, 1963.

Plotke, R.: Modern trends in the management and control of syphilis. Am. J. Nursing, 55:1482, 1955.

Randall, M. G.: Anaphylactic reactions to penicillin. Nursing Outlook, 4:617, 1956.

Rodman, M. J.: The antibiotics today. R.N., 29:45, 1966 (Nov.).

———: New drugs for fighting infections. R.N., 30:55, 1967 (June).

Sidell, S., et al.: New antistaphylococcal antibiotics. Arch. Int. Med., 112:21, 1963.

Van Arsdel, P. P., Jr.: Allergic reactions to penicillin. J.A.M.A., 191:240, 1965.

Weinstein, L., Kaplan, K., and Chang, T.: Treatment of infections in man with cephalothin. J.A.M.A., 189:829, 1964.

Westerman, G., et al.: Adverse reactions to penicillin. J.A.M.A., 198:173, 1966.

Wise, R. I.: The staphylococcus—approach to therapy. Med. Clin. N. Am., 49:1403, 1965.

Tetracyclines and Chloramphenicol

Best, W. R.: Chloramphenicol-associated blood dyscrasias. J.A.M.A., 201:181, 1967.

Burns, L. E., Hodgman, J. E., and Cass, A. B.: Fatal circulatory collapse in premature infants receiving chloramphenicol. New Eng. J. Med., 261:1318, 1959.

Collins, H. S., and Finland, M.: Treatment of typhoid fever with chloramphenicol. New Eng. J. Med., 241:556, 1949.

Dowling, H., and Lepper, M. H.: Hepatic reactions to tetracyclines. J.A.M.A., 188:307, 1964.

Frimpter, G. W., et al.: Reversible "Fanconi syndrome" caused by degraded tetracycline. J.A.M.A., 184:111, 1963.

Kunin, C. M., and Finland, M.: A new tetracycline antibiotic that yields greater and more sustained antibacterial activity. New Eng. J. Med., 259:999, 1958.

———: Clinical pharmacology of the tetracycline antibiotics. Clin. Pharmacol. Ther., 2:51, 1961.

Kutcher, A. H., et al.: Discoloration of teeth induced by tetracycline. J.A.M.A., 184:586, 1963.

McCurdy, P.: Chloramphenicol bone marrow toxicity. J.A.M.A., 176:588, 1961.

Morris, W. E.: Photosensitivity due to tetracycline derivative. J.A.M.A., 172:1155, 1960.

Vosti, G., Willett, F. M., and Jawetz, E.: Demethylchlortetracycline, a clinical evaluation. Clin. Pharmacol. Ther., 2:29, 1961.

Miscellaneous Antibiotics

Andriole, V. T., and Kravetez, M. H.: The use of amphotericin B in man. J.A.M.A., 180:269, 1962.

Blank, H., et al.: Griseofulvin for the systemic treatment of dermatomycoses. J.A.M.A., 171:2168, 1959.

Butler, W. T.: Pharmacology, toxicity and therapeutic usefulness of amphotericin B. J.A.M.A., 195:371, 1966.

DiPalma, J. R.: The antifungal drugs and their use. R.N., 30:35, 1967 (June).

Fisher, C. J., and Faloon, W. W.: Blood ammonia levels in hepatic cirrhosis. Their control by oral administration of neomycin. New Eng. J. Med., *265:*1030, 1957.

Furcelow, M. L.: The use of amphotericin B in blastomycosis, cryptococcosis and histoplasmosis. Med. Clin. N. Am., *47:*1119, 1963.

————: Histoplasmosis. Am. J. Nursing, *59:*79, 1959.

Jao, R. L., and Jackson, C. G.: Gentamicin sulfate: a new antibiotic against gram-negative bacilli. J.A.M.A., *189:* 817, 1964.

Jawetz, E.: Polymyxin, colistin and bacitracin. Ped. Clin. N. Am., *8:*1057, 1961.

Petersdorf, R. G., and Plorde, J. J.: Colistin—a reappraisal. J.A.M.A., *183:*123, 1963.

Poth, E.: Intestinal antisepsis in surgery. J.A.M.A., *183:* 123, 1963.

Rodman, M. J.: Drugs for fungal infections. R.N., *23:*37, 1960 (July).

Sweeney, F. J., and Rodgers, J. F.: Therapy of infections caused by gram-negative bacilli. Med. Clin. N. Am., *49:* 1391, 1965.

Utz, J. P.: Chemotherapeutic agents for the systemic mycoses. New Eng. J. Med., *268:*983, 1963.

· 35 ·

The Sulfonamides, Other Antibacterial
Chemotherapeutic Agents and Antiviral Agents

THE SULFONAMIDES

History and Current Status

History. Attempts to control the adverse effects of microorganisms with chemicals actually date back thousands of years. Long before men had any idea that putrefaction was caused by tiny, unseen living cells, the ancient Egyptians employed the art of embalming, which was in effect an attempt to halt the destructive effects of microbial activity on human tissues. Later, living tissues were subjected to chemical treatment when the Greeks, Romans and others poured wine and vinegar into wounds to prevent suppuration. In the 16th century, Paracelsus, the Swiss doctor and dabbler in alchemy, advocated the use of inorganic chemicals such as mercury, arsenic, iron and sulfur for treating infectious diseases.

After Koch, Pasteur and other scientists established the existence of bacteria and their significance in the pathogenesis of various diseases, others began to employ germicidal chemicals in medicine. The English surgeon Lister led the way in the 1860's with his discovery that carbolic acid, or liquid phenol, reduced surgical wound infections when applied in washes and dressings. Later, other doctors, seeking substances less likely to destroy healthy tissues along with the putrefactive microbes, introduced salts of heavy metals, such as mercury, silver, and zinc, as well as antiseptic elements—iodine and chlorine, for example—and various bactericidal dyes.

However, none of these disinfectants was safe enough to be taken internally in systemic infections. An antiseptic such as mercury bichloride was more likely to kill the patient than to wipe out the bacterial invaders responsible for blood poisoning, tetanus and similar deadly diseases. The toxicity of the available germicidal chemicals stimulated Paul Ehrlich and his successors to develop new compounds in which poisonous metals such as arsenic, mercury, bismuth and antimony were tied up in complex organic molecules that proved capable of killing pathogenic organisms when administered to patients in relatively harmless amounts (Chap. 33).

Yet, in spite of advances during the 1920's in the chemotherapy of protozoal and spirochetal diseases such as sleeping sickness, syphilis and malaria, millions of people continued to die of blood poisoning, pneumonia, meningitis and other virulent bacterial infections for which no chemical cure existed. Then, in the 1930's, one of a series of dyes that had been synthesized in Germany close to a quarter of a century before was shown to save mice injected with streptococci from an otherwise invariably fatal infection.

The drug, Prontosil, also proved effective in human patients close to death from strep and staph septicemias. Scientists soon learned that this drug's antibacterial activity depended upon its being broken down in the body to a simpler molecular fragment, which they were able to make synthetically. This substance, para-aminobenzenesulfonamide, or *sulfanilamide*, proved immediately successful in clinical trials in the late 1930's against many previously untreatable bacterial infections. Its introduction heralded the start of a new era in anti-infective chemotherapy and, in fact, stimulated research that resulted in great advances in many unrelated areas of drug therapy.

Current Status. The sulfonamide molecule was one of the first of the structures to be intensively studied and modified in efforts to develop congener compounds of even greater antimicrobial activity and safety. Among the more than 5,000 newly synthesized sulfonamides were many that possessed little or no antibacterial activity but proved to have other valuable pharmacological properties. The diuretic drugs of the acetazolamide and thiazide classes (Chap. 20)

480

and the oral antidiabetic drugs of the sulfonylurea group (Chap. 32) were discovered as the result of research leads furnished by scientists working with the related anti-infective sulfa drugs. Despite all this activity, which resulted in replacement of the first sulfonamides by safer, more effective descendants, less than a score of compounds of this class are in clinical use today (see Table 35-1).

The utility of chemotherapeutic agents of this class is now relatively limited as the result of the introduction in the intervening years of numerous antibiotics, one or another of which has proved more dependable for treating most of the infections that were once managed with sulfonamide drug therapy. Nevertheless, there are a few important infections for which these drugs are still considered the best choice (see

Table 35-2). In addition, their administration together with penicillin, tetracycline, streptomycin and other antibiotics in certain difficult-to-treat infections often produces a result superior to that attained with use of the antibiotics alone. Finally, in situations that do not permit use of the antibiotic of choice (in patients allergic to penicillin, for instance) doctors are happy to still have sulfonamide drugs in reserve to help to bring the patient's infection under control.

All of the available sulfa drugs act in essentially the same way to stop the growth of susceptible microorganisms. The major advances in sulfonamide therapy have been made mainly in the development of new drugs that, although they do not strike at a wider range of bacteria than the earlier drugs of this class, are superior by virtue of somewhat greater safety and

TABLE 35-1

SULFONAMIDE DRUGS

NONPROPRIETARY OR OFFICIAL NAME	SYNONYM OR PROPRIETARY NAME	DOSAGE
Highly Soluble, Relatively Rapidly Excreted Agents		
Sulfacetamide N.F.	Sulamyd	4 Gm., then 1 Gm. q. 4 hr.
Sulfamethizole N.F.	Thiosulfil	500 mg. 4 to 6 times daily
Sulfamethoxazole	Gantanol	2 Gm., then 1 Gm. t.i.d.
Sulfisomidine	Elkosin	2 Gm., then 1 Gm. q. 4 hr.
Sulfisoxazole U.S.P.	Gantrisin	4 Gm., then 1 Gm. q. 4 hr.
Acetyl sulfisoxazole N.F.	Gantrisin Acetyl	the equivalent of 4 Gm., then 1 Gm. q. 4 hr.
Soluble Sulfonamides for Combination Therapy		
Sulfadiazine U.S.P.		4 Gm., then 1 Gm. q. 4 hr.
Sulfamerazine U.S.P.		for use in combination
Sulfamethazine U.S.P.		for use in combination
Trisulfapyrimidines U.S.P.		4 Gm., then 1 Gm. q. 4 hr.
Slowly Excreted Sulfonamides		
Sulfadimethoxine N.F.	Madribon	2 Gm., then 1 Gm. daily
Sulfamethoxypyridazine U.S.P.	Kynex; Midicel	1 Gm., then 500 mg. daily
Poorly Absorbed Sulfonamides		
Phthalylsulfathiazole U.S.P.	Sulfathalidine	1 Gm. every 4 hrs.
Succinylsulfathiazole U.S.P.	Sulfasuxidine	1 Gm. every 4 hrs.
p-Nitrosulfathiazole	Nisulfazole	Rectally, 10 ml. of 10% sol.
Salicylazosulfapyridine	Azulfidine	4–8 Gm. daily
Injectable and/or Topical		
Mafenide HCl	Sulfamylon	Topically
Sodium sulfacetamide U.S.P.	Sulamyd sodium	Topically
Sodium sulfadiazine U.S.P.	—	I.V. 4 Gm. of a 5% sol. Repeat in 8 hrs.
Sulfisoxazole diolamine (diethanolamine)	Gantrisin diethanolamine	Topically

TABLE 35-2
ORGANISMS AND INFECTIONS SOMETIMES SUSCEPTIBLE TO SULFONAMIDE TREATMENT

SUSCEPTIBLE ORGANISMS	CURRENT STATUS OF SULFONAMIDE THERAPY
Gram-Positive Cocci	
Streptococcus pyogenes, especially Group A, Beta-Hemolytic Type	Used alone or combined with penicillin for treatment of *upper respiratory tract* infections. Sometimes used for *prophylaxis* against recurrences of *rheumatic fever,* especially in patients sensitive to penicillin.
Staphylococcus aureus	Still sometimes effective, but rarely employed alone.
Pneumococcus	Often administered in combination with penicillin for treatment of *pneumonia* and *meningitis.*
Enterococcus	Rarely employed because usually inferior to antibiotics in sensitivity tests. Ineffective against urinary tract infections caused by these organisms.
Gram-Negative Cocci	
Meningococcus	Very useful against susceptible strains of the organism causing *meningococcal meningitis.* Use of these drugs for mass prophylaxis has led to emergence of resistant strains. Penicillin is usually administered simultaneously.
Gonococcus	No longer useful against most strains of the *gonorrhea* organism after widespread use for prophylaxis during World War II.
Gram-Positive Bacilli	
Bacillus anthracis (Anthrax; "Malignant Pustule") *Clostridium tetani* (Tetanus; "Lockjaw")	Occasionally employed in treating cases of *anthrax* when penicillin cannot be used and erythromycin, tetracycline, and chloramphenicol are ineffective.
Clostridium welchii ("Gas Gangrene") *Corynebacterium diphtheriae*	No longer used for the other diseases caused by gram-positive rods; penicillin, streptomycin, erythromycin, cephalothin, and the broad-spectrum antibiotics are preferred.
Gram-Negative Bacilli	
Escherichia coli *Aerobacter aerogenes* *Aerobacter faecalis* *Klebsiella pneumoniae* Proteus species *Pseudomonas aeruginosa*	Very often useful against *urinary tract* infections by *E. coli* and susceptible strains of *A. aerogenes.* Only rarely effective in infections by other gram-negative rods, which require treatment with a variety of antibiotics.
Shigella species Salmonella species *Vibrio comma*	Sulfonamide-resistant strains have become so common that *bacillary dysentery* caused by Shigella species is rarely responsive. Used only occasionally for *acute gastroenteritis* caused by *V. comma* (*cholera*). Used rarely for salmonella infections, including *typhoid* and *paratyphoid.*
Hemophilus influenzae	Effective in *meningitis* caused by this organism, but employed mainly as adjuncts to antibiotics such as streptomycin, chloromycetin, tetracycline and ampicilllin.
Hemophilus ducreyi	Quite effective against this organism, the cause of chancroid, a venereal disease.

TABLE 35-2 (Continued)

SUSCEPTIBLE ORGANISMS	CURRENT STATUS OF SULFONAMIDE THERAPY
Gram-Negative Bacilli (*Continued*)	
Pasteurella pestis	Effective against the organism responsible for *bubonic plague*, when used alone or combined with streptomycin.
Brucella species	Now rarely used in *undulant fever*, which is treated with antibiotics.
Large Viruses	
Lymphogranuloma Venereum Agent	Effective in this *venereal disease*, but broad-spectrum antibiotics are preferred.
Trachoma Agent	Quite effective when applied topically to the *eyes* or administered orally, alone or combined with tetracycline.
Fungi	
Nocardia asteroides	Effective in the disseminated fungal infection, *nocardiosis*, alone or combined with broad-spectrum antibiotics, or with streptomycin or cycloserine.
Actinomyces	Effective only occasionally when added to penicillin, the drug of choice in *actinomycosis*.
Histoplasmosis capsulatum	An occasional alternative to the antifungal antibiotic, amphotericin B.

the ease with which they can be administered to achieve particular therapeutic purposes.

Thus, as we shall see, certain sulfonamides, such as sulfisoxazole and sulfamethizole, seem particularly suited for treating urinary tract infections, because their solubility and rapid renal excretion permits them to reach high, yet safe, bactericidal concentrations in urine. Other drugs, such as phthalylsulfathiazole and succinylsulfathiazole, have physical properties that allow them to reach high antibacterial levels in the lumen of the gastrointestinal tract. Still other sulfonamides, such as sulfadimethoxine and sulfamethoxypyridazine, stay in the tissues for relatively long periods—a property that makes them especially suitable for long-term prophylaxis programs against certain infections.

Bacterial Spectrum and Manner of Action

Antibacterial Activity. As can be seen by studying Table 35-2, the sulfonamides are effective against a wide range of microorganisms—gram-positive and gram-negative cocci and bacilli, and even some large viruses and fungi. Even though some strains of once susceptible organisms have acquired resistance to these drugs, the sulfonamides are still effective against most of the kinds of bacteria that cause the dread diseases that the first sulfonamides helped to control. These include most strains of streptococci, pneumococci, meningococci and pathogenic gram-

negative rods such as the hemophilus group of bacilli, *E. coli*, and other coliform organisms.

The sulfonamides, unlike penicillin, are mainly bacteriostatic rather than bactericidal drugs. This means that they must be given in doses large enough to keep susceptible bacteria from multiplying. Only then can the body's own defenses function effectively to destroy the pathogens by phagocytosis and other means. If sulfonamides are given in doses that deliver too little of the drug to the tissues too late, the patient may be beyond saving before the drug can stop bacterial division enough to produce a favorable effect on the infection.

Resistance. Another reason for administering sulfonamides in full therapeutic dosage is that inadequate amounts tend to aid the development of resistant strains of microorganisms. As explained in Chapter 33, administration of sulfonamides in doses that tend to leave alive even a small proportion of the more resistant members of the bacterial population favors the emergence of new families that are less susceptible than the parent strains were when they were first exposed to these antibacterial drugs. That this is more than mere theory is borne out by what has happened in clinical practice when sulfonamides have been used promiscuously in subtherapeutic doses.

Thus, the sulfonamides at first produced dramatic cures in cases of gonorrhea. Later, after the sulfonamides had been widely used for prophylaxis of venereal disease during World War II, most gonorrheal infections encountered in many areas were no longer susceptible to sulfonamide treatment. Apparently, the low dose regimens employed for preventing this disease had fostered the survival of sulfonamide-resistant strains of the gonococcus. Similarly, the routine use of sulfonamides to protect army recruits from respiratory infections soon produced sulfonamide-resistant strains of staphylococci, and the continued careless use of sulfa drugs seems even to have resulted in some resistance among the once very sensitive meningococci.

Public health authorities have urged doctors to order sulfonamides only when they are reasonably certain that the patient is suffering from an infection that is more susceptible to treatment with these drugs than to any other available anti-infective agent. Then the sulfonamides are administered in doses that hit the organisms hard, fast and continuously until long after the patient's fever or other symptoms of infection have passed. Sometimes the combination of sulfonamides with certain antibiotics (Table 35-2) is especially useful both for bringing the infection under control and for preventing development of new strains of resistant microorganisms.

Manner of Action. Scientists have sought to learn just what it is about the sulfonamide molecular structure that makes it so useful for stopping the propagation of susceptible organisms. It is apparent that the configuration of the basic molecule closely resembles that of the B-complex vitamin para-aminobenzoic acid (PABA), which many bacteria require in their diet in order to grow and reproduce. One widely held view is that the presence of the sulfa molecule in the medium keeps bacteria from using the available PABA. The drug molecule is close enough to PABA in structure to take the place of this essential metabolite in important enzyme systems. The drug fits into the place ordinarily occupied by the PABA molecule; however, it cannot perform the metabolic function of the vitamin, and its presence keeps the PABA from being utilized. As a result of such *competitive antagonism* (Chap. 2) by the sulfa drug, the bacteria are unable to synthesize substances that are necessary for further growth before they can divide and produce daughter cells.

This theory also explains both why some organisms are congenitally resistant or capable of acquiring resistance and why the sulfonamides are safe for most people to take in antibacterial doses. Susceptible bacteria require PABA in order to make another B-complex vitamin, folic acid, which serves as a component of coenzymes needed for the synthesis of nucleic acids. Blockade by sulfa molecules keeps the bacteria from incorporating PABA into the folic acid molecules that must be built before the bacterial cell nucleus can fully mature and then divide.

The cells of human beings (and of non-susceptible microorganisms) do not need to manufacture folic acid from smaller dietary fragments. They utilize dietary folic acid directly. Consequently, these drugs that "starve out" the bacterial cells, which require PABA, have no effect on mammalian cells and on microorganisms that have no similar need for PABA. The strains of organisms that become resistant to sulfonamides are thought to stem from ancestors that either learned to get along without PABA (that is, they followed a metabolic pathway different from that of most organisms of the species) or learned to make their own PABA in such abundance that its molecules can compete successfully against the sulfa drug molecules for the active centers (p. 30) in the cell's enzymatically controlled metabolic machinery.

Metabolism

The main differences between the various sulfonamide subgroups lie in the way the body handles them from the time they enter until they leave. That is, the comparative efficacy of various sulfonamides for treatment of a particular kind of infection is determined by: (1) how rapidly and completely it is *absorbed;* (2) the extent to which its molecules are *bound* to plasma proteins; (3) the way in which the free molecule is *distributed* into the infected tissues; (4) the manner in which the molecule is *inactivated* and *converted* into a more readily excreted metabolite, and (5) the rate and ease of its *excretion.* In the following discussion, we shall attempt to relate these metabolic factors to the clinical utility of various representative sulfonamide drugs.

Absorption. Most sulfonamide drugs are rapidly absorbed from the stomach and small intestine when taken by mouth. Thus, when adequate doses are administered by the convenient oral route, therapeutically effective concentrations build up quickly in the blood stream. Certain sulfonamides are also available in soluble form that permits their parenteral injection when higher tissue concentrations are required for treating severe infections in patients who may be unconscious, vomiting or unable to swallow tablets or suspensions. Sodium sulfadiazine and sulfisoxazole diethanolamine, for example, may be administered subcutaneously or intramuscularly. However, although these forms permit ready absorption of the sulfonamides into the plasma, the preferred parenteral route is by vein, which puts the sulfa drug directly into the blood stream with minimal tissue irritation when the solution is injected slowly and with care to avoid leakage into surrounding tissues.

Poorly Absorbable Sulfonamides. Certain sulfonamides (Table 35-1) are not very readily absorbed into the systemic circulation after they are swallowed. This characteristic, which keeps these drugs from reaching effective antibacterial concentrations in the tissues, makes them ideally suited for striking at susceptible organisms in the lumen of the intestinal tract. The preferred sulfonamides of this type are *phthalylsulfathiazole* and *succinylsulfathiazole* (see Drug Digest), both of which are broken down by intestinal bacteria to sulfathiazole, the active agent. The high levels of this substance that are achieved locally markedly suppress the coliform organisms of the bacterial flora.

These drugs are used mainly prior to abdominal surgery to lessen the likelihood of postoperative infections from contamination by *E. coli,* clostridia and related gram-negative cocci and rods. The usefulness of this procedure is controversial, as is indicated in the discussion of the use of certain antibiotics (Chap. 34) for the same purpose. (Neomycin is commonly combined with phthalylsulfathiazole for preoperative sterilization of the bowel.) Some of these drugs are also used in the management of ulcerative colitis and in the prophylaxis and treatment of bacillary dysentery resulting from shigella infection. However, as many as 90 per cent of strains of this organism are now said to be resistant to sulfonamides, and these drugs are rarely given alone but are used in combination with various antibiotics. In any case, sulfadiazine or other soluble sulfonamides are preferred for treatment of actual infections of the intestinal wall, through which they are excreted.

Protein binding and distribution of absorbed sulfonamides are also significant in determining the degree of utility of various compounds. Drug molecules that are tied to plasma proteins are bacteriostatically inactive, but they are also kept from being excreted by the kidneys while so attached. Portions of the drugs that are released in free form from this floating plasma depot at variable rates make their way to the fluids bathing various tissues. There, they exert their bacteriostatic effects upon pathogenic bacteria before being excreted by the kidneys. The exceptionally long-acting sulfonamides, *sulfamethoxypyridazine* (see Drug Digest) and *sulfadimethoxine* (Table 35-1) are said to owe part of their prolonged antibacterial effects to the fact that they are largely bound to blood proteins from which they are only very slowly released.

The freed fractions of all the sulfa drugs diffuse very readily into body fluids including the cerebrospinal fluid. Thus, when *sulfadiazine* (see Drug Digest) is administered by mouth or intravenously to patients with meningococcal or *Hemophilus influenzae* meningitis, it readily reaches therapeutic levels in the cerebrospinal fluid. Because of its ability to penetrate the inflamed meninges so readily, it does not have to be given by intrathecal injection, and, in fact, its instillation by this relatively dangerous subarachnoid route is contraindicated. The first dose of sulfadiazine sodium is given by vein in a saline infusion and followed by oral doses, if the patient is able to swallow. Penicillin is often administered simultaneously in meningococcal and pneumococcal meningitis, and streptomycin or chloramphenicol are given with full doses of sulfadiazine for meningitis caused by *Hemophilus influenzae.*

Biotransformations of sulfonamides are carried out mainly in the liver. Enzymatically catalyzed reactions occur in which some sulfonamide molecules are oxidized, but most are conjugated with acetic acid or with glucuronic acid. The resulting acetyl sulfonamide derivatives and glucuronides are no longer active against bacteria and are excreted in the urine.

Glucuronide derivatives are always quite soluble in the urine. Thus, a compound such as sulfadimethoxine (Table 35-1), which is largely converted to its glucuronide, is unlikely to precipitate out as crystals (see p. 486). On the other hand, early sulfonamides such as sulfanilamide and sulfathiazole are transformed into acetyl derivatives which are actually *less* soluble in acid urine than the parent compound, thus increasing the danger of crystalluria. The newer, highly soluble sulfonamides (Table 35-1) are converted to acetyl derivatives that are usually even *more* soluble than the parent compound—a factor in their detoxification which adds to their safety.

Renal Excretion. Free, or unbound, sulfonamide molecules are filtered through the kidney glomeruli, and the fraction that is not reabsorbed by the renal tubules appears in the urine. With some of the rapidly excreted sulfonamides, such as sulfadiazine (see Drug Digest), sulfisomidine, sulfamethizole, sulfacetamide (Table 35-1), and sulfisoxazole (see Drug Digest), concentrations of free drug may be so high that microorganisms in the urinary tract are not merely kept from reproducing—they are actually killed. That is, the drugs are concentrated in the urine to levels that are bacteri*cidal* rather than just bacterio*static.* This is the basis for the use of these and other sulfonamides in the treatment of acute pyelonephritis, cystitis, urethritis and also sometimes for control of chronic and recurrent urinary tract infections.

The rapidly excreted drugs are preferred for treatment of acute urinary tract infections; the long-lasting sulfonamides that need be taken only once daily have been recommended for long-term treatment and for prophylaxis. Thus, *sulfadimethoxypyridazine* (see Drug Digest) has been used for prevention of urinary tract infections in paraplegics and in patients with multiple sclerosis and others with a neurogenic bladder disorder. (Patients with structural and functional difficulties that lead to stagnation of urine in which bacteria may rapidly multiply are most subject to chronic urinary tract infections.)

The desirability of administering rapidly excreted sulfonamides on a short-term basis for prophylactic purposes during catheterization is at the present time undecided. Some authorities have suggested that all women who have to be catheterized following delivery be given sulfonamides routinely. They argue that postpartum catheterization—and, indeed, pregnancy itself

—predisposes women to bacterial contamination of the urinary tract. Such bacteriuria, often asymptomatic at first, may be the cause of chronic infections marked by frequent flare-ups of kidney-damaging pyelonephritis that can eventually lead to kidney failure. Thus, some doctors administer sulfisoxazole, sulfadiazine, trisulfapyrimidines, or other soluble sulfonamides for a few days before and after childbirth and to all patients with indwelling catheters. Other doctors feel that the indiscriminate routine administration of these and other anti-infective drugs is undesirable, since it may result in overgrowth of resistant organisms or the patient may become sensitized to sulfonamides and unnecessarily suffer a toxic reaction (see below).

Side Effects and Toxicity

Although most patients suffer no ill effects from short courses of the more recently developed sulfonamides, these drugs still possess considerable potential for causing very dangerous reactions. Broadly speaking, these are of two kinds: (1) urinary tract damage as a result of crystalluria, and (2) hypersensitivity reactions involving the bone marrow, blood, liver, skin and peripheral nervous system.

Reactions of the first type occur much less frequently with today's more soluble sulfonamides than in the early days of sulfa drug therapy. However, the incidence of sensitivity-type reactions is as high as ever. Thus, patients on sulfonamide drugs must be closely observed for signs of adverse reactions that will require immediate discontinuance of these agents and prompt employment of measures to minimize further toxicity.

Renal damage and injury to other urinary tract tissues results mainly from the formation of sulfonamide drug crystals in the kidneys, ureters or bladder. It may be manifested by hematuria, oliguria and, finally, anuria, azotemia and a sometimes fatal uremia. Because some of the earlier sulfonamides and their acetyl derivatives tended especially to precipitate in acid urine, it became customary to try to alkalinize the patient's urine by having him take a teaspoonful of sodium bicarbonate or some other systemic alkalinizer with each dose of sulfa drug. This is rarely necessary today with drugs such as sulfacetamide (Table 35-1), sulfamethizole, sulfisomidine, and sulfisoxazole, which are much more soluble in acid urine than the older drugs. Nevertheless, even with these drugs, the other measure that became routine—i.e., maintenance of a high fluid intake—must never be neglected. Patients should be encouraged to drink enough fluids to produce at least 1,200 ml. of urine daily, and, of course, the amount of urine eliminated should be measured and recorded. The doctor may also want each urine sample examined for the presence of crystals in the sediment that forms on standing.

Even before the development of the newest highly soluble sulfonamides, an interesting discovery had helped to reduce the danger of crystalluria. It was found that a solution of urine (or other aqueous liquid) that is saturated with one sulfonamide can dissolve a second, a third and even a fourth sulfonamide in amounts up to the saturation point of each because the presence of one sulfa drug in solution does not alter the solubility of other chemically related agents. Therefore, instead of administering a full therapeutic dose of *sulfadiazine,* one third of the dose of this drug is combined with equal fractions of the full dose of *sulfamerazine* and *sulfamethazine,* two related pyrimidine-type sulfonamides. The mixture, called *trisulfapyrimidines* (Table 35-1), contains a total dose of sulfonamides capable of controlling susceptible bacteria. Yet it is only about one third as likely to cause crystalluria and kidney complications as an equally effective amount of a single sulfonamide. The solubility of the mixture in urine can be further enhanced by administering a systemic alkalinizer such as lactate, acetate, citrate or bicarbonate, but this is seldom considered necessary today, and most doctors prefer to avoid the complications that could occur from too vigorous attempts to make the urine more alkaline.

Crystalluria is uncommon when the long-acting sulfonamides are administered in proper dosage, because only a small part of the daily dosage of these slowly excreted drugs appears in the urine at any one time. Most of the free molecules that are slowly released from plasma proteins and filtered by the glomeruli are reabsorbed by the renal tubules and find their way back into the blood stream. The acetylated derivative of sulfamethoxypyridazine and the glucuronide metabolite of sulfadimethoxine, which are not so readily reabsorbed as the free forms of these drugs, are even more soluble in acid urine than the parent compound.

The risk of kidney damage by these prolonged-action drugs lies only in the chance of overdosage administered through error. Unlike the earlier sulfonamides, which were given in initial doses of as much as 4 grams, followed by another gram every 4 hours around the clock, a single daily dose of 0.5 Gm. of the slowly excreted sulfonamides is usually enough to keep the drug at the bacteriostatic levels reached on the first day of treatment with a priming or loading dose of only 1.0 Gm. Sometimes initial doses of 2 Gm. may be followed by 1 Gm. every 24 hours. Higher doses are unnecessary and potentially dangerous. Thus, if a full daily dose of a long-acting agent—often a single tablet—were mistakenly ordered on the same dosage schedule as some of the earlier drugs, disastrously high levels could quickly accumulate in the patient's blood and kidneys. The nurse must be ready to question any unusual order for the low-dose sulfonamides, and the doctor often orders that the patient's blood be checked periodically by the laboratory to see that sulfonamide levels are maintained in the safe therapeutic range and that they neither fall below nor rise alarmingly above it.

Sulfonamide sensitization and direct toxicity occur less often with today's drugs than with such earlier agents as sulfanilamide, sulfapyridine, and sulfathiazole. The incidence of side effects such as nausea, vomiting, dizziness, and headache has dropped from close to 30 per cent with the earlier sulfonamides to under 10 per cent with those most frequently employed today. Nevertheless, patients who have an idiosyncrasy to sulfonamides or who become sensitized to them can sometimes suffer from various kinds of potentially dangerous reactions.

Blood dyscrasias of various kinds, including acute hemolytic anemia, thrombocytopenia, agranulocytosis and aplastic anemia have been reported. Although these do not occur frequently, patients are watched closely because of the seriousness of such reactions. The occurrence of hepatitis, also, which is a relatively rare complication of sulfonamide therapy, has led to death. Thus, these drugs are contraindicated in patients with a history of blood disorders and liver damage, as well as those with renal insufficiency.

Dermatological reactions of various kinds have been reported. Sometimes urticaria has occurred as part of an anaphylactoid reaction in sensitized individuals. Eruptions of various other types also are seen, often in patients who have exposed themselves to sunlight during treatment (photosensitivity). Most serious of all has been the development of severe exfoliative dermatitis and of bullous (blistery) eruptions, which have occurred both with and without episodes of drug fever.

Stevens-Johnson syndrome, a serious non-specific reaction involving the skin, mucous membranes, respiratory tract and other organs, has recently been associated with the administration of the long-acting sulfonamides. The Food and Drug Administration considers the danger so serious that they have required such sulfonamides to be labeled to indicate that the shorter-acting drugs be used in preference to the longer-acting drugs wherever possible. The reason for this is that the latter agents, because of their slow excretion, may continue to produce adverse effects long after they have been discontinued at the first sign of a bullous rash. Actually, however, this serious condition can occur with the shorter-acting drugs and, indeed, in many other circumstances.

Topical Application and Special Uses

Topically applied sulfonamide ointments and creams were once used indiscriminately in prevention and treatment of skin infections. These drugs are rarely used in this way today because it has become clear that topical application of the sulfonamides is a common cause of allergic sensitization and that these drugs are not very effective in the presence of pus and tissue debris on the skin and mucous membranes.

However, certain sulfonamides are employed topically in eye and ear infections and to prevent sepsis in extensive burns, as well as in certain vaginal and intestinal disorders. Sulfacetamide sodium (see Drug Digest) and sulfisoxazole diolamine, for example, have some properties that favor their use as bactericidal agents in eye infections such as conjunctivitis, blepharitis and keratitis, as well as in trachoma. Sulfisoxazole diolamine is sometimes also applied topically in external ear infections and for chronic sinus infections.

Some sulfonamides are available in cream form for use in treating vaginal and cervical infections, including senile vaginitis, in which these agents are applied topically in conjunction with estrogens. The poorly soluble sulfonamide, para-nitrosulfathiazole, is sometimes instilled rectally for its local effects in ulcerative colitis. Another agent, Sulfamylon, has recently been reported effective for preventing infections by pseudomonas and other gram-negative bacteria when applied in ointment form to deep burns covering 30 to 50 per cent of the body. Despite side effects from systemic absorption, the drug was considered beneficial because it prevented septic extension of the skin damage and reduced the amount of surface area requiring grafts.

Sulfapyridine, a drug largely discarded since the development of safer sulfonamides, is employed empirically by dermatologists in the treatment of dermatitis herpetiformis. For reasons as obscure as the cause of the condition itself, administration of sulfapyridine often stops vesiculation, itching and burning within a few days. Because it must be administered daily for months in smaller doses for maintenance of the improvement, some doctors have tried transferring patients to treatment with the more convenient long-acting agent, sulfamethoxypyridazine. The latter drug has also been advocated as a substitute for dapsone (see p. 493) in the management of leprosy, and other sulfonamides are being reinvestigated for treating resistant types of malaria.

OTHER ANTI-INFECTIVE AGENTS USED IN URINARY TRACT INFECTIONS

The usefulness of sulfonamide therapy of urinary tract infections is sometimes limited by: (1) emergence of resistant strains of gram-negative bacteria, and (2) development of sensitization to sulfonamides and subsequent allergy requiring the withdrawal of the drug. Fortunately, various old and new chemotherapeutic agents and antibiotics are available for treating acute and chronic infections of urinary tract tissues.

Methenamine mandelate (see Drug Digest) is an interesting combination of two older urinary tract antiseptics, the urinary acidifier mandelic acid and methenamine, a substance that is converted to formaldehyde in an acid urine. The concentration of formaldehyde in the urine is non-irritating to the tissues over which it washes, but it exerts a bactericidal effect upon various pathogens including some resistant to the sulfonamides.

However, the effectiveness of this antiseptic is limited to the mucosal surfaces, and it does not reach the deeper tissues. Thus, it is sometimes combined with antibiotics or sulfonamides that do affect infections in the interstitial kidney tissues. In pyelitis, for example, methenamine mandelate is sometimes administered together with the sulfonamide sulfamethizole. Unlike other less soluble sulfa drugs, this one stays in solution in acid urine and does not require administration of supplementary urinary alkalinizers to increase its solubility. These would, of course, interfere with the conversion of methenamine mandelate to mandelic acid and formaldehyde.

Occasionally, methenamine mandelate must itself be supplemented with urinary acidifiers in order to make the patient's urine sufficiently acid to form formaldehyde. Ammonium chloride and the amino acid methionine are sometimes employed for this purpose. The danger of systemic acidosis in such situations makes the administration of such combinations undesirable in patients with renal insufficiency. The combination of methenamine mandelate with sulfamethizole often turns the patient's urine turbid, presumably because the freed formaldehyde combines with the sulfonamide in the urine to form a precipitate. This is said not to be dangerous, but it is wise to warn the patient not to worry about such sedimentation.

Other chemotherapeutic agents sometimes substituted for sulfonamides in treating urinary tract infections are *nitrofurantoin* (see Drug Digest) and *nalidixic acid*. The former is a member of the furan family of antimicrobial chemicals, and the latter is a new synthetic antibacterial that is especially effective against gram-negative urinary tract invaders. Both these drugs are said to cause fewer side effects than the sulfonamides while exerting antibacterial effects against sulfonamide-resistant organisms.

The main advantage of nalidixic acid at present lies in its capacity to strike at many strains of Proteus species that are not controlled by other urinary antiseptics. However, it has already been noted that, contrary to the case with methenamine mandelate and nitrofurantoin, many urinary tract pathogens quickly develop a high degree of resistance to this antibacterial drug. In addition, although the incidence of side effects seems low, the drug has occasionally caused neurological disturbances, including convulsions, in children. Care is required in patients with renal and hepatic impairment and in those with nervous system disorders.

Another agent that is commonly combined with sulfonamides is the azo dye, *phenazopyridine*. Although introduced originally as a urinary antiseptic, this sub-stance exerts little antibacterial activity. It is said, however, to have a soothing topical anesthetic effect upon the urinary tract mucosa when excreted in the patient's urine. This tends to relieve the burning pain and the feeling of urgency which lead to the patient's frequent desire to void; it thus helps to reduce the patient's restlessness and wakefulness. (Anticholinergic drugs (Chap. 17) also are often administered in cystitis to relieve the reflex bladder muscle spasm of cystitis, which is a cause of pain, urgency and frequency.) Patients taking preparations containing this azo dye are warned that their urine may be colored orange or red, lest they worry about "blood" in the urine.

Antibiotic drugs are often effective for treating infections of urinary tract tissues caused by strains of organisms resistant to the sulfonamides and other chemotherapeutic agents. Infections caused by *Pseudomonas aeruginosa,* an organism that is difficult to eradicate, are best treated with the antibiotics polymyxin B sulfate, colistimethate sodium, and the experimental antibiotic, gentamycin (see Chap. 34). However, these antibiotics, like kanamycin and neomycin, which are especially effective against Proteus and Klebsiella species, must be used with great care because of their potential toxicity. They may cause kidney damage, and this, in turn, may result in tissue accumulation, with damage to the auditory nerve and possible permanent deafness.

Recently, neomycin and polymyxin have been employed in a solution which is used to irrigate the G.U. tract topically, in order to prevent infections following the use of an indwelling catheter, which is a very frequent cause of gram-negative bacteriuria and bacteremia. This method of administration is, of course, safer than the parenteral route for these drugs.

THE CHEMOTHERAPY OF TUBERCULOSIS

Current Status of Tuberculosis

Tuberculosis has long been one of the most prevalent of the infectious diseases that afflict man. Bones found in archeological diggings show evidence of tuberculous damage, thus indicating the presence of the disease even among prehistoric peoples. The earliest Egyptian and Greek medical writers describe the course and clinical features of the pulmonary form of this disease. During the last century, pulmonary tuberculosis—or consumption, as it was called on account of the wasting away of its victims—still remained the greatest killer of young men and women in their twenties and thirties.

Actually, the rod-shaped tubercule bacillus, *Mycobacterium tuberculosis,* attacks not only the lungs but body tissue of all types. Crippling can occur as a result of invasion of the bones and joints. The kidneys, bladder and other tissues of the genitourinary tract are subject to progressive destruction by tuberculous lesions. Children are especially subject to tuberculosis of the meninges and the central nervous system, as well as to generalized, or miliary, tuberculosis in which bacteria are seeded all through the body. These forms of the disease once had a mortality rate of close to 100 per cent.

The death rate from tuberculosis had dropped remarkably in most countries during this century. At first, this was probably the result of better sanitation, improved living conditions and more wholesome nutrition—factors which helped to reduce the spread of infection and to raise people's resistance to bacterial invasion. The even more dramatic drop in tuberculosis mortality since World War II—a reduction of 75 per cent—can be traced directly to the introduction since that time of a number of chemotherapeutic agents capable of arresting the infection.

The development of drugs effective against tuberculosis has brought about many changes in the management of this condition. For example, patients are no longer confined to sanatoria for very long periods. More and more, people are first being treated in general hospitals where they receive intensive drug therapy for perhaps four to six weeks. Then they most often continue to take their medication at home, returning to the hospital periodically as outpatients for follow-up studies during the next year or two.

Some patients are still sent to a sanatorium for six months or so, if there is fear that they might infect children or other highly susceptible people at home, or if their infection is considered especially serious. Such cases include those marked by the presence of open cavities that fail to close despite drug-induced relief of most symptoms. Even in such patients, the ability of tuberculostatic drug therapy to halt tissue destruction has been helpful. The surgical procedures employed today for the removal of unhealed tissues are far less extensive than they once were, because chemotherapy keeps pulmonary and other lesions more localized.

Despite the decrease in the death rate and the relative ease of controlling the disease with drugs, tuberculosis is still an important public health problem. Millions of people in this country and throughout the world are infected, even though they may show no clinical symptoms. Many former patients whose disease has been arrested carry living tubercle bacilli in walled-off lesions. Thus, drugs have not lessened the need to continue traditional measures employed to prevent infection or detect its presence.

Chemotherapy of Tuberculosis

First-Line Drugs. *The drugs most effective* in the treatment of tuberculosis today are the antibiotic streptomycin and the synthetic chemicals isoniazid and aminosalicylic acid (see Drug Digests). These drugs are rarely administered singly. They are instead given in various kinds of combinations, because their tuberculostatic action is somewhat increased and their toxicity to the patient lessened to some extent, when two or more agents are given together. A more important advantage is that combination therapy seems to slow the rate at which resistant strains of tubercle bacilli develop.

Resistance to antituberculosis drugs is not only a public health problem but one which often threatens the patient himself during his treatment course.

Most short-term acute infections are cleared up by drug treatment before emerging resistant microbes can harm the patient. The slowly growing tuberculosis organisms, however, are not rapidly eradicated by chemotherapy. Protected by the necrotic tissue of the tubercles in which they are lodged, many bacteria remain alive for long periods. Some of these undergo mutations (Chap. 33) that produce new strains which are insensitive to concentrations of the chemotherapeutic agents that had at first stopped the growth of earlier strains of the organism.

Thus, when streptomycin is administered alone, as it once was, it at first stops the growth of all the susceptible tubercle bacilli that it reaches. The patient's fever falls, he coughs less often and feels less fatigued. Within a month, however, if he still has open lesions, many bacteria isolated from his sputum prove to be resistant to streptomycin in laboratory tests. After just a few months of treatment, most of the patient's bacteria no longer respond to even extremely high concentrations of the antibiotic. The patient treated only with streptomycin soon suffers a severe relapse. His fever, cough, and feelings of weariness return; he begins to lose weight again; worst of all, X-ray reveals a widening of the open cavities in his lungs or an extension of necrotic areas in other tissues.

Fortunately, most patients today do not take this downhill course. The present availability of isoniazid (INH) and of para-aminosalicylic acid (PAS) for administration with streptomycin or with one another has helped control most infections before resistant strains can develop in numbers large enough to overwhelm the patient's defenses. Somehow, the combined actions of any two or of all three of these drugs delays the development of strains of tubercle bacilli resistant to chemotherapy.

Combined Therapy. The synthetic chemicals themselves are not capable of continued effectiveness against the tuberculosis organism for long periods. On the contrary, even though isoniazid is a very effective tuberculostat at the start of treatment, organisms soon emerge that are much less sensitive to this drug. Similarly, resistance develops to PAS, which is a much weaker anti-infective agent to begin with. Yet, when the two are given together, their combined effects somehow allow a much longer period of successful treatment. Administered together with streptomycin, these synthetic chemotherapeutic agents also add to the effectiveness of the antibiotic.

Thus, doctors often give these three drugs together for treating tuberculous meningitis and miliary tuberculosis. When such a regimen is begun early enough and kept up for as long as two or three years, the development of new strains of virulent organisms does not usually occur, and these infections once almost inevitably fatal, are brought under control.

In other, less immediately serious but more chronic tuberculosis infections, most patients continue to maintain their early improvement.

Response. Patients with pulmonary tuberculosis who are treated with combinations of INH and PAS, or of INH and streptomycin, for example, frequently follow the following response pattern:

1. Temperature returns to normal; coughing is less severe; appetite improves and there is a gain in weight and a general feeling of well-being.

2. Sputum is reduced in amount, and the number of bacteria that can be cultured is steadily reduced until, finally, all cultures are negative.

3. X-ray findings indicate improvement of an objective type, as lesions regress in size, stabilize, and undergo gradual healing.

Such improvement does not mean that the patient is cured. Often, caseous (cheesy) lesions harbor tubercle bacilli resistant to all three primary drugs. If the patient's natural defenses stay strong, these organisms may never break out and renew their attack, the lesions may become fibrotic and eventually they may calcify completely. This is a very slow process, during which surviving bacilli may at any time become active again and cause an extension of the disease. (This is why one speaks of tuberculosis as being "arrested" rather than "cured.")

The nurse can help prevent such relapses by encouraging the patient to continue with his drug regimen and follow all of the doctor's orders. Patients who feel remarkably better may want to stop taking the drugs, especially if—as with PAS—these agents cause stomach upset or other discomfort. It must be made clear to the patient that dropping his chemotherapeutic regimen can lead to a flare-up of infection by lurking microorganisms. The patient must be made to understand that he is compromising not only his own welfare but the welfare of others whom he could infect. Thus, the nurse's teaching should stress the value of the treatment both in hastening the patient's recovery and preventing tubercular complications, but also the importance of protecting his family—including especially susceptible children—his co-workers and others. If there is reason to believe that the patient is not taking his drugs, periodic checks of his urine

should be made for the presence of the medication and its metabolites.

Isoniazid (see Drug Digest) is the most generally useful of the three primary tuberculostatic drugs. This is, in part, because of the ease with which it is able to make its way into the fluids bathing all body tissues including the cerebrospinal and pleural fluids. This property plus its ability to penetrate into the necrotic center of infected tubercles enable it to reach bacteriostatic levels in the affected tissues of patients with all forms of the disease, including tuberculous meningitis. This drug is so useful that it may not be withdrawn even when organisms resistant to it begin to develop because its presence may still somehow synergize the action of the streptomycin with which it is commonly combined in the treatment of infections of the more serious kinds.

Streptomycin (see Drug Digest) is today often reserved for use, in combination with isoniazid, in the more complicated cases. These include tuberculous pneumonia, tuberculous meningitis, genitourinary, and miliary, or disseminated, tuberculosis, as well as in advanced cases of cavitary pulmonary tuberculosis. In bone and joint disease, the INH and streptomycin are sometimes instilled directly into infected joints and bone sinuses, after the bony lesions have been freed of necrotic tissue by débridement and the sinuses have been surgically drained.

Such local instillation of streptomycin helps also to keep its systemic toxicity to a minimum. The main difficulty with this drug—besides the rapidity with which tubercle bacilli tend to develop resistance—is the adverse effect of continuous treatment on the auditory nerve and the labyrinth of the inner ear. Patients taking the large daily doses needed for weeks or months in tuberculous meningitis often suffer from vertigo, ringing in the ears and, finally, hearing impairment that may end in permanent deafness.

Doctors try to avoid this by administering the drug only two or three times a week instead of every day, once the patient's worst symptoms are brought under control. Another measure that was once tried was to combine it in fractional amounts with the related drug, dihydrostreptomycin, on the theory that this would reduce the potential toxicity of each, while their bacteriostatic effects would be additive. This did not work out very well, and dihydrostreptomycin is used today in tuberculosis only when patients are allergic to streptomycin but not yet sensitive to its derivative. Bacteria that become resistant to one of these drugs are also insensitive to the other.

Aminosalicylic acid (PAS; see Drug Digest) is not as active as streptomycin or isoniazid in halting the growth of tubercle bacilli. Yet it is so valuable for improving the effectiveness of the latter drugs that patients must be encouraged to take the large daily doses that are needed, even when they complain of heartburn, nausea and other drug-induced gastrointestinal discomfort. The drug's usefulness as a supplement to isoniazid and streptomycin has led to efforts to prepare more palatable and less irritating derivatives.

In addition to the sodium, potassium and calcium salts, which are said to produce less gastric irritation than the parent acid, there are now available an ester derivative, phenyl aminosalicylate, and calcium benzoylpas, the calcium salt of a benzamido derivative. Both drugs are more palatable than the earlier ones and may produce less gastrointestinal distress; and the lack of soluble ions such as sodium and potassium in these compounds may make them preferable in the treatment of tuberculous patients who suffer from cardiac, kidney or liver disorders. Of course, other patients may react unfavorably to these calcium and phenyl derivatives.

Second-Line Drugs. The difficulties often encountered in the long-term use of the most effective tuberculostatic chemotherapeutic combination have stimulated a continuing search for new drugs with which to treat tuberculosis. None of the newer agents available has proved superior to the first-line drugs. However, they may be useful and, indeed, even lifesaving in some circumstances.

These secondary drugs are sometimes substituted when (1) one of the major drugs, such as isoniazid, PAS, or streptomycin, must be dropped from a patient's regimen because of his adverse reactions to it, or (2) the development of bacterial resistance to a drug like streptomycin has made it worthless for further control of a particular patient's infection. The difficulty with all of these second-choice drugs (as will be apparent from even the brief summaries below) is that they are in many cases much more toxic than the first-line drugs and, in some cases, much less effective than the latter and just as likely to encounter bacterial resistance before long.

Antibiotic substitutes include cycloserine, viomycin, and kanamycin (Table 35-3), which are usually more toxic to the patient than the streptomycin that they were intended to displace, and the tetracyclines (Chap. 34), which are less effective than the others against this organism.

Cycloserine is an antibiotic effective against a wide variety of microorganisms but one which is used clinically mainly for treating tuberculosis cases refractory to other drugs and for stubborn urinary tract infections. Its utility is limited by its capacity to cause convulsive seizures in a sizable percentage of patients receiving full daily doses. The chances of such adverse effects occurring are lessened if this drug is administered in combination with adjunctive anticonvulsant drugs or with pyridoxine, or if its dosage is reduced to half that required in severe cases. It is contraindicated in patients with a history of epilepsy.

Patients taking cycloserine in combination with other tuberculostatic drugs must be watched carefully for early signs of toxicity. These include sleepiness, headache, dizziness, speech difficulties, confusion, tremors and changes in behavior (the drug has sometimes precipitated acute psychotic reactions). The doctor should be informed of such signs so that he may order dosage reduced or even withdraw the drug before more severe toxicity develops.

Viomycin is an antibiotic similar to streptomycin and kanamycin in its antibacterial spectrum. It is sometimes effective in treating severe infections by streptomycin-resistant tubercle bacilli when administered in combination with PAS, isoniazid or other chemotherapeutic agents. Its toxic effects are similar to those of streptomycin but occur more frequently. Patients must be watched for signs of kidney damage, hearing loss, and allergy to this drug.

Synthetic chemotherapeutic agents sometimes substituted in special circumstances include pyrazinamide, ethionamide, and ethambutol (Table 35-3). *Pyrazinamide* is used mainly for short-term treatment prior to lung surgery in patients with open lesions from which bacteria have been cultured that show resistance to the first-line drugs. Its use in combination with INS for a couple of weeks before the operation and a month afterward is often effective against further spread of infection and is relatively safe. However, hepatotoxicity prevents the use of this drug for very much longer periods. Patients are watched for signs of liver function abnormality that require withdrawal of the drug.

Ethionamide is a new synthetic tuberculostatic agent which seems less toxic than most other second-line drugs in combination with other active agents. However, annoying side effects are numerous and tend to discourage ambulatory patients from continuing treatment. The drug is given after meals to reduce the gastrointestinal irritation that commonly occurs. Other side effects include sensitivity-type skin rash, drowsiness, dizziness and weakness. Tuberculous patients who are also diabetic may have increased difficulty in controlling blood sugar levels. Some of these patients have also shown signs of liver damage. Tests of liver, kidney and bone marrow function must be made frequently.

Ethambutol, a recently introduced chemotherapeutic agent, may also be useful for treating cases of pulmonary tuberculosis caused by strains of the tubercle bacillus resistant to the first-line agents. In addition, ethambutol is recommended for routine early use as a substitute for the first-line drug PAS. It is advocated for use in combination with INH for initiating therapy of previously untreated patients as well as in combination with certain second-line drugs in the management of relapsing chronic cases in which the microorganism resists INH, PAS or streptomycin.

The main advantage claimed for ethambutol over

PAS is that it may be given in a single relatively low daily dose that does not cause the kind of G.I. discomfort often brought about by the much larger amounts of PAS that must be administered. However, nausea, headache and dizziness occasionally have been reported, and this drug has sometimes caused a reduction in visual acuity. If this occurs, the drug must be discontinued in order to reverse the visual disturbance. It is also contraindicated for tuberculosis patients with a history of optic neuritis.

Prophylaxis. Children and others, including doctors and nurses, who have been exposed to people infected with tuberculosis and who show a positive tuberculin test may be treated with isoniazid or with INH-PAS combinations even though they themselves have no signs or symptoms of the disease. Such preventive medication is taken for at least a year after the last exposure to diseased patients.

Similarly, chemoprophylaxis is sometimes employed in patients who had tuberculosis before the era of modern drug therapy. Even though they may seem fully recovered, these patients whose cases were arrested by rest in a sanatorium or by pneumothorax and other surgery are considered subject to reinfection by bacteria contained within old lesions. Such a break-out of virulent organisms might, for example, occur during a severe illness for which the patient was forced to take corticosteroid medication in high dosages.

CHEMOTHERAPY OF LEPROSY

Leprosy

This disease may cause facial disfigurement and deformity of the limbs. It was so feared and loathed

TABLE 35-3
ANTIBIOTIC AND CHEMOTHERAPEUTIC AGENTS USED FOR TUBERCULOSIS TREATMENT

Official, Nonproprietary, or USAN Name	Synonym or Proprietary Name	Dosage
First-Line Drugs		
Aminosalicylic acid U.S.P.	(para-aminosalicylic acid; PAS, etc.)	12 Gm. daily in 4 divided doses after meals
Calcium aminosalicylate N.F.	—	3 Gm. 4 times a day with meals
Calcium benzoylpas	Benzapas	10 to 15 Gm. daily in divided doses after meals
Isoniazid	INH; Nydrazid; Rimifon; etc.	300 mg. daily
Phenyl aminosalicylate	Pheny-PAS-Tebamin	4 Gm. 3 times daily with meals
Potassium aminosalicylate	Paskalium; Neopasalate-K; Parasal Potassium; Potaba, etc.	12 Gm. daily in divided dosage
Sodium aminosalicylate U.S.P.	Pamisyl Sodium; Para-Pas; Pasem; Pasmed; Pasna; etc.	12 Gm. daily in 4 divided doses
Streptomycin U.S.P.	—	1 Gm. daily
Second-Line Drugs		
Cycloserine	Seromycin; Oxamycin	250 mg. twice daily
Ethambutol	Myambutol	400 mg. to 1 Gm. daily in a single dose
Ethionamide	Trecator	500 mg. to 1 Gm. daily in divided doses with meals
Kanamycin sulfate	Kanacin	1 Gm. daily I.M.
Neomycin sulfate U.S.P.	Mycifradin	4 to 12 Gm. daily
Oxytetracycline	Terramycin	2 to 5 Gm. daily
Pyrazinamide	Aldinamide; Tebrazid	20 to 35 mg./Kg. orally in 3 or 4 divided doses
Viomycin sulfate	Vinactane; Viocin	1 Gm. every 12 hours every third day

that, in times past, its victims were cast out of the community. The Bible indicates that "lepers" approaching others were required to call out that they were "Unclean!" In the Middle Ages, when the disease was widely prevalent in Europe, the Church set up special hospitals, or lazarettos, to care for lepers. Even today most patients are segregated in leprosaria.

Leprosy is believed to be caused by an acid-fast bacillus, *Mycobacterium leprae,* which is related to the organism responsible for tuberculosis infections. Because it was isolated by Dr. Hansen from the lesions of patients during an outbreak in Norway in the last century, the condition is often called Hansen's disease. Although the organism is found in infected humans in any climate, the disease is today seen mainly in the warmer parts of the world. In the United States, it is endemic mainly in Hawaii and the states bordering the Gulf of Mexico. (The U. S. Public Health Service has operated a hospital for treatment of leprosy at Carville, Louisiana.)

Drug Treatment

Many drugs have been tried and found wanting in effectiveness against leprosy. Any successes reported in the distant past were probably an indication that the patient's condition was probably not leprosy at all but some other disorder with skin symptoms. (No doubt, people were often banished as leprous when they actually had some noninfectious skin lesions.) Until just a few years ago, the only generally available drug for treating leprosy was chaulmoogra oil, a 3,000-year-old Indian remedy, and its esters including ethyl chaulmoograte—all irritating agents of dubious value.

Synthesis of the sulfones, a class of antibacterial agents with properties similar to those of the sulfonamides, led to the first truly successful treatment of leprosy in the early 1940's. Dapsone (see Drug Digest) and its derivatives (Table 35-4) were tried first in the treatment of streptococcal infections and later for tuberculosis. Although they were effective in some cases of both these infections, the sulfones proved to be more toxic than other drugs which were equally effective or superior. However, when tried against leprosy, dapsone proved superior to any other available drug. Its successors have not been shown to be more effective than the parent compound.

Taken by mouth in small doses, these drugs stop any further advance of the leprous lesions that can destroy the nose, cause blindness, damage nerves, and turn hands into claws. Healing of skin and nasal mucous membrane lesions is usually complete in two or three years, if the condition is caught early. Maintenance therapy to prevent relapse is probably desirable in most cases, even after the lesions are bacteriologically negative.

Small doses cause few side effects other than anorexia, nausea, headache and dizziness. Larger doses may result in hemolytic anemia, hematuria, and toxic psychosis. Hemoglobin determinations are made weekly at first, and later, monthly. Some patients suffer reactions during sulfone drug therapy, that are marked by fever, malaise and erythematous or bullous skin lesions. Even though these so-called lepra reactions may not be drug-induced, drug dosage must be markedly reduced. Aspirin and antihistamines are used for symptomatic relief. Patients unable to tolerate sulfones are sometimes treated with streptomycin or long-acting sulfonamides.

ANTIVIRAL CHEMOTHERAPY

Current Status

Recent advances in molecular biology have led to a more rational approach toward the development of chemicals capable of affecting virus activities without injuring the cells of the human host. Several drugs for prevention and treatment of viral infections have received clinical trials, and two have been marketed in this country up to this time (1968). One of these antiviral chemicals is idoxuridine, or IDU (see Drug

TABLE 35-4
SULFONE DERIVATIVES

Nonproprietary, Official or USAN Name	Synonym or Proprietary Name	Dosage Range
Dapsone U.S.P.	Avlosulfon; DDS	Oral 25 to 400 mg.
Sodium glucosulfone U.S.P.	Promin	I.V. 2 Gm. daily for 6 days of each week (2 to 5 Gm.)
Sodium sulfoxone U.S.P.	Diasone	Oral 330 mg. to 1 Gm.
Thiazolesulfone	Promizole	Oral 1 to 4 Gm.

Digest), which is discussed in Chapter 42. The other is a new virustatic chemoprophylactic agent, *amantadine* (Symmetrel).

Amantadine is indicated only for the *prevention* of respiratory infections by the A₂ type influenza virus, the cause of Asian influenza. It is *not* useful for *treating* infections by this or any of the other viruses responsible for respiratory tract infections. The viruses that cause influenza are continually changing antigenically. This constitutes a constant threat to the continued effectiveness of current vaccines. Despite its potential toxicity, amantadine may prove especially useful for protecting particularly vulnerable patients, especially in the event of an epidemic caused by some newly emerging strain of the A₂ virus.

Unfortunately, the high risk patients for whom this drug is intended are the very ones most susceptible to the C.N.S. side effects that have been reported during its use. Elderly patients and those with debilitating diseases, such as cardiovascular, pulmonary, renal, or metabolic disorders, may profit from prophylaxis with this drug when they are known to have been exposed to people infected with Asian influenza. However, such patients have sometimes suffered motor system side effects and psychic reactions after receiving amantadine.

Ill effects from prophylactic doses of this drug that have been occasionally reported include difficulty in concentrating, ataxia; and complaints of a lightheaded, giddy, or drunken feeling. Patients whose vision becomes blurred or whose speech is slurred while taking this drug are warned against driving or working with dangerous machinery. More serious reactions reported in experimental subjects taking somewhat higher doses include insomnia, nervousness, depression, feelings of depersonalization, hallucinations, and convulsions.

Since such reactions are especially likely to occur in elderly patients with a history of cerebral arteriosclerosis, this may limit the utility of the drug. However, when such patients, who also run a high risk of infection by influenzal respiratory viruses, are known to have been in contact with a definitely diagnosed case of Asian flu, doctors may order the drug rather than depend solely upon the effectiveness of previous vaccination.

Amantadine must be taken as soon as possible after contact with an infected individual if it is to be effective. The drug molecules are thought to act by occupying certain cellular receptors, thus preventing penetration of the cell by virus particles. Once the virus has entered the cells, however, this drug cannot prevent the replication and release of new cell-destroying virus particles.

Future Prospects

Other drugs have had some success in clinical trials against virus infections. *Beta-thiosemicarbazone* (Isatin) has proved effective for preventing smallpox infections in patients exposed to the virus during small local epidemics in India. *Cytosine arabinoside*, another antiviral agent, may act, like IDU, against the herpes virus that causes keratitis, as well as against a variety of other DNA viruses.

Interferon is a protein produced by cells infected by viruses. It apparently acts, even before formation of antibodies, to protect uninfected cells from further invasion by virus particles. Such an aid to host resistance could, of course, possess therapeutic utility. Unfortunately, it has not been possible to devise a safe and economically practical way to use interferon in humans.

Scientists are searching for a substance capable of stimulating cells to produce and release interferon. However, none of the agents tried up to now has proved sufficiently free of toxicity or antigenicity to be of clinical utility.

The problems associated with vaccination for respiratory tract infections make antiviral therapy a potentially more feasible approach than immunization against the common cold and other acute viral respiratory ailments. The rhinoviruses responsible for the common cold appear to be numbered in the hundreds. The vast number of distinct serotypes of these viruses makes the development of an effective polyvalent vaccine against the common cold seem remote at this time. Other problems also tend to limit the immediate likelihood of developing adequately safe adenovirus vaccines. Thus, the chemotherapeutic attack against the problem of viral URI infections is being actively pressed.

SULFONAMIDE TOXICITY

• *Urinary Tract Disorders*

Crystalluria in the kidneys and other G.U. tract organs may lead to pain, obstruction and tubular necrosis, with hematuria, oliguria, anuria, azotemia and uremia.

In addition to maintaining adequate fluid intake, the doctor may order renal function tests, especially if these drugs must be administered to patients whose renal function is already impaired.

- *Sensitization-type Reactions*

    Stevens-Johnson syndrome (erythema multiforme exudativum), a condition marked by crops of blisters on the skin and mucous membranes of the mouth, nose and other parts of the respiratory tract, has occurred during administration of both long- and short-acting sulfonamides.

    Other skin reactions are marked by eruptions of the urticarial, morbilliform, or scarlatiniform types. Severe exfoliative dermatitis, petechiae, purpura and photosensitivity sometimes occur. Sulfonamide therapy should be discontinued upon development of skin rashes and pruritus.

    Drug fever sometimes develops during the second week of treatment, along with headache, chills and general malaise. Discontinuation of sulfonamide therapy results in return to normal temperature. Joint pains, bronchospasm, conjunctivitis, and other indications of serum sickness reaction may occur.

- *Blood and Bone Marrow Disorders*

    Acute hemolytic anemia, thrombocytopenia, agranulocytosis, and aplastic anemia have occurred. Periodic blood tests are desirable, with discontinuance of sulfonamide therapy if changes in hematopoietic function or peripheral blood components are noted.

- *Gastrointestinal Side Effects and Toxicity*

    Anorexia, nausea, vomiting, abdominal pain, diarrhea, jaundice, liver enlargement; rarely, hepatitis and fatal acute yellow atrophy of the liver.

- *Neurological and Psychiatric Complications*

    Psychiatric disturbances, including confusion, depression, drowsiness may occur with or without signs of ataxia and vertigo, as a result of electrolyte imbalances, vasculitis, or direct drug effects. Peripheral neuritis has occasionally developed.

CAUTIONS AND CONTRAINDICATIONS

- Patients with a history of sulfa sensitivity should not be treated with sulfonamides.
- Advanced kidney disease manifested by elevated blood urea nitrogen levels is a contraindication to the use of sulfonamides.
- Caution is required in patients with liver disease, blood dyscrasias and impaired liver function.
- Sulfonamides should not be administered to infants under one month of age, since they lack the detoxifying enzymes required for elimination of sulfonamides.
- Pregnant women near term should not receive sulfonamides because of possible placental transmission to the fetus.
- Caution is required in all women who are or may become pregnant.

SULFONAMIDE THERAPY: SUMMARY OF POINTS FOR THE NURSE TO REMEMBER

- Although crystalluria resulting from sulfonamide therapy is less common now than formerly, fluid intake should be encouraged in order to prevent its occurrence. The amount of urine excreted should be noted, and the urine should be examined for signs of hematuria.

- Observe the patient for other toxic effects of sulfonamides, such as skin rash, fever, chills, sore throat.

- Remember that the dosage of the slowly excreted sulfonamides is much less than that of the more rapidly eliminated drugs. Be aware of the usual dosage range of each sulfa drug that is administered.

- Patients receiving drugs containing the azo dye, phenazopyridine, will have an orange-red hue to their urine. This should not be mistaken for blood, and the patient should be reassured that the unusual color of his urine is a harmless result of drug therapy.

TUBERCULOSIS DRUG THERAPY: SUMMARY OF POINTS FOR THE NURSE TO REMEMBER

• Administer these drugs in ways which minimize the likelihood of unpleasant side effects that may make the patient reluctant to keep taking the medication. For example, see that PAS is given after meals in divided dosage to lessen gastric irritation.

• Observe the patient carefully for signs and symptoms of potentially severe reactions. Some of the tuberculostatic drugs may be highly toxic when taken over the long periods that are required. Streptomycin, for example, can cause deafness; therefore, watch for any sign of hearing loss.

• Report promptly to the doctor any condition that may make it difficult or impossible for the patient to continue taking his medication with the essential regularity. Thus, if the patient becomes nauseated and tends to vomit an orally administered medication, the

physician should be made aware of this. Also, advise the patient to report promptly any unusual symptoms to his physician.

• Encourage the patient, who often is being treated at home for prolonged periods, to continue taking his medication despite discomforts such as gastric distress. Stress the value of drug treatment which shortens the period of his disability, prevents possible complications, and reduces substantially the chance of his transmitting his infection to others in the family or at work.

• Advise the patient, who may feel remarkably better after an initial course of therapy has reduced his fever and coughing and helped him regain his strength and appetite, not to exceed the limits of the physical activity prescribed by his physician.

CLINICAL PROBLEMS

Mr. Leslie, 52 years old, has been admitted to the hospital with a diagnosis of pulmonary tuberculosis and chronic alcoholism. He is receiving streptomycin 0.5 Gm. I.M. twice weekly; isoniazid 50 mg. q.i.d.; and pyridoxine 25 mg. q.i.d. Mr. Leslie has gastritis resulting from alcoholism, and experiences periods of nausea and vomiting.

• What observations would you make for toxic reactions Mr. Leslie may have, related to the prescribed drug therapy?

• What nursing actions are indicated when Mr. Leslie is unable to take his oral medications, because of nausea and vomiting?

• It is anticipated that Mr. Leslie, who lives alone, will recover sufficiently to continue his treatment on an outpatient basis. What factors will have to be considered when teaching Mr. Leslie to take isoniazid and pyridoxine at home? (If injections of streptomycin are still required, they will be administered at the clinic.)

REVIEW QUESTIONS

Sulfonamides

1. (a) What is the current status of the sulfonamide drugs? (i.e., how safe and effective are they considered to be in comparison with other available anti-infective agents and under what circumstances are they most likely to be employed?)

(b) List several specific microorganisms that are still so susceptible to sulfonamides that these drugs (which may

not necessarily be the preferred antimicrobial treatment) are often used for infections caused by these organisms.

2. (a) Discuss briefly the mechanism of antibacterial action of the sulfonamides.

(b) Why are some organisms congenitally resistant to sulfonamides and how are others believed to acquire resistance to these drugs?

3. (a) What precautions are employed to lessen the

likelihood that strains resistant to sulfonamides will emerge from previously susceptible microbial species?

(b) List at least two classes of microorganisms which were once sensitive to sulfonamides but now are found in the population mainly as sulfonamide-resistant strains.

4. (a) What is the rationale for the oral administration of poorly absorbable sulfonamides such as succinylsulfathiazole?

(b) In what clinical conditions or situations are sulfonamides such as phthalylsulfathiazole and others employed?

5. (a) Which sulfonamides are bound to plasma proteins for long periods after their absorption into the blood, and how does this property affect their antibacterial activity?

(b) Which sulfonamide diffuses most readily into the cerebrospinal fluid, and in what form and by what route is it administered in treating meningitis?

6. (a) Of what chemical classes are the most common metabolic derivatives of sulfonamides, which are formed as a result of biotransformation, or detoxication, mechanisms?

(b) How does the nature of the metabolites formed by many of the newer sulfonamides contribute to their reduced toxicity?

7. (a) Why are the rapidly excreted sulfonamides preferred in treating urinary tract infections? Why may the more slowly eliminated sulfonamides be better for prophylactic purposes?

(b) What properties of the rapidly excreted and of the slowly excreted sulfonamides decrease the likelihood of crystalluria?

8. (a) What precautions are taken to avoid renal toxicity by sulfonamide drugs?

(b) What property of trisulfapyrimidines decreases the likelihood of renal toxicity from the three components of this mixture of sulfonamides?

9. (a) How are oral sulfonamides administered in initiation and maintenance of therapeutic control of infections?

(b) How does the dosage of a long-acting agent such as sulfamethoxypyridazine differ from that of a shorter-acting drug such as sulfadiazine?

10. (a) Of what types are the sensitization reactions that may result from sulfonamide therapy?

(b) Which sulfonamides are most likely to cause the most serious kinds of sensitization reactions and why are such reactions worse than with other sulfonamides?

11. (a) What is the present status of topical sulfonamide therapy?

(b) What are some sulfonamides that are commonly employed in this manner, and for what purposes are they used?

12. (a) What substances are formed by the breakdown of methenamine mandelate in the urine?

(b) What advantage may this compound have over sulfonamides, and what property of the latter does it lack?

13. (a) What advantage may nitrofurantoin have over sulfonamides in the treatment of some urinary tract infections?

(b) What property does the azo dye phenazopyridine possess that may make it a useful additive to sulfonamides in urinary tract infections, and what property does it have, about which patients should be alerted?

14. (a) Against which urinary tract pathogens is the drug nalidixic acid at present considered particularly effective?

(b) What toxicity has been associated occasionally with the administration of this drug?

Tuberculostatic Agents

1. (a) What has been the effect of the introduction of effective chemotherapeutic agents on the overall management of tuberculosis?

(b) What are the two main reasons for administering the three primary antituberculosis drugs in combinations of various kinds?

2. (a) What improvements are seen when a patient with pulmonary tuberculosis is responding to treatment with a combination of chemotherapeutic agents?

(b) How may the nurse help a patient taking such treatment to maintain his improvement and not relapse?

3. (a) What property of isoniazid (INH) seems to make it an especially useful tuberculostatic agent?

(b) What is one way in which the addition of para-aminosalicylic acid (PAS) may add to the effectiveness of INH?

4. (a) What are some common side effects of isoniazid that stem from its blockade of autonomically innervated organs (i.e., atropinelike side effects)?

(b) More serious neurotoxicity of what types may occur with the continued use of this drug, and how may the likelihood of these toxic reactions be minimized by adjunctive medication?

5. (a) What are the most common complaints of patients who must take streptomycin in large daily doses for long periods?

(b) What are some means by which the likelihood of such toxicity may be lessened?

6. (a) What are the main side effects encountered upon administration of large daily doses of PAS and how may these be minimized?

(b) What related PAS preparations are available and in what ways are they claimed to be superior to the parent compound?

7. (a) Under what circumstances may it be necessary to substitute a secondary tuberculostatic drug for one of the first-line agents?

(b) What, in general, are the disadvantages of these drugs?

8. (a) What is the main limitation on cycloserine's usefulness as a tuberculostatic agent, and what adjunctive medication may sometimes be ordered with this antibiotic?

(b) Toxicity of what types must be watched for in patients taking viomycin?

9. (a) Under what circumstances is pyrazinamide often used?

(b) What kind of toxicity typically is associated with this drug?

10. (a) How is ethionamide best administered to avoid the side effects that occur most commonly?

(b) What kinds of laboratory tests are most commonly ordered for patients taking this drug?

11. (a) In what circumstances is the use of ethambutol advocated at the present time?

(b) What advantage may this drug have, and what adverse effect may require its withdrawal?

Antiviral Agents

1. (a) For what purpose is idoxuridine (IDU, Herplex, Stoxil) employed?

(b) For what purpose is amantadine (Symmetrel) specifically indicated, and what is the manner of its action in such circumstances?

2. (a) What side effects have been reported in the use of amantadine?

(b) Of the patients who may profit from amantadine, in which group must this drug be employed with caution?

BIBLIOGRAPHY

Sulfonamides

Carroll, O. M., Bryan, P. A., and Robinson, R. J.: Stevens-Johnson syndrome associated with long-acting sulfonamides. J.A.M.A., *195:*179, 1966.

Council on Drugs: Evaluation of a new sulfonamide, Sulfamethoxazole. J.A.M.A., *187:*142, 1964.

———: A new antibacterial agent for infections of the genitourinary tract—nalidixic acid. J.A.M.A., *192:*628, 1965.

Coursin, D. B.: Stevens-Johnson syndrome: Non-specific parasensitivity reaction. J.A.M.A., *198:*113, 1966.

Johnson, F. D., and Korst, D. R.: Pancytopenia associated with sulfamethoxypyridazine administration. J.A.M.A., *175:*967, 1961.

Janovsky, R. C.: Fatal thrombocytopenic purpura after administration of sulfamethoxypyridazine. J.A.M.A., *172:* 155, 1960.

Rallison, M. L., *et al.:* Severe reactions to long-acting sulfonamides. Pediatrics, *28:*908, 1961.

Rodman, M. J.: Drugs for urinary tract infections. R.N., *28:*61, 1965 (Aug.).

Salvaggio, J., and Gonzalez, F.: Severe toxic reactions associated with sulfamethoxypyridazine (Kynex). Am. Int. Med., *51:*60, 1959.

Stewart, B. L., and Rowe, H. J.: Nitrofurantoin (Furadantin) in treatment of urinary tract infections. J.A.M.A., *160:*1221, 1956.

Weinstein, L., *et al.:* The sulfonamides. New Eng. J. Med., *263:*793, 1960.

Antituberculosis Agents

Council on Drugs: Ethionamide—a new tuberculostatic agent. J.A.M.A., *187:*527, 1964.

Di Palma, J. R.: Drugs for tuberculosis. R.N., *29:*53, 1966 (July).

Frenay, Sr. M. A. C.: Drugs in tuberculosis control. Am. J. Nursing, *61:*82, 1961.

Lattimer, J. K., *et al.:* Treatment of renal tuberculosis with triple-drug therapy. J.A.M.A., *160:*544, 1956.

Pfuetze, K. H., and Pyle, M. M.: Recent advances in treatment of organ tuberculosis. J.A.M.A., *187:*805, 1964.

Rodman, M. J.: Drug treatment of tuberculosis. R.N., *22:* 56, 1959 (Jan.).

Ross, R. R.: Use of pyridoxine hydrochloride to prevent isoniazid toxicity. J.A.M.A., *168:*273, 1958.

Schwartz, W. S.: Developments in treatment of tuberculosis and other pulmonary diseases. J.A.M.A., *178:*43, 1961.

Weiss, M.: Chemotherapy and tuberculosis. Am. J. Nursing, *59:*1711, 1959.

Wolinsky, E.: Modern drug treatment of mycobacterial diseases. Med. Clin. N. Am., *47:*1271, 1963.

Antiviral Agents

Council on Drugs, A.M.A.: The amantadine controversy. J.A.M.A., *201:*372, 1967.

Hilleman, M. R.: Advances in control of virus infections. Clin. Pharmacol. Ther., *7:*752, 1966.

Dudgeon, J. A.: Advances in the treatment of virus diseases. Practitioner, *195:*496, 1965.

Kaufman, H. E., *et al.:* Use of idoxuridine (IDU) in the treatment of herpes simplex keratitis. Arch. Ophthal., *68:*235, 1962 (Aut.).

Rodman, M. J.: New drugs for fighting infections. R.N., *30:*55, 1967 (June).

Sabin, A.: Amantadine hydrochloride: analysis of data related to its proposed use for prevention of influenza virus disease in human beings. J.A.M.A., *200:*943, 1967.

Tamm, I., and Eggers, H. J.: Biochemistry of virus reproduction. Am. J. Med., *38:*678, 1965.

Wendell, H. A., *et al.:* Trial of amantadine in epidemic influenza. Clin. Pharmacol. Ther., *7:*38, 1966.

The Chemotherapy of Malaria and Other Parasitic Infections

Advances in chemotherapy are helping to bring many parasitic diseases under control. Infections, by protozoan organisms and metazoa such as blood flukes and filarid worms are among the so-called tropical diseases, for which relatively effective remedies have come into use during the past generation. Actually, these conditions are not limited to the tropics; in some cases, the insects and other vectors which transmit the infecting organisms can exist in temperate climates too, when sanitary conditions are poor, or people become careless.

In this chapter we shall discuss the chemotherapy of malaria and certain other parasitic diseases. Nurses are called upon to care for patients with these conditions, not only when practicing abroad (for example, as a member of the armed forces) but sometimes in this country also. In addition to the occasional patient who may become infected with malaria in the continental United States, others, traveling by jet plane from a land in which these diseases have not yet been eradicated, may come down with this or other illness with an incubation period longer than the flying time.

Malaria has killed hundreds of millions of people over the centuries and changed the course of history. The Bible speaks of the "burning ague" and Hippocrates describes fevers that flare every third or fourth day—both allusions to malaria. The disease is believed to have played a part in the decline of many early civilizations and in the fall of the Roman empire.

In the United States, malaria was once endemic in the South. However, with the wide use of insecticides and advances in sanitary engineering since World War II, the disease has been dying out here. The number of reported cases has dropped from nearly 200,000 before 1940 to less than 200 in 1965. Yet, it is significant that, at the present time, the number of cases rises as soldiers and others returning from en-

demic areas serve as sources of infection of local mosquitoes (and, subsequently, residents).

Great advances in malaria control have also been made elsewhere in the world, since the World Health Organization (W.H.O.) began its fight to eradicate the disease in 1949. Nonetheless, almost one million people still died of malaria in 1965 and perhaps one hundred million more were weakened by the infection. Thus, W.H.O. still considers malaria the most important of all communicable diseases and the world's No. 1 health problem.

The continued prevalence of malaria in many parts of the globe indicates the need to sustain a vigorous attack on the malaria parasite and on its insect vector, the Anopheles mosquito. Strains of mosquitoes that have developed resistance to DDT and other insecticides have appeared. Similarly, malaria parasites insensitive to antimalarial drugs are now a cause of disease in various parts of the world.

THE BIOLOGICAL NATURE OF MALARIA

Types of Malaria. Four species of protozoa of the genus Plasmodium cause malaria in man. The two that are of prime importance are (1) *Plasmodium vivax*, the cause of benign tertian malaria, and (2) *Plasmodium falciparum*, the cause of malignant tertian malaria. The term *tertian* refers to the fact that the attacks of chills and fever tend typically to recur every third day. The term *benign* indicates only that *P. vivax* infection is less severe than *P. falciparum* infection and less likely to kill quickly. The malignant disease, though relatively easy to cure in most cases with modern drugs, may start explosively and end fatally, with its victims following a rapidly progressive downhill course.

Life Cycle of the Plasmodium (Fig. 36-1). The drugs that are used in the control of malaria have variable effects on the different stages of the parasite as well as on the different species and strains. Thus, in order to understand how the drugs act and how this determines their clinical uses and limitations, we must know something about the life cycle of plasmodial organisms. The following brief review will emphasize the terms and concepts necessary for our later discussion of the several classes of drugs and their clinical uses.

The plasmodia spend part of their lives in the blood and other tissues of the human body and another part in the body of the female Anopheles mosquito. In the human, the plasmodia reproduce by *asexual* division, or *schizogony;* their reproduction while in the mosquito is through the mating of male and female parasites—that is, a *sexual* phase, which is followed by a process called *sporogony.*

The sexual phase begins when a mosquito bites a person with malaria and sucks up a drop of his blood. This blood meal contains mature male and female *gametocytes,* the sexually differentiated forms of the plasmodium. In the mosquito's stomach, these gametocytes mate to form a zygote. This product of fertilization of the female then goes through the several

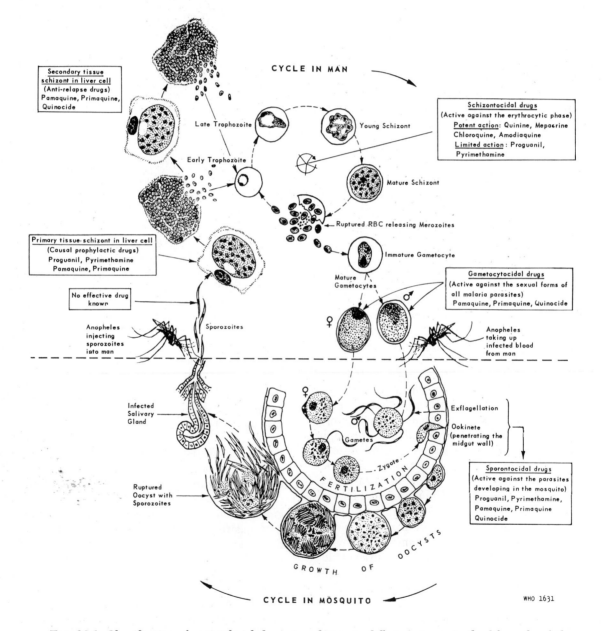

FIG. 36-1. Classification of antimalarial drugs in relation to different stages in the life-cycle of the parasite. (Bruce-Chwatt, L. J.: W.H.O. Bull. No. 27, p. 287, 1962)

stages of sporogony, finally forming numerous *sporo-zoites* (spore animals), some of which migrate to the mosquito's salivary glands.

The asexual phase has its start when the sporozoites are injected into the next human that the infected mosquito bites. The thousands of sporozoites that pour into the person's blood do not linger long in the circulation; some lodge in the liver, where they begin the process of schizogony in fixed tissue cells. This phase, which takes place before the invasion of the red blood cells, is termed the *primary tissue phase,* or the *pre-erythrocytic* or *primary exo-erythrocytic* phase, of the asexual cycle.

During the next week to ten days, these *primary tissue schizonts* grow and multiply by simple division within the liver cells. Finally, *merozoites* are formed by malarial schizonts and burst forth when the liver cells that had been parasitized are ruptured. Most of the merozoites enter the circulation and invade red blood cells, thus initiating the *erythrocytic schizogony phase* of the *asexual cycle.*

Once established in the red blood cells, more young schizonts are formed from *trophozoites* by the same process that had occurred in the liver. Periodically, mature erythrocytic schizonts rupture and the merozoites break out of ruptured red cells; these liberated merozoites invade still more erythrocytes. After several such cycles, some of the merozoites do not turn into the usual asexual trophozoites that parasitize red blood cells. Instead, they form a number of gametocytes—the same kind of sexually differentiated plasmodia with which the life cycle started and, therefore, an important link in the chain of *transmission* of the infection.

Clinical Course of Malaria. More important to the infected person himself is what happens when a large enough number of red cells have been parasitized. The sudden release of swarms of malaria parasites from millions of destroyed red cells sets off the chills and fever that mark the beginning of the clinical attack. The *chill* is caused by the break-up of the erythrocytes; the *fever* is the result of a reaction to the freed foreign protein and cellular debris.

Each time a new mass of erythrocytic schizonts bursts, releasing toxins into the circulation (about every 48 hours in the tertian malarias), the patient suffers a paroxysm of chills and fever. In *P. vivax malaria,* such attacks continue for a long time if untreated. Even after the body's defense mechanisms have brought the infection more or less under control, the patient is subject to periodic relapses. This occurs because some of the merozoites from primary tissue schizonts make their way back into liver cells where they are safe from the body's defending macrophages. Then, periodically, these *secondary tissue schizonts* or *exo-erythrocytic* forms send forth more red cell in-

vaders. These, in time, produce relapses, marked again by a series of recurrent attacks.

In the case of *P. falciparum malaria,* no such secondary exo-erythrocytic schizonts persist in the tissues. Thus, provided that the patient survives the first series of attacks, he will suffer no further relapses. However, this form of malaria is often fatal, because the parasite-damaged red cells tend to clog the patient's capillaries and thus cut off the circulation in vital organs.

THE CHEMOTHERAPY OF MALARIA

The available antimalarial drugs may be classified in accordance with the stages of the parasitic life cycle against which they are most effective. This, in turn, determines whether a particular drug can be expected to prevent an attack or to be useful in treating one, or whether it will actually cure the infection completely by wiping out all of the plasmodia in both the blood and the tissues of the patient. In the following discussion, we shall indicate which of the drugs in Table 36-1 are effective against the various phases of the different species of parasites responsible for malaria infections. We shall also introduce the terms that are used to describe the drugs' actions.

Gametocytocides are drugs that destroy the gametocytes, or sexual forms, of the parasite (the phase with which we began our discussion of the life cycle of the malaria parasite). Drugs such as *primaquine* (see Drug Digest) which kill the gametocytes in a patient's blood, or *chloroguanide* and *pyrimethamine* (see Drug Digests), which somehow keep these sexual forms from mating when they are sucked up into the mosquito's stomach, are capable of preventing transmission of the disease. That is, they break the man-mosquito-man chain by which the infection is spread.

Unfortunately, these drugs are considered too toxic and too expensive for routine administration to all people in endemic areas. Thus control of the spread of infection is today based not on drugs but on schemes for elimination of mosquitoes and their breeding places, and on the use of protective screening and insect repellents in attempts to keep people from being bitten. Of course, drugs that can eradicate the asexual forms of the parasite in the blood and tissues before they give rise to gametocytes do play a part in preventing the further spread of infection.

Prophylaxis. In theory, drugs that kill the sporozoites as soon as the infected mosquito has injected them into a person's blood stream in the act of biting should prevent infection. In practice, there are no drugs that can be given in safe doses that build up a blood concentration high enough to destroy sporozoites as soon as they enter the circulation. Thus, there are *no true causal prophylactics.*

However, once the sporozoites have made their way

to the liver and begun to develop into primary tissue schizonts, they can be destroyed there by *schizonticidal* drugs. Chemicals such as *primaquine, chloroguanide* and *pyrimethamine* can reach concentrations in the tissues that kill the parasite in this pre-erythrocytic stage, so that it never gets a chance to invade and destroy red blood cells. However, this action (which is termed *causal prophylaxis*) is not considered a practical approach. As previously indicated, these drugs are considered too toxic and expensive for mass administration to uninfected individuals in endemic areas.

Suppressive treatment, rather than causal prophylaxis, is the main approach to control of the disease with antimalarial drugs. Such treatment makes use of the capacity of some drugs to keep an infected person from coming down with an actual attack of malaria. *Chloroquine* (see Drug Digest) and related synthetic chemicals, and the cinchona alkaloid *quinine* (see

Drug Digest) act to suppress the signs and symptoms of malaria paroxysms. They do so by destroying the asexual erythrocytic forms (trophozoites, schizonts, and merozoites) or by inhibiting their further growth and development within the circulating red blood cells.

P. falciparum infections can be completely eliminated by treatment with these suppressive drugs, or with *chloroguanide* or *pyrimethamine*. When all the primary tissue schizonts of this organism have liberated merozoites into a person's blood to make their all-out attack on the red cells, no parasites are left in reserve in the liver, and the merozoites of *P. falciparum* do not reinvade liver cells. Thus, when the erythrocytic forms are wiped out by suppressive drug therapy, no secondary tissue schizonts of *P. falciparum* remain to cause later relapses.

With *P. vivax* infections, however, an infected person will eventually relapse after suppressive treat-

TABLE 36-1
ANTIMALARIAL DRUGS

Nonproprietary or Official Name	Synonym or Proprietary Name	Dosage
Amodiaquine HCl N.F.	Camoquin	Suppressive: 520 mg. every 2 weeks Therapeutic: 780 mg.
Chloroquine phosphate U.S.P.	Aralen	Suppressive: 500 mg. weekly Therapeutic: 1 Gm. initial, then 500 mg. in 6 hrs. and 500 mg. on second and third days
Chloroguanide HCl	Proguanil; Paludrine	Suppressive: 100 mg. daily Therapeutic: 600 mg. followed by 300 mg. daily as needed
Hydroxychloroquine sulfate U.S.P.	Plaquenil	Suppressive: 400 mg. weekly Therapeutic: 800 mg. a day for three days
Primaquine phosphate U.S.P.	—	26.3 mg. (the equivalent of 15 mg. of the base) daily for 14 days to achieve a radical cure
Pyrimethamine U.S.P.	Daraprim	Suppressive: 25 mg. weekly Therapeutic: 25 mg. daily for 2 days
Quinacrine HCl U.S.P.	Atabrine	Suppressive: 0.1 Gm. daily, beginning 2 weeks in advance of exposure Therapeutic: 0.2 Gm. repeated every 4 to 6 hours; then 0.1 Gm. t.i.d. for 6 days
Quinine sulfate N.F.	—	Therapeutic: 1 Gm. daily for 2 days, then 600 mg. daily for 5 days

ment is stopped. These drugs are not able to keep secondary tissue schizonts, or exo-erythrocytic forms, of this plasmodial species from becoming established in the person's liver. When the suppressive drugs that so successfully eradicated the erythrocytic schizonts are no longer maintained in the patient's blood, the *tissue forms* of *P. vivax* serve as a reservoir for formation of blood cell invaders. Thus, the nurse must encourage people to continue taking these drugs even when they are symptom-free.

Clinical cure, the relief of an actual attack, can be brought about by the same drugs that are used for suppressive treatment. They act, of course, by stopping the cycles of erythrocytic schizogony through which more and more red blood cells are parasitized by waves of liberated merozoites. By calling a halt to the periodic release of toxins responsible for paroxysms of chills and fever, drugs such as *chloroquine* and the other synthetic successors to quinine quickly terminate the attacks. They do not, however, completely eliminate the parasite from the patient's body. Thus, although his attack is clinically cured, he himself is not truly cured and is subject to relapses of *P. vivax* malaria.

Radical cure of *P. vivax* infection can, however, be brought about by chemotherapy. This is accomplished with drugs such as *primaquine*, which wipe out the secondary tissue forms of *P. vivax*. By acting to kill these exo-erythrocytic schizonts produced by merozoites that have made their way back into liver cells, primaquine prevents the red blood cell parasitizers from ever again emerging. Simultaneous *suppressive therapy* is, of course, needed to keep blood forms from continuing to survive.

In the case of *P. falciparum*, as previously indicated, suppressive treatment alone is adequate, since this organism possesses no persisting secondary exo-erythrocytic tissue forms. Sometimes vivax malaria may be cured by the use of the long-acting suppressive drug, *pyrimethamine*. Such so-called *suppressive cure* can be accomplished by continuing to treat the patient with pyrimethamine for close to three months after he has left the region where malaria is endemic. By that time all the parasites have been eliminated as they emerge from the tissues only to meet this erythrocytic schizonticide waiting for them in the blood.

More commonly, however, people leaving a malarious area are today treated with a *combination* of *primaquine* and *chloroquine*. The latter kills the schizonts in the red blood cells while the former is wiping out the exo-erythrocytic tissue forms of the parasite. Thus, *suppressive treatment* and *radical cure* are carried out simultaneously in a person who is leaving the land in which *P. vivax* and other malarias are endemic, so that he will never suffer a later attack of the disease. Of course, if a person stays on in a malarious

area, he is likely to keep being reinfected by being bitten by mosquitoes carrying plasmodial sporozoites. Thus, the authorities on malaria control do not advocate the use of drugs as radical cures in such cases, just as they do not advise their use as gametocides or as casual prophylactics.

HISTORY AND CURRENT STATUS OF ANTIMALARIAL DRUGS

The most important of the antimalarial drugs presently in use are discussed in the Drug Digests in terms of their actions, uses, adverse effects, and dosage and administration. In addition to these practical facts, the reader may gain some worthwhile insights into the nature of malaria chemotherapy by briefly reviewing the story of how these drugs came to be created and developed.

Cinchona and Quinine. The substance first employed for the specific treatment of malaria was the bark of the cinchona tree, a South American evergreen. Spanish Jesuit missionaries in Peru learned about the fever-reducing remedy from the Indians and brought samples of the bark back to Spain around 1630. Soon the Jesuit's bark, or Peruvian bark, as it was called, was being used all over Europe for treating cases of malaria, which was then an endemic disease there.

The only advance in malaria treatment during the next three hundred years came close to two centuries later with the isolation of the active principles of cinchona. In 1820, the French pharmacists Pelletier and Caventou succeeded in isolating quinine, which soon displaced decoctions of the crude bark as the main treatment for malaria. Quinine became a monopoly of the Dutch East Indian planters who cultivated cinchona trees on their plantations. When this source of the drug was cut off from the Germans during World War I and from the Allies during World War II, chemists in Germany, France, Britain and the United States launched an intensive search for synthetic substitutes for quinine.

Pamaquine. The research that began in Germany during World War I bore fruit in the mid 1920's when pamaquine (Plasmochin), the first synthetic antimalarial, was tried in human patients. This compound contained a quinoline ring like that in quinine plus an aminoalkyl chain. Pamaquine did not prove to be a practicable substitute for quinine, but the *aminoquinolines* which were later prepared turned out to be more useful and less toxic than quinine.

Quinacrine (Atabrine). This drug, developed in the 1930's as part of the continuing German research program, was used by the Allies in World War II to keep their troops in fighting shape in the malaria-infested South Pacific and in Asia. Although this drug was finally proved to be safer and more active than quinine, early fears that it might be too toxic stimulated wartime synthesis and screening of thousands of new chemicals. Today, quinacrine, which had certain drawbacks, is no longer used to any extent in malaria. It is, however, still considered extremely useful as a treatment for tapeworm (Chap. 37).

Chloroquine (Aralen; see Drug Digest), one of a series of 4-aminoquinoline compounds that had first been synthesized by the Germans in the early 1930's, was re-evaluated in the massive wartime program and proved to be superior to any of the previously available drugs. A single small oral dose taken only once weekly as suppressive therapy protected soldiers from coming down with incapacitating malaria symptoms. Administered in larger doses to patients suffering an acute attack, chloroquine promptly effected a clinical cure. It is today considered the most dependable of the blood schizontocides.

Primaquine. Effective as chloroquine was against schizonts in the red blood cells, the drug did not eradicate the exo-erythrocytic form of the parasite in the patient's liver. Thus, when soldiers as well as others who had received suppressive therapy left the malarious area and stopped taking chloroquine, they often came down with a case of clinical malaria.

This focused scientific interest once more on pamaquine and the several hundred other compounds of the 8-aminoquinoline class that had been studied in the wartime crash program. For, although pamaquine had been more toxic than quinine and weaker in its activity against blood schizonts, the early studies had shown that this drug often prevented relapses in patients with vivax malaria. Several compounds of this same series, including pentaquine, isopentaquine, and primaquine, were intensively studied and proved to be capable of destroying the form of the malaria parasite that persisted in the patient's tissue after treatment with blood schizonticides such as chloroquine and the other 4-aminoquinoline compounds.

Primaquine, the least toxic of these curative antimalarials, has found an important place in the present-day management of malaria. It both prevents relapses and brings about a radical cure. Thus, when a person is leaving a malarious region, he takes a small daily dose of primaquine for two weeks. By wiping out any malaria parasites still lurking in the liver, the drug keeps the patient from coming down with malaria even after he stops taking the weekly dose of chloroquine that had protected him from attacks but not from infection of his tissues.

Pyrimethamine (Daraprim). This drug was developed after World War II, as a result of studies on hundreds of compounds that interfere with the cell division of reproducing malarial parasites. A very small non-toxic dose has inhibiting effects on several stages of the sexual and asexual cycles of the plasmodial organisms. In addition to suppressing blood cell schizont reproduction, the drug may also keep some tissue forms from developing, and it seems to sterilize the gametocytes floating in the infected patient's blood. Thus, when a mosquito bites such a person, the sexual forms of the parasite that she picks up are unable to mate successfully, which blocks sporozoite formation. This, of course, keeps the disease from being transmitted to people whom the mosquito bites next.

In practice, this broad spectrum antimalarial has proved somewhat disappointing. Although pyrimethamine is an excellent suppressant for the warding off of malaria symptoms, its relatively slow action against blood parasites makes it less useful than chloroquine for treatment of attacks. In programs of mass prophylaxis intended to eradicate malaria in endemic areas, the drug had proved to be effective until resistant strains of parasites began to emerge. Thus, its use for this purpose is now considered unwise.

Recently, an active metabolite of this agent, cycloguanil pamoate, has been employed to produce long-lasting protection in malarious areas. Injected intramuscularly, this drug forms a depot from which only very small amounts are gradually released into the blood over a period of several months. Such very low levels of the drug in the blood seem capable of keeping both blood and tissue forms of the parasite from surviving and reproducing. This may prove to be very useful in programs of mass prophylaxis aimed at eradication of the parasites in an endemic area. Certainly, it would be easier for public health officials to see that people were injected once or twice a year than to get them to take a drug by mouth daily or even weekly.

Development of Resistance

Recently, reports have become more frequent of infections by strains of parasites able to survive and multiply in the presence of plasma concentrations of drugs that once wiped out the organisms. This has caused a good deal of concern that the usefulness of presently available drugs might be compromised.

The problem first arose in the case of chloroguanide and led to its being abandoned in many areas. A few years later, resistance to pyrimethamine was reported from various areas in which it had been tried for mass prophylaxis. Most recently, malaria infections resistant to chloroquine, the drug most widely used for suppressant therapy and clinical cure, has created real alarm.

Soldiers in Vietnam, for example, have come down with attacks caused by chloroquine-resistant strains of *P. falciparum*. Often these infections have shown cross-resistance to other synthetic antimalarial drugs that, ordinarily, are quite effective. In some of these cases, the doctors, in desperation, have resorted to courses of quinine. Fortunately, this drug—the oldest of the antimalarials and seemingly outmoded—has usually proved successful.

It is still uncertain how far the chloroquine-resistant malarial strains found in Southeast Asia are likely to spread. However, the mere threat that present drugs, though still generally effective, might prove inadequate for future control of malaria has stimulated another round of intensive scientific studies. These investigations are aimed at the development of new antimalarial drugs and the discovery of ways to increase the activity of older drugs that had been tried and discarded. Most recently, for example, scientists have returned to the sulfonamide drugs and to the sulfone, dapsone (see Chap. 35)—drugs once tried and found less useful in malaria than chloroquine and the other 4-aminoquinoline compounds. Reports from Vietnam indicating that combination of these older drugs with new ones has resulted in potentiated antimalarial activity have rekindled scientific interest in the sulfonamides and the sulfones.

OTHER PARASITIC INFECTIONS

Protozoan organisms other than plasmodia are a frequent cause of infection. Amebic infections of the intestine are taken up in the next chapter, together with a discussion of treatment of most intestinal worm infections. Here we shall discuss briefly the chemotherapy of protozoan infections such as trypanosomiasis and leishmaniasis and of infections caused by trematode-type worms, or flukes, and by nematode-type filarid worms.

Schistosomiasis is, next to malaria, the world's most important parasitic infection. More than one hundred million people are believed to be infected with blood flukes of this trematode genus. Infections are often acquired by bathing in water infested with certain species of snails, which are the intermediate host that releases the free-swimming larval form of the organism. These forked-tailed cercariae, as they are called, burrow down through the skin and are carried by the blood to the liver where they feed, grow and mature.

The person may have a passing itch and rash shortly after the larvae penetrate the skin from the film of evaporating or draining water. Allergic reactions may follow invasion of his liver. However, acute symptoms begin only after the schistosomes begin laying their masses of eggs. It is the accumulation and migration of these eggs that accounts for the many varied symptoms of this infection. Liver damage leading to cirrhosis is the most serious result of acute exacerbations of chronic infections.

Specific chemotherapy requires the use of relatively toxic drugs of two types: (1) organic antimony compounds, and (2) nonmetallic chemicals of the class known as miracils, xanthones, or thioxanthones.

Thus, it is desirable to build up the debilitated patient with dietary and anti-anemia treatments before subjecting him to drug therapy. Injections of antimonials such as *stibophen* (see Drug Digest) are considered the most effective treatment; however, nonmetallic agents such as *lucanthone* (see Drug Digest) have certain advantages. For example, the latter drug may be given by the more convenient oral route. Although often less effective than antimony, its less severe toxicity permits repeated treatment, which may finally prove successful in many cases.

Leishmaniasis is a term used to describe several diseases caused by infection with protozoan parasites of the Leishmania genus. These include kala-azar, or visceral leishmaniasis; oriental sore, or cutaneous leishmaniasis; and American mucocutaneous leishmaniasis. Kala-azar is a generalized infection with signs and symptoms involving the liver, spleen and bone marrow and ranging from vague pains in muscles, bones and joints to common complications such as bronchitis and pneumonia. The other leishmania infections are limited—to the skin, in oriental sore, and to the skin, mouth, nose and throat in mucocutaneous leishmaniasis.

Once the diagnosis is definitely established treatment of kala-azar with an organic antimonial is usually undertaken. The early forms of antimony, including antimony and potassium tartrate (Tartar Emetic) and stibophen (see Drug Digest) or related trivalent antimonials, have largely been superseded by the safer and more effective pentavalent antimonials. These include stibamine glucoside (Neostam), ethylstibamine (Neostibosan), and sodium stibogluconate (Pentostam; Solustibosan). A course of treatment with the last-named drug is said to cure most cases of kala-azar after six injections on consecutive days. Local intralesional injection of these compounds often clears oriental sore; mucosal lesions require parenteral therapy.

Resistant cases of kala-azar, such as are often encountered in the Sudan, have recently been treated with the diamidines, *pentamidine isethionate* and *hydroxystilbamidine isethionate* (see Drug Digest).

Trypanosomiasis is a protozoal infection transmitted by insects—the biting tsetse fly, in the case of African sleeping sickness, and the bedbug-like insect vector of Chagas' disease in the Americas. African trypanosomiasis is marked mainly by brain damage; American trypanosomiasis causes cardiac complications. The prognosis for patients with Chagas' disease is poor, for no satisfactory chemotherapeutic agent has as yet been discovered. Fortunately, drugs are now available for use in both the treatment and prevention of African sleeping sickness.

In general, compounds of two types are employed in African trypanosomiasis: (1) organic arsenicals such as *tryparsamide* (see Drug Digest) and *melarso-*

prol, and (2) nonmetallic trypanocides such as *suramin sodium* (see Drug Digest), *pentamidine*, and *hydroxystilbamidine* (see Drug Digest). The arsenicals, which pass the blood-brain barrier and penetrate into the central nervous system, are essential when there is C.N.S. involvement and urgent treatment is required. The less toxic nonmetallic compounds are employed for prophylaxis and in the treatment of early infections.

Pentamidine has proved especially useful as a chemoprophylactic agent against African sleeping sickness. Injected intramuscularly, the drug is apparently stored in the patient's tissues, releasing small amounts of the trypanocide over a period of months. Residents of endemic areas can be protected for long periods, thus markedly reducing the infection rate in the exposed population. Neither this drug nor suramin is given in this manner for treatment of already infected patients. In such cases, these drugs are administered intravenously in larger and more frequent doses, which are often followed by a course of tryparsamide or melarsoprol.

Filariasis is a parasitic disease caused by the presence of tiny roundworms in body tissues. A person becomes infected by being bitten by a mosquito (Culex species especially) that deposits larvae in the skin. Later, the adult females give birth to thin threadlike microfilariae which migrate into the lymphatics and the blood stream. Symptoms are the result of inflammatory reactions to the presence of living and dead worms. Obstruction of the lymphatic system by inflammatory lesions may lead to elephantiasis—gross enlargement of the legs, arms, scrotum, or breast by edema fluid.

Actually, this grim complication is a rare one that develops only in patients who have been continuously infected for many years and have had a series of acute inflammatory attacks and have suffered from chronic edema. Thus, although thousands of American servicemen were infected in the Western Pacific during World War II, none is known to have developed elephantiasis, and only a few suffered severe symptoms.

Until relatively recent years no safe drug was available for treatment of filariasis, and, in fact, there is still no chemical that can be taken to prevent infection upon entering an endemic area. Prevention involves mosquito control by means of insecticides aimed at breeding places, as well as special efforts to avoid being bitten. The relatively toxic arsenical and antimony compounds once employed with only fair success have now been largely displaced by two nonmetallic compounds diethylcarbamazine and suramin sodium (see Drug Digests).

SUMMARY OF ANTIMALARIAL DRUG THERAPY

- *Drugs for Use in Suppressive Treatment [1] and for Clinical Cure [2]*

    Amodiaquine HCl (Camoquin)
    Chloroquine phosphate (Aralen)
    Chloroguanide (Paludrine)
    Cycloguanil pamoate (Camolar) [3]
    Hydroxychloroquine (Plaquenil)
    Pyrimethamine (Daraprim)

    Quinacrine (Atabrine)
    Quinine and its salts [4]

- *Drugs [5] for Use in Radical Cure and for Causal Prophylaxis etc.*

    Isopentaquine
    Pamaquine (Plasmochin)
    Primaquine phosphate [6]
    Pentaquine

[1] These drugs are used in small doses at stated intervals for suppressing development of clinical signs and symptoms.

[2] Larger doses of the same drugs are administered (after beginning treatment with a priming dose) until all signs and symptoms have disappeared.

[3] This drug is being tried experimentally for long-term suppressive action when administered in a single parenteral repository dose.

[4] This drug is sometimes still employed for treating severe, complicated infections by organisms resistant to other drugs.

[5] Chemically, these are all 8-aminoquinoline compounds.

[6] This is the only drug of this group in actual use today; the others are mainly of historical interest. It is used in combination with a drug of Group 1 for treating severe infections and prevention of further relapses; it is ordinarily not taken routinely as causal prophylaxis or to prevent transmission of the disease, even though it is capable of doing so.

REVIEW QUESTIONS

1. Indicate the role of each of the following forms of the plasmodial parasite in the transmission of malaria or in causing clinical signs and symptoms of the disease: (1) gametocytes; (2) erythrocytic schizonts; (3) primary tissue schizonts, i.e. *pre*-erythrocytic schizonts; (4) secondary tissue schizonts, or *exo*-erythrocytic forms.

2. What is meant by each of the following terms, and which of the available antimalarial drugs, if any, may act, in theory or in practice, to produce each result?

(1) true causal prophylaxis and causal prophylaxis

(2) suppressive treatment

(3) clinical cure and radical cure

3. (a) For what two purposes is chloroquine used in antimalarial therapy, and what dosage schedules are used typically in each case?

(b) What are two (or more) conditions other than malaria for which chloroquine is employed?

4. (a) What side effects may occur when chloroquine is employed in the doses required for clinical cure?

(b) Toxicity of what types has occurred during long-term administration of chloroquine in chronic conditions or as a result of acute overdosage?

5. (a) For what purpose is primaquine used in malaria, and with what other drug is it ordinarily administered?

(b) Of potential toxicity from primaquine what sort is the most serious and what measures may the nurse and the doctor take to detect it in its early stages?

6. (a) For what purposes is pyrimethamine potentially useful, and for what purpose is it actually largely employed?

(b) What type of toxicity is possible when pyrimethamine is employed in very much larger doses than ordinarily?

7. (a) What is the source of *quinine*? For what purpose was it formerly used as an antimalarial and for what kind of cases is it largely reserved today?

(b) What are some clinical conditions besides malaria for which quinine may sometimes be ordered or taken?

8. (a) What are the characteristic signs and symptoms of overdosage with quinine (cinchonism)?

(b) What dangerous toxic reactions may result from massive overdosage of quinine?

9. (a) For what condition is stibophen a drug of choice?

(b) Toxicity of what type may occur from this antimony compound?

10. (a) For what conditions is hydroxystilbamidine employed?

(b) For what conditions is suramin sodium employed?

11. (a) What property of tryparsamide makes it particularly useful for treating cases of African sleeping sickness?

(b) What kinds of toxicity are possible with this organic arsenical drug?

BIBLIOGRAPHY

Bruce-Chwatt, L. J.: Changing tides of chemotherapy of malaria. Brit. Med. J., *1*:581, 1964.

Di Palma, J. R.: Drugs for malaria. R.N., *30*:77, 1967 (Jan.).

Gabriel, H. S.: Beware those jet-borne diseases. R.N., *30*:37, 1967 (April).

Hockwald, R. S., *et al.*: Toxicity of primaquine in Negroes. J.A.M.A., *149*:1568, 1952.

Hoskins, D. W., and Kean, B. H.: Drugs for travelers. Clin. Pharmacol. Ther., *4*:673, 1963.

Huff, C. G.: Man against malaria. Am. J. Trop. Med., *14*:339, 1965.

Most, H., *et al.*: Chloroquine for acute attacks of malaria. J.A.M.A., *131*:963, 1946.

Most, H.: The pendulum in malaria chemotherapy: From quinine to chloroquine and back to quinine? Mil. Med., *129*:587, 1964.

Powell, R. D.: The chemotherapy of malaria. Clin. Pharmacol. Ther., *7*:48, 1966.

Powell, R. D., *et al.*: Studies on a strain of chloroquine-resistant Plasmodium falciparum from Vietnam. Bull. WHO, *31*:379, 1964.

· 37 ·

The Chemotherapy of Amebiasis
and of Intestinal Helminthiasis

AMEBIASIS

Amebiasis, a condition caused by the protozoan organism, *Entamoeba histolytica,* is endemic in tropical lands. However, contrary to popular opinion, amebic infection is not limited to the tropics but may develop wherever sanitary conditions are substandard. In this country, the intestinal disease sometimes spreads among patients in mental hospitals or in institutions for elderly patients or children. Although the condition is most common in the rural South, epidemics also occur in metropolitan areas.

The life cycle of *E. histolytica* takes place in two stages in the human G.I. tract: (1) a *cyst* form and, (2) a *trophozoite* phase. An understanding of the nature of these stages is necessary, in order to comprehend the uses and limitations of the antiamebic agents employed in the management of amebiasis.

The cystic stage is the one in which this microorganism is transmitted from one person to another. This form is very resistant to adverse environmental conditions. Passed in the formed feces of infected individuals, the cysts can survive outside the body for several weeks, enduring drying, freezing, chemicals, and high heat. Water containing amebic cysts requires prolonged boiling before it is safe for drinking. Contact with the ordinary concentrations of chlorine employed in water purification does not destroy the cysts.

The amebic cysts are transmitted from person to person by ingestion of contaminated food and drink. Flies moving from filth to food are a common source of contamination as are the fingers of food handlers. These workers, who are themselves often free of intestinal symptoms, can spread the cysts if they do not wash their hands thoroughly after going to the toilet. The swallowed cysts then pass through the stomach unaffected by acid gastric juices. When they reach

the lower levels of the small intestine, some of the amebic cysts are activated there by digestive secretions and break out of the enveloping cystic wall. They then divide to form tiny trophozoites. Other amebae from the intestinal lumen never excyst and are passed in the patient's feces, thus continuing the transmission chain.

The trophozoites, the active motile forms of the amebae, move down into the cecum, where they feed, grow and produce large colonies of daughter trophozoites. These then spread to other parts of the large bowel, especially the sigmoid colon and the rectum. Although these trophozoites are able to dissolve mucosal cells and penetrate intestinal wall tissues, no evidence of pathologic changes may appear. This may be because the host's intestinal bacterial flora is of a kind that does not adequately support the amebae or aid their invasiveness. However, after a period varying from days to months, conditions finally become right for the amebae, and they begin to produce their effects.

Intestinal symptoms may be mild and consist mainly of flatulence and passing of soft stools. On the other hand, severe mucous diarrhea may develop quite suddenly in a minority of patients in whom the amebae have produced extensive necrotic ulceration of the intestinal mucosa. The abdominal pain and tenderness of acute intestinal amebiasis may concentrate in the lower right abdomen and be mistaken for appendicitis. The symptoms have also been diagnosed as those of peptic ulcer or cholecystitis. In cases marked by frequent bowel movements (as many as twenty to forty daily), untreated patients may quickly become dehydrated and prostrated, and death may follow in a few days.

Extraintestinal effects occur when the trophozoites make their way into tiny mesenteric venules and are

508

then carried by the blood to the liver and other tissues including the brain, lungs, skin and heart. Liver lesions are most common, occurring when the trophozoites lodge in thrombosed hepatic veins and colonize there. This often leads to development of one or more hepatic abscesses, which may rupture with serious results and serve as foci for the further spread of amebae through the body.

Disease states and their treatment vary very considerably. Patients range from (1) those who are *asymptomatic*, (2) those with *mild* cases of *amebic colitis* with only occasional diarrhea alternating with longer periods of constipation, (3) those with *acute amebic dysentery*, to (4) those with *amebic hepatitis* and *liver abscesses*, or with damage to other extraintestinal organs. No single drug is capable of curing *both* the intestinal and the systemic tissue forms of amebic infection; also, drugs effective in mild cases may act too slowly to be truly useful in very severe acute cases, and the most effective drug for controlling acute amebic dysentery is too dangerous for routine use in chronic cases. Thus, the treatment of amebiasis usually requires the use of amebicidal drugs of more than one class.

Types of Anti-Amebic Agents (Table 37-1)

The anti-amebic agents may be broadly subdivided into: (1) drugs that are effective *only* against *intestinal* amebiasis and (2) drugs that are capable of killing trophozoites that have invaded *extraintestinal* tissues. Only *chloroquine* and *emetine* are in the latter category. Emetine (see Drug Digest) is also effective for controlling the trophozoite-induced intestinal symptoms of *acute* amebic dysentery and in acute exacerbations of chronic ulcerative colitis of amebic origin. Chloroquine, on the other hand, is an effective hepatic amebicide but is relatively ineffective for treatment of the intestinal symptoms of amebiasis.

The drugs useful against *intestinal* amebic infections are subdivided into the following types:

1. **Arsonic acid derivatives**—organic arsenic compounds, including *carbarsone* (see Drug Digest). These are useful for controlling *mild* to *moderately severe flare-ups* of amebic dysentery in *chronic* cases but are not as reliable as emetine for treating patients critically ill with acute dysentery.

2. **Halogenated hydroxyquinolines**, including *iodochlorhydroxyquin* (see Drug Digest). These are used in the same circumstances as the organic arsenicals. However, these drugs are considered safe enough and free enough of severe side effects to be used in treating *asymptomatic* carriers, and they are, in fact, often used for *prophylaxis* of uninfected individuals traveling in countries where amebic and bacillary intestinal infections are endemic.

3. **Antibiotics** of various types. These are used to eradicate the trophozoites in the intestine, but it is doubtful that most of these drugs act specifically on the amebae themselves. It is thought that, for the most part, the antibiotics affect the amebae by altering the bacterial flora and thus depriving the amebae of essential nutrients. Broad-spectrum antibiotics of the tetracycline type, such as *oxytetracycline*, are often administered in combination with emetine to patients critically ill with acute amebic dysentery; other antibiotics, such as *paromomycin* (see Drug Digest), are used mainly in less serious situations, similar to those in which the quinoline compounds (see above) are administered.

4. **Miscellaneous amebicides** include synthetic direct-acting drugs, such as the chloracetanilide derivative *diloxanide furoate*, and a plant derivative, the glycoside *glaucarubin*, which also possesses a direct amebicidal action on the intestinal form of the parasite.

Chemotherapy of Various Stages of Amebiasis

Acute amebic dysentery is marked by the sometimes sudden development of symptoms such as severe diarrhea with blood-streaked mucus, intestinal spasm, painful anal straining (tenesmus), and colicky abdominal pains that may sometimes suggest acute appendicitis. Many patients can, of course, have their symptoms brought under control by the oral administration of carbarsone combined with antidiarrheal medications such as paregoric and adsorbent drugs (see Chap. 38). However, parenteral administration of emetine is preferred for seriously ill patients who require more prompt cessation of symptoms.

Emetine Therapy. In such cases, emetine often brings about dramatic control of acute symptoms quite rapidly. It is, however, potentially a very toxic drug capable of causing severe systemic and local reactions. Aching is common at the muscular injection site. Much more serious is the possible development of cardiovascular toxicity. For this reason, patients receiving emetine are hospitalized and kept at rest in bed.

The nurse may be required to take the patient's pulse and blood pressure several times daily during a course of treatment with emetine. If tachycardia occurs or the patient's pressure falls, the nurse should report this to the doctor who may then order electrocardiographic tracings. The appearance of ECG abnormalities together with a rise in pulse rate of over 110 beats per minute may require emetine medication to be discontinued. Sometimes the drug's ill effects on the heart develop late; therefore patients are warned not to exert themselves for weeks after a course of therapy is completed.

The nurse should discuss with the doctor his specific recommendations in regard to how much activity the patient can safely undertake following a course of emetine treatment. She can then instruct the patient on how he should plan his activities, with something more specific than a vague "you'll have to take it easy for a while." The patient should also be warned to report promptly any symptoms that he experiences during the post-treatment period.

Useful as emetine is for rapidly eradicating the trophozoites invading the bowel wall, and thus controlling the symptoms of severe amebic dysentery, this drug alone does not cure amebiasis. Emetine has no capacity to kill amebic cysts in the doses that are ordinarily employed. Thus, when the drug is discontinued shortly after the acute symptoms are brought under control, the cysts will once more begin to produce invasive trophozoites.

Adjunctive Antibiotics. In order to prevent relapses in such cases, doctors commonly administer a second, safer drug along with emetine for about 10 days, to control excysting intestinal trophozoites. The antibiotic oxytetracycline, for example, is a common choice for this purpose. Administered in daily doses of about one or two grams orally, or half those amounts parenterally, this broad-spectrum antibiotic often helps to hasten the patient's recovery.

This substance and most of the other antibiotics employed in amebiasis (Table 37-1) are thought not to act directly on the amebae. They are believed to bring about their effects indirectly by affecting the bacterial flora of the intestine. The relations between bacterial organisms and pathogenic protozoa in the bowel are not very well understood; however, it has been suggested that colonic bacteria play a part in providing the nutritional requirements of the amebae. Thus, broad-spectrum antibiotics may exert their antiamebic effects mainly by altering the bacterial flora of the intestine. Of course, their antibacterial action is also desirable for controlling secondary infections of a kind that often make it easier for amebae to burrow down into the bowel wall.

Follow-up Therapy. Once acute intestinal symptoms are brought under control by such emetine-antibiotic combinations, and the patient is out of immediate danger, a follow-up treatment plan is often put into effect. This involves the use of yet another drug combination, consisting of an intestinal chemotherapeutic amebicidal agent, such as carbarsone or diiodohydroxyquin, and an agent that is effective against *extra*intestinal protozoa. Chloroquine (see Drug Digest) is preferred for this purpose, because it is much safer than emetine for use in the several weeks of post-attack therapy that is required.

Amebic hepatitis and liver abscesses are possible complications in any patient who has had an attack of acute amebic dysentery. These extraintestinal after-effects can, in fact, develop even in infected cyst-passing individuals who have never developed diarrhea or other intestinal symptoms. For this reason most authorities feel that even asymptomatic patients who are taking courses of treatment with intestinal amebicides (see below) should receive chloroquine routinely at the same time.

Chloroquine is, fortunately, a relatively safe drug in the doses that are administered for eliminating any amebic trophozoites that may have made their way from the intestine to the liver. Chloroquine is absorbed from the small intestine and carried to the liver, where it reaches amebicidal concentrations. Thus, it often clears up symptoms of amebic hepatitis as readily as does the much more dangerous drug, emetine. Unlike emetine, however, chloroquine is ineffective against amebic dysentery, because it fails to reach the colon in adequate amounts. Thus chloroquine therapy is supplemented with a simultaneously administered intestinal amebicide such as carbarsone or diiodohydroxyquin, or one of the newer drugs of this kind (see below).

When employed in the doses used in amebiasis, chloroquine is a drug of relatively low toxicity. It is not likely to cause the kinds of disturbances reported during prolonged therapy of arthritis (see Chap. 41). However, if the patient complains of epigastric distress, the doctor may order that the drug be given after meals, even though it is more completely absorbed from the upper intestinal tract when taken on an empty stomach.

Amebic colitis of a chronic nature, with relatively mild enteric symptoms, should also be treated in an effort to rid the intestine of amebae. For such patients, however, drugs safer than emetine are usually preferred. Emetine is, in fact, not nearly as useful as the safer arsenicals and hydroxyquinolines for eliminating intestinal amebae. On the other hand, carbarsone and similar drugs sometimes produce a true cure of amebiasis by eliminating both the cyst and the trophozoite forms from the intestine.

Doctors differ in the particular intestinal amebicides that they prefer for this purpose. Sometimes, they try a course of an arsenical such as carbarsone or glycobiarsol and follow the first agent with one of the hydroxyquinolines, such as iodochlorhydroxyquin or diiodohydroxyquin. In some cases, the choice depends upon whether the patient is able to tolerate a drug of one type better than another.

Occasionally, if patients of this type react poorly to the more commonly employed intestinal amebicides, the doctor may try one of the anti-amebic antibiotics (Table 37-1). Unfortunately, these drugs also are not entirely devoid of toxicity. In fact, fumagillin, which is the only antibiotic with a directly lethal action on intestinal amebae specifically, was withdrawn from the market in this country because of the frequent side effects of some severity that it caused. The other antibiotics, including paromomycin, which affect the bacterial flora as well as amebae, may cause overgrowths of fungal or of resistant staphylococcal organisms with possible superinfections. Thus, patients being treated with these agents must be observed for signs of any new infections that may be developing.

Asymptomatic cyst passers should also receive treatment with intestinal amebicides whenever discovered. One reason is that, even though they may themselves be suffering from no symptoms, their infected condition may make them a menace to other, less resistant people whom they may infect. In addition, as long as a person has amebae in his intestinal tract, he is always subject to acute attacks whenever his resistance is lowered or the organism becomes more virulent.

TABLE 37-1
ANTI-AMEBIC AGENTS

Nonproprietary or Official Name	Proprietary Name or Synonym	Dosage
Drugs Effective in Extra-intestinal Amebiasis		
Chloroquine phosphate U.S.P.	Aralen	For amebic abscess: 250 mg. 2 or 3 times a day for 2 weeks up to a total dose of 11 Gm.
Emetine Bismuth Iodide	—	200 mg. once daily for 12 days
Emetine HCl U.S.P.	—	1 mg. per Kg. up to 60 mg. daily for 10 days
Drugs Effective in Intestinal Amebiasis		
Arsonic acid derivatives		
Carbarsone U.S.P.	—	250 mg. 2 or 3 times daily for 10 days
Glycobiarsol N.F.	Milibis	500 mg. 3 times a day for 10 days
Halogenated oxyquinoline derivatives		
Diiodohydroxyquin U.S.P.	Diodoquin; Yodoxin	650 mg. 3 times a day for 20 days
Iodochlorhydroxyquin U.S.P.	Vioform	250 mg. 3 times a day for 10 days
Iodohydroxyquinoline	Chiniofon; Yatren; Quinoxyl	250 mg. 3 times a day for 8 to 10 days
Chloracetanilide derivatives		
Diloxanide	Entamide	12 mg. per Kg. daily for 10 days
Diloxanide furoate	Furamide	500 mg. 3 times a day for 10 days
Glycoside		
Glaucarubin	Glarubin	3 mg. per Kg. orally for 5 to 10 days
Antibiotics		
Bacitracin U.S.P.	Baciguent	80,000 to 120,000 u. every 6 hours for 2 weeks
Erythromycin U.S.P.	Erythrocin; Ilotycin	1 to 2 Gm. daily
Fumagillin	Fumidil	40 mg. a day in 4 divided doses for 10 to 14 days
Oxytetracycline N.F.	Terramycin	250 mg. 4 times a day for 5 days
Paromomycin	Humatin	25 mg. per Kg. in divided doses at mealtime for at least 5 days

Although treatment is desirable for both public health and personal reasons, a carrier who has suffered no symptoms is not likely to continue taking an amebicidal drug if its side effects are disturbing. Despite explanations that he is a possible source of infection to himself and others, a patient who has never even had loose stools often is not willing to keep on taking a preventive drug—paramomycin, for example—if the drug itself causes diarrhea or nausea.

Asymptomatic carriers are treated with the least toxic of the intestinal amebicides. Most doctors consider these to be iodochlorhydroxyquin and diiodohydroxyquin—agents that are often taken without any ill effects by healthy travelers in areas where intestinal infections are endemic. Sometimes, however, patients sensitive to iodine may suffer ill effects from these drugs. A new intestinal amebicide, used up to now mainly in British Commonwealth nations where amebiasis is endemic, is diloxanide furoate. It is said to be free of side effects and thus suitable for routine use by asymptomatic but infected patients.

The nurse should encourage carriers to continue with drug therapy. However, her attitude should not take on a lofty moral tone full of reminders about remembering one's responsibility to society. Instead, the benefits to the individual should be stressed, together with the need to protect his family and co-workers. The nurse employed in industry, schools, and other institutions should teach the necessity for thorough hand-washing and recommend that all washrooms—especially those used by food handlers—be equipped with plenty of soap and towels.

Recurrences are possible, if only a single cystic ameba remained alive after the patient had been clinically "cured." However, not all former patients are necessarily suffering from amebiasis when they have an attack of diarrhea at a later time. A relapse or reinfection can be proved only by stool specimen examinations that actually detect the presence of *Entamoeba histolytica*. Only then do the authorities on the treatment of this disease recommend administration of amebicidal drugs.

In practice, however, many doctors may order amebicidal drugs for a patient with a history of amebiasis who develops diarrhea. Rather than wait for the results of the complicated laboratory procedures by which the parasitologist confirms the diagnosis, the doctor may prescribe an intestinal amebicide such as carbarsone or diiodohydroxyquin. He may also order chloroquine—but never emetine—in order to strike at any amebae lurking in the liver of the patient with only mild intestinal symptoms.

HELMINTHIASIS

Helminthiasis, invasion of the human body by parasitic worms, is prevalent throughout the world. An estimated billion human beings are believed to harbor helminths of one kind or another. In some tropical countries more than 90 per cent of the population plays host to worms. Helminthiasis is not, however, limited to tropical climates. A recent survey of hospital employees in New York City revealed that nearly one in three had parasites in his intestine. The number of Americans with pinworms is estimated at 20 millions, and several million more are infected with roundworms and other helminths.

The drugs used for removing worms from the intestinal tract are called *anthelmintics* (Table 37-2). The presently available agents of this class can be depended upon to expel these parasites with relatively little risk to the patient. Proper treatment must, however, be based upon accurate diagnosis, in which the doctor is aided by the laboratory findings of parasitologists skilled in identifying adult worms as well as eggs and larvae.

This is necessary because the choice of the best drug with which to treat a particular patient requires exact knowledge of the nature of the parasites. In addition, the use of the various anthelmintic drugs often calls for the application of pre- and post-treatment measures intended to assure maximum contact of the chemical with the worm and minimal toxicity to the patient. The nurse must be aware of these specialized techniques and the other adjunctive measures required for most effective use of the various anthelmintics employed in the treatment of the common intestinal parasitic infestations.

In this section, we shall discuss the drug treatment of infection by those worms that can be readily reached by drugs acting within the intestine. The treatment of certain helminthic invaders of extraintestinal tissues, such as the blood flukes, or trematodes, is taken up in Chapter 36. Here, we shall be concerned mainly with the nematodes (round, unsegmented worms) and, to a lesser extent, with the platyhelminths (flatworms) of the tapeworm, or cestode, type.

The nematodes of medical interest are the following: (1) *Enterobius vermicularis*—also called oxyuriads—which we shall call by their common name, i.e., *pinworms*; (2) *Ascaris lumbricoides*, the *roundworm*; (3) *Strongyloides stercoralis*, the cause of the infection called *strongyloidiasis*, or threadworm disease; (4) *Trichuris trichiura*, the *whipworm*, and (5) two species of *hookworm*, *Necator americanus* and *Ancylostoma duodenale*.

Four species of tapeworm are involved in common infestations: (1) *Taenia saginata*, the beef tapeworm, (2) *Taenia solium*, the pork tapeworm, (3) *Diphyllobrothium latum*, the fish tapeworm, and (4) *Hymenolepis nana*, the dwarf tapeworm.

Pinworms, also known as seatworms and threadworms, are the intestinal helminths most prevalent among school children in the United States. Fortunately, they are also the worms least likely to cause serious complications and the parasites most readily eradicated by certain quite safe drugs now available. The main difficulty in dealing with pinworm infestations is the ease with which children can become reinfected and spread the organism through the whole family.

Two excellent anthelmintic drugs, the piperazine salts (see Table 37-2 and Drug Digest) and pyrvinium pamoate (see Drug Digest), are available for treating pinworm infestations. Both drugs are safe, effective, and easy to take. Most authorities appear to favor a one-week course of treatment with piperazine citrate over the single-dose pyrvinium therapy now available —perhaps because of their greater familiarity with the former treatment and the staining capacity of the latter.

In addition, the need to take a daily dose of the piperazine preparation for 7 days may serve to emphasize the importance of the patient's paying strict attention to supportive hygienic measures to prevent reinfection. These include:

1. Keeping the child's nails cut short and his hands well-scrubbed, since reinfection results from the worm's eggs being carried back to the mouth after becoming lodged under the fingernails during scratching of the pruritic perianal area.

2. Giving the child a shower in the morning to wash away any ova deposited in the anal area during the night.

3. Disinfecting toilet seats daily and the floors of bathroom and bedroom periodically.

Actually, it may not always be advisable to make a fuss about a child's having worms, because overemphasis of the topic may do more harm psychologically than these parasites are ordinarily likely to do physically. Most light pinworm infestations need no treatment at all, and reinfection need not be discouraging, since treatment is now so relatively simple. On the other hand, it does no harm to take the opportunity to inculcate the desirability of washing the hands after each use of the toilet while treating a child whose symptoms have brought him to medical attention.

Itching in the area of the anus and perineum may be the only symptom. If severe, it may cause scratching and secondary infection. Thus, application of an antipruritic ointment may be a desirable adjunct to anthelmintic drug therapy. Since more severe symptoms such as abdominal pain, loss of weight, nervousness and insomnia are most likely to occur in patients who are in generally poor health, the doctor will also often order drugs and dietary measures for the management of other medical conditions simultaneously.

Pediatricians, directors of institutions, school officials and other concerned authorities have the responsibility of deciding how far to go in the direction of instituting special public health measures for coping with pinworm infestations in the family, school and community. Often suppression of symptoms in the more heavily infected individuals is more sensible and likely to succeed than are attempts to eradicate the worms in all possible contacts or to effect a complete cure in everyone. The measures required to prove that the patient is completely cured involve swabbing of the anal area with Scotch tape until no eggs are found on a microscope slide for 7 consecutive mornings. In view

TABLE 37-2
ANTHELMINTIC DRUGS

Generic or Official Name	Synonym or Proprietary Name	Dosage
Aspidium oleoresin	Male fern	5 Gm. for adults
Bephenium hydroxynaphthoate	Alcopar	5 Gm. for adults
Dichlorophen	Anthiphen	2 to 3 Gm. q. 8 hr. t.i.d.
Dithiazanine iodide U.S.P.	Delvex	100 to 200 mg. t.i.d.
Hexylresorcinol N.F.	Crystoids	1 Gm.
Piperazine citrate U.S.P.	Antepar; Multifuge	50 mg. per Kg. daily for 7 days
Pyrvinium pamoate U.S.P.	Povan	7.5 mg. per Kg. taken once
Quinacrine HCl U.S.P.	Atabrine	800 mg. in 4 divided doses
Tetrachloroethylene U.S.P.	—	0.12 ml. per Kg. up to 5 ml. total dose
Thiabendazole N.F.	Mintezol	10 mg. per lb. up to 3 Gm. daily dosage

of the lack of complications in most cases, such a program seems burdensome.

Roundworm infestation may produce no symptoms at all in many people. Yet, they are potentially so serious that doctors feel it desirable to treat any person who passes even a single worm. Even one worm may do damage in its migrations about the body, and the masses of worms likely to be produced from fertilized eggs may cause intestinal and respiratory tract obstruction.

This is especially true in children, since they are prone to become feverish, and the worms, which are sensitive to changes in body temperature, may then be stirred into activity. During such movements, the worms may block the bile duct or appendix or even occasionally break into the abdominal cavity and cause peritonitis. Thus, to avoid these and other rare but possible complications such as liver or lung abscesses, drug treatment must be promptly undertaken.

Fortunately, the roundworm is very susceptible to the paralyzing action of piperazine. Administered daily for a week, this relatively safe and easy-to-take chemical quickly clears the intestinal tract of these worms, which are readily swept out with the fecal stream even without the aid of a laxative. Piperazine ordinarily has little or no effect on the host. However, large amounts, if accidentally ingested, may be systemically absorbed and produce signs of skeletal muscle weakness. Although no fatalities have been reported and symptoms tend to disappear in a day or two, the child's stomach should be emptied and he should be kept under observation. Parents should be warned to keep the pleasantly flavored piperazine syrups or wafers out of reach of children.

Occasionally, in some areas patients are infected with other worms as well as with roundworms. In such cases, it is important that the roundworms be removed before trying to eradicate the other parasites. This is because anthelmintic medications such as tetrachlorethylene (see Drug Digest), which is used against hookworms, may activate the roundworms to make the kind of migrations that can lead to dangerous complications. Hexylresorcinol (see Drug Digest) is sometimes preferred in such cases, since it is capable of eliminating *both* roundworms and hookworms. Among other drugs occasionally employed against round worms are dithiazanine (see Drug Digest), bephenium (p. 515), diethylcarbamazine (see Drug Digest), and oil of chenopodium.

Strongyloides persistently infests the upper gastrointestinal tract and resembles hookworm in its capacity to cause weight loss and debility. Strongyloidiasis is seen in the southern United States as well as in the tropics. Light infection that results in no symptoms requires no treatment. However, heavily infected patients, such as those sometimes seen in mental hospitals and other institutions, are treated to avoid development of malabsorption syndromes as well as for relief of diarrhea and upper abdominal discomfort.

Earlier treatment with gentian violet was unsatisfactory as a cure for the condition, although it often offered temporary symptomatic relief. The newer drug, dithiazanine, has proved highly effective for eliminating Strongyloides worms in the intestine. Because the drug does not affect the larvae in the lungs and elsewhere, it is given in repeated courses in order to kill the worms when they reach the small intestine. However, this drug is reserved for the relatively rare patient with disabling symptoms. Thiabendazole (see Drug Digest), a recently introduced broad spectrum anthelmintic, is claimed more than 95 per cent effective in the treatment of threadworm disease.

Whipworms are tiny threadlike parasites that become engaged in the mucosa of the cecum but rarely burrow deeper. No treatment is necessary in lightly infected patients, and drugs may even be withheld in many cases marked by only mild, occasional diarrhea. However, if the infection is a heavy one with many eggs in the stool and prolapse of the rectum, the doctor may undertake treatment with dithiazanine or hexylresorcinol.

Hexylresorcinol, the less toxic agent, may be given by mouth and by rectum simultaneously. Because the concentrated drug is irritating, patients are told not to chew the pills, and precautions are taken to prevent burns of the skin, of the buttocks, and thighs. The mucus secreted in response to the presence of masses of attached worms protects the rectal membranes from irritation by a 1:500 retention enema, to which kaolin is added to reduce colonic cramps. Petroleum jelly is applied to protect the skin from the irritating effects of any solution that may leak during the retention period of two or three hours.

Dithiazanine is proving the most effective agent for clearing up heavily infected cases of whipworm infection. It is given for shorter periods than in the treatment of Strongyloides, but the larger doses that are required cause nausea and vomiting in as many as a third of the patients taking the drug. Such gastrointestinal upset may be minimized by administering the drug in half the recommended dose for twice as long a period. An antiemetic agent such as prochlorperazine (see Drug Digest) may be helpful in reducing drug-induced nausea. Dithiazanine is contraindicated in patients with ulcerative disease of the G.I. tract and with renal insufficiency, because of its potential systemic toxicity.

Hookworm infection, though less common in the United States than it once was, is one of the world's most common helminthic diseases. Heavy infestations are debilitating, because the worms not only damage intestinal mucosa but cause an iron deficiency anemia, with symptoms such as chronic fatigue and apathy. Such patients require treatment with oral or parenteral iron salts (see Chap. 25) or even prompt transfusion of whole blood or packed red cells. Correction of fluid and electrolyte imbalance is desirable before administration of anthelmintic drug therapy.

Infection with *Necator americanus,* the organism most common in the Western hemisphere, is readily controlled by treatment with tetrachloroethylene (see Drug Digest), taken in the morning following a fasting period or no more than a fat-free, largely liquid meal the night before. The drug is safe, inexpensive, and effective in four out of five cases. In cases in which the presence of roundworms is suspected, tetrachloroethylene is given only after the roundworms have been eliminated.

Tetrachloroethylene is not nearly so effective in hookworm infections caused by the so-called Old World hookworm, *Ancylostoma duodenale.* For treating infections by this organism a new agent, bephenium hydroxynaphthoate, is now preferred. This drug is almost equally effective in *Necator americanus* infections and can be given in cases complicated by the presence of roundworms, which it also readily removes. The new agent is nontoxic and requires no preliminary fasting or post-treatment purging. The drug's only drawback seems to be a bitter taste which requires partial masking in order to avoid gagging and possible nausea and vomiting.

Tapeworms are segmented flatworms, consisting of a scolex, or head, which attaches itself to the intestinal wall, and a variable number of segments that grow from the head, sometimes forming a worm several yards long. However, the presence of lengthy beef or fish tapeworms is not truly serious. The patient may have some mild abdominal symptoms and suffer some weight loss occasionally, but treatment is sought more for psychological than physical reasons. That is, the patient may be frightened by finding worm segments in his stool, even though their passage causes little discomfort.

The pork tapeworm, which is rare in this country, can, however, cause a more serious condition called cysticercosis. In such cases, the larval form of the worm makes its way into the blood stream and may be carried to the muscles, lungs, liver, or brain. Since no specific treatment is available for cysticercosis, it is important to remove the adult worm while it is in the intestinal tract. The once widely used vermifuge, oleoresin of aspidium, has been largely replaced for this purpose by the safer synthetic chemotherapeutic agent, quinacrine (see Drug Digest).

Whichever drug is employed to make the head of the worm loosen its hold on the intestinal wall, it is desirable to empty the patient's intestine first, in order to ensure contact between the chemical and the scolex. Drug treatment is followed by a saline purge and careful examination of all stool specimens until the worm is evacuated. Identification of the head of the worm is relatively easy after treatment with quinacrine, which stains the scolex a bright yellow.

Trichinosis is infection with the worm *Trichinella spiralis* and is caused by eating raw or poorly cooked pork containing the encysted larvae. Although the adult worms develop in the duodenum, the main damage is done by larvae that make their way through the intestine into the blood stream to skeletal muscles where they induce inflammatory reactions.

Corticosteroid drugs have been used to counteract the acute inflammatory reactions caused by larval invasion of the tissues. No chemotherapeutic agent has proved effective for killing the larvae. Thiabendazole (p. 514) is said to relieve symptoms in some patients, but its effect upon larvae that have already migrated to muscles remains uncertain at this time.

AMEBIASIS: SUMMARY OF POINTS FOR THE NURSE TO REMEMBER

- Teach carriers of amebic cysts the need to wash hands thoroughly after visiting the toilet. Recommend that washrooms of schools, factories and institutions be stocked with soap and towels as an aid to prevention of spread of infection.

- Encourage carriers to continue with drug therapy by stressing the benefits to themselves, family and coworkers rather than by adopting a punitive attitude in regard to their duty to protect the public's health.

- Take special care in administering emetine to see that injections are made in a manner that will prevent local and systemic reactions.

- See that the patient on emetine therapy stays in bed; observe him carefully for signs such as an increase in pulse rate or fall in blood pressure and inform the physician promptly of such symptoms.

- Instruct the patient to rest in the weeks following a course of emetine treatment. Advise the patient in accordance with the views expressed by the doctor as to how much activity he may safely undertake.

HELMINTHIASIS: SUMMARY OF POINTS
FOR THE NURSE TO REMEMBER

• Remember to instruct the patient and family in measures to help prevent pinworm reinfection, such as careful handwashing after using the toilet, and keeping the fingernails short.

• Be consistent in applying necessary hygienic measures for preventing spread of worms from one person to another. However, in emphasizing the need to use such precautions, do not convey a punitive attitude nor imply that you are afraid of acquiring the infection.

• Although some worm infestations are more physically harmful than others, all can be humiliating to the patient. Show the patient, by your manner when caring for him, that you accept his illness, and that you are willing to care for him.

• Suggest measures for allaying itching of the anal region, such as gentle cleansing followed by application of antipruritic ointments. These are likely to prove more effective in reducing scratching than merely reminding the patient not to scratch.

• Remember to warn patients to take anthelmintic drugs as directed, in order to avoid injury to themselves and to prevent treatment failure. Warn them also of any possible fecal discolorations, in order to avoid unnecessary concern, and advise them to keep these medications out of the reach of children.

REVIEW QUESTIONS

Amebiasis

1. (a) What characteristics of amebic cysts make this form of the pathogenic protozoa important in the transmission of *E. histolytica?*

(b) What characteristics of the trophozoite form of the organism account for its capacity to produce acute intestinal and extraintestinal symptoms of amebiasis?

2. (a) In what phases of amebiasis is emetine considered a very useful drug, and in which phases is its use considered undesirable?

(b) What are the most serious potentially toxic effects of emetine and what precautions are taken to minimize the occurrence of such toxicity?

(c) Under what circumstances is the use of emetine contraindicated?

3. (a) What observations must the nurse make of any patient who is receiving emetine?

(b) What precautions must be used when giving injections of emetine, and why are these precautions necessary?

4. (a) What is the main way in which antibiotics such as oxytetracycline, erythromycin and paromomycin etc., are believed to bring about their anti-amebic effects?

(b) In what phases of amebiasis are such antibiotics ordinarily employed?

5. (a) Toxicity of what types may occur as a result of treatment of amebiasis with a broad-spectrum intestinal antibiotic such as paromomycin?

(b) Against what organisms besides amebae is this antibiotic effective, and for what other clinical conditions may it consequently be employed?

6. (a) In what phase of amebiasis is chloroquine particularly useful, and in which phases is its use without supplementation by other anti-amebic drugs ineffective?

(b) List several clinical conditions other than amebiasis in which chloroquine therapy is sometimes indicated.

(c) What are the symptoms which the nurse should look for in the patient who is taking chloroquine?

7. (a) In what phases of amebiasis is an arsenical such as carbarsone employed?

(b) What symptoms of arsenic toxicity may develop in sensitive individuals during treatment with this drug, and under what circumstances may its use be contraindicated?

8. (a) What are two reasons for treating persons found to be cyst passers, even if they show no symptoms of amebiasis?

(b) Which drugs are considered among the safest for use in asymptomatic carriers?

(c) In what ways can the nurse help to prevent the spread of infection by carriers?

9. (a) In what phases of intestinal amebiasis are drugs such as diiodohydroxyquin and iodochlorhydroxyquin employed?

(b) What other protozoan organism may be controlled by topical application of these drugs in suppository form or by insufflation of a powder?

10. (a) For what purpose besides treatment of amebiasis is iodochlorhydroxyquin sometimes taken internally, and what type of toxicity may occur in people sensitive to it?

(b) For what purposes is this chemical sometimes applied topically in the form of an ointment or cream?

Helminthiasis

1. (a) What are the advantages of the two drugs most effective in the treatment of pinworm infections?

(b) What supportive measures of a hygienic nature are required to prevent reinfection of the patient and spread of the condition to others?

2. (a) What advice or warning should the nurse give to patients who are going to use pyrvinium pamoate?

(b) What advice or warning should the nurse give to the parents of young children who are receiving piperazine citrate medications?

3. (a) What complications might occur in a patient with roundworms who was treated with a drug that is not specific for ascarids (e.g., tetrachlorethylene)?

(b) What is the drug of choice in roundworm infections, and what is an alternative drug with a relatively wide spectrum?

4. (a) What advice or warning should be given to patients taking hexylresorcinol pills?

(b) What measures may be taken to protect the patient's skin when this substance is administered by enema?

5. (a) For infections with what kinds of worms is the dye dithiazanine employed?

(b) What side effect is common with this anthelmintic, and for what kinds of patients is it contraindicated?

6. (a) Which two anthelmintics are preferred for treating infections by the two main species of hookworms, and how must they be administered for greatest effectiveness?

(b) What adjunctive measures are often desirable in patients debilitated by hookworm infection?

7. (a) What procedures are required to prepare a patient with tapeworm for treatment with quinacrine?

(b) What is the most commonly encountered side effect of quinacrine, and what is occasionally a toxic effect of this drug?

8. (a) What kinds of helminthic conditions are claimed to respond to treatment with thiabendazole?

(b) What side effects sometimes occur during thiabendazole treatment and what warnings should patients be given?

BIBLIOGRAPHY

Amebiasis

Anderson, H. H.: Newer drugs in amebiasis. Clin. Pharmacol. Ther., *1*:78, 1960.

Berberian, D. A., *et al.*: Drug prophylaxis of amebiasis. J.A.M.A., *148*:700, 1952.

Conna, N. J.: Chloroquine in amebiasis. Am. J. Trop. Med., *28*:107, 1948.

Faust, E. C.: Amebiasis. Am. J. Nursing, *54*:1507, 1954.

Gholz, L. M., and Arons, W. L.: Prophylaxis and therapy of amebiasis and shigellosis with iodochlorhydroxyquin. Am. J. Trop. Med. Hyg., *13*:396, 1964.

Juniper, K.: Treatment of amebiasis. Modern Treatment, *3*:1016, 1966 (Sept.).

McHardy, G., and Frye, W. W.: Antibiotics in the management of amebiasis. J.A.M.A., *154*:646, 1954.

Rodman, M. J.: Antifungal and antiparasitic drugs. R.N., *25*:71, 1962 (Nov.).

————: New drugs for fighting infection. R.N., *30*:55, 1967 (June).

Helminthiasis

Brown, H. W.: The actions and uses of anthelmintics. Clin. Pharmacol. Ther., *1*:78, 1960.

Kean, B. H., and Hoskins, D. W.: Treatment of trichinosis with thiabendazole. A preliminary report. J.A.M.A., *190*:852, 1964.

Manson-Bahr, P. E. C.: Treatment of parasitic infections (excluding amebiasis). Modern Treatment, *3*:1031, 1966.

Most, H.: Treatment of the more common worm infections. J.A.M.A., *185*:874, 1963.

Rodman, M. J.: Drugs in the management of worms. R.N., *22*:47, 1959 (Aug.).

Sodeman, W. A., and Jung, R. C.: Treatment of taeniasis with quinacrine HCl. J.A.M.A., *148*:285, 1952.

Drugs Used in the Management of Common Medical Conditions

Drugs Acting on the Gastrointestinal Tract

Gastrointestinal disorders are among the most common of human ailments. The cause and cure of certain chronic G.I. conditions—ulcerative colitis, for example —still elude physicians. Fortunately, however, many kinds of drugs are now available for relief of the distress of acute and chronic G.I. disturbances as well as to retard the progress and reduce the complications of the chronic stomach and intestinal illnesses.

In this chapter, various types of agents employed to counteract common symptoms such as nausea, vomiting, painful spasms, burning sensations, bloating, belching and diarrhea will be discussed. Special emphasis will be placed upon the antacids and antispasmodics employed against the acid peptic disorders, which are said to affect as many as 10 per cent of the population of the United States. In addition, drugs used to treat motion sickness and other conditions, which are not actually G.I. ailments but manifest themselves, in part, in stomach upsets, will also be taken up here.

However, not all drugs that have desirable or adverse effects on the G.I. tract are treated in this chapter. The cholinergic drugs, which are among the most potent stimulants of gastrointestinal motility, are discussed in Chapter 15. Although the effects of opiates and anticholinergic agents on the G.I. tract receive some mention here, their actions are discussed more fully elsewhere in the book, as are the actions of the corticosteroids, which can both cause and relieve G.I. symptoms.

DRUGS USED IN THE MANAGEMENT OF ACID-PEPTIC DISORDERS

Hyperacidity and Gastric Distress

Hydrochloric acid is a natural constituent of gastric juice. Secreted by certain stomach cells in response to nervous and hormonal stimuli, this acid plays an important part in initiating the digestion of food. Ordinarily,

the mucous membranes of the gastrointestinal tract resist this digestive action, and the presence of highly concentrated acid in the stomach evokes no discomfort. In some circumstances, however, people suffer from distressing and painful symptoms caused by the action of their own acid gastric juices.

Acid-peptic disease (a term that broadly designates these conditions) may produce only minor periodic discomfort or extremely serious and life-threatening complications. Among the minor ailments related to gastric acidity is pyrosis, or, as it is commonly called "heartburn." The distress of this condition, often described as a "burning" or "warm" feeling in the epigastrium, is probably caused by acid stomach juices bubbling up into the lower esophagus to irritate its mucosal lining. If long continued, such acid irritation may lead to the chronic inflammation of peptic esophagitis. In the related condition, gastritis, the inflammation of the stomach lining is not necessarily caused by acid. However, the sourness, bloating, and belching —symptoms that laymen call "indigestion" or "dyspepsia"—are often relieved by measures for neutralizing gastric acid.

Peptic Ulcer. Most serious of the acid-related gastrointestinal disorders is peptic ulcer, a condition in which localized areas of the stomach and duodenum become eroded by the corrosive action of acid gastric juices. Sometimes only the mucosal lining is eaten away, and the tissues may in time be repaired by the body's own healing processes. In some cases, however, the crater may deepen and extend down through the underlying layers of connective tissue and smooth muscle. This may cause some occult bleeding that can be detected only by special tests. On the other hand, if the erosive process finally breaks through a large blood vessel, massive hemorrhaging may occur, and perforation of the stomach or duodenal wall may lead to peritonitis. Either of these conditions can, of course, cause circulatory collapse and death.

Hydrochloric acid is essential to the development of a peptic ulcer. The acid need not be present in excessive amounts. Patients with gastric ulcers, for example, do not ordinarily have any abnormal increase in their acid production. Thus, some gastroenterologists suggest that such ulcers are probably the result of a reduction in the resistance of the stomach tissues. The causes of this postulated loss of the normal capacity to resist the digestive action of gastric juice are not well understood. In duodenal ulcers, on the other hand, the quantity of acid produced by the stomach's secretory cells is often two to four times higher than normal. So abnormally large an amount of acid, constantly pouring down into the first couple of inches of the small intestine, can evidently wear away even normally resistant tissues. It has been suggested that the very reactions to emotional stress that possibly produce this excess acid may also lead to mucosal changes which make that tissue more vulnerable to acid-peptic digestion, but this is not yet proved.

Protection of the irritated or eroded gastrointestinal mucosa from acid gastric juices is the main objective of drug therapy in peptic ulcer. Reduction of the amount of acid present both relieves the boring, burning, or gnawing sensation and, in time, allows natural healing of the ulcer to take place. The pain of the ulcer is caused by the hydrochloric acid impinging upon nerve fibers in the base and margin of the ulcer; this, in turn, produces reflex spasm of the surrounding smooth muscles. The ulcer itself is the result of the digestive action of the proteolytic enzyme, pepsin. However, hydrochloric acid is required for this enzyme's catalytic action, which occurs most efficiently when the pH of the gastric contents falls between 1.0 and 2.0. Patients with achlorhydria never suffer from peptic ulcers.

Antacid Therapy

Relief of peptic pain and eventual healing of the ulcer usually requires a vigorously pursued program of dietary treatment and drug therapy. Various kinds of drugs are employed, including the anticholinergic-antispasmodic-antisecretory agents (see Chap. 17 and below), sedatives and tranquilizers, and various other adjunctive medications. However, the mainstay of acid-peptic disease management is antacid therapy.

The gastric antacids are an unglamorous group of chemicals that work to counteract hydrochloric acid that has been already secreted by stomach cells. They do this in several ways. Some act by a direct *double-decomposition* type chemical reaction to *neutralize* all the acid with which they come in contact. Sodium bicarbonate, calcium carbonate, and magnesium oxide are examples of such neutralizers. Others act mainly by a combination of *buffering* (a chemical counteraction less intense than the one mentioned above) and *adsorption,* a physical property of colloidal chemicals

that tends to tie hydrogen ions and other particles to their surface and thus remove them. The aluminum and magnesium compounds act in this way, as well as by chemical neutralization.

The antacids are sometimes further subdivided into those that are capable of being absorbed into the systemic circulation (e.g., sodium bicarbonate) and those that act locally without being able to enter the blood stream to any extent. Most of the antacids in current medical use are of the latter *non*absorbable type, but sodium bicarbonate is still the substance most widely used by the public for "settling a sour stomach" or for "getting rid of gas pains."

Sodium Bicarbonate. This mildly alkaline substance is a rapidly effective and generally harmless acid neutralizer when used only occasionally for relief of feelings of fullness and uncomfortable burning sensations in the stomach. Other actions besides rapid acid neutralization are thought to play a part in relieving such symptoms. First, the carbon dioxide gas that is rapidly evolved when bicarbonate comes in contact with acid usually gives rise to an eructation (i.e., a belch). This may be both psychologically satisfying to the layman and a means of removing other gases, including swallowed air, that may have distended his stomach. In addition, the sudden increase in alkalinity tends to hasten the gastric contents down into the duodenum, thus further reducing the feeling of stomach fullness.

Both of these local actions and other properties of sodium bicarbonate, including the ease with which it is systemically absorbed, make it quite undesirable for routine use in the treatment of peptic ulcer. Sudden distention of the stomach by carbon dioxide could, for example, lead to a break in an ulcer crater that was already close to perforation by putting pressure on the weak spot. Other carbonates also cause evolution of this gas, but because calcium and magnesium carbonates, for example, are less soluble and reactive, the danger of excessive distention and perforation is much less.

The decrease in gastric emptying time brought about by bicarbonate speeds the removal of the antacid itself from the sites of its action. This is undesirable because antacids are useful only as long as they are acting locally. Once the bicarbonate has been swept out of the stomach and past the first few inches of the duodenum, it is subject to absorption into the blood stream. This is undesirable in long-term ulcer therapy, because of the possible occurrence of systemic alkalosis.

The neutralizing action of bicarbonate not only is short-lived but also seems often to be followed by an actual increase in acid secretion. This so-called acid rebound may be the result of an effort by the gastric glands to compensate for the actual alkalinity (pH higher than 7) produced by sodium bicarbonate and other strong alkalinizers such as magnesium oxide. On the other hand, the rapid return of acidity may be only a natural result of the early disappearance of the neutralizing alkali from the stomach. In any case, its short duration of antacid action makes necessary extremely frequent administration of huge amounts of bicarbonate in order to keep ulcer pain under control. This, in turn, could overload the blood stream with bicarbonate in amounts greater than the patient's kidneys can eliminate.

Systemic Alkalosis. Ordinarily, the kidneys compensate for any rise in plasma alkalinity by increasing the rate of bicarbonate removal. If, however, the patient's kidney function is too impaired to get rid of the extra load of alkali, an insidious metabolic alkalosis may develop. Probably, this condition often goes unrecognized. The accumulation of excessive blood alkali may be accompanied by various vague signs and symptoms involving the gastrointestinal, neuromuscular, and central nervous systems. The patient tends first to lose his taste for food, and this is often followed by nausea, vomiting and an increase in stomach pain. He may show increased irritability and complain of dizziness, headache, and muscular pain. Later, muscle twitching and cramps may occur; the patient may become increasingly weak and finally lapse into a fatal coma.

Systemic electrolyte disturbance of another type is sometimes observed in ulcer patients taking large quantities of calcium carbonate and other alkalinizers combined with milk. This condition, called Burnett's milk-alkali syndrome, tends to occur most commonly in patients with kidney function impairment. The excess calcium settling out in the renal tissues may cause still further kidney damage, which leads, in turn, to alkalosis, potassium loss, and increased nitrogen retention in the blood and tissues.

The doctor can help counteract the hypercalcemia, hypotassemia, and alkalosis—once the condition is recognized—by having the patient discontinue his heavy milk and alkali intake and by correcting the electrolyte balance with saline and other infusions. Obviously, it is better to prevent this potentially dangerous syndrome from occurring in the first place by warning peptic ulcer sufferers against drinking several quarts of milk daily and taking large quantities of systemically absorbable alkali without medical advice.

Nonabsorbable Antacids. Because of the disadvantages discussed above, sodium bicarbonate, which was the basis of the once widely used Sippy powder ulcer treatment, has been largely displaced by various nonabsorbable antacid substances. The products most commonly employed contain aluminum and magnesium compounds alone or in combination. These substances do not have as high a neutralizing action as bicarbonate, but their ability to buffer the gastric contents to a pH of between 3.0 and 5.0 is entirely adequate to prevent pepsin from exerting its digestive action on the gastroduodenal mucosa. Indeed, because they do not actually alkalinize the gastric contents, these antacids stay in the stomach somewhat longer and do not set off the acid rebound phenomenon. Rarely are their ions absorbed into the blood in amounts that exert systemic effects. In addition, many of these compounds possess other properties considered desirable in the treatment of peptic ulcer.

Protective Action. It is generally considered desirable to coat the ulcer crater with substances similar to the mucus that ordinarily helps to protect the gastrointestinal lining. Gastric mucin obtained from hog stomachs was once widely employed for this purpose, but its unpalatability made it unpopular. Synthetic substitutes, such as sodium carboxymethylcellulose and protopectin, lack the nasty odor and saline taste of natural gastric mucus, while retaining some ability to form a tenacious coating over the irritated mucosa. Magnesium trisilicate, which becomes jellyish in gastric juice, is said to possess desirable demulcent and protective effects. Aluminum hydroxide gel, in addition to its other properties, has some tendency to form a physical barrier over the naked nerve endings of eroded areas.

Side Effects. The chief difficulty with these drugs is that they tend to cause certain gastrointestinal side effects when used in large amounts for long periods, as is so often necessary in peptic ulcer management. The aluminum, calcium, and bismuth compounds, for example, are constipating, and the magnesium ion exerts a laxative action which may lead to diarrhea. Of the two difficulties, constipation is the more common. The tendency toward formation of a hard stool is compounded by the bland ulcer diet, and in elderly patients confined to bed, uncorrected constipation may even progress to intestinal obstruction or to perforation by stony masses. Thus, the addition of a bedtime dose of magnesium hydroxide is considered desirable for most peptic ulcer patients.

These digestive problems are most commonly overcome by combining both constipating and laxative type antacids in the same physical mixture. Thus, an aluminum compound such as the hydroxide, phosphate, or carbonate may often be mixed in a single suspension with magnesium oxide, hydroxide, or trisilicate. The result is a product with additive antacid actions, in which the constipating and diarrhea-inducing effects have largely neutralized one another. Occasionally, the doctor may alternate an antacid with constipating tendencies, such as calcium carbonate, with another—magnesium oxide, for instance—which has laxative properties. One product, magaldrate (monalium hydrate; Riopan) combines aluminum and magnesium hydroxides in a single chemical union rather than as a simple physical mixture of two antacids. This complex is claimed to be not only free of local intestinal side effects (like the combination products), but also low in the residual sodium ions that sometime remain as an impurity when antacids of the two different types are prepared separately and then mixed together in a single suspension. This may be an advantage for patients requiring a low sodium intake.

Administration of Antacids

The patient with an acute bleeding ulcer may require almost continuous medication. Sometimes an antacid suspension is dripped steadily into his stomach through an intragastric tube. This medication may be alternated with milk and cream mixtures to which a hemostatic powder has been added to counteract local bleeding. Even after bleeding is controlled, the patient may still need hourly feedings, followed every half hour by an antacid mixture. Later, however, when his illness is less severe and he does not require as much care, observation, and emotional support, the patient can be taught to take over a good deal of his own treatment.

As part of his preparation for leaving the hospital, the patient should be helped to set up a schedule of medication and taught that he must adhere to this schedule rigorously. He should be made to understand that, to be truly effective, antacids must be kept in the stomach continuously, because this both prevents pain and helps the ulcer to heal. Thus, it is not only permissible but actually desirable that the patient take his own medicine during his convalescence.

To help the convalescent patient assume this responsibility, he should be furnished with a bedside supply of antacid tablets or suspension and told how

to take it. Some tablets need to be chewed or sucked slowly; others can be swallowed whole. If a suspension is employed, the patient should be instructed to shake the bottle each time before pouring his dose of the sticky stuff and washing it down the esophagus and into his stomach with a little water. He should be supplied with paper cups and a wastebasket to avoid the discouraging prospect of being surrounded by a growing mound of dirty glasses. If the disposable cups are not calibrated, a clearly marked measuring cup should be furnished to ensure ease in pouring an accurate dose even when the patient's eyesight is poor.

The nurse can reinforce the doctor's instruction to the patient and his family. She should stress the importance of timing his daily medication precisely, help him to understand why he must continue his ulcer treatment on his own for several months, and warn against giving in to any temptation to switch to some other type of antacid without consulting his doctor. Patients may sometimes read in a newspaper or magazine article about some new "wonder drug" or fad diet for curing ulcers quickly and effortlessly. These ulcer "cures" usually injure only his pocketbook, but their real danger is that the patient may be persuaded to drop the more burdensome but incomparably more effective antacid-diet regimen prescribed by his doctor.

Other Medications for Ulcer Therapy

Many kinds of drugs besides antacids have been advocated for the management of patients with peptic ulcer. Several types, including gastric antisecretory agents, sedatives, and tranquilizers have a well estab-

TABLE 38-1

GASTRIC ANTACIDS

OFFICIAL CHEMICAL OR NONPROPRIETARY NAME	SYNONYM OR TRADE NAME	DOSAGE
Aluminum hydroxide gel U.S.P.	Amphojel; Creamalin, etc.	5 to 30 ml.
Aluminum phosphate gel N.F.	Phosphalgel	15 ml.
Calcium carbonate, precipitated U.S.P.	Precipitated Chalk	1 to 2 Gm.
Dihydroxyaluminum aminoacetate N.F.	Algyln, etc.	500 to 1,000 mg.
Magaldrate (monalium hydrate)	Riopan	400 to 800 mg.
Magnesium carbonate N.F.	—	600 mg.
Magnesium hydroxide N.F.	—	300 mg.
Magnesium oxide U.S.P.	—	250 to 1,500 mg.
Magnesium trisilicate U.S.P.	—	1 to 4 Gm.
Milk of Magnesia U.S.P.	Magnesia Nagma	5 to 30 ml.
Polyamine-methylene resin	Resinat	500 to 1,000 mg.
Potassium bicarbonate U.S.P.	—	500 to 2,000 mg.
Sodium bicarbonate U.S.P.	Baking Soda	100 to 4,000 mg.
Sodium carboxymethylcellulose U.S.P.	in Carmethose	225 to 450 mg.

lished place as adjunctive medications. Others, including various plant and animal tissue extracts, have not earned an important place in ulcer therapy.

Gastric Antisecretory Agents. The anticholinergic drugs (Chap. 17) are commonly employed in ulcer regimens. These drugs block the effects of vagus nerve impulses on the gastric secretory cells and the smooth muscles of the upper gastrointestinal tract. In practice, atropine and the other belladonna alkaloids are not very effective for reducing the secretion of gastric acid, especially when administered by mouth in safe doses. Administered intramuscularly, atropine and the synthetic anticholinergic drugs of the quaternary ammonium class of compounds (e.g., methantheline, propantheline) often decrease the amount of acid secreted; but this effect is frequently bought at a price of severe side effects.

Recently, certain anticholinergic drugs have been introduced which are claimed to possess antisecretory effects more powerful and more prolonged than those of the natural belladonna extract or earlier synthetic agents. These newer drugs, including glycopyrollate (Robanul), oxyphencyclamine (Daricon), and isopropamide (Darbid), are said to reduce acid secretion for up to 12 hours, even when given orally. This would make these drugs especially useful against night-time gastric secretion. However, some authorities among gastroenterologists are not convinced that any anticholinergic drug has yet been proved to be markedly superior for reducing stomach acid secretion.

The effects of the anticholinergic drugs on gastrointestinal smooth muscle are much more marked than their actions on secretory cells. For example, they may relax spasm of visceral muscles and thus relieve pain produced reflexly when gastric acid stimulates sensory nerve endings in the ulcer crater. These drugs also reduce gastrointestinal motility, an effect which sometimes tends to prolong the effects of concurrently administered gastric antacid compounds. By prolonging the time required for the stomach to empty its contents, the vagus-blocking anticholinergic drugs let the ingested alkalinizing and buffering agents interact for a longer period with the acid that is secreted into the stomach. However, this same slowing of gastric emptying which permits the antacids to neutralize acids more efficiently may also be a source of danger for some patients. Those with partial pyloric obstruction caused by a stenosing ulcer may, for example, suffer complete blockage and gastric retention.

Sedatives and Tranquilizers. Sedatives such as phenobarbital may help to promote the rest and sleep that should be part of every regimen for preventing recurrences of ulcers. Minor tranquilizers such as meprobamate and chlordiazepoxide may also have a place in lessening the ulcer patient's responses to the emotional stresses that often play a part in precipitating an ulcer attack. These drugs do nothing to alter the underlying personality factors that are sometimes said to make people ulcer-prone; they do, however, tend to reduce the tensions that seem to set off gastric secretion and spasm. Also, ulcer pain is somewhat less upsetting to the patient under tranquilizer therapy.

Locally Acting Agents. Substances sometimes added to suspensions of nonabsorbable aluminum-magnesium antacids are: *topical anesthetics* and *antiflatulence chemicals*. The local anesthetic oxethazine (Oxaine), for example, is said to soothe the irritated gastrointestinal mucosa. By dulling the responses of nerve endings this drug is said not only to deaden pain perception directly but also to abolish certain reflexes that cause both painful smooth muscle spasm and further secretion of gastric acid. An example of a substance that is being used to help relieve the distress caused by gas retention is simethicone (Mylicon). This drug is said to possess a defoaming action that keeps air bubbles from forming painful gas pockets. Trapped gases are then freed and more easily eliminated by belching or by the passing of flatus, thus relieving pressures that often add to peptic pain.

Certain substances are periodically claimed to be useful in ulcer therapy. Some, such as the hormone enterogastrone and its urinary derivative urogastrone, are said to act as physiological inhibitors of acid secretion. Others, including a seaweed-derived material, carrageenin, and a synthetic substance, amylopectin sulfate, are claimed to possess antipeptic actions that inhibit the activity of the enzyme pepsin. Still other, and obscure, materials—cabbage juice, licorice extract, and others—are claimed to increase the resistance of the gastroduodenal mucosa to ulceration. None of these relatively expensive experimental substances can be considered to be as useful as the simple antacid chemicals in the management of peptic ulcer.

No single antacid is ideal in all respects. The properties that are considered desirable in an antacid combination product are as follows:

1. The ability to neutralize, buffer, or otherwise counteract free acid efficiently, rapidly, and for prolonged periods

2. The ability to form a mechanically protective coating capable of adhering tenaciously to the sides of a naked ulcer crater

3. Freedom from systemic toxicity, such as alkalosis and hypercalcemia, and from local side effects such as constipation, diarrhea, and gas distention

4. Ideally, antacids should also be palatable and inexpensive.

DRUGS WITH CATHARTIC ACTION

The Uses and Misuses of Cathartic Drugs

Cathartics are drugs used to bring about emptying of the bowel. They do so by speeding the passage of the intestinal contents through the gastrointestinal tract. Some substances act chemically to stimulate intestinal smooth muscles to contract more forcefully and frequently. Other agents cause an increase in intestinal bulk, which acts as a mechanical stimulus to the motor activity of the gut. The effects of other laxatives are exerted less on the G.I. tract itself than on its fecal contents. That is, they soften hardened masses and ease their passage through the lower portion of the large intestine.

Intestinal Motility

Individuals vary widely in the time it takes for food to be digested and for its residues to leave the intestinal tract. Most of the nutrients and fluid from a meal are absorbed from the small intestine in a few hours. However, indigestible particles require at least a day and sometimes several to make their way to the rectum, from which they leave the body during the act of defecation.

Of the several kinds of complex muscular contractions that churn, mix and move the intestinal contents along, the most important is *peristalsis,* a series of coordinated contractions and relaxations. In the small intestine these wavelike movements go on at a slow, steady rate that allows time for food to be digested and assimilated and for fluids to be absorbed. In the large intestine, peristaltic activity takes place only periodically at an irregular rate. During periods of inactivity fluid absorption continues, so that the liquid chyme is gradually converted to a semisolid mass by the time it reaches the transverse colon. Occasionally, strong peristaltic contractions shift this mass ahead for a considerable distance along the descending colon. Finally, one of these movements forces the fecal matter into the rectum, distending it and setting off the reflexes that lead to the desire to defecate.

Ordinarily, when we stay in good health and follow a regular routine, we remain for the most part unaware of all these goings-on in the gut, and bowel movements occur at a rate normal for the individual, whether it is several times a day or only once every two or more days. However, this rhythmic pattern may be broken by various factors that influence a person's living habits. Nervous tension, for example, may either accelerate or markedly slow down the rate of peristaltic activity.

Diarrhea results when a person's intestinal contents are rushed through the bowel too rapidly, so that the person is discomforted by many small, fluid movements daily. Constipation occurs when a person's intestinal sluggishness causes him to have relatively few, infrequent and incomplete movements.

Constipation

Not all cases of constipation require treatment with cathartics. A person may remain in good health even though his bowel movements are relatively infrequent.

Even when better bowel motility may be desirable cathartics need not be employed to bring this about. For, contrary to what most laymen have been lead to believe, cathartics have little place in the management of constipation. Actually, the habitual misuse of cathartics is one of the common *causes* of chronic constipation. The nurse, in talking to patients and other people, can do a great deal to counteract the false propaganda for proprietary laxative products, which continues to foster ancient misunderstandings that lead to the abuse of these drugs.

The most common of these misconceptions is the idea that a person has to have a daily bowel movement to keep in good health. Many people still believe that failure to empty the colon results in "poisons" being absorbed into the blood. Although this myth of autointoxication was long ago laid to rest, some advertising for laxatives continues to play on the popular fear of it. Actually, the person who misses one or more bowel movements is in no dire danger.

The kind of person who gets unduly upset when he fails to move his bowels tends to treat himself with cathartics in a way that leads to chronic constipation. This is what happens: first, the person takes a cathartic that stimulates peristalsis strongly enough to empty the entire intestinal tract. This, of course, keeps the colon from filling normally for several days. Since the desire to defecate arises only when the lower colon becomes packed with a fecal mass, the normal stimulus that sets off the defecation reflex is lacking, and so a day or two may pass without a bowel movement. This alarms the bowel-oriented person and often leads him to take a still stronger cathartic to overcome his drug-induced constipation.

Instead of restoring the "normal regularity," which is so prized by those who prepare TV commercials for these products, the continued use of cathartics soon makes it difficult for the laxative abuser ever to achieve a natural movement. He comes to depend upon the drugs' action rather than on the natural defecation reflex. Such dependence is both psychic and physical and, in one sense, does not differ a great deal from what takes place when people become addicted to drugs that act on the central nervous system!

What can the nurse do to help prevent such cathartic addiction? First, of course, she should advise people with intestinal complaints to see a physician. For, even though most constipation is caused by poor dietary and living habits, a sudden change in bowel function sometimes signals the presence of intestinal pathology. Once the doctor has ruled out such organic lesions, he may put the patient on a program aimed at correction of the causes of chronic constipation and, thus, reestablishing normal bowel movements. The nurse can help here by teaching people the need to follow the rules of hygiene upon which all such regimens are based.

Treatment of Chronic Constipation. The first thing the doctor ordinarily does for the person whose constipation stems from habituation to cathartics is to have him stop taking laxatives. As in any other addiction, this is likely to lead to what has with some justice been termed a "withdrawal syndrome" because of the patient's complaints of discomfort. These are usually treated symptomatically, with aspirin for his headaches and general malaise, sedatives for anxiety and tension and, perhaps, mild mental stimulants to overcome lethargy, weakness and mental depression.

More important are measures intended to replace the patient's faulty habits with habits conducive to good hygiene. These include trying to guide patients to reduce tension in their daily lives and getting them to set regular times for going to the toilet each day. The patient is put on a diet that includes foods that leave a bulky residue. These, taken together with plenty of fluids, help to build up the intestinal contents, so that normal defecation reflexes can be initiated. The attainment of this objective is sometimes aided by the judicious use of one type of nonirritating laxative. Bulk-producing substances such as psyllium seeds, methylcellulose and similar hydrophilic (literally, "water-loving") colloids (Table 38-2) sometimes help to form a bulkier stool. Taken daily with plenty of water, they act much as do the natural fibers in foods such as carrots, beets and cabbage. These colloid laxatives are gradually discontinued after a few weeks, when the patient's bowels have begun to function normally. If the patient succeeds, with his doctor's help, in learning to live under less emotional tension and in establishing proper habits and patterns, he will have no further need for cathartics.

It is not easy, however, for an elderly person to break the cathartic habit. A constipated patient, who has learned to lean on cathartic medication for emotional reasons, will not readily give up this crutch. Thus, lecturing the patient or scolding him will work no better here than do attempts to humiliate an alcoholic or to shame a narcotics addict. As in any situations involving a long-term habit, the doctor and nurse have to proceed slowly and gently, so that the patient senses that he has their support in his efforts to help himself. With such sympathetic aid, the patient is much more likely to do what his misused bowel requires for recovery than he would when subjected to a stern, moralistic lecture delivered in a brusque, mechanical manner.

Indications for Cathartics

Doctors order laxatives far less frequently than they used to in the days when they shared with the layman a misguided belief in the desirability of keeping the patient's bowel "open" with a daily purge. There are, however, some clinical situations in which it is considered desirable to induce defecation with drugs or to alter the consistency of the patient's stool. The few conditions in which the use of cathartics is considered valid are as follows:

Patients who are confined to bed often tend to become constipated. This is understandable, since lack of exercise, loss of appetite, and the effects of the person's illness and of the drugs used to treat it—narcotic pain relievers, such as codeine, morphine and meperidine, for example—all conspire to reduce intestinal motility. For this reason, it was once a regular practice for the doctor to order milk of magnesia, cascara or other cathartics for all his hospitalized patients.

Recently, however, the routine use of cathartics has declined, as doctors have recognized their undesirability and turned to more natural measures for maintaining bowel function. The nurse, whose request or suggestions the busy physician often follows in matters of routine patient care, should use her influence in the situation to accelerate this trend away from regular orders for cathartic medication and toward more physiologic means of keeping the patient's bowel open.

Among the most important of the measures that help avoid the need for cathartics is seeing that the patient is taken to the bathroom or is given the opportunity to use a commode at his bedside at a regular time each day. This is often possible and permissible today because of the present emphasis on early ambulation. Freed of the need to use the bedpan, the patient can assume a more normal and comfortable position and should be encouraged to do so. He should also be left alone, if possible, since lack of privacy often inhibits defecation.

Another desirable development is the fact that patients often not only are allowed to get out of bed but also are encouraged to begin eating a regular, varied diet, including fresh fruits and vegetables, on the day after surgery if their condition permits, instead of being kept on liquids for days as they once were. Of course, to avoid constipation it is also important to keep the patient well hydrated, and doctors are doing this by ordering the use of intravenous fluids postoperatively when this seems desirable or necessary.

Laxatives, suppositories and enemas may still have a place in the care of bedridden patients. In such cases these medications are used not merely to relieve the patient's discomfort but also to avoid possible fecal impaction and other dangerous complications, such as those that might result if a patient with an aneurism, embolism or myocardial infarction were to strain at stool.

Anorectal Lesions. Patients with *hemorrhoids* or other anorectal lesions should not strain in order to remove retained feces. Thus, measures for promoting a soft stool that can be passed without pain seem desirable. These include the regular use of the lubricat-

TABLE 38-2
CATHARTIC DRUGS

Nonproprietary or Official Name	Trade Name or Synonym	Dosage
Drugs Stimulating Motility by Chemical Irritation		
Acetphenolisatin	(Oxyphenisatin; isacen)	2 to 5 mg.
Aloe U.S.P.		0.250 Gm.
Bisacodyl	(Dulcolax)	10 to 15 mg.
Calomel N.F.	(mercurous chloride)	120 mg.
Cascara sagrada		
Cascara sagrada, aromatic extract U.S.P.		2 ml.
Cascara sagrada, extract N.F.		0.3 Gm.
Cascara sagrada, fluidextract N.F.		1 ml.
Castor Oil U.S.P.		15 to 30 ml.
Castor Oil, aromatic N.F.		15 ml.
Danthron N.F.	(Dorbane)	75 to 150 mg.
Phenolphthalein N.F.		60 mg.
Podophyllum		5 mg.
Senna N.F.		2.0 Gm.
Senna, fluidextract N.F.		2 ml.
Senna, syrup N.F.		8 ml.
Drugs Stimulating Motility by Increasing Physical Bulk		
Saline cathartics		
Magnesium citrate solution N.F.		200 ml.
Magnesium sulfate U.S.P.	(Epsom Salt)	15 Gm.
Potassium phosphate N.F.		4 Gm.
Potassium sodium tartrate N.F.	(Rochelle salt)	10 Gm.
Seidlitz Powders N.F.	(Compound effervescent powders)	Contents of a white and a blue paper mixed in water.
Sodium phosphate N.F.		4 Gm.
Sodium phosphate, effervescent N.F.		10 Gm.
Sodium phosphate, exsiccated N.F.		2 Gm.
Sodium phosphate, solution F.N.		10 ml.
Sodium sulfate N.F.	(Glauber's salt)	15 Gm.
Hydrophilic colloids and indigestible fibers		
Agar U.S.P.		4 to 16 Gm.
Methylcellulose U.S.P.		1.0 Gm.
Plantago Seed N.F.		7.5 Gm.
Psyllium hydrophilic muciloid	(Metamucil)	4 to 10 Gm.
Sodium carboxymethylcellulose U.S.P.		1.5 Gm.
Emollient or Lubricant Cathartics		
Liquid Petrolatum Emulsion N.F.		30 ml.
Mineral Oil U.S.P.		15 to 45 ml.
Olive Oil U.S.P.		30 ml.
Fecal softeners (Surface-active or wetting agents)		
Calcium bis-dioctyl sodium sulfosuccinate	(Doxical)	60 mg.
Dioctyl sodium sulfosuccinate N.F.	(Colace; Doxinate etc.)	100 mg.
Poloxalkol	(Polykol)	200 mg.

ing type of laxatives and the wetting agents (Table 38-2).

Diagnostic Procedures and Surgery. Cathartics are employed prior to various diagnostic or surgical procedures—before bowel surgery, for example. Sometimes the entire intestine is emptied before abdominal X-rays; at other times only the colon need be cleared—e.g., for proctosigmoidoscopy.

Anthelmintics. The treatment of intestinal *worm infestations* with anthelmintics often requires administration of a cathartic both before and after therapy. Some anthelmintics act more effectively when the bowel has first been cleared; other medications for killing worms are potentially toxic to the patient if too much is absorbed. These are often swept out of the G.I. tract by a cathartic as soon as they have had time to do their work on the worms.

Chemical Poisoning. In cases of poisoning by ingested chemicals, poisons that have passed the pylorus and can no longer be eliminated by gastric lavage are often flushed from the intestine by purgative drugs. This tends both to reduce local tissue damage by corrosive chemicals and to limit the systemic absorption of other toxic agents. Laxatives are also sometimes given routinely with constipating drugs, including especially those that may cause dangerous systemic effects when their evacuation is delayed (for example, the ganglionic blocking agents).

For each of the various indications, some cathartics are considered superior to others. This depends in part upon where and how each type of drug acts in the intestinal tract and upon the speed and degree of thoroughness with which it acts. The reasons for preferring one kind of cathartic over another will become apparent when we discuss the properties of the several classes of cathartic drugs.

Contraindications

Cathartics, as we have seen, should never be used habitually as a routine measure for inducing a daily bowel movement. Such use not only leads to chronic constipation but may produce local and systemic disturbances. The habitual use of purgatives and stimulants of intestinal motility has been held responsible for many cases of chronic colitis and other intestinal disorders that are the direct or indirect result of continued irritation of the intestinal mucosa. In addition, repeated purgation can result in dehydration and cause electrolyte imbalances similar to those that result from severe diarrhea due to gastrointestinal infections.

More serious than the effects of the long-term misuse of cathartics is the damage that can be done by giving even a single dose of a cathartic to a person with acute appendicitis. The drug-induced increase in gastrointestinal motility may lead to perforation of the inflamed intestinal wall. Such rupture of the appendix then spews pathogenic bacteria into the abdominal cavity.

Before the advent of antibiotics and other modern anti-infective drugs, the death rate from peritonitis in patients who had taken cathartics for treating painful cramps was very high. Even today, peritonitis is a serious condition. Thus, people should be warned never to medicate themselves with cathartics when they have abdominal pain and cramps or are nauseated and vomiting. These drugs are never given before adequate diagnosis has ruled out appendicitis, enteritis, ulcerative colitis, diverticulitis or the presence of organic obstructions.

The Types of Cathartic Drugs

Many materials capable of producing increased intestinal motility exist in nature. Primitive people who tasted parts of plants or drank waters from certain springs were no doubt the first discoverers of the diarrhea-producing capacity of these natural products. The shaman or medicine man made use of these natural cathartics in his practice, as a means of ridding patients of "evil spirits."

Irritant Resins and Oils

Until rather recently, many modern equivalents of the witch doctor continued to use powerful purgatives of vegetable and mineral origin. Among the strongest of these were an oil from croton seeds and the parts of several plants containing resinous principles, including, among others, podophyllum, colocynth, and jalap. All these substances stimulate peristaltic activity by irritating the mucosal lining of the intestinal tract. Their harsh irritant action is followed promptly by production of abundant watery stools.

These irritant cathartics have no place in modern medicine. Croton oil, the most dangerous of all, has the capacity to burn and blister the skin. A single drop taken internally on a lump of sugar causes cramps, and as little as 20 drops has led to death from prostration following profuse bloody diarrhea. This oil is no longer used, but small doses of the so-called drastic resinous cathartics can still be found in some proprietary products marketed for constipation treatment. Podophyllum, for example, is frequently found in combination with aloin in products that cause colicky intestinal contractions. The continued use of such irritant cathartics may also cause a loss of water and of important electrolytes such as potassium. Such dehydration and hypokalemia may prove to be even more dangerous than their undesirable local effects.

Castor oil, also classified as an irritant cathartic, is not irritating in quite the same sense. For one thing, unlike croton oil and the resins, it does not damage delicate tissues. As a matter of fact, it is bland enough to be dropped in a patient's eye as an emollient after removal of a foreign body. In the intestine, however, the oil is broken down by fat-splitting enzymes to release ricinoleic acid, a substance that strongly stimulates gastrointestinal motility.

The habitual use of castor oil is certainly undesirable. It causes the kind of complete evacuation of both the small and the large bowel that leads to a period during which there is no natural stimulus to defecation. Thus, its frequent use can, in the manner previously indicated, lead to production of chronic constipation. On the other hand, the comparatively prompt and complete action of castor oil makes its occasional use desirable in some situations. Thus, it is still used in certain hospital procedures, though much less often than it once was. Castor oil is still employed prior to X-ray examination of abdominal organs, for example, to empty the intestine and thus eliminate interfering shadows. It is usually given on an empty stomach in the late afternoon, so that it will not interfere with digestion or with sleep. It should never be taken at bedtime, because its strong action coming on in a couple of hours or so will cause a restless night.

Castor oil has been made available in more palatable pharmaceutical formulations to overcome the taste of the oil, which tends to nauseate some people.

Other Irritant Laxatives

A large number of natural and synthetic substances are classified as irritant cathartics because they stimulate peristalsis by chemical actions on the mucosa and smooth muscle walls of the intestine. These substances, including the anthraquinone compounds and phenolphthalein and related drugs, differ from castor oil and other strong irritants in one important respect: their action is limited mainly to the large intestine. Thus, they are not useful when the doctor desires rapid emptying of the entire G.I. tract. They are used, instead, to aid evacuation of the lower bowel in bedridden patients and others for whom a slow, steady action is considered more suitable than prompt purgation.

Anthraquinones. Cathartics of this class, including cascara, senna, aloe and rhubarb, contain plant principles that are converted to peristalsis-stimulating chemicals in the large intestine. These drugs travel through the small intestine and by way of the blood stream, after absorption, to reach the large intestine. Their action therefore requires six or eight hours or more, since it takes that long for the anthraquinone derivatives to build up in the large bowel in sufficient amounts. Thus, they are best given at bedtime in order to bring about a bowel movement in the morning.

Cascara and *senna* are considered the most dependable of these plant products for producing a single soft or semiliquid stool when desired. Rhubarb is often constipating because of its tannin content, and

aloe tends to cause griping pains, or colic. Like castor oil, aloe has sometimes been used in misguided attempts to produce an abortion. The use of strong irritant cathartics in late pregnancy is undesirable, because of possible reflex stimulation of uterine contractions, however, these drugs have no ability to act in this way early in pregnancy.

Pills containing aloe combined with belladonna and strychnine are still available despite their having long been stigmatized as dangerous and irrational. The amount of strychnine in a single pill has no effect upon peristalsis. However, when a child swallows a handful of the candy coated tablets, he may ingest enough strychnine to cause fatal convulsions (see Chap. 13). The belladonna alkaloids in such A.S.B. pills are supposed to reduce aloe-induced cramps by their antispasmodic action. Actually, this relaxant action on intestinal smooth muscle will have worn off long before the time the griping action of the cathartic begins to make itself felt.

Various preparations of these plant products are available, both official and in proprietary remedies. These include (1) extracted principles in liquid form, i.e., fluidextracts, tinctures, and syrups; (2) the whole ground seed, root or leaf in the form of powders, pills and tablets, and (3) in some cases, pure crystalline glycosides such as those extracted from senna. Such concentrated laxative components are probably more dependable than the galenical preparations because of their better stability, but it is doubtful that they are less likely to cause cramps.

Phenolphthalein and Its Relatives. This synthetic substance exerts most of its stimulant action in the colon after being broken down to an irritant principle by bile salts and alkali in the upper small intestine. It is a common component of many proprietary laxative preparations, including some of the most popular chocolate and gum medications. These forms of phenolphthalein are often eaten by children in large amounts, but severe toxicity is rare and is limited mainly to a dehydrating diarrhea. However, hypersensitivity reactions are not uncommon. These often take the form of a characteristically colorful dermatitis. Sometimes, the itchy, burning patches blister and become ulcerated; occasionally, the involved patches of skin stay pink or purplish for many months, and, long after the condition has cleared up, identical lesions may appear in the same places on subsequent exposure to the drug—a so-called fixed eruption.

Bisacodyl (Dulcolax) is a chemically related compound with a similar action on the large intestine. It may be given by mouth at night to produce a morning bowel movement. The drug is also available in suppository form for faster action. Rectal administration brings the chemical in contact with the mucosa and stimulates contraction of the colon within a few minutes. It has been employed in this way in preparing the lower bowel for a barium enema and prior to proctoscopy.

In general, rectal administration is a desirable way to evacuate the lower bowel without causing side effects such as small-intestine colic or running the risk of systemic absorption. Another phenolphthalein relative, *oxyphenisatin,* is an ingredient of an enema powder that is used to clean the large bowel, either prior to abdominal surgery or to aid visualization of abdominal viscera. The limiting of cathartic action to the lower colon and rectum produces relatively normal bowel movements.

Saline Cathartics

Among the most rapid-acting and powerful of cathartics are various salts that are given in solution in large amounts of water. They produce their effects by increasing the bulk of the intestinal contents, thus distending the colon and stimulating contractions by a mechanical rather than a chemical action. Because they often act in only an hour or two, salts such as *sodium sulfate* and *magnesium sulfate* are preferred for clearing the entire intestinal tract in poisonings. In general, they are used whenever a complete purge is desired—in worm treatments, for example, or to obtain stool specimens. They are usually given in the morning or in mid-afternoon, never in the evening.

The salty taste of some of these drugs makes them unpalatable. Thus, Epsom Salt or Glauber's salt should be given in cold fruit juices to mask the taste. Magnesium citrate is available in a lemon-flavored carbonated liquid that is pleasant-tasting but relatively expensive. Various salts are often presented as extemporaneously prepared effervescent liquids which also have greater palatability but are more costly. Palatability is, of course, no problem when various of these salts (sodium phosphate, for example) are given by enema.

The more concentrated solutions exert greater osmotic activity but also cause more nausea. Thus, the salts are given as well diluted isotonic solutions when only their cathartic action is desired. Sometimes hypertonic solutions are employed to reduce edema, by pulling fluid from the blood and into the gut by an osmotic action. Less concentrated solutions not only are adequate for catharsis but actually are preferred. Taken on an empty stomach, such solutions pass the pylorus more readily and enter the intestine where the unabsorbed ions retain enough fluid to initiate peristaltic activity.

Ordinarily, so little of these salts makes its way through the semipermeable intestinal membrane that there is little likelihood of systemic toxicity. Poisoning has occurred, however, when the patient's kidneys were functioning poorly and failed to clear absorbed magnesium ions from the circulation. Accumulation of magnesium may cause coma as a result of the central nervous system depressant effect of this ion. The sodium-containing cathartic salts are undesirable for treating edematous patients with cardiovascular disorders.

Other Bulk-Producing Laxatives

Another kind of mechanically acting cathartic is quite different from the saline type in actions and uses. This group includes the hydrophilic colloids and other indigestible fibers, mentioned earlier as useful adjuncts in the treatment of chronic constipation. Natural substances, such as psyllium seeds and agar, and semisynthetic materials, such as methylcellulose, produce their desired action by forming a bulky jellyish mass in the intestine. This resembles in its effects the food residues that normally stimulate peristalsis and defecation.

These bulk-formers are the most natural and least irritating of laxatives. They should not, however, be taken habitually any more than any other cathartic. Patients should be told never to take these products without water. This is important, not merely because their effectiveness depends in large part on their ability to absorb enough fluid to make a gelatinous mass. When swallowed dry, these fibers, seeds and granules may pick up just enough moisture in the esophagus to swell and obstruct that food passageway. Thus, these materials are to be both mixed with water and followed by plenty of fluid.

Lubricating Laxatives and Stool Softeners

It is often desirable to make defecation easier, not by stimulating peristalsis but by changing the consistency of the patient's stool. Sometimes this is best done with retention enemas of olive oil or cottonseed oil, which turn hard, dry fecal "stones" into soft moist masses. These can then be readily passed by the patient or washed out with cleansing tap-water or soapsuds enemas.

Occasionally these emollient oils are taken orally. However, *liquid petrolatum,* an indigestible oil that does not add to the patient's caloric intake, is much more widely used in this way for lubricating and softening the stool. It is employed mainly for patients with hemorrhoids or other painful anal lesions and for others who must avoid straining at stool. By coating the fecal contents, mineral oil also tends to reduce fluid absorption from the feces and thus prevents their becoming excessively dry.

Mineral oil is itself bland and chemically inert. However, irritant cathartics such as cascara and phenolphthalein are sometimes combined with it in irrational mixtures. People should be advised to use plain liquid petrolatum; the added irritant may be undesirable for patients who need only a lubricant. Flavored mineral oil emulsions are available—at extra cost—for people who dislike the feel of the plain oil on the tongue. (The oily aftertaste can be cut by sucking on an orange slice.)

Liquid petrolatum should not be taken for long periods both because dependence on it may deaden natural defecation reflexes and on account of possibly adverse effects. Some authorities suggest that this oil may remove fat-soluble vitamins from the body before they can be absorbed. In theory, this could lead to deficiencies of carotene and of vitamins A, D, E, and K. Loss of the last-named vitamin (for example, by a pregnant woman taking liquid petrolatum all through pregnancy) could lead to a reduction in prothrombin synthesis and development of hypoprothrombinemic bleeding (Chap. 24).

To avoid possible interference with digestion and absorption of food, liquid petrolatum is not taken with meals and is taken preferably at bedtime. A dose of 15 to 30 ml. is usually effective; larger amounts may lead to leakage through the anal sphincter and soiling of clothes or bedding. In addition to this esthetic disadvantage, excessive amounts of the oil may cause anal itching and slow the healing of surgical wounds—after hemorrhoidectomy, for example.

Surface-active agents, inert chemicals that act like detergents, are also used to soften the stool. *Dioctyl sodium sulfosuccinate,* the most widely used of these substances, is available for oral administration and in enemas. It is thought to act by reducing the surface tension of the fecal contents of the rectum. This permits water and fatty materials to penetrate and make a more moist and bulky mass. This action occurs when wetting agent solutions are administered as retention enemas; however, there is some doubt that small oral doses have the desired effect.

The surface active agents, which, in themselves, seem safe enough, are sometimes offered in proprietary combinations with irritant cathartics, which are considered much less desirable for long-term use. It may also be undesirable to administer mineral oil together with these wetting agents, because they may tend to facilitate passage of the inert oil through the intestinal mucosa. Once the liquid petrolatum, which is ordinarily unabsorbable, gets into the tissues, it cannot be eliminated and may act as a foreign body in the lymph nodes, liver and spleen.

Other Intestinal Stimulants

Among many other substances claimed to increase gastrointestinal motility are the *bile salts* and certain derivatives of the B complex vitamin pantothenic acid. Neither of these is believed to be truly effective for counteracting constipation and preventing or correcting a lack of intestinal muscle tone, especially when the patient has no deficiency of bile or vitamins. One particular derivative of pantothenic acid, *dexpanthenol,* has been widely promoted for parenteral use postoperatively for reduction of abdominal distention

and prevention of paralytic ileus. Although this drug appears to be nontoxic, most doctors prefer to use better established remedies for this potentially serious condition, which can lead to circulatory collapse if uncorrected. These include the potent enterokinetic cholinergic drugs, *neostigmine, bethanechol* and *urecholine* (Chap. 15), together with intubation and other physical measures for removing retained gas and feces.

DRUGS USED IN THE MANAGEMENT OF DIARRHEA

Diarrhea may be a symptom of many different diseases or disorders. Most commonly, it is an acute and self-limiting condition—the result of the intestine's attempt to rid itself of an irritant. On the other hand, diarrhea caused by chronic inflammation or overstimulation of the intestine can be most persistent and difficult to treat. Besides treating the symptom, the doctor tries to determine its cause. Usually, this is easily accomplished—for example, when a pathogenic microorganism susceptible to a specific anti-infective agent can be cultured and eliminated. Sometimes, however, the cause of a patient's diarrhea may be very difficult to discover and overcome. For example, in psychogenic diarrhea, the emotional factors underlying an autonomic nervous system imbalance may be quite obscure.

In any case, even when the cause of diarrhea cannot be readily found and rooted out, it is usually possible to give the patient some symptomatic relief. Certain systemically acting drugs often help to reduce intestinal hypermotility. These agents include the opiates (Chap. 9), which act directly on the intestinal smooth muscle to slow excessive peristaltic activity, and the anticholinergic drugs (Chap. 17), which relax spasm caused by parasympathetic nervous system stimulation.

Various locally acting substances are also said to provide relief of diarrhea by their physical effects on the intestine and its contents. Some doctors doubt that these chemicals actually duplicate their test tube actions within the intestinal tract. However, these substances are safe and inexpensive. Thus, they are widely employed as vehicles for the systemically active agents, on the assumption that, if nothing else, they may provide desirable placebo effects for the distressed patient.

Locally Acting Materials

Adsorbents, Astringents, and Demulcents. Among the most commonly employed of the antidiarrheal drugs are *kaolin* and *pectin*, agents often given together several times daily in acute cases of diarrhea. Kaolin, an aluminum silicate clay is an *ads*orbent, a substance capable of holding on its surface other chemicals with which it comes in contact. This, it is thought, is responsible for its ability to pick up, bind, and remove bacteria, toxins, and other irritants from the intestine. It is also claimed to form a coating over the mucosa which both protects it against irritation and filters out toxins that might otherwise be absorbed into the blood. The pectin component of such products is a plant derivative that is said to provide a demulcent or soothing effect on the irritated bowel lining in addition to aiding in adsorption. Other agents also offer these desirable mechanical actions. *Attapulgite,* a silicate clay like kaolin, is claimed to be several times more effective than the latter in its endotoxin-adsorptive action. It comes in the form of an ultrafine powder said to offer a vast surface area. (The particles in 1 pound of powder, it is claimed, could cover 13 acres of surface!) A heat-treated form, *activated attapulgite* (Claysorb), possesses an increased adsorptive capacity. It is sometimes suspended in alumina gel, a substance with adsorbent, demulcent, and astringent properties of its own. Other minerals claimed to act as intestinal astringents include bismuth and calcium salts. These and the vegetable product, tannic acid, are thought to precipitate cellular proteins and mucus and to shrink local swelling caused by dilated capillaries in the inflamed mucosa.

Hydroabsorptive Substances. The watery, unformed stools characteristic of diarrhea are the result of the rapidity with which the chyme or liquid digestive mass is rushed through the intestine. Ordinarily, most of the fluids in the intestinal contents are reabsorbed into the blood by way of the large bowel wall. However, excessive peristaltic activity permits little time for such absorption by the colon, and, as a result, unusually liquid stools are passed. This loss of fluid, if severe and long-continued, can lead to serious dehydration and electrolyte imbalances, which may be made even more serious if the diarrhea is accompanied by vomiting. Fatalities from the infantile diarrheas that sometimes still spread through hospital nurseries are often the result of unrelieved dehydration, alkalosis or acidosis, hemocentration, and terminal cardiac irregularities.

Such serious complications of diarrhea require intensive treatment to rehydrate the patient and replenish lost electrolytes. However, much simpler measures may be employed in most cases to increase the consistency of the stools. Various hydrophilic (literally, "water-loving") substances may be used to absorb some of the intestinal moisture. The *pectins* act, in part, in this manner, as do *methylcellulose* and *psyllium seed mucilloids* (see the section on bulk laxatives in this chapter). Another hydroabsorptive substance, called *polycarbophil,* is claimed to possess certain advantages over the latter agents. This synthetic substance does not swell in the stomach to cause an uncomfortable feeling of fullness. It is said to exert its

TABLE 38-3

LOCALLY ACTING ANTIDIARRHEAL DRUGS
(Adsorbents, Astringents, Demulcents, Protectives, etc.)

	DOSAGE
Activated Attapulgite (Claysorb)	2 to 5 Gm.
Activated Charcoal U.S.P.	10 Gm.
Bismuth subcarbonate U.S.P.	1 to 4 Gm.
Bismuth subnitrate N.F.	1 to 4 Gm.
Calcium carbonate, precipitated (Chalk) U.S.P.	1 to 2 Gm.
Kaolin N.F.	2 to 5 Gm.
Kaolin mixture with pectin N.F. (Kaopectate)	30 ml.
Pectin N.F.	50 to 300 mg.
Polycarbophil	0.5 to 1 Gm.
Tannic acid N.F.	1 Gm.

water-binding action only upon reaching the alkaline medium of the small intestine and colon.

Systemically Acting Drugs

Antiperistaltic-Antispasmodic Agents

Although the locally active drugs discussed above are used widely, certain systemically acting agents are much more effective for the management of the symptoms of simple diarrhea. Mainly, two types of drugs are employed for reducing acute intestinal hypermotility and spasm: (1) the opiates, and (2) the anticholinergic agents.

Opium Preparations. The alkaloids of opium—morphine, codeine, and papaverine—act in several ways to cause constipation. This action, which is considered an undesirable side effect when opiates are being employed for relief of pain, is, of course, extremely useful for controlling conditions marked by excessive propulsive movements of the intestine. *Paregoric* (camphorated tincture of opium) is given in doses of one or two teaspoonfuls several times daily during acute diarrhea. *Deodorized tincture of opium* (laudanum), which contains a higher concentration of alkaloids, may be administered in drop dosage for the same purpose. In an emergency, morphine itself may be injected to stop a diarrheal state that has brought the patient to the brink of exhaustion and collapse.

Unfortunately, because of their potential for causing addiction, the opiates cannot be used routinely in chronically diarrheal conditions such as ulcerative colitis. Although they may be used to initiate treatment of such patients, the opiates must be gradually discontinued after a few weeks. For this reason, they have recently been largely replaced by the relatively nonaddictive antiperistaltic drug, *diphenoxylate* (Lomotil) in the treatment of long-continued functional diarrhea. This synthetic substance (see Drug Digest) is a derivative of the narcotic analgesic meperidine (Demerol), but it does not share the pain-relieving property of the parent compound, and, unlike the latter, it has rarely been abused by addiction-prone individuals. However, it shares the ability of the opioids to produce constipation by slowing the motility of the intestinal tract and increasing the tone of smooth muscles.

Anticholinergic Agents. The belladonna alkaloids—atropine, hyoscine, and hyoscyamine—and certain synthetic anticholinergic drugs are commonly employed to help relieve painful smooth muscle spasm and retard peristalsis in diarrheas of varied origin. These drugs are most effective when the condition is accompanied by excessive parasympathetic nerve activity, as sometimes occurs in the irritable colon syndrome. This gastrointestinal disturbance (also called spastic colitis, mucous colitis, etc.) has many causes, among which are emotional difficulties.

In some people, emotional tension is thought to cause intensified cholinergic nerve activity, with a resultant increase in the motility of the colon. By blocking acetylcholine, the neurohormone released by cholinergic nerves, the belladonna extracts and synthetic antispasmodics such as dicyclomine (Bentyl), mepenzolate (Cantil), methscopolamine bromide (Pamine), and propantheline (Pro-Banthine) often offer relief of this functional bowel disorder. These drugs are relatively ineffective against diarrhea resulting from regional enteritis and other inflammatory disorders, including ulcerative colitis, and they may, in fact, be contraindicated because of the danger of producing paralytic ileus and bowel obstruction in patients whose intestines have been scarred and narrowed by disease.

The anticholinergic agents are frequently combined with phenobarbital or other sedatives and tranquilizers that tend to relieve the tension that is thought to cause as well as accompany the diarrhea of the irritable bowel syndrome. Rest and relaxation is an important part of the treatment of these patients, and, indeed, bed rest is desirable for *all* patients with acute diarrhea. Patients are usually put to bed for 24 hours and are not permitted to take solid foods by mouth, because materials entering the stomach tend to set off gastrocolic reflexes which intensify lower bowel motility. The anticholinergic drugs diminish the lower motor portion of this reflex, just as topical mucosal anesthetics such as *oxethazine* (Oxaine) help to cut the upper, or afferent, portion of this reflex arc.

The main difficulty in regard to the use of the anticholinergic agents to reduce gastrointestinal motility in diarrhea is they must be given in doses which almost invariably produce side effects because of blockade at other cholinergic sites. Dryness of the mouth, nose, and skin are common but not serious side effects. On the other hand, the effects of these drugs on the eye, heart, and urinary bladder may be dangerous in some patients. Thus, where possible, the doctor may avoid use of these drugs and depend instead upon simple measures such as heat applications to the abdomen during the period of bed rest previously mentioned.

The patient may receive supportive psychotherapy as well as drugs. Such support sometimes helps the patient to overcome his distressing symptoms. It often provides the patient with an opportunity to talk about his worries and concerns and may, perhaps, help him to recognize possible relationships between his emotional problems and his intestinal symptoms.

An effort may also be made to divert the patient's attention from his symptoms, which tend to be aggravated when a patient pays too much attention to them. Diversion can be useful as an adjunct to the drug therapy of diarrhea in those patients who concentrate on the number and frequency of their bowel movements.

Infectious Diarrhea

Acute diarrhea often results from bacterial, viral, or amebic infection, following ingestion of contaminated food or water. Staphylococcal bacteria, the most common cause of food-poisoning diarrhea, produce a toxin which makes its victim violently ill. However, the symptoms usually subside in a few hours, and no specific antibacterial therapy is necessary. Viral gastroenteritis and diarrhea is also of brief duration and readily controlled by symptomatic treatment measures. On the other hand, in diarrhea resulting from salmonellosis, bacillary dysentery (shigellosis), and amebiasis, the doctor may have to resort to treatment with specific antibiotic and chemotherapeutic agents (Chaps. 34, 35 and 37), once the diagnosis has been confirmed by stool cultures and other means.

Most often, however, no specific pathogenic bacteria or protozoan parasites can be found in the stools. This is generally true of the so-called "turista," or tourist diarrhea, which so often affects international travelers. The exact cause of this common condition is still unknown, but some authorities suggest that it is the result, not of an acquired infection at all but of a change in the bowel's bacterial population. That is, the change in the traveler's dietary and water intake is thought to cause new strains of certain pathogenic residents of the traveler's own intestine to begin to grow explosively. The prophylactic employment of certain anti-infective chemicals and antibiotics has been recommended to prevent the emergence of such strains of intestinal organisms in people traveling to foreign lands.

Among the agents most commonly recommended

both for prophylaxis and for treatment of bacterial diarrheas are certain poorly absorbable sulfonamides and antibiotics. The former include phthalylsulfathiazole (Sulfathalide) etc. (Chap. 35), and the latter are mainly the neomycin-streptomycin-kanamycin group of antibiotics and polymyxin (Chap. 34). Because the anti-infective agents of both types tend to stay in the intestine when administered orally, they accumulate there to keep diarrhea-inducing bacteria under control and produce few systemic side effects.

Some authorities are opposed to the prophylactic use of gastrointestinal antiseptics routinely because acute diarrhea has often actually resulted from changes in the intestinal bacterial flora brought about by orally administered antibiotics. This has occurred most commonly following the administration of the tetracycline-type of broad-spectrum antibiotics (Chap. 34). By killing off many of the *non*pathogenic organisms that normally keep certain pathogens under control, these antibiotics sometimes cause the emergence of certain resistant strains of staphylococci and fungi.

The diarrhea that results from such microbial overgrowths is usually mild, but staphylococcal enterocolitis can be quite serious. Such superinfections, as they are called, may require prompt and vigorous treatment with other antibiotics to which the tetracycline-resistant organisms are susceptible, including the newer semisynthetic penicillins oxacillin (Prostaphlin) and methacillin (Staphcillin), and the broad-spectrum agent chloramphenicol (Chloromycetin). In diarrhea caused by overgrowths of the monilial organism *Candida albicans,* the antifungal antibiotic nystatin (Mycostatin) is often employed for prevention and treatment.

ANTIEMETIC DRUGS

Nausea and Vomiting

Nausea is one of the most commonly reported symptoms. This feeling of being "sick in the stomach" is often followed by retching and vomiting, the complex reflex act by which the stomach's contents are ejected. Vomiting serves a useful purpose when it removes toxic irritants from the stomach before they can be absorbed into the systemic circulation. (The use of emetics to induce vomiting and thus help rid the stomach of ingested poisons is discussed in Chap. 3.)

Unfortunately, vomiting occurs most often in situations which do not require emptying of the stomach. Thus, there is no protective value in the vomiting that is part of the body's response to certain types of motion. Similarly, the nausea of early pregnancy does not serve as a useful warning signal in any way, and vomiting that persists may actually endanger the mother by causing a severe fluid-electrolyte imbalance and interfering with her nutrition.

The stimuli that set off the vomiting reflex may originate not only in the gastrointestinal tract but anywhere in the body. Such stimuli may be physical, chemical, or psychological. Thus, it is not surprising that nausea and vomiting should be part of the picture in so many clinical conditions, ranging from minor infections to metastatic carcinoma. The doctor therefore first tries to determine the *cause* of the vomiting and then takes steps to eliminate it, if possible.

Once the cause has been recognized, however, symptomatic relief is desirable to reduce the patient's discomfort and prevent the possibly dangerous consequences of persistent vomiting. Sometimes, relief requires only simple nursing care measures, such as providing a quiet, restful environment and seeing that the patient gets ice to suck or a cold carbonated drink or hot tea to sip. On the other hand, effective antiemetic drugs may also be ordered, which act by dampening hyperactive vomiting reflex activity.

Vomiting Reflex Mechanisms

Vomiting, like most other reflexes, requires the presence of receptors that react to stimuli and send nerve impulses centrally via afferent pathways. Such sensory stimuli may stream in from anywhere in the body, including not only the mucosa of the gastrointestinal tract but also the labyrinth of the inner ear, as well as the cerebral cortex and other brain areas involved in emotional responses. Another group of nerve cells located beneath the cortex—the chemoreceptor trigger zone (CTZ)—also relays afferent impulses toward the vomiting center.

The center that receives these incoming impulses and reacts by transmitting messages to the muscles involved in the vomiting act is located deep in the medulla oblongata. It lies close to the nerve nuclei that control cardiovascular, respiratory and other autonomic functions. Thus, when this area is being bombarded by excessive numbers of nerve impulses from overexcited receptors anywhere in the body, some of these impulses spill over onto these adjacent areas. This accounts for signs and symptoms such as salivation, sweating, pallor and slowing of the heart rate in the nauseated, vomiting person.

Drug Treatment of Nausea and Vomiting

All of the drugs used in the management of nausea and vomiting act by reducing hyperactive reflex activity in one way or another. Some do so by dulling the reactivity of the receptors to stimuli, thus lessening the rate at which impulses pass centrally from peripheral sites such as the stomach. Others make the chemoreceptor trigger zone less sensitive to emetic chemicals circulating in the blood stream or to nerve impulses arriving at this relay station from motion receptors in the inner ear. Occasionally, the threshold of the vomiting center itself may be raised by drugs that depress its neurons.

The drugs used in the management of nausea and vomiting may be classified as (1) *locally acting,* and (2) *centrally acting* (Table 36-4). Substances of the first type include topical mucosal anesthetics, antacids and adsorbents, demulcent-protective agents, and drugs that reduce distention of the stomach by retained gases (e.g., simethicone, and the carminatives).

The centrally acting antiemetics may be further subdivided into (1) the *phenothiazine* and (2) *non-phenothiazine* compounds. The former include many agents also used as major tranquilizers (Chap. 7), as well as some chemicals of this class that are not used in mental illness. The nonphenothiazines are often employed as antihistaminic and anticholinergic agents also.

Locally Acting Agents

Vomiting caused by local irritation of the gastro-intestinal tract is usually self-limited, because, once the stomach rids itself of the troublesome irritant, the source of the person's difficulty is gone, and the mucosal receptors stop sending their distress signals centrally. In some cases of acute gastroenteritis, however, the inflamed membranes continue to bombard the vomiting center with messages that trigger nausea and emesis. Drugs that reduce the reactivity of these receptors may be helpful in overcoming these manifestations of stomach upset while the patient's condition is being gradually cleared up by other measures aimed at removing its cause.

Topical Anesthetics. Various local anesthetics are sometimes administered orally in an attempt to raise the threshold of receptor responsiveness to local irritants. Among the topically active agents often taken by mouth to reduce the number of afferent impulses originating in the G.I. tract are *benzocaine* and *procaine.* It is doubtful, however, that these short-acting substances have much effect on vomiting. The longer-acting local anesthetic, *lidocaine,* is available as a viscous solution which is said to control severe reflex vomiting for several hours when taken orally in tablespoon doses. Another agent, *oxethazine,* which is suspended in an antacid alumina gel, is said to afford prolonged topical anesthesia because it is present in an adherent coating that protects the irritated gastric mucosa.

Among other locally acting agents are various volatile oils, including *peppermint, clove, ginger,* and *cinnamon.* Administered as alcoholic solutions (spirits) or as waters, these carminatives often give a feeling of warmth in the stomach and sometimes seem to help expel gas by causing a reflex increase in gastro-intestinal motility. It is difficult to say whether the carminatives act chemically or psychologically (i.e., through a desirable placebo effect, as discussed in Chapter 2). In any case, removal of accumulated gas is thought to lessen local stimuli that lead to discomfort and nausea.

The psychological effects of some agents used for stomach upset should not be ignored. Although scientific proof of their effectiveness is usually lacking, the placebo response is often a desirable one. Thus, if a patient who takes something occasionally to "settle the stomach" gets from it the comfortable feeling that he is doing himself some good, the nurse should not shatter his confidence in the medication that he finds

TABLE 38-4
CENTRALLY ACTING ANTIEMETIC AGENTS

Nonproprietary or Official Name	Trade Name	Antiemetic Dose (Single, Oral, Adult)
Chlorpromazine HCl U.S.P.	Thorazine	10 to 25 mg.
Cyclizine HCl U.S.P.	Marezine	50 mg.
Chlorcyclizine HCl U.S.P.	Diparalene	50 mg.
Dimenhydrinate U.S.P.	Dramamine	50 mg.
Diphenhydramine U.S.P.	Benadryl	50 mg.
Meclizine HCl U.S.P.	Bonine	25 to 50 mg.
Perphenazine	Trilafon	4 to 8 mg.
Prochlorperazine maleate U.S.P.	Compazine	5 to 10 mg.
Promethazine HCl U.S.P.	Phenergan	25 to 50 mg.
Scopolamine HBr U.S.P.	Hyoscine	0.5 to 1.0 mg.
Thiethylperazine maleate	Torecan	10 to 20 mg.
Triflupromazine HCl	Vesprin	10 to 20 mg.
Trimethobenzamide HCl	Tigan	250 mg.

helpful. If, as in this case, the remedies are considered harmless, it may be wise to stay silent about the worthlessness of a "cure for sour stomach" that makes a person feel better or more comfortable.

Other commonly employed antinauseants that are claimed to work for some people include *Coca Cola syrup* and a product with essentially similar properties, *phosphorylated carbohydrate solution* (Emetrol). These liquids are taken in tablespoonful doses without any other fluids. Although there is little scientific evidence of how they act, these substances are said to relax G.I. muscle spasms by a local effect, thus reducing afferent impulses to the vomiting center.

Centrally Acting Agents

The first of the systemically acting drugs used to depress the central portion of the vomiting mechanism were sedatives, such as *chloral hydrate* and the *barbiturates,* and the centrally acting anticholinergic drug, *scopolamine.* Combinations of barbiturates and scopolamine were widely used by the armed forces during World War II for preventing the nausea and vomiting induced by the motion of ships at sea, airplanes, and other vehicles.

Although scopolamine is still considered an excellent motion sickness preventive, the drowsiness often induced by these early nonspecific antiemetic combinations frequently was a drawback, especially when the operator of a plane, tank, jeep or car had to stay alert. In addition, the cycloplegic action of scopolamine sometimes causes blurring of vision, and the mouth dryness induced by this drug is a somewhat uncomfortable side effect. Thus, the advent of the newer phenothiazine and *non*phenothiazine derivatives, which act more specifically on the nervous pathways involved in vomiting from various causes, has been a boon to many patients. For, though the calming effect of many of these drugs probably plays some part in their antiemetic action, their most important advantage lies in their ability to prevent or relieve vomiting without making most patients excessively drowsy or otherwise distressing them.

The Nonphenothiazines. The effectiveness of the first modern antiemetic drug, *dimenhydrinate* (Dramamine), was discovered accidentally. This agent, which is a close chemical relative of the antihistaminic agent diphenhydramine (Benadryl, Chap. 40), was first tested for efficacy in treating allergic reactions. A patient who was susceptible to motion sickness noted that she did not become carsick on the trolley ride home from the clinic to which she went for treatment of hives with this drug. The doctors to whom she reported this were quick to follow up the lead. They tested dimenhydrinate on soldiers making a rough midwinter ocean voyage to Europe and found the drug to be a relatively effective antinauseant, with fewer side effects than the belladonna derivatives and barbiturates previously employed.

Later, other drugs were introduced which were said to have an even lower incidence of side effects such as drowsiness, mouth dryness and visual blurring. These include *cyclizine* (Marezine) and *meclizine* (Bonine). The latter is claimed to have an especially long duration of action—a single small dose is said to produce prophylactic effects against motion-induced nausea for up to 24 hours.

These drugs and *trimethobenzamide* (Tigan), a more recently introduced *non*phenothiazine, are thought to act mainly by blocking transmission of nerve impulses along the long nervous pathways passing from the inner ear to the vomiting center via the vestibular portion of the 8th cranial nerve, the vestibular nuclei, the cerebellum and the chemoreceptor trigger zone. This is said to account for their special effectiveness in motion sickness and in ailments such as labyrinthitis, Meniere's disease and the dizziness and nausea that often follow surgical procedures involving the inner ear.

In all of these conditions, receptors within the inner ear that have to do with maintaining body balance are overstimulated by motion, inflammation, or trauma. As a result, unusually large numbers of nerve impulses are relayed centrally from these receptor sites. Impulses passing to various nerve nuclei set off the sickening sensation of dizziness or giddiness called vertigo, as well as nausea and vomiting.

These drugs are thought to act mainly by their ability to interrupt transmission of such impulses from the labyrinth of the inner ear to the various responsive central sites. However, the fact that they sometimes cause drowsiness indicates that sedation may also play a part in reducing the patient's sensitivity to disturbing impulses. Thus, people who intend to operate a motor vehicle should be told that these centrally acting antihistaminic-anticholinergic agents may tend to reduce their alertness.

Antiemetics of this type have been considered safe enough to be sold without prescription, but recent reports that some of these drugs have caused developmental defects in animals have led to restrictions in their sale. The Food and Drug Administration has warned against the use of the antinauseant drugs *meclizine, cyclizine* and *chlorcyclizine* during pregnancy. The manufacturers of these products argue that millions of doses have been taken without causing any increase in the incidence of malformations among newborn babies. All agree, however, that pregnant women should use caution in taking *any* drugs. (The difficulty is, of course, that congenital damage to the embryo from any adverse environmental influence is most likely to occur in the first six to eight weeks, before most women are aware that they are pregnant.)

The Phenothiazine Antiemetics. Many of the major tranquilizers, including *chlorpromazine, prochlorperazine* and *perphenazine* also possess potent antiemetic activity. Although they are not as effective against motion-sickness vomiting as are the nonphenothiazines, these drugs seem superior in most other types of severe vomiting. They appear to act by reducing the responsiveness of the chemoreceptor trigger zone to circulating emetic substances.

This action accounts for the usefulness of the phenothiazines not only against drug-induced vomiting but in various clinical conditions marked by changes in hormonal levels or metabolic state. This is very likely the case in pregnancy, for example, in which nausea is probably related to the high levels of estrogens and gonadotropins in the patient's plasma. Most women become tolerant to such hormonal alterations after the early months of pregnancy. Ideally, they should be able to pass through the period of morning nausea without taking any drugs at all or with only occasional use of one of the safer *non*phenothiazine drugs. However, in cases of severe hyperemesis gravidorum not controlled by such measures, the phenothiazine antiemetics are often effective. By their ability to block the sensitive C.T.Z., these drugs keep the circulating hormones and toxins from stimulating the C.T.Z. to send impulses to the vomiting center.

Antineoplastic Chemotherapy and Irradiation. The phenothiazine antiemetics are often useful for cancer patients who are receiving treatment with drugs or irradiation (Chap. 44). Nausea and vomiting are common in these patients, both because of the malignancy itself and because of the toxins released by the tissue-destroying effects of radiation and cytotoxic drugs.

The phenothiazine antiemetics often help to reduce vomiting in patients with uremia, liver and gallbladder disease, and severe infections such as meningitis.

The calming action of many of the phenothiazines undoubtedly adds to their effectiveness by reducing the anxiety and tension that play a part in increasing the patient's susceptibility to other stimuli that cause vomiting.

The nurse should be aware of the importance of psychological factors in nausea and vomiting. Thus, in administering these drugs, she should take advantage of the power of positive suggestion by saying something like, "This medication is going to make you feel better." Similarly, it is desirable to avoid upsetting the nauseated patient in any way. Noise, vibrations and, of course, odors tend to induce vomiting in an already queasy patient, and for example, the aide should be instructed not to bring a food tray into the patient's room. Later, when he feels better, the patient may be given frequent, small meals rich in nutritive substances. In general, it is desirable to keep the patient quiet and to offer psychological and physical support. For example, help the vomiting patient assume a comfortable position.

Postoperative Vomiting. The phenothiazine antiemetics are effective for relief of postoperative vomiting that may threaten the success of the surgery—for example, in patients who have had eye operations or extensive abdominal incisions. Although phenothiazines are often administered *pre*operatively for various purposes, their routine use before the operation in order to reduce later vomiting is considered unwise when weighed against the possible adverse effects of these depressant drugs. (See Chap. 7.)

Some antiemetics of this class are claimed to cause fewer phenothiazine-type side effects than those agents that are also used as tranquilizers. One of these drugs, *thiethylperazine* (Torecan), is claimed to block the vomiting center itself as well as the chemoreceptor trigger zone, and this supposed specificity of action is said to account for a lower incidence of side effects with this agent, compared to other phenothiazine derivatives.

However, the administration of this drug to children under 12 years old is not recommended, because young children are susceptible to central nervous system stimulation by drugs of this class. For example, children receiving the chemically related agent *prochlorperazine* (Compazine) for vomiting have sometimes suffered convulsive spasms as a result of extrapyramidal motor system stimulation. For this reason, doctors prescribe the smallest effective doses, and the nurse should tell parents not to give the child any more than the doctor ordered, because the chances of such side effects rise sharply when the dose is raised.

DIGESTANTS AND RELATED DRUGS

Digestion and Indigestion

In order to be utilized by the body, food must be broken down into simple, soluble molecules that can be absorbed into the blood and can enter into cellular metabolic reactions. The many mechanical and chemical processes to which food is subjected in the mouth, esophagus, stomach and intestines comprise *digestion.* The terms *indigestion* and *dyspepsia* are not as readily defined. They are usually used by laymen to describe any one of a number of vague abdominal symptoms, including feelings of flatulence or bloating, burning epigastric pain, and acidic belching.

Such symptoms may be caused by gastrointestinal inflammatory ailments, including gastritis and peptic ulcer, or they may be the result of a functional reaction to emotional tension. Only rarely are they caused by an actual lack of the chemical substances secreted into the G.I. tract during the digestive processes. Yet, many pharmaceutical preparations containing *digestive enzymes, bile salts,* and sources of *hydrochloric acid* are marketed for the management of indigestion.

Most people who take such products do not actually have any deficiency of digestant chemicals, and the pharmaceutical digestants are usually present in amounts too small to substitute for any actual lack if it existed. However, a relatively few patients—mostly elderly or suffering from organic digestive tract ailments or the aftereffects of gastrointestinal surgery—do have a deficiency of one or more digestive chemicals. In such cases, the administration of such substances in adequate amounts constitutes a rational form of replacement therapy.

Hydrochloric Acid

A deficiency of gastric acid occurs in various conditions, including pernicious anemia (Chap. 25) and stomach cancer, as well as in elderly people and others who have no such serious diseases. Oddly, patients with an almost complete absence of free hydrochloric acid (*achlorhydria*) may have few gastrointestinal complaints, whereas others, with a relatively small deficiency of gastric acid (*hypochlorhydria*), may be bothered by bloating and other symptoms of dyspeptic distress.

The administration of *diluted (10%) hydrochloric acid* often benefits the digestion of patients of both types. Sometimes, amounts of acid too small to seem useful appear to relieve some patient's complaints, possibly by a placebo effect. Best results are obtained, however, when the patient takes repeated doses in amounts that actually leave free acid in the stomach. Thus, although the average dose is only about one teaspoonful (4 ml.) of the dilute acid, further diluted in several ounces of water, some doctors prescribe a total of about 10 milliliters of dilute acid. This is watered down about 10 to 20 times and taken in several divided doses at intervals during and after each meal.

The patient's teeth should be protected from the action of the acid by having him sip the well diluted solution through a glass tube and then take some food or wash his mouth with a mildly alkaline solution.

Also available as a source of hydrochloric acid are *betaine hydrochloride* and *glutamic acid hydrochloride* (Acidulin). These are powders that, when taken in capsules or tablets, release hydrochloric acid in the stomach. They do not yield large quantities of free acid, but they offer a safe, convenient, and often adequate treatment in many cases of gastric achlorhydria.

Digestive Enzymes

Pepsin. The hydrochloric acid is provided in order to furnish an optimal medium for the action of pepsin, the gastric enzyme that begins the breakdown of proteins into smaller fragments. Some patients with *gastric achylia* lack both acid and pepsin. Thus, this enzyme is often administered alone or combined with

sources of hydrochloric acid to aid the digestion of patients with gastric hypoacidity or anacidity. Actually, however, pepsin is not ordinarily lacking, even in patients with achlorhydria, and, in any case, the proteolytic enzymes of the pancreas and intestine can break down protein, even when it has not previously been acted upon by pepsin.

Pancreatic Enzymes. The juice secreted into the duodenum by the pancreas contains enzymes capable of attacking starches (amylases) and fats (lipases), as well as the enzymes trypsin and chymotrypsin, which aid in the breakdown of the polypeptide products of peptic digestion to amino acids. Many digestant products that are available contain these enzymes in the form of *pancreatin*, a substance prepared from hog pancreas. The amounts of pancreatin usually present ordinarily are not adequate for aiding digestion.

For patients with cystic fibrosis and chronic pancreatitis, gastroenterologists often prefer to administer much larger amounts of more concentrated preparations of pancreatic enzymes. For example, a product called *pancrelipase* contains much more lipase, amylase and trypsin activity per unit of weight than the official preparation. Such enzyme concentrates are also used for patients with steatorrhea and other malabsorption syndromes marked by inadequate digestion of fat. Because these enzymes (like all others) are largely protein, they may themselves be partially digested in the stomach. Thus they are often administered in enteric-coated capsules that protect them from acid-peptic digestion and later release them lower in the G.I. tract. However, they are also available in gelatin capsules that are taken with meals. It is claimed that the food-filled stomach affords protection to the enzymes, which are then transported to the proper place for maximum digestive activity.

Bile Salts and Other Choleretics

Bile is secreted by liver cells, stored and concentrated in the gallbladder, and released into the duodenum via the common bile duct. Bile, although it contains no enzymes, plays an important part in the digestion of fats and is essential for absorption of the vitamins—A, D, E, and K—that dissolve in fat.

Natural bile contains organic acids which are, in part, combined into complex salts—for example, *sodium glycocholate* and *taurocholate*. These bile salts have detergent properties that account for their ability to aid in fat digestion and absorption. That is, they act like soaps to lower the surface tension of the large fat globules in food and break them down into tiny droplets. This emulsifying effect exposes a much larger surface area of the lipids to attack by pancreatic lipases. By this enzymatic action the solubilized fat is rapidly converted to readily absorbable fatty acids.

Bile salts are sometimes useful as replacement therapy for patients with partial biliary obstruction or biliary fistulas, and after cholecystectomy or other surgical operations on the biliary system which have led to a deficiency of natural bile. In such patients, administration of natural bile salts in the form of *ox bile extract,* for example, aids in the digestion of fat and in absorption of fatty acids and fat soluble food factors. It is also claimed to have a mildly stimulating effect on the smooth muscle of the gastrointestinal tract that helps to keep peristaltic activity normal. These digestive actions are often useful for patients with a lack of bile; however, the administration of bile salts to individuals without such a deficiency probably produces no significant digestant or laxative actions. Various substances, including the laxatives, aloe and podophyllum, have been claimed to stimulate a flow of laxative bile. It is doubtful that they do, indeed, cause an increased flow of what the TV commercials call "golden" liver bile or that bile would add any desirable action, if it were actually produced in larger amounts.

Choleretic Activity. Bile salts have other pharmacological effects besides those discussed above. For example, after they have been absorbed from the gastrointestinal tract, they tend to stimulate the liver to secrete increased quantities of whole bile. This so-called *choleretic* action, which is shared by certain natural and synthetic substances, including *tocamphyl,* is believed to serve little useful purpose in therapy and may even be undesirable for patients with liver and biliary tract disorders. Patients suffering from *complete* biliary obstruction, for example, should not receive bile salts or tocamphyl, since their action adds to the bile already backing up into the patient's blood

stream to produce jaundice and other toxic effects. Such products are also avoided in patients with acute hepatitis and gallstone colic.

However, certain substances that stimulate an increased flow of a thin, fluid bile seem to have some clinical utility. One of the best of these *hydrocholeretics,* as the agents that promote secretion of dilute bile are called, is *dehydrocholic acid,* a semisynthetic substance produced by oxidation of natural cholic acid. It is used to help flush out the biliary tract when it is only *partially* obstructed by mucus and small stones. This is supposed to keep the bile passages free of infections and calculi.

The sodium salt of this substance, sodium dehydrocholate, is sometimes injected by vein to help outline the gallbladder with X-ray contrast media (see Chap. 45) and to remove such chemicals after biliary tract roentgenography. Such injections are also used for an entirely different purpose—the determination of circulation time. When the solution that is injected into the patient's cubital vein reaches his tongue, he becomes aware of its bitter taste, and the time it took to travel from arm to mouth is recorded as an index of circulation time.

Cholagogues. When fatty food enters the first portion of the small intestine, a hormone called *cholecystokinin* is released and causes the gallbladder to contract and force its contents into the duodenum. This hormone and other substances that stimulate evacuation of the gallbladder are called *cholagogues.* They have little or no therapeutic value but are sometimes employed in the diagnosis of cholelithiasis, as a means of obtaining samples of the gallbladder's contents for microscopic examination. Among other substances

TABLE 38-5
DIGESTANTS AND RELATED DRUGS

Nonproprietary or Official Name	Trade Name	Dosage Range
Betaine HCl	Normacid	500 to 1,000 mg.
Cellulase	—	2 to 8 mg.
Dehydrocholic acid N.F.	Decholin	250 to 500 mg.
Diluted hydrochloric acid N.F.	—	4 to 10 ml., diluted
Florantyrone	Zanchol	250 to 1,000 mg.
Glutamic acid HCl N.F.	Acidulin	300 to 600 mg.
Ox bile extract	—	300 to 600 mg.
Pepsin N.F.	—	500 to 1,000 mg.
Pancreatin N.F.	—	500 to 1,000 mg.
Pancrelipase	Concentrated pancreatic enzymes	150 to 300 mg.
Sodium dehydrocholate injection N.F.	—	2 Gm. I.V.
Tocamphyl	Gallogen; Syncuma	75 to 225 mg.

used for this purpose are *olive oil* and *magnesium sulfate*. Taken on an empty stomach, the latter relaxes the tonically contracted sphincter of Oddi, the ring of smooth muscle that normally keeps bile from flowing out of the common bile duct into the duodenum.

Reduction of Blood Bile Levels

Jaundice is often accompanied by severe pruritus. This is thought to be caused by the bile acids that have backed up into the blood. One of the drawbacks of administration of bile salts to patients with partial biliary tract obstruction is the tendency to aggravate the severe itching. Thus, some doctors avoid their use

in this condition and administer vitamin K and other fat-soluble food factors *parenterally*.

Recently attempts have been made to lower plasma bile acid levels of jaundiced patients by administration of an ion-exchange resin that binds these acids in the intestine before they can be reabsorbed. This substance, called *cholestyramine resin* (Cuemid, Questran) is said to relieve pruritus in patients with partial obstructive jaundice and primary biliary cirrhosis. Unfortunately, it has a fishy odor and gritty taste and has to be taken by mouth in large daily doses. Patients have to be watched for possible hypoprothrombinemic bleeding resulting from interference with vitamin K absorption.

SUMMARY OF POINTS FOR NURSES TO REMEMBER CONCERNING DRUGS USED IN TREATING ACID-PEPTIC DISEASE

- The nurse must use good judgment in determining whether a patient may be permitted to medicate himself with antacid drugs or whether he requires their regular administration by herself.

- The acutely ill peptic ulcer patient requires the nurse's physical care and emotional support and thus should be observed frequently and have his medication administered by the nurse.

- During his recovery, the patient should be taught to measure and take his own ulcer medications at the proper times, since he will have to do this when he returns home.

- The patient should be supplied with waxed paper cups and a container for disposing of them to avoid having

a disorderly array of used medicine glasses collect on his bedside stand.

- When antacids are being administered by continuous drip through a stomach tube, the nurse must regulate the flow of medicine in accordance with the doctor's orders and provide all the care the patient requires for minimizing the discomfort of this procedure.

- Patients taking drugs by mouth should be told to chew antacid tablets before swallowing them but to avoid chewing anticholinergic antispasmodic drugs. The antacids should be washed down with a little milk or water, and hard candies or fluids supplied for counteracting mouth dryness from antisecretory drugs.

SUMMARY OF POINTS FOR THE NURSE TO REMEMBER CONCERNING CATHARTIC DRUGS

- The nurse should suggest that the person who habitually takes any cathartic seek a physician's advice about his problem.

- The nurse should instruct the constipated patient in the hygienic measures that will aid in re-establishing normal bowel function.

- Remember that it is not enough merely to lecture the patient on the desirability of eating a proper diet, drinking plenty of fluids, learning to handle his tensions, establishing a "habit time," etc. It is also necessary to recognize the patient's problem in misusing cathartics and to offer him your support in changing habit patterns which may have existed for many years.

- Observe the bowel function of all patients and particularly those whose conditions may lead to fecal impaction. Remember to ask the patient specific questions, when it is not possible to inspect his stool personally.

- Carefully note the patient's response to any cathartic that he receives. Note, for example, how soon the drug acted and the number and character of the stools that occurred as a result of its action.

SUMMARY OF INDICATIONS AND CONTRAINDICATIONS OF CATHARTICS

- *Indications*
  Prevention of fecal impaction in bedridden patients
  Reduction in straining at stool,
  a. in patients with cardiovascular complications such as aneurism, embolism, and myocardial infarction
  b. in patients with hemorrhoids and other anorectal lesions
  Emptying the G.I. tract prior to diagnostic procedures such as abdominal roentgenography, proctosigmoidoscopy, etc.
  Removal of ingested poisons from lower G.I. tract

  Adjunctive uses in anthelmintic therapy
  Adjunctive use in correction of constipation

- *Contraindications*
  Habitual use for forcing bowel movements in constipation
  Acute appendicitis and other causes of abdominal pain and cramps, including regional enteritis, diverticulitis, and ulcerative colitis
  Pregnancy, late in third trimester
  During menstrual periods, possibly

REVIEW QUESTIONS

Drugs vs. Acid-Peptic Disorders

1. (a) Indicate the postulated role of hydrochloric acid in producing discomfort, pain, and ulcerations in acid-peptic disease.

(b) Indicate the main objective of drug treatment in acid-peptic disease, and list several classes of drugs commonly employed for this purpose.

2. (a) List several ways in which certain chemicals counteract hydrochloric acid in the upper gastrointestinal tract.

(b) Another property besides acid-building capacity that is considered desirable in a product designed to relieve ulcer pain is a protective action. List several substances that possess such an ability to coat the ulcer crater.

3. (a) What actions of sodium bicarbonate account for its ability to relieve certain upper G.I. symptoms?

(b) Why do these same properties make this antacid undesirable for long-term treatment of peptic ulcer?

4. (a) Describe two types of systemic imbalance which may occur as a result of the excessive intake of absorbable antacids.

(b) How may these potentially dangerous conditions be prevented or counteracted?

5. (a) Indicate two types of digestive difficulties which may develop as a result of long-term use of large amounts of antacids of the *non*absorbable type.

(b) Indicate how such difficulties are most commonly overcome, and state an advantage claimed for one particular product over the many others in which the same principle is employed.

6. (a) List several ways in which the nurse can help the convalescent ulcer patient take care of himself during his convalescence.

(b) List some advice which the nurse may offer to the ulcer patient who is about to leave the hospital.

7. (a) List two kinds of systemically acting medications and two kinds of locally acting agents that are employed as adjuncts to antacids in peptic ulcer treatment.

(b) How may administration of anticholinergic drugs aid the effectiveness of antacid therapy in acid-peptic disease?

8. List several properties considered desirable in antacid products.

Drugs with Cathartic Action

1. (a) Explain how the misuse of cathartics may lead to development of chronic constipation.

(b) What advice can the nurse give a person who complains of constipation, in regard to establishment of physiological habit patterns?

2. (a) List two general classes of medical patients for whom the use of laxatives may be indicated.

(b) List three other clinical situations in which cathartics are sometimes employed.

(c) List two general situations in which the use of cathartics is contraindicated.

3. (a) List some undesirable local and systemic effects of the continued use of strongly irritant cathartics such as podophyllum and aloin.

(b) What is the likely result of too frequent use of castor oil?

4. (a) For what valid use is castor oil most commonly employed in hospital practice?

(b) At what time of day is castor oil commonly given and at what times is its use avoided?

5. (a) At what time of day are cathartics such as cascara sagrada and senna best administered?

(b) For patients of what types is cascara sagrada considered a desirable laxative?

6. (a) How serious is the potential toxicity of cathartic candies and gums containing phenolphthalein?

(b) What characteristic hypersensitivity reaction is sometimes seen in patients taking laxatives that contain phenolphthalein?

7. (a) At what time of day and in what form are saline cathartics usually administered?

(b) In what patients may magnesium and sodium salt cathartics be contraindicated because of possible systemic effects?

8. (a) For what purpose may laxatives of the hydrophilic colloid type such as psyllium seeds be employed?

(b) How are these substances best administered?

9. (a) For what patients is liquid petrolatum often preferred over other laxatives?

(b) What are some possible disadvantages of liquid petrolatum and how may some of these be minimized?

10. (a) What is the manner of action of dioctyl sodium sulfosuccinate?

(b) List several drugs that are employed to increase peristaltic activity postoperatively in patients with abdominal distention?

Antidiarrheal Drugs

1. (a) How are substances such as kaolin and activated attapulgite thought to aid in controlling diarrhea?

(b) What additional local effect is pectin believed to have?

2. (a) List several chemicals that are classified as intestinal astringents.

(b) List several substances used in the treatment of diarrhea because of their hydroabsorptive properties.

3. (a) Name two opiate preparations that are used to control diarrhea.

(b) What is the main advantage of the synthetic antidiarrheal agent diphenoxylate over the natural opiate preparations?

4. (a) Name several natural and synthetic drugs with anticholinergic activity that may help to control diarrhea.

(b) What is the manner in which these drugs are thought to provide relief of the irritable bowel syndrome?

5. (a) List a sulfonamide drug and several antibiotics that are used to treat infectious diarrhea because they are able to accumulate in the intestinal tract in concentrations that control various pathogenic microorganisms.

(b) How does the use of certain antibiotics sometimes lead to infectious diarrhea, and what other antibiotics are sometimes used to combat diarrhea of this kind?

Antiemetic Drugs

1. (a) List several receptor sites for stimuli capable of setting off the vomiting reflex mechanism.

(b) Where is the *vomiting center* located and what other coordinating centers lie close to it?

2. (a) In what general way do locally acting antiemetics act to relieve nausea and vomiting?

(b) In what general ways do the centrally acting drugs act?

3. (a) How are drugs such as lidocaine claimed to act as antinauseant-antiemetics?

(b) What should the nurse's attitude be toward patients who take carminatives, Coca-Cola syrup and other "nonscientific" substances that they find useful for relief of stomach upsets?

4. (a) What disadvantages limited the utility of the older motion sickness products containing barbiturates and scopolamine?

(b) What are the advantages claimed for dimenhydrinate, cyclizine and, especially, meclizine?

5. (a) What property of these and other *nonphenothiazine* drugs is said to make them especially useful for clinical conditions in which nausea and vomiting are accompanied by vertigo?

(b) List several such clinical conditions for which drugs of this type are commonly prescribed.

6. (a) What warning may be desirable for drivers taking drugs against motion sickness?

(b) What facts require consideration in determining whether to take an antiemetic drug for the nausea of pregnancy?

7. (a) What are mainly the site and manner of action of the phenothiazine-type antiemetic agents?

(b) List several clinical conditions in which these drugs are preferred for control of vomiting.

8. (a) What measures may the nurse take to add to the effectiveness of an antiemetic drug?

(b) What advice may the nurse give the parents of a vomiting child for whom the doctor had ordered small doses of a phenothiazine-type antiemetic?

Digestants and Related Drugs

1. (a) How is hydrochloric acid usually administered?

(b) What other preparations may be employed to yield acid?

2. (a) Which digestive enzyme is activated by the presence of hydrochloric acid?

(b) What are the conditions that are treated with this enzyme-acid combination called?

3. (a) List the several kinds of enzymatic activity that a product such as pancreatin possesses.

(b) List several conditions in which adequate dosage of pancreatic enzymes may prove desirable as replacement therapy.

4. (a) Name two bile salts and indicate how they aid the digestion and absorption of food fats.

(b) In what conditions are natural bile salts such as those in ox bile extract administered orally as replacement therapy?

5. (a) Explain the meaning of the terms *choleretic, hy-*

drocholeretic and *cholagogue;* for each type of action list one representative drug.

(b) For what purposes are hydrocholeretic drugs sometimes administered?

(c) In what conditions are choleretic and hydrocholeretic drugs contraindicated?

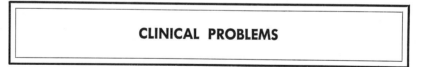

CLINICAL PROBLEMS

Mr. West's physician is treating him at home for peptic ulcer. In addition to rest and a bland diet, the doctor has ordered Amphogel 8 cc. every hour, Prantal 50 mg. t.i.d., a.c., and at h.s., and Librium 10 mg. t.i.d.

- What directions should the public health nurse give Mr. West about taking his Amphogel?

- Mr. West mentions that his mouth is very dry. What suggestions could the nurse make to him for relieving the dryness?

BIBLIOGRAPHY

Acid-Peptic Disease

Di Palma, J. R.: Drugs in the management of peptic ulcer. R.N., *26*:71, 1963 (April).

Epstein, F. H.: Treatment of the milk-alkali syndrome. *In* symposium on treatment of acid peptic disease. Modern Treatment, *1*:1507, 1964 (Nov.).

Goldstein, F.: Newer approaches to the management of peptic ulcer. Med. Clin. North Am., *49*:1253, 1965.

Kirsner, J. B.: Facts and fallacies of current medical therapy for uncomplicated duodenal ulcer. J.A.M.A., *187*: 423, 1964.

Kirsner, J. B., and Palmer, W. L.: Treatment of peptic ulcer, current comments. Am. J. Med., *29*:793, 1960.

Kushlan, S. D.: Diet and drug therapy in peptic ulcer. *In* symposium on treatment of acid peptic disease. Modern Treatment, *1*:1450, 1964 (Nov.).

Law, D. H., *et al.:* Drug therapy of gastrointestinal disease. Am. J. Med. Sci., *238*:160, 1959.

Rodman, M. J.: Drugs for peptic pain. R.N., *21*:64, 1958 (May).

Sun, D. H., and Shay, H.: Optimal effective dose of anticholinergic drugs in peptic ulcer therapy. Arch. Int. Med., *97*:442, 1956.

Winklestein, A.: The clinical evaluation of oxyphencyclamine (Daricon) in patients with peptic ulcer. Am. J. Gastroenterol., *32*:66, 1959.

Woldman, E. E.: Peptic ulcer: current medical treatment. Am. J. Nursing, *59*:222, 1959.

Drugs with Cathartic Action

Abramowitz, E. W.: Phenolphthalein today: a critical review. Am. J. Diges. Dis., *17*:79, 1950.

Becker, G. L.: The case against mineral oil. Am. J. Diges. Dis., *19*:344, 1952.

Dreiling, D. A., Fischl, R. A., and Fernandez, O.: Dulcolax (Bisacodyl), a new nonpurgative laxative. Am. J. Diges. Dis., *4*:311, 1959.

Frohman, I. P.: Constipation. Am. J. Nursing, *55*:65, 1955.

Gray, G., and Tainter, M. L.: Colloid laxatives available for clinical use. Am. J. Diges. Dis., *8*:130, 1941.

Morgan, J. W.: The harmful effects of mineral oil (liquid petrolatum) purgatives. J.A.M.A., *117*:1335, 1941.

Munch, J. C., and Calesnick, B.: Laxative studies. I. Human threshold studies of white and yellow phenolphthalein. Clin. Pharmacol. Ther., *1*:311, 1960.

Rodman, M. J.: The use and misuse of cathartics. R.N., *21*:48, 1958 (July); *21*:49, 1958 (Aug.).

Steignamm, F.: Are laxatives necessary? Am. J. Nursing, *62*:90, 1962.

Wilson, J. L., and Dickinson, D. G.: Use of dioctyl sodium sulfosuccinate (Aerosol O.T.) for severe constipation. J.A.M.A., *158*:261, 1955.

Antidiarrheal Drugs

Barowsky, H., and Schwartz, S. A.: Comparison of the antidiarrheal effect of diphenoxylate with that of camphorated tincture of opium. J.A.M.A., *180*:1058, 1962.

Cooke, R. E.: Current status of therapy in infantile diarrhea. J.A.M.A., *167*:1243, 1958.

Hoskins, D. W., and Kean, B. H.: Drugs for travelers. Clin. Pharmacol. Ther., *4*:673, 1963.

Kean, B. H., *et al.:* The diarrhea of travelers. J.A.M.A., *180*:367, 1962.

Low, D. H., *et al.:* Drug therapy of gastrointestinal disease. Am. J. Med. Sci., *238*:638, 1959.

Rodman, M. J.: Drugs for vacation ills. R.N., *25*:73, 1962 (June).

———: Drugs for G.I. distress. R.N., *28*:49, 1965 (June).

Antiemetic Drugs

Belleville, J. W., Bross, I. D. J., and Howland, W. S.: Postoperative nausea and vomiting; evaluation of antiemetic drugs. J.A.M.A., *172*:1488, 1960.

Borison, H. L., and Wang, S. C.: Physiology and pharmacology of vomiting. Pharmacol. Rev., *5*:193, 1953.

Boyd, E. M.: Antiemetic action of prochlorperazine (Compazine). Canad. M. A. J., *76*:286, 1957.

Chinn, H. I., and Smith, P. K.: Motion sickness. Pharmacol. Rev., *7*:33, 1955.

Doyle, O. W.: Evaluation of trimethobenzamide as an antiemetic in nausea and vomiting associated with neoplasms. Clin. Med., *7*:43, 1960.

Hoskins, D. W., and Kean, B. H.: Drugs for travelers. Clin. Pharmacol. Ther., *4*:673, 1963.

North, W. C., *et al.*: Factors concerned with postoperative emesis and its prevention with thiethylperazine. J.A.M.A., *183*:656, 1963.

Rodman, M. J.: Drugs for upset stomach. R.N., *21*:56, 1958 (Sept.).

———: Drugs for gastrointestinal distress. R.N., *28*:49, 1965 (June).

Trumbull, R., *et al.*: Effect of certain drugs on the incidence of seasickness. Clin. Pharmacol. Ther., *1*:280, 1960.

Winters, H. S.: Antiemetics in nausea and vomiting of pregnancy. Obstet. Gynec., *18*:753, 1961.

Drugs Acting on the Muscles of the Uterus

STRUCTURE AND FUNCTION OF THE UTERUS

The uterus is a hollow organ in which the fertilized ovum develops into the embryo and fetus. Its rounded upper part, the *fundus*, is joined at its two sides by the fallopian tubes, through which ova pass from the ovary to the main body of the uterus. The lower part—the neck, or *cervix*—tapers to the *external os*, or mouth, which opens into the vaginal tract. The uterus of a nonpregnant nulliparous woman is only about 3 inches long, but it grows enormously during pregnancy. This organ is made up mainly of two kinds of tissue: (1) the *endometrium*, a layer of mucous membrane that lines its inner surface, and (2) the *myometrium*, a thick wall of muscle that constitutes the bulk of the uterus.

Uterine tissue of both kinds responds to circulating chemical substances. The glandular epithelium of the endometrium undergoes continual changes during the menstrual month and in pregnancy in response to steroid hormones secreted by the ovaries. The nature and significance of these changes are discussed in Chapter 29, the Female Sex Hormones. We shall limit this review to the myometrium, since the drugs discussed in this chapter act directly upon its smooth muscle cells to contract or relax them.

The *myometrium* is made up of interlacing bands of muscle fibers that circle the uterus on the inside and run lengthwise and obliquely in its outer layers. Blood vessels pass between the intertwining fibers, bringing a rich flow of nutrient fluids to the placenta, the organ formed from fetal and maternal tissues in the pregnant uterus. The inner surface of the placenta sends fingerlike projections into openings, or *sinuses*, in the wall of the uterus. The blood in the sinuses bathes the placental extensions and thus transfers oxygen and nutrients to the fetal circulation. The mother's vessels and those of the developing fetus are not directly connected; materials contained in the blood supply of both—including carbon dioxide and other wastes from the fetus—*diffuse* across the vascular membranes of the placenta and the umbilical cord which passes from the placenta's outer surface to the fetus.

The size and weight of the uterus increase greatly during pregnancy. It grows from only a couple of ounces to two pounds or more, exclusive of its contents. The fiber bundles stretch to accommodate the rapidly growing fetus. Their contractions, which are weak in early pregnancy, become stronger and occur more often as pregnancy advances. Finally, at term myometrial irritability is markedly increased, presumably because of sudden changes in the levels of various circulating hormones, and the contractions of labor begin.

PARTURITION (LABOR) AND DELIVERY

The exact nature of the complex chemical and physical changes that initiate labor is not fully established. A sudden increase in estrogen secretion and a decrease in progesterone production seem to play a part. In addition, when the uterus distends beyond a certain point, nerve impulses passing from it to the brain and the posterior pituitary gland are believed to bring about the reflex release of *oxytocin*. This hormone induces strong rhythmic contractions in the muscles of the uterus. The pressure built up in this way helps to dilate the cervix, the narrow neck of the uterus leading into the vaginal tract. Such cervical dilation increases the transmission of stimuli to the brain that cause more oxytocin to pour out of the pituitary and pass to the uterus by way of the blood stream.

Labor, or parturition (the process by which the baby is delivered), is divided into three stages. The first stage begins with the onset of strong contractions of the fundus, the rounded upper portion of the uterus, and continues until the opening of the cervix is fully dilated. In the second stage, mounting contractions, becoming stronger and occurring more frequently, propel the infant's head through the open cervical mouth, or os, into the vaginal tract and continue to push the child along the birth canal until delivery is completed. The third stage is marked by separation of the placenta from the wall of the uterus and the expulsion of the so-called afterbirth. This stage is followed by the *puerperium*, the period during which the uterus gradually returns to its pregravid state.

Immediately after the delivery of the baby and the placenta, the uterus becomes completely relaxed. During this period of uterine atony, the mother may lose a good deal of blood through the sinuses in the uterine wall where the placenta tore away. A pint or more of blood may be lost before the flaccid myometrium begins to contract again spontaneously and becomes firm once more. Once such contractions start, the muscle fibers clamp down on the blood vessels like living ligatures. This shuts off the flow of blood from the uterus, thus halting any further significant hemorrhaging. During the next few days of the puerperium, the uterus regains much of its tone, and in the next eight or ten weeks *involution*—a reduction in size—gradually takes place. These natural processes can often be speeded by the administration of certain pharmacological agents that are widely employed in obstetrics.

OXYTOCIC DRUGS

The response of the uterus to drugs depends upon when they are given. The myometrium responds to drugs most strongly late in pregnancy and early in the postpartum period. The agents that are used clinically to stimulate uterine motility are called *oxytocics*. These chemicals fall mainly into two classes: (1) *ergot* de-

rivatives, and (2) the natural or synthetic posterior pituitary gland hormone, *oxytocin*. Both these substances share a similar property—the ability to set off strong myometrial contractions. However, certain differences in some of their properties make oxytocics of one or the other type better suited to various clinical situations.

Thus, ergot and oxytocin are equally useful when administered during the third stage of labor or in the puerperium to control bleeding after the birth of the baby or following an abortion; only oxytocin, however, is used *before* labor or during its earlier stages. Ergot derivatives are never used to bring about the onset of labor or during its first and second stages. Unlike oxytocin, which is rapidly inactivated, ergot has a long-lasting action upon the myometrium. If, by chance, the uterus were to go into a prolonged, powerful tetanic contraction before the baby was born, both baby and mother might be seriously endangered before the myometrium could be made to relax. On the other hand, many obstetricians prefer ergot for daily use during the postpartum period, because orally administered doses have a long action which helps to bring the uterus back to its normal size and tone.

Ergot Alkaloids

Ergot is a parasitic fungus that grows on rye and other cereal grains. It contains many potent chemical substances, including the alkaloids ergotamine and ergonovine, which are widely used in modern medicine for their dependable actions in certain clinical conditions. The use of ergotamine in the management of migraine headache is discussed in Chapter 41. *Ergonovine* and a semisynthetic derivative, *methyl-*

TABLE 39-1
OXYTOCIC AGENTS

Nonproprietary or Official Name	Trade Name	Dosage
Ergonovine maleate U.S.P.	Ergotrate	0.2 mg. (200 mcg.) orally 3 or 4 times a day, or by I.M. or S.C. injection.
Methylergonovine maleate U.S.P.	Methergine	0.2 mg. (200 mcg.) orally 3 or 4 times a day, or by I.M. or I.V. injection.
Oxytocin Injection U.S.P.	Pitocin; Syntocinon; Uteracon	1 ml. (10 units) I.M., repeated in 30 minutes if necessary.
Oxytocin citrate	Pitocin citrate	200 to 3,000 units parabuccally.
Sparteine sulfate	Spartocin; Tocosamine	150 to 600 mg. I.M.

ergonovine, are used in obstetrics because of their relatively selective action on the uterus at term.

Effects on the Uterus. Small doses of these two drugs act directly upon the smooth muscle fibers of the uterus and cause them to contract. To prevent *postpartum hemorrhage,* they are most commonly administered intramuscularly or by vein.

Some obstetricians prefer to give ergonovine toward the end of the second stage of labor when the baby's head and one of its shoulders have appeared. Injected intravenously, it begins to make the uterus contract within one minute. This helps to complete the delivery of the infant and placenta. The uterus remains hard and firm following ergot-aided delivery, instead of becoming naturally soft and flaccid. This keeps bleeding to a minimum by clamping the uterine fibers down on the open arterioles.

Other doctors prefer to wait until the placenta has been expelled before administering an oxytocic drug. They feel that premature contraction of the uterus may trap the afterbirth in the womb. If the placenta does not separate spontaneously, the doctor may have to detach and remove it manually—a complicated maneuver. Thus, these obstetricians may decide to make their injections intramuscularly just as the baby is being born, in order to obtain the desired uterine contractions about two to five minutes later, during the third stage of labor when the placenta is delivered and blood begins to flow from the open uterine sinuses.

Whichever method is preferred, the nurse must be ready to administer the oxytocic as soon as the doctor orders it. To minimize maternal blood loss and danger to the baby it is important to give the drug neither too late nor too soon. Thus, when she is assisting in the delivery room, the nurse should see that the right dose of the oxytocic drug is made ready, along with the needles and syringes for administering it exactly when the doctor desires. His directions for timing the administration of ergot should be followed precisely.

Ergot is often ordered for purposes other than prevention of postpartum hemorrhage. Even doctors who prefer to employ the pituitary-type oxytocics at the time of delivery often order oral ergonovine or methylergonovine for the next several days. The drugs are quickly and completely absorbed from the G.I. tract to produce long-lasting uterine contractions. Given several times a day for a few days, the drug helps to hasten the return of the uterus to its normal tone. Some obstetricians believe that ergot administration also lessens the likelihood of infection, by closing the gaping uterine sinuses through which bacteria might enter to spread infection.

Ergot is sometimes ordered after a spontaneous partial abortion. Whereas oxytocin is often considered superior for initiation of contractions, ergonovine may be more effective for reducing the bleeding that follows expulsion of the dead fetus and the membranes. If hemorrhage persists, the doctor may have to do a dilatation and curettage of the womb. Surgical repair is necessary for control of hemorrhage from cervical tears or lacerations of the birth canal, since ergot alone does not stop bleeding from trauma to such sites.

Side Effects and Toxicity. Ergonovine is a remarkably safe drug when given in proper dosage, because its effects are largely limited to myometrial smooth muscle. Occasionally, however, it may raise a patient's blood pressure to abnormally high levels. Injection of chlorpromazine by vein counteracts this reaction quite readily. The synthetic derivative, methylergonovine, is said not to produce such pressure rises and may therefore be preferred for patients with high blood pressure. Both of these drugs are best avoided in patients with peripheral vascular diseases, although they have very little of the vasoconstrictor activity of other ergot alkaloids such as ergotamine.

The main danger of overdosage with ergot products is that the patient's peripheral circulation may be severely impaired. Narrowing of the vessels and damage to the inner lining of the arterioles may lead to the formation of blood clots and finally to gangrene of the toes, fingers and other parts. During the Middle Ages, epidemics of gangrene occurred periodically, as a result of eating bread made with ergot-contaminated grain. Because the limbs of its victims became horribly blackened, the condition was called Holy Fire. Peasants who left their homes and made a pilgrimage to the shrine of St. Anthony often improved. Thus, the name "St. Anthony's fire" is also associated with this disease. Modern milling methods have largely eliminated such episodes of ergotism; however, a short-lived outbreak occurred in France in recent years.

Today, cases of ergot poisoning are relatively rare and are most often the result of a rash attempt to produce an abortion by taking large doses of preparations such as the fluidextract, which contain vasoconstrictive alkaloids. Such efforts are misguided at best and are especially dangerous because, in the early months of pregnancy, a woman's blood vessels are much more reactive to these drugs than is her uterus. Although ergot is contraindicated throughout pregnancy, the myometrium is very much less responsive to ergot at first than it becomes during the third trimester and at term.

Signs and symptoms of ergotism include itching, tingling, numbness and cold in the fingers and toes. Such signs of circulatory stasis call for treatment measures similar to those used in peripheral vascular diseases (Chap. 26). The worst sequelae of ergot toxicity may often be prevented by the administration of vasodilator and anticoagulant drugs, application of heat to the abdomen to induce reflex vasodilation, and by careful skin care. However, it is also important to pay attention to the patient's mental state.

In dealing with a patient recovering from an unsuccessful attempt at abortion, the nurse should concentrate on her care and not attempt to judge her. A kind and considerate attitude by the nurse can play an important part—together with support from her family, the doctor, or a clergyman—in helping her to get well and go through with her pregnancy.

The nurse can also often help to prevent abortion attempts in the first place: women who want to terminate a pregnancy will often approach a nurse, rather than a doctor, for information about abortifacient drugs. It is important to listen patiently and carefully to these questions and to encourage the woman to talk about her problems. The patient may then be encouraged to seek the help of her physician or her clergyman. These measures can often help the patient to carry through with her pregnancy.

The nurse also recognizes more subtle clues that may suggest that a pregnant woman may be planning to take an oxytocic drug. In teaching a mothers' class, for example, the nurse should be alert for the occasional woman who seems upset and depressed or who asks more or less pointed questions about drugs for inducing uterine contractions. The nurse should allow time after the group session for an individual conference with such a patient, to give her an opportunity to express some of her fears or worries in regard to her pregnancy. The doctor can then be notified or an arrangement made for him to see her promptly so that the woman can get further assistance with her problems.

Accidental ergotism is most likely to occur in women who are taking ergot postpartum for slow involution of the uterus. Early side effects to watch for in such cases include nausea, vomiting, cramps, and diarrhea. Drowsiness, dizziness and headache, as well as confusion and, sometimes, psychotic reactions are central effects that may occur with this lysergic acid amide derivative (ergonovine is *lysergic acid dihydroxypropylamide*). Occasionally these gastrointestinal signs and symptoms and central effects may develop before the signs of circulatory disturbances in hands and feet appear.

Oxytocin, Natural and Synthetic

The posterior pituitary gland, or neurohypophysis, secretes hormones of two kinds. One of these is *vasopressin,* the antidiuretic hormone (ADH), which is discussed in detail in Chapter 27. The other pituitary principle is *oxytocin,* which probably plays a part in initiating natural labor. Oxytocin has been extracted in relatively pure form and is also available as a synthetically prepared compound. These preparations are used in obstetrics both for prevention of postpartum hemorrhage and for other purposes in which their relative safety makes them superior to the ergot derivatives.

Indications and Dangers. Oxytocin is often used today to induce labor as well as to check postpartum and postabortal hemorrhage. However, its dosage, concentration and method of administration differ considerably when it is given *before* rather than after labor.

In the second stage of labor, for example, 3 to 10 units are usually given intramuscularly when the anterior shoulder appears; on the other hand, no more than *one* unit at a time is injected by this route when the doctor desires to induce labor or when he wants to stimulate it after it has started and then stalled. Similarly, one unit of oxytocin may occasionally be mixed with a few milliliters of saline solution and injected by vein to check severe postpartum hemorrhage; however, that amount is *never* injected intravenously in so concentrated a solution *prior* to the onset of labor. It is instead diluted a thousandfold (see below) and then dripped into the vein very slowly and cautiously.

A large dose of oxytocin is not given before delivery or early in labor for the same reason that ergot is never given at all at such times—i.e., to avoid the danger of causing serious injury to both mother and baby. Sometimes the nurse needs to explain this to the patient who asks why she can't be given a large dose of a drug that will get labor started or make it proceed more rapidly. Powerful spasms induced by drugs before the cervix is adequately softened and dilated may result in the death of the fetus and possibly in fatal trauma to the mother.

Strong contractions that force the fetus against a hard, unyielding and only partially dilated cervix can tear the cervical tissues or even rupture the muscles of the fundus itself. The infant's head or other parts may be damaged when shoved against the unripe cervix in this way. Sustained uterine spasms may also choke off the child's only source of oxygen—the blood that flows from the mother's arteries into the placenta during periods of relaxation. Thus, tetanic contractions of the uterus can kill the unborn baby or cause serious birth defects.

Induction of Labor. Despite these dangers from too early administration of oxytocic agents, most obstetricians now believe that the cautious use of oxytocin is sometimes desirable to induce labor or restart it in cases of uterine inertia. However, the doctors still disagree as to just when this potentially dangerous procedure is entirely justified. Many argue that oxytocin should be administered before and during early labor only for a sound obstetrical reason—for example, when delay occasioned by the wait for contractions to start or to resume spontaneously might result in a stillbirth. Other physicians are so confident of the safety of oxytocin (when it is properly employed and certain criteria are met) that they use the drug routinely to induce labor whenever it suits their personal convenience or that of the patient.

Both those who have gone along with the fad for having "babies by appointment" and the doctors who deplore this elective use of oxytocin agree that the drug should be used only when the patient can be kept under close observation and there are no contraindications to its use. For example, oxytocin is used to induce labor only when the head of the fetus and the mother's pelvic outlet are in proper proportion and the baby's head is in position for normal delivery, as determined by X-ray. Drug-induced labor is not recommended for patients predisposed to uterine rupture, including those who have had four or more children or previous deliveries by cesarian section.

Administration for Induction. One of the safest ways to give oxytocin is by slow intravenous infusion of a very dilute solution. One unit of the drug is added to 1,000 ml. of a glucose solution and dripped into a vein at a rate of only about 15 drops per minute. Later, if contractions are slow in coming, the flow of the dilute solution is gradually raised to up to 2 ml. per minute and continued until regular contractions begin. Too strong spasms must be avoided, lest they interfere with blood flow to the fetus. When caring for any patient who is receiving oxytocin for induction, the nurse carefully observes the frequency, strength and duration of uterine contractions and listens to the fetal heart sounds.

Less efficient but more convenient ways of administering oxytocin are by buccal tablets and by application of a solution to the nasal mucosa. A tablet that contains pitocin citrate is placed between the patient's cheek and gum. Tablets are added every half hour until labor begins, and the number of tablets needed to maintain moderate contractions is kept at that level. If contractions become too strong, the tablets may be spat out, or even swallowed, since they are inactivated in the G.I. tract. All the usual precautions, including medical supervision in a hospital, are required, even when the drug is given by the buccal or intranasal routes, because tetanic contractions of the uterus and fetal heart irregularities have been reported even with this relatively safe route of administration.

The synthetic form of oxytocin (see Table 39-1) is reported to be superior to the natural glandular extract. Unlike the latter, it is free from contamination by the other pituitary principle, vasopressin, as well as by animal proteins. The presence of vasopressin in natural posterior pituitary extracts is said to cause constriction of coronary arteries occasionally—a reaction that can cause cardiac ischemia and death from cardiovascular collapse. Animal protein has caused anaphylactoid reactions. Neither of these adverse effects of natural contaminants is observed with the synthetic oxytocin injection.

Other Uses. Ordinarily, oxytocin is given only at term in small doses and when the patient's cervix is soft and dilated. Sometimes, much larger doses are administered earlier in pregnancy to induce a therapeutic abortion or to rid the uterus of a fetus that has died. Infused by vein, these large doses of oxytocin help to expel the products of a failed pregnancy or an incomplete abortion. Even when the cervix fails to dilate adequately, the drug's firming action makes surgical curettage easier to perform and reduces postoperative and postabortive bleeding.

Oxytocin has an interesting effect on certain muscular elements in the breasts. It makes these muscle cells contract around the milk-containing alveoli to squeeze the milk out. This action is used to relieve painful engorgement of the breasts post partum and to aid in breast feeding. A nasal spray of synthetic oxytocin is available for instillation into the nostrils a couple of minutes before nursing. Its effects imitate those of the natural hormone released reflexly when a baby suckles. When the natural stimulus for ejecting the milk so that the baby can draw it from the nipple is inadequate, the drug's action helps to make up for the inefficient reflex. Oxytocin is, of course, not responsible for milk production, which is under the influence of prolactin (Chap. 27).

Sparteine Sulfate

A third type of oxytocic drug, the plant derivative sparteine sulfate, has recently been introduced into American obstetrical practice. The drug is claimed to have certain advantages over oxytocin for the induction of labor and for overcoming uterine inertia. However, the place of sparteine still remains to be determined through fuller evaluation than it has thus far received.

Actually, this alkaloid has been known for nearly a century. It was introduced originally for the treatment of cardiac arrhythmias. However, quinidine and procainamide HCl (Chap. 21), which are much more dependable antiarrhythmic drugs, have completely replaced sparteine in the treatment of tachycardia. Sparteine is now recommended only for its oxytocic action.

The main advantage originally claimed for sparteine was that patients receiving it did not require the degree of supervision that is needed when an intravenous oxytocin drip is being employed for elective induction of labor. The drug was claimed to cause only contractions similar to those encountered in normal labor, and it was suggested that sparteine was especially desirable when nurses were too busy to stay with patients continuously, as they must during an infusion of oxytocin.

Recent reports of cases in which the use of sparteine has been followed by rupture of the patient's uterus, lacerations of the cervix, and fetal trauma indicate that the use of this drug requires all the precautions that are ordinarily taken with other oxytocic agents. Thus, patients must be carefully selected by the usual criteria for safe induction and carefully observed throughout the period of developing contractions. In addition to the usual contraindications—cephalopelvic disproportion, previous abdominal deliveries, and other unfavorable obstetrical conditions—sparteine is considered undesirable for patients with a history of heart disease because of possibly adverse effects upon cardiac function.

Sparteine has also been advocated for restoring rhythmic contractions in cases of arrested labor. Administered intramuscularly, the drug is said to overcome such uterine inertia and to speed the first and second stages of desultory labor. A dose of 1 ml. (150 mg.) is injected initially and repeated hourly, if necessary, up to a total of four doses. By restarting a stalled labor in this way, sparteine is said to aid the nearly exhausted mother and avoid stillbirth. However, contrary to earlier claims that this drug caused only regular contractions followed by complete relaxation, it is now known that tetanic contractions are an ever-present danger even when sparteine is used judiciously.

With this agent, as with other oxytocics, the degree to which the uterus will respond is always unpredictable. A small dose, administered after a couple of ineffective earlier ones, may sometimes cause sudden precipitate labor. Similarly, when patients fail to respond to sparteine, several hours must be allowed to elapse before employing oxytocin because the two drugs often act synergistically in a way which may result in tetanic contractions of the uterus.

UTERINE RELAXANTS

Relatively few drugs are available specifically for relaxing spasm of the uterus as dependably as the oxytocics contract it. The means by which the obstetrician most commonly attempts to overcome premature labor contractions and threatened abortion are bed rest and sedation with barbiturates and opiates. The main purpose in giving these drugs is to keep the patient calm rather than to relax the uterus directly.

The nurse does not, of course, rely on drugs alone to help the patient relax but tries to make her feel more secure so that she will let herself rest and receive the full benefits of the drugs. The patient is often apprehensive both for her own welfare and that of the baby. Observing the patient frequently or, preferably, remaining with her, can convey to the woman that she is being cared for by a careful, competent nurse who is really concerned about what happens to her and her baby.

In addition to their use for calming the patient and reducing uterine motility during premature labor, nervous system depressants are sometimes employed to relax contraction rings in abnormal labor or following oxytocic-induced uterine reactions. Although large doses of morphine and meperidine (Demerol) may be useful for allaying the patient's pain and anxiety, the inhalation of ether is probably the most reliable means of relaxing the uterus. However, when excessive relaxation of the postpartum myometrium is brought about by this anesthetic, the mother may be exposed to the danger of excessive bleeding.

Ovarian Hormones. Certain female sex hormones have been employed clinically for reduction of uterine motility. The use of the sex steroid *progesterone* and its derivatives in the treatment of threatened abortion is discussed in Chapter 29. Two other ovarian principles, which are not steroids, also have uterus-relaxing activity. These substances, *relaxin* and *lututrin,* have been used clinically in attempts to lessen uterine spasms, but their value in the various clinical situations for which they have been used has not been established.

Relaxin (Releasin; Cervilaxin), a mixture of polypeptides found in the blood of pregnant women, has been extracted in relatively purified form from animal ovaries and made available for use in counteracting premature labor. Administered by frequent intramuscular injections or by slow intravenous drip, this substance reportedly halted labor when it began prematurely in some women between the 29th and 36th weeks of pregnancy. This kept the babies from being born too soon and aided their chances of survival. However, the true value of relaxin has not yet been established. Because the drug is expensive and capable of causing severe foreign protein reactions, it is rarely used today, and most cases of premature labor are still managed with bed rest and sedation.

Relaxin has another interesting action, which has led to its being tried as an adjunct to oxytocin in the induction of labor. Administered at term by intravenous drip after rupture of the membranes, relaxin has a softening action on the cervix. When oxytocin is then added to the I.V. drip, the softened cervix is more readily effaced and dilated by the resulting contractions. The combined effects of the two hormones is said to speed the course of labor.

Lututrin (Lutrexin), another uterine relaxing factor, has been used in the treatment of dysmenorrhea as well as in threatened abortion and premature labor. For the relief of menstrual pain this substance is administered orally, beginning the day before menstruation is expected, since it is said to be more effective when given *before* uterine cramps have become severe. This hormone seems to be free of toxicity even when taken in large daily doses.

Antispasmodic drugs have been advocated for relaxation of myometrial spasms in various conditions. Thus, atropine and other belladonna derivatives, which possess spasmolytic effects on gastrointestinal smooth muscle, are often added to mixtures of analgesic drugs for dysmenorrhea. These anticholinergic agents have not, however, proved very useful for relieving uterine menstrual cramps.

A synthetic antispasmodic drug, *isoxsuprine* (see Chap. 26), has been employed recently to relax uterine contractions in premature labor. It reportedly arrested excessive motility when injected before the patient's membranes have ruptured. However, if given later in labor, the drug is usually ineffective and may tend to increase postpartum bleeding, because of its vasodilator effects. Some patients who received high doses parenterally have suffered hypotensive reactions and reflex tachycardia, which required treatment with vasopressor drugs. When administered orally in the treatment of dysmenorrhea, this drug has little effect on the heart or blood pressure—but, unfortunately, it also has relatively little effect on painful menstrual cramps either. (See Chap. 29 for a further discussion of drugs used in treating dysmenorrhea.)

OXYTOCIC DRUGS: SUMMARY OF THERAPEUTIC USES, SIDE EFFECTS, TOXICITY, CAUTIONS AND CONTRAINDICATIONS

- **Therapeutic Uses**
  1. Control of postpartum hemorrhage
  2. Control of postabortal bleeding after therapeutic or spontaneous abortion
  3. Induction of labor at term
  4. Management of uterine inertia during labor
  5. Hasten involution of an atonic uterus during the puerperium and reduce chances of bleeding and infection at that time

- **Side Effects and Toxicity**
  1. *Ergot derivatives*
     Nausea, vomiting; rise in blood pressure; excitement, confusion, tremors, convulsions; itching, tingling, numbness and cold in fingers and toes; thrombophlebitis, necrosis and gangrene of the feet, hands, etc.
  2. *Oxytocin and Posterior Pituitary extract*
     Nausea, intestinal cramps; urticaria and angioneurotic edema; bronchial and vascular constriction, leading to asthmatic and coronary attacks and cardiovascular collapse
  3. *Sparteine sulfate*
     Cardiac arrhythmias

  4. *ALL oxytocics*
     Uterine rupture, cervical lacerations, trauma to or asphyxiation of the fetus

- **Cautions and Contraindications**
  1. *Ergot derivatives*
     Patients with peripheral vascular disease; coronary artery disease, arteriosclerosis, arteritis; liver or kidney disease; sepsis
  2. *Oxytocin and posterior Pituitary Extract*
     Patients with coronary vascular disease or toxemia of pregnancy
  3. *Sparteine sulfate*
     Patients with a history of cardiac disease
  4. *ALL oxytocics*
     Should not be used unless patients can be kept under continuous observation
     Should not be used for induction of labor unless various criteria are met which indicate that an entirely normal delivery can be expected (e.g., *No* cephalopelvic disproportion nor malpresentation; no uterine scarring, etc.)

SUMMARY OF POINTS FOR NURSES TO REMEMBER CONCERNING OXYTOCIC DRUGS

- The nurse must follow meticulously the obstetrician's orders in regard to the *timing* of administration of oxytocic drugs in the delivery room. She should prepare the required drugs and equipment and acquire the knowledge needed to administer these drugs promptly and accurately, in advance, as part of her preparation for assisting in delivery.

- The nurse should warn women against the use of oxytocic drugs when they approach her to discuss ways of terminating an unwanted pregnancy. She should listen to the patient's views with understanding and compassion, and arrange an opportunity for her to talk further with a physician and, perhaps, a social worker.

- The nurse should be aware of the toxic symptoms of ergotism in order to be able to recognize quickly that a patient may have accidentally or deliberately taken a toxic overdose of an ergot preparation.

- The nurse should concentrate her attention exclusively on the all-important aspects of the care required when a woman is suffering the effects of an attempted drug-induced abortion. She should be aware of the complex emotional and social factors which may have precipitated such an action. A helpful, non-judgmental attitude on the part of the nurse and others is desirable for the patient's recovery, and for the sake of the unborn baby if the abortion attempt was (as is usual) unsuccessful and the fetus was not expelled.

- The nurse should be able to explain to the patient in labor why her doctor has not ordered medication to make it proceed more quickly—i.e., that such drugs are too dangerous to be used to speed up an otherwise normal labor as a way of lessening the normal distress and discomfort of this period.

- The nurse keeps under constant observation the patient in whom labor is being induced with the aid of oxytocin. She checks the patient's blood pressure and the fetal heart sounds as well as the frequency, strength and duration of uterine contractions. If relatively prolonged uterine contractions occur, the intravenous drip of dilute oxytoxin solution is temporarily cut off and other necessary measures are taken.

- The nurse helps to calm patients with premature labor contractions who are receiving sedatives and opiates to reduce uterine motility. By staying with the patient or observing her frequently, the nurse can add to her sense of security and thus help to relax both the patient and her uterine contractions.

REVIEW QUESTIONS

1. (a) What is meant by the following terms pertaining to the *structure* of the uterus: (1) endometrium; (2) myometrium); (3) cervical os; (4) uterine sinuses?

(b) What is meant by the following terms pertaining to uterine *function:* (1) The three stages of parturition; (2) the puerperium; (3) involution of the uterus?

2. (a) Define the term *oxytocic* and give examples of the two main types.

(b) In which stage of labor are oxytocics of *both* types employed, and when is one *or* the other type preferred?

3. (a) *When* are the ergot derivatives administered in order to check postpartum hemorrhage, and *how* do they act to do so?

(b) What is the most important nursing consideration when oxytocic drugs are to be administered for this purpose?

4. (a) For what other purposes besides control of postpartum hemorrhage are the ergot alkaloids ergonovine and methylergonovine often administered?

(b) For what obstetrical indications for other oxytocic drugs are these ergot derivatives *never* employed?

5. (a) In patients of what types would the use of ergonovine and methylergonovine probably be contraindicated, and in what type patient may the latter derivative be preferred?

(b) What are some of the signs and symptoms of ergot overdosage and what is the main danger in ergot poisoning?

6. (a) Why is oxytocin administered in only small amounts of a highly diluted solution when used for induction of labor?

(b) What are some circumstances in which the use of even such relatively safe doses of oxytocin for inducing labor is considered undesirable (i.e., what criteria must be met before labor can be induced with drugs)?

7. (a) What are some of the nurse's duties during the administration of oxytocin for induction of labor?

(b) Describe three ways in which oxytocin may be given to induce labor and indicate how these differ from the way this drug is administered for control of postpartum hemorrhage.

8. (a) List at least two other clinical uses of natural or synthetic oxytocin and indicate how the hormone acts in each case to bring about the desired effect (e.g., what are its effects on the lactating breast?).

(b) What advantage is claimed for the synthetic oxytocin over the natural extract of the posterior pituitary gland?

9. (a) For what purposes is sparteine sulfate employed?

(b) What are two different kinds of adverse effects which may occur with this drug and what are some precautions that must be taken when it is used in obstetrics?

10. (a) What *non-specific* drugs are sometimes used for relaxing spasms of the uterus?

(b) What may the nurse do to aid the effectiveness of such uterine relaxant drugs?

11. (a) What are two different obstetrical uses of *relaxin?*

(b) What is the main clinical use of the related ovarian hormone *lututrin?*

(c) Name two antispasmodics of different types which are used to relax uterine spasms.

BIBLIOGRAPHY

Boysen, H.: Sparteine sulfate and rupture of the uterus: report of a case. Obstet. Gynecol., *21:*403, 1963.

Cramer, W. C., Reeves, B. D., and Danforth, D. N.: Sparteine sulfate in the conduct of labor. Am. J. Obstet. Gynecol., *89:*268, 1964.

Davis, M. E., Adair, F. L., and Pearl, S.: The present status of oxytocics in obstetrics. J.A.M.A., *107:*261, 1936.

Dillon, T. F., Douglas, R. G., and du Vigneud, V.: Observations on transbuccal administration of Pitocin for induction and stimulation of labor. Obstet. Gynecol., *20:* 434, 1962.

Kobak, A. J.: Intravenous pitocin infusion in obstetrics. Am. J. Obst. Gynec., *71:*1272, 1956.

Moir, J. C.: The history and present day use of ergot. Canad. M. A. J., *72:*727, 1955.

Rodman, M. J.: Drugs for childbirth. R.N., *21:*67, 1958 (March).

———: Drugs for labor and delivery. R.N., *24:*41, 1961 (May).

———: Drugs used in labor and delivery. R.N., *28:*81, 1965 (Sept.).

Schade, F. F., and Gernand, H. C.: Clinical evaluation of methylergonovine (Methergine). Am. J. Obst. Gynec., *71:*37, 1956.

Drugs Used in Allergy, Cough, and Asthma

ALLERGY, HYPERSENSITIVITY AND ANAPHYLAXIS

Allergy is a common cause of chronic and acute illness. Allergic disorders result when a person comes in contact with some substance to which his tissues are especially sensitive. This contact leads to discomforting, disabling, or even fatal reactions. Although no drug can cure allergy, various types of pharmacological agents can counteract the allergic patient's signs and symptoms.

In order to understand how these drugs protect the patient from the effects of an allergic reaction, we must review briefly what is believed to occur in the cells and tissues when an *antigen* and *antibody* react there. An antigen is a substance foreign to the body, which by its presence stimulates the production of specific antibodies that counteract it. In immunity, antibodies that the body has developed as a result of previous exposure to an antigen, react with the antigen to neutralize its toxicity or infectiousness, and thus protect the body from harm.

In allergy, on the other hand, the reaction between the antibodies of the previously sensitized person and the antigen to which his body is once more being exposed is harmful. Such hypersensitivity reactions are generally classified as (1) the *immediate,* or *anaphylactic, type* which develop within seconds or minutes, and (2) the *delayed,* or *tuberculin, type* which may take hours or days to develop. We will emphasize here the immediate antigen-antibody reaction, involving chemical changes that can best be counteracted by the several classes of anti-allergy drugs available at present.

Antigen-antibody reactions in hypersensitive persons result in damage to cells in a way which is still not well understood. The two substances seem to combine in a manner that somehow triggers the release of highly active chemicals from certain cells. These chemical mediators then combine with receptors in the cells of certain other target, or shock, tissues. This, in turn, produces profound changes in the physiological functioning of these tissues. The effects of these functional changes contribute to the development of the different allergic reactions that are seen clinically, including those caused by sensitivity to drugs (Chap. 3).

The *chemical mediators* that are released as the result of an antigen-antibody reaction in the tissues of a sensitized person are: histamine; heparin; serotonin; acetylcholine; a chemical called the slow-reacting substance (SRS); and perhaps others.

HISTAMINE

Histamine, the substance that causes many allergic symptoms in humans, is present in bound form in most tissues, especially in the skin, lungs, and gastrointestinal tract. Actually, much of the histamine in these tissues is contained in and around the blood vessels that run through them. It is present in high concentration (1) in the *mast cells,* which are located just underneath the inner lining of the capillaries, and (2) in the *basophils,* a type of white cell circulating in the blood stream. The part played by the histamine released physiologically in small quantities by such cells under ordinary conditions is still not understood. However, the role of histamine released from these and other cells damaged in an antigen-antibody reaction of the immediate type seems clear. Many, though not all, of the pathological effects of both mild and severe allergic reactions can be traced to the pharmacological effects of suddenly released histamine on the hypersensitive person's blood vessels, bronchial muscles, and exocrine gland cells.

Pharmacological Effects of Histamine

The vascular system is markedly affected by histamine released endogenously or injected from an outside source. These effects are most clearly seen in the skin, which immediately becomes red at the spot of injection or release of histamine. Then a diffuse flush develops around the original area, and, finally, a wheal of edema fluid localizes at the site at which the first red spot appeared. Such hives, or acute urticarial lesions, are marked by intense itching which stems from the action of histamine on sensory nerve endings in the skin.

This reaction, which is not limited to the skin, is the result of the dilating action of histamine on tiny arterioles, venules, and capillaries. The same sort of small arteriole dilation that causes flushing of the face occurs in the cerebral, or cranial, vessels and accounts for the vascular headache that often accompanies generalized allergic reactions. Similarly, the same histamine-induced increase in capillary permeability that accounts for the outward flow of fluid into the subcutaneous spaces is the cause of the laryngeal edema that can lead to asphyxia in a severe anaphylactic reaction. It is also the cause of nasal congestion in allergic rhinitis.

Also, in acute anaphylactic reactions, released histamine may cause the blood pressure to fall rapidly to shock levels. Blood trapped in the dilated terminal arterioles adds to the pressure that forces protein-containing fluids into the extravascular spaces. The loss of plasma proteins from the circulation, together with the reduced resistance of the arterioles, results in a steady fall in blood pressure. If blood continues to pool in the peripheral vessels, the venous return to the heart is reduced. This leads in turn to decreased cardiac output, despite reflex responses which increase the rate and contractile strength of the myocardium. The resulting reduction in blood flow to the brain can cause loss of consciousness and failure of nervous control over respiration and other vital functions.

Smooth muscles, other than those of the small arterioles, are contracted by contact with released histamine. This is most significant in the bronchioles, which are constricted, with a resulting reduction in vital capacity. This action of histamine is thought to account in large part for the breathing difficulties of the patient with bronchial asthma. However, other substances released simultaneously during an antigen-antibody reaction may also account for the respiratory embarrassment. For example, the slow-reacting substance (SRS) is also said to exert a potent constricting action on the bronchioles.

Exocrine glands of the gastrointestinal and respiratory systems, and others (the lacrimal glands, for example), are stimulated by histamine. The stomach cells that secrete hydrochloric acid are most powerfully activated. This action, together with the contractile effects of histamine on smooth muscle of the gastrointestinal tract, probably plays a part in producing the epigastric distress, nausea and vomiting, and diarrhea that are often the first warning of an oncoming anaphylactic reaction. The sensitivity of the gastric glands to injected histamine is the basis for a commonly employed test of stomach secretory function (see Drug Digests for histamine phosphate and for betazole). The increased secretion by the lacrimal glands seen in hay fever patients and at least part of the increase in bronchial secretion in asthmatics probably stem from the stimulating action of histamine on exocrine gland cells.

Histamine Antagonists

The histamine theory of allergic reactions has stimulated a search for drugs that can antagonize this chemical and its effects. In theory, there are many ways of doing this.

The most specific allergy treatment is *desensitization,* a procedure intended to prevent tissue-damaging antigen-antibody reactions and thus keep histamine and other chemical mediators from being released in the first place. In this non-pharmacological approach, the allergist tries to build up the patient's immunity to a troublesome allergen by injecting dilute extracts of it, until the allergen finally fails to elicit adverse reactions. Other treatments have been based on attempts to increase the rate of histamine detoxication by the enzyme histaminase.

Various drugs have been employed to counteract the effects of released histamine. Adrenergic drugs, such as epinephrine and other sympathomimetic agents, act by producing pharmacological effects that directly oppose those of histamine. As indicated in Chapter 16 and later in this chapter, these drugs have vascular and bronchial effects exactly opposite to those of histamine. By constricting the arterioles and dilating the bronchioles, epinephrine-type drugs counteract the actions of histamine responsible for many allergic signs and symptoms.

Other classes of drugs with anti-allergy effects include the corticosteroids (Chap. 28), which somehow dampen the responsiveness of the patient's tissues to released histamine, and the expectorant drugs that counteract certain allergic symptoms.

THE ANTIHISTAMINE DRUGS

Manner of Action. The so-called antihistamine agents do not act in any of the ways mentioned above. That is, they do not prevent histamine from being liberated as does successful desensitization therapy; they do not speed the breakdown of the released histamine as histaminase therapy might, if it were feasible; nor do these drugs exert pharmacological effects that reverse those of histamine, as do epinephrine, ephedrine, and other drugs.

These histamine-antagonizing agents compete with the natural amine for certain reactive sites, or receptors, in the cells of the target tissues. That is, the molecules of these drugs, which resemble those of histamine in certain respects, occupy the receptors to which the released histamine molecule must attach itself in order to elicit its effects on vascular and other smooth muscles, and on exocrine glands. Although the antihistamine drug molecules themselves have no effect on these structures, their presence on the histaminergic receptors prevents histamine from producing many of the signs and symptoms of allergic disorders.

Other Pharmacological Effects. The antihistamine drugs not only block the effects of histamine, but can elicit various pharmacological effects of their own on peripheral tissues and on the central nervous system. Some of these secondary effects of the various chemical classes of antihistamine drugs may be useful in the total management of allergic patients; others are a source of undesired side effects that limit the usefulness of these drugs for some patients (see p. 558).

Certain central effects of the antihistamine drugs are more important clinically than their histamine-blocking action. Thus, these drugs are used for purposes other than allergy treatment. Some, such as dimenhydrinate, are employed mainly to manage motion sickness and other conditions marked by nausea, vertigo, and vomiting (Chap. 38). Others, including orphenadrine as well as its relative diphenhydramine (see Drug Digest), are used for treating patients with parkinsonism (Chap. 8). The sedative-hypnotic actions of some of these drugs have led to their being advocated as substitutes for the barbiturates in the management of anxiety and insomnia (Chap. 6). In fact, the first drugs introduced as major tranquilizers (Chap. 7) were originally discovered and developed in the search for new antihistaminic agents for treating allergy.

None of these central effects of the antihistamines has anything to do with their ability to block the effects of histamine in peripheral vascular tissues, nor with the local anesthetic actions that some of these compounds exert on peripheral sensory nerve fibers. There may possibly be a relationship, however, between the atropine-like, or acetylcholine-blocking, effects of some of these drugs on smooth muscle and a similar central anticholinergic activity.

Allergy Treatment

The antihistamine drugs are used to relieve the symptoms of various allergic disorders. In such conditions, these drugs are more effective against some types of symptoms than others. Reactions resulting from the effects of histamine upon capillaries and arterioles are best blocked by antihistamine drug treatment. Thus, such allergic symptoms as itchy skin wheals and edematous congestion of the nasal mucosa are often well controlled by low, safe doses of antihistamines, such as chlorpheniramine (see Drug Digest) and other drugs listed in Table 40-1.

On the other hand, these drugs have little or no ability to antagonize histamine-induced gastric gland secretion of acid. They are also relatively ineffective for relief of the dyspnea of acute asthma, and may make breathing more difficult by drying the mucous secretions within the bronchial tubes, thus hampering productive coughing. Scientists do not know exactly why histamine antagonists are ineffective in human asthma, for these drugs can protect guinea pigs from the effects of *inhaled* histamine in one commonly employed test for finding drugs with histamine-antagonizing ability.

One explanation of this is that the histamine released in the lungs during an asthmatic antigen-antibody reaction attaches itself immediately to the smooth muscle cell receptors of the bronchioles. The molecules of antihistamine drugs cannot then compete successfully with the histamine that is released in high concentrations in such close contact with the bronchial muscles. However, another view holds that in asthma bronchoconstriction is brought about, not by histamine, but by some other mediator, such as the slow-reacting substance (SRS), which is not readily antagonized by histamine-blocking drugs.

Allergic dermatoses are variably responsive to treatment with antihistamine drugs. *Acute urticaria* is the condition best controlled by these drugs, which block histamine and other substances released from mast cells in the vessels of the skin. This keeps protein-containing fluid from leaking into the dermis to form itchy wheals. Of course, in a severe anaphylactic reaction that also causes giant urticaria, or angioneurotic edema of the mucous membranes of the lips, mouth, and larynx, epinephrine is the preferred emergency measure. Injected parenterally, it counteracts the swellings of the larynx which might cause fatal choking before an antihistamine drug could take effect. However, the parenteral administration of antihistamines is also desirable, after epinephrine has had its life-saving effect, for antagonizing tissue histamine.

Chronic urticaria is more complicated and more difficult to treat than acute urticaria, requiring many medical measures. Even here, however, the antihistamines help relieve itching in about half the patients, while the doctor is seeking the cause of the continuing condition. Antihistaminic drugs that are relatively strong sedatives, such as diphenhydramine (see Drug Digest), are often preferred for bedtime administration, in order to help the patient to get a night's rest. The tranquilizing action of certain other antihistamines is also considered desirable for patients suffering from the pruritus of atopic dermatitis (see Chap. 43).

Certain antihistamines, such as tripelennamine (see Drug Digest), exert a local anesthetic effect on sensory nerve endings when applied topically to the abraded skin or to the mucous membranes of patients with contact dermatitis and in other forms of pruritus that may not necessarily be allergic in origin. However, the local application of antihistamine drugs may actually prove sensitizing to the skin of atopic individuals. Thus, the use, in eczematous dermatoses, of creams and ointments containing antihistamines is best limited to short periods, lest the drugs themselves cause contact dermatitis and other allergic reactions. In such cases topically applied corticosteroids are preferred to antihistamines for relief of the pruritus.

The dermal aspects of serum sickness and blood transfusion reactions are sometimes controlled by administration of antihistamines. These drugs are occasionally employed prophylactically prior to the administration of penicillin, fibrinolysin, and other drugs known to cause urticarial and febrile reactions, especially in patients with a history of allergy. However, the prior or simultaneous administration of an antihistaminic agent is not a dependable means of preventing anaphylactic reactions to drugs such as penicillin. Similarly, antihistamine prophylaxis does not prevent reactions resulting from transfusion of incompatible blood, or fever-producing (pyrogenic) reactions to sera, enzymes, and other substances containing, or derived from, animal protein. Even in the urticarial-type reactions, antihistamines may only postpone rather than prevent the discomfort.

Upper respiratory tract allergies, such as those caused by contact with pollen, are often treated effectively with antihistamine drugs. By blocking the actions of the histamine that is released by the antigen-antibody reaction, these drugs protect the nasal arterioles, capillaries, and glands from its effects. This keeps the nasal mucosa from becoming congested with the blood in dilated arterioles and boggy with edema fluid leaking from the capillaries. Such symptoms as sneezing, running nose and eyes, and itching of the nasal and ocular mucosa are relieved.

Antihistamine therapy of pollinosis, or seasonal hay fever, is most effective in the early edematous stage of the condition. The antihistamines are less likely to prove useful for patients with perennial vasomotor rhinitis caused by ingested, rather than inhaled, allergens. Similarly, hay fever symptoms are more readily controlled early in the season when the inhaled air contains heavy concentrations of the allergen.

Antihistamine drugs are, of course, often combined with adrenergic decongestant drugs in nose drops, sprays, and tablets sold without prescription for the symptomatic relief of the common cold. In theory, the antihistamines are supposed to protect the nasal tissue from histamine liberated by the viruses responsible for colds. In practice, for reducing rhinorrhea the atropine-like drying action of some of these drugs on nasal gland secretions may be more helpful than their histamine-blocking action. In any case, these drugs do not "cure" a cold, as was originally claimed.

Rhinitis treatment with combinations of antihistamines, anticholinergic drying agents, and adrenergic vasoconstrictor-decongestant agents (Chap. 16) offers desirable symptomatic relief. Such drug mixtures are applied topically or orally for systemic effects. Topical application is preferred for controlling acute nasal and sinus symptoms, but the systemically acting products may have advantages for maintenance therapy. Whereas the orally administered drugs take longer to exert their effects, they can reach parts of the nasal and sinus mucosa that are not readily accessible to topical therapy. Carried to these sites by way of the blood stream, the antihistamines block the effects of released histamine on the mucosal capillaries, and the adrenergic drugs constrict the dilated arterioles in the same congested area. As a result, the patient may get relatively longer relief and better aeration and drainage than when nose drops are employed. In addition, such reactions to overuse of topical therapy as secondary, or rebound, congestion, decreased ciliary motility, and increased mucus secretion are claimed less likely to occur with the orally administered products.

Some authorities suggest that systemic side effects are more likely to occur with the dosage forms that are taken by mouth. Yet improperly administered topical products that trickle down the throat are as likely to produce systemic effects after being absorbed. (To avoid this, keep the patient's head down below the side of the bed when applying nose drops.) The combined central side effects of simultaneously administered antihistamine and adrenergic drugs may tend to cancel each other out. That is, when these agents are taken together for their desired effects on the nasal mucosa, the slight central depressant action of some of the antihistamines may counteract the restlessness and insomnia that may be induced by the central stimulating action of certain adrenergic decongestants. Similarly, the alerting effects of the latter drugs may help to counteract the antihistamine-type side effects.

Side Effects and Precautions. The most common side effect of antihistamine drugs is their tendency to cause drowsiness. This action is more marked with some chemical classes of antihistamines than with others. However, sedation can occur in some patients with almost any of these drugs. Thus, the nurse should advise the patient not to drive if he becomes sleepy when he begins to take a new allergy medication, nor to engage in other activities that require alertness and motor coordination.

Tell the patient to inform the doctor if he experiences sleepiness or ataxia, rather than simply stop taking the medication as some do. The doctor can order another antihistamine that may prove less likely to cause drowsiness in that particular patient.

Patients are often told not to drink alcoholic beverages or take barbiturates during the early days of treatment with antihistamines, for synergistic depressant effects are believed to have contributed to motor vehicle accidents and other mishaps. The doctor may, instead, prescribe the antihistamine drug in combination with a mild psychomotor stimulant such as caffeine, methylphenidate, or an amphetamine (Chap. 13).

Toxicity. Children who accidentally ingest large amounts of antihistamine drugs in the form of a pleasantly flavored cough syrup or cold capsules may suffer acute poisoning. In such cases, early sedation may be followed by restlessness, increasing irritability, and muscular twitching. Occasionally, convulsive seizures may develop, and, finally, coma, cardiovascular collapse, and respiratory failure may occur.

Treatment of poisoning by antihistamine products is difficult on account of this odd mixture of central depressant and stimulating features. It may be further complicated by the presence of salicylates and adrenergic drugs in the "cold" capsule. Prevention is, of course, the best approach to the problem. The nurse can make parents aware that these seemingly safe products, so widely advertised on television and elsewhere, contain potentially dangerous drugs and should be stored where young children could not get at them.

If convulsions occur during the management of a case of antihistamine overdosage, an anticonvulsant barbiturate of the quick and short-acting type such as thiopental, may be carefully administered in amounts just sufficient to control muscle spasms. Overdosage of this antidote may synergize the underlying depressant effect of the antihistamine, thus causing coma and respiratory failure.

The use of a mechanical respirator may be required for ventilating the patient, if his breathing becomes too slow and shallow. The use of analeptic drugs to stimulate respiration in such situations is considered undesirable, for these C.N.S. stimulants may precipitate convulsive activity in an unconscious victim of antihistamine drug overdosage.

THE USE OF DRUGS IN THE MANAGEMENT OF COUGHING

The Nature and Significance of Coughing

A cough is a reflex mechanism that helps to protect the respiratory tract from foreign particles and retained secretions. Ordinarily a stream of mucus covering the respiratory tract membranes traps dust particles and bacteria and moves them up toward the throat along with the debris of cellular breakdown. Sometimes, however, some of this mucus may tend to collect in the tracheobronchial tree and obstruct the air passages, especially if it becomes infected. A productive cough prevents this by driving the debris-laden mucus up toward the pharynx from which it can then be expectorated or removed by swallowing.

TABLE 40-1

OFFICIAL ANTIHISTAMINE DRUGS *

Nonproprietary or Official Name	Synonym or Proprietary Name	Dosage
Antazoline phosphate N.F.	Antistine	100 mg.
Carbinoxamine maleate N.F.	Clistin	4 mg.
Chlorcyclizine HCl U.S.P.	Di-Paralene; Perazil	50 mg.
Chlorothen citrate N.F.	Tagathen	25 mg.
Chlorpheniramine maleate U.S.P.	Chlor-Trimeton; Teldrin	4 mg.
Diphenhydramine HCl U.S.P.	Benadryl	oral 25 mg. parenteral 50 mg.
Doxylamine succinate N.F.	Decapryn	25 mg.
Methapyrilene HCl N.F.	Histadyl, Semikon, etc.	50 mg.
Promethazine HCl U.S.P.	Phenergan	oral 25 mg. parenteral 50 mg.
Pyrilamine maleate N.F.	Neo-Antergan, etc.	25 mg.
Thenyldiamine HCl N.F.	Thenfadil	15 mg.
Thonzylamine HCl N.F.	Anahist; Neohetramine	50 mg.
Tripelennamine citrate U.S.P.	Pyribenzamine citrate	oral 50 mg.
Tripelennamine HCl U.S.P.	Pyribenzamine HCl	oral 50 mg. parenteral 25 mg.

* Others are listed in Chapter 38 as motion sickness remedies and antiemetics.

The cough reflex is normally set off by the stimulus of mucus accumulating at sensitive sites in the bronchi, trachea, or pharynx. Nerve impulses travel from these peripheral receptors by way of afferent fibers of the vagus and glossopharyngeal nerves to the so-called "cough center" in the medulla oblongata. Certain nerve cells in this brain stem area respond by sending out motor messages by way of efferent fibers. These impulses then cause contractions of the diaphragm and of the muscles in the chest and abdominal wall. At the same time, the vocal cords and epiglottis close shut over the top of the respiratory tree. When they snap open again an instant later the air that had been confined and compressed within the passages is hurled forth at close to hurricane wind velocity. This helps to eject the mucous mass that had precipitated the reflex by irritating the sensitive receptors.

Although coughing is a protective mechanism, the use of *antitussive*—or cough-combating—agents is indicated when the patient is plagued by *excessive coughing* of a *non*-productive nature. This can, at the very least, cause discomfort and interfere with rest and sleep. At its worst, persistent coughing causes permanent damage to delicate respiratory tract structures. In *chronic bronchitis,* for example, coughing that fails to move thick mucopurulent plaques may weaken the walls of the bronchioles. Pockets of infection may then form in the dilated bronchial tubes (*bronchiectasis*), and this sets off still more useless coughing as the patient tries to dislodge the infected mucus.

With continued unproductive coughing, the walls of the alveoli, where the actual exchanges of oxygen and carbon dioxide take place, may thicken, lose their elasticity, and become torn. Air then becomes trapped in these enlarged spaces, and the patient suffering from such *emphysema* cannot adequately empty his lungs of accumulated carbon dioxide or breathe in enough oxygen to satisfy the needs of his tissues.

Indications for Drug Treatment

Drugs of various kinds are available for the symptomatic management of coughing. However, before the doctor orders any cough medication, he must first find out what is causing the cough. Some coughs may not require treatment, whereas others are so serious that they require much more than a mere cough-relieving medication.

A cough resulting from fluid dripping into the throat from nasal passages irritated by a common cold virus usually clears up spontaneously as the upper respiratory symptoms subside. On the other hand, the cause of a persistent cough may be the pressure of a growth —in bronchial carcinoma, for example—that requires surgical excision rather than antitussive therapy. A cough that stems from lung congestion—as in heart failure or pneumonia—needs, not cough-suppressing palliative drugs, but treatment with such life-saving agents as digitalis, diuretics, or antibiotics.

For some coughs, such as those resulting from a nasal virus infection, the patient needs no more than a candy cough drop for relief during the few days of postnasal drip before the cold clears up or is controlled by nasal medication. Coughs caused by stimuli arising from a dry, irritated mucous surface are best controlled by a centrally acting cough suppressant such as codeine. Such an antitussive agent raises the threshold of the cough center, so that fewer afferent impulses break through to trigger volleys of unproductive coughs that further irritate an already inflamed surface.

Patients with chronic obstructive diseases of the respiratory tract, such as bronchial asthma, usually require a mucus-liquefying expectorant drug, which makes it easier to cough up material blocking the air passages. A mild, centrally acting antitussive may be added to reduce the number of cough volleys. The coughs that then occur are fewer but stronger and more effective in bringing material up from deep within the chest.

TYPES OF COUGH MEDICATIONS

Coughs have been treated traditionally with complex mixtures of many drugs. Such "shotgun" prescriptions, which spray medical buckshot with the hope that one of the many ingredients may hit the mark, have no place in modern therapeutics. Yet, even today, many commercially available cough mixtures contain as many as a half dozen drugs, most of which are worthless. Most coughs can be treated adequately by a combination of no more than two types of agents which may or may not be aided in their action by being offered in the form of a syrupy liquid.

All known cough medications act essentially in one of two major ways: They may act *centrally* to reduce the sensitivity of the medullary cough center to sensory impulses arriving from respiratory tract receptors by way of afferent nerve fibers. They may act *peripherally* to reduce the number of afferent nerve impulses that pass up to the cough coordinating center. Drugs do this in any of several ways. Some may lessen local irritation and thus reduce the rate at which receptors in the respiratory tract mucosa are stimulated. Others may depress the receptors so that they become less responsive to irritating stimuli. Most commonly, many peripherally acting drugs bring about changes in the viscosity of the mucus and thus make it easier to remove this source of irritation. Some substances act by a combination of central and peripheral actions.

Centrally Acting Antitussives

Almost any drug that depresses the central nervous system can reduce coughing or the discomfort that it causes. However, these central depressants are not all equally useful. Whereas sedative-hypnotics such as the barbiturates may, for example, help a person sleep better by lessening his coughing, the drowsiness that these drugs tend to produce makes them undesirable for daytime use. Similarly, although such potent pain-relievers as morphine, methadone, and hydromorphone can effectively control coughing by depressing the cough center, these analgesic-antitussives sometimes cause a degree of respiratory depression that makes their use in many patients dangerous. Thus, medical scientists have been seeking cough suppressants that act specifically on the cough center with minimal actions at other central and peripheral sites and preferably without any abuse potential. We shall compare, here, three types of presently available cough center depressants.

Analgesic-Antitussives. These potent drugs, such as the opium alkaloid *morphine* and its derivatives *hydromorphone* and *heroin,* are *not* commonly employed to control coughing. This is because these drugs or certain synthetic agents with similar properties, such as *methadone* and *phenazocine,* are *too* effective and thus reduce the capacity to cough to such an extent that secretions are not cleared adequately from the lower respiratory tract. The accumulating secretions may then keep the lungs from expanding properly or may cause them to collapse at some points (*atalectasis*). This is one of the reasons why the nurse often has to make special efforts to induce coughing in postoperative patients who have received such potent analgesics.

These drugs have a variety of effects that account for their being *contraindicated* in such chronic obstructive diseases of the pulmonary passages as bronchial asthma, bronchiectasis, and emphysema. For one thing, these potent antitussives tend to interfere with ventilation of the lungs by depressing the respiratory center almost as readily as they do the cough center.

In addition to this and to their capacity to keep the patient from coughing productively by excessively depressing the cough reflex, morphine and its relatives may have various adverse effects on other parts of the natural protective mechanism of the respiratory tract. For example, they may slow the activity of the cilia—hair-like processes that keep the mucous covering moving up toward the pharynx. The mucous stream may then stop flowing and become dried out, and thus permit microorganisms to penetrate into the underlying tissues. At the same time, the bronchial smooth muscle, which ordinarily contracts in a series of upward-sweeping peristaltic movements, may be sent into spasm by these drugs. The end result of all these adverse actions may be formation of hard mucous plugs in the constricted bronchiolar tubes and increased difficulty in breathing.

For these and other reasons, including their poten-

tial for causing addiction, these potent but dangerous antitussives are employed for cough control in only a limited number of special clinical situations. For example, they are best suited for use in conditions marked by *both* cough and pain, such as fractures of ribs, pleurisy, and lung cancer. Similarly, in situations requiring relief from anxiety as well as reduction of pain and coughing, morphine, methadone, and similar drugs are sometimes ordered. For example, cough caused by pulmonary congestion following an acute coronary attack may be controlled by low, carefully adjusted doses of morphine, which at the same time acts to relieve pain and apprehension. Some doctors also order morphine-type antitussives for patients in respiratory distress following a pulmonary embolism. In all such cases, care is required to keep these drugs from further reducing ventilation of the lungs by depression of the respiratory center.

Codeine and Hydrocodone. These are considered the most generally useful analgesic-antitussives available. Although these drugs are related to morphine and hydromorphone and are less effective antitussives than those more potent agents, they are relatively free of the main drawbacks of the latter. Codeine does not, for example, usually depress the respiratory center significantly, nor is it likely to suppress the cough reflex completely. Thus, while codeine reduces the reactivity of the cough center to some of the incoming afferent impulses, enough sensory stimuli still break through to permit productive coughing (see Drug Digest).

In practice, this means that drugs such as codeine and hydrocodone may be especially useful in coughs caused by irritation of an inflamed respiratory mucous membrane. In such cases, coughing is described as "dry" or "unproductive" and further inflames and irritates the respiratory mucosa. Thus, these drugs, which reduce the responsiveness of the cough center to streams of sensory impulses from the irritated receptors, help to cut down considerably the volleys of useless, annoying coughs.

The *adverse effects* of codeine are *not* a drawback to its use as a palliative for brief periods, despite the implications of television advertising for non-codeine cough medications. Such commercials commonly imply that persons who use a codeine-based product for cough control are well on their way toward drug addiction. Actually, codeine does not have a high capacity for producing dependence. While prolonged abuse of products containing such substances as codeine and hydrocodone may occasionally be the prelude to the misuse of such powerfully addicting drugs as morphine and heroin, this road to narcotic addiction is rarely taken by potential addicts.

Codeine may, however, cause some undesirable effects in patients who are especially sensitive to it. Some people, for example, suffer *gastrointestinal* upset manifested by nausea, vomiting, and constipation. Adverse *central* effects include dizziness, headache, and drowsiness. Massive overdoses may cause respiratory depression, but this does not ordinarily become severe, apparently because high doses of codeine tend to stimulate the central nervous system. Nevertheless, all cough medications containing codeine should be kept out of the reach of children, as high overdoses of this drug can cause delirium, muscular tremors and convulsions as well as coma. Most cough medications are attractive to children because of their flavoring and sweetness. Thus the nurse should suggest to parents that they take special care in the handling and storage of *any* antitussive product.

Non-narcotic Antitussives. These drugs, which constitute the third type of centrally acting cough suppressants, are said to depress the central cough control mechanism in doses that do not affect other parts of the brain. Thus these relatively selective cough suppressants do not produce the euphoria or pain relief that often occurs with the opiate and opioid antitussives, and so they are unlikely to be abused by addiction-prone persons. These non-narcotic cough suppressants are claimed not to cause the drowsiness and constipation or other central and peripheral effects sometimes seen in patients taking the opiate type antitussives.

Dextromethorphan (see Drug Digest) is by far the most widely employed antitussive of this type. It is available under a variety of trade names in many widely advertised cough medications. The drug seems both safe enough to warrant its availability in non-prescription products and effective enough to reduce the mild coughs due to colds for which it is advocated. However, it is not as effective in controlling the more severe chronic coughing of patients with respiratory tract disorders.

Most of the other available cough center suppressants are also claimed to possess peripheral actions which add to their effectiveness for cough control. Some such as *carbetapentane* and *caramiphen* (Table 40-2) are said to exert a desirable bronchial antispasmodic action. Others, including *chlophedianol* and *pipazethate,* exert topical anesthetic effects. However, the practical usefulness of such peripheral actions has not been properly evaluated.

One agent, *benzonatate,* is thought to act not only by depressing the cough center but by an interesting peripheral effect. When absorbed into the systemic circulation, this chemical relative of the local anesthetic tetracaine is thought to deaden the sensitivity of stretch receptors in the lungs. This is said to help relieve the sensation of tightness in the chest often felt by asthmatic coughers. However, the drug's action is not strong enough to make it useful when given by mouth prior to such procedures as bronchoscopy and laryngoscopy. In such cases, it is still customary to spray or instill topical anesthetic solutions to suppress the cough reflex and prevent gagging and bucking.

Peripherally Acting Antitussives

Many soothing substances act in the throat or deeper in the respiratory tract to counteract local irritation. For example, candy cough drops can be helpful in reducing coughs resulting from pharyngeal irritation. The sugary, spicy confection tends to stimulate a flow of saliva, which acts as a natural demulcent to protect the dry or inflamed membranes. Then, too, the person sucking on a cough lozenge is keeping his mouth shut, thus preventing further drying of the membrane through the evaporation of moisture. The addition of a topical anesthetic such as *benzocaine* or other medications adds little to the effectiveness of such lozenges.

Cough syrups containing such flavorful substances as wild cherry and licorice are of limited effectiveness. Little of their local demulcent-protective action in the throat persists, once these sugary solutions are swallowed, and they do not, of course, reach the parts of the respiratory tract below the epiglottis. Thus, such syrups are used mainly as pleasantly flavored vehicles for other peripherally acting drugs, such as the expectorants.

The expectorants—the term means, literally, "out of the chest"—make coughing more productive by stimulating the secretion of the natural lubricant fluid of the lower respiratory tract (RTF). This flow of natural secretions also helps to liquefy any thick mucous masses that may plug the narrow bronchioles. By decreasing the viscosity of such mucous plugs, the drug-induced secretion of RTF aids in removing mucus from the chest. Administration of a drug such as potassium iodide (see Drug Digest) makes it easier for patients with bronchial asthma to cough up the dry, hardened mucus blocking the bronchial tubes. In addition, the reduced tenacity of respiratory tract secretions increases the efficiency of the ciliated mucous blanket and the bronchiolar muscle peristaltic activity that also act to move thickened secretions toward the pharynx from the depths of the respiratory tract.

The expectorants do not enter the respiratory tract immediately upon being swallowed. Instead, they act by one or both of two main mechanisms to stimulate the flow of RTF: (1) Some substances, such as syrup of ipecac (administered in subemetic doses) and ammonium chloride, or other strongly saline substances, irritate the stomach lining. This sets off the same sort of reflex activity that occurs during nausea. That is, nerve impulses pass to the medullary area to stimulate the reflex secretion of bronchial fluids and saliva. (2) Other agents are thought to act after being absorbed into the blood stream. Substances such as glyceryl

TABLE 40-2
DRUGS USED IN THE MANAGEMENT OF COUGHING

Nonproprietary or Official Name	Proprietary Name or Synonym	Usual Adult Antitussive Dosage
Centrally Acting Antitussives		
Narcotic Antitussive-Analgesics		
Codeine N.F.	Methylmorphine	15–30 mg.
Codeine phosphate U.S.P.	Methylmorphine phosphate	15–30 mg.
Codeine sulfate N.F.	Methylmorphine sulfate	15–30 mg.
Dihydrocodeine bitartrate	Drocode; Rapacodin; Paracodin	10–20 mg.
Hydrocodone bitartrate N.F.	Dihydrocodeinone; in Hycodan, etc.	5–10 mg.
Hydromorphone N.F.	Dihydromorphinone; Dilaudid	2 mg.
Levorphanol tartrate N.F.	Levo-Dromoran	2 mg.
Meperidine HCl N.F.	Demerol	50 mg.
Methadone HCl U.S.P.	Adanon; Amidon; Dolophine	1.5–2 mg.
Morphine sulfate U.S.P.	—	2–3 mg.
Purified opium alkaloids	Omnopon; Pantopon	2–3 mg.
Non-narcotic Antitussives		
Benzonatate	Tessalon	100 mg.
Caramiphen ethanedisulfonate	Toryn	10–20 mg.
Carbetapentane citrate N.F.	Toclase	15–30 mg.
Chlophedianol HCl	Ulo	25 mg.
Dextromethorphan HBr N.F.	Romilar, etc.	10–20 mg.
Dihyprylone	Piperidione; Sedulon	60–120 mg.
Dimethoxanate HCl	Cothera	25–50 mg.
Levopropoxyphene napsylate	Novrad	50–100 mg.
Noscapine U.S.P.	Narcotine; Nectadon	15–30 mg.
Noscapine HCl N.F.	Narcotine; Nectadon	15–30 mg.
Pipazethate	Theratuss	20–40 mg.
Locally Acting Antitussives		
Expectorants, Demulcents, and Vehicles		
Acacia Syrup		
Ammonium chloride U.S.P.		300 mg.–1 Gm.
Calcium iodide	in Calcidrine Syrup	150 mg.
Glycyrrhiza Syrup	Licorice Syrup	
Honey N.F.		
Hydriodic Acid Syrup N.F.		5 ml.
Glyceryl guaiacolate	in Robitussin, Quibron, etc.	100 mg.
Ipecac Syrup U.S.P.	in Ipsatol, etc.	5 ml.
Potassium guaiacolsulfonate N.F.		500 mg.
Potassium iodide U.S.P.		300 mg.
Sodium iodide U.S.P.		100 mg.
Terpin hydrate N.F.		85 mg.
Tolu Balsam Syrup N.F.		
White Pine Syrup		
Wild Cherry Syrup U.S.P.		

guaiacolate and potassium guaiacolsulfonate are then excreted into the sputum by the bronchial glands. In the process of being eliminated by this route, they are thought to stimulate secretion of RTF by the mucosal glandular cells. Some expectorants such as potassium iodide, which also appears in the sputum after being swallowed, are thought to act by a combination of both mechanisms.

Other agents for liquefying mucus are discussed in the following section of this chapter.

DRUG THERAPY IN THE MANAGEMENT OF BRONCHIAL ASTHMA

Bronchial asthma is a chronic respiratory disorder marked by recurrent attacks of dyspnea. About half the cases occur in persons known to be allergic to material that they inhale or ingest. Other patients can not be readily proved sensitive to specific allergens such as house dusts, pollens, food, or drugs. In such cases, respiratory tract infections often play an important part in triggering such asthmatic symptoms as wheezing and dyspnea.

Several classes of drugs are employed for the symptomatic relief of asthma. These include the adrenergic bronchodilator and vasoconstrictor drugs (Chap. 16); the adrenocorticosteroid drugs (Chap. 28); certain sedatives, tranquilizers, and antibiotics (Chaps. 6, 7, and 34); and the expectorants taken up in the preceding section of this chapter.

In this section we shall discuss in some detail the manner in which these and certain other drugs are employed in the management of asthmatic patients. Because this depends upon the severity of the symptoms, we shall describe two different situations: first, the emergency care of severely ill patients hospitalized with status asthmaticus, the most severe form of the disorder; second, the drug therapy of milder chronic cases that are marked by only occasional acute asthmatic attacks.

Status Asthmaticus

An asthmatic patient who arrives at the hospital after suffering repeated severe attacks is as acutely ill as his appearance indicates. His pale face often mirrors his fright, as he struggles to draw air through bronchial tubes narrowed by smooth muscle spasm and clogged with thick, tenacious secretions. Relief of the patient's distress requires prompt medical action and intelligent nursing care.

Among the *general measures* routinely employed are the following: (1) Protect the patient from exposure to the allergens that may have set off his attacks in the first place and that may continue to perpetuate them. (2) Overcome his dehydration and the malnutrition which may have developed during the previous days of increasingly severe and unremitting attacks. (3) Relieve the fear that typically accompanies severe attacks, not only to lessen emotional strain and provide rest, but to prevent the anxiety and apprehension that make the patient's condition worse and tend to set off new attacks.

Sedative and tranquilizing drugs are often ordered to calm the agitated asthmatic patient. These include such older *sedatives* as phenobarbital and chloral hydrate and the newer minor *tranquilizers* chlordiazepoxide (Librium) and meprobamate (Equanil; Miltown). More potent depressants such as morphine and meperidine (Demerol) are generally avoided, because they tend to reduce the rate and depth of the already inadequate respiration.

Continued use of these drugs in this chronic condition could result in dependence upon them. If the physician's orders give some choice in the matter, administer sedatives only when essential for securing the mental and physical rest that the patient requires. Never employ depressant drugs merely to quiet the querulous complaints of a difficult patient.

Sympathetic and skillful nursing care is often more effective than drugs for reducing anxiety. Among the nursing measures that help to lessen apprehension are simply staying with the patient and listening to his personal concerns. If the nurse cannot stay with the patient, she should provide him with a way to signal, and answer his calls promptly. Even if he does not call, she should look in on him often to note his condition and his response to drug therapy.

When administering medication, the nurse can often add to a drug's effectiveness by expressing confidence that it will shortly relieve the symptoms. When the nurse conveys to the patient the feeling that she is not frightened by his condition, the patient feels more secure.

The nurse should cultivate an awareness of her own reactions to the patient's condition, because if severe dyspnea makes her fearful, she can readily intensify the patient's nervousness. Nothing should be said within the patient's hearing to indicate that his attack is unusually severe or that his condition is a cause for concern, for this would alarm him and thus deprive him of the rest and relaxation that the drugs are intended to give him. The nurse's actions and words should indicate that his condition does not unduly alarm the persons who are now assuming responsibility for his care. He should be made to feel that they understand his illness and know how to help him.

Liquefying the patient's sputum is perhaps the most important measure in the emergency treatment of the severely ill asthmatic patient, for respiratory distress stems mainly from obstruction of the terminal bronchial tubes by plugs of hardened mucus. Presumably these plugs in status asthmaticus prevent the patient from responding to injections of epinephrine or to the administration of ephedrine and the other adrenergic bronchodilator drugs that would ordinarily relieve his distress.

Thus, before treating the bronchospasm itself, the doctor usually orders medication that thins the tenacious bronchial secretions so that the patient can clear his lungs by coughing productively. The first step for loosening such secretions is to administer intravenous fluids to make up for those probably lost in the days prior to hospitalization. When the patient can drink again, oral fluids may be forced; and the nurse must see to it that he drinks the dozen or so glasses of water that he needs each day.

Once the patient has been rehydrated, *expectorant drugs* are administered to stimulate the secretion of respiratory tract fluids. Inorganic iodide salts have been traditionally employed for this purpose, and they do indeed seem effective for liquefying hardened mucous casts, provided that the patient's body fluids have first been fully restored and that he continues to receive fruit juices or milk with each dose. This measure also helps to disguise the saline taste and lessens gastric irritation caused by iodides and large doses of most other expectorants, including ammonium chloride and ipecac.

Potassium iodide (see Drug Digest) is still the most popular drug of this class, despite the introduction of organic iodide compounds that are claimed to be less irritating to the stomach. All the iodides are, however, undesirable for patients who are sensitive to them. Such sensitivity may become manifest as an acnelike skin eruption, which may spread from the sebaceous areas and become a generalized, potentially fatal furunculosis. Thus expectorants containing potassium, sodium, or calcium iodide or iodinated glycerol should be withdrawn if a skin eruption appears shortly after treatment is started. A mumps-like, painful swelling of the parotid gland also sometimes develops early in treatment, but it is less likely to occur if the patient has been receiving plenty of fluids.

Other measures must be employed for loosening bronchial secretions in patients who have an idiosyncracy to iodides, thyroid disease, or tuberculosis, and in those who develop signs of iodism during long-term iodide therapy. Substitution of expectorants such as ammonium chloride or glyceryl guaiacolate may be helpful for milder chronic cases during continued therapy. However, in acute cases the doctor may choose syrup of ipecac. Administered in subemetic doses, this drug stimulates the same secretory reflexes as do iodides. Although overdosage often induces voming, which is undesirable in infants and weakened elderly patients, some patients even benefit by this because retching helps to dislodge and expel mucus obstructions of the bronchi.

Mucolytic—mucus-dissolving—drugs may be administered as nebulized aerosol mists or occasionally as solutions that are carefully instilled into the tracheo-bronchial tree by special techniques. Among the substances sometimes employed as mucolytic agents are certain *enzymes, detergents,* and miscellaneous substances such as purified *propylene glycol,* and *acetylcysteine.* Some authorities doubt that these substances are any more beneficial than nebulized warm water or salt solution, which have been found useful for keeping the respiratory passages humidified without causing the irritation sometimes seen with these chemicals.

Patients with bronchial asthma are especially susceptible to the adverse effects of such enzymes as *trypsin, chymotrypsin,* and *pancreatic dornase* which are, of course, obtained from animal sources. Acetylcysteine (Mucomyst), an amino acid derivative that splits the sulfide linkages of mucoproteins, has also sometimes caused serious bronchospasm in asthmatic patients. Such detergents as *tyloxypal* and *sodium ethasulfate,* which exert a physical rather than a chemical effect, seem less irritating, but require prolonged aerosolization and are less effective for reducing the viscosity of thick mucopurulent pulmonary plaques than the agents that act chemically.

With any drug that produces an increased volume of thinned sputum, prompt removal of the liquefied secretions is important, lest the patient drown in his own fluids. Elderly and weakened patients must be closely watched and encouraged to cough productively. The nurse should examine the sputum cup contents and report its appearance and amount to the doctor, who will use this information along with his own observations in evaluating the patient's progress. Postural drainage and mechanical suction are also employed to keep the airway clear after the administration of expectorants or nebulization or instillation of mucolytic agents.

Bronchodilator drugs to control bronchospasm and allow adequate oxygenation may be effective once the pulmonary passages have been partially cleared of clogging secretions. Often, however, epinephrine is ineffective in status asthmaticus. Part of the seriously ill patient's nervousness may result from the central effects of the high doses of this drug that have been administered in efforts to relax bronchial spasm.

Sometimes patients refractory to epinephrine respond to the bronchodilating action of *aminophylline* (see Drug Digest) administered by vein or rectally. The intravenous drip of this drug must be adjusted to a proper speed—about 250 mg. per 15 minutes—for too slow an infusion may fail to produce bronchodilation and too rapid a rate of absorption may cause cardiovascular and central nervous system toxicity. The I.V. infusion is often repeated twice more in 24 hours; or the drug may be administered as a retention enema. When the acute phase is over, aminophylline may be given by mouth or as suppositories.

Oxygen may be administered by mask, nasal catheter, or tent to overcome anoxemia. However, patients who already fear suffocation may feel so closed-in by a tent or mask that they may be made worse by the procedure. To reduce his nervousness and to increase the value of oxygen treatment, it is necessary to explain the purpose of the therapy to the patient. It is important to stress that the oxygen is going to let him breathe easier, and to stay with the patient until he gets used to the equipment and sees that the stream coming out of the opening does indeed aid his breathing.

Too high a concentration of oxygen may, of course, be dangerous, for it tends to lessen hypoxic stimulation of the respiratory center and thus permits the build-up of excessive serum carbon dioxide. Thus, the oxygen content of the mixture is ordinarily kept well below 50 per cent, except for brief periods. If anoxia is severe, positive-pressure devices may be used for a few minutes several times daily and 100 per cent oxygen administered for a short time.

Other measures have been suggested recently for counteracting the effects of an undesirable build-up of carbon dioxide in the blood in acute pulmonary insufficiency. Certain of the newer analeptic drugs (Chap. 13), such as *ethamivan (Emivan) and doxapram (Dopram)*, have been used to stimulate ventilation and reduce respiratory depression in patients suffering from carbon dioxide narcosis marked by mental confusion, sleepiness, and lethargy. However, the use of such drugs in severe asthma, acute flare-ups of chronic bronchitis, emphysema, and other obstructive pulmonary diseases requires great care to avoid excessive respiratory stimulation, for this adds to the work of breathing in a way that may actually increase hypercapnia. Similarly, the infusion of the new systemic alkalinizer *tromethamine (talatrol; Tham E)* for correcting the sometimes severe acidosis of respiratory failure requires close supervision.

Corticosteroid drugs are often administered in high doses to acutely ill patients who do not seem to respond well to other measures during the first day of hospitalization. The way in which these drugs help the patient is still not understood, but their benefits become so obvious several hours following intravenous or oral administration that all authorities now advocate the use of steroid therapy in life-threatening status asthmaticus.

A presently preferred preparation is the soluble ester *hydrocortisone sodium succinate* (see Drug Digest). Injected intravenously in 100 to 200 mg. doses, a single steroid treatment sometimes remarkably improves the exhausted patient's condition. If the response is less dramatic, the drug is repeated every six hours until his labored breathing becomes easier. Then steroid therapy is continued with orally administered drugs, until the chest is practically clear. Corticosteroid drug dosage is reduced rapidly and discontinued in four or five days, or dropped back to maintenance levels if the patient had been taking steroids before the acute attacks began.

Chronic Asthma

Most patients with mild chronic asthma remain relatively comfortable for long periods when they learn to avoid exposing themselves to the secondary stresses that aggravate their condition. Even those who are subject to frequently recurring attacks can usually gain quick symptomatic relief with bronchodilator drugs or can keep persistent pulmonary symptoms under control with combinations of bronchodilators and expectorants. Corticosteroid drugs are usually reserved for those chronic cases that cannot be adequately controlled by these more conventional measures.

Corticosteroids. *Oral corticosteroid* drug administration for prolonged periods is considered warranted when chronic asthma continues to disable the patient despite his steady use of bronchodilators. Once the doctor has weighed the possible dangers of continued steroid therapy and has decided to employ these drugs, he tries to choose a drug and dosage regimen that will keep adverse effects to a minimum (see p. 394).

One of the synthetic steroids (Table 28-1) is usually preferred to the natural hormones, cortisone and hydrocortisone, which are more likely to cause fluid retention difficulties. Dosage regimens of these drugs vary, but in general an attempt is made to maintain the patient on the minimal dose that will control his symptoms. This may be accomplished in some cases by beginning with a low dose and raising it gradually. Some patients when first seen during an attack may get a high initial dose that is then reduced until wheezing begins to recur. Then that dose level is maintained for a while, but attempts are made periodically to reduce steroid dosage, or to withdraw the drug entirely. (The difficulty of doing this and the nurse's role in helping patients stick to a steroid treatment plan are discussed in Chapter 28.)

Aerosol steroid therapy is sometimes employed to attain a high local concentration in the lungs with lower total doses than when these drugs are given orally. Many patients do seem to require less steroids when treated with inhalation of *dexamethasone* phosphate sodium (Decadron Phosphate). Some patients with severe chronic asthma have then even been able to discontinue oral steroids entirely. However, the dosage of nebulized dexamethasone must be as carefully adjusted as that of the oral steroids, to avoid overdosage. The aerosol is never ordered on an "as needed" basis during periods of acute exacerbation, as patients may quickly develop cushingoid symptoms (p. 391). In any case, the use of aerosolized steroids for immediate relief is pointless, since they are not effective for several hours.

The anterior pituitary hormone _corticotropin_ (Chap. 27) is used today much less often than it once was. This substance, which is derived from animals, sometimes sets off severe anaphylactic reactions in allergic patients. It must be injected, and depends for its action on the responsiveness of the patient's own adrenals, and is often slow and unreliable in eliciting desirable responses. Doctors now doubt that corticotropin protects the patient's own adrenal glands from suppression by prolonged steroid medication. Thus, instead of administering corticotropin periodically to stimulate the production of natural steroids, doctors are striving to devise dosage schedules of the synthetic steroids with minimal adverse effects on the chronic asthmatic patient.

One recent finding indicates that the steroids are best given in a single morning dose to minimize their adverse effects on the patient's own pituitary-adrenal function. Another suggestion for avoiding cushingoid effects and reducing drug-induced suppression of the patient's adrenal function is that the drugs be given intermittently. On such regimens, the chronic asthmatic patient gets three days of medication followed by four days without it; or he may get his total two day steroid dosage on alternate days.

Bronchodilator drugs of the *adrenergic* and *xanthine* types are widely used in mild to moderately severe chronic asthma, in order to relax contracted bronchial muscles and thus widen the air passages in a way that increases the patient's vital capacity. The _adrenergic drugs_ most commonly employed for this purpose—epinephrine, isoproterenol, and ephedrine—are discussed in detail in Chapter 16 (see also Drug Digests). Thus, we shall note here only a few points pertinent to the use of the several available dosage forms—aerosols for inhalation, injectable solutions, and orally administered products.

Patients who suffer relatively mild but recurrent attacks of chronic asthma can often get rapid relief by inhaling an aerosol containing epinephrine, isoproterenol, or other adrenergic drugs. It is important to teach the patient to use the nebulizer properly, lest the mist be lost. Thus, he should be told to press his lips tightly around the plastic mouthpiece before beginning to release the medicated mist that is then inhaled deep into the bronchi.

The nurse may also teach the patient how to inject his own epinephrine subcutaneously for coping with more acute attacks. He should get many opportunities to practice, using a sterile saline solution, so that in an actual attack he can perform the injection in spite of haste, nervousness, and dyspnea. It is desirable to teach the injection technique to a member of the patient's family, who can help when an attack comes

TABLE 40-3

SOME DRUGS USED IN THE MANAGEMENT OF ASTHMA

	DOSE
Bronchodilator Drugs	
Adrenergic Type (see also Chap. 16)	
Ephedrine sulfate U.S.P.	Oral 25 mg. q. 4 hrs.
Epinephrine U.S.P.	1:100 sol. for inhalation; 1:1,000 sol. of 0.3–0.5 ml. S.C. for inj.
Isoproterenol HCl U.S.P.	Sublingual 10 mg. q. 4 hrs.; Inhalation 1:100 and 1:200 sol.; Subcutaneously 0.06 mg. in a 0.02% sol.
Methoxyphenamine (Orthoxine)	50–100 mg. q. 3–4 hrs.
Xanthine Type	
Aminophylline U.S.P. (Theophylline ethylenediamine)	Oral 200 mg. t.i.d.; I.V. slowly 500 mg. up to t.i.d.; Rectal 500 mg. one or two times a day
Oxtriphylline (Choline theophyllinate; Choledyl)	100–200 mg.
Theophylline sodium acetate N.F.	200 mg.
Theophylline sodium glycinate N.F.	300 mg.
Expectorants (see also Table 40-2)	
Glyceryl guaiacolate	100–200 mg.
Ipecac Syrup	0.5–2.0 ml.
Potassium guaiacolsulfonate N.F.	500 mg.
Potassium iodide U.S.P.	300 mg. up to q.i.d.
Potassium iodide solution N.F.	0.3 ml. containing 300 mg.
Adrenocorticosteroids (see also Chap. 28)	
Dexamethasone phosphate sodium N.F. (Decadron Phosphate)	18 mg. per spray of inhalation
Hydrocortisone sodium succinate U.S.P. (Solu-Cortef)	50–300 mg. daily I.V. or I.M.
Methylprednisolone sodium succinate N.F. (Solu-Medrol)	10–40 mg. I.V. or I.M.

on too quickly for the patient to prepare the injection himself.

The orally administered adrenergic bronchodilators give more prolonged relief of mild asthmatic attacks and are also useful for reducing the frequency of paroxysmal episodes. Ephedrine is most often found combined with a barbiturate, which helps to counteract its tendency to make some patients jittery. Another common ingredient of such combinations is theophylline or one of its derivatives, for drugs of the xanthine class seem to delay development of tolerance to ephedrine and tend to increase the effectiveness of the adrenergic bronchospasmolytic agents.

Theophylline and its various derivatives are often administered orally or by rectum in the management of patients with chronic bronchial asthma. These drugs act to relax smooth muscle which is in a spastic state, including that of the blood vessels and biliary system as well as the bronchial tubes. Thus, these drugs, and particularly the soluble salt aminophylline, have been advocated for use as vasodilators in coronary insufficiency and for relief of acute biliary colic. In both conditions, as well as in status asthmaticus, best results are obtained when these drugs are given by parenteral routes that permit attainment of effective tissue levels.

Most theophylline preparations are poorly absorbed when taken by mouth. When the dose is raised in order to increase the amount absorbed systemically, these drugs often cause gastrointestinal irritation resulting in nausea, vomiting, and epigastric pain. The various double salts and complexes of theophylline (Table 40-3) are claimed to be more soluble and absorbable and less likely to cause gastrointestinal irritation than the parent compound. An alcoholic solution of theophylline, Elixophylline, is said to reach high levels in the blood and tissues shortly after oral administration. The rectal route is often employed as a means of avoiding upper G.I. distress. However, since continued use of aminophylline suppositories may cause anorectal irritation, the nurse should look for signs of such irritation and report their presence.

Administration of aminophylline suppositories to children has resulted in overdosage and dangerous reactions. Apparently, young children are sensitive to the central stimulating action of theophylline derivatives and tend to become restless and agitated when they receive only moderately excessive amounts. Fatalities following drug-induced vomiting, fever, and convulsions have been reported. Special low-dosage pediatric suppositories are now available, but as much care should be taken to avoid overdosage with them as with the administration of adult-dosage suppositories. If a child appears to be restless, dehydrated, and feverish, the nurse should consult the physician before routinely administering an ordered dose of aminophylline.

Adjunctive Therapy. *Respiratory tract infections* can be both a precipitating cause of a bronchial asthma attack and a dangerous complication in status asthmaticus. In the latter case, the doctor ordinarily orders one of the *tetracycline*-type antibiotics or *erythromycin* to be administered daily until the purulent sputum is free of pathogenic bacteria. If laboratory culture tests indicate that the particular pathogenic microorganism is more susceptible to some other antibiotic, the physician will administer that agent, provided that the patient is not allergic to it. One of the new semisynthetic penicillins such as *oxacillin* may, for example, be preferred for respiratory infections caused by resistant staphylococci, unless, of course, the patient is sensitive to penicillin.

Preventive Therapy. *General and specific measures* for the prevention of asthma are beyond the scope of this discussion. We may note here, however, that patients undergoing desensitization therapy may suffer reactions that require drug therapy.

Desensitization or hyposensitization is a form of immunization in which the patient receives a series of gradually increasing doses of an extract of the allergen to which he has been found sensitive. Patients undergoing such treatment should be asked to stay in the clinic or doctor's office for 20 or 30 minutes during which they are carefully observed for signs of a reaction. If a sudden, severe reaction develops, the doctor should be notified immediately. The nurse then quickly prepares an injection of epinephrine and assists in its administration.

If the patient has suffered an anaphylactic reaction, the physician may want to give epinephrine by vein as rapidly as possible. Thus, a 1:1,000 solution of epinephrine HCl and physiologic saline solution for diluting it to a safe concentration for slow intravenous solution should always be readily available. Tourniquets should be kept handy, to reduce further absorption of the allergen from the extremity, if anaphylaxis develops.

Patients should be instructed in regard to what measures to take if a reaction to an allergic extract develops later at home. For example, they should be told to apply a cold compress to the injection site to slow further absorption, and to take a dose of an antihistaminic drug. Whereas these agents are not very effective in chronic asthma, they may counteract the ill-effects of a mild reaction to hyposensitization therapy with allergic extracts.

SUMMARY OF POINTS FOR THE NURSE TO REMEMBER CONCERNING COUGH CONTROL

- Encourage persons with persistent coughs to seek medical attention rather than treat themselves with non-prescription cough remedies. They must find out what is causing the cough to continue and stop taking drugs that may cause allergic hypersensitization or habituation.

- Carefully observe any patient who is receiving morphine or other analgesic-antitussives for relief of cough, in order to detect any excessive slowing of respiration or interference with his ability to cough up secretions.

- Use adjunctive nursing measures to help patients who are receiving expectorants. For example, assist the patient to a sitting position when he must cough, and encourage him to maintain a high fluid intake, for this helps to lessen the viscosity of bronchial secretions.

- Help the patient to control an irritating, nonproductive cough that interferes with sleep. Helpful measures are: raise his head by elevating the bed, offer him beverages to sip such as tea or ginger ale, or instruct him to take a few deep breaths and to try to relax when he feels that he is about to resume coughing.

- Remember that some medications have a desirable local effect on the pharyngeal mucosa, that is brief at best, and should not be further shortened by giving the patient something to eat or drink shortly after he has swallowed the syrupy liquid or sucked a demulcent, topical anesthetic lozenge.

SUMMARY OF POINTS FOR THE NURSE TO REMEMBER CONCERNING THE MANAGEMENT OF ASTHMA

- Nursing measures to relieve apprehension are important. For example, provide a call bell and promptly answer it, and remain with the patient.

- Convey calmness and confidence in the value of the drugs administered, not only to ease the patient's emotional strain but to increase the likelihood that he will benefit from treatment.

- Observe the patient frequently to note his response to drug therapy. Observe whether and to what extent symptoms are relieved, and whether the patient shows symptoms of adverse reactions to medications, such as anorectal irritation from aminophylline suppositories, and nervousness and trembling due to epinephrine.

- Encourage the intake of fluids and nourishing foods that are easy to eat in order to reverse dehydration and malnutrition.

- Note whether the patient is known to be allergic to any substances in his environment, and if so, remove them.

- Because asthma is usually a chronic condition, teach the patient and his family how to give medications such as those administered by aerosol and injection.

CLINICAL PROBLEM

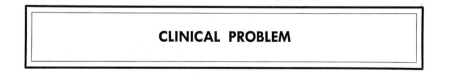

Mrs. Waterbury has been brought to the hospital for treatment of an acute asthmatic attack. Her physician has ordered 0.5 cc. of a 1:1,000 solution of Adrenalin stat. After the injection, the nurse notices that Mrs. Waterbury's pulse rate has increased from 96 to 120; she has trembling hands and is more restless and apprehensive. She can breathe somewhat more easily after the injection.

• Explain the probable reason for the patient's increased pulse rate, tremors, and restlessness.

• What nursing actions would be necessary in this situation?

REVIEW QUESTIONS

Allergy, Hypersensitivity, and Anaphylaxis

1. (a) What is thought to happen at the cellular level to trigger a hypersensitivity reaction?

(b) What chemicals are believed to be released when a reaction of this kind occurs?

2. (a) What are the main tissue sources of histamine? (That is, in what tissues is it bound until released in a reaction?)

(b) What types of tissues are the chief targets of released histamine?

3. (a) What is the effect of histamine upon the small blood vessels of the skin and mucous membranes throughout the body?

(b) By what symptoms are such histamine-induced vascular changes manifested in: (1) the skin, (2) the cranial vessels, (3) the nasal and laryngeal mucosa?

(c) What are two ways in which a severe anaphylactic reaction can lead to fatal circulatory or respiratory failure?

(d) How do the effects of histamine and other substances released in an allergic reaction account for the breathing difficulties of a patient who suffers an asthmatic attack?

4. (a) What is the effect of histamine upon the gastric glands and how is this employed diagnostically?

(b) What is the advantage of employing the histamine analogue betazole for this purpose, and what precautions should be taken in administering either drug?

5. (a) List at least two types of drugs that counteract allergy symptoms by exerting pharmacological effects that counteract those of released histamine.

(b) How do the so-called antihistamine drugs differ from the latter in the manner of their action?

(c) What kinds of allergy symptoms induced by histamine are most effectively counteracted by treatment with antihistamine drugs?

(d) In which allergic conditions are the antihistamine drugs considered least effective?

6. (a) List some types of allergic dermatoses in which administration of the antihistaminic drugs may give symptomatic relief.

(b) What central and peripheral actions of certain antihistamine drugs, besides their histamine-antagonizing effects, may play a part in the relief of allergic pruritus?

7. (a) List some types of upper respiratory tract conditions and symptoms that are counteracted by antihistamine drugs.

(b) What advantages over topical therapy may there be—in terms of increased effectiveness and reduced toxicity—when antihistamine and adrenergic drugs are combined in products for oral administration in the symptomatic treatment of rhinitis, sinusitis, and other upper respiratory tract disorders?

8. (a) What is the most common side effect of many antihistamine drugs and what warning should be given to patients relative to its possible occurrence?

(b) How may this side effect of antihistamines be prevented, counteracted, or minimized?

9. (a) What type of clinical picture may appear in a child who has accidentally ingested a massive overdose of antihistamine drugs?

(b) What measures may the doctor take to manage a case of antihistamine drug poisoning?

Management of Cough

1. (a) What is the ordinary function of a cough?

(b) What complications of excessive coughing may be prevented by treatment?

2. (a) What are some serious conditions in which the control of coughing by antitussive therapy is less important than diagnosis of the cause of the cough and treatment of the causative factors?

(b) What are some relatively minor respiratory tract disorders in which cough medications of various types may be indicated?

3. (a) What is the manner in which centrally acting antitussives suppress coughs?

(b) What are some of the ways drugs act peripherally (i.e., in the respiratory tract) to reduce coughing?

4. (a) What difficulties limit the utility of such potent analgesic-antitussives as morphine, methadone, and hydromorphone?

(b) For what types of coughing are these agents best indicated and for what kinds of patients are they ordinarily contraindicated?

5. (a) What advantages does codeine have over morphine for the control of coughing in most patients?

(b) What are some adverse effects of codeine in patients sensitive to that drug?

6. (a) What advantages may a typical non-narcotic antitussive such as dextromethorphan have over codeine-based cough medications?

(b) What are some of the peripheral effects that are claimed to add to the effectiveness of certain centrally acting antitussives?

7. (a) How do cough lozenges act to reduce coughing?

(b) What purposes are served by flavored cough syrups, such as Wild Cherry, White Pine, and Licorice?

8. (a) What purpose is served by stimulating the production of respiratory tract fluid through the oral administration of expectorant agents?

(b) By what two main mechanisms are the expectorant drugs thought to stimulate increased secretion of the mucus-liquefying respiratory tract fluids?

Management of Bronchial Asthma

1. (a) List several types of drugs that are sometimes employed to manage patients with bronchial asthma.

(b) List three general measures that are routinely employed in the early management of patients suffering from status asthmaticus.

2. (a) List some central depressant drugs that may be used to calm an anxious asthmatic patient and indicate some others that are generally avoided. Why should all such drugs be used with caution?

(b) List briefly some ways in which the nurse can help allay anxiety in the severely ill asthmatic patient.

3. (a) Why should the asthmatic patient receive fluids intravenously and later in the form of oral water, fruit juice, or milk prior to and during the administration of expectorant drugs?

(b) What is the reason for administering expectorant drugs and how, in general, do they bring about their desired effects?

4. (a) List some common early side effects caused by iodides and some early signs of hypersensitivity which may necessitate discontinuing the drug.

(b) List some signs of chronic iodide poisoning, or iodism.

5. (a) What is meant by the term "mucolytic agent" and what are some examples of the several types and drugs that are classed in this category?

(b) What are some measures that are commonly employed following the use of mucolytic agents?

6. (a) What action of aminophylline accounts for its usefulness in the management of bronchial asthma?

(b) List several other pharmacological actions of aminophylline and indicate how these account for some of its side effects and for its potential usefulness in conditions other than bronchial asthma.

7. (a) What are some nursing considerations concerning the administration of oxygen to hypoxic asthmatic patients?

(b) List several drugs that have recently been employed experimentally in the treatment of hypoxia, hypercapnia, and acidosis in acutely ill patients with bronchial asthma and other severe respiratory disorders.

8. (a) List a natural corticosteroid preparation that is commonly employed in status asthmaticus and indicate the manner in which it is administered.

(b) What are some other life-threatening emergencies in which this and similar synthetic corticosteroids may be employed?

9. (a) Under what circumstances may corticosteroid drugs be employed in the management of chronic bronchial asthma, and what means are employed to minimize the likelihood that steroid toxicity would develop?

(b) What advantage may there be in administering steroid drugs by inhalation of an aerosol, and what precaution is required when they are given in this way?

10. (a) What practical points about the use of certain dosage forms of adrenergic drugs may the nurse teach patients and their families?

(b) What precautions should be observed in the rectal administration of theophylline and its derivatives to adults and to children?

11. (a) List several antibiotics that are commonly employed for counteracting respiratory tract infections in asthmatic patients?

(b) List several measures that may be employed to minimize the effects of a reaction that develops as a result of desensitization therapy. What is the nurse's role when the patient has such a reaction?

BIBLIOGRAPHY

Allergy, Hypersensitivity, and Anaphylaxis

Council on Drugs: Status report on antihistaminic agents in the prophylaxis and treatment of the common cold. J.A.M.A., *142*:566, 1950.

Denny, F. W., Jr., and Dingle, J. H.: Current status of therapy in upper respiratory tract infections. J.A.M.A., *166*:1595, 1958.

Dragstedt, C. A.: Histamine, its pharmacology and role in anaphylaxis. J. Allergy, *26*:287, 1955.

Eisenberg, B. C.: Management of chronic urticaria. J.A.M.A., *169*:82, 1959.

Friend, D. G.: The antihistamines. Clin. Pharmacol. Ther., *1*:5, 1960.

Heatly, C. A.: Current status of therapy in paranasal sinusitis. J.A.M.A., *178*:1021, 1961.

Jillson, O. F.: Treatment of urticaria and contact dermatitis. Modern Treatment, *2*:895, 1965 (Sept.).

Michelson, A. L., and Lowell, F. C.: Antihistaminic drugs. New Eng. J. Med., *258*:994, 1958.

Patterson, R.: Allergic emergencies. J.A.M.A., *172*:303, 1960.

Rodman, M. J.: Drugs for allergic reactions. R.N., *29*:61, 1966 (Feb.).

———: Drugs for treating coughs and colds. R.N., *27*:85, 1964 (March).

———: Pollinosis. R.N., *19*:50, 1956 (Aug.).

———: The common cold. R.N., *19*:74, 1956 (Nov.).

West, G. B.: Studies on the mechanism of anaphylaxis: a possible basis for a pharmacologic approach to allergy. Clin. Pharmacol. Ther., *4*:749, 1963.

Wilhelm, R. E.: The newer anti-allergic agents. Med. Clin. N. Amer., *45*:887, 1961.

Wyngarden, J. B., and Seevers, M. H.: The toxic effects of antihistaminic drugs. J.A.M.A., *145*:277, 1951.

Management of Coughing

Bickerman, H. A.: Clinical pharmacology of antitussive agents. Clin. Pharmacol. Ther., *3*:353, 1962.

————: The newer antitussive agents. Med. Clin. N. Amer., *45*:805, 1961.

Boyd, E. M.: Respiratory tract fluid and expectorants. Pharmacol. Rev., *6*:521, 1954.

Bucher, K.: Pathophysiology and pharmacology of cough. Pharmacol. Rev., *10*:43, 1958.

Douglass, B. E.: Causes and therapy of cough. Med. Clin. N. Amer., *38*:949, 1954.

Ebert, R. V., and Pierce, J. A.: Therapy in chronic bronchitis and pulmonary emphysema. J.A.M.A., *184*:490, 1963.

Rodman, M. J.: Drugs that curb coughing. R.N., *21*:33, 1958 (Dec.).

Management of Asthma

Bickerman, H. A., and Itkin, S. E.: Aerosol steroid therapy and chronic bronchial asthma. J.A.M.A., *184*:533, 1963.

Ebert, R. V., and Pierce, J. A.: Therapy in chronic bronchitis and pulmonary emphysema. J.A.M.A., *184*:490, 1963.

Hildreth, E. A.: Some common allergic emergencies. Med. Clin. N. Amer., *50*:1313, 1966.

Jorgensen, J. R., and Falliers, C. J.: A rational approach to corticosteroid therapy for asthma in children. J.A.M.A., *198*:197, 1966.

Koelsche, G. A., and Henderson, L. L.: Bronchial asthma—the acute attack. Med. Clin. N. Amer., *48*:851, 1964.

McKee, M., and Haggerty, R. J.: Aminophylline poisoning. New Eng. J. Med., *256*:956, 1957.

Rodman, M. J.: Drugs for the relief of asthma. R.N., *30*:35, 1967 (March).

————: Drugs in the management of bronchial asthma. R.N., *24*:73, 1961 (Oct.).

Rowe, A. H., and Rowe, A. H., Jr.: Bronchial asthma—its treatment and control. J.A.M.A., *172*:1734, 1960.

Sherman, W. B.: Bronchial asthma. Modern Treatment, *1*:255, 1964 (March).

Unger, A. H., and Unger, L.: Modern treatment of bronchial asthma. Am. J. Nurs., *54*:1367, 1954.

Drugs Used in the Management
of Rheumatic Disorders and Headache

Pain and discomfort arising in the head and musculoskeletal tissues constitute the most common of all complaints. Many different types of drugs are employed to relieve symptoms stemming from such sites. This chapter summarizes the status of drug treatment in various conditions of this kind. Detailed discussions of some of the most important drugs used in the treatment of rheumatic diseases and headaches are found elsewhere in this book. For example, the *salicylates*, the agents most widely used in treating arthritic disorders and headaches, are taken up in Chapter 10; and the *corticosteroids*, which are important in the management of acute rheumatic fever and severe rheumatoid arthritis, are treated in detail in Chapter 28.

Here, we only point out the place of these two classes of drugs in the total management of joint and head pain. Groups of drugs that are *not* dealt with elsewhere, such as agents specific for gout and for migraine headaches, and others that are used occasionally in arthritic conditions resistant to the salicylates and corticosteroids, are discussed mainly in this chapter, both in the narrative text and in individual Drug Digests.

THE RHEUMATIC DISEASES

More than 12 million Americans are victims of arthritis and related rheumatic disorders, of which about 80 separate entities are now recognized. All are characterized by chronic musculoskeletal pain, soreness, or stiffness—symptoms often described by the layman with the catch-all term "rheumatism." We shall focus our attention here mainly on drugs used to reduce inflammation and pain in four types of conditions: rheumatoid arthritis, osteoarthritis, ankylosing spondylitis, and gout.

Although there are no true cures and hardly any specific drug treatments for these conditions, doctors can now do a great deal to relieve pain and to slow the progress of these chronic, potentially crippling diseases. Many measures besides drug administration are part of the doctor's total treatment program for patients with rheumatic diseases. These include physical therapy, orthopedic procedures and operations, special exercises for maintaining joint mobility, and measures for resting both inflamed joints and the whole body.

The successful application of all these types of care requires the active cooperation of the rheumatic patient. Unfortunately, persons suffering from rheumatoid arthritis and related conditions often become impatient with the slow progress that they seem to be making. Losing faith in the program that the doctor has laid out for them, they may look for some dramatic "miracle cure." Scorning salicylates as too familiar to be effective, people may spend large sums for medicines that are much less useful than aspirin, the drug that is still the cornerstone of arthritis treatment. Elderly people, who can least afford it, are among those who are said to spend more than $250 million annually on needlessly expensive and even worthless drugs, devices, and dietary treatments for arthritis. By delaying to undertake a medically supervised program, many expose themselves to unnecessary crippling.

The nurse can, of course, help steer these people away from the purveyors of worthless, money-wasting remedies. She can also advise the patient to stay with his treatment program when he gets discouraged and wants to quit. The nurse who understands the true status of the antiarthritic drugs currently available can encourage the patient by pointing out that the chances of arresting the disease and avoiding crippling are enhanced by starting treatment early and continuing with it faithfully.

The Salicylates in Rheumatic Diseases

Aspirin and its sister salicylates (Chap. 10) are still considered the safest and most effective drugs for most patients with all types of rheumatic diseases. The central analgesic and antipyretic action of these drugs, together with their local anti-inflammatory actions in the joints and in *non*-articular musculoskeletal tissues, makes them useful for relief of pain, fever, and swelling and stiffness of the joints.

Among the disorders whose symptoms usually respond to aspirin are: *osteoarthritis,* a degenerative joint disease that often develops with advancing age or as a result of trauma; *bursitis,* a condition marked by sometimes severe pain in the shoulder and elsewhere; and other inflammatory connective tissue disorders such as *fibrositis, tendinitis,* and *myositis.* The salicylates are most useful in the management of acute *rheumatic fever* and in *rheumatoid arthritis,* a chronic condition marked by acute flare-ups.

In the acute phases of rheumatoid arthritis and in rheumatic fever, the doctor orders aspirin or sodium salicylate in doses as high as 5 to 10 Gm. daily. The dose is often deliberately raised to the point of producing symptoms of minor salicylate toxicity (salicylism). The nurse listens for complaints of ringing in the ears, for such tinnitus is an early sign that the limits of safe dosage are being reached and that the doctor should reduce the dosage to a somewhat safer level. The patient's stomach distress may be minimized by giving him his salicylates after meals or with milk and crackers, or the doctor may order that some sodium bicarbonate be taken with each dose of the antirheumatic agent.

Keeping the plasma levels of salicylate high in this way often results in dramatic improvement in a few days. In rheumatic fever, for example, the temperature frequently falls and general discomfort is reduced. Here, and in acute flare-ups of rheumatoid arthritis too, the hot, red, swollen joints may soon return to close to normal appearance, and the patient becomes willing and able to move them. This allows the physiotherapist to maintain joint mobility with special exercises and gentle massage, thus preventing crippling contractures.

After the acute phase is over, the patient who has been advised to rest the affected joints is encouraged to move them. He continues to take salicylates in moderately large doses even when he is not in great pain, because aspirin is not only an analgesic-antipyretic but also a continuously acting anti-inflammatory agent. Most patients can take this relatively safe drug daily for years without suffering any toxic effects except for the mild salicylism that develops when the

dosage is raised occasionally in order to cope with exacerbations of the arthritic condition.

Although the salicylates can bring such acute episodes under control, neither they nor the even more potent and more toxic corticosteroids are capable of curbing rheumatoid disorders by overcoming the underlying disease process.

The Corticosteroids in Rheumatic Disorders

When they were first introduced, the corticosteroids were hailed with high enthusiasm as a "cure" for rheumatoid arthritis. Unfortunately, the dramatic relief often brought about by administration of these drugs was not accompanied by arrest of the joint disease. In fact, some authorities believe that the use of these steroids sometimes accelerates destruction of joint tissue. Nevertheless, when properly employed, these potent anti-inflammatory agents may prove very valuable in certain forms of arthritis.

As indicated in Chapter 28, corticosteroids are never used in chronic rheumatoid arthritis until the advancing condition no longer responds to more conservative management with salicylates and other less dangerous drugs (see below) together with a carefully planned program of rest, exercise, and physical therapy. Even then, corticosteroids do not replace salicylates but are *added* to the patient's regimen in low doses. If, as often happens in arthritis, the patient's condition goes into spontaneous remission, the doctor tries to reduce and even eliminate steroid dosage during the inactive phase of the disease.

Corticosteroid dosage is kept at the lowest levels compatible with control of crippling, because chronic steroid toxicity may develop. If a potentially dangerous reaction develops, these drugs are discontinued. Patients who have benefited from these drugs are often unwilling to give them up, especially when withdrawal leads to a return of even more intense pain than previously. Thus, the doctor tries to hold corticosteroid therapy in reserve, until he judges that these drugs are absolutely necessary to keep the patient from becoming incapacitated and losing his livelihood as a result of crippling by rheumatoid arthritis.

Corticosteroids are not ordinarily administered at all to patients with osteoarthritis. However, when this condition is especially severe and limited to only one or two weight-bearing joints such as the hip or knees, steroids are sometimes injected directly into the inflamed joints. Sometimes a single injection of a relatively long-lasting steroid salt or ester, such as betamethasone acetate or prednisolone butylacetate (see Drug Digest), may give relief lasting for several weeks without causing any systemic side effects.

Such intra-articular steroid administration may be used in rheumatoid arthritis that involves only a few joints, such as those of the spine. Patients are warned not to undertake too much activity, because this may speed the rate of joint destruction by the underlying disease process which continues despite relative freedom from pain and swelling in the joint. With the relatively insoluble esters, relief may sometimes be slow in onset, and local discomfort may increase for a day or two, as a result of so-called "postinjection flare." Thus, oral salicylates and other measures are also continued.

Corticosteroids are most valuable and least likely to cause complications when administered for short periods to control acute rheumatic symptoms that have not been overcome by massive doses of salicylates. In cases of acute rheumatic fever, for example, the doctor may order quite high doses of corticosteroids, especially if the patient shows signs of cardiac complications. Whether such steroid treatment protects the heart from the residual effects of myocarditis has not been resolved. However, intensive steroid therapy certainly brings about control of signs of systemic toxicity as well as local inflammation in most cases of this disabling and dangerous condition; and the drugs do so while producing few, if any, of the signs of hypercorticism that develop during prolonged therapy of chronic arthritic diseases.

Miscellaneous Anti-Arthritic Agents

Many patients with rheumatoid arthritis and related arthritic diseases are adequately managed by programs based upon salicylate therapy with the occasional judicious addition of corticosteroids. As indicated, these anti-inflammatory agents do not affect the unknown underlying disease mechanisms. Sometimes, patients suffer from rapidly progressive rheumatic diseases that do not yield to treatment with safe doses of salicylates and steroids. Thus, researchers are continually trying to discover new anti-inflammatory agents and other drugs that might actually *cure* arthritis by overcoming the rheumatic disease process. The status of the presently available nonsalicylate, nonsteroid antirheumatic drugs is discussed below.

Indomethacin (Indocin) is a nonsteroid anti-inflammatory agent that has proved beneficial for patients who cannot take salicylates or are no longer aided by aspirin. In many cases of rheumatoid arthritis, for example, joint pain, swelling, and stiffness are reduced after a few days of treatment, and the patient may regain the use of a previously immobilized limb. Although indomethacin is not as effective as the corticosteroids in severe cases, its administration often permits withdrawal of steroids or, at least, a substantial reduction in dosage of these potentially dangerous agents.

The use of indomethacin often permits elimination of phenylbutazone (see Drug Digest) from the regimen of patients with ankylosing spondylitis. This condition, also known as Marie-Strümpell disease, is a form of arthritis that affects the small joints of the

spinal column. It attacks young men mainly, beginning with low-back and leg pain and progressing to a point at which the spine is bent into a bow, or rendered completely rigid. Until recently, phenylbutazone was the best agent for slowing the progress of this condition. However, as indicated in the Drug Digest, prolonged use of phenylbutazone may be potentially toxic to the bone marrow and in various other ways. Indomethacin, on the other hand, has caused no hematological reactions or other dangerous toxic reactions.

Indomethacin does, however, produce side effects of some severity in many patients, especially at the start of treatment. About one out of four patients complains of symptoms of central origin, including headaches, vertigo, light-headedness, and, occasionally, mental confusion. These reactions make it undesirable for the patient to drive during the early weeks of treatment. About 10 to 15 per cent of patients taking indomethacin are forced to discontinue the drug because of headaches and other central symptoms.

As is the case with phenylbutazone and other anti-inflammatory agents, indomethacin often causes epigastric distress. While this may be minimized by giving the drug after meals or with a glass of milk, some patients must stop taking the drug on account of continuing nausea, indigestion, burning stomach pain, and diarrhea. The drug is contraindicated in patients with active peptic ulcers and is employed only with caution in those with a history of ulcerative gastrointestinal disease.

Adverse reactions of the central and G.I. types occur less frequently with the presently available capsules than with the tablets employed in early clinical trials. Administration of the drug in low doses—25 mg. two or three times daily—at first, followed by a gradual increase at weekly intervals, tends to help keep reactions to a minimum. Dosage larger than 150 to 200 mg. are not recommended, and, in any case, the doses required for controlling acute states should be reduced to a lower maintenance level during periods of relative remission.

Gold Salts. Treatment with the heavy metals listed in Table 41-1 is sometimes beneficial in the early stages of rheumatoid arthritis, when the progress of the condition is not being arrested by salicylates or corticosteroids. It seems likely, however, that favorable responses to gold salts require administration of doses close to the toxic level. Since some types of toxic reactions to gold are potentially serious, patients are carefully observed to detect early signs of adverse effects.

As indicated in the Drug Digest for gold sodium thiomalate, the most common reactions are dermatoses and those involving the mucosa of the G.I. tract. Less frequent but more dangerous are renal damage, blood dyscrasias, and reactions affecting the central and peripheral nervous systems. To minimize toxicity, treatment is initiated with small doses and discontinued if urinalyses, blood counts, or physical examination indicate the development of abnormalities.

Chrysotherapy (treatment with gold salts) of arthritis now seems to be established as effective in selected patients when administered by rheumatologists who are very familiar with the administration of courses of treatment with the available salts. (For a while, treatment with gold salts was out of favor, when its usefulness appeared to be outweighed by its toxicity.) Although the advocates of gold therapy suggest that

TABLE 41-1

DRUGS USED IN THE MANAGEMENT OF ARTHRITIS AND GOUT

Nonproprietary or Official Name	Proprietary Name or Synonym	Dosage
Allopurinol [1]	Zyloprim	200–600 mg. daily
Aurothioglucose [2]	Solganal; gold thioglucose	10 to 50 mg. weekly I.M. up to a total dose of 1.5 Gm. per course of treatment
Aurothioglycanide [2]	Lauron	25 mg. I.M. initially; gradually increased by increments of no more than 25 mg. at weekly intervals for 22 weeks to a maximum single dose of 150 mg.
Chloroquine phosphate [3] U.S.P.	Aralen, etc.	250 mg. daily
Colchicine U.S.P. [1]	—	1 mg. q. 2 hrs. for 6–8 doses as suppressant; 0.5 mg. maintenance
Gold sodium thiomalate [2] U.S.P.	Myochrysine	10 mg. I.M. initially, increasing to 50 mg. per week to a *total* dose of 750 to 1,500 mg.
Gold sodium thiosulfate [2] N.F.	Sanochrysine	5 to 75 mg. weekly dosage range, to a *total* dose of 500 to 1,000 mg. per course
Hydroxychloroquine sulfate [3] U.S.P.	Plaquenil	200–600 mg. daily
Indomethacin [4]	Indocin	50–150 mg.
Oxyphenbutazone [4]	Tandearil	300–600 mg. daily
Phenylbutazone [4] N.F.	Butazolidin	300–600 mg. daily
Probenecid U.S.P. [5]	Benemid	500 mg.–2 Gm. daily
Quinacrine HCl [3] U.S.P.	Atabrine	200–800 mg. daily
Sulfinpyrazone [5]	Anturan	200–800 mg. daily

[1] Gout treatment, miscellaneous.
[2] Gold salts for rheumatoid arthritis.
[3] Antimalarial-type antiarthritic.
[4] Antirheumatic–anti-inflammatory.
[5] Gout treatment, uricosuric.

it counteracts the causes of arthritis, the occurrence of relapses upon withdrawal of these drugs indicates that the progress of the underlying disease is not really affected.

Antimalarial Drugs for Arthritis (Table 41-1). Certain of the drugs originally discovered in the search for synthetic substitutes for quinine in malaria suppression (Chap. 36) are being employed in the management of selected patients with rheumatoid arthritis and in cases of the related collagen disease, discoid lupus erythematosus. Like the gold salts, these drugs are sometimes claimed to arrest the arthritic process by some sort of specific rather than merely symptomatic action. What is certainly true is that chloroquine and hydroxychloroquine (see Drug Digest) possess no immediate analgesic or anti-inflammatory activity. Thus, during the weeks or months in which these drugs must sometimes be administered, before a remission occurs, salicylates and corticosteroids must be administered simultaneously for relief of pain and other joint symptoms.

When taken in the large daily doses required, these drugs cause a high incidence of minor side effects, including gastrointestinal disturbances and skin eruptions. More serious are visual symptoms resulting from retinal damage. Unless detected early by ophthalmological tests, these ocular lesions can cause blindness. Somewhat less serious are symptoms caused by deposits of chloroquine and its metabolites in the cornea. Patients with this condition may complain of seeing halos around lights. This calls for reduction of dosage or withdrawal of the drugs, after which the keratopathy usually disappears within a few months.

Mefenamic Acid (Ponstel). This recently introduced drug is one of a series of anthranilic acid derivatives with analgesic-antipyretic and anti-inflammatory properties. It has been found useful for some patients who are unable to take aspirin, and, although it is non-narcotic, it is said to be superior to codeine for relief of pain following dental extractions. However, the usefulness of mefenamic acid in chronic disorders such as arthritis appears limited by the fact that it may be administered at present for periods of no more than one week.

This limitation stems, apparently, from studies indicating that the drug's safety margin is reduced when it is taken over longer periods and in higher than presently recommended doses. Side effects from small doses taken in a short term treatment regimen are said to be relatively mild and infrequent. Most commonly reported are drowsiness, dizziness, nervousness, headache, nausea and G.I. distress. Upper tract upset can be reduced by taking the drug during meals. Development of diarrhea is a sign that the medication must be discontinued. Caution is required in patients with G.I. tract inflammation and the drug is contraindicated when intestinal ulceration is already present.

THE NATURE AND TREATMENT OF GOUT

Gout is a form of arthritis with distinctive features which made it one of the earliest diseases recorded by the ancients and the first kind of arthritis to be differentiated from other forms of rheumatic disease. Among its characteristic features is the sudden, severe attack involving only a single joint, most often that of the big toe. The joint becomes swollen, hot, and extremely tender. Even the skin overlying the joint turns an angry red. In the intervals between attacks, the gouty joint is *not* nearly as sore and stiff as would be the case in rheumatoid arthritis, in which many joints are usually affected at once and painful symptoms of the underlying progressive rheumatic process persist for long periods.

Another characteristic of gout is abnormally high blood levels of uric acid—that is, serum uric acid concentrations of from 7 to 14 mg. per cent compared to normal levels of less than 6 mg. per cent. Such hyperuricemia is most often the result of a metabolic disorder, involving the purine portion of the nucleoproteins present in all body cells.

Primary gout of this type affects men much more often than women and is rare in children. However, hyperuricemia may also develop secondary to certain neoplastic diseases, including the acute leukemia of childhood, as a result of the large amounts of nucleic acids and purines that are produced by the abnormal numbers of growing and disintegrating cells. Drugs that increase the rate of tumor tissue destruction can, of course, add to the hyperuricemia. Thus, gout attacks may be a complication of cancer treatment.

Pathogenesis of Gout. Patients with persistent hyperuricemia may be symptom-free for many years. However, at serum levels higher than 8 mg. per cent, uric acid salts begin to settle out in the tissues. Such urate deposits, known as tophi, appear in the cartilage of joints, tendons, bursae, and elsewhere, including even the ears. These foreign bodies may cause local tissue necrosis and inflammatory reactions followed by fibrous tissue formation. Sometimes such tophaceous nodules may ulcerate and drain by way of discharging sinuses. Uric acid and urate salts precipitating out in the kidneys and urinary tract can cause insidious damage, so that well-advanced nephropathy may be present in a painless form, long before the patient has an attack of joint pain.

Acute gout attacks develop in only a small percentage of persons with high uric acid blood levels. In fact, urate crystals may even form in joints without causing arthritic reactions. Nevertheless, crystal formation in joint tissues is the first step in the process that leads to an attack. Local factors then determine whether or not an inflammatory reaction to the urate deposits will occur.

One such factor seems to be the extent of tissue acidity. Uric acid tends to crystallize out most readily in the presence of acids. When leukocytes infiltrate areas containing uric acid crystals and attempt to remove these foreign bodies by phagocytosis, the reaction leads to a local increase in lactic acid. As a result, still more uric acid settles out in the joint and these crystals call forth a further inflammatory reaction. Thus, treatment is based on attempts to (1) lower blood and tissue levels of uric acid, and (2) lessen local leukocytosis, phagocytosis, and inflammatory responses to crystals of uric acid.

Drug treatment of gout involves the use of three types of agents: (1) Those that control the inflammatory reactions responsible for the acute attacks—for example, colchicine (see Drug Digest), phenylbutazone (see Drug Digest), indomethacin, and corticotropin and the corticosteroids (Chaps. 27 and 28). (2) Uricosuric agents—drugs such as probenecid (see Drug Digest) and sulfinpyrazone, which increase the renal excretion of uric acid, thus lowering its serum level. (3) Allopurinol (Zyloprim), a unique drug at present, in that it reduces uric acid blood levels by blocking the biosynthesis of some part of the total amount of uric acid that would otherwise be produced by the body.

Acute attacks may be aborted in most cases if the patient begins to take colchicine tablets when he feels the first painful premonitory signs. No gout patient should ever be without this drug, which is so specific for control of attacks that its failure to do so makes the doctor doubt his original diagnosis. Oddly, the way in which this old plant derivative produces its effects is still not well understood. It does not reduce pain perception by a central action; that is, it is not an analgesic. Nor does colchicine increase uric acid excretion—and, indeed, the uricosuric drugs that do so do not halt the attack and may even sometimes start one.

Colchicine has no antirheumatic action against *other* inflammatory joint diseases. Its anti-inflammatory effect in an acute gout attack may result from an ability to keep granulocytes from migrating into the joints to engulf urate crystals. In doing so and thus reducing phagocytosis and associated lactic acid production, colchicine may break the cycle of increased tissue acidity, greater amounts of uric acid precipitation, and increased inflammatory responses of the tissues to these irritating foreign particles.

Colchicine must be taken in a special way, in order to attain maximal benefits with minimal ill effects. The patient takes one or two 0.5 or 0.6 mg. tablets every hour or two, until the gout symptoms subside or symptoms of drug toxicity appear. Toxicity is manifested by the onset of gastrointestinal distress, including diarrhea. The patient may have to take paregoric, alone or combined with kaolin-pectin or attapulgite,

for control of this symptom. Actually, most mild gout attacks can be controlled at early stages, before the patient has taken amounts of colchicine that he cannot tolerate.

Occasionally, however, when an acute attack flares up after smoldering for several days, the inflammatory response may be too far advanced for safe control by colchicine. In such cases, indomethacin may help to relieve pain through its nonspecific anti-inflammatory action. Corticosteroids injected directly into the joint may give some relief after an initial delay in onset. Corticotropin (ACTH) injections sometimes terminate acute attacks after a while. Phenylbutazone and oxyphenbutazone may be administered in gout attacks for their anti-inflammatory effects. These agents also have a uricosuric action.

Chronic gouty arthritic processes can continue in the absence of acute attacks. Continued deposition of uric acid crystals may disable the patient by destroying cartilage, joints, and bone epiphyses. Thus, although continued administration of small daily doses helps to lengthen the periods between acute attacks, other drugs are needed for preventing tophaceous structural changes in the intervals between attacks.

Fortunately, drugs that are both effective for reducing the size of articular uric acid deposits and safe enough to be taken for the many years of treatment required, without causing severe toxicity, are available. Administered daily in doses tailored to individual needs, the uricosuric agents (Table 41-1) not only serve as prophylactics against attacks but also help to improve joint function by eventually eliminating tophi and reversing local lesions.

Probenecid and sulfinpyrazone, a derivative of phenylbutazone that has a greater uricosuric action than the parent compound but none of its anti-inflammatory action, both act in essentially the same way. They prevent uric acid that has entered the lumen of the renal tubules from being reabsorbed into the blood. Thus greater amounts of uric acid are eliminated in the urine; the concentration of urates in the plasma falls gradually to normal levels; and the size of tophaceous deposits is gradually reduced. Sulfinpyrazone is more potent than probenecid but causes a greater amount of gastrointestinal upset and may even reactivate peptic ulcers in susceptible patients.

Neither drug relieves pain or reduces inflammation. Thus, one would assume that salicylates would be administered simultaneously. Unfortunately, salicylates interfere with the uricosuric effects of these drugs, and so, aspirin must *not* be taken at the same time. Probenecid and sulfinpyrazone may be given together, however, for producing additive effects in patients resistant to either drug alone. However, patients with advanced gouty nephropathy may not respond to treatment even with these combined uricosuric agents, because of the decreased capacity to excrete uric acid by way of their damaged kidneys.

Sometimes, especially at the start of treatment, these drugs themselves set off an acute gout attack or cause the formation of urate kidney stones. To prevent precipitation of uric acid in the urinary tract during its increased excretion as a result of the action of these drugs, certain precautions are necessary: (1) The uricosuric drugs are given in repeated low doses at first, rather than in single high doses; (2) fluids are forced to produce a large volume of less concentrated urine, and (3) the solubility of the uric acid in this dilute urine may be further increased by alkalinizing it through concurrent administration of small amounts of sodium bicarbonate or citrate.

Because of these and other disadvantages of the uricosuric agents, scientists have long sought for drugs that would lower the blood levels of uric acid, without simultaneously raising urinary uric acid to too high concentrations. Recently, a drug has been discovered that does this by reducing the rate at which the body produces uric acid, rather than by increasing its rate of excretion. This drug, allopurinol, may thus prove especially useful for patients with gouty nephropathy and a tendency to produce further renal urate stones when treated with uricosuric agents alone.

Allopurinol is a close chemical relative of the purine bases xanthine and hypoxanthine, the substances from which uric acid is formed in the last step of the series of reactions by which the body catabolizes cellular nucleoproteins. When allopurinol is administered it interferes with the breakdown of these precursor substances by inhibiting the enzyme xanthine oxidase, which ordinarily converts these substances to uric acid. This, of course, leads to a *decrease* in uric acid formation and in its urinary excretion, and to an increased production and excretion of xanthine and hypoxanthine. These substances are much more soluble than uric acid in serum and urine and do not crystallize out in body fluids and tissues as uric acid does. However, a fluid intake of 2 to 4 liters daily is recommended for patients taking allopurinol alone as well as when it is administered in combination with uricosuric agents in the treatment of resistant hyperuricemia.

Such a combined attack on hyperuricemia and on resistant tophaceous uric acid tissue deposits is especially effective and is proving helpful to patients with severe gouty arthritis, whose high uric-acid production had previously prevented complete control of their condition. With the simultaneous administration of low daily doses of colchicine to prevent acute inflammatory reactions, most patients who are promptly treated with the presently available drugs have an excellent prognosis. The nurse can confidently assure patients with gout that their condition is the best controlled of all the rheumatic disorders.

DRUGS USED IN THE MANAGEMENT OF HEADACHE

Headache is one of the most frequently reported symptoms. Almost everyone has a headache at some time, either when coming down with a cold or other viral respiratory illness or as a result of a transient period of emotional tension. Such occasional headaches are of minor significance. They ordinarily need neither special medical diagnosis nor intensive drug treatment. On the other hand, patients who complain of chronically recurring headaches should be advised to visit a physician, for chronic headaches may be a symptom of some serious organic disorder or emotional problem.

The doctor studies such patients carefully, to find the underlying disturbance. Occasionally, for example, headaches indicate the presence of intracranial structural changes caused by brain tumors, or serious cerebral vascular disorders such as aneurysms or angiomas. Ocular disturbances such as glaucoma may first be made manifest by headaches. Other organic disorders marked by the occurrence of frequent headaches include hypertension, chronic sinusitis caused by infection or allergy, and pressure on nerves in the region of the cervical spine. Thus, the patient who complains frequently of recurrent headaches should be urged to seek medical advice.

Usually headaches are not a sign of organic disease. They stem from psychophysiologic reactions to stressful situations. Some persons, for example, cannot express emotions such as anger. Sometimes such patterns of overcontrolled behavior established in childhood seem to precipitate reactions in skeletal muscles and in vascular smooth muscles that result in periodic, incapacitating head pain. Personality factors of this kind appear to play a part in the most common kinds of chronic headaches. These are: (1) *tension*, or *muscular contraction*, headaches and (2) *vascular headaches*, such as the morning headaches of *hypertension* and *migraine attacks*. While we naturally emphasize drug therapy here, the nurse should recognize that treatment is also directed toward helping the patient deal with his emotional problems.

Tension, or Muscular Contraction, Headaches

The physiologic mechanism responsible for the development of these so-called "tension" headaches is a sustained state of contraction of the muscles of the neck and scalp. The tensing of these muscles often results from an unconscious reaction to stress—much as we set our jaw when reacting to a situation that calls forth a fighting response. Recurring headaches of this type may also be the result of other factors. For example, persons whose occupations require them to keep the head in a set position—in typing, watch-repairing, etc.—may develop muscle tension headaches.

Headaches of this kind occur more commonly than the more severe vascular type. Because the pain is more bearable than that of the truly incapacitating vascular-type headache, people with tension headaches often try to treat themselves with widely advertised headache remedies. This is unfortunate—first, because failure to consult a physician while covering up this symptom with analgesic drugs may result in the advance of some serious undetected illness. In addition, the repeated use of drugs for self-treatment of persistent headaches may lead to dependence upon them and to chronic toxicity.

The nurse can help the patient to recognize the boundary between appropriate self-medication, such as the use of aspirin for an occasional headache, and undesirable "aspirin eating." Certainly, when the patient is suffering the side effects of excessive analgesic medication—including drug-induced headaches—the source of his symptoms should be tactfully pointed out to him. In teaching proper health practices such as this, the nurse takes care not to look down on the patient and upbraid or blame him.

Often the headache problem of a patient can be solved by a simple physical change in his work routine. Even when the main cause of his headaches is emotional and muscle tensions stemming from psychological pressures, *non*-pharmacological measures may relieve discomfort. Often, the nurse can suggest some safe, everyday measures such as gentle massage of the back of the neck and setting aside some time for a quiet rest period or even for taking a warm, relaxing bath. She can point out that pampering oneself in this way is certainly better than becoming a pill-taker.

However, when the drugs that are most commonly used for tension headache are employed only occasionally, they, too, can be helpful and completely safe. The several most useful classes of pharmacological agents, all of which are discussed in more detail elsewhere in this book, are: (1) the non-narcotic analgesics, (2) the sedatives and minor tranquilizers, and (3) the centrally acting muscle relaxant agents.

The *non-narcotic analgesics* of the salicylate and para-aminophenol or coal tar types (Table 10-1) are most widely used for pain relief, both as self-medication and on a doctor's prescription. Salicylates such as aspirin probably relieve headaches just as effectively when administered alone as when they are combined with a variety of other drugs. Thus, most mild to moderate tension headaches yield to treatment with a couple of 5-grain aspirin tablets. This amount, repeated in two to four hours if necessary, is harmless to most people.

Some sensitive individuals, however, cannot tolerate aspirin. In some cases it causes gastric irritation when taken in doses as low as 10 grains. In theory, such stomach upset may be avoided in two ways: (1) the aspirin can be combined with alkalinizing and solubilizing agents, or (2) the total dose of aspirin may be reduced and replaced in part by an analgesic of another class such as phenacetin. These methods form the pharmacological basis for many of the headache products on the market.

As indicated in Chapter 10, the advantages of both such types of more expensive products are doubtful. The headache patient who is sensitive to salicylates should probably avoid them entirely and use an agent of another chemical class such as acetaminophen (see Drug Digest). This is certainly true for patients who are hypersensitive to the salicylates, since they may suffer severe allergic reactions from taking as little as one aspirin tablet.

Occasionally, headaches of more than normal severity may require the use of an analgesic more potent than aspirin, phenacetin, or acetaminophen. The opiate-type analgesics codeine and oxycodone, which are available in combination with the non-narcotic agents, are often ordered in such situations. The doctor tries to use narcotic-containing analgesics only sparingly, for, although codeine is not a strongly addicting drug, its routine use by patients with chronic head pain is not considered desirable because some patients become psychologically dependent on it.

Many persons with chronic headaches tend to become "pill-takers" even when the drugs involved are not opiates. That is, they begin to take aspirin indiscriminately, alone or combined with phenacetin and caffeine, for relief of head pain. As with anything else that produces a feeling of relative well-being, such tablet-taking soon becomes a habit; and the habitual ingestion of large amounts of even these relatively safe drugs can have serious results. (See Chap. 10 for a discussion of acetanilid-induced blood disorders and the occurrence of nephritis following prolonged abuse of phenacetin.)

Several non-narcotic analgesics that are claimed to equal codeine in pain-relieving potency have come into use in recent years as substitutes for salicylates in sensitive patients. These include propoxyphene (see Drug Digest) and ethoheptazine (Chap. 10) and certain agents that also help to relax skeletal muscle spasm, such as phenyramidol and orphenadrine (Chap. 8). A number of other such agents are also on clinical trial, alone or combined with the traditional drugs.

Other types of drugs often found in commonly prescribed remedies for tension headaches include the classic sedatives such as the barbiturates and the newer minor tranquilizers. While barbiturates in low doses are not themselves analgesics—that is, they do not appreciably raise the pain threshold—their addition to an aspirin-phenacetin combination is said to lessen the patient's emotional reaction to his head pain.

Minor tranquilizers that have a muscle relaxant

component are often preferred for tension headache treatment. These so-called "tranquilaxants" include meprobamate (Equanil, Miltown), phenaglycodal (Ultran), and chlormezanone (Trancopal). On the other hand, sometimes a mild psychomotor stimulant such as dextroamphetamine (see Drug Digest) added to the standard analgesic combination may be better for reducing the patient's distress through its mild mood-elevating effect.

Most patients with tension headaches manage to control their symptoms reasonably well by modifying somewhat their responses to stress and by using the simple physical and pharmacological measures mentioned above. Sometimes, however, muscle contraction headaches are only one symptom of a severe depressive syndrome. The doctor who detects this does not treat such symptoms with mere analgesics, minor tranquilizers, or mild stimulants, or even with superficial psychotherapeutic supportive measures. Instead, he refers patients with serious unconscious psychological conflicts to a psychiatrist. If such a psychotherapist believes in the use of any drugs at all for treating recurrent tension headaches, he will probably order one of the major tranquilizers or antidepressant drugs as an adjunct to psychotherapeutic measures (Chap. 7).

Vascular Headaches

The most severe kinds of headaches develop when blood vessels in the tissues surrounding the brain become excessively dilated and begin to throb painfully. Although the tissues of the brain are themselves insensitive to painful stimuli, the pulsating cranial and extracranial arterioles apparently pull upon pain-sensitive structures in the head. This, and possibly the local release of certain pain-provoking chemicals, is thought to account for most of the patient's distress in headaches of this type. In addition, a late muscle-contraction type headache may result if the patient keeps his neck stiff in an effort to maintain his head in one position. This involuntary effort to avoid pain thus superimposes a tension headache on the one that stems from distended cranial blood vessels.

Vascular headaches are sometimes classed as migraine and *non*-migrainous types. In non-migrainous headaches the doctor tries to find the underlying cause and deals with it directly rather than only through the use of analgesic and sedative drugs. For example, if cranial vasodilation stems from infection and fever, the remedy may be an antibiotic rather than aspirin alone. Similarly, even in more chronic conditions such as essential hypertension, the hypertensive vascular headaches with which the patient commonly wakens in the morning are best dealt with by controlling high blood pressure with antihypertensive agents (Chap. 23).

Migraine headaches, on the other hand, have more complex causes that cannot be so readily counteracted. Thus, the aim of pharmacotherapy has been mainly to control the discomfort of the immediate migraine attack with specific drugs. Until recently, attempts to prevent attacks involved psychological rather than pharmacological approaches—that is, investigation of personality, environment, and emotional conflicts and problems, followed by efforts to eliminate the stresses that trigger the attacks.

Migraine Headaches

Treatment of an Acute Attack. Migraine patients are fortunate in having available a relatively specific agent for treating acute attacks—the ergot derivative *ergotamine tartrate* (see Drug Digest), which acts mainly to contract the smooth muscle walls of cerebral blood vessels. This action on dilated, pulsating cranial arterioles, directly counteracts the mechanism thought to cause the pain of vascular headaches. Interruption of vasodilation and distention stops any further pulling on pain-sensitive cranial structures and probably prevents leakage of inflammatory substances into the area. This often leads to dramatic relief of the attack.

Administration of Ergotamine. Doctors have learned a great deal in recent years about how best to give ergotamine. More than 90 per cent of patients can be helped by prompt administration of an adequate dose; failure to halt an attack is usually the result of giving too little of the drug too late. Thus headache specialists advocate the use of full doses of ergotamine. Caution is needed too, because overdosage can cause ergotism (Chap. 39), a condition in which excessive constriction of peripheral vessels can lead to circulatory obstruction and gangrene. Fortunately, the safety margin for this ergot alkaloid is fairly wide. Thus the doctor can find a dose that causes the desired cranial artery constriction without affecting the circulation to other parts of the body.

First the doctor determines the lowest dose of ergotamine needed to abort the attacks. Then the patient is taught to take that amount of ergotamine as soon as he feels an attack coming on. At first, the patient takes the drug by mouth in divided doses—usually two 1-milligram tablets at once, and then another 1-mg. tablet every half hour up to a maximum of 6 mg. Once a patient knows how much ergotamine it takes to abort his attacks, he may take that entire amount at once and then rest quietly in a darkened room for a few hours.

The oral route is the slowest-acting and least effective way to take ergotamine. Rectal administration by suppository or retention enema is somewhat more rapid and avoids loss of the drug by vomiting, which often occurs both as part of the migraine syndrome and as a side effect of ergotamine. The surest and swiftest action occurs when ergotamine is injected intramuscularly. Often this aborts the attack in a few minutes, especially if the injection is given soon after the first symptoms appear.

Side Effects. Nausea and vomiting, which are the result of central stimulation rather than irritation of the G.I. tract, occur even more frequently upon parenteral administration of ergotamine than when it is taken by mouth. This does not, however, keep the injected drug from exerting its full effects on the cranial vessels. When the drug is given orally, it is often combined with belladonna-type antispasmodics, barbiturate sedatives, and antiemetics such as cyclizine (Chap. 38). If vomiting persists, a phenothiazine-type antiemetic (e.g., chlorpromazine) may be administered.

More serious than these gastrointestinal complaints are signs of peripheral vasoconstriction, such as sensations of coldness, numbness, and tingling in the patient's toes and fingers. His leg muscles may become painfully cramped due to ischemia caused by partial shutdown of circulation. Such potentially dangerous reactions are said to occur only rarely in most patients. However, the possible occurrence of excessive vasoconstriction makes the use of ergotamine undesirable in patients sensitive to anything that reduces local blood flow.

Contraindications. Ergotamine is contraindicated in peripheral vascular diseases such as intermittent claudication (Chap. 26) and various other vascular diseases marked by atherosclerosis. Patients with a history of coronary disease, for example, may complain of chest pains similar to those of an attack of angina pectoris; in hypertensive patients blood pressure may rise as a result of drug-induced generalized vasoconstriction. The drug is not given to patients with sepsis and liver or kidney disease. Because of its potential oxytocic effect on the uterine musculature, ergotamine is contraindicated during pregnancy. (For a discussion of the treatment of acute ergot toxicity, see Chap. 39.)

Other Antimigraine Agents. The oxytocic ergot alkaloid ergonovine (Chap. 39), though less effective than parenterally administered ergotamine, is at least equal to it in activity when given by mouth. It is said to afford adequate relief for some patients while causing less nausea and gastric distress than ergotamine. Another derivative, dihydroergotamine methanesulfonate (DHE-45), may cause even less systemic vasoconstriction than ergotamine, but because its cranial constrictor action is weaker too, it must be injected in larger doses than the latter.

Few other drugs are sufficiently specific for the cerebral arteriolar walls. *Caffeine* is claimed to exert a mild constrictor effect on the cranial arteries, which is said to add to the effectiveness of ergotamine when combined with it. An adrenergic drug, *isometheptene,* is also said to act with relative specificity upon the cranial vessels without affecting the systemic circulation. However, caution is indicated when it is used for migraine patients who have cardiovascular diseases.

Because vascular headaches sometimes lead to muscle-contraction headaches, and vice versa, the doctor sometimes orders non-narcotic analgesics such as aspirin and propoxyphene (Chap. 10), or tranquilizing muscle relaxing agents such as meprobamate, phenaglycodol, and chlormezanone (Chap. 7). While these drugs are ineffective against severe migraine, they tend to counteract the tension component of such so-called "combined headaches." Although the ergot drug dosage should not be repeated, the analgesics and tranquilizers can be given every three or four hours when late head pain persists. Codeine may be given occasionally, but such narcotic analgesics as meperidine (Demerol) are considered undesirable in recurrent headaches because of the danger of addiction.

Prevention of Migraine. Ideally, the best way to prevent migraine attacks is through a therapeutic regimen designed to minimize fatigue and stress and to aid the patient in coping more effectively with his emotional problems. Drugs such as the tranquilizers are sometimes used to reduce emotional tension. However, some patients with migraine do not benefit significantly from tranquilizer therapy, perhaps because they resist the effects of agents that tend to reduce their energy and drive.

Minor tranquilizers such as meprobamate and chlordiazepoxide are sometimes employed as adjuncts to psychotherapy, which is considered the most constructive approach to migraine management. Ergotamine has proved ineffective and potentially dangerous as a prophylactic. However, another ergot derivative introduced recently has apparently proved useful for this purpose.

Methysergide (see Drug Digest), a drug closely related to the ergot alkaloid methylergonovine, appears to have some value as a prophylactic agent, not only in migraine but also in other types of vascular headaches. This agent is neither a sedative-tranquilizer nor a potent vasoconstrictor like ergotamine. The mechanism of its preventive action is not understood. However, it antagonizes serotonin, histamine, and other body chemicals that are thought to play a part in producing the cranial vasodilation, local edema, and tenderness that develop during a migraine attack.

This drug is said to reduce the frequency and severity of migraine attacks. It is sometimes given for many months to patients who had been having one or more incapacitating attacks each week. Patients with histamine headaches of the cluster type have also been helped. They usually take the drug only during the periods when their headaches begin to come in bunches. (This drug does not, however, stop any specific attack once it has started.)

Methysergide is somewhat safer than ergotamine, but it shares some of the pharmacological actions, side effects, and potential toxicity of the latter. Patients are observed periodically while on long-term maintenance therapy. They are warned to report any signs of vasospasm, such as cold or numbness in the hands, cramping leg pains, or constricting chest pain. These reactions are most likely to occur in patients who already have some tendency toward vascular obstruction. Thus, methysergide is, like ergotamine, contraindicated in peripheral vascular disease or phlebitis. Evidence of arteriosclerosis or of coronary artery disease or severe hypertension also indicates that this drug should be avoided. It is withdrawn periodically to prevent possible fibrous growth formation, which has been reported in some patients.

Although methysergide seems to have even less effect on uterine than on vascular smooth muscle, the use during pregnancy of a drug so closely related to the oxytocic agent methylergonovine (Chap. 39) is considered undesirable. The epigastric distress, nausea, and vomiting sometimes seen with ergotamine are likely to occur early in treatment with methysergide. To minimize such gastrointestinal side effects, the drug is ordinarily taken with meals. Patients sometimes start on one tablet a day, taken at bedtime with food or liquid. Then a second dose is added at breakfast, and after several days of observation, postluncheon and, finally, after-dinner doses are added to the patient's regimen.

SUMMARY OF POINTS FOR THE NURSE TO REMEMBER

- Carefully observe patients receiving high doses of salicylates for such symptoms as ringing of the ears, and promptly report this to the physician.

- Observe the patient who receives corticosteroids for such symptoms as edema and moon-face. Help the patient to understand why the dosage of corticosteroids must be reduced once his acute attack is over.

- Emphasize a regimen that helps reduce the likelihood of exacerbations of rheumatoid arthritis. Such measures as lessening fatigue and emotional strain and preventing infection are important; help the patient to learn how he can implement such health measures.

- The patient with gout requires specific detailed instruction concerning the dosage and timing of the varied medications that are prescribed. Make certain that the patient understands the way he is to use the drugs, and the possible side effects of drug therapy.

REVIEW QUESTIONS

Management of Rheumatic Disorders

1. (a) What advice can the nurse give an arthritic patient who is discouraged by his failure to be free of discomfort and is fearful of becoming disabled while following a conservative treatment based on salicylates, rest, exercise, and physical therapeutic measures?

(b) What advice can she give the patient who inquires about the value of widely publicized drugs, dietary schemes, and devices that he can purchase directly?

2. (a) List some common rheumatic conditions involving the joints that are relieved by adequate doses of salicylates.

(b) List some *non*-articular musculoskeletal conditions for which the salicylates also offer symptomatic relief.

3. (a) What is a common sign of the limit of safe dosage of salicylates in patients with acute rheumatic fever in whom these drugs may be being pushed to the limit of tolerance?

(b) How can one minimize the symptoms of gastric irritation from the high doses of salicylates often given to arthritics?

4. (a) Why does the doctor withhold corticosteroids until he is forced to use them in patients with chronic arthritis, and how does he try to regulate their dosage in such cases?

(b) What are two ways in which corticosteroids may sometimes be administered with relative safety?

5. (a) What advantages may indomethacin have over salicylates, corticosteroids, or phenylbutazone for some patients?

(b) What types of side effects sometimes occur with indomethacin and how may they be minimized?

6. (a) What are some early signs of toxic reactions caused by therapeutic doses of gold salts?

(b) What types of precautions are taken to avoid gold salt overdosage, and in what types of patients are they employed with extreme caution, if at all?

7. (a) Why are the antimalarial-type antiarthritic drugs often administered in combination with aspirin?

(b) What are the potentially most serious toxic reactions caused by chloroquine when it is administered in high daily doses in the long-term treatment of arthritis?

8. (a) How is a patient advised to take colchicine for aborting an acute attack of gout?

(b) What type of side effects may develop during the use of colchicine in this manner and what medication may be administered for relief of some of the symptoms of overdosage?

9. (a) In what way is colchicine thought to affect the underlying pathogenic mechanism responsible for an acute gout attack?

(b) What drugs besides colchicine sometimes shorten the duration of an acute gout attack?

10. (a) In what manner do uricosuric agents such as probenecid and sulfinpyrazone bring about their desired effects upon the levels of uric acid in the gout patient's blood and tophaceous tissues?

(b) Why is the use of aspirin contraindicated in gout patients who are receiving uricosuric agents?

11. (a) What difficulties may arise early in the administration of probenecid and other uricosuric agents?

(b) What precautions are suggested to prevent an undesired side effect of the uricosuric activity of these drugs?

12. (a) How does the drug allopurinol counteract hyperuricemia without at the same time raising the concentration of uric acid in the urine to excessively high levels?

(b) What types of gout patients may benefit from the use of allopurinol alone in place of uricosuric agents?

(c) What types of gout patients may benefit especially from combined treatment with allopurinol, probenecid, and low daily doses of colchicine?

Management of Headache

1. (a) What are some serious conditions that may first be manifested by an acute headache or chronically recurring headaches?

(b) What sort of personality factors are said to play a part in the recurrence of headaches in people without organic disorders?

2. (a) What is the mechanism of the tension, or muscle contraction, type of headache?

(b) What should the nurse suggest to persons who are obviously taking excessive amounts of analgesics in an unwise attempt to treat recurrent tension headaches?

3. (a) List three types of drugs that are often ordered for the symptomatic relief of recurring tension headaches.

(b) What is the most commonly employed agent for treating tension headache, and with what other substance is it sometimes combined for reducing side effects and increasing its effectiveness?

4. (a) Why do some persons become habituated to headache remedies containing non-narcotic analgesics, as well as to those that contain codeine?

(b) List several non-narcotic analgesics that are claimed to be equal to codeine in relieving headache pain.

(c) What *non*-analgesic drugs are often added to headache remedies for their effects on emotional or muscular tension?

5. (a) What type of treatment besides analgesics may be required to control vascular headaches accompanying infection and fever?

(b) What type of treatment is best for hypertensive-type vascular headaches?

6. (a) For what specific purpose is ergotamine tartrate employed, and in what manner does it bring about its desired effect in this clinical condition?

(b) What effect is caffeine thought to have when added to ergotamine in products for treating this condition?

7. (a) What instructions should the nurse give the patient for taking ergotamine by mouth when he feels an attack coming on?

(b) By what other routes may ergotamine be administered, particularly by the doctor or nurse when rapid onset of action is desired?

8. (a) What is a common side effect of ergotamine as well as part of the migraine syndrome?

(b) What drugs may be administered together with or after ergotamine to control this symptom or side effect?

9. (a) What are some symptoms of excessive vasoconstriction caused by ergotamine?

(b) For what types of patients is use of ergotamine contraindicated?

10. (a) For what specific purpose is methysergide employed?

(b) What type of side effects from methysergide should the nurse tell patients to report?

BIBLIOGRAPHY

Management of Rheumatic Disorders

Bartels, E. C.: Allopurinol (xanthine oxidase inhibitor) in the treatment of resistant gout. J.A.M.A., *198*:708, 1966.

Batterman, R. C., and Hagemann, P. O.: Treatment of rheumatoid arthritis: salicylates, corticosteroids. Postgrad. Med., *25*:96, 1959.

Cooperating Clinics Committee, American Rheum. Assoc.: A three month trial of indomethacin in rheumatoid arthritis. Clin. Pharmacol. Ther., 8:11, 1967 (Jan.–Feb.).

Katz, A. M., Pearson, C. M., and Kennedy, J. M.: A clinical trial of indomethacin in rheumatoid arthritis. Clin. Pharmacol. Ther., *6*:25, 1965 (Jan.–Feb.).

Lockie, L. M., Norcross, B. M., and Riordin, D. J.: Gold in the treatment of rheumatoid arthritis. J.A.M.A., *167*: 1204, 1958.

McEwen, C.: Management of rheumatoid arthritis. Symposium on treatment of arthritis. Modern Treatment, *1*:1041, 1964 (Sept.).

Pearson, C. M.: Management of ankylosing spondylitis. Symposium on treatment of arthritis. Modern Treatment, *1*:1221, 1964 (Sept.).

Rodman, M. J.: Drug treatment of gouty arthritis. R.N., *23*:33, 1960 (Dec.).

————: Drugs for the relief of arthritis. R.N., *24*:68, 1961 (Nov.).

————: Drugs to help the arthritic. R.N., *28*:69, 1965 (Dec.).

Rothermich, M. O.: An extended study of indomethacin. J.A.M.A., *195*:531, 1966; *195*:1102, 1966.

Sataline, L. R., and Farmer, H.: Impaired vision after prolonged chloroquine therapy. New Eng. J. Med., *266*: 346, 1962.

Seegmiller, J. E., and Grayzel, A. I.: Use of the newer uricosuric agents in the management of gout. J.A.M.A., *173*:106, 1960.

Management of Headache

Friedman, A. P.: Treatment of migraine. Symposium on the treatment of headache. *In* Modern Treatment, *6*: 1363, 1964 (Nov.).

Friedman, A. P., and Etkind, A. H.: Appraisal of methysergide in treatment of vascular headaches of migraine type. J.A.M.A., *184*:125, 1963.

Graham, J. R.: Treatment of muscle-contraction headache. Symposium on the treatment of headache. *In* Modern Treatment, *6*:1399, 1964 (Nov.).

Graham, J. R., et al.: Fibrotic disorders associated with methysergide therapy for headache. New Eng. J. Med., *274*:359, 1966.

Hale, A. R., and Reed, A. F.: Prophylaxis of frequent vascular headache with methysergide. Am. J. Med. Sci., *243*:92, 1962.

Katz, J.: Abdominal angina as a complication of methysergide maleate therapy. J.A.M.A., *199*:124, 1967.

Ostfeld, A. M.: Migraine headache, its physiology and biochemistry. J.A.M.A., *174*:1188, 1960.

Rodman, M. J.: Drugs for recurring headache. R.N., *29*: 65, 1966 (June).

————: New drugs for headache. R.N., *25*:47, 1962 (July).

· 42 ·

Drugs Used in the Treatment and Diagnosis of Eye Disorders

More than half our population is plagued to some extent by impaired vision. Most of these ocular defects can be readily corrected with eyeglasses or contact lenses. More than a million Americans, however, are completely sightless, and two million more are all but blind.

In this chapter we shall discuss some of the most important drugs used to control glaucoma and ocular inflammatory disorders, as well as agents that are employed in the diagnosis of eye defects and as adjuncts to the surgical correction of cataracts and other conditions. Most of these drugs belong to groups that are discussed elsewhere in this book. However, emphasis here is on the particular agents of each class that are reserved mainly for use in ophthalmic therapy.

Nurses can do a great deal to advise patients in the proper use of drugs that are prescribed in eye disorders. They can perform an important public service by influencing people to give up self-medication for eye discomforts and by suggesting that they have their eyes examined by an ophthalmologist. Although eye medications that are available without a prescription are harmless—except to people sensitive to some of their ingredients—they are ineffective in such specific conditions as ocular infections and allergy and are useless in such serious disorders as cataracts and glaucoma. Many people who suffer from chronic glaucoma, for example, can be spared the gradual but inevitable loss of vision, if the condition is detected early enough, through a simple test.

GLAUCOMA

Glaucoma comprises a number of disorders that have in common an abnormally high intraocular pressure. The build-up of excessive pressure within the eye leads to progressive loss of vision resulting from damage to the optic nerve. Once the doctor makes a diagnosis of glaucoma, he tries to limit the extent of nerve fiber destruction and atrophy by ordering treatment measures that are aimed at lowering the intraocular tension. Such treatment may be surgical or medical or a combination of both, depending on the kind of glaucoma with which the patient is afflicted.

Types of Glaucoma

Normal intraocular pressure (about 20 mm. of mercury) reflects the presence and push of fluid that forms naturally within the eye. Ordinarily the amount of this aqueous exudate that enters the eye by diffusion from the ciliary body equals that which leaves it through thin channels in the angle of the eye connecting with the blood stream. Any abnormality that interferes with the normal functioning of this ocular hydraulic system, so that more fluid enters the eye than can leave it, leads to an increase in intraocular pressure.

Sometimes, such a rise in pressure within the eye occurs during an infection as a result of inflammatory processes that close off the drainage channels. This type of *secondary glaucoma* usually responds to treatment with *corticosteroid* and *anti-infective agents*. Once this and other temporary causes of a mechanical drainage block are eliminated, secondary glaucoma usually clears up promptly.

A more common cause of glaucoma is some basic structural defect in the anterior chamber of the eye. Such so-called *primary glaucoma* takes two forms: (1) the *narrow*, or *closed, angle* and (2) the *wide*, or *open, angle* type. The angle referred to is the space between the base of the iris and the place where the cornea comes in contact with the scleral coat, or outside layer, of the eye (Fig. 42-1). This angle contains

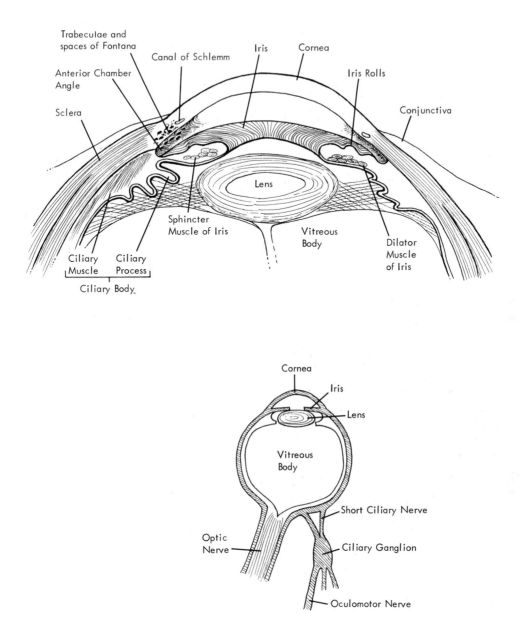

FIG. 42-1. (*Top*) The angle of the eye. An attack of glaucoma can occur when the folds of the iris and the ciliary processes crowd into the angle and block the outflow of fluid from the eye. (*Bottom*) Innervation of the eye.

the canal of Schlemm, a large outflow channel, and the spaces of Fontana—a meshwork of smaller openings.

Narrow-Angle Glaucoma. Some people are born with shallow angles, which can be detected with an instrument called a *gonioscope* which allows the doctor to look directly into the angle of the anterior eye chambers by means of a mirror. Circumstances sometimes cause a narrow angle to become even more crowded, resulting in partial or complete blockage of fluid outflow and a sharp rise in intraocular tension. This can be measured by another instrument, the *tonometer,* which may show an abnormally high pressure—30 or more mm. of mercury.

A common cause of excessive crowding of the angle, leading to acute blockage, is dilation of the pupil. When this window in the iris widens, the folds of that colored curtain (Fig. 42-1) roll back into the already narrow angle and cut off fluid outflow. This is why *acute attacks* are sometimes set off by emotional disturbances, in which, as we know, sympatho-adrenal discharge leads to pupillary dilation. For this reason *mydriatic* (pupil-dilating) drugs such as *atropine* are *always contraindicated* in glaucoma.

The nurse makes every effort to reduce the chance that a mydriatic drug solution may be instilled accidentally into the eye of a patient with narrow-angle glaucoma. The resulting pupillary dilation and blockade of the drainage canals by the thickening root of the iris and by the relaxing (or paralyzed) ciliary muscle (Fig. 42-1) can set off an acute glaucoma attack. This is not only extremely painful but can lead to permanent blindness, unless the high intraocular pressure is promptly reduced by surgical or medical measures (see below).

Open-Angle (Chronic, Simple) Glaucoma. In this form of glaucoma, the angle of the anterior chamber is normally deep, or wide. It is thought, however, that the network of pores in the sclerocorneal structure somehow becomes blocked, thus reducing the rate of drainage into Schlemm's canal. In any case, intraocular pressure gradually increases. This often occurs so slowly and painlessly that most persons are unaware of any loss of vision until late in the course of the disease. By that time, steady pressure may have pushed the center of the optic nerve, as well as its peripheral fibers, so far out of shape that the nerve no longer conducts visual impulses.

Approximately 50,000 people in this country are completely blind from chronic, simple glaucoma. Another 150,000 have lost the sight of one eye and live in fear of total blindness. An estimated one million more have this condition without being aware of it. Since they are mostly over 40 years old, the *routine use* of *mydriatic drugs* is *contraindicated* in patients of this age group, for these agents may precipitate acute attacks in these especially susceptible people. Such

attacks are similar to those seen in narrow-angle glaucoma.

Drug Treatment of Glaucoma

Early detection is important, because the longer the process goes on, the greater is the extent of visual loss. However, the progress of this blinding disease is often halted by drug treatment or by a relatively simple surgical procedure called *iridectomy,* in which a new drainage channel for intraocular fluid is made by cutting out a part of the iris.

The ophthalmologist must differentiate between narrow-angle and open-angle glaucoma, since treatment in the two conditions is usually quite different. Open-angle glaucoma is often controlled for long periods by the use of *miotic agents*—drugs that *constrict* the *pupil.* In narrow-angle glaucoma, on the other hand, treatment with miotics is a stopgap prior to surgery, which is the best treatment for most such patients. The weak miotics discussed in the next section do not offer adequate control of pressure in narrow-angle glaucoma, and the more powerful drugs of this type may sometimes cause a paradoxical *rise* in pressure in these patients.

Miotic Drugs

Manner of Action. The drugs most commonly employed to increase the rate of fluid drainage in glaucoma are the miotics. These are mainly *cholinergic agents* (Chap. 15) that directly or indirectly cause the sphincter muscles of the iris and of the ciliary body to contract. This pulls these structures away from the angle and seems to open up the meshwork of small channels that drain into Schlemm's canal. Constriction of the pupil also tends to thin the iris and pull its folds and its root out of the angle. These and other local ocular actions lead to the desired reduction in intraocular pressure.

Types of Miotics. These drugs can be classified as *direct-acting* cholinergic drugs and as *indirect-acting,* or *anticholinesterase,* agents (Table 42-1). The latter type of drugs (Chap. 15) brings about an increased local concentration of the neurohormone acetylcholine by inhibiting the activity of cholinesterase, the enzyme that promptly destroys it. The resulting accumulation of acetylcholine at postganglionic cholinergic neuro-effectors in the iris and ciliary body causes these smooth-muscle ocular structures to contract.

The direct-acting drugs such as *pilocarpine* (see Drug Digest) are relatively short-acting and must be instilled repeatedly. Most of the cholinesterase inhibitors—for example, *demecarium* and *echothiophate* (see Drug Digest)—produce much longer muscle-contracting effects. While their prolonged effects are often desirable in selected cases of chronic glaucoma, these potent miotics can cause many local and systemic side effects (see below). Thus, the less efficient but better tolerated agent, pilocarpine, may be more widely useful than these newer, more potent miotics.

Pilocarpine is used both to begin the treatment of open-angle glaucoma and to lower intraocular pressure in narrow-angle and secondary glaucoma. It is safe enough for use during acute attacks, in which it is sometimes instilled with solutions of *physostigmine* (see Drug Digest), another natural alkaloid, which is relatively weak but safe compared to the potent synthetic cholinesterase inhibitors.

The latter long-acting anticholinesterase compounds —*demecarium, echothiophate,* and *isoflurophate*—are *not* ordinarily administered in narrow-angle glaucoma or used to reduce the rise in pressure that often develops during inflammatory eye disorders (e.g., secondary glaucoma of iritis). Their powerful and prolonged contracting action on the sphincter of the iris and ciliary body may cause congestion and push these muscles against other ocular structures in ways that can actually *decrease* the *outward flow* of fluid from the overcrowded angle. In addition, these cholinesterase inhibitors dilate the ocular blood vessels, which can lead to an increase in *fluid formation,* another factor in the paradoxical and potentially dangerous rise in intraocular pressure that these drugs may set off in eyes with narrow angles.

There seems little need to use these new drugs in cases of chronic simple glaucoma that are adequately controlled by pilocarpine, physostigmine, or carbachol. However, some specialists claim that these potent drugs are useful in the management of patients whose eyes no longer respond to the weaker miotics. When the doctor orders these potent miotics, the patient must be taught how to use them so that the danger of adverse local and systemic effects is minimized.

Adverse Effects. Most miotics cause some degree of discomfort on initial use. The doctor tries to avoid local irritation by ordering dilute solutions initially and increasing the strength gradually as needed. However, even the lowest concentrations that control intraocular pressure are likely to cause some annoyance. For example, the patient may complain of darkened vision—a natural result of the diminished amount of light entering the constricted pupils.

Contraction of the ciliary muscle—another expected and desired action of cholinergic eye drops—is often a source of inconvenience or pain. For instance, distant vision becomes blurred. This stems from spasm of accommodation, a condition caused by the sustained contraction of the ciliary muscles. When these lens-controlling muscles fail to relax, the suspensory ligaments around the lens loosen. The lens becomes more globular and is forced forward. It is then fixed for near vision and fails to flatten out, as it must to bring distant objects into focus. Long-continued contraction of the ciliary muscles by the potent cholinesterase inhibitors often leads to aching in the eye, brow, and head.

The stimulating effect of anticholinesterase-type miotics upon skeletal muscles sometimes causes the eyelids to twitch. Occasionally, enough of these drugs is absorbed into the systemic circulation to cause signs and symptoms similar to some of those that occur in myasthenic patients in cholinergic crises or in persons exposed to certain poisonous insecticides. Thus the nurse should, with glaucoma patients, listen for complaints of salivation, nausea and vomiting, and abdominal cramps or diarrhea, and report them to the doctor.

Ophthalmic Administration

When treatment involves the use of miotics or of any topical medication discussed below the patient should be instructed in their proper use, in order to avoid adverse local and systemic effects. Some points to consider are summarized here and at the end of the chapter.

To avoid adverse effects on other body organs and systems from such potent drugs as the cholinergic miotics discussed above or from atropine, measures must be taken to minimize the systemic absorption of drug solutions that are dropped in the patient's eyes. This is best done by applying slight pressure to the inner canthus. This area near the nose contains the lacrimal ducts, through which the solution may otherwise rapidly run into the upper respiratory tract and be absorbed into the blood stream. Keeping the patient's lids apart for several seconds while applying such pressure tends to retain the drug solution on the surface of the eye and to prolong the action on eye structures. (Some eye drops contain adjunctive thickening agents such as methylcellulose and its derivatives, which also tend to delay absorption and enhance local activity of topically applied ophthalmic solutions.)

To avoid loss of the medication and lessen the likelihood of local irritation, the patient should be taught how to instill eye drops and apply ophthalmic ointments. One or two drops are placed carefully in a sac made by gently everting the lower lid, instead of dropping the drug directly on the sensitive cornea. The patient then closes his eyelids gently instead of squeezing them tightly together. Ointments are squeezed in a thin ribbon onto the inner surface of the lower lid which is then gently massaged.

All equipment for administering ophthalmic medications, including droppers, tubes, or plastic containers, must be sterile. The tip of the tube or dropper is not permitted to touch the eye, for the container may then become a vehicle for the spread of infection. To prevent the container from being thrust into his eye if the patient moves, it is good practice to support your hand by placing a finger on his forehead.

In administering ophthalmic products, it is important to read the label carefully and comply with all instructions for storage. Physostigmine solutions, for

TABLE 42-1
DRUGS USED IN THE DIAGNOSIS AND TREATMENT
OF EYE DISORDERS

Nonproprietary or Official Name	Trade Name or Synonym	Dosage and Administration
Miotic Agents (Ophthalmic Cholinergic Drug Solutions)		
Direct-Acting Drugs		
Carbachol	Carcholin; Doryl	0.1 ml. of 0.75, 1.5, or 3.0% sol. 1 to 4 times daily
Pilocarpine HCl U.S.P.	—	0.1 ml. of 0.5 to 4% sol.
Pilocarpine nitrate U.S.P.	—	1 to 6 times daily
Indirect-Acting Drugs (Anticholinesterase Agents)		
Demecarium bromide	Humorsol	1 to 2 drops of 0.25% sol. once or twice daily, or less often
Echothiophate iodide U.S.P.	Phospholine	1 drop of 0.06 to 0.25% sol. once or twice a day
Isoflurophate N.F.	Floropryl; DFP	1 drop of 0.1% sol. every 12 to 72 hrs. Also available as ointment
Neostigmine bromide U.S.P.	Prostigmin	1 or 2 drops of 0.25 to 5% sol. 2 to 6 times daily
Physostigmine U.S.P.	Eserine	0.25% ointment applied topically to conjunctiva up to 4 times a day
Physostigmine salicylate U.S.P.	Eserine salicylate	0.1 ml. of 0.02 to 1% sol.
Physostigmine sulfate U.S.P.	Eserine sulfate	0.1 ml. of 0.25 to 1 % sol. instilled up to 4 times a day
Mydriatic Drugs		
Anticholinergic Mydriatic-Cycloplegic Agents		
Atropine sulfate U.S.P.	—	0.5 to 1% sol. or oint. up to 6 times a day
Cyclopentolate HCl U.S.P.	Cyclogyl	0.1 ml. of 0.5 to 1% sol. 1 to 6 times a day
Eucatropine HCl U.S.P.	Euphthalmine	0.1 ml. of 2 to 5% sol. on the conjunctiva
Homatropine HBr U.S.P.	—	0.1 ml. of 1 to 2% sol. 1 to 6 times a day
Tropicamide	Mydriacil	For mydriasis 1 or 2 drops of 0.5% sol.; for refraction 1% sol. and repeat in 5 min.
Adrenergic Mydriatics and Decongestants		
Epinephrine U.S.P.	Eppy	0.1 ml. of 1 to 2% sol. applied as required (e.g., repeated every 5 to 15 min. if necessary)
Epinephrine bitartrate U.S.P.	Epitrate; Mytrate	
Epinephrine HCl	Glaucon	

TABLE 42-1 (Continued)

Nonproprietary or Official Name	Trade Name or Synonym	Dosage and Administration
Mydriatic Drugs (*Continued*)		
Adrenergic Mydriatics and Decongestants (Continued)		
Hydroxyamphetamine HBr U.S.P.	Paredrine	0.1 ml. of a 0.25 to 1% sol.
Phenylephrine HCl U.S.P.	Neo-Synephrine	0.1 ml. of a 0.125 to 10% sol.
Carbonic Anhydrase Inhibitors		
Acetazolamide U.S.P.	Diamox	500 mg. initially oral or parenteral, then 125 to 250 mg. orally 2 to 4 times a day
Acetazolamide sodium U.S.P.	Diamox sodium	
Dichlorphenamide U.S.P.	Daranide; Oratrol	Initially 100 to 200 mg.; maintenance 25 to 150 mg.
Ethoxzolamide	Cardrase	62.5 to 125 mg. 2 to 4 times daily
Methazolamide U.S.P.	Neptazane	50 mg. every 8 to 24 hrs.
Corticosteroids for Topical Ophthalmic Use		
Cortisone acetate N.F.	Cortogen acetate; Cortone acetate	0.5 to 2.5% suspension
Dexamethasone sodium phosphate N.F.	Decadron phosphate	0.05% oint. or 0.1% sol.
Fludrocortisone acetate	Florinef	0.1% sol.
Fludrocortisone hemisuccinate	Florinef ophthalmic	0.1% sol.
Hydrocortisone acetate U.S.P.	Cortef; Cortril; Hydrocortone acetate	0.5 to 2.5% suspension; 1.5% oint.
Prednisolone acetate U.S.P.	in Metimyd; Metreton, etc.	0.2 to 0.5% suspension
Prednisolone sodium phosphate U.S.P.	Hydeltrasol, etc.	0.5% sol. and oint.
Topical Ophthalmic Anti-Infective Agents		
Bacitracin U.S.P.	Baciguent	500 units 1 Gm. oint.
Chloramphenicol U.S.P.	Chloromycetin	1% oint.
Chlortetracycline N.F.	Aureomycin	0.5% sol. 1% oint.
Erythromycin	Ilotycin	0.5% oint.
Idoxuridine	Herplex; IDU; Stoxil	0.1% sol.
Neomycin sulfate U.S.P.	Myciguent	0.5% oint.
Oxytetracycline N.F.	Terramycin	0.5% sol. 1% oint.
Polymyxin B sulfate U.S.P.	Aerosporin	20,000 units 1 Gm. oint.
Sulfacetamide sodium U.S.P.	Sulamyd	10 to 30% sol. 10% oint.
Topical Ophthalmic Anesthetics		
Benoxinate HCl	Dorsacaine, etc.	1 to 3 drops, 0.4% sol.
Butacaine sulfate	Butyn	2% oint.
Cocaine N.F.	—	2 to 4% sol.
Lidocaine U.S.P.	Xylocaine	4% sol.
Phenacaine HCl N.F.	Holocaine	2% oint.
Piperocaine HCl	Metycaine	4% oint.
Proparacaine	Ophthaine	1 to 2 drops of a 0.5% sol.

example, should be stored in a cool place and protected from light to reduce the rate of deterioration. Solutions should be checked before they are used, for physical changes may make them ineffective or irritating. Cloudy or discolored solutions may have to be discarded. (For example, physostigmine tends to turn pink or red; epinephrine turns brown; and phenylephrine becomes cloudy.)

Adrenergic Agents

In some patients with open-angle glaucoma, intraocular pressure cannot be controlled completely with miotics and certain sympathomimetic, or adrenergic, agents must be used. Instillation of such substances as *epinephrine bitartrate* (see Drug Digest) and *phenylephrine* shortly after the use of a miotic such as pilocarpine often produces an additive drop of pressure within the eye.

It may seem odd that a cholinergic and an adrenergic drug should have additive effects, for they are usually antagonists. Indeed, the adrenergic drugs *do* tend to dilate the pupil (Chap. 16), whereas miotics constrict it. However, it is the effect of adrenergic drugs on the ocular *blood vessels* rather than on the iris that accounts for most of their therapeutically desirable effects in glaucoma.

Topical administration of epinephrine constricts the vessels of the eye. This is thought to reduce the rate at which aqueous fluid is formed within the eye. In addition, the outflow of fluid may be increased by adrenergic drugs, in a manner that is not well understood. In any case, the *reduced* fluid *inflow* brought about by these drugs, together with the miotic-induced *increase* in *outflow*, helps to lower the intraocular pressure further. The miotic is always administered first to counteract any mydriatic action of the adrenergic drug. The latter, pupil-dilating action, which tends to force the root of the iris into the angle, is especially undesirable in narrow-angle glaucoma. Thus the use of adrenergic drugs is contraindicated in such cases.

The topical application of epinephrine often causes a stinging sensation in the eye. It is desirable to warn the patient of this in advance and assure him that the discomfort will not last long and usually does not occur at all with continued treatment. Sometimes, however, prolonged use of sympathomimetic drug solutions results in redness, itching, and burning of the eye. Such acquired sensitivity makes it necessary to discontinue the use of the adrenergic drug.

Carbonic Anhydrase Inhibitors

Sometimes the pressure continues to rise despite combined treatment with cholinergic miotics and adrenergic vasoconstrictors. This is especially likely to happen during an acute attack of glaucoma. Until recent years, the excruciating pain of this condition was relieved only by morphine, followed by mandatory surgery. Now, the pressure is often controlled by administering a carbonic anhydrase inhibitor (Table 42-1) such as *acetazolamide* (Chap. 20) or *dichlorphenamide* (see Drug Digest).

Drugs of this class were introduced as diuretics for treating edema but have been largely replaced for that purpose by the newer thiazide-type diuretics. They are, however, uniquely useful for reducing the rate at which fluid is secreted into the eye. This is thought to result somehow from their ability to inhibit the activity of the enzyme carbonic anhydrase (CA) which apparently plays a role in the control of ocular fluid formation, as it does in urinary acid secretion.

In an emergency, acetazolamide is given by vein, while miotics such as pilocarpine and physostigmine are being applied topically in repeated attempts to constrict the pupil. Often this reduces the intraocular pressure within a few minutes, and the effect may be sustained by additional oral doses. The oral route is employed during the long-term treatment of chronic simple glaucoma.

The adverse effects of these drugs are of two types. Some signs and symptoms are secondary to the dehydration and excessive electrolyte loss that follows continued diuretic therapy. These include such gastrointestinal effects as anorexia, nausea, and vomiting, and nervous system difficulties including dizziness, headache, drowsiness, mental confusion, and numbness and tingling of the skin in various areas.

Other toxic reactions seem to be of the sulfonamide-sensitivity type. These include blood dyscrasias such as agranulocytosis and thrombocytopenia, and skin rashes. Patients should be watched for early signs of these conditions which require discontinuance of CA inhibitor drug therapy. The drugs are not employed in patients with acid-base imbalances or kidney and liver difficulties. Potassium salt supplements may be required to overcome drug-induced hypopotassemia.

Adjuncts to Ocular Surgery

Most cases of narrow-angle glaucoma sooner or later require surgery. Even though acute attacks usually respond to treatment with the combinations of drugs described above, the condition tends to worsen with each attack that causes adhesions to form in the angle. When done early, as an elective procedure, a peripheral iridectomy is relatively simple and usually successful.

In patients who require an emergency iridectomy, the high intraocular pressure must be reduced to safer levels. This is sometimes brought about by the intravenous administration of the *osmotic diuretics, mannitol* and *urea* (Chap. 20). Recently, because of various adverse effects of these parenteral drugs, some ophthalmologists have employed high oral doses of a 50 per cent *glycerin* solution preoperatively. This is said to bring about a prompt drop in the intraocular pressure of most patients.

Oral glycerin solutions are also used in preoperative preparation of patients who are to undergo cataract surgery. A cataract is a cloudiness of the lens, most commonly seen in elderly patients but, often, also in children and young adults. There is no medical treatment for this condition, and surgical removal of the opaque lens is usually recommended as soon as the condition begins to interfere with vision. In such cases, the intraocular pressure is not usually high. However, surgery is safer when the pressure within the eye is reduced *below* normal.

The operation for cataract removal is relatively simple and highly successful. When it is recommended by an ophthalmologist, patients should be encouraged to undergo the procedure rather than to hope in vain for some new medical treatment. (Charlatans have sometimes taken advantage of people's fears of eye surgery by selling them prolonged, expensive and useless drug therapy.) Drugs that produce proper anesthesia and fight infection have, of course, proved valuable in increasing the safety and success of surgery for cataracts.

Another agent, the enzyme *alpha-chymotrypsin* (*Alpha-Chymar*), has simplified removal of some types of cataracts. This proteolytic enzyme dissolves the lens ligaments or zonules, a procedure that is particularly desirable in young patients with relatively resistant ligaments. The area is washed with a weak solution of the enzyme to loosen the cataract so that it can be lifted or suctioned out without mechanical manipulation. Removal of the lens without force is said to shorten convalescence.

Local Anesthetics. Ocular surgery is usually carried out under local anesthesia. Some procedures require retrobulbar infiltration anesthesia (Chap. 11), but others can be carried out solely by surface anesthesia with topically applied agents. In any case, retrobulbar anesthesia for orbital surgery is more readily accomplished after the conjunctiva and cornea are first desensitized by topical application of local anesthetics. In addition to their use during iridectomy and in cataract anesthesia, surface anesthetics are employed prior to removal of foreign bodies and sutures, and for facilitating such diagnostic procedures as tonometry and gonioscopy.

At one time, *cocaine* was most commonly used for ocular surface anesthesia, but it has been largely replaced by drugs that have fewer local and systemic side effects. *Benoxinate* (*Dorsacaine*) and *proparacaine* (*Ophthaine*) are examples of such widely accepted newer agents. Both produce relatively rapid anesthesia of short duration. With proparacaine, for example, enough anesthesia develops within a half minute of instillation of a drop or two to permit placement of a tonometer on the eye surface and measure-

ment of intraocular tension. The relatively short effect (15 to 20 minutes) of these drugs is said to reduce the risk of corneal irritation and keratitis in short procedures; for longer procedures, adequate depth and duration of anesthesia is maintained by repeated instillation.

Unlike cocaine, these better suited ocular anesthetics do not cause much early stinging, burning, tearing or redness, and dryness and pitting (stippling) of the corneal epithelium do not develop later. Cocaine's sympathomimetic action causes the radial muscle of the iris to contract, with resultant pupillary dilation, which can, of course, precipitate an acute attack of narrow-angle glaucoma. The more ideal ocular topical anesthetics do not affect pupillary size or intraocular pressure.

OCULAR INFLAMMATION

The eyes, like other body tissues, become inflamed when irritated by allergy, infection, trauma, or exposure to toxic chemicals. Ocular inflammation is not only discomforting but can result in blindness. Inflammatory reactions in some structures, such as the conjunctiva, usually clear up readily without residual effects. However, the cornea and certain parts of the inner eye such as the iris and the ciliary body, may be so badly damaged by inflammatory swelling and scar tissue formation that blindness results.

Before treating an eye inflammation, the doctor tries to determine its cause. Some reactions—for example, most conjunctival inflammations—subside spontaneously. Potent medication administered here merely to "do something" may only further irritate the eye or even interfere with its natural defenses against disease. When the specific cause has not been determined, simple *saline irrigation* or at most mild *antiseptic-astringent solutions* such as boric acid or zinc sulfate are considered the safest and least expensive remedies.

Certain more modern medications have helped to save the sight of many patients who might once have been left blinded by serious inflammatory eye disorders. The most useful of these drugs have been the *corticosteroids.* They are most commonly employed in combination with *antibiotics* and other *anti-infective agents,* or with *antihistamine drugs.*

Corticosteroid Therapy

Once the doctor decides to employ steroid drugs to suppress inflammation in an ocular structure, he chooses the type of preparation best suited for the particular condition. If the inflamed tissues lie close enough to the surface to be seen without special instruments, *topically applied steroids* are used (see Table 42-1). Deep-seated disorders—for example, conditions involving structures behind the iris, such as choroiditis and optic neuritis—require administration of *systemic steroid* medication orally or by injection.

Systemic administration of high doses of corticosteroids or of corticotropin (ACTH) for a few days often relieves pain and discomfort dramatically. More important, steroids suppress the adverse early and late effects of ocular inflammation. By preventing the proliferation of tiny new blood vessels that leak edema fluid, these drugs reduce the swelling that can severely distort eye structures. They also interfere with fibroblast formation and thus lessen late scarring and synechiae (the adhesions that tend to form between parts of the eye pressed together by inflammation). These inflammation-suppressing actions of the steroids in such sight-threatening disorders as posterior uveitis, choroiditis, optic and retrobulbar neuritis, and sympathetic ophthalmia have done much to help reduce the incidence of blindness in recent years.

Although high steroid doses are relatively safe for short periods, long-term use of these drugs for chronic intraocular inflammatory disorders can cause serious side effects (see Chap. 28). The ophthalmologist who undertakes the treatment of a smoldering infection of the internal eye has to weigh the dangers of prolonged systemic steroid therapy against the chance that his patient may be blinded if the drugs are withheld. If he decides on long-term steroid administration, the same precautions are required as in other serious, chronic conditions of a *non*-ocular nature that are treated with steroids.

Topical application of steroids rarely gives rise to reactions. High local concentrations can be attained in the anterior chamber of the eye without causing systemic steroid side effects. However, because long-term use of topical steroids for external eye infections sometimes raises the intraocular pressure, frequent tonometric checks are advised. (Ordinarily, steroids *prevent* the kinds of adhesions or synechiae that may lead to secondary glaucoma.)

Steroid–Anti-Infective Combinations

Steroids do *not* counteract the *causes* of ocular diseases any more than they get at the underlying difficulty in other inflammatory disorders. Thus, they are often combined with drugs that *do* affect the source of the inflammatory reaction. This is especially important in infections, because steroid therapy tends to make it easier for the causative bacteria, fungi, or viruses to spread and invade deeper ocular tissues. For this reason, steroids are commonly prescribed in combination with antibiotics and chemotherapeutic agents for combating inflammatory eye infections.

Among the anti-infective agents most commonly combined with corticosteroids for treating infections of *external* eye structures are the nonirritating topical sulfonamide *sulfacetamide* (see Drug Digest) and the antibiotics *neomycin, bacitracin,* or *polymyxin.*

The serious bacterial infections of *inner* eye structures, which were once a leading cause of blindness in children, are now largely controlled by parenteral administration of *penicillin, chloramphenicol,* or the *tetracycline*-type antibiotics (Chap. 34) along with high doses of corticosteroids.

Infections of the cornea caused by fungi and viruses—including *herpes simplex,* an acute virus disease marked by cold sores on the lips and face—are *not* ordinarily treated with topical corticosteroids. This is because—until recently at least—no specific chemotherapeutic agents could halt these organisms. Thus steroids might speed the spread of unchecked herpes virus particles and lead to deep corneal ulcers with eventual loss of vision.

The recent introduction of *idoxuridine* (see Drug Digest), an antiviral chemotherapeutic agent specific for herpes simplex, has led some ophthalmologists to employ it along with steroid therapy in treating certain eye infections in which the virus is well established. Ordinarily, in superficial herpes simplex keratitis, corticosteroid therapy is contraindicated. Another eye infection in which steroids are not employed is active tuberculosis of the anterior chamber.

Steroid-Antihistamine Combinations

Allergic eye disorders marked by itching, burning, and tearing are often treated with corticosteroids combined with antihistamine agents. The latter type of drug reduces the effects of free histamine released in ocular tissues by the antigen-antibody reaction (Chap. 40). The steroids help to control the exudative phase of the reaction—for example, the pale, milky edema of allergic conjunctivitis is counteracted. Combined treatment with a topical steroid such as prednisolone phosphate or acetate (see Drug Digest) and an antihistamine drug like chlorpheniramine often relieves the ocular symptoms of hay fever and of seasonal eye allergies such as vernal conjunctivitis, blepharitis, and keratitis.

CHEMICAL BURNS OF THE EYE

Corticosteroids are sometimes successfully employed in some kinds of chemical and heat burns to reduce scarring and keep the cornea from becoming opaque. However, steroids and all other medication are not nearly as important in chemical burns as is quick, copious, and continuous irrigation with water (or any other available bland liquid).

Industrial nurses are often called upon to meet such emergencies or to advise workers on what to do in case of eye injury. Although first-aid manuals often list neutralizing agents for counteracting acid or alkali burns, time should not be wasted trying to obtain such substances. Instead each eyelid should be gently pulled away from the eyeball and each pouch made in this way thoroughly irrigated to remove all traces of the irritant. It is important, too, to look closely for any particles—of plaster or lime, for example—and remove them carefully.

Later, to keep adhesions from forming during healing of denuded areas, boric acid or other bland ointments may be placed between the lids. Other medications are applied sparingly, if at all, for they tend to delay healing. Topical anesthetics and antibiotics, for example, are not used routinely but only to treat pain and infection, and are usually promptly discontinued when no longer necessary. Steroids and atropine-type mydriatics (see below) may reduce inflammation and adhesions.

OPHTHALMOLOGIC DIAGNOSTIC AIDS

Mydriatic-Cycloplegic Agents. The ophthalmologist often employs drugs to facilitate his examination of the structure and function of the patient's eyes. The agents most commonly employed for such purposes are the anticholinergic drugs (Chap. 17), which are applied topically to produce *mydriasis* and *cycloplegia*. *Atropine*, the most potent agent of this type, has been largely replaced for diagnostic purposes by other agents such as *cyclopentolate, homatropine,* and *eucatropine* (see Drug Digests), and by a more recently introduced anticholinergic drug, *tropicamide* (*Mydriacil*).

The main advantage of these drugs over atropine is that their disabling effects on vision wear off much more rapidly. With the long-lasting cycloplegic action of atropine the patient's near vision may be blurred for days; on the other hand, drugs such as eucatropine and tropicamide, which—in low concentrations at least—have little or no cycloplegic activity, permit the patient to read and to see close objects normally within a few hours. Thus these drugs, or certain adrenergic mydriatics such as *hydroxyamphetamine* and *phenylephrine* (Chap. 16), are preferred when the doctor wants to produce *only* mydriasis, in order to examine internal eye structures.

However, for attaining the degree of cycloplegia required for refractive purposes, cyclopentolate and homatropine are usually preferred. Their effects upon accommodation are neither too transient nor too prolonged ordinarily. However, it is important to explain to the patient that his near vision may remain somewhat blurred for the rest of the day. Also, he should be advised to wear dark glasses when outdoors to avoid discomfort caused by sunlight that enters the dilated pupils which cannot constrict reflexly as readily as usual.

Atropine is preferred when the doctor wishes deliberately to induce prolonged rest, relaxation, and even paralysis of the sphincter muscles of the iris and the ciliary body. This is often desirable in treating inflammatory disorders of the inner eye, for it helps to relieve painful reflex spasm of these smooth muscle structures. It also tends to prevent contact and subsequent formation of adhesions between these and other ocular structures such as the lens and cornea. (Sometimes combinations of shorter-acting mydriatic-cycloplegic drugs are alternated with miotics in an effort to break up adhesions that have begun to form.)

All of these anticholinergic drugs are contraindicated in patients with glaucoma, and eye drops containing them are never used routinely without the doctor's permission, particularly in patients over 40 years old. Children tend to be quite susceptible to the systemic action of atropinelike drugs. Thus special efforts are made to prevent topically applied drugs of this type from being absorbed. The nurse should be alert for signs of local hypersensitivity and systemic toxicity induced by these drugs.

Disclosing Dyes. Certain dyes are often applied topically to stain ocular tissues and thus disclose the presence of local damage. *Fluorescein sodium,* for example, enters the cornea but leaves a greenish yellow stain only on those areas in which there is a break in the epithelial coat. For this reason it is used to find foreign bodies, locate abrasions, and reveal the characteristic branching pattern of a herpes simplex lesion on the cornea. The dye is also used as part of other diagnostic procedures including applanation tonometry, and in contact lens fitting.

While fluorescein and other dyes such as *merbromin* and *rose bengal* are themselves harmless, bacterial contamination of their solutions can cause infection. Thus freshly prepared solutions for individual use are preferred to stock solutions for general use, which might become contaminated with pseudomonas and other pathogenic organisms. Sterile filter paper strips impregnated with fluorescein are available for insertion into the space under the lids. Left in place for a few seconds and then flushed out with sterile saline, these fluorescein papers leave a greenish discoloration on denuded areas that can be readily detected by the examiner.

SUMMARY OF POINTS FOR THE NURSE
TO REMEMBER

- Advise patients who are trying to treat themselves for eye discomfort to visit their physicians, for the use of nonprescription medications without medical advice leads to delay in getting proper examination and treatment, and overuse of eye drops or sensitization to them may prove harmful.

- Be aware of the potential seriousness of accidentally administering a mydriatic instead of a miotic to a patient with narrow-angle glaucoma. (It may precipitate an acute attack which could lead to blindness.)

- Never administer mydriatics routinely when eye examinations are being performed. Always ask the physician which patients are to receive mydriatics prior to the examination.

- If hospital policy permits, let each patient keep the bottle of eye drops ordered for him at his own bedside. This reduces the chance of confusion and errors that may occur when medications are dispensed from a central station or assembled on a common tray.

- Keep ophthalmic solutions and their containers sterile when being used for treating a traumatized eye. This is difficult to do in the absence of single dose dispensers. Plastic containers for repeated use are not permitted to touch the patient's eye, for they may then spread infection.

- Place eye drops gently into the sac made by everting the lower lid, while taking care not to thrust the point of the dropper or other container into the eye. Avoid dropping the solution on the sensitive cornea. When instilling drops containing potent cholinergic miotics or anticholinergic agents such as atropine, apply pressure at the inner canthus to lessen systemic absorption of these drugs.

- In applying ophthalmic ointments, have the patient look up while a thin ribbon of medication is placed on the inner surface of the lower lid. Then have the patient close his eyes without squeezing the lids together tightly, and massage the area gently to spread the medication around.

- If the ophthalmic medication is likely to cause initial stinging or discomfort, let the patient know this and assure him that the irritation will subside shortly.

- In cases of chemical injury to the eye, do not take time to obtain or prepare acid or alkali neutralizing solutions, but, instead, see that the victim's eyes are thoroughly washed with large quantities of tap water.

REVIEW QUESTIONS

1. (a) What advice should the nurse offer persons who are purchasing nonprescription medications for relief of eye discomfort?

(b) What precautions are taken to avoid medication errors involving eye drops?

2. (a) Explain briefly how instillation of a mydriatic drug in an eye with a narrow angle may set off an acute attack of glaucoma.

(b) Explain briefly how the instillation of miotic drugs in open-angle glaucoma helps to reduce intraocular pressure.

3. (a) What is the main advantage of the synthetic miotic drugs demecarium and echothiophate?

(b) What disadvantages make these drugs less generally useful than the weaker alkaloidal miotics pilocarpine and physostigmine, and actually contraindicated in narrow-angle glaucoma?

4. (a) What are two types of complaints that result from the actions of miotic drugs that are desired in treating glaucoma? (That is, what complaints can be ignored because they are a natural accompaniment of the therapeutic action of these drugs?)

(b) List some local and systemic adverse effects of cholinergic miotic drugs.

5. (a) What measure may be taken to minimize the systemic absorption of potent cholinergic miotics?

(b) What are some technical measures to be observed in instilling eye drops?

6. (a) In what main manner are adrenergic drugs believed to reduce intraocular pressure in open-angle glaucoma?

(b) What other action of these drugs in the eyes makes their use undesirable for patients with narrow-angle glaucoma?

(c) What warning and reassurance may be given to a patient who is about to use eye drops containing epinephrine for the first time?

7. (a) In what manner are the carbonic anhydrase inhibitor drugs believed to lower intraocular pressure in glaucoma?

(b) List some side effects of two types that sometimes occur in patients taking CA inhibitors.

8. (a) What type of drugs is commonly employed to reduce abnormally high intraocular pressure prior to surgical intervention?

(b) What enzyme is sometimes applied locally during surgery for cataract removal and how is it said to facilitate the procedure?

9. (a) List several ocular procedures in which prior instillation of a surface anesthetic is commonly employed.

(b) Name a couple of topical ophthalmic anesthetics and indicate some of the ways in which they are superior to cocaine for use in the eye.

10. (a) List some inflammatory disorders of the external eye in which topical corticosteroids are employed; also some internal eye disorders in which systemic administration of these drugs is beneficial.

(b) What actions of the steroid drugs within the inflamed eye account for their usefulness?

11. (a) Why is the simultaneous administration of an anti-infective agent especially important when steriods are employed to combat ocular inflammation caused by infection?

(b) In what types of corneal infections is the use of corticosteriods ordinarily contraindicated?

12. (a) Name a topical sulfonamide and several antibiotics commonly employed in the local management of bacterial eye infections.

(b) Name an antiviral ocular chemotherapeutic agent and indicate the current status of its simultaneous use with steroids in treating herpes simplex keratitis.

13. (a) What combination of topically applied agents is most useful for controlling ocular allergy inflammatory reactions?

(b) What is the most important measure for dealing with chemical contamination of the eyes?

14. (a) What are the pharmacological effects of anticholinergic drugs on the eye, and for what clinical *diagnostic* purposes are these actions commonly employed?

(b) What are the advantages of such agents as eucatropine and homatropine over atropine itself?

15. (a) What measures may the nurse take to avoid chances of error or undesirable effects in older patients and in children in situations involving anticholinergic ocular solutions?

(b) For what *therapeutic* purposes are atropinelike drugs sometimes employed in managing ocular disorders, and how may their adverse effects be counteracted pharmacologically to some extent?

BIBLIOGRAPHY

Becker, B., and Gage, T.: Demecarium bromide and echothiophate iodide in chronic glaucoma. Arch. Ophth., *63:* 102, 1960.

Council on Drugs: Evaluation of idoxuridine (IDU). J.A.M.A., *190:*535, 1964.

Gordon, D. M.: Use of dexamethasone in eye disease. J.A.M.A., *172:*311, 1960.

Kaufman, H. E., Nesburn, A. B., and Maloney, E. D.: Treatment of herpes simplex keratitis with IDU. Arch. Ophth., *67:*583, 1962.

Leopold, I. H.: Steroid therapy in ophthalmic lesions. J.A.M.A., *170:*1547, 1959.

Leopold, I. H., and Keates, E.: Drugs used in the treatment of glaucoma. Clin. Pharmacol. Ther., *6:*130, 262, 1965.

Rizzuti, A. B.: Alpha-chymotrypsin in cataract surgery. Arch. Ophth., *61:*135, 1959.

Rodman, M. J.: Drugs used in eye diseases and injuries. R.N., *24:*63, 1961 (March).

———: Drugs used in eye disorders. R.N., *30:*63, 1967 (Feb.).

Vaughn, D. A., Jr.: Contamination of fluorescein solution. Am. J. Ophth., *39:*55, 1955.

· 43 ·

Drugs Used in Dermatology

Skin disorders are among the most common and certainly the most visible medical conditions. Many people with skin lesions are never seen by a doctor because they treat themselves with one or more of the hundreds of skin remedies that are so heavily promoted in all types of advertising media. Although self-medication is not always harmful, people with chronic skin complaints should see a doctor. After the condition has been diagnosed, it may be controlled with simple nonprescription remedies, but some skin lesions are signs of serious systemic disorders that require more specific treatment. Then, too, overtreatment with topically applied drugs sometimes leads to sensitivity reactions that are much worse than the original dermatological disorder.

In this chapter, we shall touch on many different types of drugs that are used to treat and prevent various skin diseases. Space permits detailed discussion of only a few representative drugs. We will, however, classify and list in tabular form the most commonly employed agents. In addition, we shall discuss the pharmacological management of a few of the most common of the more than 600 known skin conditions.

Before we begin to discuss drugs, we shall review briefly the structure and function of the skin and indicate some of the ways in which the skin reacts pathologically in the more common dermatological disorders.

ANATOMY AND PHYSIOLOGY OF THE SKIN

The structure of skin differs greatly in different parts of the body. The various regions differ in thickness, hairiness, oiliness, and the amounts of moisture that collect on the surface, and thus respond differently to disease-producing stresses and drug treatments. Certain generalizations help us to understand how the skin is affected by stress and what measures help it to return to normal.

The skin is made up of a series of strata, or layers (Fig. 43-1). At the base is a layer of fatty subcutaneous tissue upon which rests the *dermis,* or *corium,* which is made up mainly of connective tissues. On this layer is a thin cellular membrane, the *epidermis,* which consists of several strata; the most important strata are: an inner layer of living cells called the *germinative stratum* because it is the source of all the other epidermal cells, and the *stratum corneum,* a closely packed layer of flat, hard cells that have died during their gradual rise from the basal layer.

The epidermis contains two kinds of cells: (1) those that manufacture a protein called *keratin* which accounts for the hard, horny protective outer layer of the skin, as well as for the toughness of the hair and nails, and (2) those that manufacture *melanin,* a dark pigment that accounts for skin color—the more melanin, the darker the skin. Only if the melanocytes fail to make any melanin at all is a person's skin truly colorless (albino).

The epidermis is nourished by the underlying skin structures. The corium, or true skin, contains blood vessels, including the capillaries that carry nutritive materials and remove wastes. It is also supplied with a network of sensory and motor nerve fibers. In contrast to the keratin-containing epidermis, the corium is made up of bundles of fibers consisting mainly of another protein—collagen—through which run the vessels and nerves.

The sweat glands, sebaceous glands, and hair follicles originate in the epidermis and grow down into the corium. The sweat glands are of two types: (1) the *eccrine* glands, which respond to heat by secreting a dilute, salty fluid into ducts that lead up to the surface of the skin, and (2) the *apocrine* glands, which are not nearly so widely distributed and which produce a different type of fluid under the influence of emotional stress. This milky secretion is odorless when it reaches the skin surface in the axilla and elsewhere, but bacterial decomposition of its chemical constituents produces its distinctive odor.

The sebaceous glands secrete a mixture of fatty substances known as sebum which spreads out over the skin surface, after reaching it by way of the hair follicles. The face and scalp contain many of these fat-secreting glands, whereas the palms and soles contain none. Excessive skin oiliness—seborrhea—is seen most frequently on the face and scalp and to a lesser extent on the chest and upper back. Oiliness is greatest during puberty, for hormones stimulate the sebaceous glands to heightened activity. The skin of elderly people is dry, for sebaceous function fails.

PATHOLOGICAL REACTION PATTERNS OF THE SKIN

The hundreds of different dermatological ailments are caused by varied combinations of functional or structural changes in one or more of the skin elements mentioned above. All the bewildering combinations of signs and symptoms of these skin disorders are the result of relatively few kinds of reactions. These include: (1) inflammatory responses to injury, (2) acceleration, slowing, or even complete failure of a normal function, and (3) changes in the growth rate of glands and other types of cells.

Inflammatory responses to trauma of all kinds are characterized by early redness and edema. Fluid may then accumulate in the dermis to form wheals, or it may collect within the epidermis as *vesicles* (blebs) and *bullae* (blisters). Sometimes pus is trapped in these raised, thin-walled areas, and when such pustules rupture, their contents form yellowish seropurulent crusts, or scabs, over the eroded areas. Deep erosions into the dermis in the form of denuding ulcers tend to develop into small pitted scars as they heal. When even deeper damage destroys the fatty subcutaneous tissue stratum, the destroyed areas are replaced by overgrowths of fibrous connective tissue. Such scars may even become tumorlike keloids.

Abnormal growth rates of various skin elements and structures are often apparent. Sometimes, for example, the basal layer of epidermal cells develops daughter cells so rapidly that the dead cells of the stratum corneum pile up in high layers that come off in shreds, instead of just flaking off invisibly as they ordinarily do. This leads to *scaling*, or *desquamation*, a condition that varies in degree from formation of a relatively few light dandruff flakes to the disfiguring papulosquamous lesions sometimes seen in chronic psoriasis. This scaly skin debris may form dry and powdery flakes or thick, greasy plaques.

In other conditions, the outer layer of keratin-containing skin cells may be pressed into hard, horny masses, such as corns or calluses, or viruses may mysteriously set off spurts of hyperkeratotic growth, re-

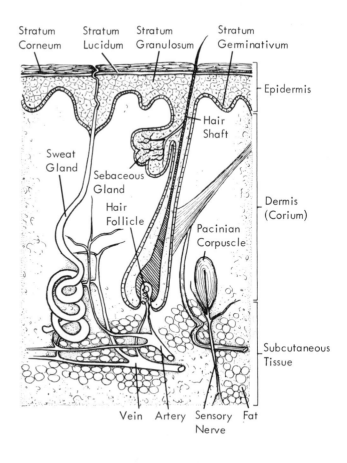

Fig. 43-1. The structure of the skin.

sulting in crops of warts. Rarely, instead of such benign tumors, the uncontrolled growth of epidermal cells leads to epitheliomata or to malignant melanoma. Fortunately, hyperfunction of the basal cell melanocytes usually takes the form of moles and freckles. Failure of function in some of these cells occasionally results in loss of skin pigment in irregular patches, a condition called vitiligo.

Increased keratin formation at the mouth of the hair follicles combined with increased outpouring of sebum by the underlying sebaceous glands can plug the pores and lead to the characteristic lesions of acne. On the other hand, these fat-secreting glands may atrophy in some circumstances. Similarly, the sweat glands often pour out excessive secretions that fail to evaporate. This then softens the skin and makes it subject to invasion by pathogenic microorganisms. In other circumstances, many of the sweat ducts become blocked, resulting in the inflammatory epidermal reactions known as "prickly heat."

TYPES OF DRUG ACTION ON THE SKIN

Many chemicals act locally when applied to the skin and produce effects that may be either beneficial or harmful. When we have studied these effects we shall be able to understand better how such drugs are employed in the treatment of skin conditions.

Broadly speaking, chemicals affect the skin in two main ways: (1) They may *cause irritation* of varying degrees. Depending upon the degree of irritation and the extent to which it is kept under control, the actions of drugs may be mild and useful for treating certain skin symptoms, or they may be destructive and cause deep scarring. (2) Chemicals may *prevent irritation* of the skin or reduce pathologic reactions to skin-damaging chemical and physical factors. Some substances of this sort mechanically cover the skin, others act to make it softer, more pliable, and less subject to excessive dryness; and agents such as the topically applied corticosteroids reduce inflammatory reactions and the discomforting itching, or even pain, that are often part of such excessive responses to skin trauma.

Local Irritants. The extent to which chemicals induce inflammatory reactions when applied to the skin usually depends on how dilute or concentrated they are. A chemical may produce only faint redness— a rubefacient effect—in low concentration, whereas stronger solutions may lead to swelling and blistering, or vesication, and finally to a caustic, or corrosive, action that kills the tissue and results in scarring. Some drugs have only limited irritating properties, even when applied to the skin in full strength.

*Keratolytic Agents.** These are the most mild skin irritants. Some, such as sulfur, tars, and ammoniated mercury, are so mild that there is even some doubt that they help to speed the rate of peeling of keratin-containing cells when they are applied in acne, seborrheic dermatitis, or psoriasis. On the other hand, the desquamating action of salicylic acid is quite clear cut when it is combined in moderately high concentrations with resorcinol or other antifungal agents for treating athlete's foot, or when its keratolytic action is used to help remove corns and calluses. In fact, in peripheral vascular diseases or diabetes self-medication with products containing such keratolytic substances is dangerous, for they are sufficiently irritating to cause skin ulcers if local circulation is poor.

Depilatories, which have somewhat stronger keratolytic action, are used for removing superfluous hair, or, occasionally, in place of shaving in preparing patients for surgical procedures. Alkaline sulfides once used for this purpose have been largely replaced by mixtures of calcium and strontium hydroxide and calcium thioglycollate. The creams and lotions containing such substances are left on the skin for a specified

---

* Literally, keratin-dissolving.

time and then removed by thorough washing to prevent irritation. Even so, some people's skin tends to redden before the hair shafts soften and dissolve. Patients who have a history of allergy are cautioned against trying out many new products of this type, or for that matter, *any* product, including even deodorants, that may contain potential skin sensitizers.

Caustics are corrosive chemicals that are sometimes carefully applied in order to destroy hyperkeratotic tissues. Substances such as glacial acetic acid, trichloroacetic acid, liquefied phenol, and podophyllum resin are sometimes used to destroy warts. Silver nitrate sticks are used on granulomatous tissues. Nitric acid has been used to cauterize animal bites when it is feared that rabies virus may have been implanted in the wound. In all such cases, care is required to see that these chemicals come in contact only with the areas to be treated. Surrounding normal tissues must be protected from contact with the caustic chemicals.

Astringents are chemicals that cause a slight protein-coagulating effect. Since the action is usually mild and the coagulum forms a protective film over the skin and mucous membrane surface, these drugs are hardly considered irritants at all. The aluminum salt solutions that are applied to oozing skin areas in poison ivy, athlete's foot, and acute eczematous states act in this way to aid in reducing inflammation. Yet other aluminum salts may cause axillary skin irritation in some persons using antiperspirant and deodorant creams containing these substances. Similarly, some zinc salts have a desirable healing action when applied in dilutions with mild astringent activity, whereas stronger solutions are dangerously irritating.

Mechanical and Physical Protectives. Many types of topically applied agents soothe the skin. They either prevent loss of moisture or keep irritating substances from coming in contact with the skin. These protective chemicals come in the form of ointments, pastes, creams, lotions, and dusting powders. Sometimes they are added to bath water so that a protective residue forms on the skin. In general, such preparations are applied sparingly, for otherwise they are both messy and wasteful.

Dusting powders, including starch, talc, and stearates of magnesium and zinc, absorb moisture as it forms on the skin and reduce rubbing between adjacent irritated skin surfaces, or soothe diaper-irritated skin. Such skin surfaces are dried before the dusting powder is applied, for caking of powder leads to further irritation. Cornstarch and magnesium oxide are the constituents of an absorbable dusting powder used to lubricate surgeon's gloves.

Protective dressings are made of layers of gauze containing petrolatum, or bandages covered with a gelatin-zinc oxide jelly. Collodion, a viscous liquid containing pyroxylin dissolved in an ether-alcohol mixture, makes a flexible protective covering for sealing small wounds. Dimethicone, a more modern water-repelling silicone oil, is sometimes used in ointment form to protect skin from external irritants such as soap, detergents, acids, and alkalis. It may also help to prevent diaper rash, bed sores, and chapping.

Emollients are oily or fatty substances that are applied to the skin to keep it soft and to prevent or counteract dryness. Among the most important emollients are petrolatum and lanolin, substances that form the basis for many ointment bases that serve as vehicles for other soothing agents. These substances are most useful when applied to dry, cracked skin, especially on the hands and feet. Other nongreasy ointments, such as hydrophilic ointment, are preferred for application to hairy areas. Pastes are not suited for hairy sites but are most useful for soothing subacute skin lesions, as are emulsion creams.

Corticosteroid drugs, which have proved valuable for relieving symptoms stemming from skin inflammation, have become an important part of dermatologic therapy. About half the prescriptions that doctors write for treating skin disorders contain these drugs, and patients often require advice about them. Patients with atopic dermatitis, for example, who often have to apply large quantities of topical steroid preparations for long periods, may express concern about possible toxicity. The nurse can assure these persons that steroids are safe when applied topically, for little is absorbed into the systemic circulation from the types of products ordinarily used.

Many different types of vehicles are employed for delivering topical steroids. Cream-based steroids are preferred for reducing redness, swelling, and oozing from the denuded epidermis. Lotions containing steroids counteract inflammation and itching in hairy areas and on the face. Greasy ointment bases are not used on hairy areas and are mainly reserved for dry, scaly lesions, such as those of psoriasis. In psoriasis, steroids are frequently applied under airtight dressings, in order to promote deeper penetration of these drugs. Even in such cases, systemic absorption and subsequent development of hypercorticism is unlikely.

THE TREATMENT OF SPECIFIC SKIN DISORDERS

Acne

Acne is one of the most common of all skin disorders. An estimated 80 to 90 per cent of all adolescents are affected to some extent. Many youngsters need no special treatment besides faithful use of simple hygienic measures for cleansing the skin. Other teen-agers cannot control the spread of acne by ordinary skin-care measures. They should be urged to seek medical attention rather than use the products widely advertised for self-medication. Severe, uncontrolled acne causes scarring, which may adversely affect the emotional health and developing personality structure in young people.

The lesions of acne develop at puberty and during adolescence as the result of hormone-induced changes in the skin of people predisposed to react adversely to such stimulation. Androgens secreted by the sex and adrenal glands stimulate the sebaceous glands to increase in size, and to increase the production of sebum. Such fatty secretions are kept from reaching the skin surface by excessive numbers of keratin-containing cells around the outlet of the follicle. Blockage of the opening and narrowing of the follicular passageway by sloughed off epithelial cells causes the backed-up sebum to change in physical consistency and chemical composition.

Plugs of cellular debris containing keratin, trapped bacteria, and hardened sebum are called comedones, or, more commonly, "blackheads" and "whiteheads." Closed comedones blocking follicular openings act like foreign bodies to provoke inflammatory reactions which often lead to the formation of pustules and—in severe cases—cysts or deep abscesses. Crops of recurrent pustules are, of course, psychologically distressing, and cystic destruction in the dermis or corium can eventually cause extensive skin scarring.

Topical treatment of acne is aimed mainly at keeping the pores open by eliminating comedones. Attempts are made to control skin bacteria by scrupulous cleanliness. In many mild cases, cleansing the skin well with hot, soapy water keeps the condition under control. Soaps and detergent liquids containing *hexachlorophene* (see Drug Digest) keep the cutaneous bacterial count at a low level. Gentle washing tends to remove sebum and keratin from the skin surface. It may be followed by the application of alcohol, which has desirable antiseptic and drying actions.

More persistent acneform eruptions are treated with preparations containing keratolytic agents that speed drying and desquamation (scaling) of the superficial skin layers. Sulfur and resorcinol (see Drug Digest) are the most popular peeling agents employed in acne preparations. Low concentrations of these chemicals help to reduce sebaceous oiliness and to remove keratin plugs when applied as lotions and creams. These products are usually skin colored for cosmetic purposes.

Pustular and cystic acne often must be treated with more potent products. A time-honored remedy is *Vleminckx' solution,* a sulfurated lime solution which is applied in the form of hot compresses for 10 or 15 minutes once or twice daily. If the dermatologist desires even more vigorous desquamation, he may employ a mixture of *carbon dioxide ("dry") ice* crushed into a slush with a small quantity of acetone. This material is brushed over the eruption once a week and then washed off. The degree of desquamation that develops depends on how long the medication is kept in contact with the skin.

Systemic treatment of severe acne involves mainly the administration of antibiotics such as the *tetracyclines* and *erythromycin* and of hormones of the estrogenic type. The use of vitamins in large doses, especially *vitamin A,* is often advocated, but results are not impressive. Systemic *corticosteroids* are sometimes desirable anti-inflammatory agents, but these potentially dangerous drugs have reportedly caused acne to flare up.

Antibiotics were originally administered in full therapeutic doses—for example, 1 Gm. of tetracycline daily—to control pustular and cystic forms of acne. It has been suggested that maintenance therapy with much smaller amounts—as low as 250 mg. daily—may control the condition, and is safer for the patient. The rationale for such therapy is that once secondary infections by pathogens such as staphylococci are controlled, low daily doses of the antibiotics can suppress other, more susceptible skin bacteria.

Although the latter are not true pathogens, they are thought to play an indirect role in causing acne inflammation. These bacterial skin residents tend to become trapped in the cellular debris blocking the follicles. They then exert an enzymatic action that converts the bland sebaceous fats of the plug into free fatty acids. Such fatty acids, including propionic acid, irritate the dermis, which then responds with a typical inflammatory reaction. Thus, when low doses of broad-spectrum antibiotics suppress these seemingly harmless skin dwellers, one of the main factors responsible for formation of acne lesions is removed.

Estrogen therapy antagonizes the stimulating effect of androgenic hormones upon sebaceous gland secretion. The doses that are required to do so cannot be given to boys without running the risk of causing feminizing effects. The female hormones do, however, sometimes control severe acne in girls without producing adverse effects, except for occasional menstrual irregularities. It has been suggested that even this side effect can be eliminated by combining the estrogens with progestins. Thus, some of the same formulations that are employed as oral contraceptives are occasionally prescribed for acne in young women, because progestin administration and withdrawal regularizes the menstrual cycle.

Psoriasis

Psoriasis is a chronic skin eruption of the papulosquamous type. That is, its characteristic lesions are reddish papules, or raised areas, that are covered by dry, silvery scales, or squamae. Although this condition often seems to respond readily to treatment, the lesions almost inevitably tend to recur.

Topical Treatment. Though psoriasis is usually a lifetime disease, it can be controlled for long periods in most cases by the judicious use of topical therapy, which involves the application of various substances that are mildly or strongly irritating. These are thought to slow down the rapid production of epidermal cells and thus to reduce psoriatic scaling. Some of these substances are said to stimulate healing of the underlying papular lesion. It is customary for dermatologists to begin therapy with mild preparations such as ammoniated mercury ointment (see Drug Digest) and then to add to it certain more irritating substances such as salicylic acid and coal tar, if the scaly lesions fail to clear up.

The plant-derived exfoliative principle chrysarobin has been largely replaced in recent years by a synthetic skin irritant, anthralin, which is said to be a safer antipsoriatic agent and less likely to stain the skin and clothing. Another antipsoriatic substance, allantoin, is claimed to both break down the keratin of scaly psoriatic lesions and help restore the skin beneath to a healthy condition.

The *acute stages* of psoriasis may be made worse by smearing the rapidly spreading eruption with these traditional irritating coal tar–keratolytic combinations. Instead the doctor orders skin-soothing emollient baths followed by frequently applied lubricant ointments. This treatment keeps the skin hydrated and softened, while potent systemically acting agents are being administered in an attempt to control the condition.

Systemic therapy of psoriasis includes the use of antimetabolites, such as the folic acid antagonists, which have otherwise been used only in neoplastic diseases. The antifolic drugs *aminopterin* and *methotrexate* (see Drug Digest) have been used in relatively small doses (compared to those used in leukemia) in efforts to reduce the rapid rate at which the skin cells are reproducing and forming scales in acute psoriasis. Unfortunately, even when carefully administered in low doses and for short courses, these potent drugs sometimes cause dangerous toxic reactions that make it necessary to discontinue treatment.

Corticosteroid Therapy. *Systemic* corticosteroid therapy is sometimes employed to control extensively spreading acute psoriasis. The high doses that are required often cause hypercorticism, and when the steroids are finally withdrawn, the condition may become worse than before. Continued use of corticosteroids in a chronic condition such as psoriasis is undesirable. Though the use of long-term steroids to control skin symptoms may be justified in potentially fatal conditions such as pemphigus and disseminated lupus, psoriasis is, after all, essentially benign and never fatal.

Steroids are applied *topically* to psoriatic lesions in new ways which often produce remissions. Whereas merely massaging steroid creams into psoriatic plaques had proved relatively ineffective, the new methods of administration seem to deliver large local quantities of the drugs down into the deeper layers of the skin. These more successful methods of administration involve: (1) the use of occlusive dressings and (2) intralesional injections.

Occlusive dressings made of polyethylene plastic film—for example, Saran Wrap or Handiwrap—are wrapped around the parts to which the topical steroids have been lightly applied at bedtime or after a morning bath, and the edges are taped down. This keeps moisture from evaporating and raises the temperature of the skin. The resultant softening of the scaly layers permits the steroid to penetrate deeply in large amounts overnight or during an eight-hour daytime application. Remarkable remissions have been reported after courses of this type of treatment, but the lesions usually return before long, after it is discontinued.

Intralesional injection of corticosteroids, such as triamcinolone acetonide (see Drug Digest), reportedly produces long-lasting remissions. Suspensions of such steroids (Table 43-1) infiltrated into unsightly psoriatic lesions at monthly intervals often eliminate unsightly plaques on the patient's arms, legs, and body. Since steroids are not systemically absorbed from these superficial injection sites, hypercorticism has not occurred. However, the high local concentrations of corticosteroids have sometimes caused shrinkage of the skin tissues at the injection site. Such pseudoatrophy is itself disfiguring but is only temporary.

Dermatitis

Dermatitis is a general term that is used for all the varied dermatologic disorders in which inflammation occurs during the course of the condition. An inflammatory reaction, ranging from mild to severe, is the characteristic response of the epidermis to damage by chemical and mechanical irritation or by heat. Such injuries may cause skin changes ranging from only slight erythema, or redness, through formation of massive bullae, or blisters, with deep destruction in the underlying dermal layer. Usually, these changes are temporary. If the patient does not scratch and rub the itchy areas or pick at the protective crusts that form over oozing blebs or blisters, the inflamed skin ordinarily heals completely.

The general purpose of all types of treatment of dermatitis is to aid the natural recovery mechanisms. Dermatoses of quite different causes and with varied clinical courses are treated with many of the same types of topically applied agents, because the acute, subacute, or chronic stages of all types of dermatitis are essentially the same. Thus, the same drugs may be used to relieve itching, dry up oozing areas, or soothe and protect excessively dry, cracked skin, no matter what type of dermatitis is encountered. In the following discussions of the treatment of several representative dermatoses, the manner of use of the most important types of dermatologic therapeutic agents is illustrated by examples.

Seborrheic dermatitis is one of the least severe dermatoses ordinarily. In its mildest forms—ordinary dandruff, for example—hardly any inflammation is detectable. Instead, the main sign is an excessive scaliness of the scalp and of the skin around the ears, eyes, and nose. Such scales usually differ clearly from those of psoriasis, being greasy and yellowish rather than dry and silvery. Although the condition is never severely disabling (unless complicated by secondary infections), seborrheic itching is often annoying and the unsightly scaling is sometimes embarrassing.

The more severe forms of chronic seborrheic dermatitis are often treated with the same sort of irritant-keratolytic combinations that are employed against psoriatic scaliness. Thus antiseborrheic ointments containing coal tar, precipitated sulfur, resorcinol, and salicylic acid are often rubbed into the scalp at bedtime and kept on overnight. The head is shampooed on the following morning. When such substances are used in lotion form, care is required to keep them from running into the eyes and ears.

Ordinary soap and water or commercial cosmetic shampoos may be used for washing the head. Often, however, if the scales recur too promptly, special medicated shampoos are used. One of the most popular of these is selenium sulfide detergent suspension (see Drug Digest). Selenium is similar to arsenic in toxicity when taken internally, and may irritate the eyes and sometimes increases the oiliness of the hair. Another antiseborrheic substance, cadmium sulfide, is available as a shampoo that is claimed not to cause systemic toxicity, nor conjunctivitis or contact dermatitis.

Acute contact dermatitis results from exposure of the skin to chemical substances that elicit inflammatory responses. The reaction may range from a slight redness and itching to severe swelling and blistering of the skin. The chemical cause may be either a primary irritant or a substance to which a particular individual has become allergic through prior exposure and sensitization. Although almost any chemical can cause allergic contact dermatitis, some substances are relatively stronger sensitizers than others.

One of the most familiar skin sensitizers in this country is the plant we call "poison ivy." Like its relatives of the *Rhus* genus, poison oak and poison sumac, it contains a sensitizing oil, called urushiol, to which most Americans react positively in skin tests. Exposure of the skin to this allergen leads to a dermatitis marked by development of groups or lines of vesicles containing serous fluid.

Contrary to what is commonly supposed, the fluid from broken blebs is not a source of further quantities of allergen. Although the original allergen that was picked up on the fingers from contact with the plant itself may be quickly spread to parts of the body that the person touches or scratches, lesions that appear late in an attack of poison ivy may result from further exposure to the plant or may simply have developed more slowly on account of local differences in the susceptibility of the skin.

Topical treatment is aimed primarily at relieving itching and thus stopping the urge to scratch. Scratching is undesirable, *not* because it "spreads the poison," but because pathogenic bacteria may enter breaks made in the skin by the fingernails. The secondary bacterial infections that often follow such scratching tend to keep the skin from recovering its normal state of health.

In addition to antipruritic action, topically applied medications help the skin to heal itself. *Soaks, compresses, and lotions* encourage drying and crusting of the oozing areas in the acute stages of contact dermatitis. When applied to weeping blebs and blisters, substances such as aluminum acetate solution and dilute potassium permanganate solution (see Drug Digests) tend to stop further flow of serous fluid. Such solutions are applied for about 20 minutes, and then the area is daubed with a drying lotion that is shaken before use. The thin layer of skin protectant, such as zinc oxide, that is left on the denuded areas soothes the skin and relieves itching. The addition of phenol, menthol, or camphor to calamine lotions (see Drug Digest) adds to the antipruritic action of such preparations. In the later stages, when the skin may be dry and cracked, the doctor may switch to calamine ointment or some other greasy emollient substance.

Steroids. Topical steroid application is not very useful until the acute stage has subsided. Steroids do not penetrate the epithelium of vesicles and bullae, and when such blisters break, the flow of serous fluid simply washes away the drug. Later, however, when applied in the periods between wet dressings, creams containing hydrocortisone or other steroids sometimes help to relieve inflammatory itching. However, topically applied steroids are not as necessary here as in other pruritic dermatoses, and may be too expensive to use if the eruption covers large areas of the body.

Systemic steroids are preferred in extensive and severe contact dermatitis. Large doses of these drugs, administered immediately and then rapidly reduced and finally withdrawn over a period of several days or a week, are indicated in the management of acute, self-limited conditions such as poison ivy. This type of steroid treatment is relatively safe, as it does not lead to hypercorticism or significantly depress adrenal cortical function, as is inevitably the case in more chronic conditions (Chap. 28).

Antihistamine drugs taken by mouth are not considered very useful in acute contact dermatitis. Even though this condition is often brought about by an antigen-antibody reaction, the skin changes do not result from release of substances such as histamine, serotonin, or acetylcholine—the agents that are antagonized by antihistamine drugs (Chap. 40). Except when secondary urticarial reactions develop, a histamine-blocking effect in the peripheral tissues is not needed. On the other hand, the sedative side effects of certain antihistamine agents (Table 40-1) may make the patient less aware of itching.

Topical application of creams containing antihistamine drugs that act as local anesthetics on open skin lesions sometimes helps to relieve *Rhus* dermatitis itching. However, these antipruritic drugs, including tripelennamine (see Drug Digest), may themselves be sensitizing and thus cause contact dermatitis. The risk of such sensitization probably increases when products containing antihistamine agents combined with skin protectants such as zirconium oxide are applied regularly for prophylaxis against contact with *Rhus* plants.

Protection against further exposure is essential for recovery from an attack of contact dermatitis. Although creams containing certain chemicals, such as silicone oils (dimethicone), are claimed to offer some protection from contact irritants, elimination of the offending substance from the environment is a more sure measure. Persons with poison ivy should stay away from fields, garden, or woods; if they do expose themselves, the skin should be washed repeatedly with a strongly alkaline soap solution followed by rinsing with alcohol.

Atopic dermatitis is a chronic skin condition that often appears in infancy and lasts through childhood into adult life. Like other chronic dermatoses that are often lumped under the vague term "eczema," its basic cause is not known. There are indications that a predisposition to these skin lesions is inherited. Often the patient or members of his family suffer from hay fever, asthma, or a tendency toward urticarial reactions. Allergy is not always present, however. Similarly, although many patients with this condition seem to have psychological problems, it is not certain that psychic factors always play a part.

The lesions of this disorder do, however, seem to be the result of one primary condition—a skin that is extremely sensitive to stimuli that are interpreted as itchiness. Apparently, either the sensory nerve network in the skin of these patients is excessively reactive, or their psychic make-up is such as to make them highly sensitive to afferent impulses of low intensity. In any case, slight sensations originating in the skin seem to be amplified and felt as pruritus, and this, in turn, sets off bouts of scratching.

Scratching the skin with the nails seems to help suppress itching by substituting a stronger stimulus that breaks up the pattern of itch impulses traveling up to the brain. However, scratching gives only temporary relief, and may even increase the hyperexcitability of the skin by setting free certain itch-producing proteolytic enzymes. Just how these protein-splitting enzymes precipitate itching is not well understood. They may act directly on the subepidermal receptors or indirectly by releasing an itch-provoking agent from the protein of epidermal skin cells. In either case, patients with atopic dermatitis seem to be victims of an itch-scratch-itch cycle that subjects their skin to physical damage and secondary bacterial infections.

Treatment of atopic dermatitis is based on the need to relieve itching and inflammation by means of topical and systemic medication. The most effective agents are topical corticosteroids in creams, lotions, or ointments. Hydrocortisone is the least expensive of these compounds, but triamcinolone acetonide (see Drug Digest) and other new synthetic steroids such as betamethasone valerate, fluocinoline and flurandrenolone (Table 43-1) are much more potent. All are equally free of primary irritancy or of any tendency to produce sensitization.

Sometimes local anesthetic creams are employed to relieve itching, burning, and pain stemming from lesions of the skin and mucous membranes. Substances such as cyclomethycaine, lidocaine, pramoxine, and dimethisoquin (Table 11-2) often provide relief by deadening sensory nerve endings in abraded skin. However, dermatologists do not advise the routine use of these drugs for long periods in patients with a definite history of allergy, for they are likely to become sensitized to them.

Claims are often made that such sensitization is unlikely with a particular product, because it differs chemically from benzocaine, a well-known sensitizer, or because it is a so-called "non-caine" anesthetic. Actually, patients whose skins are predisposed to react to chemicals tend to develop allergic-type reactions to almost anything that is smeared on the skin often enough. Thus, if any of these drugs are employed as antipruritics, including the antihistamine agents with local anesthetic properties, the patient's skin should be carefully watched for signs of allergic reactions.

Antihistamine drugs administered by mouth are considered more useful for relieving pruritus in atopic dermatitis than in contact dermatitis. This may stem, in part, from their ability to block histamine, serotonin, and other chemicals released in the tissues by antigen-antibody reactions, in much the manner that antihistamine drugs act in urticaria. On the other hand, the role of allergy in atopic dermatitis is not always clear. Relief of pruritus by antihistamine drugs may be centrally mediated, much as is the drowsiness that often accompanies their use.

In this regard, two antihistamine agents effective against itching—*methdilazine* and *trimeprazine*—are phenothiazine compounds with probable tranquilizing properties similar to those of the related drugs that are employed in emotional and mental disorders (Chap. 7). Thus, their effectiveness against pruritus in atopic dermatitis may stem from the ability to reduce the patient's perception of itch stimuli and lessen his emotional reaction to the kinds of psychologically stressful situations that tend to precipitate itching and scratching in a tense person. This may also account for the antipruritic activity of a minor tranquilizer such as *hydroxyzine* (Chap. 7), which also possesses antihistaminic and anticholinergic properties, and of *cyproheptadine* (see Drug Digest), a central depressant that also has potent histamine and serotonin antagonizing peripheral effects.

PREVENTION AND TREATMENT OF SKIN INFECTION

Many products containing antiseptic chemicals are available for topical application to the skin and mucous membranes to prevent infection or, at least, limit its spread. Most commercial antiseptic products that are offered to the public for daubing at cuts have little value. On the other hand, the proper use of skin antiseptics by medical personnel is an important part of patient care.

Most skin scratches and abrasions are best dealt with by washing the skin around the wound with soap and water, drying gently with a clear towel or tissue, and, perhaps, covering the area with a simple dressing to keep out dirt and lessen local irritation. Such simple measures help the healthy skin's own natural defenses. Strong antiseptic solutions may injure healthy tissues and interfere with the body's own ways for keeping pathogenic organisms from becoming established in a break in the skin.

Most species of microorganisms among the transients that are always pouring onto the skin from the surrounding air do not survive for long. The outer layer of skin cells is low in moisture and relatively high in organic acids. This apparently offers a hostile environment in which bacteria quickly dry out and die. Some species can survive and colonize in the skin. These residents then apparently prevent colonization by other species, including potential pathogenic invaders.

Skin Cleansing and Disinfection

Many factors lower the skin's resistance to bacterial invasion. When the host's defenses are weakened by injury or disease, even ordinarily harmless residents of the skin's bacterial flora can become pathogenic. Such opportunistic microbial infections are especially common in patients with leukemia, diabetes, and various debilitating diseases. Patients taking high doses of corticosteroid drugs or broad-spectrum antibiotics for long-term treatment of chronic ailments are also subject to superinfections.

The surgical patient is, of course, exposed to an unusual risk of infection. Wound infections following surgery cannot be eliminated entirely. Even if bacterial contamination from the environment could be entirely prevented, the effects of anesthesia, trauma, and other factors that shock the system and upset normal biochemical balances would so lower the tissues' defenses that organisms already present could become invasive. This should not discourage efforts to keep contaminating skin bacteria to a minimum; rather, it should spur greater effort in that direction.

Surgical Scrubbing. Recent evidence reconfirms what has been known since the time of Lister in the last century: the development of postoperative skin infections is much less likely when every effort is made to reduce the numbers of microorganisms on the skin in the area of the surgical incision and on the hands of attending medical personnel. Surgical scrubbing is performed in many different ways and with the use of a wide variety of antiseptic chemicals. We can discuss here only certain widely used substances and how these are best employed for full effectiveness and safety.

Scrubbing the skin of the hands with soap and water and long-continued, vigorous friction for relatively prolonged periods is a standard preliminary procedure. Soap has little effect as an antibacterial agent, but as a detergent it removes such skin debris as keratin and natural fats. At the same time most of the contaminating bacteria contained in such surface substances is removed. Soaps and certain synthetic anionic surfactants, or "wetting agents," permit water to penetrate better and thus help to float out some of the flora that reside deep in the crypts, crevices, pits, and ridges of the skin.

Alcohols, such as ethyl and isopropyl alcohols, are often used to rinse residual soap from the skin. Both can kill bacteria but not their spores. For best results, a 70 per cent concentration by weight of ethyl alcohol is recommended, whereas isopropyl alcohol is used full strength. The longer these alcohols are in contact with the skin, the greater the germicidal effect. However, even briefly swabbing the skin with an alcohol-soaked cotton sponge just before inserting a hypodermic needle has some utility. This is because the solvent action of alcohol on the sebaceous secretions helps to clean the skin of surface bacteria.

The cleaning, drying, and hardening actions of alcohol may account for its ability to prevent bed sores in some patients prone to decubital ulceration. However, emollients are preferred if the skin is dry and may be irritated and become fissured from alcohol rubs. Alcohol rubs, of course, have other desirable effects. When massaged into the skin, alcohol is mildly irritating and aids the local flow of blood, as is seen in the increased redness of the skin surface. Such rubefacient and counterirritant activity often helps to relieve muscle aches and pains in a manner that may be more a psychological response than the result of the

vasodilation itself. In addition, alcohol sponging is a desirable way to remove heat from the body surface by evaporation and thus temporarily reduce the body temperature of feverish patients.

Hexachlorophene and benzalkonium chloride (see Drug Digests) are among the many substances used for disinfecting the patient's skin and the surgeon's hands preoperatively. The latter agent, like other quaternary ammonium compounds (Table 43-2), has valuable detergent and keratolytic properties in addition to its antiseptic action. However, it is important to remember that the antibacterial action of these *cationic* substances is almost completely neutralized by the presence on the skin of even small traces of soaps, which are *anionic* in nature. The surgical field is rinsed thoroughly with water and then is swabbed with alcohol before benzalkonium or other cationic detergent antiseptics are applied.

Hexachlorophene can be combined with soaps without losing its antiseptic activity. When a liquid or solid soap or a detergent cream or suspension containing this phenolic chemical is used routinely as a hand antiseptic, the bacterial skin population is reduced well below normal. Patients may be instructed to wash the area to be operated on several times daily for four days to a week before surgery. Such home scrubs with hexachlorophene-containing products are also recommended after surgery and for families infected by staphylococcal organisms. In such situations, patients should be told *not* to rinse the skin with alcohol, for this removes from the skin the hexachlorophene film that is being built up by the daily washings.

Although such soaps containing hexachlorophene, trichlorocarbanilide, or other antiseptic additives may have been used preoperatively by the patient in this manner, it is still necessary to apply strong antiseptic solutions in preparing the operative site just prior to surgery. Rapid-acting chemicals that kill microbes, rather than merely suppress their growth, are required. Such skin disinfectants must not cause primary irritation or be strong sensitizers.

Iodine dissolved in diluted alcohol, which was introduced for use in preoperative skin preparation at the end of the last century, is widely used in preoperative preparation (see Drug Digest). The modern Tincture of Iodine irritates the skin less than the strong solutions that were previously employed. The iodine-stained skin site is swabbed with alcohol before the operative area is draped, for residual iodine may damage the epidermis. Some individuals are sensitive to even small amounts of iodine and severe skin reactions may result.

Recently, iodine has been combined with various organic substances to form complexes that release elemental iodine when in contact with the skin. These so-called *iodophors* are free enough of the irritating properties of iodine to be safely used on mucous membranes as well as on skin. However, their effectiveness for preoperative preparation of the skin is controversial. Some reports state that solutions of elemental iodine in alcohol are far superior to iodophors such as undecoylium chloride-iodine (Virac) or povidone iodine (see Drug Digest); others claim that povidone iodine is more effective for surgical scrubbing than the older, more widely used agents.

Topical application of even the most modern chemical antiseptics is not desirable for *treating infected wounds.* Such substances are usually inactivated by contact with serum and pus in suppurating wounds. The antibiotics of the bacitracin, tyrothricin, neomycin type (Chap. 34), which are not broken down in this way, are preferred. However, *systemic* administration of properly selected antibiotics is considered the best medical measure. Surgical drainage, removal of foreign bodies, and debridement of dead tissues are also, of course, essential to avoid development of infection in wounds incurred as a result of violence.

Bacterial skin infections may occur if the underlying areas are invaded through the follicles or by way of breaks in the skin. More than 90 per cent of infections are caused by gram-positive organisms (staphylococci and streptococci). The rest are the result of the pathogenic activity of gram-negative rods, such as pseudomonas, which invade moist areas when local or systemic skin defenses are weakened.

The pus-provoking gram-positive organisms cause various primary or secondary pyodermas, such as impetigo, ecthyma, folliculitis, and furunculosis (boils). Boils are best allowed to localize with the aid of hot compresses or soaks. After they have "pointed" and have been incised and drained by the doctor, the skin is kept clean with alcohol swabs and is washed with hexachlorophene preparations to minimize further spread of infection. Systemic and topical antibiotic therapy is usually reserved for cases of recurrent furuncles and carbuncles.

Antibiotic therapy has, however, helped to reduce the seriousness of cellulitis and to make control of impetigo-type infections easier. In severe cellulitic infections, such as erysipelas, a diffusely spreading inflammatory skin infection caused by streptococci, penicillin injections have, for example, improved the formerly grave prognosis. Impetigo and folliculitis respond readily to topical treatment with ointments containing bacitracin, polymyxin, and neomycin (Chap. 34).

Prevention of infection by the routine application of these antibiotics is ordinarily not considered desirable, because such use may encourage emergence of resistant bacterial strains or cause allergic sensitization. The various chemical disinfectants long used to prevent and control superficial infections of the skin and mucous membranes are, in general, either too weak to be effective or so strong as to be potentially harmful to the tissues.

Some *mercury compounds,* for example, are too irritating to be used on tissues, whereas others are too mild to be useful. Mercury bichloride is best reserved for disinfecting inanimate objects. On the other hand, organic mercurials such as merbromin (Mercurochrome)—which, when applied to broken skin, stain the tissues brilliant red—are relatively inactive and lack penetrating power. Certain insoluble mercurial compounds, such as the yellow oxide of mercury and ammoniated mercury (see Drug Digest), are used in ointment form for special purposes. The small amounts of active mercury that are slowly released are, at least, relatively harmless, and may be slightly antiseptic.

Silver salts, on the other hand, are highly germicidal in relatively low concentrations. Silver nitrate (see Drug Digest) in a 1 per cent solution prevents gonorrheal infections of the eyes of newborn infants by wiping out organisms that may have been acquired during birth. While it is certainly effective for this purpose, silver nitrate itself may irritate the ocular tissues in this concentration. For this reason, various authorities advocate replacing it for routine use by antibiotics, such as penicillin or erythromycin or by the sulfonamide sulfacetamide (see Drug Digest). However, the use of silver nitrate solutions has long been codified in state laws which will probably not yield readily to the march of medical progress.

Boric acid (see Drug Digest) is also widely used by force of tradition rather than proved effectiveness. It presumably does no harm, at least when applied to skin and mucous membranes in adequate dilutions. Yet its use in solutions for self-application to the eyes may keep a person from seeking proper medical care and even serve as a means of spreading infection. Similarly, as one ingredient of a talcum-based dusting powder for babies' skin, boric acid is harmless. However, the continued application of *full strength* boric acid powder to abraded skin surfaces in treating diaper rash has led to absorption of toxic quantities and caused deaths.

Substances such as *phenol* (carbolic acid) and *formaldehyde* have little place in modern skin antisepsis. Phenol, the disinfectant first employed by Lister, long served as the standard by which other germicides were measured. However, it is too irritating to human tissues when used in germicidal concentrations. Phenol and formaldehyde are best reserved for disinfecting inanimate objects, and are used on the skin only in dilute solutions intended for other purposes. Thus, as indicated elsewhere, formaldehyde is sometimes used as a foot soak for reducing sweating, and low concentrations of phenol (1% or less) are added to skin lotions to relieve itching. Full strength phenol solutions are occasionally used for cauterizing wounds.

Fungal infections of the skin, or dermatophytoses, are caused by organisms whose enzyme systems can digest the keratin of the stratum corneum and of the hair and nails, also. As they burrow into the epidermis, such ringworm fungi cause characteristic itchy lesions in various areas, including the scalp (tinea capitis), the feet (tinea pedis), the groin (tinea cruris).

The availability of griseofulvin (see Drug Digest) has made control of these conditions much easier. Taken by mouth, this antifungal antibiotic effectively overcomes fungal infections which were once marked by prolonged chronicity and frequent recurrences. Tineal infections tend to recur in susceptible individuals, some time after they stop taking griseofulvin. Thus, they should use dusting powders and other topical measures to keep the skin of interdigital and intertriginous areas dry and relatively free of fungi.

Since sweating of the feet favors the spread of athlete's foot, formaldehyde solution soaks are sometimes ordered to reduce perspiration. Elsewhere on the body, "antiperspirant" creams containing aluminum compounds are applied in attempts to reduce the flow of fluids from the sweat glands. Actually, such metallic salts act mainly as deodorants, by reducing the number of local bacterial organisms whose action makes sweat odorous. Thus, in severe hyperhidrosis that leads to softening of the skin and aids fungal invasiveness, the doctor may prescribe an atropine-type anhidrotic drug (Chap. 17).

Other topical treatments for fungal infections involve combinations of chemicals that act in various ways to relieve symptoms and to attack superficial skin fungi (Table 43-2). Carbol-fuchsin solution (see Drug Digest), for example, combines several agents that relieve pruritus, dry the area, and directly stop further fungal growth. Whitfield's ointment is a classic combination of keratolytic salicylic acid with benzoic acid, an antifungal agent that reaches the microorganisms more readily as a result of the other chemical's keratin-softening action. Less irritating than the latter are certain antifungal fatty acids including undecylenic acid and its salts, and caprylic and propionic acid compounds (Table 43-2).

Sometimes the skin is invaded by fungi that do not respond to treatment with griseofulvin—for example, *Candida albicans* infections and tinea versicolor. Fortunately, other antifungal drugs are available. The antifungal antibiotics (Chap. 34), for example, are applied topically to the skin to control candidal infections. (See Drug Digests for nystatin and for amphotericin B.) A new chemical, acrisorcin (Akrinol), is claimed to control tinea versicolor, a condition in which the skin becomes covered with spots of varied color, including depigmented areas that fail to tan.

Vaginal infections by fungal, bacterial, and protozoal organisms can be controlled by a variety of new drugs that are applied topically or administered by mouth. Vaginal candidiasis, a fungal infection sometimes seen during pregnancy or after broad-spectrum antibiotic therapy, was, for example, traditionally treated with applications of gentian violet solution, which was often effective but somewhat messy. A new antibiotic, *candicidin,* with an antifungal spectrum similar to that of nystatin and amphotericin, is claimed to bring about cures in close to 100 per cent of cases. It is administered in the form of vaginal tablets during a 14-day course of therapy.

Infections caused by the protozoan parasite *Trichomonas vaginalis* are controlled effectively by a trichomonadicidal drug. Since its introduction in 1963, this agent, metronidazole (Flagyl), has completely changed the outlook in this distressing condition. Taken by mouth in a 10-day course, the drug is carried by the blood stream to areas not accessible to the previously available drugs that had to be applied topically. Thus, it eradicates reservoirs of the organisms which once could not be reached. The source of reinfection—the male partner—can also be treated with oral tablets.

Despite early fears, metronidazole seems to be safe. Side effects are few and minor, i.e., anorexia and an unpleasant taste. Although the drug is transported through the placenta, there are no reports of fetal damage. However, some doctors prescribe the drug in vaginal tablet form in the first trimester of pregnancy. Topical therapy alone is less effective than when the drug is given by mouth at the same time.

As is the case in skin infections, measures that reinforce the body's own defense mechanisms are desirable adjuncts to the antimicrobial therapy of vaginitis. For example, the doctor orders mildly acid douches if the vaginal secretions are approaching alkalinity. A relatively high pH favors the growth of the flagellated parasite of trichomoniasis and of the fungal organism that causes mycotic vulvovaginitis. Similarly, in the treatment of nonspecific bacterial infections, it is often considered desirable to strengthen the vaginal mucosal defenses by administering another agent besides the topically applied sulfonamide antibacterial drugs commonly employed. Vaginal suppositories containing estrogenic substances are inserted, in order to bring about hormone-induced thickening of the mucosa as well as other local changes in postmenopausal (senile) and prepubertal vaginitis.

Parasitic infestations by mites and lice lead to itching and to scratching that often results in secondary skin infections which cause oozing and crusting of the skin and scalp. These conditions—scabies and pediculosis—occur when people live under conditions of crowding and particularly when they have little or no opportunity or desire to bathe. Alcoholics on skid row, for instance, sometimes suffer from scabies and lousi-

TABLE 43-1

CLASSES OF DRUGS THAT ACT LOCALLY ON THE SKIN OR MUCOUS MEMBRANES

Local Irritants

Keratolytics; Antieczematic; Antipsoriatic; Antiseborrheics

Allantoin; Anthralin N.F.; Cadmium sulfide; Chrysarobin; Ichthammol N.F.; Resorcinol U.S.P.; Resorcinol monoacetate N.F.; Salicylic acid U.S.P.; Selenium sulfide U.S.P.; Sulfur sublimed N.F.; Sulfurated lime solution N.F.; Tar, coal U.S.P.

Depilatories

Alkaline sulfides; Calcium hydroxide; Calcium thioglycollate; Strontium hydroxide.

Caustics

Acetic acid, glacial; Nitric acid, concentrated; Phenol, liquefied U.S.P.; Podophyllum resin U.S.P.; Silver nitrate, toughened U.S.P.; Trichloroacetic acid U.S.P.

Astringents and Antiperspirants

Alum N.F.; Exsiccated alum N.F.; Aluminum acetate solution U.S.P.; Aluminum chloride N.F.; Aluminum subacetate solution U.S.P.; Calcium hydroxide U.S.P.; Formaldehyde solution U.S.P.; Tannic acid N.F.; Zinc chloride U.S.P.; Zinc oxide paste with salicylic acid N.F.; Zinc sulfate U.S.P.

Counterirritants

Camphor liniment N.F.; Camphor and soap liniment N.F.; Chloroform liniment N.F.; Methyl salicylate U.S.P.

Local Agents That Counteract Irritation and Inflammation

Emollients and Demulcents

Acacia U.S.P.; Acacia mucilage N.F.; Acacia syrup N.F.; Cold cream U.S.P.; Glycerin U.S.P.; Glycyrrhiza elixir N.F.; Glycyrrhiza fluidextract & syrup U.S.P.; Lanolin U.S.P.; Lanolin anhydrous U.S.P.; Olive oil U.S.P.; Paraffin N.F.; Petrolatum N.F.; Petrolatum, hydrophilic U.S.P.; Petrolatum, liquid U.S.P.; Petrolatum white U.S.P.; Rose water ointment N.F.; Starch glycerite N.F.; White ointment U.S.P.; Yellow ointment N.F.

Protectants; Adsorbents; Dusting Powders

Absorbable dusting powder U.S.P.; Aluminum U.S.P.; Aluminum paste U.S.P.; Benzoin, compound tincture U.S.P.; Bismuth subcarbonate U.S.P.; Bismuth subnitrate N.F.; Boric acid U.S.P.; Calamine U.S.P.; Calamine ointment N.F.; Collodion, flexible; Dimethicone; Magnesium stearate U.S.P.; Starch U.S.P.; Talc U.S.P.; Zinc gelatin U.S.P.; Zinc oxide U.S.P.; Zinc stearate U.S.P.; Zirconium oxide.

Topical Corticosteroids

Betamethasone N.F.; betamethasone valerate; Dexamethasone N.F.; Fludrocortisone acetate; Fluocinolone acetonide; Fluoromethalone; Flurandrenolone; Hydrocortisone acetate U.S.P.; Triamcinolone acetonide.

Sunscreens and Skin Pigmentation Stimulants

Methoxsalen; Para-aminobenzoic acid; Titanium dioxide U.S.P.; Trioxsalen; Zinc oxide.

Depigmentation Agents

Hydroquinone; monobenzone N.F. (monobenzyl ether of hydroquinone)

---

ness requiring the attention of medical personnel. These conditions are also still all too frequently seen in the slum areas of our cities.

Safe and effective insecticides, including chlorophenothane (DDT), benzyl benzoate, and gamma benzene hexachloride (see Drug Digest), can quickly overcome these conditions. Scabies lesions, which are caused by the burrowing of a female mite in the stratum corneum of the skin, are found in the spaces between fingers, on the wrists, waistline, buttocks, axillae, and breasts. The tunneling mite can be seen with a hand lens when the upper layer of skin is lifted gently with a needle. Lice are not readily seen, but pediculosis is recognized by the presence of nits, or eggs, attached to the patient's hair or clothing.

Scabies and pediculosis are readily controlled by application of creams and lotions containing the new scabicides and pediculocides in regimens that also employ prolonged bathing in warm, soapy water and vigorous shampooing. It is also important, however, that clothing and bedding be laundered, sterilized, or fumigated in order to avoid prompt re-exposure to the vermin.

SUBSTANCES THAT AFFECT SKIN PIGMENTATION

The color of the skin depends mainly on its melanin content. This pigment, made by the melanocytes in the lowest stratum of the epidermis, protects the skin from excessive sunlight. Tanning results from stimulation of the melanocytes by ultraviolet light. The pigment produced migrates to the upper layers of the epidermis over a period of several days. This, together with simultaneous thickening of the stratum corneum, increases the skin's tolerance to sunlight and protects it from further sunburn.

TABLE 43-2
LOCAL ANTI-INFECTIVES (ANTIBACTERIAL, ANTIFUNGAL, ETC.) AND DISINFECTANTS

Nonproprietary or Official Name	Synonym or Proprietary Name	Nonproprietary or Official Name	Synonym or Proprietary Name
Acrisorcin	Akrinol	Methylbenzethonium chloride N.F.	Diaparene
Alcohol U.S.P.	Ethanol	Metronidazole	Flagyl
Bacitracin U.S.P.	—	Neomycin sulfate U.S.P.	Mycifradin
Benzalkonium chloride U.S.P.	Zephiran	Nifuroxime N.F.	Micofur
Benzethonium chloride N.F.	Phemerol	Nitrofurazone N.F.	Furacin
Benzyl benzoate U.S.P.	in Albacide; Benylate, etc.	Nitromersol N.F.	Metaphen
Bithional N.F.	Actinol; Actamer	Phenol liquefied U.S.P.	Carbolic acid
Boric acid U.S.P.	—	Phenylmercuric nitrate N.F.	Merphenyl
Calcium undecylenate	in Caldesene	Polymyxin sulfate U.S.P.	Aerosporin
Candicidin	Candeptin	Potassium permanganate U.S.P.	—
Carbol-fuchsin solution N.F.	Castellani's paint	Povidone-iodine N.F.	Betadine; Isodine
Cetylpyridinium chloride N.F.	Ceepryn	Resorcinol U.S.P.	—
Chlorothymol N.F.	—	Resorcinol monoacetate N.F.	—
Cresol N.F.	—	Salicylanilide N.F.	Ansadol; Salinidol
Furazolidone N.F.	Furoxone	Silver nitrate U.S.P.	
Gamma benzene hexachloride	in Kwell	Silver protein, mild N.F.	Argyrol
Gentian violet U.S.P.	Methylrosaniline HCl	Sodium hypochlorite solution, dilute N.F.	Dakin's Solution, Modified
Halazone N.F.	—	Sodium perborate N.F.	—
Hexachlorophene U.S.P.	pHisoHex; Gamophen, etc.	Sodium propionate N.F.	—
Hydrogen peroxide U.S.P.	—	Thimerosal N.F.	Merthiolate
Ichthammol N.F.	Ichthyol	Thiram	Tetramethylthiuram disulfide
Iodine tincture U.S.P.	—	Thymol N.F.	—
Iodochlorhydroxyquin U.S.P.	Vioform	Triclobisonium chloride	Triburon; Trib
Iodoform N.F.	Triiodomethane	Tyrothricin N.F.	—
Isopropyl alcohol N.F.	—	Undecoylium chloride-iodine	Virac
Merbromin N.F.	Mercurochrome	Undecylenic acid N.F.	in Desenex, etc.
Mercuric oxide, yellow N.F.	—	Zinc peroxide, medicinal U.S.P.	—
Mercury, ammoniated U.S.P.	—	Zinc undecylenate U.S.P.	in Desenex, etc.
Mercury bichloride N.F.	Mercuric chloride; corrosive sublimate		

Drugs are available for treating the major types of skin pigment disorders: *hypo-* and *hyper*pigmentation. Other agents protect both normal and abnormal skin from sunburn and photodermatitis eruptions.

Vitiligo is a condition marked by loss of melanin in scattered patches of skin. The cause of this disfiguring hypopigmentary disorder is unknown, and it cannot be treated satisfactorily. In one approach the depigmented areas are covered with cosmetics or walnut juice stains. A chemical called dihydroxyacetone, which reacts with skin proteins when applied topically, colors the skin reddish-brown. This is often satisfactory in white persons, but the stain produced is not dark enough to cover vitiliginous patches in Negroes.

Repigmentation is sometimes achieved in vitiligo with the aid of photodynamic drugs—agents that sensitize the skin to ultraviolet light when applied topically or taken by mouth. The use of the two available drugs of this type, methoxsalen and trioxsalen (see Drug Digest), requires the patient's close cooperation if adverse effects are to be avoided. If drug-photosensitized skin is exposed to too much sunlight, severe sunburn may result.

These drugs often are photoprotective for some fair-skinned persons who normally suffer painful burns or peel without burning when exposed to sunlight. Used carefully, these photosensitizing agents stimulate production of protective pigment and increase the thickness of the stratum corneum—that is, they aid the tanning process.

Sunscreen chemicals are much more commonly employed than the latter drugs by persons with normal skin who wish to encourage tanning and avoid burning. These substances (Table 43-1) absorb some of the sun's burning rays when applied to the skin in the form of lotions, creams, and ointments. Although people who use these products can stand exposure to the sun for longer periods, such chemicals do not completely protect against sunburn. For that purpose, opaque barriers of red veterinary petrolatum, zinc oxide, titanium oxide, and so forth are required, but are cosmetically less acceptable. They are often employed along with protective clothing, parasols, and even systemically administered drugs by persons with skin disorders that require complete avoidance of sunlight.

Photosensitive eruptions and discoid lupus erythematosus (DLE) lesions, which develop on skin areas exposed to the sun, often require the use of the so-called "antimalarial" drugs (Table 36-1) that are sometimes employed in treating rheumatoid arthritis (Chap. 41). These agents were once thought to act by filtering out the light rays that activate DLE lesions and polymorphic light eruptions (PLE), but it is now believed that they exert a steroid-like anti-inflammatory effect in these skin disorders. Although the newer agents of this type do not stain the skin yellow as the earliest agent, quinacrine, did, all can adversely affect the skin, hair, eyes, and other organs. If these reactions develop, the antimalarial drugs are withdrawn.

Hyperpigmentation ranges in degree from simple freckles and moles to the deep darkening of the skin that sometimes develops in patients with pituitary–adrenal gland disorders. Another condition of this kind, chloasma, sometimes occurs during pregnancy. It has recently been found in women who take oral contraceptive products containing synthetic progestins. A chemical called monobenzone, which is applied in lotion or ointment form, is often used to lighten the skin in such conditions or at least to prevent further darkening. Applied daily over a period of several months, these preparations sometimes depigment the darkened areas. Care is required to avoid depigmentation of normal skin. Sensitization and irritation sometimes result in contact dermatitis.

SUMMARY OF POINTS FOR THE NURSE TO REMEMBER

- Note the reaction of the skin to locally applied medications and bring to the doctor's attention any signs of irritation that may indicate primary irritancy or a sensitization reaction.

- Avoid applying all ointments, creams, lotions and so forth (especially those containing corticosteroids) in too copious quantities, for this is messy and unnecessarily expensive. (Check with the physician as to whether he wants previously applied topical medication removed before applying a new layer.)

- Apply liquids sparingly to the scalp for treating seborrhea, to prevent the liquid from running into the eyes or ears. (In general, products containing keratolytic agents require care to prevent contact of the medication with the eyes.)

- Shake heavy lotions such as calamine before using. Apply them with a firm touch, for light dabbing can increase the sensation of itching.

- Dry the skin surface before applying a powder, for caking caused by moisture may lead to irritation.

- Use an emollient rather than alcohol for back care if the skin is excessively dry, for alcohol can cause decubiti by irritating and cracking the already dry skin.

- Remove any blood or pus that might interfere with contact. When using silver nitrate sticks, apply the medication only to the area being treated. (In general, when caustic chemicals are applied to hyperkeratotic and other areas, protect adjacent areas with petrolatum or by other means.)

- Know which skin lesions are infectious and take all appropriate precautions. Explain the need for such measures to the patient but avoid the gingerly touch when applying medications, which may make him feel that his condition is unacceptable to others.

- In scrubbing, remember that friction is important in preoperative preparation for surgery, regardless of which germicides or regimens are employed.

- Advise patients with a history of allergy against trying a variety of skin products, such as deodorants or depilatories, for they may become sensitized to new chemicals. They should stick to the few products that they know by experience cause them no adverse reactions.

- Advise patients who have peripheral vascular disease against self-medication with products containing keratolytic agents, such as plasters for removal of corns and calluses. Such products may be irritating and lead to formation of skin ulcerations in persons with poor circulation.

- Advise people not to worry about the possibility of systemic absorption of corticosteroids and consequent dangerous systemic reactions, for this is unlikely in most circumstances. (On the other hand, women sometimes overestimate the usefulness of cosmetic creams containing estrogens, on the erroneous assumption that these hormones are absorbed systemically to produce desirable feminizing effects, including a more youthful skin.)

REVIEW QUESTIONS

1. (a) What kinds of cells are found in the lower layers of the epidermis and what is the function of each type?

(b) What types of tissues are found in the dermis, or corium, and what are some of the functions of these various structures?

2. (a) What are some objective results of inflammatory skin reactions? (That is, what may we *see* during and after mild to severe reactions?)

(b) What signs of abnormal growth are sometimes seen on the skin?

3. (a) What is a keratolytic agent, and in what skin conditions is keratolytic action considered desirable?

(b) What warnings are suitable when patients wish to employ products containing keratolytic chemicals? What precaution is required when caustic chemicals are to be applied for medical purposes?

4. (a) What are some dermatologic agents of several different types that are used to protect the skin from irritation?

(b) What is the status of dermatologic treatment with topically applied steroids? (That is, how useful and safe are they in skin disorders?)

5. (a) List some mild, moderate and strong irritant substances that are applied topically in acne treatment, and indicate what actions are desired.

(b) What two types of systemically acting drugs are sometimes administered to acne patients, and what are the rationales for such treatments?

6. (a) List several substances employed in chronic psoriasis to stop scaling and stimulate healing of the papulosquamous skin lesions.

(b) What are two types of systemically acting drugs sometimes administered in attempts to control psoriasis in its most acute stages?

(c) By what two special methods are topical corticosteroids often administered in psoriasis, and what is the purpose of such special ways of delivering these drugs?

7. (a) What precautions are desirable during use of selenium sulfide suspensions as shampoos in seborrheic dermatitis of the scalp?

(b) What other antiseborrheic agents are often employed in ointments to stop excessive scaling in seborrheic dermatitis?

8. (a) Why are soaks with solutions of aluminum acetate or potassium permanganate desirable in the "weeping" stages of poison ivy and other dermatoses?

(b) What is the purpose of applying calamine lotion-type preparations, and what precautions should the nurse or patient be aware of and take in applying even such simple preparations?

9. (a) What two other types of drugs are sometimes applied topically in poison ivy, and what is their current status?

(b) What two types of systemically acting drugs are sometimes administered in poison ivy and other contact dermatoses and what is their current status?

10. (a) What two types of drugs are often applied topically in cases of atopic dermatitis, and what are their current status?

(b) In what ways do certain so-called antihistamine drugs relieve itching when taken by mouth in treating atopic dermatitis and other pruritic skin disorders?

11. (a) What properties of ethyl and isopropyl alcohols make their application to the skin useful in surgical and medical situations?

(b) Why is it desirable to wash with alcohol the iodine-stained skin of patients being prepared for surgery?

12. (a) Under what circumstances are hexachlorophene-containing soaps and detergents of maximal benefit?

(b) What precaution is required in order to retain the antiseptic effectiveness of benzalkonium-type preparations in preoperative skin preparation?

13. (a) Which antibiotics are most commonly applied topically for treating secondary bacterial skin infections?

(b) Which antibiotic is most effective for systemic administration in cellulitis (e.g., in the streptococcal infection erysipelas)?

14. (a) For what purpose is silver nitrate (1% solution) commonly employed?

(b) For what purpose is silver nitrate used in solid form or as a concentrated solution?

15. (a) What antibiotic is administered by mouth for treating fungal infections of the skin, and which antibiotics are applied topically in candidal infections of the skin and mucous membranes?

(b) What are some substances applied topically for their antifungal, antipruritic, and keratolytic effects in tinea-type (ringworm) dermatophytoses?

16. (a) What substance is administered by mouth to both women and men for treating *Trichomonas vaginalis* vaginitis?

(b) What new antibiotic and what old dye are employed in treating mycotic vulvovaginitis?

(c) What adjunctive measures are often employed to increase the effectiveness of antifungal and antibacterial drugs in vaginal infections?

17. (a) List three drugs used in the management of scabies and pediculosis.

(b) What precautions and adjunctive measures must be employed along with scabicide and pesticide drugs?

18. (a) List two photosensitizing-photoprotective drugs used in the management of vitiligo for repigmentation and for aiding tanning.

(b) In what manner are these drugs thought to act and what precautions are required to avoid toxicity?

19. (a) List some sunscreen substances used in cosmetic products intended to aid tanning and prevent burning.

(b) List some substances that are opaque barriers in conditions that require complete avoidance of sunlight.

20. (a) What drugs are sometimes taken internally by patients with discoid lupus erythematosus and polymorphic light eruptions?

(b) What drug is applied topically in hyperpigmentary disorders such as chloasma?

BIBLIOGRAPHY

Blank, I. H.: Action of emollient creams and their additives. J.A.M.A., *164:*412, 1957.

Carney, R. G.: Topical use of antibiotics. J.A.M.A., *186:* 646, 1963.

Council on Drugs: An agent for stimulating pigmentation or tolerance to sunlight, trioxsalen. J.A.M.A., *197:*43, 1966.

Demis, D. J., and Gass, H. H.: Treatment of psoriasis, lichen planus, and seborrheic dermatitis. Modern Treatment, *2:*873, 1965 (Sept.).

Heseltine, H. C., and Lefebre, I.: Treating vaginal trichomoniasis with metronidazole. J.A.M.A., *184:*1011, 1963.

Lerner, A. E.: Treatment of disorders of pigmentation. Modern Treatment, *2:*927, 1965 (Sept.).

Lobitz, W. C., and Learner, A. E.: Psoriasis 1961. G.P., *23:*109, 1961.

Pochi, P. E., and Strauss, J. S.: Treatment of acne vulgaris and acne rosacea. Modern Treatment, *2:*847, 1965 (Sept.).

Richards, R. C.: Some practical aspects of surgical skin preparation. Am. J. Surg., *106:*575, 1963.

Rodman, M. J.: Acne—an adolescent problem. R.N., *19:* 42, 1956 (April).

——: Facts about the itch mechanism. R.N., *22:*41, 1959 (Aug.).

——: Drugs for treating skin infections. R.N., *28:*77, 1965 (Feb.).

——: Drugs used in skin diseases. R.N., *31:*53, 1968 (March).

Sulzberger, M. B., and Witten, V. H.: Some useful procedures in office dermatology. Med. Clin. N. Amer., *45:* 1577, 1961.

Sulzberger, M. B., et al.: Treatment of acne vulgaris. J.A.M.A., *173:*1911, 1960.

Witten, V. H., and Sulzberger, M. B.: Newer dermatologic methods for using corticosteroids more efficaciously. Med. Clin. N. Amer., *45:*857, 1961.

Drug Treatment of Neoplastic Diseases

THE NATURE AND TREATMENT OF NEOPLASTIC DISEASES

Cancer kills close to 300,000 people annually in the United States. This condition—or, more accurately, the hundred or more different diseases classified as cancer—is second only to cardiovascular disorders as a cause of death. The death rate—about 155 per 100,000 people—is approximately the same as that of those other lands where deaths from infection have dropped dramatically in recent years and where people no longer die of malnutrition. Although the total number of persons dying of cancer has increased—especially in certain categories such as lung cancer—the rate is about the same as it was 50 years ago, when it is adjusted in terms of the increased proportion of older people in the population. That is, more people survive infections to become part of the older age group, in which malignant tumors most commonly occur.

Surgery or Radiation. Treatment of cancer is most successful when the malignancy is discovered early while it is localized. The malignant tumor may then be removed completely by *surgery* or destroyed by *radiation*. Cancer experts claim that half of the close to one half million persons who develop cancer each year could be cured by these means, if their condition were detected early enough. Thus, nurses and others in the health professions should educate the public about cancer. The nurse in her daily contacts with people, can conduct a quiet campaign to promote periodic physical examinations, for cancers often can be detected before they have produced any symptoms at all. (Office diagnostic measures such as the "Pap smear" test, which has helped bring about an almost 50 per cent drop in deaths from uterine cancer, may also aid in detecting breast and rectal cancers in their early stages.) Similarly, if she recognizes a warning sign of cancer, she often can persuade the person to visit a physician. He may find a mass or other lesion and can confirm the presence of cancer by biopsy.

Chemotherapy. Not all cancers are curable by surgery or irradiation. Some malignancies cannot be completely excised because they are located in a vital organ; others are resistant to safe doses of radiation. Malignancies that have metastasized widely and those which, like leukemia, are generalized to begin with are not curable by surgery and radiation. In advanced cancers of these kinds, chemicals that seek out and destroy the disseminated cancer cells offer the main means of treatment.

The current status of cancer chemotherapy is not satisfactory in terms of the cure rate by drugs. No kind of cancer—except possibly one unusual type of neoplasm—has been eradicated totally by drugs that destroy malignant cells selectively. However, new drugs and new ways of delivering them to the diseased areas are constantly being developed; these advances have helped to lengthen the lives of some patients, and brought subjective relief to others. There is reason to hope that increased research in molecular biology may lead to an understanding of what causes cancer, which, in turn, will result in the tailoring of new drug molecules that can kill cancer cells without harming normal tissues.

The selective toxicity of chemicals for cancer cells is much more limited than that of the antimicrobial drugs which are used for treating infections. Penicillin, for example, attacks bacterial cells without harming those of the infected human host, because it blocks certain biochemical pathways essential for building the microbial cell wall without at all affecting the essential metabolism of mammalian cells. The metabolism of neoplastic cells, on the other hand, is essentially similar to that of the normal tissues in which the cancer began to grow. Thus, drugs that damage malignant tissues are likely to interfere with the functioning of healthy, rapidly growing cells.

Another factor that limits the effectiveness of cancer

chemotherapy is that body defense mechanisms do not work with antineoplastic drugs to eradicate the neoplastic cells in the way that they aid antibacterial drugs. For example, when bacteriostatic agents such as the sulfonamides and the tetracycline-type antibiotics halt the growth of microbial cells, the phagocytes of the body finish the task of destroying the invaders; but because cancer cells, on the other hand, are not truly foreign, they are not very vulnerable to attack by antibodies, and, indeed, cancer chemotherapeutic agents often suppress natural immune mechanisms.

The toxicity of antineoplastic drugs is manifested mainly by their effects on such rapidly metabolizing tissues as the *bone marrow* and the *G.I. mucosal epithelium*. The margin between the dose of an antileukemic drug that destroys the neoplastic cell population of the bone marrow and that which is detrimental to healthy hemopoietic elements is narrow. For instance, drugs that attack the myeloid elements involved in granulocytic leukemia are likely to injure the erythroid elements that manufacture red blood cells and the primitive cells from which blood platelets or thrombocytes are being formed.

Drugs that attack solid tissue tumors and lymphatic cancers tend to depress bone marrow function in only slight overdoses. Consequently, all patients who are treated with anticancer chemicals are watched closely for clinical signs of anemia and bleeding tendencies. Frequent laboratory blood tests detect early microscopic signs of drug-induced hematopoietic toxicity. A sudden excessive fall in white blood cell counts calls for prompt withdrawal of the drug, because the adverse effects of depression of other bone marrow elements, such as erythrocytes and thrombocytes, usually appear only much later, even though the damage may already have been done.

The drugs sometimes must be discontinued because of trauma to the G.I. tract lining. Unlike such early signs of G.I. tract irritation as anorexia, nausea, and vomiting, the development of oral ulcers and intestinal bleeding and diarrhea is potentially dangerous. Destruction of the mucosal lining indicates that these drugs are affecting the development of these fast-growing cells almost as readily as they are damaging those of the malignant neoplasm. Patients should be warned to report any such signs, for they may indicate that the bone marrow is being affected excessively and that drug dosage should be reduced.

The nurse does all she can to lessen the discomfort induced by cancer chemotherapy. Food is not served, for example, until the patient's nausea following administration of certain of these drugs has subsided. When the patient is feeling better, the nurse can find out what he wants to eat. If oral ulceration develops, the patient will require mouth care and a diet of soft, bland foods. The patient whose white blood cell counts have dropped precipitously must be protected from infection, during this period of reduced resistance, by special precautions. For example, the nurse should put a clean gown over her uniform and wash her hands carefully before caring for the patient.

Special techniques for administering anticancer chemicals to minimize toxicity are being tested. The objective is to bring a high concentration of the chemical into local contact with the malignant tissues, while keeping the amount of drug in the systemic circulation as low as possible. In the isolation-perfusion method some drugs are circulated only through local areas, thus by-passing the general blood stream. The blood supply of the diseased body part is shunted through a heart-lung machine, where it receives a high dose of the drug. The blood is returned to the involved area by the extracorporeal oxygenator pump. The resultant concentration of the drug in the neoplasm tends to destroy tumor tissue more readily and at the same time avoid damage to healthy cells elsewhere in the body.

Resistance to anticancer drugs is inevitable eventually, no matter how well the patient responds to treatment at first. Apparently, as these drugs eliminate the susceptible neoplastic cells, new populations of cells arise that are so different in some aspect of their metabolism that they are no longer readily destroyed. In time, strains of cancer cells take over which are unaffected by drug concentrations that are prohibitively damaging to normal tissues. The patient then no longer improves but suffers severe side effects if higher doses are administered.

Dealing with the patient and his family under such circumstances often requires mature judgment and tact, in order not to raise false hopes, on the one hand, or, on the other, to discourage the continuation of drug treatment that can help to slow the progress of the disease. What the patient and his family can be told about the drug he is receiving depends on various individual circumstances. In any case, it is important that everyone—doctor, nurse, and other staff personnel—give the patient the same explanations concerning the purposes, advantages, limitations, and potential toxicity of the drugs employed.

Once the nurse knows what the patient and his family have been told about the nature of his condition and the reason for treating it with drugs that can cause so much discomfort, she can listen to their expressions of hope or their complaints and then help to make the difficult situation more bearable for all concerned.

The patient who knows he has cancer may be more willing to bear the miseries of drug toxicity, and will probably be more receptive to the nurse's suggestion that the benefits of drug therapy outweigh the nausea that he may be experiencing. On the other hand, the nurse may have to help the patient and his family by not letting their hopes for a drug-induced miracle rise too high, only to have these hopes dashed later. For

TABLE 44-1

ANTINEOPLASTIC AGENTS

GENERIC OR OFFICIAL NAME	SYNONYM OR PROPRIETARY NAME	USUAL DOSAGE RANGE
Alkylating Agents		
Busulfan U.S.P.	Myleran	1 to 6 mg. orally
Chlorambucil U.S.P.	Leukeran	2 to 12 mg. orally
Cyclophosphamide N.F.	Cytoxan	100 mg. orally maintenance
Mechlorethamine U.S.P.	Mustargen; Nitrogen mustard	200 to 600 mcg./Kg. I.V.
Melphalan	Alkeran; l-Phenylalanine mustard	6 mg. orally; then regulated in accordance with weekly blood counts
Pipobroman	Vercyte	1 mg./Kg. per day orally initially; 0.1 to 0.2 mg. per day maintenance
Thiotepa U.S.P.	Thio-TEPA; TESPA, etc.	Up to 200 mcg./Kg. parenterally
Triethylenemelamine N.F.	TEM	2.5 mg. daily for 2 or 3 days; then 0.5 to 5 mg. weekly
Uracil mustard	—	1 mg. daily orally maintenance
Antimetabolites		
Fluorouracil	—	7.5 to 15 mg./Kg. by intravenous infusion, up to a maximum daily dose of 1 Gm.
Mercaptopurine	Purinethol	2.5 mg./Kg. orally
Methotrexate	Amethopterin	Children 2.5 to 5.0 mg./Kg. orally or parenterally. Adults 5 to 30 mg./Kg. orally or parenterally
Thioguanine	—	2 to 3 mg./Kg. orally per day
Alkaloids and Antibiotics		
Dactinomycin	Actinomycin D; Cosmegen	Adults 0.5 mg. I.V. daily for up to 5 days. Children 15 mcg./Kg. daily for 5 days
Vinblastine sulfate	Velban	0.1 mg./Kg. increased up to 0.5 mg./Kg. I.V. no oftener than once every 7 days
Vincristine sulfate	Oncovin	2 mg./sq. meter of body surface per week intravenously
Hormones		
Adrenocorticosteroids Androgens Estrogens		See text of this chapter and of Chapters 28, 29, and 30 for lists of available compounds, and dosage-administration data.
Radioactive Isotopes		
Radio-gold Solution Au198	Aurocoloid; Aureotope	35 to 150 millicuries parenterally
Sodium Iodide I 131 Capsules and Solution U.S.P.	Theriodide; Oriodide; Radiocaps; Tracervial	Oral or I.V., the equivalent of 1 to 100 *milli*curies for therapy, or 1 to 100 *micro*curies for diagnosis

TABLE 44-1 (Continued)

GENERIC OR OFFICIAL NAME	SYNONYM OR PROPRIETARY NAME	USUAL DOSAGE RANGE
Radioactive Isotopes (Continued)		
Sodium Phosphate P 32 Solution U.S.P.	—	Oral or I.V., the equivalent of 1 to 5 *milli*curies for therapy, or 250 *micro*curies to 1 millicurie for diagnosis
Miscellaneous		
Hydroxyurea	Hydrea	*Intermittent therapy:* 80 mg./Kg. orally as a single dose every third day. *Continuous therapy:* 20 to 30 mg. orally as a single dose daily
Quinacrine HCl U.S.P.	Atabrine	200 to 1,000 mg. daily by intracavitary (intrapleural or intraperitoneal instillation)
Urethan	Ethyl carbamate	3 to 6 Gm. orally daily

example, when a leukemia patient goes into remission or a patient with bone metastases becomes pain free during a course of drug therapy, the nurse can share the patient's pleasure without contributing to the development of any unrealistic attitudes about the final outcome. It is, in fact, desirable to correct any misinformed views that may be voiced by members of the family. The patient, on the other hand, should be permitted to cling to hope, no matter how unrealistic, if his physician feels that this is psychologically desirable.

CLASSES OF CHEMOTHERAPEUTIC AGENTS

Several classes of cancer drugs have been developed through trial-and-error screening of thousands of compounds and by the recent application of the fruits of research on possible differences between normal cells and malignant tissues. Many of these drugs are classified according to how they affect cancer cell reproduction. Others are grouped in terms of the natural sources from which they are obtained—for example, the plant alkaloids and the antineoplastic antibiotics derived from fungi.

We shall discuss these agents in general terms under the following classification: alkylating agents, antimetabolites, alkaloids and antibiotics, hormones, radioactive isotopes, and miscellaneous. (For details concerning the most important representative agents of each class, see the Drug Digests.)

Alkylating Agents (Table 44-1)

Several highly reactive kinds of chemicals are termed alkylating agents, because they are able to combine with cellular substances by means of certain chemical groups called alkyl radicals. Although the chemical reactions differ, the result of such alkylation of intracellular molecules by all these kinds of drugs is the same: the cells fail to divide to form daughter cells. The chemical attack alters molecules of deoxyribonucleic acid (DNA), a substance essential to cell division. In their ability to interfere with mitosis and in other respects, some of these drugs resemble ionizing radiation which also adversely affects chromosomal activity and cell division. (Thus, the biological actions of these drugs are sometimes termed *radiomimetic,* or radiation-imitating.)

These drugs affect *all* cells adversely, but those that are growing and dividing most rapidly are most prone to injury. With carefully individualized dosage, various types of rapidly proliferating cancer cells often can be destroyed without doing excessive damage to the more slowly growing normal cells. However, the safety margin is usually so narrow that even slight overdosage often may injure those human tissues that have the highest turnover rate—for example, the blood-forming cells of the bone marrow, the epithelium of the intestinal mucosa, and sperm cells. Naturally, when strains of more resistant cells emerge that yield to only high doses of these cytotoxic drugs, much greater damage is done to healthy rapidly multiplying cells also.

Nitrogen Mustards. *Mechlorethamine* (see Drug Digest) was the first drug of this class found useful for treating cancers. Studies of the mustard gases used in chemical warfare revealed that this compound and other nitrogen mustards are selectively cytotoxic to lymphoid tissues. Tried in patients in the terminal stages of malignant lymphoma, mechlorethamine provided dramatic, though temporary, remission. It is considered useful for treating lymphomas such as Hodgkin's disease, despite certain severe drawbacks. (For example, this blister-gas derivative has the same vesicant action as the chemical warfare agents from which it is derived.)

Hodgkin's disease causes about 3,200 deaths annually in the United States. When detected early, this malignancy of the lymph nodes is best treated by *radiotherapy*, which is claimed actually to cure the condition. Once it has spread to other regions of the body, however, systemic chemotherapy is required. Of the various drugs available, including the *Vinca* alkaloids and the corticosteroids, mechlorethamine seems to produce the most rapid remissions. Administered by vein in patients with disseminated disease, it often promptly relieves symptoms such as high fever, drenching sweats, and extreme weakness. The patient's appetite is restored, and he regains much of the weight that he had lost while the disease was untreated.

Such improvement is usually preceded, however, by a period of nausea and vomiting, and is sometimes followed by thrombocytic bleeding for a while. Patients should be assured that these signs and symptoms of drug toxicity are transient and not serious. Women may be warned that menstrual periods may be absent temporarily and that the cycles may be irregular for a while. If the injection solution leaks out of the vein and into adjacent tissues, application of ice compresses is often ordered. (Occasionally, the doctor may order that the area be infiltrated with a chemical antidote to local irritation, such as sodium thiosulfate solution.)

Other nitrogen mustards that have been developed are preferable to mechlorethamine in various types of neoplastic diseases. For example, *cyclophosphamide* (see Drug Digest) does not cause local tissue damage when injected. It can be given by mouth without excessively irritating the G.I. tract. Although nausea and vomiting occur sometimes, such symptoms are milder than those caused by the parent compound.

This mustard derivative has reportedly produced remissions of acute lymphocytic leukemia, and like another agent of this class, *chlorambucil* (see Drug Digest), is beneficial in some cases of chronic lymphocytic leukemia. Cyclophosphamide is useful mainly in Hodgkin's disease patients who can take the drug on maintenance dosage schedules without having to be hospitalized. Frequent blood tests detect any developing bone marrow depression. Patients should be warned that alopecia could result, and, at the same time, they can be reassured that their hair will grow in again. (Another drug of this class, *uracil mustard,* which can be taken by mouth like cyclophosphamide, does not cause baldness, but is potentially as toxic as the older mustards.)

Melphalan, or *l*-phenylalanine mustard, the latest of these agents to be introduced, is used mainly in multiple myeloma. In this malignancy, tumors scattered throughout the bone marrow eventually destroy the skeleton after depressing formation of the formed elements of the blood. Low oral doses often relieve pain and permit the patient to move about more comfortably. Half the patients in some series have shown objective improvement for a time.

The relative utility of melphalan in other conditions in which nitrogen mustards are employed has not been studied in adequate numbers of patients. However, it apparently helps some patients with metastatic melanoma, the rapidly spreading black-pigmented skin tumor. Best results have been attained in melanomas localized in the lower extremities. The isolated perfusion procedure allows high concentrations of this mustard-type chemical to be recirculated through the main artery and vein of an extremity. Since little seeps into the systemic circulation, the toxic effects typical of drugs of this class are unlikely. (When administered orally, the drug can produce characteristic toxicity, and like the other mustards, it is contraindicated in patients who show signs of bone marrow toxicity such as anemia, leukopenia, and thrombocytopenia.)

Other alkylating agents, which have properties similar to those of the nitrogen mustards, are used in specific types of neoplasms. *Busulfan* (see Drug Digest) is relatively selective for the bone marrow elements that manufacture granulocytes. Thus, it is the drug of choice for control of chronic granulocytic leukemia. Low doses that rarely cause the G.I. upsets characteristic of the nitrogen mustards often bring about remissions in this condition. Overdosage can affect other bone marrow elements besides the myeloid cells. Thus, the usual precautions are required to avoid adverse effects upon platelet and red blood cell production.

Pipobroman (Vercyte), a new nonmustard alkylating agent, is, like busulfan, used in treating chronic granulocytic leukemia. However, it is primarily indicated in polycythemia vera. In this condition, which is believed to result from a neoplasm of erythroid bone marrow tissue, hemoglobin and red blood cell levels are high. Because of the increased viscosity of the blood, thrombotic complications and bleeding episodes may result. Treatment is directed at reducing blood volume by bleeding at regular intervals. In addition to frequent phlebotomy, radioactive phosphorus has been administered to reduce erythropoiesis. From recent experience in the use of pipobroman on hundreds of polycythemia patients, some hematologists state that it may soon become the drug of choice for treating this condition.

Thiotepa (see Drug Digest) and the related drug *triethylenemelamine* (TEM) are alkylating agents that produce effects similar to those of the nitrogen mustards but do not cause as much G.I. upset. Thiotepa, which, unlike mechlorethamine, is not locally irritating, is often injected directly into tumors. It is also injected directly into body cavities to stop the flow of serous fluids from metastatic neoplasms. It is said by some to be better than radioactive gold when administered in this manner to relieve the symptoms caused by such effusions. Relief of pleural cavity edema following thiotepa treatment alleviates breathing difficulty and coughing. Similarly, when administered after paracentesis, it slows the accumulation of peritoneal cavity fluids. When used in conjunction with surgery, thiotepa is thought to destroy loose cancer cells dislodged during the operation before they take root elsewhere in the body.

Antimetabolites (Table 44-1)

This group of antineoplastic agents stops the production of rapidly growing neoplasms, not by damaging DNA already formed in cancer cells, but by interfering with its formation in various ways. The molecular structures of these drugs resemble those of various substances that the cells require for carrying on essential biochemical reactions. The drug molecules displace those of the metabolite that they closely resemble. The false metabolite blocks the cells' biosynthesis of important enzymes, and eventually of DNA itself. Among the metabolites blocked by these drugs are folic acid and various purines, pyrimidines, and amino acids.

The *folic acid antagonist methotrexate* (see Drug Digest) competes with folic acid for a place in an enzyme system that forms a substance required for cellular reproduction. Competitive inhibition of this enzyme by methotrexate keeps the cancer cells from forming a coenzyme needed for making the chemical materials of which DNA is built. As a result, these cells stop reproducing, and a remission of the disease soon follows.

Methotrexate and its predecessor aminopterin were the first drugs to bring about remissions of acute leukemia in children. More recently, methotrexate has been used successfully for treating choriocarcinoma, a relatively rare neoplasm that originates in placental tissues and ordinarily spreads swiftly to the lungs and other organs. Some women are alive so many years after treatment with methotrexate, that their doctors feel safe in calling them "cured." Although this constitutes the first chemical cure of a cancer, choriocarcinoma is not a typical neoplasm, since it originates in the fetal membranes rather than the uterus. (Thus,

the drug's action may be aided by some immune mechanism that rejects the foreign fetal tissues.)

Other solid tumors have not been eradicated by treatment with methotrexate when the drug has been tried in breast, testicular, and other cancers. Recently, doctors have tried to treat inoperable head and neck tumors by infusing high concentrations of the drug directly into the carotid artery. The drug that eventually reaches other body tissues is, of course, diluted to less toxic concentrations by the blood. Ill effects are prevented by periodic intramuscular injection of the antidotal drug *leucovorin*. (This antidote may be administered promptly in case of accidental overdosage with methotrexate.)

Although courses of methotrexate sometimes stop the rapid progress of acute childhood leukemia for many months, the cancer cells finally become resistant to this folic acid analogue. In such cases, the doctor may substitute combinations of various other drugs including the *corticosteroids, vincristine,* and another antimetabolite, *mercaptopurine* (see Drug Digest). Mercaptopurine, an analogue of the purine precursors of various important cellular constituents, including DNA, often brings about further remissions in children whose disease has become resistant to other drugs. Another newer antimetabolite, *thioguanine,* is sometimes substituted for mercaptopurine in acute leukemia patients who cannot tolerate mercaptopurine.

Fluorouracil, another useful antimetabolite-type cancer treatment agent, is a fluorinated form of the pyrimidine uracil, which plays an important part in the biosynthesis of DNA. Administered by vein to patients with malignant solid tissue tumors of many kinds, including carcinomas of the large bowel and the bladder, this drug is sometimes beneficial. Unfortunately, effective doses often cause severe G.I. side effects; patients are watched closely for development of oral inflammation, mouth ulcers, and diarrhea. In efforts to reduce its general toxicity, various methods have been devised for administering this drug to attain high local concentrations in the tumor and minimal amounts elsewhere in the body. Fluorouracil has, for example, been infused directly into liver cancers by a tiny portable pump that keeps the liver saturated with the drug continuously for days and weeks, during which time the patient is often ambulatory.

Plant Alkaloids and Antibiotics

Certain natural products, including antibiotics synthesized by species of fungi, and alkaloids extracted from an ornamental shrub, are being used as anticancer chemicals. For example, the antibiotic *dactinomycin* is effective against cancers that attack children under five years old, including Wilms' tumor, a growth that originates in the kidneys and spreads to the lungs and other tissues. Dactinomycin, administered alone or combined with other drugs as an adjunct to surgery and ionizing radiation, has brought about remissions in this condition and in rhabdosarcoma. It is said to add to the effectiveness of x-rays in some pulmonary metastases.

In addition to its usefulness for treating these nephroblastomas and skeletal muscle sarcomas, dactinomycin has proved effective against trophoblastic tumors such as choriocarcinoma and metastatic tumors of the testes, such as seminoma. In these conditions it is commonly combined with methotrexate and chlorambucil. However, it sometimes has been successful when used by itself in treatment of tumors that had become resistant to methotrexate or in patients for whom that drug was contraindicated because of liver damage or kidney function impairment. (Dactinomycin is itself quite toxic, and the danger of blood, G.I. tract, and skin reactions is often increased when it is combined with other anticancer drugs.)

Vinblastine and vincristine (Table 44-1) are alkaloids extracted from the periwinkle plant *Vinca rosea*. Scientists first studied the properties of this garden ornamental when their curiosity was aroused by its reputation in folk medicine as a diabetes cure. The several purified alkaloids that they extracted showed no hypoglycemic activity, but instead proved toxic to the bone marrow of experimental animals. The alkaloids were then screened for antineoplastic activity and found to stop the growth of tumor transplants. Although these and the other alkaloids of this plant differ only slightly in chemical structures, they are quite different from one another in the relative selectivity for various types of tumors. Thus, they are used clinically in treating different types of malignancies.

Vinblastine is used mainly in the treatment of advanced Hodgkin's disease when x-ray therapy or such alkylating agents as mechlorethamine and cyclophosphamide are no longer effective. It has been tried for treating choriocarcinoma that has become resistant to the first line drugs methotrexate and dactinomycin. This drug is locally and systemically toxic, and so it requires extreme care in adjustment of dosage and during injection. (If it leaks into tissues surrounding the vein, the doctor orders ice packs or cold compresses to be promptly applied to help relieve pain and prevent cellulitis.)

Vincristine shares its sister alkaloid's toxicity on the G.I. tract and nervous system. However, it is less toxic to the bone marrow in general. Thus, though effective in Hodgkin's disease, it is used mainly to manage acute leukemia in children. In such cases, it is reserved usually for patients who no longer respond to the less toxic antimetabolites methotrexate and mercaptopurine, which produce longer-lasting remissions. (This alkaloid can cause severe peripheral neuropathy resulting in long-lasting pain and even paralysis and atrophy of skeletal muscles.)

These new drugs are in no sense superior to other available agents. Yet they not only may extend life for a brief period, but also may add to the effectiveness of the other drugs when combined with them. For example, recent reports indicate that some leukemia patients had much longer lasting remissions when treated not with one compound, but with a combination of four called VAMP—*v*incristine, Amethopterin (methotrexate), *m*ercaptopurine, and *p*rednisone.

Hormone Therapy

Certain hormones, including the adrenocorticosteroids and their synthetic derivatives, and the male and female sex steroids, are effective for palliation of certain specific types of neoplastic diseases. These agents are discussed in detail in Chapters 28, 29, and 30. Thus, we shall mention here only some points concerning their use in the management of cancerous conditions.

Corticosteroids often bring about prompt remissions in children acutely ill with leukemia. These drugs somehow cause the dissolution of the primitive lymphocyte-like cells in leukemic bone marrow. As a result, normal cells regenerate rapidly, and the patient feels and acts much better. *Prednisone* is the steroid most commonly used for this purpose. Relatively low doses that produce few signs of hypercorticism in a short course are adequate at first. After later relapses, the much higher doses that are needed can cause all the complications characteristic of steroids. The doctor may decide that the benefits are worth the risk. (In terminal stages, steroids no longer produce remissions, but may reduce fever and lessen bleeding.)

Corticosteroid therapy sometimes relieves symptoms and reduces complications in other kinds of cancer. These drugs, for example, often improve the hematologic status when the blood picture has been adversely affected both by the neoplasm and the other antineoplastic drugs that have been used to treat it. Thus, in chronic lymphocytic leukemia, Hodgkin's disease and other lymphomas, as well as in hemolytic anemia, corticosteroids often raise lowered hemoglobin and platelet levels. Patients with solid tumors sometimes receive symptomatic relief with steroid administration. Thus, in advanced breast cancer with metastases to bones and brain, steroids sometimes help to lower the high blood calcium levels and to counteract the effects of brain tissue compression.

Androgens. The male sex hormone testosterone often temporarily improves the condition of women with advanced breast cancer. This hormone and its derivatives counteract the effects of estrogens on this hormone-dependent neoplasm. They do so, in part, by directly antagonizing the growth-stimulating effects of the female hormone on the metastatic mammary tissues. In addition, they may act by suppressing pituitary secretion of gonadotropin. (These desirable effects of hormone therapy are often achieved surgically by castration, hypophysectomy, and adrenalectomy.)

In about 20 per cent of such patients, cancerous lesions in the bones and elsewhere regress under androgen therapy. Even when the osseous and soft tissue tumors do not grow smaller and the patient's life is not lengthened, hormone therapy often relieves pain and improves appetite, strength, and well-being. These subjective benefits may stem from the anabolic effects of the male hormone.

The *adverse effects* of androgen therapy are in general much less severe than those of other anticancer drugs. However, while there is no danger of bone marrow damage or G.I. ulceration and bleeding, the masculinizing effects of the high doses that are often required pose a psychological difficulty. The nurse should be aware of not only the physical effects but also of possible emotional reactions. Another possible complication is the sudden development of hypercalcemia, which requires prompt withdrawal of androgen therapy. Thus, the short-acting ester testosterone propionate is preferred to the longer-acting esters in treating disseminated mammary carcinoma.

Estrogens are sometimes used in treating metastatic breast cancer—but *only* in women who are five years or more past the menopause. In such patients, remissions are probably brought about by the sex hormones' suppression of pituitary gonadotropins. More important is the use of estrogens in the management of metastatic prostate carcinoma in men, a procedure that has had beneficial palliative effects in many thousands of men.

Diethylstilbestrol administration by mouth is the most common treatment for suppressing the growth-stimulating effect of endogenous androgens on the disseminated prostatic neoplasm. Often this promptly relieves pain and later reduces osseous and soft tissue lesions. Patients who do not benefit from estrogens or who become resistant to them require castration to achieve similar effects. In many cases, the disease is best controlled by a combinaton of castration and estrogens. Although patients eventually relapse, as new populations of resistant prostatic cancer cells emerge, this treatment often prolongs life and alleviates severe suffering.

Although the feminizing effects of estrogens are physically and psychologically undesirable, patients usually prefer such adverse effects to the pain of the prostatic metastases to bone and elsewhere. The nurse, of course, takes every opportunity to offer emotional support to men disturbed by side effects such as gynecomastia and other changes in secondary sex characteristics.

Radioactive Isotopes

A few radioactive elements are used to treat certain types of neoplasms. Ideally, such a substance concentrates in the cancer and selectively damages its cells without affecting normal tissues. In practice, such selective toxicity does not occur with any isotope. Thus, although some do destroy tumor tissues, they also damage normal cells.

Two official radioisotopes in common use in cancer treatment are sodium phosphate P 32 (see Drug Digest) and radio-gold (^{198}Au). A third isotope employed to deliberately damage human tissues is sodium iodide I 131, which is discussed in Chapter 31. In adequate doses, all emit *beta particles* or "radiations" in amounts that destroy living tissues in the immediate vicinity. Radioactive gold produces, in addition, the more penetrating gamma rays that are effective at a considerable distance from the patient.

^{32}P incorporated in sodium phosphate is taken up to some extent by all body tissues when the solution of this salt is taken internally. However, because bone marrow neoplasms utilize phosphorus rapidly, the radioactive element is relatively more damaging to any cancer cells in this tissue. Although beta radiations penetrate only a short distance, they can damage enough erythroid or myeloid cells to produce remissions in polycythemia vera and to a lesser extent in chronic granulocytic anemia.

If overdosage permits too much radioactive phosphate to accumulate in the bone marrow, normal hematopoietic tissues may also be damaged. This can result in leukopenia, thrombocytopenia, and anemia as a result of excessive reduction in all the formed elements of the peripheral blood. Thus, the less toxic alkylating agent busulfan is usually preferred for chronic leukemia treatment, and the new alkylating agent pipobroman may be preferable to ^{32}P in polycythemia vera treatment.

Radio-gold 198 (gold Au 198 solution) injected into certain body cavities brings about changes in the tissues that help to reduce the effusion of edema fluids from solid tumor tissues. Although the effects of such radiation do often result in less fluid formation from malignancies in the pleural spaces and in reduced abdominal cavity ascites, the danger to the patient and possibly to nurses and the attending staff makes this a difficult substance to deal with. It is essential to learn the necessary precautions required for one's safety in caring for the patient, changing his bedclothes, and disposing of his excreta.

Miscellaneous

Since radioactive gold therapy is hazardous, many authorities prefer thiotepa for this purpose. Recently, *quinacrine* (see Drug Digest), which was introduced as an antimalarial agent and is used for treating tapeworm infections and other conditions, has been used to control the effusions from metastatic malignancies in the pleural and peritoneal cavities. Instilled into these serous cavities, quinacrine—which is *not* radioactive—sets off an inflammatory reaction on the membranous lining. This is followed by a fibrous proliferation which somehow improves symptoms without modifying the metastatic breast cancer or other carcinomatous tumors at all.

Quinacrine is not without toxicity when administered in this way. The inflammatory reaction causes pain in the chest and sometimes dyspnea after intrapleural instillation. Abdominal pain may follow intraperitoneal instillation and inflammation of the serous lining of that cavity (peritonitis). Systemic side effects and toxicity include fever, nausea and vomiting, possible yellow skin pigmentation, and occasional transient hallucinations.

Urethan is occasionally used in the management of multiple myeloma. However, the G.I. upset induced by the high oral doses that are required limits its usefulness. With the recent introduction of the much more potent agent melphalan for treating this condition, urethan will probably have little future use. The drug is mentioned here mainly to indicate the sad fact that cancers must be treated by drugs that are too toxic to be used for other clinical purposes.

Urethan was introduced into medicine many years ago as a hypnotic and sedative. Such a drug would not pass modern toxicity testing procedures. Yet, this drug and others that are damaging to bone marrow and other vital tissues are precisely those sought in cancer drug screening programs. This indicates the main problem with antineoplastic agents: their toxicity for cancer cells is not sufficiently selective; thus, they damage normal tissues when administered in the doses needed to eradicate tumor tissues.

PRESENT STATUS AND FUTURE PROSPECTS IN CANCER CHEMOTHERAPY

Most authorities think that real advances will come only after much more is known about the biochemical differences between normal cells and tumor tissues and their metastases. Scientists are searching for the kinds of metabolic alterations from normal that make cancer cells more vulnerable to specially constructed chemotherapeutic drug molecules. Such agents could be concentrated exclusively in the tumor and its metastases and act there to destroy the malignant tissues without harming even immediately adjacent and rapidly reproducing cells with normal metabolic activity.

Until such knowledge is acquired and exploited, doctors are trying to learn how to make the most of the chemical weapons at hand. As indicated, they must: (1) attain and maintain a dosage level of the antineoplastic drug that is most effective and least toxic for each patient and type of neoplasm, (2) employ several drugs in the best possible sequences or combinations to attain remissions of maximal length, (3) use techniques of administration—for example, intra-arterial infusion and isolation-perfusion—that tend to concentrate the antineoplastic agent in the tumor, while protecting normal, rapidly growing cells, such as those in healthy bone marrow, from injury and destruction.

Cancer patients require especially skillful nursing care and supportive therapy. The nurse can, for example, use special precautions to protect the patient with leukopenia from infection. She can lessen the discomfort of drug-induced oral inflammation and ulceration by providing the patient with frequent mouth care and serving him bland foods that are neither too hot nor too cold.

The nurse also has an important role in implementing and assisting with the various supportive treatments that the doctor orders, such as transfusions and administration of medications to relieve pain. The patient who receives radioisotope therapy requires special safety precautions. (For information of this kind, see Chap. 8 of *Care of the Adult Patient* by Smith and Gips.*)

* Published by J. B. Lippincott Co., Philadelphia, 1966.

SUMMARY OF POINTS FOR THE NURSE TO REMEMBER

- Most drugs used in cancer chemotherapy are potentially toxic. Observe the patient's reaction carefully and report any new symptoms promptly to the physician; it may be necessary to alter the dosage or to discontinue the drug.

- Make every effort to lessen the discomfort brought about by drug therapy, thus helping the patient to tolerate treatment which can relieve some of the distressing symptoms of his disease and prolong his life.

- Find out what the physician has told the patient about the purpose and expected action of the drug, so that you do not inadvertently give the patient conflicting information.

- Encourage the patient to take his medication, and show him that you share his satisfaction when he shows symptomatic improvement. Avoid comments that may lead the patient and his family to develop unrealistic hopes of cure by drug therapy.

- Be available to the patient and his family if they wish to talk with you about the drug therapy. Often they feel caught between the ravages of the disease and the distressing effects of its treatment.

- Find out what precautions are necessary when working with patients who are treated with radioisotopes, in order to protect yourself and others.

REVIEW QUESTIONS

1. (a) What kinds of malignancies are treated with chemotherapeutic agents?

(b) What, in brief, is the current status of cancer chemotherapy?

2. (a) What are the two main types of toxicity caused by antineoplastic drugs?

(b) What kinds of signs of toxicity are watched for most closely in patients being treated with antineoplastic agents?

3. (a) What are some measures that the nurse may take to help reduce discomfort and the danger of infection in patients receiving cancer chemotherapeutic agents?

(b) What technique is sometimes employed in administering anticancer drugs to minimize systemic toxicity while achieving the full effects of high local concentrations in the tumor tissues?

4. (a) What should the nurse do before discussing a cancer patient's drug therapy with him and his family?

(b) What attitudes may it be desirable for the nurse to take toward the comments that the cancer patient or his family may make concerning his responses to drug therapy?

5. (a) What, in general, is the manner of action of the class of antineoplastic drugs called alkylating agents?

(b) What types of healthy tissues are most susceptible to damage by these drugs when the emergence of cancer cells resistant to the alkylating agents requires the dose to be raised?

6. (a) What kinds of neoplastic conditions respond best to treatment with mechlorethamine and other nitrogen mustards?

(b) What type of local toxicity may occur with mechlorethamine and what precautions are required in administering it in order to avoid or minimize such reactions?

7. (a) What advantages does cyclophosphamide have over mechlorethamine in the management of certain types of neoplastic conditions?

(b) What assurance can the patient be given concerning the most common adverse effect of this drug?

8. (a) What type of leukemia is most responsive to chlorambucil?

(b) What type of leukemia is most responsive to busulfan?

9. (a) In what types of neoplastic conditions has melphalan proved especially useful?

(b) For what purpose is pipobroman proving especially effective?

10. (a) For what purposes is thiotepa mainly employed?

(b) By what methods is this drug administered?

11. (a) In what general way do antimetabolite-type of antineoplastic agents interfere with the growth and reproduction of cancer cells?

(b) In what specific manner does methotrexate interfere with the reproduction of leukemic cells and with that of normal tissues and of other types of neoplasms?

12. (a) What neoplastic conditions commonly respond to treatment with methotrexate?

(b) What signs of toxicity must be watched for with methotrexate and in what types of patients is it employed with caution, if at all?

13. Against what specific types of neoplasms is each of the following drugs particularly effective?

(1) mercaptopurine
(2) dactinomycin
(3) fluorouracil
(4) vinblastine
(5) vincristine
(6) prednisone and other corticosteroids
(7) androgens such as testosterone and its derivatives
(8) estrogens such as diethylstilbestrol

14. (a) For what purposes are radioactive phosphate and gold isotopes employed?

(b) What type of toxicity is watched for in patients receiving sodium phosphate P^{32}, and what are some other safety considerations in caring for patients who are receiving radioisotope therapy?

15. (a) What are some aspects of nursing care of the cancer patient who is receiving drug therapy?

(b) What are some factors that the physician considers in using chemotherapeutic agents in order to gain their maximum effectiveness and minimal toxic effects?

BIBLIOGRAPHY

Ansfield, F. J., Schroeder, J. M., and Curreri, A. R.: Five years clinical experience with 5-fluorouracil. J.A.M.A., *181*:295, 1962.

Calabresi, P., and Welch, A. D.: Chemotherapy of neoplastic diseases. Ann. Rev. Med., *13*:147, 1962.

Ellison, R. R.: Treating cancer with antimetabolites. Am. J. Nurs., *62*:79, 1962.

Gelhorn, A.: Management with chemotherapeutic agents. J.A.M.A., *191*:315, 1965.

Golbey, R. B.: Chemotherapy of cancer. Am. J. Nurs., *60*:521, 1960.

Hall, T. C.: Chemotherapy of cancer. New Eng. J. Med., *266*:129; 178; 238; 289; 1962.

Hammack, W. J.: Chemotherapy of metastatic malignancy. G.P., *31*:121, 1965.

Li, M. C.: Management of choriocarcinoma and related tumors of the uterus and testis. Med. Clin. N. Amer., *45*:661, 1961.

Monto, R. W., et al.: A-8103 (pipobroman) in polycythemia. J.A.M.A., *190*:833, 1964.

Rodman, M. J.: Chemicals against cancer (Part I). R.N., *23*:63, 1960 (May); (Part II) R.N., *23*:49, 1960 (June).

————: New drugs in the fight against cancer. R.N., *27*:79, 1964 (Nov.).

Welch, A. D.: The problem of drug resistance in cancer chemotherapy. Cancer Res., *19*:359, 1959.

Wilson, H. E., and Price, G.: Leukemia. Am. J. Nurs., *59*:601, 1956.

Wimer, B. M., and Maycock, P. P.: Further comment on busulfan. New Eng. J. Med., *273*:226, 1965.

· 45 ·

Miscellaneous Therapeutic and Diagnostic Agents

Up to now, this text has dealt only with drugs. However, substances that are not so classified because they do not possess pharmacological actions useful in therapy are often used in the treatment and diagnosis of disease. In this chapter, we shall discuss several unrelated types of natural and synthetic substances that the nurse is often called upon to administer, or about which she is called upon to advise people.

The therapeutic and diagnostic agents taken up in this final chapter are:

- Substances that correct body fluid disturbances;
- Drugs used for diagnosis, especially in roentgenography;
- Vitamins and minerals;
- Immunologic agents.

The nurse who, in her practice, has occasion to make frequent use of these substances should, of course, also consult more specialized texts for the details of administration of these non-pharmacological agents.

SUBSTANCES THAT CORRECT BODY FLUID DISTURBANCES

The proper functioning of every cell in the body depends on the composition of the fluids that surround it. If the volume and composition of this internal environment are drastically altered and allowed to stay that way, severe functional disturbances soon develop. Thus, when the body's defense mechanisms fail to maintain internal homeostasis, medical measures must be taken.

Most important are measures that correct the primary causes of the homeostatic disorder—disease, trauma, and poisoning, for example. It is often necessary to correct the abnormality by supplying missing minerals, water, and nutrients. Some substances commonly employed to overcome fluid and electrolyte deficiencies are listed in Table 45-1.

The fluids that bathe the tissues retain their steady state as a result of exchanges of materials with the blood. Any disturbance in the blood supply is soon reflected in changes in the volume and composition of the interstitial fluids and development of abnormalities in cellular function. Though the principles of fluid and electrolyte therapy are not discussed in this text, we shall say something about some substances that are employed when blood volume becomes abnormally low.

Fluid Replacement in Hemorrhage and Shock

As indicated in Chapters 18 and 25, the blood which the heart pumps through the vascular tree is the source of the oxygen, salts, and nutrients needed by the cells. Loss of red blood cells through heavy bleeding interferes with oxygen transport to the tissues. The fall in blood pressure as fluid leaves the circulatory system, either through hemorrhage or by other means, also interferes with the exchanges by which the tissues receive essential elements and rid themselves of excretory products of metabolism. Thus, it is important in hemorrhage and in shock from other causes both to correct the cause of the condition and to make up for deficiencies in red blood cells and plasma, or both.

Whole Blood. In shock resulting from severe hemorrhage, the best treatment is the infusion of an adequate quantity of compatible whole blood obtained from another individual. Such transfusions correct not only hypovolemia, or low blood volume, within

TABLE 45-1

BODY FLUID REPLENISHERS AND BLOOD VOLUME SUPPORTERS

Official Name	Dosage and Administration
Blood Replenishers and Blood Volume Supporters	
Albumin, Normal Human Serum U.S.P.	Volume equivalent to 25 to 75 Gm. of albumin I.V.
Blood Cells, Packed Human U.S.P.	Equivalent of 1 unit (500 ml.) I.V. of whole blood, repeated as necessary
Blood, Citrated Whole Human U.S.P.	1 unit (500 ml.) I.V. repeated as necessary
Plasma, Normal Human U.S.P.	500 ml. I.V. repeated as necessary
Plasma Protein Fraction (Human) U.S.P.	500 ml. I.V.
Fluid and Electrolyte Replenishers and Plasma Expanders	
Dextran Injection (Expandex; Gentran; Macrodex; Plavolex)	250 to 500 ml. I.V.
Dextran 40 Solution (Rheomacrodex; LMD 10%)	As required; total dose should not exceed 2 Gm. (20 ml.) per Kg. of body weight
Dextrose Injection U.S.P.	I.V. as required
Dextrose and Sodium Chloride Injection U.S.P.	I.V. or S.C. as required
Fructose Injection N.F.	I.V. or S.C. as required
Fructose and Sodium Chloride Injection N.F.	I.V. or S.C. as required
Lactated Potassic Saline Injection N.F.	40 to 80 ml./Kg. of body weight I.V. or S.C.
Lactated Ringer's Injection U.S.P.	500 to 1,000 ml. I.V.
Protein Hydrolysate Injection U.S.P.	500 ml. of a 5% solution I.V.
Ringer's Injection U.S.P.	500–1,000 ml. I.V.
Sodium Chloride Injection U.S.P.	500 ml. I.V. as an isotonic solution
Sodium Lactate Injection U.S.P.	1,000 ml. of a ⅙ molar solution I.V.

the vascular tree, but also the anemia resulting from red cell loss. Thus, provided that the source of the bleeding is located and repaired, whole blood transfusions usually overcome both the dangerous hemodynamic disturbances of shock (Chap. 16), and the low oxygen tension of the tissues. However, transfusions are not lightly undertaken. Whole blood is ordered only when definitely needed, for serious and even fatal reactions of various kinds can occur. Some of these are the result of errors in blood typing and administration. Thus, the nurse must exercise the greatest care to help prevent transfusion reactions.

She cannot, of course, avert ill effects brought about by the carelessness of someone else during the collection, labeling, handling, and storage of whole blood. However, the nurse takes every precaution to avoid administering blood to any individual other than the one for whom it is intended. It is her responsibility, as well as that of the person who starts the infusion, to check the labels on the blood carefully and identify the patient correctly, in order to avoid the very serious error of the patient's receiving mismatched blood.

During the administration of blood, the patient is watched carefully for signs of hemolytic or allergic reactions. The blood is transfused at a slow rate at first, and the patient is observed for signs such as flushing, chills, fever, restlessness, and complaints of headache, back pain, and nausea. If these signs of transfusion reactions or the itching, urticarial rashes, or bronchospastic reactions of allergy occur, the transfusion is stopped and measures are taken to prevent more serious effects from developing.

Blood Fractions. In some circumstances, the administration of a portion of the blood is preferable to whole blood itself. For example, if there is danger that the fluid portion of administered blood might overload the circulation, the doctor may order a transfusion of only *packed red cells* to overcome anemia. This is especially desirable in elderly patients or infants, and in persons with normal blood volume, especially in the presence of cardiac, pulmonary, or renal disease. On the other hand, if the blood is highly concentrated—in shock following burns, for example—plasma transfusion is preferred for raising the blood volume, for the administration of red cells is best avoided. In fact, if all that is required is additional fluid to raise the blood volume, the doctor may order only saline solutions or plasma expanders rather than whole blood or any of its components.

Plasma, the liquid part of uncoagulated blood, has certain advantages over whole blood when red cells are not required. Blood typing is not needed, for the risk of hemolytic reactions from pooled plasma is negligible. Plasma is usually preserved and made available more readily than whole blood, which can be kept for only about 21 days. (However, the frozen blood now becoming available can be kept for more than a year.) Unfortunately, while pooling the plasma of several donors reduces the risk of reactions from agglutinins, it increases the possibility of transmitting serum hepatitis virus. The hazard of hepatitis is lessened by subjecting plasma to heat during processing or by prolonged storage.

Serum albumin, the chief protein of plasma, presents no hepatitis hazard. A 5 per cent solution raises the blood volume in the emergency treatment of shock. A 25 per cent solution overcomes hypoproteinemia in nutritional deficiency states and in nephrotic and cirrhotic edema. (The salt-poor, or low sodium, form of albumin is employed in the management of edema stemming from reduced blood proteins secondary to kidney or liver disorders.)

Plasma protein fraction is a solution of a mixture of albumin and globulins, which overcomes low blood volume in shock. It is sometimes administered together with saline solutions for treating shock in infants dehydrated by diarrhea. Like albumin, this blood fraction does not cause hepatitis. The absence of the third type of plasma protein, fibrinogen, means that this plasma protein fraction cannot correct coagulation defects, though it may be substituted for whole blood for a time when the latter is unavailable for treating hypovolemic shock from hemorrhage.

Plasma Protein Substitutes. Many substances have been studied as possible substitutes for plasma proteins in overcoming low blood volume. *Gelatin,* specially modified and dissolved in saline solution, is sometimes used to raise the circulatory volume in shock states. Such solutions as lactated Ringer's and isotonic saline and glucose solutions have been used with safety when blood, plasma, and plasma proteins were not available. The main difficulties with these small, diffusible molecules is that they leak out of the capillaries too rapidly, when sustained action is needed.

Nonprotein plasma substitutes of a colloidal rather than a crystalloid kind have long been sought for helping to expand plasma volume in hypovolemia. One such substance of synthetic origin is *polyvinyl-pyrrolidone* (PVP). It has been largely replaced by solutions of dextrans. Crude dextran is prepared by the action of a specific microorganism upon a sucrose-containing medium. This bacterial action links glucose units up into lengthly branched-chain molecules of high molecular weight. For use as a plasma expander, the crude dextran is then treated chemically to break it up into smaller molecules.

Dextran 70 (Macrodex, etc.) has a molecular weight close to that of serum albumin—about 70,000. Thus, when a solution of this substance is injected intravenously, it shares many of the properties of the natural plasma proteins. For example, it can draw fluid from the extravascular spaces into the blood, thus expanding the plasma volume. Unlike saline and glucose solutions, dextran does not readily leak out of the vessels; so it affects osmotic pressure and vascular volume for long periods.

Although dextran—like plasma and serum albumin—is no substitute for whole blood when a large quantity of red cells have been lost, it does help to overcome hypovolemic shock, whether caused by hemorrhage or by trauma or burns. Because it is safer than plasma (no hepatitis hazard) and cheaper than serum albumin, dextran solution is often used to prevent shock during surgery. Care must be taken, of course, to avoid overloading the circulation in kidney shut down, for this may precipitate congestive heart failure and pulmonary edema.

Dextran may act as an allergen and occasionally causes antigen-antibody reactions of varying degrees of severity. Thus, the nurse watches patients for signs such as urticaria and wheezing during dextran administration, so that the infusion can be stopped promptly if necessary. Patients are also observed for any signs of bleeding tendencies, for a transient increase in bleeding time is sometimes seen several hours following dextran infusion.

A dextran of lower molecular weight—about 40,000—has been developed. Although more readily excreted and shorter in action, it has properties that make it superior in some situations. A 10 per cent solution of this dextran 40 (Rheomacrodex; LMD 10%) has a low viscosity which makes it advantageous as a priming fluid in heart-lung pump procedures (extracorporeal circulation). Used in this way as a hemodiluent, it tends to keep blood cells from sludging within small vessels. This action, which protects capillaries from being blocked by clumped red cells, may prove especially useful in traumatic shock.

However, when a dextran 40 solution is administered I.V. to a poorly hydrated patient, there is some danger that it may further dehydrate him by drawing water from the extravascular, or tissue, fluids into the plasma. Thus, to avoid this and possible renal failure, patients who show signs of dehydration should receive additional fluid—perhaps in the form of an infusion of an osmotic diuretic such as mannitol (see Chap. 20 and Drug Digest).

DRUGS USED FOR DIAGNOSIS

Drugs are sometimes administered not to treat diseases, but to detect them. Diseases often elicit unusual responses to ordinary doses of drugs—in fact, in certain illnesses the reaction is so strong that even low doses of drugs cannot be administered safely. It is on the basis of such reactions (the same basis on which certain drugs may be contraindicated in patients with various disorders) that certain drugs are used as diagnostic tools.

We have seen, in previous chapters, several examples of drugs that produce effects so different in some patients that the presence of a suspected disease is verified—or the suspicion is, at least, strengthened. For example, low doses of edrophonium or curare are used in the detection and differential diagnosis of myasthenia gravis; histamine or its analogue betazole is administered in order to test the secretory capacity of the patient's gastric glands; and the injection of various drugs which provoke or prevent unusual cardiovascular responses in patients with pheochromocytomata (Chap. 17) is a standard part of the battery of tests for detecting such catecholamine-secreting tumors.

Other tests are based on differences in the ways in which drugs are handled by the body in the presence of disease. This is best seen in liver and kidney function tests in which are detected differences from normal in the rate and completeness of excretion of chemicals such as sulfobromophthalein in the bile and phenolsulfonphthalein in the urine.

Radioactive isotopes are often given for diagnostic purposes because of the ease of detecting them even when widely distributed throughout the body. Even extremely low concentrations of isotopically labeled chemicals can be detected externally by instruments that pick up gamma rays emitted from organs in which the isotope is concentrated. For example, we have seen how radioactive iodine is used to diagnose thyroid gland disorders. Radioactive phosphorus is similarly employed for localizing brain tumors.

Other isotopes are sometimes used to trace the absorption of tiny amounts of vitamin B_{12}; to measure blood flow through the heart, kidneys, and elsewhere; and to visualize internal organs by holding a scintillation scanner over the body and determining the distribution of gamma ray–emitting radio isotopes. However, x-rays are often preferred for this, because they give clearer pictures of organ contours and motility and because the use of radiopharmaceuticals for diagnosis poses many pharmaceutical problems and requires considerable care to avoid exposure of patients and personnel to radiation.

Radiopaque Contrast Media. In order to visualize internal structures other than bones and air-containing regions such as the lungs, contrast media are employed. These are chemicals through which x-rays cannot penetrate. As a result of this radiopacity, organs in which these chemicals concentrate can be differentiated from their surroundings and made visible by the shadow that they cast upon the x-ray plate. To be useful as contrast media, chemicals must contain atoms that completely absorb roentgen rays. At the same time, the relatively toxic heavy atoms that best absorb x-rays must be combined chemically into complexes that keep them from injuring body tissues. All presently available contrast media, except barium sulfate, contain iodine in organically combined form.

Some of these substances are taken by mouth either for local radiopaque effects in the intestinal tract or for their effects after they are absorbed and excreted into organs such as the gallbladder. Other contrast media are instilled directly into the organ that is to be visualized—the bronchial tree, uterus, or spinal tract,

for example. The most recently developed contrast media are safe enough to be injected intravenously, or even intra-arterially.

However, safety is not always assured, and while the contrast media seem to be substances of low direct tissue toxicity, reactions of several kinds are common and sometimes prove serious or even fatal. Thus, the nurse who assists in such diagnostic procedures watches the patient closely for early signs of drug reactions, so that treatment measures can be instituted immediately. The patient is also observed for delayed reactions after he returns to the ward.

Barium sulfate is the most commonly used substance for outlining the viscera of the G.I. tract. It is administered orally as a thick paste for esophageal studies or as a dilute suspension prior to searching for peptic ulcerations or upper G.I. tract lesions. Lower bowel lesions are looked for following a cleansing enema and instillation of a large amount of a warmed barium sulfate retention enema.

Barium that is not completely expelled from the G.I. tract may be constipating. Thus, the doctor often orders a cleansing enema after completing the procedure. In any case, it is important for the nurse to note the state of bowel motility and report this to the doctor. Other than for the tendency to cause constipation, barium sulfate itself is an entirely safe substance pharmacologically. It does not irritate the G.I. mucosa and is not absorbed into the systemic circulation. However, accidents and complications have been reported following barium ingestion and enemas.

If, for example, the patient has a tiny, undetected perforation in the wall of the gut, some barium may leak into the abdominal cavity and may even carry bacteria with it. This can cause painful adhesions, abscesses, and even peritonitis. Occasionally, barium *sulfite* or *sulfide*—both of which are soluble, absorbable, and extremely toxic salts—has been dispensed, by error, instead of the innocuous barium *sulfate*. The addition of tannic acid to barium enemas has occasionally been the cause of severe complications also. Apparently tannic acid can be absorbed through damaged areas of the colonic mucosa. Fatal necrosis of the liver has resulted from systemic absorption of this antidiarrheal astringent following its use as an adjunct to barium enema.

Iodinated compounds of two general types are used in diagnostic roentgenography. One kind consists of compounds that are *lipid-soluble*. These are absorbable from the G.I. tract when taken by mouth; oily iodized solutions are also instilled locally. The other kind of organic iodine compounds are *water-soluble*. Solutions of these substances are injected for visualizing the vascular structures of various regions and the excretory organs in which they concentrate.

Cholecystography—the use of radiopaque substances for visualizing the biliary system—may be carried out with both orally administered and injectable iodinated organic compounds. Among the most commonly employed oral contrast media for the diagnosis of gallbladder disease are iodoalphionic acid and iopanoic acid (Table 45-2). When taken by mouth, these substances are rapidly absorbed into the portal vein and carried to the liver, which soon excretes them in the bile. They concentrate in the gallbladder and to a lesser extent in the bile ducts, where they help to cast dense shadows during the making of roentgenograms.

If the gallbladder is in relatively good condition, the x-ray picture is clear and the presence or absence of stones is readily detected. A badly inflamed gallbladder usually shows up faintly or may not be seen at all. In such a case, the doctor may take further x-ray pictures after administering intravenously a water-soluble agent, such as iodipamide meglumine or sodium (Cholografin). Such intravenously administered salts also allow clearer visualization of the bile ducts than do the orally administered iodine compounds.

The tablets are given with several glasses of water or after a light (and fat-free) meal, in order to minimize G.I. irritation and to lessen the likelihood of side effects, such as nausea, vomiting, and diarrhea. They are usually taken in the late afternoon, and the patient is told not to eat until after the x-ray procedure on the following morning. Occasionally, a new compound for oral use such as calcium ipodate is used in faster procedures in which the biliary system is visualized within only a few hours after the patient has taken the tablets —that is, on the same day.

Adverse Reactions. When, as often happens, the latter test is unsuccessful, the doctor may try the more effective intravenous technique. However, the danger of reactions and complications is greater when iodinated contrast media are administered by this route.

TABLE 45-2
RADIOGRAPHIC DIAGNOSTIC AGENTS
(RADIOPAQUE MEDIA)

Nonproprietary or Official Name	Proprietary or Trade Name	Dosage and Administration
Barium Sulfate U.S.P.	—	300 Gm. orally or 400 Gm. rectally in suitable suspension
Iodized Oil N.F.	Lipiodol	10 ml. by special injection
Iodoalphionic Acid N.F.	Priodax	3 Gm.
Iodopyracet Injection N.F.	Diatrast	20 ml. I.M. or I.V.
Iopanoic Acid U.S.P.	Telepaque	3 Gm.
Iophendylate Injection U.S.P.	Pantopaque	6 ml. by special injection or intrathecally
Meglumine Diatrizoate Injection U.S.P.	Cardiografin; Gastrografin; Renografin	25 ml. I.V. of a 60% solution
Meglumine Iodipamide Injection U.S.P.	Cholografin Meglumine	20 ml. of a 52% solution
Meglumine Iothalamate Injection U.S.P.	Conray	30 ml. of a 60% solution I.V.
Propyliodone, Sterile Suspension U.S.P.	Dionosil	0.2 ml./Kg. of body weight intratracheal to a maximum of 18 ml.
Sodium Diatrizoate Injection U.S.P.	Hypaque Sodium	30 ml. of a 50% solution I.V.
Sodium Iodomethamate Injection N.F.	Neo-Iopax	10 Gm. I.V. and by special injection
Sodium Iodipamide Injection U.S.P.	Cholografin Sodium	20 ml. I.V. of a 20% solution
Sodium Iothalamate Injection U.S.P.	Angio-Conray; Conray-400	0.5 ml. of a 66.8 or 80% solution per Kg. of body weight I.V. or intra-arterial
Sodium Methiodal Injection N.F.	Skiodan	20 Gm. I.V. in 50 ml.

These adverse effects are especially likely to occur in patients with liver and kidney disease, for these organs do not readily excrete the injected dose of the drug when damaged by disease. Thus, procedures employing iodinated radiopaque compounds are contraindicated in patients with a history of hepatic or renal insufficiency resulting from acute injury of these organs. Patients whose history reveals hypersensitivity to iodine are also not good candidates for diagnostic procedures employing these agents.

During the first 15 to 30 minutes after injection of an iodinated diagnostic agent, the nurse should watch the patient carefully for signs of histamine-release reactions and other possible ill effects. Sneezing, wheezing, and skin swellings may be the first indications of even more severe anaphylactoid reactions. Thus, the nurse sees to it that the drugs and equipment for dealing with this dangerous emergency (Chaps. 34 and 40) are always readily available during radiographic procedures employing parenterally administered radiographic drugs.

Some patients seem to be especially susceptible to cardiovascular effects that do not occur in the majority of people who receive ordinary injectable diagnostic doses. These reactions are often manifested by a fall in blood pressure and reflex tachycardia. Thus, it is desirable to check the patient's blood pressure periodically. Failure to detect and treat severe hypotension has been followed by myocardial infarction, renal failure, and other complications.

Urography—x-ray visualization of the urinary tract—is carried out shortly after intravenous injection of one of the water-soluble organic iodine contrast media, such as meglumine diatrizoate (Renografin) or sodium diatrizoate (Hypaque sodium). Soon after these materials are slowly infused, they are carried to the kidneys and begin to appear in the urine. Serial x-rays are taken beginning about five minutes after the contrast medium has been injected completely, when dense shadows develop in the urinary collecting system.

Retrograde Urography. In this procedure the contrast medium is instilled into the kidneys through catheters placed by cystoscopy. Thus, the kidneys and the urinary collecting system are outlined without spreading the chemical throughout the body via the circulation. In both this and the above procedures, it is customary to administer a laxative about 12 hours before the administration of the contrast medium. This, and the subsequent withholding of food, empties the bowel and thus minimizes development of abdominal shadows that might make it difficult to interpret the urographic roentgenograms.

Renal arteriography delivers the contrast medium solution directly into the kidney arteries through rapid injection into the abdominal aorta. Although this procedure often reveals defects in the renal circulation

better than any other test, it is relatively hazardous. Two new agents, meglumine and sodium iothalamate, are said to be safer than earlier contrast media for carrying out this test and such other angiographic procedures as cardiac, aortic, and cerebral circulatory x-ray studies. In such studies, the solutions are injected swiftly into the vessels of the organ that is to be visualized. For example, dilute solutions are injected directly into the carotid and vertebral arteries before x-rays of brain blood circulation are taken.

Instillation of oily or viscous iodized contrast media directly into hollow organs, rather than via the blood, is often employed for visualizing certain areas. For example, the uterine cavity and fallopian tubes are visualized by introducing iodized oil (Lipiodol), ethiodized oil (Ethiodol), or one of the water-soluble iodine preparations made suitably viscous by the addition of a thickening agent. This procedure, hysterosalpingography, is used in sterility studies to determine the patency of the tubes and in the diagnosis of other gynecological conditions.

Bronchography is carried out by introducing similar agents, including propyliodone (Dionosil), directly into the trachea, from which they spread down the tracheobronchial tree along the walls of this tract. After the roentgenograms are made, most of the material is removed by having the patient sit up and cough forcibly. Most of the rest of the chemical is apparently absorbed slowly and eliminated from the respiratory tract by other routes. However, some may remain in the lower lungs for long periods and cause chronic inflammatory reactions.

Myelography, visualization of the spinal cord, is carried out by instillation of an iodinated contrast medium into the subarachnoid space. This procedure is widely used for finding evidence of herniated intervertebral discs and other sources of spinal cord compression. Iophendylate, the agent most often used for myelography, is said to be better tolerated than the agents previously employed. Like the others, however, it is aspirated from the spinal fluid immediately after the fluoroscopic or roentgenographic examination.

VITAMINS AND MINERALS

The Physiological Function of Vitamins

Vitamins are substances that the body requires for carrying out essential metabolic reactions. Because the body cannot biosynthesize enough of these compounds to meet all its needs, preformed vitamins must be obtained from vegetable and animal tissues taken in as foodstuffs.

The body needs only small amounts of vitamins because they function mainly as *coenzymes*—substances that activate the protein portion of enzymes. Small quantities of enzymes catalyze a great deal of biochemical activity. Thus, tiny amounts of vitamins go a long way, and any excess of these nonprotein co-factors is either rapidly excreted by the kidneys or gradually broken down to inactive fragments after storage in the tissues.

Dietary Deficiencies

Ordinarily, a person who eats a well-balanced diet takes in enough of these natural nutrients to meet the everyday needs of his body. In such circumstances, there is no need to supplement his intake with purified vitamin concentrates in pharmaceutical form. To take vitamins in amounts that exceed the body's requirements is a needless expense, and, occasionally, the ingestion of excessive amounts of vitamins may prove toxic.

There are, however, various situations in which supplemental vitamins may be of value to avoid development of multiple deficiencies of these nutrients. Even people who are in good health and eat an adequate diet sometimes need extra nutrients, including vitamins, at certain periods of their lives. This is true, for example, of infants fed by formula, as well as women during pregnancy and lactation. Children often require some supplementation of their dietary vitamin intake during periods of rapid growth.

Vitamin supplementation is desirable for the many people who do not eat properly. Some have developed poor eating habits; others have never learned what foods are needed for a balanced diet containing adequate quantities of all the vitamins. Poverty keeps some people from purchasing enough of the foods needed for good nutrition.

Yet many people who can well afford to purchase a full quota of nutritionally desirable foods often fail to do so. For example, alcoholics and other emotionally disturbed people are likely to eat foods that do not supply adequate amounts of vitamins. People who adhere to faddish diets may develop deficiencies of several vitamins found together in the foods that are absent from their diets. Occasionally, a person adheres too strictly to a religious code regulating diet.

In all such cases, patients should be helped to get adequate amounts of vitamins through better dietary planning or from supplementary vitamin concentrates. The doctor determines how the patient's diet should best be supplemented, while the nurse concentrates on helping the patient realize the need for a properly balanced diet and on teaching him what he should know about proper eating. Such help should be offered with due respect for the patient's religious beliefs and the practices of his ethnic group in regard to diet.

The nurse is more likely to succeed in the difficult task of getting people to change their dietary habits if she shows respect for their particular background and practices, and tries to work within the existing framework instead of fighting it. She may, for instance, suggest that the patient check with his religious adviser concerning the interpretation of the rules in his case, since some people deprive themselves unnecessarily because they misunderstand the meaning of a stricture or adhere to it too rigidly.

Patients with certain types of pathology are among those most likely to develop vitamin deficiencies. In various G.I. disorders, for example, vitamins may not be absorbed from food. If parenteral feeding is necessary vitamin supplementation is almost certainly required. During prolonged chronic illnesses, most patients lose their appetites and become unwilling or unable to eat well. The nurse then does all she can to encourage the patient to eat properly, and the doctor often orders vitamins added to the patient's diet in amounts calculated to make up for those he fails to get from food. He usually prescribes high potency pills—that is, *therapeutic* vitamin formulations—when deficiencies of one or more vitamins are evident or seem likely. The nurse should stay alert for signs such as glossitis (inflamed tongue) and fissures in the corners of the mouth, especially in elderly people and those who she knows to be on a borderline diet, so that they can be referred to a physician or to a clinic.)

Excess Vitamins

Most people do not need therapeutic multivitamin formulations and should be advised not to spend their money on such high-potency vitamins. An excessive intake of the water-soluble vitamins, which are promptly voided in the urine, is wasteful; and if overdoses of the fat-soluble vitamins are steadily ingested they may accumulate to toxic levels in body tissues. Thus, for persons in normal health who feel the need for nutritional insurance, products containing only low doses of vitamins are adequate. Provided the person does not overpay for what should be available at moderate cost, such supplementation is harmless; and, in view of the proved value of placebos in many medical situations, vitamins may even provide psychological benefits far beyond their actual physiological effects for those who believe in their value. The nurse, however, does not recommend specific vitamin formulations; rather, she concentrates on teaching people to eat a diet adequate in vitamin content. Determining whether a patient needs a vitamin supplement and, if so, which vitamins and in what amounts, is the physician's function.

Vitamin Allowances

Although the nurse does not tell people what vitamins to purchase, she may well advise them to look for the least expensive product that will meet their needs. She may suggest that they read the labels to compare the formulas and prices of competing products, which sometimes vary considerably in cost. The

Food and Drug Administration requires that the labels of all vitamin products indicate the amounts of each ingredient and the proportion of the *Minimum Daily Requirement* (*MDR*) represented. The MDR is the amount of the nutrient needed to *prevent deficiency symptoms* from developing.

The MDR differs from the *Recommended Daily Dietary Allowances* (*RDDA*), which are standards set and periodically revised by the Food and Nutrition Board of the National Research Council. The RDDA, which indicates the quantity of a nutrient needed to *keep most healthy people* in *good nutritional status*, is always substantially higher than the MDA, for it provides a margin of nutritional safety over and above the minimum needed to stave off deficiency states. Thus, even individuals whose needs are well above those of the majority of normal people are nutritionally safe, if their total intake of vitamins from food and other sources is equal to the RDDA.

A vitamin supplement need not, of course, meet the RDDA, or even the MDR, since people who eat less than an adequate diet still fulfill many or most of their vitamin needs. People tend to think that if a little is good, more is that much better. Actually, it has never been shown that larger amounts of vitamins are ordinarily more beneficial. Thus, products that are labeled to indicate relatively low MDRs are adequate, if priced proportionately low. Products containing many times the MDR are best purchased only after consultation with a physician.

Water-Soluble Vitamins

Certain vitamins are commonly considered together because they are all water soluble, and most are found in the same kinds of foods. They are subdivided into vitamin C and the B complex group. The latter include thiamine, riboflavin, nicotinic acid, pyridoxine, pantothenic acid, folic acid, cyanocobalamin (B_{12}), and possibly biotin, choline, inositol, and para-aminobenzoic acid (PABA). Two of these—folic acid and cyanocobalamin—are discussed in Chapter 25 because they are best reserved for the treatment of macrocytic anemias resulting from deficiencies of one or another or both of these blood-building B vitamins.

Thiamine

Thiamine was the first of the B complex vitamin group to be isolated and chemically identified. Thus, it is also known as *vitamin B_1* and—because it counteracts the neurological signs and symptoms of beriberi—as the *antineuritic* and *antiberiberi* vitamin. Its natural sources include meats, whole cereal grains, and yeast.

When ingested with foods that contain it, thiamine is converted to a coenzyme that plays an important part in carbohydrate metabolism. A lack of thiamine results in a reduction in numerous biochemical reactions that are essential to the normal functioning of all living cells. However, overt symptoms of thiamine deficiency appear most commonly in the form of malfunctioning of nerve cells and as G.I. and cardiovascular system disabilities.

The *neurological difficulties*—seen today in this country mostly in alcoholic patients (Chap. 12)—are manifested mainly in complaints stemming from peripheral neuritis. These include sensory nerve signs such as tingling, burning, and aching, and motor nerve disabilities leading to muscle weakness and paralysis. C.N.S. function is often disturbed by a lack of thiamine, as indicated by irritability, depression, inability to concentrate, and loss of memory.

Cardiovascular complications of thiamine deficiency include signs of congestive heart failure such as edema, dyspnea, and tachycardia, together with a variety of cardiac irregularities. *G.I.* ill effects include loss of appetite, vomiting, and chronic diarrhea.

The MDR of thiamine for adults is about 1 mg., and the RDDA is approximately 1.5 mg. No more than 2 mg. a day is ever needed as a vitamin supplement in normally healthy people who have an ordinary diet. However, patients with diagnosed thiamine deficiency may require as much as 30 mg. daily. This is best administered parenterally in the form of several spaced fractional doses. Once the thiamine stores return to normal in this way, low oral doses are sufficient.

Thiamine replacement therapy usually produces prompt improvement in patients suffering from beriberi, alcoholic neuritis, and the neuritic and cardiovascular complications that sometimes occur in pregnant women and others whose diets lack this vitamin. Patients with similar symptoms that, however, do *not* stem from a deficiency of thiamine cannot be expected to improve. Yet thiamine injections are often part of the management of trigeminal neuralgia and other types of neuritis, as well as ulcerative colitis and other conditions marked by chronic diarrhea. Any improvement that follows such thiamine therapy is probably the result of a placebo reaction or is purely coincidental.

Riboflavin

This substance, vitamin B_2, gets its name from the presence of the sugar ribose and from its yellow color (Latin *flavus* yellow). It is converted in the body to two coenzymes that work together with a wide variety of proteins to catalyze many of the cellular respiratory reactions by which the body derives its energy. Rich dietary sources of riboflavin include dairy products (milk and cheese), eggs, meats, green vegetables, beans, and whole cereal grains.

Deficiency of riboflavin does *not* result in a definite disease such as beriberi, but is accompanied by a variety of typical lesions. Ocular symptoms include itching, burning, photophobia, and tearing. The cornea may show signs of invasion by tiny capillaries (vascularization). A typical lesion of the lips and angles of the mouth (cheilosis) is characterized by development of deep fissures in the mucous membranes and skin, together with inflammation of the tongue (glossitis).

The MDR for preventing the development of characteristic riboflavin deficiency lesions is about 1.2 mg. for adults. The RDDA is close to 2 mg. Riboflavin deficiency states may be treated with injections totaling up to 10 mg. daily, followed by oral doses of 1 to 5 mg. daily for maintenance, together with an adequate diet. Actually, ariboflavinosis rarely occurs alone, and patients who require treatment usually receive thiamine, niacin, and other B complex vitamins simultaneously.

Niacin (Nicotinic Acid)

Nicotinic acid has only slight chemical resemblance to nicotine and none of that potent alkaloid's widespread pharmacological actions (Chap. 17). Thus the official name *niacin* is preferred; the term *niacinamide* is used for its amide derivative which is equally effective in a variety of essential metabolic reactions. Both dietary substances, as well as the essential amino acid *tryptophan* which is derived from dietary protein, are converted into two coenzymes that play a vital role in many enzyme-catalyzed biochemical reactions.

These coenzymes into which niacin, niacinamide, and tryptophan are built are: (1) nicotinamide adenine dinucleotide (NAD), formerly known as diphosphopyridine nucleotide (DPN), and (2) nicotinamide adenine dinucleotide phosphate (NADP), once called triphosphopyridine nucleotide (TPN). These substances, the physiologically active forms of niacin, take part in many important cellular oxidation-reduction reactions. Specifically, they act as hydrogen acceptors for dehydrogenase enzymes in many steps of intermediary metabolism. When the hydrogen is transferred to flavin-containing enzymes, these pyridine nucleotides become available once more in oxidized form for further reactions.

A lack of these metabolically essential substances results finally in *pellagra,* a nutritional deficiency disorder affecting the skin, digestive tract, and nervous system. In its milder form, subclinical pellagra—as seen sometimes in chronic alcoholics, for example—is manifested by nervousness, insomnia, headache, itching-burning skin sensations, and G.I. upset. The full-blown pellagra syndrome, now relatively rare as a result of niacin-enrichment of diets in endemic areas, includes the following characteristic changes: (1) Symmetrical skin eruptions resembling sunburn—on the backs of both hands, for example—tend to heal as darkened scars. (2) A characteristically bright red swollen tongue together with other oral lesions and heavy salivation. (3) Mental disturbances ranging from confusion, depression, and memory loss to psychosis marked by dementia, hallucinations, and delusions.

Pellagra occurs most commonly when diets are low not only in niacin but also in dietary protein containing tryptophan (of which 60 mg. is equal to 1 mg. of niacin). Thus, people whose protein comes mainly from corn meal instead of meat, milk, and eggs are especially susceptible to pellagra, for corn products are deficient in the amino acid tryptophan. Niacin itself is found in only low quantities in corn, whereas large amounts are present in lean meats, liver, peas, beans, potatoes, and fish.

Pellagra responds readily to high oral doses of niacin (50 mg. up to 10 times daily); much lower doses are adequate for maintenance therapy. Occasionally, psychotic patients and those suffering from G.I. malabsorption syndromes require parenteral therapy.

Niacin often causes flushing of the skin, and sometimes—especially following injections—a fall in blood pressure. The nurse should explain to the patient that the flushing is a natural reaction, so that he will not worry unnecessarily that he is suffering an allergic reaction. Patients who complain of weakness or dizziness from niacin are advised to lie down until the discomfort passes and to tell their doctor about the reaction. He may then substitute nicotinamide, which is the preferred form of the vitamin because it does not cause these local and systemic circulatory effects. Unlike niacin itself, however, this amide derivative cannot, of course, be used clinically as a vasodilator, nor is it effective for reducing serum cholesterol levels (see Chap. 22).

Pyridoxine

This substance and the related compounds pyridoxal and pyridoxamine make up the essential dietary factor called *vitamin B₆*. All are enzymatically converted in the body to the coenzyme pyridoxal phosphate. This physiologically active form of the vitamin then combines with various proteins to catalyze many different types of metabolic reactions. It is necessary, for example, for the biosynthesis of NAD from tryptophan. In addition, this biologically active form of the vitamin plays an important part in amino acid metabolism and in certain fatty acid syntheses.

Pyridoxine is found naturally in the same dietary sources as thiamine. The RDDA is 1.5 to 2 mg., but more is probably required during pregnancy and when the intake of protein—and the subsequent rate of reactions involving amino acids—is unusually high. Although no specific disease is associated with pyridoxine deficiency, skin and mucosal lesions and convulsions have occurred in individuals deprived of the vitamin.

A syndrome resulting in convulsive seizures was once seen, for example, in some infants fed a modified milk formula deficient in pyridoxine. The peripheral neuritis that sometimes develops during isoniazid therapy in tuberculosis (Chap. 35) is believed to result because this drug can block the conversion of dietary pyridoxine to the biologically active form. To overcome this competitive blockade and prevent the resulting peripheral neuritis, pyridoxine supplements are commonly administered for prophylaxis together with the daily dosage of the antituberculosis drug.

Pyridoxine has been combined with the antiemetic meclizine to prevent nausea and vomiting of pregnancy. It has been suggested that emesis and other disturbances during pregnancy result from a relative lack of this vitamin at a time of increased protein metabolism. There is, however, no objective proof of the effectiveness of pyridoxine for this purpose. In view of questions recently raised concerning whether the meclizine component of such combinations harms the fetus (Chap. 38), it would seem preferable for supplemental pyridoxine to be supplied to pregnant women separately, or in the form of foods containing it, rather than as part of such an antiemetic product.

Pantothenic Acid

This organic acid is so widely distributed in natural foods that specific deficiencies are unlikely to occur. An ordinary American diet containing about 10 mg. of pantothenic acid provides an adequate intake of this vitamin. Deficiencies produced experimentally by administration of an antivitamin compound are marked by G.I. disturbances, headache, and fatigue.

Pantothenic acid is converted in the body to the metabolically important coenzyme A, which takes part in a variety of vital biochemical reactions. The acetylated form of this enzyme is involved in carbohydrate and fatty acid metabolism and in the formation of the neurohormone acetylcholine. A derivative, *dexpanthenol* (Chap. 38), has been advocated for relief and prevention of paralytic ileus, on the apparent assumption that this substance increases biosynthesis of the neurohormone which helps to regulate the motility of the gut. There is no adequate evidence that postoperative paralytic ileus is related to a deficiency of pantothenic acid or to a resulting lack of acetylcholine.

Although the daily requirement for this vitamin is not known, and no RDDA is established, it is considered an essential substance, and its salt, calcium pantothenate, is a common constituent of many multivitamin preparations, including the official Decavitamin capsules and tablets.

Miscellaneous Water-Soluble Food Factors

Several substances widely distributed in nature are believed to be important nutrients, but how much, if any, is required by humans is not established. These include biotin, para-aminobenzoic acid, inositol, and choline.

Choline is a lipotropic agent sometimes employed therapeutically to reduce the fat content of the liver in the treatment of Laennec's cirrhosis in chronic alco-

holics and in other patients (Chap. 12). However, it is doubtful whether supplementary choline is required by patients with hepatic cirrhosis who can eat a high protein diet. Meat, milk, and eggs supply enough choline and the amino acid methionine (which can substitute for choline) to meet the needs for fat-transporting substances. Choline is also combined with acetylcoenzyme A in the enzymatically catalyzed biosynthesis of acetylcholine (Chap. 14). However, there is no evidence that a lack of dietary choline ever leads to a deficiency of this important neurohormone.

Ascorbic Acid

This essential dietary substance is water soluble but so different in its natural distribution in foods from the vitamin B complex group that it was given the separate designation *vitamin C*. The term *ascorbic acid* stems from its ability to prevent the deficiency disease scurvy (i.e., it is the *antiscurvy* or *antiscorbutic vitamin*). It is found in fruits such as oranges, lemons, and limes and in vegetables, including cabbage, tomatoes, and potatoes.

Ascorbic acid plays an important part in biological oxidation-reduction reactions. Unlike the B vitamins, it is not converted into a coenzyme which then combines with proteins to catalyze metabolic steps. Instead, vitamin C acts in various other ways to aid the activity of many different types of enzyme systems, including especially sulfhydryl systems which it helps to keep in the activated reduced form.

Deficiency of vitamin C interferes with the formation of the connective ground tissue substance that cements cells together. Loss of collagenous fibers from this bed of intracellular connective tissues leads to development of widespread lesions. Local bleeding, for example, is believed to be the result of excessive fragility of the capillary walls. In scurvy, the gums become red and swollen and bleed readily. The teeth are loosened and bone is lost from the jaws. Joints and growing long bones are also subject to hemorrhages. All such symptoms of vitamin C deficiency are relieved in a few days by the administration of about 200 mg. of ascorbic acid daily, divided into several fractional doses. Once healing becomes apparent, dosage can be lowered gradually to 100 mg. or less.

The MDR of ascorbic acid is 30 mg. for adults, and the RDDA is normally 75 mg. An intake of such amounts ordinarily makes up for the amounts of the vitamin that the body uses each day. However, the rate of oxidation of vitamin C may markedly increase in tuberculosis or other infectious diseases. The requirements of such patients may be met by raising the daily intake of ascorbic acid to about 120 mg. There is no evidence that this vitamin has any therapeutic value for patients not suffering from an overt deficiency of ascorbic acid. Yet its administration is advocated for treating a wide variety of clinical conditions, including especially some that are characterized by scurvylike symptoms.

Fat-Soluble Vitamins

Vitamins A, D, E, and K, the fat-soluble essential food factors, tend to stay in the body for much longer periods than the water-soluble B vitamins and ascorbic acid. Absorption of these vitamins requires the presence of adequate amounts of digestible fat and bile salts in the intestinal tract. Once absorbed, little is lost by way of the kidneys, and considerable amounts of these vitamins may be stored in body fat, muscles, and liver. Because small amounts may be released from such reservoirs as required to meet metabolic needs, symptoms of deficiency are slow to develop even during long periods of inadequate dietary intake. On the other hand, the lack of efficient excretory mechanisms may lead to accumulation of some of the vitamins to toxic levels, if excessive amounts are ingested.

Vitamin A

This essential dietary substance is found in the fat of milk, yolk of eggs, and in liver. Although it does not occur as such in plants, vitamin A is formed in the body from carotene, the plant pigment responsible for the color of carrots and other deep-yellow and dark-green vegetables. When carotene rather than already formed vitamin A is the main dietary source of the vitamin, the daily requirement of 4,000 to 5,000 units of vitamin A may double.

Deficiency of vitamin A may develop as a result of a prolonged intake of an inadequate diet. More commonly, it occurs in patients with certain chronic digestive diseases that interfere with absorption of fats and the vitamins dissolved in them. Patients with obstructive biliary disease, hepatitis, cirrhosis, steatorrhea, and chronic diarrhea are most likely to develop this type of avitaminosis as a result of inadequate absorption even when the diet contains adequate amounts of the vitamin.

Signs and symptoms of vitamin A deficiency are manifested mainly in changes in ocular structure and function and in other epithelial tissue abnormalities. Night blindness, a decreased ability to adapt to darkness or dim light, is an early deficiency symptom. Dryness and then deformity of the cornea may lead to permanent visual impairment if not quickly detected and corrected by administration of vitamin A. The skin may become dry and keratinized. Diarrhea may follow pathological changes in the epithelial lining of the G.I. tract; and in the urinary tract, stones may form around pieces of shedding epithelium. Growth and development of infants and children is slowed by persistent, uncorrected dietary lack of vitamin A.

Treatment. Once diagnosed, a deficiency state is treated with high daily doses—25,000 to 50,000 units—of vitamin A. Even higher parenteral doses may be ad-ministered for a few days to correct corneal and other ocular lesions quickly. The daily dose is then reduced to that employed as a dietary supplement during pregnancy, lactation, and in infants—that is, about 5,000 units daily.

People with vitamin A deficiencies are especially susceptible to infections of the eyes, skin, and respiratory tract. This does not mean, however, that administration of vitamin A supplements to those whose dietary intake is adequate will lessen susceptibility to infections. Yet vitamin A is frequently taken in large amounts with the idea that this so-called "anti-infective vitamin" prevents colds. As is true with other vitamins, there is no evidence that intake of vitamin A in excess of ordinary requirements helps to prevent or relieve colds, speeds the healing of skin infections, or in any way overcomes symptoms that are similar to those seen in deficiency states but not caused by a lack of the vitamin.

Chronic overdosage with vitamin A products has resulted in hypervitaminosis A, a toxic state marked mainly by bone and skin lesions. If the condition is correctly diagnosed and the vitamin withdrawn immediately, recovery usually occurs before long. Acute poisoning in infants has followed ingestion of massive overdoses. The illness that results from eating polar bear liver is believed to be the result of its high vitamin A content. The manner in which excesses of this vitamin cause poisoning is not well understood.

Vitamin D

Vitamin D is actually two related substances with similar biological activity: *ergocalciferol* (vitamin D_2), and cholecalciferol (vitamin D_3). (The original vitamin D, or D_1, was found to be a mixture of D_2 and D_3.) Ergocalciferol is obtained by irradiating the plant sterol ergosterol with ultraviolet rays. Similar irradiation of the skin sterol 7-dehydrocholesterol by sunlight results in its activation and formation of vitamin D_3. The latter is also obtained by irradiating other sterols of animal origin—those in milk fat, for example—and is also the form present in fish liver oils.

Dietary sources of vitamin D are relatively limited. Egg yolk and milk contain small amounts but other foods eaten by Americans do not adequately satisfy even minimal needs. (Eskimos meet their needs by eating fish livers rich in this vitamin.) A significant proportion of most peoples' need for vitamin D is met by exposing the skin to sunlight, since ultraviolet rays stimulate the synthesis of this vitamin from skin sterols. The main sources of this vitamin in the American diet are in milk and other foods that have been enriched by ultraviolet irradiation or by the addition of vitamin D concentrates. When such fortified products are unavailable, the diets of infants, rapidly growing children, and pregnant or lactating women are supplemented with 400 units of this vitamin daily, especially during the winter months in temperate zones.

The main action of vitamin D is to aid the absorption of ingested calcium from the G.I. tract. By raising the blood levels of calcium and of the phosphate that moves with it, vitamin D tends to facilitate the deposition of these minerals in bone. Thus, a deficiency of vitamin D in infants and children can quickly lead to rickets, and adults may develop osteomalacia.

Once these metabolic bone disorders have developed, rapid administration of relatively high doses of vitamin D is required to heal the bone lesions and prevent permanent deformity of skeletal structures. Infants with rickets may receive about 10 times the daily prophylactic dose, or about 4,000 units, each day for several weeks or until bone x-rays reveal adequate mineralization; dosage is then reduced to 1,000 or 2,000 units daily and finally to the 400 unit maintenance level. Adults with softening and malformation of the bones (resulting from lack of vitamin D and *not* due to osteoporosis) may receive up to 50,000 units of this vitamin for a time.

Toxicity is, however, a definite threat when this vitamin is taken in excessive doses for more than a few weeks or months. Hypervitaminosis D, as this condition is called, results in the movement of calcium from bones to blood (hypercalcemia). This mineral may then be deposited in such tissues as the kidneys. heart, and blood vessels. Fatalities have resulted from impaired renal function. However, the condition is readily reversible, if further administration of the vitamin is stopped, and the patient is put on a low calcium–high fluid regimen.

In summary, vitamin D supplementation requires more careful attention to dosage than any other nutrient. It is more difficult to get enough of this vitamin naturally than any other, and at the same time it is easy to get too much. Thus infants receive vitamin D supplements promptly when artificial feeding is begun; yet care is required to keep the daily dosage at a safe level. Adults who have an adequate diet ordinarily need no vitamin supplementation; yet vitamin D deficiencies are likely to develop during prolonged periods of physiological stress. Thus, the addition of 400 units of vitamin D daily is certainly desirable during pregnancy and lactation.

Vitamin E

Several natural substances called tocopherols possess biological activity of the vitamin E type. Of these, *alpha-tocopherol* most potently counteracts the effects of vitamin E deficiency in experimental animals whose diet lacks this vitamin. This substance is available in synthetic form and in wheat germ oil, the main natural source. Fresh lettuce leaves and the fat of milk and eggs are other foods in which vitamin E is found.

Deficiency of this vitamin for long periods in several animal species results in effects that resemble certain clinical disorders in humans. For example, rats are rendered sterile, rabbits and guinea pigs develop skeletal muscular dystrophy, and several species suffer various kinds of cardiac muscle lesions.

In humans there is no reliable evidence that vitamin E therapy cures sterility, strengthens muscles in dystrophic patients, or is of benefit in cardiovascular disorders. There is, in fact, no proof that humans require this vitamin and that its absence results in any clinical syndrome that is counteracted by tocopherol administration. Nevertheless, many products containing vitamin E are marketed and advocated for treating a number of conditions, including sterility, habitual abortion, muscular dystrophy and peripheral vascular diseases.

Multiple Vitamin Combinations

As mentioned, a deficiency of only one vitamin is rare. More likely is a deficiency of combinations of vitamins that are found together in the same kinds of foods, when the dietary intake of these foods is inadequate or when some G.I. disorder interferes with their absorption. Thus, it is customary to combine several of the B complex vitamins, alone or with ascorbic acid; or the fat-soluble vitamins A, D, and K may be combined. For full supplementation both water-soluble and fat-soluble vitamins are often administered together.

Decavitamin capsules and tablets, the only officially recognized multivitamin preparations, contain the following: vitamin A, 4,000 units; vitamin D, 400 units; ascorbic acid, 75 mg.; thiamine HCl or mononitrate, 1 mg.; riboflavin, 1.2 mg.; pyridoxine HCl, 2 mg.; calcium pantothenate, 5 mg.; nicotinamide, 10 mg.; cyanocobalamin, 2 mcg.; folic acid, 0.25 mg. (vitamin K is not included, because dietary deficiency rarely occurs, and this vitamin has special uses for which it is best administered alone rather than in combination.

Many multivitamin preparations contain only half the RDDA. These relatively low dosages adequately supplement the amounts of natural vitamins in a diet that the doctor considers to be somewhat less than adequate. Other multivitamin products contain about one and a half times the RDDA. Such preparations are preferred if prolonged illness has resulted in a marked reduction in food intake, or if a therapeutic diet is not adequate in nutritional factors—in allergic states, for instance, or in chronic disease of some portion of the digestive tract. A third type of multivitamin product containing three to five times the RDDA is for patients who require specific vitamin therapy or supportive therapy in pathological conditions in which vitamin requirements are markedly increased.

Minerals

Many minerals play important parts in maintaining body function and structure. For example, we have seen that homeostatic mechanisms that control the concentrations of *sodium* and *potassium* in body fluids play a vital role in the functioning of all body cells. Drugs that affect the metabolism of these key minerals are often employed to counteract pathophysiological states (e.g., the mineralocorticoid-type of adrenal hormones and the saluretic, or sodium-removing, diuretics used in congestive heart failure); yet drugs can also cause excessive loss of these important minerals with adverse effects on the function of the heart, nervous system, and various other vital organs. Thus, deficiency states such as hypokalemia and hyponatremia often require careful replacement of potassium or sodium parenterally.

Another mineral, the importance of which was noted, is *iron,* an essential element in the manufacture of red blood cells (Chap. 25). Traces of iron are necessary for the proper functioning of various vital enzyme systems. Other trace elements believed to be important in body metabolism include *copper, cobalt, magnesium, manganese, molybdenum,* and *zinc.* As noted, however, contrary to the case of iron, deficiencies of these plentiful elements are not known to occur or to cause any human disorders. Thus the practice of including them in polypharmacal vitamin-mineral products is irrational and economically wasteful even though it is physiologically harmless.

The halogen elements in the form of their salts—the *chlorides, bromides, iodides,* and *fluorides*—have important physiological and pharmacological, and sometimes toxicological, properties, aspects of which have been touched upon elsewhere in this text. *Fluorides* are of particular interest not only because they are potentially toxic (Chap. 3), but because they are beneficial to teeth and bones.

The addition of fluorides to pediatric vitamin supplements in minute amounts appears justified in some circumstances because they aid the development of teeth that are more than normally resistant to dental caries. Fluoride salts are often incorporated into commercial dentifrices and their solutions are sometimes applied directly to teeth to reduce decay. Actually, fluoridation of community water supplies to bring the fluoride concentration up to one part per million seems to be the best way to decrease the percentage of tooth decay in the local population. This concentration makes the enamel more resistant without causing any excessive mottling of the tooth surfaces.

Calcium, in the form of its phosphate and carbonate salts, makes up a major part of the skeletal system. It plays an important part in maintaining neuromuscular activity in a normal state, and in regulating the rhythm of the heart; it is an essential factor in the series of complex steps leading to blood coagulation.

The body's stores of this mineral must be replenished through ingestion of foods that are high in calcium—for example, milk and products made from it. Children and pregnant women need more dietary calcium than others and their diets may have to be supplemented with calcium salts.

Hypocalcemia, a reduction in calcium levels of the blood below the normal 10 mg./100 ml., may occur as a result of a dietary deficiency of this mineral. A lack of vitamin D and of the hormone of the parathyroid glands, both of which help to regulate the body's complex calcium economy, may also lead to a drop in blood calcium. When these substances are lacking, dietary calcium is inadequately absorbed from the upper G.I. tract, and calcium tends to move from bone to the blood. This can cause rickets and osteomalacia.

Despite this drain of the calcium stored in bone, blood levels may finally fall so far below normal that signs of excessive neuromuscular excitability appear. This is manifested by muscular fibrillations, twitching, tetanic spasms, and finally exhausting convulsions. The main treatment of *hypocalcemic tetany,* no matter what the underlying cause, is to raise the blood level of the mineral back to normal. In an emergency, this is best accomplished by a slow and careful intravenous injection of available soluble salts, such as *calcium chloride* or *gluconate.*

These salts are injected slowly in order to avoid the adverse effects of high calcium concentrations upon the heart. Care is required, especially with the acidic and highly irritating chloride salt, to avoid leakage into extravascular tissues. Calcium gluconate injection may also cause abscess formation in infants when given intramuscularly. Both these drugs may be administered by mouth for milder states of tetany, but less irritating salts such as *calcium lactate* and *levulinate* are often preferred for this purpose. When hypocalcemic tetany is the result of hypoparathyroidism, calcium injections may be supplemented by administering parathyroid hormone extracts parenterally.

During pregnancy and lactation, the demands of the fetus or infant may double the mother's daily requirement for calcium. Dietary calcium in milk is supplemented by preparations containing calcium salts alone or combined with vitamin D. The ordinary multivitamin and mineral supplements are relatively low in calcium. (A one-a-day capsule containing a dozen or more different vitamins and minerals but only about 250 mg. of a calcium salt does not go very far toward satisfying a daily requirement of close to 2 Gm. of elemental calcium.)

Because the bulky salts of calcium are not easily put into capsules or tablets convenient for swallowing, other dosage forms are often preferred. Unless the patient doesn't mind swallowing a dozen or so tablets a day containing *calcium carbonate* or *calcium phosphate,* the nurse may suggest that the powdered min-

TABLE 45-3
VITAMINS

Nonproprietary or Official Name	Synonym or Proprietary Name	Daily Dosage
Ascorbic acid U.S.P.	Vitamin C	75 mg. requirement; 500 mg. therapeutic
Calcium pantothenate U.S.P.	—	10 to 50 mg.
Cholecalciferol U.S.P.	Vitamin D_3	400 units
Cyanocobalamin U.S.P.	Vitamin B_{12}	10 to 100 mcg. I.M. at weekly to monthly intervals
Ergocalciferol U.S.P.	Vitamin D_2	10 mcg. (400 units) daily; 30 mcg. therapeutic
Folic acid U.S.P.	Pteroylglutamic acid	0.1 mg. daily requirement; 10 mg. daily therapeutic orally or I.M.
Menadiol sodium diphosphate U.S.P.	Kappadione; Synkayvite	5 mg. daily parenterally
Menadione U.S.P.	Vitamin K_3	2 mg. daily
Menadione sodium bisulfate N.F.	Hykinone	2 mg. I.V. or S.C.
Niacin N.F.	Nicotinic acid	20 mg. requirement; 50 mg. therapeutic
Niacinamide U.S.P.	Nicotinamide	20 mg. prophylactic, 50 mg. therapeutic three to ten times daily orally or parenterally
Phytonadione U.S.P.	Vitamin K_1; Konakion; Mephyton	20 mg. orally; 5 mg. I.M. or I.V.
Pyridoxine HCl U.S.P.	Vitamin B_6	1 or 2 mg. prophylactic; 5 to 150 mg. therapeutic
Riboflavin U.S.P.	Vitamin B_2	2 mg. daily
Sodium ascorbate U.S.P.	Vitamin C salt	100 mg. parenterally
Thiamine HCl U.S.P.	Vitamin B_1	2 mg. daily
Vitamin A	Retinol; anti-xerophthalmic vitamin	1.5 mg. (5,000 units) daily prophylactic; 7.5 to 60 mg. (25 to 200 thousand units) therapeutic

eral be sprinkled on food or that a watery suspension that is prepared cheaply by a pharmacist be swallowed at each meal. Flavored wafers that contain a good quantity of a calcium salt are also available. In any event, patients should be told that—as is the case with iron salts—adequate quantities of calcium are best obtained in cheaply prepared dosage forms containing a single ingredient rather than in expensive—and nutritionally inadequate—polypharmacal combinations. This applies also to elderly patients who may require calcium for osteoporosis and to families with several growing children, though their daily requirements are best satisfied by drinking a quart of vitamin D enriched milk.

IMMUNOLOGIC AGENTS

Active and Passive Immunity

Immunity is a state of relative resistance to disease that develops after exposure to the specific agent responsible for an infection. Some individuals or species are born with an innate ability to resist certain diseases. Most people, however, are not congenitally immune to the common infectious diseases. Instead, they *acquire* immunity in the process of fighting off the foreign microbial invaders.

Active immunity of this kind is brought about by the body's response to proteins and polysaccharides in the invading viruses and bacteria. These chemicals foreign to the individual's tissues act as an *antigen*. That is, they stimulate the gradual formation of immune *antibodies* by the reticuloendothelial and lymphoid tissues. These specifically structured protective protein molecules then circulate in the serum, particularly in its gamma globulin fraction. Then, whenever the same foreign substance enters the body in the future, the antibodies of the immune serum combine with the antigen and neutralize it.

Passive immunity is the transfer of immune serum from an animal or a human who has been actively immunized to a person who has not been previously exposed to the pathogen and thus must borrow antibodies in order to combat or ward off an infection caused by that organism. These borrowed antibodies begin immediately to attack the invaders or to neutralize their toxins exactly as would antibodies made by the patient's own tissues, if there had been time enough for them to have been formed in adequate amounts.

Actively or passively acquired antibodies act in the same ways. They may make bacteria clump together (agglutinate), precipitate, or break up before they can gain a foothold in the body and begin to grow and multiply. Some antibodies (antitoxins) keep the poisons produced by tetanus or diphtheria bacilli from becoming fixed to body tissues, thus forestalling the worst effects of infections by these pathogens.

Immunization. Active immunization can also be *artificially acquired* without the need to suffer an actual clinical or subclinical infection through exposure to the pathogens. That is, a person may be inoculated with products derived from microorganisms, or their toxins, that have lost their pathogenic power but still retain the ability to stimulate antibody production. The amount of antigen *primarily* produced in this way may not be great compared to that formed during a spontaneous infection. However, in artificially acquired active immunity, as in natural active immunity, later exposure to the same antigen somehow stimulates the rapid production of large quantities of antibody.

This so-called *secondary response* in an actively immunized individual accounts, in part, for the relatively long duration of active immunity compared to passive immunity. The latter lasts only a few weeks and then disappears as the borrowed antibody is broken down and removed from the body. Active immunity, on the other hand, may last a lifetime, especially if reinforced by periodic administration of booster inoculations to stimulate a rapid secondary rebound of antibody levels. Thus, passive immunity, though useful in an emergency because of the immediate protection it provides, is less desirable in the long run than the more slow to develop but longer lasting and reinforceable active immune state.

IMMUNOPROPHYLAXIS has been one of the most important of the medical advances that have lengthened life expectancy from about 35 to 70 years during the last hundred years. Children have been the chief beneficiaries, for infectious diseases killed two out of five born in this country late in the last century. Today, routine immunizations in infancy against smallpox, diphtheria, tetanus, and whooping cough have caused deaths from these diseases to drop to the vanishing point.

Attempts to protect people by artificial immunization date back to ancient times. The Chinese tried to produce mild cases of smallpox by exposing people to material taken from patients with relatively light cases. They hoped in this way to prevent more serious infections during epidemics of more virulent forms of this potentially deadly disease. However, the use of fluids and scabs taken directly from smallpox patients had inherent dangers that limited the usefulness of this procedure. (Though usually mild, the contagious disease spread in this way may sometimes cause virulent smallpox.)

Thus, millions of people continued to die of smallpox even after the introduction of artificial inoculation into Europe about 1720. The first truly successful procedure was developed late in the same century following Dr. Edward Jenner's discovery that people could be protected against smallpox by infecting them with *cowpox*, a related but much milder bovine disease.

This procedure—called *vaccination* from the Latin *vacca*, a cow, and *vaccinia*, the term for cowpox—could completely eradicate smallpox if universally practiced. Its widespread use in this country and Europe during the last century all but wiped out this scourge that had killed hundreds of millions and blinded or disabled countless others. People inoculated with fluid harvested from cowpox vesicles usually develop only a localized lesion but the antibodies induced by this antigenic stimulus can protect them completely against smallpox.

Immunization is now employed to prevent various other infections besides smallpox. In this country, infants are now commonly immunized against diphtheria, tetanus and pertussis (whooping cough) with a "triple antigen" vaccine administered during their first six months. Today, they are also inoculated against poliomyelitis. Since the introduction of Salk vaccine in 1955, and later, the Sabin oral polio vaccine, the incidence of this crippling and frequently fatal disease has dropped from close to 60,000 cases in this country in 1952 to only 65 cases in 1966. Most recently, measles vaccines have been introduced for protecting against this very common and sometimes serious childhood disease. Vaccination (the term is sometimes used for inoculations against other diseases besides smallpox) may also be employed in special circumstances against influenza, typhoid and other infections including, most recently, mumps.

Products for Active Immunity

Antigenic products employed for conferring active immunity artificially are mainly of two types: *Vaccines* are made from the microorganisms—viruses, bacteria and rickettsia—responsible for various diseases. *Toxoids* are made from the toxins, or poisons, secreted by certain bacteria. It is the toxins that are responsible for the most devastating effects of diseases caused by these organisms, such as diphtheria and tetanus.

Vaccines may contain either the "killed" (or, more correctly, chemically inactivated) microorganisms, or live viruses or bacteria that have been treated to reduce their virulence. Both kinds of vaccines are safe, since special handling has destroyed their capacity to cause disease without affecting their ability to stimulate production of antibodies. Vaccines made from bacteria grown in artificial media and then killed are said to be somewhat safer because they are relatively free of foreign protein that might cause allergic reactions.

VIRUS VACCINES, on the other hand, cannot be washed free of the foreign protein of the living animal tissues in which viruses must be grown and made to reproduce. Thus, patients known to be sensitive to egg protein, for example, could suffer an allergic reaction when immunized with a vaccine that contains virus grown in chick embryos. Live virus vaccines are, however, no more dangerous than those containing "dead" virus; and viruses that are alive but weakened in pathogenic potency are claimed to produce immunity of longer duration. This is related to the greater amounts of antibody produced by introducing harmless virus particles that have retained some ability to reproduce in body tissues. Also, such so called *live, attenuated virus vaccines* often produce immunity after a single dose, whereas killed virus vaccines usually require administration of several doses at properly spaced intervals. Both types of virus vaccines require the periodic administration of boosters in order to keep antibodies at high protective levels.

Toxoids are vaccines made by modifying the toxins secreted by certain bacteria so that they are no longer poisonous but are still able to stimulate production of antibodies by the tissues of the inoculated individual. That is, careful treatment with heat or chemicals such as formaldehyde destroys their poisonous qualities without affecting their capacity to act as antigens that confer long-lasting immunity.

The duration of the immunizing effects of toxoids may be lengthened by precipitating or adsorbing the toxoids by various methods in which chemicals such as alum, aluminum hydroxide or aluminum phosphate

are employed. Such adsorbed toxoids persist in the tissues for longer periods, after injection, and so, they stimulate greater quantities of protective antibodies. However, the relatively insoluble adsorbed toxoids also tend to cause more frequent local reactions such as redness and swelling. These reactions may be more painful and disabling in older children and adults. Thus, adults are often started on even smaller immunizing doses of these products than are young children.

Products for Passive Immunity

Immune sera (antisera) are products obtained from the blood of animals (usually horses) or humans who have been exposed to infectious organisms or to their toxic secretions. These antisera may contain antitoxins, antivenins, and—today, only occasionally—antibacterial and antiviral antibodies. The character of the antibodies depends upon the nature of the antigen with which the donor was naturally or artificially inoculated.

For example, horses may be hyperimmunized by being injected repeatedly with diphtheria or tetanus toxoids or with pit viper or black widow spider venom. At first, very small doses are administered, and the amount of antigen given is then gradually raised. After a period of weeks, when tests indicate that the toxin-neutralizing antibodies have reached a maximum level, the animals are bled. After removal of the red cells, the separated serum is purified and concentrated. This involves precipitation of the globulin fraction of the blood to rid it of other plasma proteins and of non-protein impurities, leaving mainly the antibody-containing fraction.

Despite such purification procedures, these products obtained from animal blood may still cause allergic reactions in some people. That is, the animal protein may act as an allergen, a substance that causes *hypersensitization* (see Chap. 40), the other of the two basic types of biological immune reactions. This phenomenon differs from that which produces protective antibodies against infection. The patient is, instead, made prone to suffer allergic reactions.

Such serum sickness reaction may be delayed for several days, until the patient's tissues build up antibodies that react with the foreign protein still in the patient's circulation. The delayed reaction may be marked by general discomfort, fever, hives, swollen glands and joint pains. A patient previously sensitized to horse serum may suffer an immediate and more severe anaphylactoid reaction (see Chap. 3).

Patients who require passive immunization must be closely questioned about possible previous exposures to horse serum or past allergic reactions. To avoid setting off serious serum reactions, the doctor may decide to withhold the immune serum from patients with a history of earlier allergy episodes, particularly when they show a strong positive reaction to skin or ophthalmic tests for sensitivity to horse serum. If the seriousness of the patient's infection warrants the risk of treatment with antisera, the materials required for managing an acute allergic reaction must be kept readily available. These include epinephrine, oxygen, corticosteroids and antihistamines and the equipment for administering these agents.

Human blood serum also serves as a source of immune globulins containing antibodies against various bacterial and viral infections. Such homologous sera have the advantage of being free of the foreign allergenic proteins that are responsible for horse serum reactions. *Immune serum globulin,* a product obtained from the pooled plasma of human donors, contains antibodies against various common infectious diseases including measles, German measles, poliomyelitis and infectious hepatitis. It has been most frequently employed to prevent or modify the severity of measles and infectious hepatitis in individuals known to have been exposed to other persons with these infections. This product is sometimes also administered to women of child-bearing age who have been exposed to the rubella virus of German measles. This virus can cause congenital malformations in infants exposed to it in utero during the first 12 weeks of pregnancy. Administration of immune globulin is recommended when tests indicate that a woman may be both pregnant and susceptible to rubella.

Other human immune globulin products containing antibodies against specific diseases are also now available. These products are especially prepared from the blood of patients who have recently recovered from a particular infection such as measles, pertussis or polio. They may also be made from the plasma of hyperimmunized human volunteer donors in whom high counts of measles or tetanus antibodies have been built up from gradual administration of graded doses of the infectious agent or toxoid. Such products are especially useful when tests reveal that the patient is both susceptible to the pathogenic organism and highly sensitive to horse serum. Although the use of such homologous serum products in an emergency is safe and usually effective, such passive immunization is no substitute for active immunoprophylaxis employed long before exposure to disease.

Immunologic Products in Individual Infections

The most important immunologic products currently employed in the prevention and treatment of disease will now be discussed below in the context of the conditions against which they are used. That is, rather than discuss these agents in the traditional grouping as active or passive immunizing agents, we shall instead review briefly the various infectious diseases in which these products are employed and indicate the place of such products in the prevention and treatment of these diseases. (See also Table 45-4 for dosage and administration data concerning these products.)

Botulism

Botulism is a frequently fatal disease caused by eating home-canned foods contaminated by the rod-shaped bacillus *Clostridium botulinus*. This organism produces an exotoxin that has been called "the most poisonous poison" because of the minute amounts required to disrupt nerve impulse transmission to skeletal muscles and produce fatal respiratory failure.

Botulism antitoxin containing antitoxic antibodies obtained from the serum of horses inoculated with the two most common strains of the organism, may be life-saving if injected I.V. early enough. Once the ingested toxin has become fixed to the victim's tissues, it cannot be counteracted by even massive doses of antitoxin. However, in such cases, the antitoxin is given anyway to neutralize any still unbound toxin, while the patient is being treated supportively. The nurse encourages the patient who has suffered food-poisoning to stay quiet and calm, checks on the adequacy of parenteral fluid flow, and aids in keeping the patient's throat free of secretions that can cause bronchopneumonia if aspirated.

The antitoxin is most effective when administered to members of the family who have not yet suffered any ill effects—perhaps, because they ate less of the contaminated food than the others. The antitoxin may then prevent muscle paralysis or other severe effects of the infection from ever appearing in these individuals.

Cholera

Cholera is an acute infectious disease caused by ingesting food and drink contaminated by fecal matter containing the bacillus *Vibrio comma*. Infection is characterized by the sudden onset of severe diarrhea and vomiting. Large volumes of fluid are rapidly lost in the frequent watery stools and through heavy vomiting. Extreme dehydration can cause death from circulatory collapse within a few hours after several days of anuria and uremia.

Cholera vaccine is recommended for travelers to India and the Middle and Far East. The vaccine produces only a relatively short partial immunity; therefore, booster vaccinations are advised every four to six months for people staying in areas where cholera is endemic. Other measures for preventing infection should, of course, not be neglected. In areas where cholera is present and the quality of the water supply uncertain, water should be boiled and chlorinated. Food should not be eaten raw and should be protected from flies.

Diphtheria

Diphtheria is an acute infectious disease caused by the airborne bacillus, *Corynebacterium diphtheriae*, which produces and secretes a poisonous exotoxin. Damage to the tissues of the throat causes necrosis and an inflammatory reaction that often results in formation of a suffocating membrane. Death can occur from hypoxia unless a tracheotomy is performed. Heart failure may follow toxic myocardial damage. Paralysis of cranial and peripheral nerves may occur as late complications of diphtheria.

Diphtheria antitoxin administered immediately and in adequate quantities is the most important immediate treatment measure. Injected I.M. or I.V. before the toxin has been bound to body cells, the antitoxic antibodies combine with it and keep tissues from being injured by circulating toxin. Early treatment with antitoxin and with penicillin (to eradicate the toxin-secreting bacteria) has brought about a drop in diphtheria mortality from the former 20 to 50 per cent to only about 2 per cent.

Although the antitoxin may also be employed to protect people who have been exposed to diphtheria, even if they are asymptomatic, the danger of inducing allergic reactions in individuals sensitive to horse serum limits its utility for prophylaxis. The doctor may prefer to keep the exposed person under close observation and administer the antitoxin only at the appearance of early signs of illness. On the other hand, if passive prophylactic or therapeutic immunization seems essential, tests for horse serum sensitivity are employed, and if these are positive, the patient must first be desensitized by frequent subcutaneous injections of small doses before receiving larger amounts of antitoxin.

Diphtheria toxoid is the type of preparation preferred for long-term prophylactic immunization against diphtheria. It is available alone or combined with tetanus toxoid (DT) or with tetanus toxoid and pertussis vaccine (DTP); and all three (toxoid and combinations) are also available in the adsorbed forms which cause longer stimulation of antibody formation by the body but tend also to produce more painful local reactions.

Diagnostic Diphtheria Toxin is employed in the Schick test of the degree of a person's immunity to diphtheria. Injection of a small amount of test toxin between layers of skin on the flexor surface of the forearm produces a red, swollen area within a few days in susceptible individuals. A positive Schick test indicates the need for active immunoprophylaxis with diphtheria toxoid. If, on the other hand, an adult proves to be Schick-negative, he may be spared the series of injections of the toxoid, which sometimes causes severe local and systemic reactions in people who have become allergic to the foreign protein in it.

Influenza

Influenza is one of the common viral respiratory infections that afflict hundreds of millions of people annually. Epidemics are frequent, and even pandemics have occurred at rare intervals. The influenza pandemic of 1918–1919 led to the deaths of an estimated 20 million people, mostly from secondary bacterial infections. Local death rates tend to rise during influenza epidemics as a result of such complicating infections in elderly and debilitated patients.

Influenza virus vaccine is considered desirable for administration to adults over 45 years old and to people of all ages with conditions that might make them more likely to suffer from influenza complications—patients with chronic cardiac, lung or kidney disease, for example, or diabetics. Despite the pessimistic statements that are commonly made about their lack of effectiveness, influenza virus vaccines are frequently useful for short-term prophylaxis.

The main reason for failure of past influenza vaccines to protect against this infection is that the various viral strains tend to undergo frequent mutations. This means that the antibodies built up in an individual by prior influenza vaccination may be unable to counteract the new strain of virus to which he is now being exposed. For this reason, scientists at the National Institutes of Health (N.I.H.) try constantly to detect changes in the nature of prevailing influenza virus strains. The Division of Biologic Standards of N.I.H. then determines the strains of virus that should go into any newly formulated influenza vaccine. The products licensed for distribution each year are best administered in the autumn. Influenza vaccines containing suitably selected strains of virus should then give good protection to most people during the winter months when influenza infections most commonly occur.

Measles

Measles is mainly a childhood disease, but it can also develop in adults who had not been attacked earlier in life by the virus. Although uncomplicated measles is rarely serious, the disease is potentially fatal, especially for children under five years old and for elderly nonimmune patients. Otitis media and bronchopneumonia are among the most common complications. Encephalitis is another of the dangerous sequelae of measles that make prevention and treatment with modern immunologic agents so valuable.

Measles Immune Globulin, a product high in measles antibodies, is effective for *preventing* measles in susceptible individuals when administered soon after they have been exposed to the virus. Measles immune globulin is also used to *modify* an attack of measles so that the symptoms are relatively mild and the illness rarely followed by complications. An advantage of such modification, which is carried out by administering doses of measles antibody products much smaller than those used for complete prevention, is that it permits the invading virus to make most people permanently immune to measles. On the other hand, those who have been completely, but temporarily, protected by passive immunization will require later vaccination.

Measles vaccines of the inactivated and the live attenuated virus types are now available. Each of these products has its advocates, but both types have been shown capable of protecting at least 90 per cent of vaccinated persons against measles. Thus, every child who has not had measles should be immunized with one or another of these vaccines. Such immunization is particularly important for children with chronic cardiac or bronchopulmonary diseases.

INACTIVATED MEASLES VIRUS VACCINE is preferred for infants under one year of age and is effective and safe when administered at as early an age as three or four months. Unlike the live virus vaccines, it may be administered to patients with leukemia, lymphoma and other disseminated malignancies. Some authorities say that the killed vaccine, which is administered in three monthly doses, does not provide long-lasting protection and that it should be followed, after the patient is one year old, by a live virus vaccination.

LIVE VIRUS ATTENUATED MEASLES VACCINE of two types are now available. One contains the so-called *Edmonston B strain* of virus; the other contains the *Schwarz strain* in which the pathogenic potential of the virus has been still further reduced. Both are claimed to be effective for inducing long-lasting active immunity in about 99 per cent of nonimmune children over one year of age. Younger infants do not respond as well because antibodies passively acquired from the mother in utero and still circulating in the child's blood may destroy the live virus before it can stimulate a satisfactory response by his own tissues.

The live virus vaccines, more often than the killed vaccine, cause adverse reactions. The Edmonston B strain virus sometimes produces high fever and rash. These measles signs can be reduced—especially when the vaccine is to be given to children with a history of convulsions—by also administering a dose of measles immune globulin too small to interfere with the desired antibody response. The Schwarz strain vaccine is said not to require such supplementation ordinarily, because this more attenuated virus rarely causes febrile reactions or skin eruptions.

Children in whom the immune response has been depressed may be unable to respond to either the live or the killed virus vaccine. In the case of the latter this means only that the patient may fail to become immune. Live virus vaccines may expose such patients to infection. Thus their use is contraindicated in children who are being treated with corticosteroid drugs or with antineoplastic agents or irradiation.

Mumps

Mumps is ordinarily a minor illness of childhood marked by fever of short duration and a distinctive puffing out of the cheeks and jaw as a result of parotid gland inflammation and swelling (parotitis). Complications are very rare in young children but occur in a higher proportion of people who contract the infection as adults. These include inflammation of the testes (orchitis), a painful condition that can occasionally result in some loss of fertility. More rarely, meningo-encephalitis may complicate mumps.

Mumps Immune Globulin contains antibodies produced by hyperimmunizing human donors with mumps virus vaccine. The product is used for temporary prevention and for treatment of mumps. It reduces the severity of acute mumps and helps to prevent orchitis in susceptible males who have been exposed to the infection.

An inactivated and a live attenuated mumps virus vaccine are available. The latter, introduced in 1968, requires only a single injection to stimulate protective antibodies in most children and adults. The antibody pattern appears to be similar to that induced by a natural mumps infection, but the limited experience thus far with this vaccine does not, as yet, indicate whether vaccination confers permanent immunity. For this reason, at this time the routine use of this vaccine in all children is *not* recommended. It is reserved, instead, mainly for those who have not yet had mumps and are approaching or past puberty. Vaccination may also be indicated for children living in institutions or in other large groups where epidemics seem likely and for adults—doctors, nurses and other students, for example—who have never been exposed to mumps.

Pertussis

Pertussis (whooping cough) is a respiratory disease that occurs mainly in infants and other young children. Inadequately treated cases have a high mortality rate in infants under six months. However, the death rate has been remarkably reduced since the advent of broad-spectrum antibiotic therapy.

Pertussis Immune Globulin of human origin may be employed to reduce the severity of pertussis and for passive prevention. Serum sickness from this product is highly unlikely, and no cases of transmission of serum hepatitis by administration of this product have been reported.

Pertussis Vaccine is now part of the routine regimen of immunization in early infancy. The first injection is made at, or even before, three months of age; this is followed by at least two more monthly injections and by a booster, about one year after the last injection of the first series. Boosters may also be administered at ages three and six and at times of epidemics. Vaccination is withheld from children with nervous diseases because of their relative susceptibility to neurological reactions.

Poliomyelitis

Poliomyelitis, or infantile paralysis, is an acute viral disease that, until only a few years ago, occurred in this country as frequent sporadic epidemics. Damage to the gray matter of the spinal cord results in muscular paralysis; involvement of the medulla oblongata (bulbar polio) can cause rapidly progressive respiratory failure. Fortunately, the availability of vaccines for active immunization has remarkably reduced the incidence of this disease—until only recently common and dreaded.

Poliomyelitis vaccines are of two main types: an inactivated virus vaccine (Salk vaccine); and a live oral attenuated virus vaccine (Sabin vaccine). The Salk vaccine, introduced in 1953, was the first to be employed. Administered in a series of four injections, it stimulates antibodies against types I, II and III polio virus and thus proved highly successful for producing active immunity and protecting against paralysis. However, because this injected virus does not lead to significant resistance to growth of the virus in the intestine, it does not prevent spread of the disease by carriers.

The live oral vaccine, on the other hand, does induce resistance to viral growth in the intestine. Thus because of this and its apparent ability to produce a longer-lasting immunity, the Sabin vaccine is now generally preferred for immunizing children. Its use for vaccinating infants and preschool children in continuing community immunization programs is recommended by authorities on the control of poliomyelitis.

The three types of monovalent live oral vaccines may be given separately or together in trivalent form for the primary immunization of infants. Monovalent vaccines are given in three doses and trivalent vaccines in either two or three doses, beginning at about two months of age—that is, at the time of the first diphtheria–tetanus–pertussis inoculation. The primary series is completed with a dose of trivalent vaccine at 12 to 15 months, and an additional dose is commonly administered at the time the child enters school.

Rabies (hydrophobia)

Rabies is a virus infection of wild animals, including bats and skunks, that sometimes spreads to domestic animals, particularly dogs, which may then transmit the disease by attacking and biting humans. The disease has a relatively long incubation period, during which immunologic prophylaxis and therapy may be effective; but, once symptoms appear, the disease is inevitably fatal, following convulsions and progressive muscular paralysis that finally affects the muscles of respiration.

Antirabies serum should be administered immedi-

ately to severely bitten individuals, along with rabies vaccine. This antibody-containing passive immunization product—which provides immediate protection until the vaccine induced antibodies appear—is both injected intramuscularly and infiltrated around the bites in an effort to neutralize the virus locally before it begins to spread to the nervous system. Use of this agent is accompanied by local treatment with detergents, topical antiseptics including alcohol 70 per cent, and debridement, if necessary, under local anesthesia. Suturing of bite wounds should, if possible, be delayed.

Rabies vaccine is used in two general ways: first, as a pre-exposure immunoprophylactic agent for persons who have *not* been bitten but who run a high risk of exposure to rabies because of their occupation (e.g., dogcatchers, veterinarians) or their avocations (e.g., spelunkers who investigate bat-infested caves). Second, the vaccine is administered to people who have been bitten by an animal suspected of being rabid. Such postexposure immunoprophylaxis requires a course of daily injections under the skin of the abdomen for 14 to 21 days.

Rabies vaccine prepared from a virus grown in duck egg embryos and then inactivated is preferred to older rabies vaccines that were made from viruses grown on rabbit nervous tissue. The latter caused a relatively high incidence of neurologic or neuroparalytic reactions. Because the duck embryo vaccine is free of the so-called paralytic factor found in mammalian nervous tissue, it can be given without fear that its use might result in a fatal reaction. However, unnecessary use of rabies vaccine should be avoided, as the course of treatment is often painful and may result in severe local erythematous reactions and in abdominal distress, nausea and vomiting.

Smallpox

Smallpox, as indicated previously, was once one of the most widespread and deadly of acute infectious diseases. Although extremely rare in areas in which vaccination is mandatory, the disease is endemic in certain regions and could be carried back to the United States by an air traveler from Asia, Africa or elsewhere while still in the incubation stage. Thus, evidence of recent vaccination is required upon a person's entering this country. Most Americans who have not been vaccinated relatively recently have probably lost their primary immunity.

Smallpox vaccine is ordinarily prepared from the lymph taken from calves inoculated with vaccine virus. Recently, a smallpox vaccine prepared from infected portions of the membranes of embryonated chicken eggs has also been introduced. It is said to be fully as effective for active immunization against smallpox and less likely to cause some of the reactions occasionally seen with the older type of vaccine.

The most important consideration in vaccination is prevention of infection of the lesion that develops at the site of deposition of the virus in the deeper layers of the epidermis. Thus, the site should be cleansed with alcohol or acetone and then wiped dry before vaccination. Mothers should be advised concerning proper aftercare of the lesion to avoid contamination. Dressings are not employed, because they tend to become moist and contaminated.

The development of systemic vaccinia reactions and of postvaccinal encephalitis has occasionally been reported. However, the proportion of such dangerous reactions is extremely low compared to the vast number of vaccinations that are performed. Thus, all people except those with eczematous eruptions should be vaccinated. The procedure is first carried out in children between one and two years of age and then repeated at ages six and twelve as well as at later ages. Routine revaccination is recommended every five years, and the Surgeon General advises that doctors, nurses and other medical personnel be revaccinated every three years.

Tetanus (Lockjaw)

Tetanus is a disease caused by contamination of wounds with the bacillus *Clostridium tetani*. This organism and its spores are found most commonly in fields fertilized with animal excreta. However, ordinary soil and even dust may carry the organism, and it may even, in fact, sometimes be found on unsterilized surgical dressings to which it has been borne through the air on dust particles.

Once tetanus bacilli gain entrance to the tissues they begin to multiply and produce their toxins. The danger is greatest when the organism is driven deep into tissues that have been traumatized and contaminated by debris. Gunshot wounds, compound fractures and other injuries characterized by crushing and destruction of tissues offer favorable sites for the growth of tetanus bacilli. However, even relatively minor skin punctures may sometimes be the cause of tetanus infections.

The main symptoms of tetanus, which usually take several days and occasionally weeks to develop, involve the central nervous system. The continuing convulsions that can finally end in death of the patient are caused, not by the bacilli, but by the toxic products given off during their growth. When tetanus toxin reaches the nervous system and combines with motor nerve cells, it sets off severe convulsive spasms.

Tetanus antitoxin obtained from horse serum was until recently the only product used to neutralize the bacterial toxins before they become fixed to nervous tissue. However, *tetanus immune globulin* prepared from human blood plasma is now preferred for passive immunization procedures, because it does not cause allergic reactions like those sometimes seen after administration of the antitoxin. Another advantage of administering gamma globulin from human serum is that the antibodies stay at effective levels for three weeks or more—which is several times the duration of availability of antitoxin-induced antibodies. This gives protection for the full incubation period of most tetanus cases. However, human globulin is no substitute for tetanus toxoid, which should be administered at the same time to produce active immunization.

Tetanus toxoid is a very valuable vaccine that gives good, prolonged protection when given prior to injury. It is administered in early infancy and reinforced periodically with booster shots at intervals of about five years and after injuries that might be contaminated with tetanus organisms. The series of three subcutaneous injections rarely causes reactions other than occasional local redness and swelling. The adsorbed tetanus toxoid is somewhat more likely to cause local reactions, but its longer duration of action permits active immunization with only two injections. Both the toxoid solution and the adsorbed toxoid suspension are available combined with diphtheria toxoid and pertussis vaccine in the triple antigen (DTP) combinations that, together with oral polio vaccine, constitutes the infant's earliest series of immunizations.

Tuberculosis

The nature of this disease and its treatment with tuberculostatic chemotherapeutic agents has been discussed in Chapter 25. Here we will take up briefly only the use and status of certain diagnostic and immunoprophylactic agents.

Old Tuberculin U.S.P. and the **Purified Protein Derivative of Tuberculin U.S.P.** are preparations of the growth products of the tubercle bacillus that are used as aids in the diagnosis of tuberculosis. Injected intracutaneously, minute amounts produce positive reactions (redness, edema, etc.) in individuals who are, or had ever been, infected with the tuberculosis organism. A negative reaction indicates that the person does not have tuberculosis—and also shows that he has built up no antibodies to defend against future invasion, if he should be exposed to the risk of infection.

BCG Vaccine is an active immunizing product prepared from the living cells of the **Bacillus Calmette Guerin**, an attenuated strain of an organism that causes bovine tuberculosis. Its value for immunoprophylaxis against tuberculosis is debatable, and authoritative committees have indicated that its routine use in large scale public health tuberculosis control programs is unnecessary in this country. In fact, because its administration produces positive tuberculin test reactions and thus makes diagnosis more difficult, its widespread use is considered undesirable. Nevertheless, this immunizing agent *has* been administered

TABLE 45-4

IMMUNOLOGIC AGENTS

Disease	Organism	Products Employed for Prevention or Treatment	Dosage and Administration
Botulism	*Clostridium botulinum*	Botulism Antitoxin U.S.P. (passive immunizing agent)	I.M. or I.V. Prophylactic: 2,500 u. Therapeutic: 10,000 to 50,000 u.
Cholera	*Vibrio comma*	Cholera Vaccine U.S.P. (active immunizing agent)	S.C. or I.M. 0.5 ml.; then 1 ml. at least 7 days later. Repeat 0.5 ml. dose every 6 months if necessary
Diphtheria	*Corynebacterium diphtheriae*	Diphtheria Antitoxin U.S.P. (passive immunizing agent)	I.M. or I.V. Prophylactic: 1,000 to 10,000 u. Therapeutic: 10,000 to 80,000 u.
		Diphtheria Toxoid U.S.P. (active immunizing agent)	S.C. injections of 0.5 to 1 ml., at least 4 weeks apart
		Adsorbed Diphtheria Toxoid U.S.P. (active immunizing agent)	S.C. or I.M., 2 injections of 0.5 to 1 ml. at least 4 weeks apart; a third, reinforcing dose 6 to 12 months later
		Diagnostic Diphtheria Toxin (for Schick Test)	Intracutaneous 0.1 ml.
Influenza	Various strains of influenza virus	Influenza Virus Vaccine U.S.P. (active immunizing agent)	S.C. 2 injections of 1 ml., at least 2 months apart
Measles	Various strains of rubeola virus	Measles Virus Vaccine, Live, Attenuated (Edmonston B strain)	S.C. 0.5 ml. for active immunization
		Measles Virus Vaccine, Live, Attenuated (Schwarz strain)	S.C. 0.5 ml. for active immunization
		Measles Virus, Inactivated	I.M., 0.5 or 1 ml. in 3 doses at monthly intervals for active immunization
		Measles Immune Globulin U.S.P. (passive immunizing agent)	Prophylactic: I.M., 0.22 ml. per Kg. of body weight. Modification of measles: 0.022 to 0.045 ml. per Kg.
		Immune Serum Globulin U.S.P. (passive immunizing agent)	Prophylactic: I.M. 0.22 ml. per Kg. for measles (0.02 ml. per Kg. for infectious hepatitis). Modification of measles: 0.045 ml. per Kg.
Mumps	Various strains of epidemic parotitis virus	Mumps virus vaccine, live, attenuated (active immunizing agent)	S.C. a single dose of not less than 5,000 $TCID_{50}$ for active prophylaxis
		Mumps vaccine, inactivated virus for active prophylaxis (active immunizing agent)	S.C. or I.M. 2 injections of 1 ml. each administered at intervals of 1 to 4 weeks
		Mumps Immune Globulin Human (passive immunizing agent)	1.5 ml. to 4.5 ml., depending on body weight
Pertussis	*Bordetella pertussis*	Pertussis Vaccine U.S.P. (active immunizing agent)	S.C. 3 injections, usually of 0.5 ml., at least 4 weeks apart
		Pertussis Immune Globulin U.S.P. (passive immunizing agent)	Prophylactic: one or two I.M., injections at 1 week intervals in amounts recommended by manufacturer. Therapeutic: 2 injections at 1-day intervals
Plague	*Pasteurella pestis*	Plague Vaccine U.S.P. (active immunizing agent)	S.C. 2 injections of 0.5 to 1 ml. at least 7 days apart

TABLE 45-4 (Cont'd)

Disease	Organism	Products Employed for Prevention or Treatment	Dosage and Administration
Poliomyelitis	Various strains of polio virus	Poliomyelitis Vaccine U.S.P. (Salk Vaccine) (active immunizing agent)	S.C. 2 injections of 1 ml., 4 to 6 weeks apart, then 1 ml. at least 7 months later.
		Live Oral Poliovirus Vaccine, Monovalent U.S.P. (active immunizing agent)	Each of the monovalent vaccines is given separately at intervals of 6 to 8 weeks
		Live Oral Poliovirus Vaccine, Trivalent U.S.P. (active immunizing agent)	Two drops to 2 ml., depending upon the concentration used are administered for primary immunization in 3 doses at intervals of 8 weeks
Rabies	Various strains of rabies virus	Rabies Vaccine U.S.P. (active immunizing agent)	S.C. 2 ml. of a 5% suspension or its equivalent daily for 14 to 21 days for postexposure immunoprophylaxis
		Antirabies Serum (passive immunizing agent)	I.M. 20 u. per lb. of body weight
Smallpox	Variola virus	Smallpox Vaccine U.S.P. (active immunizing agent)	Percutaneous injection (into the skin) of the contents of one capillary tube by the multiple puncture method
Tetanus	*Clostridium tetani*	Tetanus Toxoid U.S.P. (active immunizing agent)	S.C. 3 injections of 0.5 ml. at least 4 weeks apart
		Adsorbed Tetanus Toxoid U.S.P. (active immunizing agent)	I.M. or S.C. 2 injections of 0.5 ml. at least 4 weeks apart
		Tetanus Antitoxin U.S.P. (passive immunizing agent)	I.M. or S.C. Prophylactic: 1,500 to 10,000 u. Therapeutic: 10,000 to 100,000 u.
		Tetanus Immune Globulin U.S.P. (passive immunizing agent)	I.M. Prophylactic: 250 u. Therapeutic: 1,500 u. (or more)
Tuberculosis	*Mycobacterium tuberculosis*	BCG Vaccine U.S.P. (active immunizing agent)	Intradermal, 0.1 ml. Percutaneous, 1 drop on surface of skin, administered by multiple puncture method
		Old Tuberculin U.S.P. (diagnostic aid)	Intracutaneous 0.00001 to 0.001 ml.
		Purified Protein Derivative of Tuberculin U.S.P. (diagnostic aid)	Intracutaneous, 0.02 to 5 mcg.
Typhoid	*Salmonella typhosa*	Typhoid Vaccine U.S.P. (active immunizing agent)	S.C., 3 injections of 0.5 ml. at least 7 days apart
		Typhoid and Paratyphoid Vaccine U.S.P. (active immunizing agent)	S.C. 3 injections of 0.5 ml. at least 7 days apart
Typhus	*Rickettsia prowazekii*	Typhus Vaccine U.S.P.	S.C., 2 injections of 1 ml. at least 7 days apart
Yellow fever	Virus	Yellow Fever Vaccine U.S.P. (active immunizing agent)	S.C. 0.5 ml.

to hundreds of millions of people elsewhere in the world; and its use here is recommended for tuberculin-negative individuals who are exposed to infection and cannot be readily protected by other control measures (for example, migrant workers and others often living under crowded unsanitary conditions).

Typhoid Fever

Typhoid is an acute systemic infection caused by a Salmonella organism that enters the G.I. tract through ingestion of contaminated food or water and then makes its way into the blood stream. The disease, which is marked by malaise and the gradual development of a persistent fever and a rose-colored rash resembling that of typhus (hence the name, "typhoid"), may be relatively mild or rapidly fatal. Related paratyphoid-type Salmonella organisms cause less severe infections than S. *typhosa,* the pathogen of true typhoid fever.

Typhoid vaccine and *typhoid-paratyphoid vaccine* have been less important than advances in sanitation in reducing the incidence of typhoid fever in this country. Their efficacy as active immunoprophylactic products is certainly not great enough to warrant neglect of sanitation by vaccinated individuals. However, even though protection offered by available typhoid and combination, or "triple," vaccine (containing three types of Salmonella organisms) is limited and short-lived, their use by travelers in areas where typhoid is endemic is recommended by some authorities. Vaccination against typhoid is also indicated for medical laboratory workers and others who might come in contact with fecal matter containing typhoid bacteria. The procedure should not be performed while the person is ill with an infection or if he has diabetes or nephritis. Local and systemic reactions, while not severe, occur in a high proportion of those receiving the typhoid or typhoid-paratyphoid vaccines. Passive immunization is not employed in treating typhoid, but the broad-spectrum antibiotics (Chap. 34), especially chloramphenicol, have proved highly effective.

Typhus Fever

Typhus is a disease caused by rickettsiae, microorganisms with characteristics midway between those of bacteria and viruses. Epidemic typhus has periodically swept through Asia, Europe and other areas over the centuries and decimated armies during sieges of Old World Cities and in other military campaigns. In World War II, the introduction of DDT for control of rickettsiae-bearing lice prevented the transmission of typhus on the few occasions when small outbreaks of the disease occurred. In addition to body-dusting with DDT (and other personal sanitation measures), immunoprophylaxis with typhus vaccine is desirable in areas where a reservoir of rickettsiae is known to exist. (Such vaccination is *not* effective against murine (scrub) typhus, a related rickettsiae infection endemic in North and Central America.)

Typhus vaccine is made from rickettsiae cultures grown in chick embryo membranes (like virus, these organisms require living tissues for reproduction). Thus, caution is required in vaccinating individuals known to be allergic to eggs. Otherwise, the vaccine is safe and relatively effective. Even if an immunized person does contract the disease, his symptoms are relatively mild and of short duration. (Ordinarily, typhus victims develop sudden severe headache and high, persistent fever, followed sometimes by fatal bronchopneumonia; a red, maculopapular rash appears on the back and chest around the fifth day and then extends to the extremities and abdomen, forming small hemorrhages, purple patches and, possibly, becoming gangrenous.) Immunization is carried out by administering two doses subcutaneously at an interval of 7 to 10 days. Boosters are given at the beginning of an epidemic and repeated 3 months later, and then every six months.

Summary: We have seen examples of many active and passive immunizing agents that are used for prevention and treatment of various acute infectious diseases. Since many of these infections, particularly those caused by viruses, cannot yet be effectively treated with antimicrobial chemotherapeutic agents and antibiotics, active immunoprophylaxis with viral vaccines and bacterial toxoids is still very valuable. Also, in cases of actual infection and threatened infection by dangerously virulent organisms, the early administration of antibody-containing serums may be lifesaving. In such cases, immune serums derived from *human* blood are especially effective and safe, since such homologous gamma globulin blood fractions are relatively free of the danger of sensitization reactions sometimes seen following administration of horse serum.

REVIEW QUESTIONS

Body Fluid Disturbances

1. Why is compatible whole blood preferred to other fluids in the management of severe hemorrhage?

2. What are some adverse reactions that may result from transfusion of whole blood or of blood plasma?

3. What are some of the nurse's duties and responsibilities relative to the transfusion of blood?

4. Under what circumstances may the doctor prefer plasma transfusions to whole blood, and for which patients might he order packed red cells rather than either plasma or whole blood?

5. What advantages does plasma administration sometimes have over whole blood transfusion, and what advantage do serum albumin and plasma protein fraction have over plasma itself?

6. What physical property of dextran accounts for its plasma protein–like action and makes it preferable to saline-glucose solutions in hypovolemia?

7. What observations does the nurse make during infusion of dextran in order to detect early signs of adverse effects?

Diagnosis

1. For what purpose is barium sulfate employed?

2. What observations does the nurse make and report concerning the condition of patients who have received barium sulfate orally or by enema?

3. What kinds of accidents and complications have sometimes occurred in situations in which barium ingestion or enemas have been ordered?

4. List some radiopaque substances administered orally or intravenously as contrast media in cholecystography, and indicate the manner in which these substances aid the physician in determining the condition of the biliary system.

5. What instructions does the patient receive prior to taking tablets of contrast media employed in cholecystography?

6. When is the administration of iodinated contrast media contraindicated?

7. For what signs are patients observed after they have received iodinated diagnostic agents?

8. List some new contrast media that are said to be relatively safe when injected in various arteriographic, or angiographic, diagnostic procedures.

9. List some agents instilled into the uterine cavity and fallopian tubes for hysterosalpingography in sterility studies.

10. List the preferred contrast media for bronchography and myelography.

Vitamins and Minerals

1. What is the main general function of most vitamins?

2. In what periods of life is the body's demand for extra vitamins likely to be greatest?

3. How may the nurse help people who are in danger of developing a vitamin deficiency because of poor dietary practices?

4. What is the nurse's responsibility if she suspects that a person has a vitamin deficiency or if she is asked to recommend a vitamin formulation for purchase as self-medication?

5. What is meant by the terms *Minimum Daily Requirement* (MDR) and *Recommended Daily Dietary Allowance* (RDDA)?

6. What are some signs of thiamine deficiency and in what clinical conditions is thiamine replacement therapy most likely to overcome signs of deficiency?

7. What are some signs of riboflavin deficiency?

8. What condition is associated with niacin deficiency and what are some clinical signs and symptoms that may be overcome by administration of replacement doses of niacin?

9. What side effect of niacin is the patient told to anticipate, and what derivative may the doctor substitute to avoid this effect?

10. With what medications is pyridoxine sometimes administered as an adjunct, and what signs and symptoms are sometimes seen in a deficiency state?

11. Which two dietary factors of the vitamin B complex group play a part in the biosynthesis of the important neurohormone acetylcholine?

12. What disease is associated with a deficiency of ascorbic acid, and what are some natural food sources of vitamin C?

13. What are some clinical conditions that sometimes lead to a deficiency of vitamin A or other fat-soluble vitamins, and what is a common early sign of vitamin A deficiency?

14. How are the needs of most people for vitamin D met in this country, and what deficiency disorders may develop if this vitamin is long lacking?

15. Which two vitamins cause toxicity when administered in high overdoses over a period of time?

16. What are some clinical disorders for which administration of vitamin E is sometimes advocated; and what is the status of such therapy and of the use of vitamins generally in conditions not caused by deficiencies?

17. In what circumstances are each of three different dose levels of multivitamins preferred?

18. What is the purpose of adding fluoride salt supplements to the diets of some patients?

19. What persons are most prone to develop a deficiency of calcium, and what are some of the signs of hypocalcemia?

20. What forms of calcium are administered parenterally in emergencies? In what kind of products is supplemental calcium best administered to assure a cheap and an adequate intake?

Immunologic Agents

1. List three ways in which artificial active and passive immunization differ (e.g., sources of antibodies; time of onset of antibody activity; duration of immune state).

2. What are the constituents of the triple antigen vaccine with which infants are now immunized during their first months, and what is a fourth vaccine now also frequently first administered during the early months of life?

3. What advantages may live, attenuated virus vaccines have over those made from completely inactivated (killed) viruses?

4. What advantage do adsorbed toxoids have over ordinary toxoid, and what properties of all toxoids make these chemically treated toxins effective for active immunization but free from disease-producing danger?

5. What advantage do human immune sera have over those derived from the blood of horses or other animals?

6. List some infections against which products for passive immunization are now available containing specific antibodies in the gamma globulin fraction of human serum.

7. What product is available for the passive immunization of patients suffering from botulism, and what supportive measures must be taken in such cases?

8. What product is available to prevent travelers from contracting cholera and what measures are required to control transmission of this disease?

9. What products are available for determining a person's susceptibility to diphtheria; for producing immunoprophylaxis; and for emergency treatment of individuals thought to have been infected?

10. (a) What factor limits somewhat the utility of influenza virus vaccine?

(b) For what kinds of persons is its routine use each autumn considered desirable?

11. Under what circumstances and in what two ways is measles immune globulin employed?

12. What advantages are claimed for the inactivated and the live virus measles vaccines, respectively, and how may possible reactions from inoculations with the latter be minimized?

13. What product is used to minimize complications in patients with mumps, and which of the available products is preferred for active immunization against this disease?

14. What immunologic and other important agents are employed in the prevention and treatment of pertussis?

15. What are the advantages of the live attentuated poliomyelitis vaccine over the inactivated vaccine?

16. What products and procedures are employed for treating a patient suspected of having been bitten by a rabid animal?

17. What locally adverse effects must be guarded against in vaccinating against smallpox, and what severe systemic reactions have been very rarely reported? In what type of patient may smallpox vaccination be contraindicated?

18. What is now the preferred product for passive immunization against tetanus, and in what forms is the active immunizing agent against this disease available?

19. (a) For what purpose are tuberculin products employed?

(b) What is the current status of BCG vaccine in this country?

20. (a) What is the status of typhoid and typhoid-paratyphoid vaccines in immunoprophylaxis against certain Salmonella infections?

(b) In what circumstances is typhoid vaccination contraindicated?

21. (a) What sanitation and immunoprophylactic measures are employed for control of typhus?

(b) What, in terms of its relative safety and effectiveness, is the status of typhus vaccine?

BIBLIOGRAPHY

Body Fluid Disturbances

Dutcher, I., and Fielo, S.: Water and Electrolytes. The Macmillan Co., New York, 1967.

Hamit, H. F.: Status of human plasma as a plasma volume expander. J.A.M.A., *174*:1617, 1960.

Howard, J. M.: Fluid replacement in shock and hemorrhage. J.A.M.A., *173*:516, 1960.

Metheney, N., and Snively, W. D.: Nurses' Handbook of Fluid Balance. J. B. Lippincott Co., Philadelphia, 1967.

Rasmussen, M. G., et al.: Transfusion therapy. New Eng. J. Med., *264*:1034; 1038; 1961.

Rodman, M. J.: Fluid and electrolyte balance. R.N., *22*:41, 1959 (May).

Wilson, J. S., et al.: The use of dextran in the treatment of blood loss and shock. Am. J. Med. Sci., *223*:364, 1952.

Diagnosis

Crocker, D., and Vandam, L. D.: Untoward reactions to radiopaque contrast media. Clin. Pharmacol. Ther., *4*: 654, 1963.

Hoppe, J. O.: Some pharmacological aspects of radiopaque compounds. Ann. N. Y. Acad. Sci., *78*:727, 1959.

Rodman, M. J.: Drugs used for diagnosis. R.N., *22*:43, 1959 (Dec.).

Wagner, H. N., Jr.: Radioactive pharmaceuticals. Clin. Pharmacol. Ther., *4*:351, 1963.

Vitamins and Minerals

Council on Foods and Nutrition: Deficiencies of fat-soluble vitamins. J.A.M.A., *144*:34, 1950.

———: Deficiencies of water-soluble vitamins. J.A.M.A., *144*:307, 1950.

———: Vitamin preparations as dietary supplements and as therapeutic agents. J.A.M.A., *169*:41, 1959.

Griffith, W. H.: The physiologic role of vitamins. Am. J. Med., *25*:666, 1958.

Recommended Dietary Allowances, Report of the Food and Nutrition Board, National Academy of Sciences, National Research Council, Pub. 1146, Washington, D.C. 1964.

Rodman, M. J.: Blood-building B vitamins and how they work. R.N., *22*:33, 1959 (Nov.).

Sebrell, W. H.: Some clinical aspects of vitamin B deficiencies. Am. J. Med., *25*:673, 1958.

Immunologic Agents

Blatt, N. H., and Lepper, M. H.: Reactions following antirabies prophylaxis. Am. J. Dis. Child., *86*:395, 1965.

Coriel, L. L.: Smallpox vaccination. When and whom to vaccinate. Pediatrics, *37*:493, 1966.

Donaldson, A. W.: Current status of national immunization programs. Med. Clin. N. Am., *51*:831, 1967 (May).

Eickhoff, T. C., *et al.:* Observations on excess mortality associated with epidemic influenza. J.A.M.A., *176*:776, 1961.

Hayne, A. L., and Slotowski, E. L.: Frequency of encephalitis as a complication of measles. Am. J. Dis. Child, *73*:554, 1947.

Hilleman, M. R.: Immunologic, chemotherapeutic and interferon approaches to control of viral disease. Am. J. Med., *38*:751, 1965.

Medoff, H. S., *et al.:* Epidemiologic study of inactivated measles vaccine. J.A.M.A., *189*:723, 1964.

Moffet, H. L., *et al.:* Outbreak of influenza A₂ among immunized children. J.A.M.A., *190*:806, 1964.

Peck, F. B., *et al.:* A new antirabies vaccine for human use (rabies vaccine made from embryonated duck eggs). J. Lab. Clin. Med., *45*:679, 1955.

Sabin, A. B.: Oral poliovirus vaccine. History of its development and prospects for eradication of poliomyelitis. J.A.M.A., *194*:872, 1965.

Schwarz, A. J. F.: Preliminary tests of a highly attenuated measles vaccine. Am. J. Dis. Child., *103*:386, 1962.

von Magnus, H.: Measles vaccines—present status. Med. Clin. N. Am., *51*:599, 1967 (May).

Drug
Digests

CHAPTER 3

THE TOXIC EFFECTS OF DRUGS AND CHEMICALS

CALCIUM DISODIUM EDETATE U.S.P. (CALCIUM EDTA; EDATHAMIL CALCIUM; CALCIUM VERSENATE)

Pharmacology. This antidotal chemical combines with free lead ions in body tissues to form a firm complex. Then the metal in this nonionized and inactive chelate form is excreted by the kidneys. The presence of more than 500 mcg. of lead in a 24 hour urine sample, following administration of this drug, is diagnostic of lead poisoning. A course of treatment is then indicated for mobilizing lead from the liver, bones, blood, and other body tissues. In children suffering from lead encephalopathy, dimercaprol is sometimes administered prior to edatate to speed the rate of lead excretion; supportive treatment including the use of osmotic diuretics reduces intracranial pressure in such cases; and anticonvulsant medications control seizures.

Possible side effects of edetate treatment include general malaise, lethargy, thirst, chills, and fever, followed by frontal headache, nausea, and vomiting. Thrombophlebitis is reported occasionally. In experimental animals, severe kidney damage culminating in tubular necrosis sometimes develops. Clinically in human patients, renal failure is rare if the drug is discontinued temporarily upon appearance of early signs of kidney malfunction.

Dosage and Administration. For treatment of acute and chronic lead poisoning and encephalopathy and for prophylaxis against exacerbations 1 Gm. is diluted with 250 to 500 ml. of fluid and infused I.V. over a 1-hour period. This may be repeated twice daily for up to 5 days. If a further course is required, it is administered after a 2-day interruption of edetate treatment. Parenteral therapy may be followed by 4 Gm. daily, administered orally in divided doses. Dosage for children should not exceed 1 Gm./30 lb. parenterally or 1 Gm./35 lb. orally, administered in two equal doses daily.

DIMERCAPROL U.S.P. (BAL; BRITISH ANTI-LEWISITE)

Pharmacology. This heavy metal antagonist is used in the treatment of poisoning by mercury, arsenic, and gold salts. It donates its two thiol (SH) groups, which bind the metallic ions and keep them from attacking the essential tissue sulfhydryls. As a result, cellular sulfhydryl enzyme systems are protected from poisoning by the heavy metals; if this antidotal drug is given early enough, it even removes metallic ions already bound to tissue SH groups; thus it reactivates the poisoned enzymes and restores normal cellular function.

Dimercaprol, in the form of an oily solution with a disagreeable garlicky odor, is itself potentially toxic. Common side effects include nausea and vomiting; headache; a burning sensation of the lips, mouth, throat, and eyes; tingling of the hands and feet; and a sense of tightness in the chest. Too frequent administration may cause a sharp rise in blood pressure. Children frequently become feverish during the course of continued treatment.

Dosage and Administration. A 10% solution of dimercaprol in oil is administered by deep intramuscular injection in doses of 2.5 to 5.0 mg./Kg. body weight. This dose is repeated at 4-hour intervals for the first 2 days so that an adequate quantity of this dithiol compound is in the tissues to compete there with sulfhydryl groups for the free metallic ions. After the early intensive treatment, the number of injections may be reduced to two on the third day and to once daily for the next week or until complete recovery.

CHAPTER 6

THE BARBITURATES AND OTHER SEDATIVE HYPNOTIC DRUGS

AMOBARBITAL U.S.P. (AMYTAL)

Pharmacology. This barbiturate of moderate duration is effective for 3 to 6 hours generally. This may make it more useful than the short-acting compounds for patients who tend to wake during the night or early morning, but it is more likely than the latter to cause residual drowsiness.

It has essentially the same uses as the short-acting compounds (see Pentobarbital, Drug Digest). Like certain ultra-short-acting barbiturates (see Thiopental, Drug Digest) amobarbital has been used to facilitate psychiatric interviews (narcoanalysis) and in related procedures such as narcosuggestion and narcosynthesis.

Like other barbiturates, amobarbital is contraindicated in patients with a history of addiction to drugs of this class and in elderly patients who exhibit nocturnal restlessness and confusion. The drug, like the others, is given with extreme care to patients with severe pain, anemia, fever, hyperthyroidism, and porphyria.

Dosage and Administration. Amobarbital is available in tablets of 16 to 50 mg. and elixirs of 20 to 40 mg./5-ml. teaspoon. For sedation, 16 to 50 mg. is given two or three times a day; a dose of 100 to 200 mg. is given for sleep about 20 to 60 minutes before bedtime; repeated doses of 200 to 400 mg. control convulsions.

CHLORAL HYDRATE U.S.P.

Pharmacology. This drug—the oldest sedative-hypnotic in use—is a relatively cheap, rapidly effective, and safe sleep-producer. It is not widely used because the unpleasant taste and odor is hard to disguise and it tends to cause occasional gastric irritation. However, chloral hydrate is now available in pharmaceutical forms and chemical complexes in which these disadvantages have been minimized.

Even though toxicity is low, care is required in patients with severe cardiac, renal, or hepatic disease, because the drug may be detrimental to the heart and because it is metabolized in the liver and the metabolites are excreted by the kidneys. Chloral hydrate combined with alcohol in the so-called "Mickey Finn" or "knockout drops" results in further C.N.S. depression.

Dosage and Administration. Chloral hydrate is available in soft gelatin capsules and suppositories as well as in flavored liquid preparations. Doses of 500 mg. are given three times a day for sedation; 1 Gm. or more is required for hypnotic action. Among related compounds recently prepared are chloral betaine, chlorhexadol, dichloralantipyrine, and petrichloral.

ETHINAMATE N.F. (VALMID)

Pharmacology. This is a relatively rapid-acting nonbarbiturate sedative-hypnotic of short duration. It seems weaker and less dependably effective than comparable short-acting barbiturates. Although it produces little "hangover" after one bedtime dose, it may have to be given several times nightly, and residual sedation could occur in such circumstances.

Lack of tolerance, habituation, and addiction have been claimed, but recent reports indicate that these are the effects of abuse of ethinamate. Massive overdoses can cause death, and lower overdoses may interfere with ability to drive or perform other complicated tasks.

Dosage and Administration. One or two 500-mg. tablets taken 20 minutes before retiring is the usual dose to induce sleep, but some individuals require up to 2 Gm. The drug is of least value in patients with severe insomnia, in which sleep is light at best and subject to frequent interruption.

GLUTETHIMIDE N.F. (DORIDEN)

Pharmacology. This sedative-hypnotic drug is comparable in duration of action to the intermediate-acting barbiturates. (It is not given less than 4 hours before the patient arises if residual sedation is to be avoided.)

The drug is best reserved for patients who are hypersensitive to barbiturates; otherwise, it has no special advantages in the management of elderly patients, those with liver or kidney damage, or patients prone to abuse or misuse drugs. Prolonged abuse for euphoric purposes has resulted in physical dependence, manifested by withdrawal reactions including convulsions. Fatalities have resulted from overdosage, especially in persons who have been drinking alcholic beverages.

Dosage and Administration. This drug is given only by mouth in tablets containing 125 to 500 mg. and a capsule of 500 mg. Sedation is achieved and maintained with doses of 125 to 250 mg. administered after each of the day's three meals. Sleep follows administration of 500 mg. at bedtime, or up to 1 Gm. given an hour before surgical anesthesia.

PARALDEHYDE U.S.P.

Pharmacology. This sedative-hypnotic liquid has a characteristic odor, which is detected on the breath of patients taking it. Because of this and its difficult-to-disguise and disagreeable taste it is used mainly in the management of hospitalized alcoholic patients. The unpleasant odor and taste are said to discourage habituation; however, alcoholics and other chronic drug abusers sometimes use the drug to produce euphoria.

Paraldehyde is given rectally and by intramuscular injection to overcome convulsions in eclampsia, tetanus, and strychnine poisoning. It is a basal anesthetic and produces analgesia in obstetrics. It somewhat irritates the tissues of the G.I. and respiratory tracts and the muscles at the site of injection. Otherwise, it is relatively safe in therapeutic dosage.

Dosage and Administration. The liquid is usually given by mouth after it has been poured over shaved ice or into cold flavored syrups, elixirs, or fruit juices. Doses range from 2 teaspoonfuls (10 ml.) to 2 tablespoonfuls (30 ml.) several times daily and at night. It is sometimes administered intramuscularly in a dose of 5 ml., but this may be irritating and lead to sterile abscesses. Administration by the I.V. route is considered very dangerous and should be carried out at a very slow rate (e.g., 1 ml./minute). A mixture of 15 to 30 ml. with oil may be instilled rectally as a retention enema for basal anesthesia.

Avoid exposing paraldehyde to air and sunlight, since this leads to production of toxic decomposition products.

PENTOBARBITAL SODIUM U.S.P. (NEMBUTAL)

Pharmacology. This agent and the calcium salt are short-acting compounds with sedative-hypnotic effects lasting 3 or 4 hours. Among its many uses it controls the hyperexcitability of anxiety states and simple insomnia, and—combined with aspirin, phenacetin, and other ingredients—relieves pain and discomfort. Pentobarbital is employed for preoperative sedation, in obstetrical analgesia and amnesia (alone, or combined with morphine, meperidine, or hyoscine), and as a rapid-acting anticonvulsant in tetanus, poisoning by convulsant drugs, and eclampsia.

Dosage and Administration. Oral doses are 20 to 100 mg. in tablets, capsules, and an elixir. For sedation, 30 to 60 mg. is administered several times daily; a hypnotic dose of 100 mg. is given at night in insomnia and 100 to 200 mg. is given preoperatively; in obstetrics, 200 to 300 mg. may be administered in a single dose. Dosage is reduced proportionately for children. Suppositories of 30 to 200 mg. content and solutions of 30 to 50 mg./ml. are available.

PHENOBARBITAL U.S.P. (LUMINAL ETC.)

Pharmacology. This barbiturate is relatively slow in onset of action, presumably because it crosses the blood-brain barrier rather slowly. However, it has, a relatively long duration of action; hypnotic doses produce sleep lasting at least 6 hours, with much longer periods of residual sedation. It is excreted slowly, which may lead to accumulation, especially in renal insufficiency.

Phenobarbital is preferred for long-term use as a sedative, rather than as a hypnotic in insomnia or for preoperative sedation. Its rather selective depressant action on motor neurons makes it especially useful in epilepsy. When used for this purpose and as a daytime sedative, side effects are few, except for some tendency to cause excessive drowsiness.

Dosage and Administration. The dose for adults is usually 100 to 200 mg. daily. For daytime sedation and in management of grand mal epilepsy, the drug is usually given by mouth in three or four divided doses, the last of which may be somewhat larger than the others to ensure sound sleep.

Tablets containing 15 to 100 mg. of phenobarbital or its sodium salt and an elixir containing about 20 mg./5 ml. teaspoon are available. Solutions of phenobarbital sodium of 60 to 320 mg./ml. are injected parenteraly, mainly to prevent convulsions following neurosurgery, or prior to administration of high doses of local anesthetic drugs.

CHAPTER 7

PSYCHOTHERAPEUTIC AGENTS

Major Tranquilizers

CARPHENAZINE MALEATE (PROKETAZINE)

Pharmacology. This potent, relatively short-acting phenothiazine drug is recommended mainly for the management of chronic schizophrenic reactions, including the catatonic and paranoid types. Several months may be required for maximal improvement of such chronic cases, and treatment is continued indefinitely to avoid relapses.

Extrapyramidal reactions of several types occur with relatively high doses. These include parkinson-type symptoms, such as muscular weakness, tremors, rigidity, and fatigue; sudden dystonic reactions; and akathisia, or motor restlessness. All these symptoms are controlled by reducing the dosage and administering antiparkinsonism agents. Other types of phenothiazine toxicity are rare and mild, but the usual precautions are required to prevent or overcome reactions.

Dosage and Administration. Treatment of chronic conditions is best begun with low dosage—25 to 50 mg. three times daily—which may be increased by 25 or 50 mg. daily at weekly intervals until optimal levels are attained. Other patients (e.g., those with acute schizophrenic reactions) receive lower initial doses that are then raised more rapidly, depending on the response. The maximal recommended daily dosage is 400 mg.

CHLORPROMAZINE HYDROCHLORIDE U.S.P. (THORAZINE)

Pharmacology. This was the first phenothiazine drug to be introduced, and it remains in wide use to control anxiety, tension, and excitement of varying degrees of severity. Although mainly an adjunct to psychotherapy in treatment of neuroses and psychoses, chlorpromazine is useful in many medical, surgical, and obstetrical situations. For example, it is an antiemetic and can potentiate the pain-relieving properties of narcotic-analgesic agents.

Chlorpromazine can produce a wide spectrum of C.N.S. and autonomic nervous system side effects, including drowsiness, atropinelike symptoms, and orthostatic (postural) hypotension. Hypersensitivity reactions include jaundice, blood dyscrasias, and dermatoses. Signs of such reactions require discontinuance of the drug usually.

The drug is administered with care to acutely intoxicated patients, for coma may result from potentiation of the C.N.S. depressant action of alcohol, barbiturates, or narcotics by chlorpromazine. Patients must remain lying down for some time after parenteral administration to avoid dizziness and faintness from postural hypotension.

Dosage and Administration. Chlorpromazine is available in many dosage forms for oral, rectal, and parenteral administration. Adult dosage is 30 to 1,500 mg. daily, depending on the severity of the condition. A syrup and suppositories are often employed for children. Deep intramuscular injection is the preferred route for control of hospitalized psychotic patients.

FLUPHENAZINE HYDROCHLORIDE (PERMITIL; PROLIXIN)

Pharmacology. This is one of the most potent and sustained-acting of the phenothiazines. It controls psychomotor *hyper*activity in manic states and stimulates activity in some *hypo*reactive types of chronic schizophrenics. Low, safe doses are used in children with behavioral problems, in treatment of mild to moderate degrees of anxiety-tension in psychoneuroses, and as an adjunct in controlling the emotional component complicating various somatic disorders.

Fluphenazine seems to cause less sedation and fewer autonomic blocking effects than does chlorpromazine. Although it appears less likely to potentiate the effects of depressant drugs, it is not used in patients who are taking high doses of hypnotics. Extrapyramidal neuromuscular symptoms of the dystonic type occur frequently with high doses. Dosage is reduced and antiparkinsonism drugs are administered in order to lessen the severity of such reactions.

Dosage and Administration. Oral doses as low as 1 mg. daily adequately control some mild states of anxiety and tension. Parenteral dosage for psychotic patients begins with 2.5 to 10 mg. daily and is raised or lowered as indicated by the severity of the symptoms. Oral doses of 20 mg. are the most that can usually be safely given in one day; as symptoms are controlled, improvement may be maintained by gradually reducing the dose to 1 mg. daily.

This drug is administered I.M. in doses usually not exceeding 10 mg. daily. However, *fluphenazine enanthate*—a long-acting form that is now available—is given I.M. in a dose of 25 mg., but *this dose is not repeated for 2 weeks.*

THIORIDAZINE (MELLARIL)

Pharmacology. This phenothiazine derivative of the piperidyl subgroup resembles chlorpromazine in many respects, but appears to cause a lower incidence of side effects. The drug does not possess strong antiemetic properties, nor does it commonly cause extrapyramidal motor symptoms. Thus, it has been suggested that thioridazine acts most specifically on the subcortical centers subserving emotion rather than on closely adjacent brain areas controlling other activities.

The most common side effects are of the C.N.S. depressant (e.g., drowsiness) and autonomic blockade types (e.g., mouth dryness; relatively mild and infrequent hypotension). Hypersensitivity reactions are uncommon. However, in some psychotic patients taking high daily doses one unusual reaction is reported: the development of deposits of brownish pigment in the retina. Pigmentary retinopathy is avoided when dosage is kept within the recommended limits.

Dosage and Administration. Patients with relatively mild emotional disturbances may be maintained on low oral doses—10 to 25 mg. three or four times daily. Psychotic patients require much larger amounts—from 100 mg. three or four times daily to as much as 1,600 mg. a day have been given—but 800 mg. per day is the maximum recommended dose.

Minor Tranquilizers

CHLORDIAZEPOXIDE HYDROCHLORIDE N.F. (LIBRIUM)

Pharmacology. This agent is used mainly to reduce mild to moderate degrees of anxiety and tension in various neuropsychiatric and somatic conditions in which emotional upset requires control. Higher doses, usually administered parenterally, calm acutely agitated patients. Although such high dosage helps to calm hyperactive alcoholics, addicts suffering withdrawal symptoms, and others exhibiting psychotic symptoms, the major tranquilizers are usually preferable for the long-range management of these conditions.

Side effects are limited mainly to drowsiness and motor incoordination (ataxia). These are most likely to occur in elderly and weakened patients and are usually prevented or overcome by careful dosage adjustment. However, other patients beginning chlordiazepoxide therapy are cautioned against undertaking hazardous activities that require complete alertness and rapid motor responsiveness.

Dosage and Administration. Dosage varies with the condition and response to the drug, and is adjusted for each individual. The dose for elderly patients is limited at the start to no more than 10 mg. daily. Extremely excited patients may tolerate 50 to 100 mg. parenterally, and this dose may be repeated in 4 to 6 hours.

HYDROXYZINE HYDROCHLORIDE N.F. (ATARAX); HYDROXYZINE PAMOATE (VISTARIL)

Pharmacology. This drug has, in addition to its sedative action, a number of other C.N.S. and peripheral effects. These are said to contribute to the drug's utility in a wide variety of medical conditions. The emotional component of these conditions is claimed to be favorably affected: hydroxyzine controls mild to moderate degrees of anxiety and tension. The drug's antihistaminic action may contribute to the symptomatic relief of the physical aspects of allergic disorders (e.g., itching, in chronic urticaria and other dermatoses). As an anticholinergic and antiemetic agent, it may aid in the management of G.I. upset and other conditions in which nausea and vomiting occur. Hydroxyzine also has antiarrhythmic properties which may be beneficial to some anxious cardiac patients. Transitory drowsiness and mouth dryness are the only common side effects.

Dosage and Administration. Recommended adult oral doses are 75 to 400 mg. daily, divided into three or four parts. The parenteral form may be injected intramuscularly or into a vein at a rate no faster than 25 mg./minute up to a total dose of 100 mg. Such injections are repeated every 4 to six hours as needed.

MEPROBAMATE U.S.P. (EQUANIL; MILTOWN)

Pharmacology. This prototype minor tranquilizer can: (1) control some manifestations of mild to moderate degrees of anxiety and (2) bring about skeletal muscle relaxation by a depressant action on spinal interneurons within the C.N.S. Thus, this drug is used clinically as an adjunct in the management of various somatic and neurological conditions, as well as in neuroses and other nonpsychotic emotional disturbances.

Drowsiness, the most common side effect, occurs less frequently than with equally effective sedative doses of barbiturates. Like the latter drugs, meprobamate may be abused by alcoholics and others who are likely to take excessive amounts of centrally acting drugs with disinhibiting effects. Patients with a history of drug dependence or of severe psychoneurotic instability are carefully supervised to see that they do not take excessive amounts of meprobamate. If such patients abuse the drug, it is discontinued by reducing the dosage gradually and slowly, because abrupt withdrawal may result in severe psychomotor reactions, including hallucinations and convulsions.

Dosage and Administration. The usual adult dose is 400 mg. three or four times daily by mouth. Sustained-release capsules containing 200 mg. and 400 mg. are also available for prolonged action (10 to 12 hours) and need be given only twice daily.

Antidepressant Drugs

AMITRIPTYLINE HYDROCHLORIDE (ELAVIL)

Pharmacology. This antidepressant drug does not stimulate the C.N.S.; in fact, it sedates or tranquilizes prior to improvement of mental depression. Thus, this drug has been suggested as most desirable for those depressed patients who show symptoms of anxiety, including certain psychoneurotic patients who complain volubly about their bodily ills. Amitriptyline is, however, effective in all depression states. Patients who respond to the drug become more optimistic and outgoing. Feelings of guilt, despair, and hopelessness are lifted and somatic symptoms such as headaches, lack of appetite, and insomnia are overcome.

Amitriptyline may cause a wide variety of minor side effects involving malfunction of the central and the autonomic nervous systems. Most of these effects, including drowsiness, mouth dryness, blurred vision, constipation, and tachycardia are usually overcome by reducing the daily dosage. However, the atropine-like actions may be most undesirable for patients with prostatic enlargement or glaucoma. This drug is never administered in combination with the monoamine-oxidase type of antidepressant drugs or until at least 2 weeks have elapsed after the latter agents have been discontinued.

Dosage and Administration. Amitriptyline is usually given by mouth in doses of 75 mg. daily at the start to 150 mg. later, or, rarely, as high as 300 mg. a day in hospitalized patients. The drug may be administered intramuscularly in doses of 20 to 30 mg. four times a day to initiate therapy; this is replaced by oral dosage within two weeks.

NIALAMIDE (NIAMID)

Pharmacology. This hydrazide derivative has not caused the type of liver toxicity found with earlier, related antidepressant drugs. Like other drugs of this class, including isocarboxazid and phenelzine, it is effective in treating mental depression, especially that marked by feelings of fatigue, weakness, apathy, hopelessness, or despair. Its "psychic energizer" action is manifested in the recovery of drive and of interest in the environment. The patient becomes less preoccupied with himself and more willing to take part in outgoing activities.

These desirable actions on mood, mental alertness, and physical activity may be slow in onset and require many weeks for full effect. Thus, prompt electroconvulsive therapy may be preferred for severely depressed suicidal patients. Side effects are mainly the result of C.N.S. overstimulation (e.g., restlessness, insomnia) or autonomic blockade (e.g., postural hypotension).

Remember that nialamide, like other monoamine-oxidase inhibitors, intensifies the actions of many other drugs. For example, sympathomimetic compounds, such as those often found in nose drops and other common cold remedies, may have their C.N.S.-stimulating and vasoconstrictor actions potentiated. The

depressant effects of alcohol, barbiturates, narcotics, and tranquilizers may also be increased.

Dosage and Administration. Oral dosage is 75 to 200 mg. during initiation of treatment. After a satisfactory response has been obtained, doses may be gradually reduced to as low as 12.5 mg. every other day. A period of at least 2 weeks should elapse after discontinuing this (or other MAO inhibitors) before the patient is switched to therapy with antidepressant drugs of the tricyclic type (e.g., imipramine, etc.).

IMIPRAMINE HYDROCHLORIDE (TOFRANIL)

Pharmacology. This drug is effective in endogenous depressions of various types but most especially in those marked by anxiety and complaints of mental and physical misery (i.e., dysphoric depression). Those patients who respond favorably to imipramine may begin to do so in a few days, but full effects are sometimes delayed for several weeks. Thus, in acute suicidal episodes, electroconvulsive therapy is begun immediately; the drug is given daily during the course of ECT treatments. Maintenance dosage is continued long after symptoms seem relieved, because relapses may occur if the drug is discontinued abruptly.

Minor side effects—many of them the result of autonomic nervous system blockade (see Chap. 14)—occur frequently. Neurological effects may be manifested by muscular twitching and hyperreflexia, which indicates the need for caution in epileptic patients. Convulsions have occurred; actually, however, they usually result from massive overdosage or from combined administration with an antidepressant of the monoamine-oxidase inhibitor type. Overdosage with such combinations has caused high fever, delirium, convulsions, coma, and death.

Dosage and Administration. Hospitalized patients are often started on oral doses of 100 to 150 mg. daily, which may be gradually increased over a period of several weeks to as much as 250 to 300 mg. a day given in divided doses. The dose may be reduced gradually, after the patient has improved, and many persons are maintained for long periods as outpatients on as little as 50 mg. daily.

TRANYLCYPROMINE SULFATE (PARNATE)

Pharmacology. This nonhydrazine MAO-inhibitor antidepressant has several advantages, including a relatively rapid onset of action and freedom from liver toxicity. However, it has produced side effects so serious that it is recommended only for patients who fail to respond to other antidepressant drugs and are either hospitalized or under close supervision.

The most serious reactions with this drug are hypertensive crises, some of which result in intracranial bleeding and death. Consequently, tranylcypromine is contraindicated in cerebrovascular and cardiovascular diseases including hypertension. It is not recommended for patients over 60 years old or for those with a history of liver disease.

Dosage and Administration. Patients are usually started on 10 mg. twice daily, continued for 2 weeks. If a satisfactory response occurs, dosage is reduced to a maintenance level; if no improvement is seen, dosage may be raised to 30 mg. daily—20 mg. in the morning and 10 mg. in the afternoon.

Tranylcypromine is not administered together with any *non*-MAO inhibitor. If one of the latter has been tried unsuccessfully, at least 1 week must elapse before switching to tranylcypromine.

This drug is not combined with other MAO inhibitors or with amphetamine and other adrenergic drugs.

Warn patients against self-medication with any other drug and not to eat cheese or drink alcoholic beverages while being treated with this drug. Instruct patients to report onset of headache or other unusual symptoms promptly.

CHAPTER 8

ANTICONVULSANT AND ANTISPASMODIC DRUGS

BENZTROPINE MESYLATE N.F. (COGENTIN)

Pharmacology. This synthetic centrally acting anticholinergic drug is used in all kinds of parkinsonism. It relieves rigidity and tremor and consequently reduces difficulties in walking, talking, writing, and swallowing. Side effects are atropinelike and include dryness of the mouth and skin (the latter may be dangerous in hot weather, for failure to sweat may lead to heat stroke), and nausea, vomiting, constipation, and dysuria. Blurring of vision often occurs, which indicates the possibility that glaucoma attacks may be precipitated in susceptible people.

Dosage and Administration. The daily dose of the tablets is 0.5 to 6 mg., depending on the response and tolerance of the individual. In acute dyskinetic reactions to tranquilizers, 2 mg. is injected intravenously for rapid relief. Parenteral administration is also preferred if swallowing is difficult or a more rapid response is desired, as in an oculogyric crisis.

CARISOPRODOL (RELA; SOMA)

Pharmacology. This relative of the minor tranquilizer meprobamate may have some analgesic as well as muscle relaxant action. It relieves pain and restores mobility in patients with sacroiliac strains, intervertebral disc difficulties, postoperative muscle pain, spinal osteoarthritis, and other musculoskeletal difficulties. The drug is also an adjunct to physical therapy in cerebral palsy and other neurological disorders. Side effects include drowsiness and skin rash in hypersensitive individuals. In such cases, the drug is discontinued.

Dosage and Administration. The usual adult dose is 350 mg. tablet four times a day. A 250 mg. capsule may be administered to children two or three times a day.

CHLORZOXAZONE (PARAFLEX)

Pharmacology. This C.N.S. depressant relaxes skeletal muscle spasm by reducing nerve impulse transmission through the polysynaptic reflex arcs involved in painful medical and orthopedic conditions such as: acute and chronic back disorders, arthritis, bursitis, fibrositis, spondylitis, and tendinitis.

Drowsiness, dizziness, and G.I. disturbances develop occasionally and allergic rashes rarely. The drug is stopped if skin itching and redness or signs of liver damage appear.

Dosage and Administration. The drug is given in doses of 250 to 500 mg. three or four times daily, either alone or combined with non-narcotic analgesics, such as acetaminophen.

DIAZEPAM (VALIUM)

Pharmacology. This more potent analogue of the minor tranquilizer chlordiazepoxide reportedly benefits patients with cerebral palsy and athetosis. It reduces anxiety reactions and the acute agitation of alcoholism. The drug is contraindicated in convulsive disorders and psychoses, as well as in glaucoma. Patients taking the drug must not drive an automobile or engage in other activities that require alertness and coordination.

Dosage and Administration. In muscle spasm of cerebral palsy oral doses of 2 to 10 mg. are given three or four times daily. Psychoneurotic reactions may require up to 10 mg. several times a day, and 10 mg. three or four times daily is the starting dose in acute alcoholic agitation, reduced later to 5 mg. as needed.

Diazepam is also administered parenterally in individualized dosage that should not exceed 30 mg. within an 8-hour period. In psychoneurotic reactions, 2 to 10 mg. are injected I.M. or I.V.,

repeated in 3 to 4 hours if necessary. For acute alcoholic withdrawal, 10 mg., I.M. or I.V. is followed by 5 to 10 mg. when necessary. In other acute stress reactions and for muscle spasm, 5 to 10 mg. are injected, repeated as necessary. All injections are made slowly.

DIPHENYLHYDANTOIN SODIUM U.S.P. (DILANTIN)

Pharmacology. This drug depresses the motor cortex and reduces the rate at which excessive discharges spread from focal areas to other parts of the brain. It is a drug of choice in grand mal epilepsy and is sometimes useful in convulsive episodes of other types. It has been tried experimentally in trigeminal neuralgia and a wide variety of other conditions, including cardiac arrhythmias.

Patients taking diphenylhydantoin are relatively free of the drowsiness and dullness often caused by phenobarbital; however, the drug can produce a wide variety of other side effects. Neurological complications include staggering gait, slurred speech, and blurred vision. Gastric distress, nausea, and weight loss occur early in treatment. Gingival hyperplasia, an unsightly overgrowth of the gum tissue, is a common reaction; it is best prevented by frequent cleansing of the mouth, but may require surgical excision. Skin eruptions of a morbilliform and acnelike type sometimes develop.

Dosage and Administration. Most adults are maintained on 300 to 600 mg. daily, after being started on 100 mg. three times daily. Children are started on the 30-mg. capsule twice daily and later receive this dose three or four times a day. The drug is often combined with phenobarbital, sometimes with desoxyephedrine added to combat drowsiness.

A parenteral form of diphenylhydantoin is used in status epilepticus and to prevent convulsive episodes in neurosurgery. A dose of 150 to 250 mg. may be injected by vein at a rate of no more than 50 mg./minute. If necessary, 100 to 150 mg. is given a half hour later.

ETHOSUXIMIDE (ZARONTIN)

Pharmacology. This succinimide derivative is used mainly in treating petit mal type epilepsy. It may increase the frequency of grand mal attacks if it is used alone in patients with mixed seizures. Thus, it is commonly combined with other anticonvulsants in such cases.

Various side effects involving the G.I. tract and C.N.S. have been reported. These include loss of appetite, nausea, and vomiting; headache, dizziness, and drowsiness; or insomnia, restlessness, and inability to concentrate. These symptoms usually subside during continued use of the drug.

Periodic blood counts are performed to detect leukopenia or evidence of other dangerous blood dyscrasias, since fatal pancytopenia has been reported. Urinalysis and liver function tests are advisable, because of the possibility of dysfunction of these organs, such as has been reported with other drugs of this chemical class.

Dosage and Administration. Treatment is started with a 0.25-Gm. capsule daily for children under 6 years of age or two tablets in divided dosage for older patients. The daily dosage is then raised gradually until maximal control is achieved with minimal side effects. Seizure control may require as much as 1.5 Gm. daily, an amount reached by adding 0.25 Gm. every 4 to 7 days.

METHOCARBAMOL (ROBAXIN)

Pharmacology. This relatively long-acting depressant of internuncial neurons of the spinal cord and lower brain centers reduces skeletal muscle pain and spasm in many musculoskeletal and neurological disorders. Among the acute conditions in which it is used are whiplash injuries, herniated disk syndromes, strains, sprains, and dislocations. It is used in the management of chronic myositis, fibrositis, and arthritis.

Side effects of oral administration include mild nausea. Injection, if too rapid, may be followed by dizziness, drowsiness, lightheadedness, and vertigo. Occasional hypersensitivity-type skin reactions have been reported.

Dosage and Administration. Oral dosage of 6 to 8 Gm. daily is used to initiate treatment. This may be lowered later to about 4 Gm. a day, given in three or four divided doses.

The solution is usually injected slowly by vein in undiluted form or as an intravenous drip in saline or 5% dextrose. The usual dose is 10 ml. for relief of moderate muscle spasms, but more severe cases may require 20 to 30 ml. Instruct patients to lie flat during the injection and for 10 to 15 minutes afterward. No more than 5 ml. is injected intramuscularly into each gluteal muscle at 8-hour intervals when necessary.

ORPHENADRINE HYDROCHLORIDE (DISIPAL)

Pharmacology. This relative of the antihistamine drug diphenhydramine is used mainly to relax muscular spasm and relieve other distressing symptoms of Parkinson's syndrome. It acts centrally to produce its antispasmodic and antitremor effects. In addition, this drug often has a slight cerebral stimulating action which may be helpful for parkinsonian patients who are mentally depressed or physically fatigued.

Orphenadrine sometimes causes anticholinergic, or atropine-type, side effects including mouth dryness, blurring of vision, constipation, urinary retention, and cardiac palpitations. In addition to these peripheral effects, certain adverse central actions may occur, such as headache, dizziness, drowsiness, and mental confusion. The drug is contraindicated in glaucoma, enlargement of the prostate gland, and G.I. obstruction.

Dosage and Administration. This drug is administered alone or combined with other antiparkinson agents. The usual oral dose is 50 mg. three times a day. However, higher doses (to about 300 mg. daily) may be well tolerated.

PRIMIDONE U.S.P. (MYSOLINE)

Pharmacology. This drug is used mainly as an alternative or additional agent in grand mal epilepsy and as a first line drug for preventing psychomotor seizures. It is of little value in petit mal epilepsy and its variants.

Primidone is much safer than phenacemide for psychomotor epilepsy treatment. However, it can produce various minor and some major reactions. Occasionally, the first dose of this drug causes an acute illness marked by nausea, vomiting, headache, dizziness, and drowsiness. A measleslike skin rash and a condition resembling megaloblastic anemia have been reported.

Dosage and Administration. Treatment is begun with low dosage (50 mg.) to avoid gastroenteric disturbances. This may be raised gradually to as high as 2 Gm. daily, starting with one dose given at bedtime and building up to several doses daily. The average daily dose for adults is 750 mg. to 1.5 Gm.; about half these amounts is usually adequate for children.

TRIHEXYPHENIDYL HYDROCHLORIDE U.S.P. (ARTANE; TREMIN)

Pharmacology. This central and peripherally acting synthetic antispasmodic reduces muscle rigidity in all forms of parkinsonism (idiopathic, postencephalitic, and arteriosclerotic). It often counteracts mental depression in these patients and reduces excessive salivation and sweating. The drug has been used recently to control extrapyramidal reactions induced by tranquilizers of the phenothiazine and rauwolfia types.

Side effects are similar to but less severe than those caused by belladonna alkaloids. They include blurring of vision (the drug can precipitate glaucoma attacks in susceptible individuals), and mouth dryness, nausea, dizziness, and mental confusion.

Dosage and Administration. It is customary to initiate therapy with doses as low as 1 mg. and to build up to an optimal level of 6 to 10 mg. daily divided into three or four doses taken near mealtimes. Older patients are more sensitive and require relatively small amounts; others may need and may tolerate as much as 10 to 15 mg. daily.

Sustained-release capsules containing 5 mg., given during the morning or early afternoon, provide maximum antispasmodic action during waking hours.

TRIMETHADIONE U.S.P. (TRIDIONE)

Pharmacology. This is the most effective agent available for treating seizures of the true petit mal type. It is usually ineffective for grand mal and may even increase the number of attacks. In mixed seizures, it is usually combined with a barbiturate or hydantoin drug.

A unique side effect is a photophobia called the glare phenomenon or hemeralopia, in which objects appear indistinct and look as though they were covered with snow or ice. No optic nerve damage occurs, and the condition disappears in a few days after the drug is withdrawn.

More dangerous are bone marrow effects that may result in fatal agranulocytosis or aplastic anemia. Thus, blood studies are made frequently, and patients are asked to report sore throat, fever, rash, or other unusual symptoms. Nephrosis, lymphadenopathy, and systemic lupus erythematosus also have been reported.

Dosage and Administration. The daily oral dose for adults and older children is 900 to 2,100 mg., divided into three or four equal doses. For young children, 600 mg. is divided into several doses daily. Infants are given 300 mg. daily.

CHAPTER 9

THE NARCOTIC ANALGESICS

ALPHAPRODINE HYDROCHLORIDE (NISENTIL)

Pharmacology. This relative of meperidine is marked by a rapid onset and relatively short duration of analgesic action. These properties make it useful for managing short bouts of pain brought on by painful manipulations. It is used, for example, prior to cystoscopy in patients with urethral strictures, and in procedures such as reduction of dislocations and fractures, and changing of dressings in severely burned patients. It is often combined with barbiturates and local or inhalation anesthetics to provide rapid but brief analgesia during minor surgery of the eye, nose, and throat.

An advantage of this drug is the fact that respiratory depression from overdosage is not long-lasting and so does not require prolonged supervision of the patient. However, when used for obstetrical analgesia, the drug does pass the placental barrier and has caused delay in spontaneous breathing by the newborn baby. Its effects are readily counteracted by injection of a narcotic antagonist into the umbilical vein.

Dosage and Administration. Alphaprodine is usually administered subcutaneously in a dose of 40 to 60 mg. which is repeated in 2 hours if required. Doses of 20 to 30 mg. given intravenously rapidly relieve pain. In obstetrics, the drug is administered subcutaneously after the cervix begins to dilate, but it is not given within 2 hours of the expected time of delivery, because it would depress fetal respiration.

CODEINE PHOSPHATE U.S.P. (METHYLMORPHINE)

Pharmacology. The natural opium alkaloid codeine is much less potent an analgesic and antitussive than is morphine. However, it is much less addicting than morphine and less likely to cause constipation, respiratory depression, or any of the other side effects and toxic reactions of morphine. Consequently, codeine and its salts, the phosphate and sulfate, are commonly employed to relieve moderate degrees of pain and dry, irritating, nonproductive coughs. This alkaloid causes little sedation, and overdosage is usually marked by excitement rather than depression. Convulsions have occurred in accidentally poisoned children, but fatalities are rare.

Dosage and Administration. Doses of 8 to 10 mg. (such as are contained in about one teaspoonful of Elixir of Terpin Hydrate and Codeine) are given to depress the cough reflex. Doses of 15 to 30 mg. usually relieve moderate pain. If not, the dose may be raised to 60 mg. However, if this amount offers no further relief, higher doses are unlikely to prove effective, and a more potent analgesic, such as meperidine or morphine, is employed.

HYDROMORPHONE HYDROCHLORIDE N.F. (DIHYDROMORPHINONE; DILAUDID)

Pharmacology. This semisynthetic derivative of morphine is several times more potent than the natural alkaloid in both analgesic and respiratory depressant activity. The drug is claimed to cause less constipation, nausea and vomiting, and sedation than morphine, and the duration of its analgesic action is shorter.

Dosage and Administration. The usual oral and parenteral dose to relieve moderate to severe pain is 2 mg. The drug is administered in a 3-mg. suppository for longer-lasting nocturnal analgesia. It may be combined with atropine (0.4 mg.) to relieve spastic pain in biliary and ureteral colic, acute cardiospasm, and pylorospasm. A cough syrup containing 1 mg. in each teaspoonful dose is administered every 3 or 4 hours for antitussive effects.

LEVORPHANOL TARTRATE (LEVO-DROMORAN)

Pharmacology. This synthetic analgesic is more potent than morphine and longer in the duration of its action. Its clinical uses, contraindications, and potential toxicity are similar to those of morphine. The drug is claimed less likely to cause constipation, a fact which may make it more desirable in the long-term treatment of patients who are forced to remain bedridden for long periods. Nausea, vomiting, and dizziness are less frequent in nonambulatory patients, and pruritus and sweating are rare.

Dosage and Administration. Levorphanol is promptly absorbed following oral as well as subcutaneous administration of the usual 2-mg. dose. This may be increased to 3 mg. if necessary, but ordinarily the drug is not given more frequently than every 6 to 8 hours.

MEPERIDINE HYDROCHLORIDE N.F. (DEMEROL; PETHIDINE; ETC.)

Pharmacology. This synthetic analgesic is more potent than codeine but less effective than morphine against severe pain and shorter in the duration of its action. The drug differs from morphine in several ways. For example, it is less spasmogenic and constipating. It is less likely to cause sedation and is commonly combined with sedatives, such as scopolamine, promethazine, and barbiturates, when used for preanesthetic medication or for obstetrical analgesia. Unlike the opiates, this opioid does not control coughing or diarrhea.

Side effects, which occur most commonly in ambulatory patients, include dizziness, nausea and vomiting, flushing and sweating, and mouth dryness. More acute toxicity is marked by weakness and fainting due to postural hypotension. An atropine-like component in the drug's actions may result in development of mydriasis, excitement, and delirium. High overdosage is followed by motor incoordination, tremors, convulsions, and death resulting from respiratory failure. Chronic toxicity is not uncommon, meperidine being the drug to which doctors and nurses are said to become most frequently addicted.

Dosage and Administration. Meperidine is orally effective but acts more promptly and reliably when administered parenterally. The usual oral or intramuscular dose is 50 or 100 mg., depending on the severity of the pain. Dosage is repeated at intervals of 1 to 4 hours, if needed.

METHADONE HYDROCHLORIDE U.S.P. (DOLOPHINE; ADANON; ETC.)

Pharmacology. This synthetic analgesic is equal to morphine in potency and duration of action. Because of its cumulative effects, it is preferred for patients suffering from the chronic pain of metastatic malignancy but is considered relatively undesirable for use during delivery. It is also an effective antitussive in chronic tuberculosis, whooping cough, and in less serious conditions in which coughing occurs.

Methadone produces less sedation and euphoria than morphine and, thus, is less useful for preanesthetic medication. Addiction is slow to develop, and is manifested by the development of discomfort upon withdrawal of the drug after prolonged use. This drug completely relieves the syndrome caused by withdrawal of other opiates and is used for this purpose in the management of addiction. In practice, the substitution of methadone for morphine or heroin results in a milder but more prolonged abstinence syndrome, when methadone is itself gradually withdrawn. In the still experimental "methadone maintenance" program for treating heroin addiction, this drug is continued indefinitely, because its presence in the body is believed to relieve hunger for heroin and to block the heroin "high" (the euphoric state sought by the addict).

Dosage and Administration. This drug is effective when given by mouth in doses of 5 to 15 mg., depending on the severity of the pain. One-half to 1 teaspoonful of a syrup containing about 1.5 mg./teaspoonful is given to adults every 4 to 6 hours for cough, and about half this amount is administered to children. The drug is not given by vein, but doses of 5 to no more than 10 mg. may be administered intramuscularly or by the somewhat more irritating subcutaneous route.

OXYMORPHONE HYDROCHLORIDE (NUMORPHAN)

Pharmacology. This is a semisynthetic derivative of morphine, closely related to dihydromorphinone. It is much more potent than morphine as an analgesic; however, it has a correspondingly increased respiratory depressant effect. Despite this, the drug does not depress the cough center effectively and is not useful as an antitussive. Oxymorphone is claimed to be less likely to cause constipation, nausea and vomiting, or drowsiness, but it does produce euphoria and addiction.

Dosage and Administration. The drug gives rapid and relatively long relief (3 to 6 hours) when administered by any of several routes. The oral dose is 5 to 10 mg.; rectal suppository dose, 2 to 5 mg.; intramuscularly or subcutaneously, 1.5 mg.; intravenous dose is only 0.75 mg.

PHENAZOCINE HYDROBROMIDE (PRINADOL)

Pharmacology. This synthetic analgesic was introduced with the claim that it is less addicting than morphine and less likely to produce respiratory depression. Actually, it seems essentially similar to morphine in these respects. The drug may, however, cause less drowsiness than morphine or meperidine. Thus, barbiturates are commonly administered with phenazocine when additional sedation is desired during obstetrical procedures or in preoperative use. Because the depressant effects of this drug may be potentiated by barbiturates and other hypnotics, tranquilizers, or anesthetics, such combinations are used with caution, especially in elderly or debilitated patients.

Dosage and Administration. The usual dose is 2 mg. intramuscularly every 4 to 6 hours. Lower doses (0.5 to 1 mg.) may be given by vein as an adjunct to anesthesia and followed by additional fractional doses (0.25 to 0.5 mg.) as needed. The doctor or nurse must be especially alert to signs of respiratory depression when this drug is given intravenously to patients with decreased pulmonary ventilation.

Narcotic Antagonist

NALORPHINE HYDROCHLORIDE U.S.P. (NALLINE)

Pharmacology. This synthetic morphine relative is an *antagonist* of *narcotics*. It reverses respiratory depression and other signs and symptoms of severe overdosage with opiates and opioids. It is not, however, an antidote to barbiturates or other types of central depressants. Nalorphine and other antagonists apparently act to displace narcotic molecules from the receptors of depressed nerve cells.

Nalorphine prevents depression of fetal respiration and is administered shortly before delivery of women who have received opiates for obstetrical analgesia. Injected into the umbilical vein of the newborn baby, it overcomes the apnea of asphyxia neonatorum, if it is caused by narcotics administered to the mother.

This drug is also employed in testing for the presence of physical dependence to narcotics. The nalorphine test reveals addiction by promptly eliciting signs of the opiate abstinence syndrome, such as dilation of the pupil or more severe withdrawal symptoms.

Dosage and Administration. A dose of 5 to 10 mg. administered by vein antagonizes depression of respiration and other effects of overdosage by potent natural and synthetic analgesics. The dose may be repeated twice at intervals of 10 to 15 minutes, but further dosage may be undesirable if depression has not been reduced. Intravenous administration of 5 to 10 mg. to the mother shortly before delivery prevents asphyxia of the newborn, or 0.2 mg. may be injected into the infant's umbilical vein immediately after delivery.

CHAPTER 10

ANALGESIC-ANTIPYRETICS AND OTHER NON-ADDICTING DRUGS FOR PAIN

ACETAMINOPHEN N.F.
(N-ACETYL-*p*-AMINOPHENOL; APAP)

Pharmacology. This metabolite of both acetanilid and phenacetin, has replaced these aniline derivatives in many analgesic-antipyretic products. Unlike its precursor compounds, acetaminophen does not break down in the body to form significant amounts of the chemical by-products that cause methemoglobin formation in the blood. This drug's water solubility permits its use in palatable liquid preparations that are well suited for administration to children. It relieves pain and reduces fever in infants and children with respiratory infections, postimmunization reactions, headache, earache, and toothache. It relieves post-tonsillectomy discomfort and does not tend to increase capillary bleeding, because it does not act as an anticoagulant as do the salicylates.

Dosage and Administration. Acetaminophen is administered orally as tablets or drops and in the form of a syrup. The dose of the tablets for adults and older children is 300 to 600 mg. three or four times daily. Dosage for infants and young children is 60 to 300 mg. several times daily.

ASPIRIN U.S.P. (ACETYLSALICYLIC ACID)

Pharmacology. Aspirin is more readily absorbed from the upper G.I. tract and less irritating to its mucosa than sodium salicylate. It relieves minor pain and discomfort in headaches, myalgia, neuralgia. It reduces fever and relieves the malaise often accompanying influenza and other viral infections. High doses relieve the inflammatory symptoms of acute rheumatic fever and rheumatoid arthritis.

Although the low amounts of aspirin taken to relieve most of the common painful conditions are considered harmless, severe allergic reactions sometimes occur in hypersensitive individuals. Gastric irritation is common and sometimes leads to mucosal bleeding and iron deficiency anemia. The high doses administered in acute rheumatic fever and rheumatoid arthritis often affect the central and peripheral nervous systems adversely. The symptoms of such *salicylism* include ringing in the ears (tinnitus), transient visual disturbances, confusion, and restlessness.

Aspirin is the most common cause of accidental poisoning in children. Massive overdosage causes severe acid-base imbalances, including respiratory alkalosis and metabolic acidosis. If these are not quickly corrected and blood levels of salicylate lowered, death may occur following convulsions, coma, cardiovascular collapse, and respiratory failure.

Dosage and Administration. Aspirin is most commonly taken in amounts of 600 mg. for relief of minor pain and may be repeated in 2 to 4 hours. However, as much as 10 Gm. daily may be administered in order to reach and maintain the high plasma levels required to relieve pain and joint symptoms in rheumatoid arthritis and acute rheumatic fever.

AMINOPYRINE (PYRAMIDON, ETC.)

Pharmacology. This drug is an analgesic and antipyretic with potent anti-inflammatory properties. It is rarely used in this country because it has caused severe and sometimes fatal agranulocytosis. However, it is widely used in Europe and may be prescribed by foreign physicians practicing here. It cannot be obtained in products intended for self-medication.

This drug certainly has no place in the treatment of minor aches and pains that can be readily relieved by much safer drugs such as aspirin and acetophenetidin. However, it could, conceivably, be lifesaving in cases of acute rheumatic fever in which the patient is sensitive to salicylates. In such cases, the doctor takes frequent blood counts in order to detect any drop in white blood cells.

Dosage and Administration. Aminopyrine is administered orally, one or two 0.3-Gm. tablets every 4 hours, or it may be combined with various other drugs in products for relief of mild to moderate pain. Several grams a day may be administered in the treatment of acute rheumatic fever.

PHENACETIN U.S.P. (ACETOPHENETIDIN, ETC.)

Pharmacology. This coal-tar or aniline derivative is commonly combined with aspirin in proprietary analgesic mixtures that are sold without prescription. It is similar to the salicylates in its pain-relieving and fever-reducing properties but does not share their ability to counteract rheumatic inflammation or to lower plasma uric acid levels in gout.

Phenacetin is somewhat less likely to cause methemoglobinemia than the more toxic, related drug acetanilid. It occasionally causes the breakdown of red blood cells. Such hemolytic reactions occur in sensitive individuals of two types: those whose red cells are congenitally deficient in the enzyme glucose-6-phosphate dehydrogenase; and those who develop antibodies that, in the presence of the drug, tend to make their red cells agglutinate. Recently, acetophenetidin has been linked to kidney damage in analgesic abusers (persons who habitually take excessive daily doses of nonprescription headache remedies).

Dosage and Administration. Phenacetin administered in full oral doses of 300 to 600 mg. relieves joint and muscle pain and headache. It is rarely given alone, however, except to those hypersensitive to salicylates. It is most commonly administered in a fraction of the full therapeutic dose, which is combined with a fractional dose of aspirin plus a small amount of caffeine—the common APC formulation. This is supposed to take advantage of the additive effects of the two analgesics while reducing the side effects of each. It may instead subject sensitive individuals to toxicity of two different types.

PROPOXYPHENE HYDROCHLORIDE U.S.P. (DARVON)

Pharmacology. This analgesic is about equal to codeine in pain-relieving ability, but it does not require a narcotic prescription. It also seems to cause fewer C.N.S. and G.I. side effects than the opiate. However, some patients complain of epigastric pain when the larger, more effective, dose is employed, and drowsiness and dizziness are sometimes reported. High doses have reportedly caused convulsions, which might be made worse if the depressed patient were treated with analeptics. Although the drug is not a narcotic, depression produced by massive overdosage is probably best treated by the narcotic antagonists nalorphine or levallorphan.

Dosage and Administration. This drug is administered in doses of 32 and 65 mg. It is available in combination with aspirin and phenacetin, which provide the antipyretic and anti-inflammatory actions that this analgesic lacks. It is combined with the minor tranquilizer phenaglycodol for treating painful conditions complicated by anxiety and muscle spasm. For all these products, 1 or 2 capsules are administered three or four times daily as needed to relieve pain.

SALICYLAMIDE N.F.

Pharmacology. This close chemical relative of salicylic acid is said to produce about the same degree of analgesic, antipyretic, and anti-inflammatory effects as aspirin. It may prove a useful substitute for aspirin in patients who are allergic to the latter. However, such patients may in time acquire hypersensitivity to salicylamide, also.

Massive overdosage with this compound seems less likely to cause the severe respiratory stimulation and other excitatory effects seen in poisoning by aspirin and other salicylates. This may be because the drug is a mild C.N.S. depressant. Mild sedation as well as increased analgesia may result when this drug is combined with other non-narcotic analgesics, such as acetophenetidin and acetaminophen.

Dosage and Administration. Salicylamide is given by mouth in doses of 300 to 600 mg. every 4 hours. Higher doses—1 to 2 Gm. every 4 hours or 2 to 4 Gm. three times daily—may be required in rheumatoid arthritis. To reduce gastric irritation, the drug is best given after meals or with milk. Doses for children are reduced proportionately.

CHAPTER 11

GENERAL AND LOCAL ANESTHETICS

Local Anesthetics

COCAINE HYDROCHLORIDE N.F.

Pharmacology. This alkaloid, obtained from the leaves of the coca plant or prepared synthetically, is an effective topical anesthetic that also causes local vasoconstriction at the site of application. It is used mainly to anesthetize and shrink the mucous membranes of the nose and throat. Although low dilutions are effective when applied to the eye, certain new ophthalmic agents (e.g., *proparacaine*) seem less likely to cause stinging, burning, redness, or corneal lesions.

Cocaine is not administered by injection ordinarily, because of its relatively high toxicity; toxic reactions are marked by severe C.N.S. stimulation followed by deep depression and death due to respiratory failure. Cocaine causes various sympathomimetic effects, such as pupillary dilation, increased heart rate, and hypertension—actions that, like local vasoconstriction, ordinarily do not occur with the synthetic local anesthetics.

Cocaine is sometimes abused because of its C.N.S. actions. Although physical dependence is not proved, the drug is considered an addicting agent because of the dangerous mental and physical consequences of its continued abuse, and its sale is subject to the provision of federal and state narcotics laws.

Dosage and Administration. Cocaine is applied topically to the mucosa of the nose and throat in concentrations of 5 to 10%. Lower concentrations are used in the eye. Although epinephrine may not be necessary because of cocaine's own vasoconstricting action, the two drugs combined potentiate the desired hemostatic action of each in nasal surgery. Maximum safe dosage for application to mucous membranes is 150 mg.

LIDOCAINE HYDROCHLORIDE U.S.P. (XYLOCAINE)

Pharmacology. This versatile local anesthetic is given by all routes of administration to produce prompt loss of pain perception. It is somewhat more potent and longer lasting than procaine and not significantly more toxic when employed in low concentrations. The drug penetrates to nervous tissues and diffuses readily when applied topically or injected. It is used before obstetrical, dental, and surgical procedures; for treating bursitis, fibrositis, and other painful medical conditions; and as a means of differential diagnosis in certain clinical situations. Dilute solutions are being employed experimentally to prevent and overcome postcoronary cardiac arrhythmias. Sedation is a more common systemic effect of this drug than with most local anesthetics. However, with overdosage, muscle twitching and even convulsions may occur.

Dosage and Administration. The concentrations and total amounts of lidocaine employed for various procedures should be no more than half those required when procaine is used for similar purposes. No single dose of lidocaine solutions of 2% strength or higher exceeds 300 mg., though this may be increased to 500 mg. if epinephrine is added to the solution in amounts up to 1 part in 100,000. Higher doses may be used when concentrations as low as 0.5 to 1.5% are used in continuous caudal procedures. On the other hand, with the 5% hyperbaric (high specific gravity) solution used in the saddle block technique, the single total dose should not exceed 200 mg.

PROCAINE HYDROCHLORIDE U.S.P. (NOVOCAIN)

Pharmacology. Procaine, one of the earliest local anesthetics to be synthesized, is widely used for infiltration and regional nerve block. It is relatively safe when administered by these routes, because it is rapidly destroyed by plasma esterase enzymes. This, of course, also limits its duration of action, which may, however, be extended if epinephrine and related vasoconstrictors are added to the solutions.

Because of its relatively rapid destruction, procaine occasionally is administered by slow intravenous injection to produce generalized analgesia in various painful conditions. However, the relief of pain attained in this way seems no greater than that obtained by more routine measures and does not appear to warrant the risks involved in hypersensitive patients or in the event of inadvertent overdosage.

Procaine is not an effective topical anesthetic for application to mucous membranes. However, it is given by mouth to relieve pain, nausea, and vomiting caused by irritation of the upper G.I. tract mucosa. It is considerably weaker than *oxethazaine* for this purpose in the symptomatic relief of esophagitis, gastritis, and peptic ulcer.

Dosage and Administration. Solutions of 0.25 to 1% are commonly employed for infiltration procedures and administered in single doses of up to 1,000 mg. A 2% solution is most commonly used for nerve block procedures. The total dose for spinal anesthesia and related procedures is 50 to 200 mg., injected intrathecally or peridurally. For intravenous administration, a 0.1% solution in isotonic saline is injected slowly in a dose of 4 mg./Kg. body weight given over a 20-minute period. Oral doses of 250 mg., four times a day are employed.

General and Basal Anesthetics

CYCLOPROPANE U.S.P. (TRIMETHYLENE)

Pharmacology. This gas, in concentrations that permit full oxygenation at the same time, produces complete anesthesia. Induction is easier than with ether, even when carried out with low concentrations which do not irritate mucous membranes or cause stimulation of excessive secretions; recovery is rapid and relatively free of postanesthetic complications. Cyclopropane is a preferred anesthetic for operations in which the chest is opened, because it produces quiet, regular breathing. Inhalation of low concentrations relieves labor pains; larger amounts do not interfere with uterine contractions or with the breathing of the mother or baby.

Cyclopropane has few adverse effects on the cardiovascular system when the patient is kept well oxygenated and carbon dioxide is kept from accumulating. However, cardiac arrhythmias including ventricular fibrillation have been reported. These are especially likely to occur if sympathomimetic amines are administered simultaneously; therefore these sensitizing agents are avoided.

Administration. Cyclopropane-oxygen mixtures are always given by the closed-circuit method which includes a system for absorbing carbon dioxide. It is best given by an anesthesiologist experienced in its use and in detection of danger signals, which may not be as readily observable as with other anesthetics. Premedication with atropine or scopolamine to prevent laryngospasm is desirable. This anesthetic is often combined with ether, thiopental, or local anesthesia for various procedures.

ETHYL ETHER U.S.P. (DIETHYL OXIDE)

Pharmacology. The vapors of this volatile liquid produce full anesthesia when inhaled in relatively low concentration. This allows large amounts of oxygen to be administered simulta-

neously. Other safety factors include: (1) the drug produces relatively few adverse effects involving the myocardium, liver, and kidneys; (2) it relaxes the peripheral muscles, which reduces the amount of ether needed for complete anesthesia (i.e., deep depression of spinal motor reflex centers may not be required); (3) it irritates the respiratory mucosa, which may serve to stimulate the depressed respiratory center reflexly.

Such mucous membrane irritation is, however, also a disadvantage because it tends to stimulate a copious flow of secretions that interfere with inhalation of the vapors by blocking the airway. Other drawbacks include the relatively long and sometimes stormy induction and recovery periods, the high incidence of nausea and vomiting, and the fact that ether vapors may burst into flame or be exploded by a spark.

Administration. Ether may be readily administered by the open drop method or in a closed system. Often, it is preceded by inhalation of nitrous oxide-oxygen mixtures to produce more rapid and pleasant induction; low concentrations of ether are then introduced into the system and provision is made for adequate oxygenation and for the removal of carbon dioxide to prevent hypercarbia. Atropine premedication is desirable for reducing salivary and bronchial secretions. The dose of curare-like compounds administered for an adjunctive muscle relaxing effect is reduced to about one third the usual amount, if such agents are used at all.

HALOTHANE (FLUOTHANE)

Pharmacology. The vapors of this liquid cause rapid induction of anesthesia which can be readily reversed when necessary. Among its other advantages are relative freedom from complications such as respiratory irritation, excessive secretions, and vomiting, and it is inflammable. Halothane is an effective anesthetic for operations of many different types, including chest surgery and neurosurgery. However, it is not desirable in obstetrics, because it stops uterine contractions.

Halothane often causes hypotensive reactions and slowing of the heart or other cardiac arrhythmias. Falls in blood pressure have been most severe when this anesthetic is used together with the muscle relaxant tubocurarine. Thus, succinylcholine is the preferred neuromuscular blocking agent for use with this anesthetic. Deaths from toxic hepatitis have occurred in patients who had been anesthetized with halothane. However, a direct causal relationship has not been proved.

Dosage and Administration. Special vaporizers control the concentration of this potent anesthetic. Surgical anesthesia is rapidly induced by use of about a 2% concentration which is then reduced to 1% or less for maintenance of that state. Atropine premedication prevents excessive cardiac slowing. Careful administration of certain vasopressor amines (e.g., methoxamine) helps to overcome hypotension.

SODIUM THIOPENTAL U.S.P. (PENTOTHAL SODIUM)

Pharmacology. This ultra-short-acting barbiturate is a basal anesthetic and by itself produces sleep prior to brief surgical procedures. It overcomes acute convulsions and, occasionally, is used in psychiatry for interviewing under narcosis.

Thiopental rapidly induces anesthesia, but, because it is not a good analgesic or muscle relaxant, it is not used for full anesthesia in long or complicated surgery, in which cases it is supplemented by a general anesthetic (e.g., ether) and peripherally acting muscle relaxants. Among the minor operations for which it is used are various obstetrical, orthopedic, and genitourinary procedures.

Overdosage may rapidly paralyze the medullary respiratory center. Thus, the drug is used only when facilities for assisting respiration are available. Because of the possibility of laryngospasm, atropine premedication is desirable, as is passage of an endotracheal tube after administration of a muscle relaxant. Thiopental is not recommended for patients with respiratory and circulatory difficulties.

Dosage and Administration. Dosage is determined according to individual needs. However, basal anesthesia may be induced slowly in most adults by injecting a total of 50 to 75 mg. by vein at intervals of 30 to 60 seconds (i.e., 2 or 3 ml. of the 2.5% solution). Thiopental is administered by rectum in a specially formulated injection containing 400 mg. per Gm. A dose of 1 Gm. of the suspension per 75 lb. of body weight is usually adequate for preanesthetic sedation. Deeper anesthesia is induced with doses up to 1 Gm. of suspension per 50 lb. of body weight. Total dosage should normally not exceed 1 to 1.5 Gm. for children weighing 75 pounds or more, or 3 to 4 Gm. for adults weighing 200 pounds or more.

TETRACAINE HYDROCHLORIDE U.S.P. (PONTOCAINE)

Pharmacology. This drug produces a powerful and prolonged anesthetic action by topical application, infiltration or intrathecal injection. However, its potency and relatively slow rate of elimination can lead to severe toxic reactions in the event of overdosage or hypersensitivity. Inhalation of excessive amounts, during forceful spraying, or accidental intravenous injection can cause cardiac syncope, hypotension to shock levels, and convulsions followed by coma and fatal respiratory paralysis. Consequently, precautions against rapid absorption of excessive amounts are especially important with tetracaine solutions.

Dosage and Administration. A concentration of only 0.15% is used for continuous caudal analgesia. Solutions of 0.3 to 0.5% produce long-lasting spinal analgesia. A 2% solution is used for spraying the throat in rhinolaryngology. The total amount of drug sprayed into the trachea should not exceed 20 mg.; spinal injections have a maximal safe dose of 10 to 15 mg. Higher amounts may be infiltrated or administered caudally over longer periods.

CHAPTER 12

PHARMACOLOGY OF ETHYL ALCOHOL

Drugs for Treatment of Alcoholism

DISULFIRAM (ANTABUSE; TETRAETHYLTHIU-RAM DISULFIDE; TETD)

Pharmacology. This drug is used as an adjunct to medical and psychiatric treatment of alcoholism. Patients who take it know that they will suffer an unpleasant reaction if they drink any alcohol during the time the drug is in the body. Symptoms include flushing and a feeling of heat, dizziness, nausea and vomiting, and heart palpitations. These are believed to result from vasodilatation, hypotension, and reflex tachycardia, which are pharmacological effects produced by the accumulation of acetaldehyde, a metabolite of alcohol. Disulfiram is thought to interfere with the functioning of the enzymes that normally participate in the oxidative breakdown of ethyl alcohol.

Disulfiram, itself, is of relatively low toxicity. Patients may complain occasionally of a metallic or garlicky aftertaste, headache, drowsiness, and skin eruptions, but such symptoms tend to disappear during prolonged maintenance therapy at reduced dosage. Use of this drug is undesirable in patients with heart disease, cerebral damage, and severe kidney and liver disorders, not because of adverse effects of the drug itself, but because of danger to patients who may drink despite having taken the drug.

Since the alcohol-disulfiram reaction occasionally causes violent reactions and fatal circulatory collapse, this drug is never given to patients without their knowledge and consent, or to alcoholics who are judged to be psychotic.

Dosage and Administration. Treatment is initiated with 0.5 Gm. taken once daily after a period of 12 hours or longer of abstinence from alcohol. After 2 weeks, the dose may be reduced to 0.25 Gm. or to 0.125 Gm. because of the drug's cumulative effects. Daily treatment is safely continued for months or years if the drug does deter the alcoholic from drinking while receiving psychotherapy.

CHAPTER 13

CENTRAL NERVOUS SYSTEM STIMULANTS

BEMEGRIDE U.S.P. (MEGIMIDE)

Pharmacology. This C.N.S. stimulant was originally introduced with the claim that it is a specific biochemical antagonist of the barbiturates. This proved to be incorrect, and it is now known that the drug acts only through ordinary C.N.S. stimulation. The drug's rapid analeptic action makes it useful in treating some cases of overdosage by depressant drugs. In such situations, it stimulates the depressed respiration in the same way as does pentylenetetrazol. Like the latter drug, bemegride is sometimes used in neurology to aid in the diagnosis of epilepsy.

Overdosage must be avoided to prevent the development of undesired convulsive spasms in drug-depressed patients. However, the short duration of this durg's stimulating action tends to minimize the danger of overdosage. Some patients have reportedly suffered delayed psychotic reactions after recovering from drug-induced depression when treated with this analeptic. This may not be a true toxic effect of this drug but a sign of barbiturate or alcohol withdrawal brought on more rapidly than normally by the arousal effect of this drug.

Dosage and Administration. Bemegride is given by intravenous injection or infusion in doses of 50 mg. Several such doses are ordinarily required to stimulate the respiration of deeply depressed patients or to arouse them.

CAFFEINE U.S.P.

Pharmacology. This alkaloid is one of the methylxanthine group found in the parts of various plants, including coffee, tea, and cola. Low oral doses such as those ingested in a cup or two of the beverages containing it tend to aid mental activity and to counteract sleepiness and fatigue. Somewhat higher doses may cause insomnia, irritability, and tremors. When injected in moderate amounts, caffeine stimulates not only such cerebral cortical activity but also that of the medullary respiratory center.

Caffeine is frequently combined with analgesic drugs, such as aspirin and phenacetin, in headache remedies. Its usefulness in such products, and when combined with ergotamine for treating migraine and hypertensive headaches, is believed to be the result of its constricting effect upon cerebral blood vessels. It is occasionally added to cold remedy products to counteract the sedative actions of antihistaminic drugs, and it is used by the public in tablet and beverage form to stave off drowsiness and to overcome the depressant effects of alcohol. Caffeine may be administered intramuscularly to stimulate the respiration and blood pressure of patients suffering from overdosage by depressant drugs such as morphine, the barbiturates, and alcohol.

The side effects of caffeine are mainly the result of excessive stimulation. However, some sensitive individuals may complain of heart palpitations and G.I. upset after even one cup of coffee.

Many individuals have developed a psychological dependence upon the caffeine in coffee. This is not harmful, except that they may feel irritable and have headaches when deprived of the beverage.

Dosage and Administration. A cup of coffee ordinarily contains 100 to 150 mg. of caffeine, and tea and cola beverages contain considerably less. The amount found in pharmaceutical preparations is 50 to 100 mg. ordinarily and is thus, if anything, less than that contained in one cup of coffee. The usual dose range is 100 to 500 mg. The latter amount of caffeine sodium benzoate U.S.P. is administered intramuscularly or subcutaneously as a respiratory stimulant.

DEXTROAMPHETAMINE SULFATE U.S.P. (DEXEDRINE)

Pharmacology. This psychomotor stimulant produces its desired C.N.S. action at lower doses than are required with the racemic mixture of levo- and dextro-amphetamines (i.e., Benzedrine). The dextrorotatory isomer causes fewer undesirable cardiovascular effects than the latter when administered in amounts that are effective clinically in conditions such as minor mental depressive states, obesity, narcolepsy, postencephalitic parkinsonism, petit mal epilepsy, and behavioral disorders in children. The drug is combined with antihistamine, anticonvulsant, antiparkinsonism, and other depressant drugs to counteract drowsiness. It is used occasionally as an analeptic for treating overdosage by depressant drugs.

Side effects of central origin include restlessness, irritability, tension, tremors, and insomnia. Adrenergic effects may bring about cardiac palpitation and arrhythmias with possible chest pain and elevation of blood pressure. G.I. effects include mouth dryness, loss of appetite, nausea, vomiting, cramps, and constipation *or* diarrhea. This drug, like other sympathomimetic agents, is used with caution, if at all, in patients with a history of coronary disease, moderate to severe hypertension, and hyperthyroidism. Its abuse characteristics contraindicate the use of dextroamphetamine in patients with psychopathic personalities or others known to drug abuse.

Dosage and Administration. The usual dose is 5 mg. taken in tablet form every 4 to 6 hours during the day. Sensitive patients may be limited to as little as 2.5 mg. per dose, whereas others—in narcolepsy, for example—may require and tolerate 60 mg. daily. To avoid insomnia, it is often desirable to administer the last dose of the day no later than 4 P.M.

PENTYLENETETRAZOL N.F. (METRAZOL)

Pharmacology. This brain stem stimulant is used to determine the depth of depression caused by overdoses of barbiturates and as an analeptic for stimulating the respiration and hastening the arousal of drug-depressed patients. Overdoses can cause convulsions or vomiting with danger of aspiration.

Oral doses of this drug are advocated for improving the mental functioning of confused and disoriented elderly patients, but its usefulness for this purpose is not established. The use of pentylenetetrazol as a pharmacoconvulsant in the chemoshock therapy of mental illness has diminished in favor of the use of flurothyl and electroshock therapy. Subconvulsant doses are occasionally infused by vein as an aid in the diagnosis of epilepsy. Sometimes actual convulsions are precipitated in order to determine the exact nature of the seizure pattern.

Dosage and Administration. A 10% solution is available for intravenous use in the diagnosis and treatment of drug-induced depression and for producing convulsive seizures in shock therapy. A dose of 100 to 500 mg. (1 to 5 ml.) is injected in such cases. Tablets containing 100 mg. of this drug are available for oral use in a dose of 200 mg. three times daily.

CHAPTER 15

CHOLINERGIC (PARASYMPATHOMIMETIC) DRUGS

AMBENONIUM CHLORIDE (MYTELASE)

Pharmacology. This anticholinesterase type of cholinergic drug is said to have a more sustained muscle strengthening effect than neostigmine in the treatment of myasthenia gravis. Another claimed advantage is that muscarinic side effects are fewer. However, the relatively late appearance of abdominal cramps, diarrhea, salivation, and bronchial secretions may be a disadvantage, as these serve as warning signs of more serious overdosage.

Dosage and Administration. Dosage is adjusted to individual tolerance and the extent of therapeutic response. The average dose ranges from 5 to 25 mg., three or four times daily, which is increased to 200 mg. or more daily in severe cases.

BETHANECHOL CHLORIDE U.S.P. (URECHOLINE)

Pharmacology. This parasympathomimetic choline derivative is used mainly to stimulate the G.I. tract and the urinary bladder. It is employed chiefly in treating postoperative abdominal distention and urinary retention. It has been used to overcome similar states caused by drugs such as the ganglionic blocking agents during the treatment of hypertension.

Dosage and Administration. Bethanechol is given orally or subcutaneously in doses determined by the response. Usually, oral doses of 10 to 30 mg. three or four times daily are adequate. If this treatment is not effective, 2.5 to 5 mg. is given subcutaneously. The drug is never injected intramuscularly or by vein, as excessive parasympathetic stimulation may result in abdominal cramps, asthmatic attacks, and a fall in blood pressure. Similar side effects that sometimes occur even with subcutaneous administration are overcome by injecting 0.6 mg. of atropine sulfate.

EDROPHONIUM CHLORIDE U.S.P. (TENSILON)

Pharmacology. Edrophonium is a cholinergic drug with a relatively short anticurare and antimyasthenic action. It is used occasionally as a supplement to oxygen and artificial respiration in the management of respiratory muscle weakness caused by curare overdosage or acute myasthenic crisis.

The most important use of edrophonium is in the differential diagnosis of myasthenia gravis and to determine whether the severe muscle weakness is caused by undertreatment (myasthenic crisis) or by overdosage with anticholinesterase agents (cholinergic crisis).

Dosage and Administration. For diagnosis of myasthenia, 10 mg. is injected by vein. This dose causes no change in the muscle strength of nonmyasthenics or only fasciculations of isolated fiber groups followed by transient weakness. A marked increase in muscle strength in response to edrophonium is a positive test for myasthenia gravis.

For differentiating between myasthenic crisis and cholinergic crisis only 1 to 2 mg. is injected intravenously. If the muscle weakness is not relieved or worsens, the crisis is considered cholinergic; and anticholinesterase drug medication is withdrawn. When injection of a test dose of edrophonium produces a rapid gain in muscle strength, the crisis is probably myasthenic; and administration of more of this drug or of other antimyasthenic cholinergic agents is indicated.

METHACHOLINE SALTS N.F. (MECHOLYL)

Pharmacology. This synthetic choline ester produces parasympathomimetic effects, including slowing of the heart, dilation of blood vessels, and stimulation of visceral smooth muscles. It is used sometimes to terminate attacks of paroxysmal atrial tachycardia and to increase local blood flow in various conditions that are characterized by spasm of blood vessels in the extremities, including Raynaud's disease.

Methacholine is contraindicated in patients with bronchial asthma. Excessive cholinergic side effects, including increased peristaltic activity, bradycardia, and hypotension, may be overcome by administering atropine, which should always be available in a hypodermic syringe containing 0.6 mg.

Dosage and Administration. Two salts are available, methacholine *bromide,* which may be administered orally as tablets in doses of 200 to 600 mg. two or three times daily, and methacholine *chloride,* a powder used for preparing parenteral solutions. Such solutions are injected subcutaneously only, *never* intramuscularly or intravenously, in doses of 10 to 40 mg. In the treatment of chronic skin ulcers, the drug is best administered by iontophoresis, or ion transfer, a method that limits the drug's effects to local sites, thus reducing systemic side effects.

NEOSTIGMINE SALTS U.S.P. (PROSTIGMIN)

Pharmacology. This cholinergic drug inhibits the enzyme cholinesterase, and thus increases nerve impulse transmission by acetylcholine at various neuromuscular junctions. Neostigmine increases the tone and motility of visceral smooth muscle, which prevents and overcomes postoperative distention of the intestine and urinary bladder, provided that these organs are not obstructed mechanically. Applied topically, it reduces intraocular pressure in glaucoma. It is often employed to increase skeletal muscle strength in myasthenia gravis.

Dosage and Administration. Neostigmine is available as two salts, the *bromide* (U.S.P.) and the *methylsulfate* (U.S.P.). Neostigmine bromide tablets (15 mg.) are used mainly in myasthenia gravis. Dosage depends on requirements and tolerance. A 5% ophthalmic solution of this salt in eye drops is instilled into the conjunctival sac as a miotic in glaucoma.

Neostigmine methylsulfate solution containing 0.25 mg., 0.5 mg., or 1 mg./ml. is injected subcutaneously or intramuscularly in the treatment of postoperative abdominal distention and urinary retention, and as a screening test for pregnancy in delayed menstruation. For prevention of postoperative atony, a parenteral dose of 0.25 mg. is administered immediately and repeated several times daily for two or three days. When paralytic ileus or bladder atony develop, doses of 0.5 mg. are administered every few hours as an adjunct to physical and mechanical measures, such as heat applications, enemas, and intubation, or catheterization.

PILOCARPINE AND ITS SALTS U.S.P.

Pharmacology. This plant alkaloid stimulates smooth muscles and glands that are innervated by postganglionic cholinergic nerve fibers. It is used mainly as a miotic in glaucoma and overcomes mydriasis and cycloplegia caused by atropine. It is sometimes administered alternately with mydriatic drugs to prevent adhesions from forming between the iris and the lens.

Pilocarpine often produces profuse secretion of the salivary, gastric, and sweat glands and stimulation of G.I. tone and motility. These actions are generally considered undesirable. Occasionally, however, salivation is deliberately induced with this drug to combat mouth dryness caused by overdoses of atropine or the ganglionic blocking agents.

Dosage and Administration. Pilocarpine alkaloid is available in a 2% castor oil solution for ophthalmic use. The hydrochloride (U.S.P.) and nitrate (U.S.P.) salts are available in isotonic, buffered aqueous solutions of various strengths for use in ophthalmology. Hypodermic tablets are used for preparing solutions for subcutaneous administration in doses of about 5 mg., when sweating, salivation, and increased peristaltic activity are desired.

PYRIDOSTIGMINE BROMIDE U.S.P. (MESTINON)

Pharmacology. Pyridostigmine is a cholinergic drug that overcomes the muscle weakness of myasthenia gravis. It inhibits the enzyme acetylcholinesterase, which is concentrated at nerve-muscle junctions. The resultant rise in acetylcholine levels increases the rate of transmission of nerve impulses across the neuromuscular junctions.

This agent is said to cause fewer G.I. disturbances than neostigmine. However, overdosage can cause abdominal cramps and diarrhea, as well as other muscarinic actions, such as increased bronchial secretions, sweating, and salivation. More serious effects of overdosage are nicotinic actions such as skeletal muscle cramps and twitching, which may progress to extreme weakness (cholinergic crisis) and respiratory muscle paralysis.

Dosage and Administration. Dosage is adjusted to the needs of each myasthenic patient. The drug is available in 60 mg. tablets, which are administered as needed to maintain maximum muscle strength: 1 to 25 tablets daily. Sustained-action tablets (*Timespan*) containing 180 mg. reduce the frequency of administration. These are taken no more often than every 6 hours, but may be supplemented by the more rapidly acting regular tablets as needed to maintain muscle strength.

CHAPTER 16

SYMPATHOMIMETIC (ADRENERGIC) DRUGS

ANGIOTENSIN AMIDE (HYPERTENSIN)

Pharmacology. This most potent vasopressor, though *not* an adrenergic drug, is discussed here because it is used clinically to treat acute hypotensive states just as are levarterenol and certain other sympathomimetic amines. This drug is believed to constrict splanchnic arterioles by directly stimulating their smooth muscle walls. It does not stimulate alpha adrenergic receptors or constrict venules as levarterenol does. This may account for the fact that tachyphylaxis does not develop, nor does local ischemia with consequent necrosis and sloughing occur.

Angiotensin amide is sometimes successful in cases of severe shock refractory to adrenergic pressor amines; however, the reverse has proved true occasionally.

Dosage and Administration. Five ml. of sterile distilled water is added to the contents of one vial (2.5 mg.) and this solution is added in required amounts to 500 ml. of saline solution, which is then slowly infused by vein. The rate of infusion is usually 0.5 to 20 mcg./minute, depending on the response. The rate is watched carefully and adjusted to bring the blood pressure to the desired level and to avoid dangerous degrees of hypertension. Blood pressure readings are taken frequently, and the site of injection is inspected to avoid leakage of the infusion solution into tissues adjacent to the venous insert.

EPHEDRINE SULFATE U.S.P.

Pharmacology. This sympathomimetic substance, the active principle of the Chinese plant ma huang, is available as the base and as the sulfate and hydrochloride salts. It differs from epinephrine in that it is a longer-lasting vasoconstrictor and bronchodilator, is more effective when administered by mouth, and stimulates the C.N.S.

Ephedrine is widely used to relieve bronchial spasm in asthma. It is less effective in G.I. spasm and in relaxing the urinary bladder and other genitourinary tract smooth muscle. However, it is used occasionally in nocturnal enuresis (bedwetting) to increase the tone of the trigone and sphincter muscles of the bladder while relaxing the detrusor muscle. Another unusual use is in myasthenia gravis, in which it occasionally strengthens skeletal muscles.

More commonly it is used as a nasal decongestant in the common cold, hay fever, and other acute and chronic inflammatory and allergic disorders of the upper respiratory tract. The drug is applied to the eye as a mydriatic and is sometimes administered parenterally to raise blood pressure in hypotension and to treat syncope in heart block. Its central stimulating action may overcome drowsiness in narcolepsy, but it is also a source of nervous excitement and insomnia when used for other therapeutic purposes.

Dosage and Administration. Ephedrine salts may be administered orally in doses of 25 to 50 mg. An injectable solution containing 50 mg./ml. and a 3% solution for ophthalmic use are available. The latter may be diluted with isotonic saline solution for topical application to the mucous membranes of the nose.

EPINEPHRINE U.S.P. (ADRENALIN)

Pharmacology. This adrenal hormone has many actions and uses. It promptly relieves acute asthmatic attacks and counteracts urticarial and anaphylactoid-type allergic reactions. In asthma and emphysema its combined bronchodilator and decongestant actions help to clear the clogged, constricted airway, thus facilitating pulmonary ventilation. In allergy, it constricts arterioles and reduces capillary permeability and thus prevents plasma leakage into the tissues.

Epinephrine is occasionally effective in cardiac arrest when it is injected directly into the heart or jugular vein, preferably with simultaneous clamping of the aorta and myocardial massage. However, because the drug itself may set off ventricular fibrillation, the related drug isoproterenol is preferred for treating syncopal episodes in heart block.

The local vasoconstrictor action of epinephrine is useful for stopping local bleeding from the skin and respiratory tract membranes. Dilute solutions are combined with local anesthetics to delay their systemic absorption. The drug's decongestant action on nasal and ocular mucous membranes sometimes relieves allergic rhinitis, sinusitis, and conjunctivitis. Topical application as a hemostatic is useful in epistaxis (nosebleed) and for stemming oozing of blood after some types of surgery.

Overdosage as the result of a miscalculation, the use of too strong a solution, or accidental injection of a subcutaneous dose into a vein, may cause dangerous cardiovascular effects marked by pallor, high blood pressure, cardiac arrhythmias, chest pain, and headache. Death may result from cerebrovascular accident, ventricular fibrillation, or cardiac dilation with pulmonary edema.

Dosage and Administration. Epinephrine is ineffective when given by mouth and must be administered parenterally or topically. A 1:1,000 solution (1 mg./ml.) is available for injection, usually in doses of 0.2 to 0.5 ml. subcutaneously. This strength solution and a 1:10,000 dilution are applied topically to the skin and mucous membranes for local vasoconstrictor action.

A much stronger solution (1:100) is sprayed into the respiratory tract in asthma. *It is never injected* when the 1:1,000 solution is ordered. An oily suspension (1:500) produces relatively prolonged bronchodilator effects when injected intramuscularly. A 1% ointment is available for application to the eye in ophthalmic conditions, as are several concentrations of a solution of the bitartrate salt.

ISOPROTERENOL HYDROCHLORIDE U.S.P. (ISUPREL; ISONORIN)

Pharmacology. This powerful adrenergic drug is mainly a bronchodilator and a cardiac stimulant. It relaxes bronchial smooth muscle, and thus relieves bronchial spasm in asthma,

pulmonary emphysema, and during anesthesia. It is often effective in asthmatic patients who no longer respond to epinephrine. Although these two drugs may be alternated, they are not given simultaneously because their additive effects may cause undesirable degrees of tachycardia due to excessive stimulation. Nervousness, nausea, tremor, and headache are possible side effects of isoproterenol.

Isoproterenol stimulates the ventricular rate and strengthens the beat in heart block, Stokes-Adams disease, and the carotid sinus syndrome—conditions marked by excessive cardiac slowing and periodic syncope. It is used cautiously in patients with coronary insufficiency, hypertension, hyperthyroidism, and vasomotor instability.

Dosage and Administration. This drug, available as the hydrochloride and sulfate salts, may be administered by inhalation or sublingually in doses of 10 to 20 mg. in amounts not to exceed 60 mg. a day. A 1:100 or 1:200 solution or powder is administered for oral inhalation in acute asthmatic attacks. Occasionally, a 1:5,000 solution is injected parenterally in low doses (0.02 to 0.15 mg.), which tend to stimulate the heart. The drug is available in suppository form (5 mg. dose) and as an ingredient of an antiasthmatic cough syrup (3 mg./5 ml.).

LEVARTERENOL BITARTRATE U.S.P. (LEVOPHED)

Pharmacology. This potent vasopressor, an isomer of the primary neurohormone of the sympathetic nervous system—norepinephrine—is used to treat shock and acute hypotensive states in various clinical situations. It raises blood pressure mainly by directly stimulating the alpha type receptors in the smooth muscle of the arterioles, but constriction of venules may also play a part in its pressor action. Although it does not usually increase cardiac output and may actually cause a reflex slowing of the heart, its relative lack of cardiac irritating action makes levarterenol preferable to epinephrine in the management of cardiogenic shock following a myocardial infarction.

The main danger in the use of this drug is that overdosage may raise blood pressure excessively. Patients with atherosclerotic vessels are especially prone to suffer cerebrovascular accidents in such circumstances. Headache and propulsive vomiting are early signs of drug-induced hypertension, which should be avoided by making frequent blood pressure readings during the slow intravenous infusion of the drug solution. Caution is also required to avoid leakage of the drug from the vein into surrounding tissues, as abscesses, with death of the tissue and sloughing, may develop. Patients are never left unattended during administration of this drug.

Dosage and Administration. Levarterenol is infused intravenously, preferably through a plastic tube inserted deep into a large central vein and fixed securely so that it does not become dislodged. An ampule of the 0.2% solution is added to a 5% dextrose solution, the degree of dilution depending largely on fluid requirements. Although patients may receive blood transfusions or plasma simultaneously, the drug is not added to these natural fluids, as its potency may be reduced by the destructive action of plasma enzymes.

PHENYLEPHRINE HYDROCHLORIDE U.S.P. (NEO-SYNEPHRINE)

Pharmacology. This synthetic adrenergic drug produces relatively prolonged local and systemic vasoconstrictor effects. Locally its solutions are applied topically to the nasal mucosa as a decongestant in colds, sinusitis, hay fever, and vasomotor rhinitis. Instilled in the eye, it acts as a decongestant in conjunctivitis, or, in higher concentrations, as a mydriatic to dilate the pupil for diagnostic purposes in ophthalmology.

Systemically, phenylephrine prevents or overcomes hypotensive reactions during spinal and inhalation anesthesia. Its pressor action is not accompanied by cardiac irregularities or by C.N.S. stimulation. However, it is not used in patients with hypertension, hyperthyroidism, diabetes, or heart disease.

Dosage and Administration. Phenylephrine is applied topically in the nose in a concentration of 0.25% or 0.5%, in the form of drops, sprays, jelly, and tampons. As an ocular decongestant a 0.125% solution is employed, and for mydriasis 1 or 2 drops of a 2.5% ophthalmic solution is used. A 10% solution or emulsion is sometimes employed in certain eye conditions; its use is preceded by a drop of a local anesthetic solution to prevent irritation and pain in the eye.

For shock prevention and treatment, phenylephrine is injected subcutaneously or intramuscularly in doses of 2 to 5 mg., using a 1% solution, or intravenously in a dose of 0.5 to 1 mg., using the 0.2% parenteral solution. The drug is available in oral form (dose 10 to 25 mg.) for treatment of the common cold and management of allergic rhinitis, chronic sinusitis, and other conditions in which its decongestant action on upper respiratory tract mucous membranes is desired.

CHAPTER 17

AUTONOMIC BLOCKING AGENTS

Antimuscarinic-Type Cholinergic Blocking Drugs

ATROPINE SULFATE U.S.P.

Pharmacology. This prototype anticholinergic alkaloid produces its many peripheral effects by blocking the transmission of cholinergic nerve impulses to smooth muscle, cardiac muscle, and exocrine glands. This ability to compete successfully with acetylcholine for receptor sites in these structures, tissues, and organs accounts for both its therapeutically useful actions and its many undesired side effects.

The anhidrotic action of atropine which is seen with the lowest doses, is mainly a side effect (mouth dryness; skin dry, hot, and red), but it is also used to dry the respiratory tract during acute colds and prior to inhalation anesthesia, and to reduce excessive salivation and sweating. Somewhat higher doses of this and other belladonna alkaloids reduce G.I. tone, motility, and secretions in the treatment of peptic ulcer, etc.

Topical application of atropine solutions to the eye facilitates examination of the fundus of the eye, measurement of refractive errors, and the management of various inflammatory ocular conditions. However, similar actions (i.e., mydriasis, cycloplegia, and intraocular pressure increases), which may occur upon systemic administration of atropine, may precipitate an attack of acute glaucoma. Thus, the drug is contraindicated in patients with a history of glaucoma, as well as in those with prostatic hypertrophy, heart disease, and organic pyloric stenosis.

Atropine, a mild stimulant of the medulla and higher cerebral centers, is rarely used as a respiratory or cortical stimulant. However, it affects C.N.S. motor control mechanisms to reduce the tremor and rigidity of parkinsonism. Its usefulness in this condition is limited by the development of tolerance and by side effects such as blurring of vision, constipation, and urinary retention—the latter especially in elderly males with prostatic hypertrophy.

Dosage and Administration. The usual oral or injected dose of atropine is 0.5 mg., but dosages ranging from 0.3 to 1.2 mg. may be administered. Solutions for topical application to the eye range from 0.25% (in castor oil) to 0.5, 1, 2, 3, and 4% strengths (aqueous).

DICYCLOMINE HYDROCHLORIDE (BENTYL)

Pharmacology. This antispasmodic drug has minimal acetylcholine-blocking properties and produces its effects mainly by directly relaxing the contractile mechanism of G.I. smooth muscle. This accounts both for its inability to reduce gastric secretion and for its relative lack of atropine-like side effects.

Dicyclomine controls the symptoms of functional disorders of the G.I. tract marked by hypermotility and spasm, including spastic constipation and spastic colitis. It relieves spasm secondary to peptic ulcer, but antacids must be administered at the same time to counteract acidity. Dicyclomine relieves spasm secondary to other organic conditions, such as ulcerative colitis and diverticulosis.

Although this drug is relatively safe for patients with glaucoma, it shares some of the other contraindications of the anticholinergic-type antispasmodics. For example, it is not desirable for patients who have any obstruction of the G.I. or genitourinary tract, such as pyloric stenosis or urinary retention.

Dosage and Administration. One or 2 capsules or teaspoonfuls of a syrup, each containing 10 mg., or a single 20 mg. tablet, is administered three or four times daily, either alone or combined with a sedative dose of phenobarbital. For infants, ½ teaspoonful of the syrup is diluted with an equal amount of water and given three or four times daily. For rapid action 20 mg. may be injected intramuscularly every 4 to 6 hours.

PROPANTHELINE BROMIDE U.S.P.* (PRO-BANTHINE)

Pharmacology. This synthetic cholinergic blocking drug of the quaternary ammonium class is said to be more potent than the related prototype methantheline, but it is claimed to cause fewer side effects than the latter. Drugs of this type have a double blocking action. Unlike atropine, they are thought to block impulses at parasympathetic *ganglia* as well as at the smooth muscle and gastric gland receptor sites. They also differ from the natural anticholinergic alkaloids in that they do not cause C.N.S. side effects.

In practice, propantheline and related synthetic drugs produce effects similar to those of atropine, and are used clinically for the same purposes. Thus, propantheline is employed, like the less expensive belladonna alkaloids, for its antispasmodic-antisecretory actions in the management of peptic ulcer, gastritis, pancreatitis, etc. and for reducing intestinal hypermotility in the irritable bowel syndrome, diverticulitis, etc. It helps to relax spasm of the ureters and urinary bladder.

The side effects of propantheline are essentially the same as those of atropine, and its use is contraindicated in patients who cannot take atropine because of conditions that make them intolerant of anticholinergic drug effects. Massive overdosage with this and similar drugs can block the sympathetic ganglia and the motor end-plates of skeletal muscle. This might lead to a steep drop in blood pressure and failure of respiration, such as occurs in curare poisoning.

Dosage and Administration. The usual dose of propantheline is 15 mg., but it may be given in amounts up to 60 mg. four times a day and during the night for reducing pain, spasm, and acid secretion in episodes of acute peptic ulcer. Later, lower maintenance doses are established. The drug is given orally or by injection. When given by vein, the contents of an ampule (30 mg.) are diluted in at least 10 ml. of water for injection.

SCOPOLAMINE HYDROBROMIDE U.S.P. (HYOSCINE)

Pharmacology. This solanaceous alkaloid obtained mainly from *Hyoscyamus* produces peripheral effects similar to those of atropine, and it may be used for treating many of the same

---

*See Table 17-3 for a listing of related synthetic anticholinergic agents.

clinical conditions. However, scopolamine differs from atropine in its C.N.S. effects, for it causes marked depression, especially when administered parenterally.

Scopolamine is often used alone or combined with morphine preoperatively and in obstetrics to produce sedation and amnesia. It is sometimes used as a hypnotic in insomnia and for quieting agitated patients in a manic state or alcoholics with delirium tremens. The drug is employed in parkinsonism and to prevent motion sickness. It produces all of the peripheral side effects and C.N.S. toxic reactions seen with atropine, and its use is contraindicated in the same conditions as the other solanaceous alkaloids.

Dosage and Administration. Scopolamine is administered orally or subcutaneously in doses of 300 to 800 *micro*grams (0.3 to 0.6 mg.). The usual dose is 600 mcg. (0.6 mg.). It may also be applied topically to the conjunctival sac as 0.1 ml. of a 0.2% buffered aqueous solution.

Adrenergic Blocking Agent*

PHENTOLAMINE MESYLATE U.S.P. (REGITINE)

Pharmacology. This adrenergic blocking drug is used in the diagnosis and treatment of pheochromocytoma. It prevents the rise in blood pressure that occurs in this condition as a result of the abnormally high levels of circulating catecholamines released by the chromaffin cell tumors. This form of phentolamine is preferred for preoperative preparation of the patient and during the surgical operation for removal of the tumor. Such pretreatment prevents paroxysms of hypertension and other ill effects resulting from sudden release of large amounts of epinephrine into the blood stream. This injectable form of the blocking drug is also used in a diagnostic screening test to help determine whether or not various signs and symptoms, including high blood pressure, are due to pheochromocytoma.

Dosage and Administration. In the diagnostic test, a solution of this salt is injected intravenously or intramuscularly in a dose of 5 mg. under certain standard conditions. A marked drop in blood pressure that develops shortly after the injection indicates the possible presence of pheochromocytoma; if no change or only slight changes in blood pressure occur, the prior hypertension is probably due to other causes.

A dose of 5 mg. may also be injected prior to anesthesia and surgery and repeated, if necessary, during the operation for removal of the tumor tissue. For medical management during the time between diagnosis and surgery, oral tablets containing 50 mg. of phentolamine hydrochloride N.F. are administered four to six times daily. Patients with severe cases may require higher doses, whereas children need much lower amounts.

Neuromuscular Blocking Agents

GALLAMINE TRIETHIODIDE N.F. (FLAXEDIL)

Pharmacology. This first synthetic curarelike drug is said to have several advantages over the natural alkaloids. It seems less likely, for example, to cause circulatory collapse, for it does not block sympathetic ganglia. However, its cholinergic-blocking action is not entirely limited to skeletal muscle end plates; and the drug may interfere with transmission of inhibitory impulses to the heart via the vagus nerve. This atropinelike action can cause an undesirable increase in the heart rate. Also, although this drug does not cause the release of free tissue histamine, it may produce allergic reactions in patients sensitive to iodine.

This neuromuscular blocking agent, like tubocurarine, brings

*See also Azapetine; Phenoxybenzamine; Tolazoline, Drug Digests.

about better muscular relaxation during a variety of surgical, manipulative, and intubation procedures; prevents dislocations and fractures during electroconvulsive shock therapy; and reduces muscle spasm in orthopedic procedures, such as reduction of dislocations and fractures.

Dosage and Administration. Gallamine is injected intravenously in an initial dose of about 1 mg./Kg. body weight. This may be followed during prolonged procedures by doses of 0.5 to 1 mg./Kg. at intervals of 40 to 50 minutes. As with tubocurarine, lower doses are required when it is used with ether anesthesia.

SUCCINYLCHOLINE CHLORIDE U.S.P. (ANECTINE; QUELICIN; SUCOSTRIN; ETC.)

Pharmacology. This neuromuscular blocking agent of the depolarizing type produces rapid muscular relaxation of short duration. This is said to make it especially suitable for use in procedures that require only brief muscular flaccidity, such as endotracheal intubation, orthopedic manipulation, and electroshock therapy, in which it lessens the severity of muscle spasms during the convulsive seizure. This drug is used during more prolonged surgical procedures as an adjunct to anesthesia administered by continuous intravenous drip.

Succinylcholine acts relatively specifically at the myoneural junctions in skeletal muscles; and so it is relatively free of some of the side effects occasionally seen with tubocurarine. However, sometimes patients complain of muscle soreness as a result of the initial contractions that often occur prior to the onset of paralysis. Although respiratory depression is usually of short duration, prolonged apnea sometimes occurs, especially in patients with low plasma levels of the enzyme cholinesterase, which ordinarily converts the drug to inactive metabolites rapidly. For this reason, this relaxant is contraindicated for patients with severe liver disease, anemia, or malnutrition and for those who have a hereditary deficiency of plasma cholinesterase. Facilities for artificial ventilation must always be readily available.

Dosage and Administration. Usually 10 to 40 mg. is infused intravenously as a 0.1% solution. However, although such doses produce adequate relaxation for about 2 to 5 minutes, much larger amounts may be infused over long periods, provided that the patient is watched carefully from moment to moment during the prolonged infusion, and the rate of flow is carefully adjusted in accordance with his response.

TUBOCURARINE CHLORIDE U.S.P. (TUBARINE; TUBADIL; and in INTOCOSTRIN)

Pharmacology. This salt of the active alkaloid of curare produces neuromuscular blockade: it prevents the motor end-plates of skeletal muscle fibers from being depolarized by the acetylcholine released from somatic motor nerve fiber terminals. Its main use is as an adjunct to general anesthesia, in order to produce muscular relaxation while employing relatively low, safe amounts of the anesthetic.

The margin between the amount of the drug that relaxes the muscles of the limbs and abdomen and that which paralyzes the respiratory muscles is narrow and variable. Consequently, the drug is administered only by anesthesiologists and other personnel especially trained in the use of neuromuscular blocking agents. Facilities for resuscitation in case of respiratory failure must be readily available. These include equipment for opening a free airway and for administering artificial respiration with oxygen, as well as such pharmacological anticurare agents as neostigmine or edrophonium.

Dosage and Administration. The dosage varies depending on many factors that the experienced anesthesiologist takes into consideration. However, the official dose is 6 to 9 mg. injected slowly by vein over a period of 30 to 90 seconds. This may be followed in 5 minutes by 3 to 5 mg. more, if required; and small supplements are added as needed during a prolonged operation.

CHAPTER 19

DIGITALIS AND RELATED HEART DRUGS

DIGITALIS PURPUREA – U.S.P. CRUDE PREPARATIONS

Pharmacology. Powdered digitalis leaf and the Tincture of Digitalis are essentially crude preparations of the active principle digitoxin, accompanied by various impurities. The latter tend to increase the likelihood of nausea and vomiting during early administration. The only advantage of these crude preparations has been their relative inexpensiveness, but some pure glycosides are now available at even lower prices.

Dosage and Administration. Tablets and capsules of powdered digitalis are given in divided doses over a period of 1 or 2 days in amounts totaling 1.2 to 2.0 Gm. Digitalization is maintained by single daily doses of 0.1 Gm.

The dose of Digitalis Tincture is 1 ml. This hydroalcoholic liquid is administered by means of a standardized dropper or accurately calibrated medicine glass. The standardized U.S.P. dropper provides 1 ml. or 15 minims in 40 drops of the tincture. Other droppers for measuring definitely calibrated amounts are available; they are used only for delivering these amounts and not merely any number of drops.

DIGITOXIN U.S.P. (CRYSTODIGIN; PURODIGIN, ETC.)

Pharmacology. This pure, crystalline glycoside is completely absorbed from the G.I. tract when administered by mouth. However, whether given this way or parenterally, digitoxin is relatively slow in its onset of action, and is slowly eliminated.

These factors determine the drug's utility in particular clinical situations. Because it is not fully effective for 6 to 10 hours, digitoxin cannot be used when rapid digitalization is urgently required. On the other hand, the delayed excretion makes it relatively easy to maintain effective quantities in cardiac tissues for long periods, once dosage has been properly adjusted. In the event of overdosage, however, the slow disappearance of symptoms after withdrawal of the drug is disadvantageous.

Dosage and Administration. A single dose of 1.2 mg. provides satisfactory rapid digitalization for a large proportion of patients; others may require an additional 0.2 to 0.4 mg. on the following day.

To reduce the danger of overdosage, some doctors prefer to give multiple fractional doses. An initial dose of 0.6 to 0.8 mg. may be followed by subsequent doses of 0.2 or 0.4 mg. every 3 or 4 hours until the patient is digitalized.

DIGOXIN U.S.P. (LANOXIN)

Pharmacology. This pure crystalline glycoside is relatively rapid in onset of action, especially when it is given by vein. It is eliminated much more rapidly than digitoxin.

Because its effects reach a peak about 3 hours after administration – an action rapid enough to meet most clinical needs – digoxin is employed to produce relatively prompt digitalization.

This drug's moderately rapid rate of excretion makes it safer than digitoxin in the event of overdosage. On the other hand, during maintenance, the drug's action may not remain entirely uniform throughout the period between doses. For this reason, it may be preferable to administer digoxin in several divided doses daily rather than in a single total dose intended to last for a longer period.

Dosage and Administration. Rapid oral digitalization may be achieved by administering 1.5 mg. initially, followed by additional doses of 0.25 to 0.5 mg. at 6-hour intervals. The drug may be given by vein in an initial dose of 0.5 to 1.0 mg., followed by 0.25 to 0.5 mg. at 2 to 4-hour intervals.

Slower digitalization (0.5 to 1.0 mg. by mouth, daily) may be employed; and, for infants and children, special lower dosage schedules are consulted, as indicated, for example, in the package insert of the Pediatric Elixir.

Digitalization of adults is usually maintained with oral or parenteral doses of 0.25 to 0.75 mg., or, for children, by administration of one-quarter of the total digitalizing dose in single or divided daily dosage.

Occasionally, patients are gradually digitalized by the daily administration of 0.15 to 0.2 mg. for about 3 weeks. After this, most patients are maintained by doses of 0.1 to 0.2 mg. daily, depending on individual response.

LANATOSIDE C, N.F. (DIGILANID C; CEDILANID) AND DESLANOSIDE N.F. (DESACETYL-LANATOSIDE C; CEDILANID D)

Pharmacology. These *Digitalis lanata* glycoside derivatives have approximately the same rapid onset and moderately short duration of action as digoxin. Oral administration of lanatoside C tablets is said to cause less nausea and vomiting than digoxin. The more soluble and stable desacetyl derivative deslanoside, is injected for more rapid onset of digitalizing action.

Dosage and Administration. Rapid digitalization can be achieved by parenteral administration of 1.6 mg. of deslanoside in one dose or in divided dosage within 12 hours. Lanatoside C is administered in divided oral dosage for digitalization in 48 to 72 hours. Neither product is used routinely for maintenance therapy. However, lanatoside C may be administered in daily oral doses of 0.5 to 1.5 mg. when a rapidly excreted product is deemed desirable, as in certain geriatric patients.

OUABAIN INJECTION U.S.P.

Pharmacology. This derivative of *Strophanthus gratus* is the most potent of all the digitalis-type glycosides. It is not given by mouth because it is not absorbed from the G.I. tract. However, it is readily soluble in saline solution for parenteral administration of full digitalizing doses.

The effects of ouabain begin to come on within a few minutes and reach full development in about an hour. This makes it one of the drugs of choice in emergencies. However, its short duration of action (24 hours) and its unavailability in oral form preclude its use for maintenance therapy.

Dosage and Administration. Ouabain Injection is usually administered by vein in doses of 0.25 to 0.5 mg. The latter dose is not repeated within 24 hours. The lower levels of dosage are preferred for patients who have previously taken digitalis preparation. Ouabain is said to be less irritating than other parenteral digitalis preparations and less likely to cause venous thrombosis.

GITALIN (AMORPHOUS) U.S.P. AND DIGILANID

Pharmacology. These products are mixtures of glycosides. (Gitalin is a mixture of *Digitalis purpurea* glycosides in amorphous form; Digilanid is a mixture of the crystallized *D. lanata* glycosides, lanatosides A, B, and C.)

Gitalin is claimed to have a greater safety margin than other digitalis preparations. Digilanid has actions and uses essentially the same as those of digitalis powder, U.S.P.

Dosage and Administration. Gitalin is usually administered orally over a period of several days, in scored tablets of 0.5 mg., until full digitalization is produced. This may be maintained by daily doses of one-half a scored tablet (0.25 mg.) to 2 tablets.

Digilanid may be administered in the form of two to four 0.33 mg. tablets, until digitalization is achieved in several days; or it may be administered parenterally for more rapid digitalization. Effects may be maintained with one or two tablets (0.33 to 0.66 mg.) daily.

CHAPTER 20

DIURETICS FOR EDEMA MANAGEMENT

ACETAZOLAMIDE U.S.P. (DIAMOX)

Pharmacology. This drug produces a flow of urine rich in sodium bicarbonate and, consequently, tends to cause a mild tissue acidosis. It relieves edema in various clinical conditions. It reduces intraocular pressure in glaucoma and controls seizures in selected cases of petit mal and grand mal epilepsy.

Side effects include drowsiness, paresthesias of the face and extremities, and G.I. upset. It is used cautiously in hepatic cirrhosis because drug-induced potassium loss may play a part in precipitating hepatic coma.

Dosage and Administration. The usual dose for treating edema is about 250 mg. daily. Raising the dose beyond 375 mg. a day may increase side effects without significantly enhancing the diuretic action. Supplements of potassium often counteract excessive excretion of this ion, especially in digitalized heart patients and in those with hepatic cirrhosis.

CHLOROTHIAZIDE N.F. (DIURIL)

Pharmacology. This prototype of the benzothiadiazine class of sulfonamide diuretics interferes with the renal absorption of sodium and causes the excretion of sodium and chloride ions in approximately equal proportions (saluresis). Oral doses are often nearly as effective as parenteral mercurials; yet serious side effects are less likely than with the metallic compounds, and the drug can be taken daily with little likelihood that tolerance will develop.

Chlorothiazide is widely employed, not only for treating edema, but also as an adjunct in the management of hypertension. Its use lessens the need for a rigid low-sodium dietary regimen and reduces the required dosage of specific antihypertensive drugs, such as the ganglionic blocking agents, etc.

While generally well tolerated, chlorothiazide can cause hypokalemia, hypochloremic alkalosis, and other electrolyte imbalances. Thus, patients — especially those taking digitalis for heart failure, and hepatic cirrhosis cases — are watched closely for signs of electrolyte pattern distortion, and these are corrected by administration of potassium supplements or acidifying salts.

Dosage and Administration. The usual total daily dose is 1 Gm. divided into two doses of 500 mg.; sometimes a 500 mg. dose suffices; at other times, three such daily doses are required. As little as 250 mg. twice daily may be effective for adjunctive action in hypertension. A sodium salt is available as a lyophilized powder for intravenous administration after solution in a suitable diluent.

CHLORTHALIDONE (HYGROTON)

Pharmacology. This drug is a phthalimidine-type sulfonamide diuretic, similar to chlorothiazide in its actions and uses for treating edema and hypertension. Its saluretic action is relatively prolonged, the effects of a single dose sometimes lasting as long as 2 or 3 days. Like other sulfonamide diuretics, chlorthalidone can cause hypokalemia and hypochloremic alkalosis; it is used only with caution in patients with severe renal damage, especially when blood urea nitrogen (BUN) is rising. It may be desirable to use a uricosuric agent such as probenecid to prevent hyperuricemia, since chlorthalidone therapy sometimes precipitates acute attacks of gout.

Dosage and Administration. Patients are usually started on a dose of 100 mg., taken with the morning meal, three times *a week*. Individual patients may require as much as 150 or 200 mg. three times weekly, or may need to take the 100 mg. dose *daily*

for satisfactory maintenance of "dry weight." No more than 200 mg. is ever given on a single day.

MANNITOL N.F. (OSMITROL)

Pharmacology. This sugar derivative, when filtered by the glomeruli, passes through the renal tubules without being reabsorbed. Its molecules carry through the tubules large quantities of the fluid in which they are dissolved. This osmotic action may account for the claimed protective action of injected mannitol solutions, when kidney function is threatened by conditions that cause poor renal blood flow.

This osmotic diuretic is advocated for preventing acute renal failure following severe bleeding, burns, and transfusion reactions, for use in cardiovascular surgery, including open-heart operations. Mannitol-induced diuresis has also been tried as a means of hastening the elimination of barbiturates in cases of poisoning. This diuretic lowers cerebrospinal pressure during neurosurgical procedures and reduces intraocular pressure rapidly in some cases of glaucoma. It is occasionally used as an adjunct to other diuretics in the management of resistant edema.

Dosage and Administration. Solutions of 5 to 20% are administered intravenously in different amounts and at varying rates depending on the condition being treated. About 100 Gm. may be administered cautiously in 24 hours as an adjunct to other measures for the management of oliguria. Care must be taken to avoid overloading the circulation and precipitating congestive heart failure. A low test dose is administered to determine the ability of the kidneys to respond with increased urine production.

MERALLURIDE SODIUM U.S.P. (MERCUHYDRIN)

Pharmacology. This is a mercurial compound combined with a small amount of theophylline. The addition of theophylline to organic mercurial compounds is thought to reduce local irritation by increasing the speed and completeness of the absorption of mercury from intramuscular sites. Parenteral injection usually produces profuse diuresis, but a better result is obtainable in some cases if the patient first receives ammonium chloride for several days to mobilize edema fluid. Cardiac arrhythmias and other manifestation of mercury poisoning may be treated with dimercaprol (BAL).

Dosage and Administration. One to 2 ml. of the solution (containing 130 mg./ml.) may be injected intramuscularly, or occasionally, with care, subcutaneously or intravenously. A product for oral use contains ascorbic acid to aid absorption and to minimize gastric irritation; one or two tablets containing 60 mg. of meralluride are taken daily after meals.

SODIUM MERCAPTOMERIN U.S.P. (THIOMERIN)

Pharmacology. This mercurial diuretic contains a sulfur linkage, which is claimed to reduce the local and systemic toxicity of the metal without interfering with its desired depression of renal tubular sodium ion reabsorption. The drug relieves dyspnea and pulmonary edema in heart disease and removes ascitic fluid from ·the abdomen in hepatic cirrhosis. It is used with caution in selected cases of nephrotic edema and subacute or chronic nephritis, but is never used in acute nephritis, as it may cause renal shutdown and mercury cumulation in the kidney and other body tissues.

Dosage and Administration. This drug is claimed to be free enough of local irritation to be administered subcutaneously, as well as intramuscularly and intravenously. However, care is required to place the needle beneath the subcutaneous fat and to make injections at varied sites. The dose of the solution (125 mg./ml.) is 0.2 to 2 cc., depending on the requirements of the individual. Gently massage the area of the injection site.

SPIRONOLACTONE U.S.P. (ALDACTONE)

Pharmacology. This steroid drug competes with the mineralo-cortical hormone aldosterone at its site of action in the distal renal tubules. Thus, it antagonizes the sodium-retaining effect of the adrenocortical hormone. In addition, it stops the potassium loss caused by aldosterone. The result of these two actions is often an increase in urinary excretion of sodium (natriuresis) and a tendency toward potassium retention. This double action is best exploited by combining spironolactone with a sulfonamide diuretic to potentiate the action of the latter and to counteract the potassium-excreting action of the thiazides, phthalimidines, etc. The drug is relatively safe, except in severe renal insufficiency, in which plasma potassium levels may be elevated (*hyper*kalemia).

Dosage and Administration. A new, improved dosage form, more readily absorbable from the G.I. tract, requires only one-quarter of the original dosage. Four daily doses of 25 mg. are administered, either alone or combined with a thiazide, phthalimidine, or mercurial diuretic, for more rapidly effective action. Simultaneous administration of a glucocorticoid (e.g., hydrocortisone, prednisone) may also add to the effectiveness of spironolactone, especially in edema resulting from the nephrotic syndrome.

UREA U.S.P. (CARBAMIDE; UREAPHIL; UREVERT)

Pharmacology. This osmotic diuretic may be administered orally to reduce edema, but the new lyophilized sterile powder which is dissolved in invert sugar solution and injected intravenously is preferred. A hypertonic solution, dripped slowly into a vein, often reduces intracranial pressure in patients with cerebral edema. Therefore, such products are employed during and after neurosurgical procedures, as well as following burns (to counteract oliguria) and in other types of edema.

Dosage and Administration. Freshly prepared solutions are infused slowly by intravenous drip at a rate of about 60 drops/minute, while the needle is kept securely within the vein as leakage into surrounding tissues can cause sloughing of tissues. Total daily adult dosage is 1 to 7.5 Gm./Kg. body weight, but should not exceed 120 Gm. The usual oral dose is 8 to 20 Gm. several times daily; the solutions are flavored to mask the taste and are administered after meals to minimize gastric irritation.

CHAPTER 21

ANTIARRHYTHMIC DRUGS

PROCAINAMIDE HYDROCHLORIDE (PRONESTYL) U.S.P.

Pharmacology. This derivative of the local anesthetic procaine has a much more prolonged duration of action than the latter. It is used clinically for its cardiac effects, which include reduction of myocardial excitability, and slowing of impulse conduction through the atria, nodal tissues and bundle of His, and the ventricles.

The drug is used mainly to control ventricular extrasystoles and tachycardia, and may be useful for auricular arrhythmias, especially atrial fibrillation of recent onset and paroxysmal atrial

tachycardias not benefited by other bradycrotic drugs and measures. Procainamide is especially useful for control of arrhythmias caused by cyclopropane and other anesthetics, and in chest or heart surgery.

Cardiovascular toxic reactions, including severe falls in blood pressure, and ventricular asystole or tachycardia and fibrillation, have been reported from too rapid intravenous administration and cumulative overdosage. High oral dosage may cause anorexia, nausea, and vomiting. Sensitivity reactions including agranulocytosis occur occasionally, and a history of such hypersensitivity contraindicates use of the drug.

Dosage and Administration. Oral administration of 0.5 to 1 Gm. every 4 to 6 hours is preferred for ventricular tachycardia. Low doses (0.5 Gm.) may be adequate for ventricular extrasystoles, and higher doses (1.25 Gm.) are recommended for auricular arrhythmias. Intramuscular dosage is essentially the same, but intravenous doses are usually somewhat lower.

Intravenous use is usually limited to extreme emergencies, for steep drops in blood pressure and cardiac arrhythmias may occur readily. Solutions are diluted and infused by vein slowly with electrocardiographic monitoring to detect excessive depression of conduction. Blood pressure is measured almost continuously, and the infusion is discontinued temporarily if the fall is considered too great. Levarterenol (Levophed) should be available to counteract severe hypotensive reactions.

QUINIDINE SULFATE U.S.P.

Pharmacology. This salt of the cinchona alkaloid quinidine is the form most commonly used in maintenance therapy after termination of cardiac arrhythmias such as atrial fibrillation and flutter, paroxysmal atrial and ventricular tachycardias, and extrasystoles of both atrial and ventricular origin. Like other quinidine compounds, it acts by depression of various myocardial properties including excitability, conductivity, and automatic rhythmicity. In all these heart rhythm disorders, the drug lengthens the period during which cardiac tissues are refractory to ectopic stimuli.

Quinidine causes toxic cardiac and extracardiac effects. Overdosage may result in reduced contractile strength of the heart, complete A-V block, and even fatal cardiac arrest. However, these dangerous reactions and sudden sharp falls in blood pressure are more likely to occur when soluble salts such as quinidine gluconate are being injected rapidly during an emergency than when this salt is being given by mouth in gradually increasing dosage with electrocardiographic monitoring of heart function.

Quinidine salts can cause cinchonism, a characteristic syndrome also often seen when the closely related alkaloid quinine is employed in treating malaria. Signs and symptoms include tinnitus (ringing in the ears), blurring of vision, dizziness, light-headedness, and nausea, vomiting, and diarrhea. Such G.I. distress is said to be lessened when quinine polygalacturonate is employed, since that salt is less irritating to the gastric mucosa.

Quinidine is contraindicated in patients with a history of allergic hypersensitivity to it. In addition to urticarial skin reactions, angioneurotic edema, and asthma, petechial hemorrhages of the mucous membranes of the mouth may develop. Such bleeding is a manifestation of thrombocytic purpura, a condition in which blood platelets are destroyed by an antigen-antibody reaction precipitated by quinidine.

Dosage and Administration. Quinidine sulfate is administered orally in individualized dosage schedules. If an initial dose of 0.1 to 0.2 Gm. causes no indications of sensitivity, 0.2 to 0.6 Gm. is given every 2 to 4 hours, until the arrhythmia is terminated or toxic symptoms develop. A 300 mg. extended-action tablet is available for administration in doses of 2 tablets every 8 to 12 hours for maintenance therapy. Other soluble salts of quinidine are available for parenteral use in emergencies or when the patient cannot tolerate oral administration.

CHAPTER 22

DRUGS USED IN CORONARY ARTERY DISEASE

GLYCERYL TRINITRATE U.S.P. (NITROGLYCERIN)

Pharmacology. This drug is the prototype of the rapid-acting nitrites that terminate acute anginal attacks. It is often taken prior to physical exertion to prevent attacks, and is sometimes included in long-term prophylactic regimens. Upon sublingual administration, it promptly improves blood flow through the hypoxic heart muscle. Its main action is most probably the result of a direct relaxing effect on the smooth muscle walls of the coronary vessels, especially that portion which is in spasm. However, it may also affect neighboring vessels that are not in spasm, thus increasing blood flow through the collateral circulation. Nitroglycerin may also reduce the work load of the heart by decreasing peripheral resistance and possibly by reducing the oxygen consumption of the heart.

A throbbing headache is a common side effect. Potentially more serious is a sharp drop in blood pressure which leads to faintness, dizziness, and flushing. Nitrite syncope, a severe shocklike state, has occurred in some patients, especially when they have drunk alcoholic beverages while taking nitroglycerin.

Dosage and Administration. For aborting attacks, tablets of 0.3 to 0.6 mg. are placed under the tongue at the first sign of anginal symptoms. Patients may also use a sublingual tablet about 15 minutes before expected physical exertion. Nitroglycerin is also available as sustained-action tablets of 1.3 to 6.5 mg.; these are swallowed at 8 to 10-hour intervals for prolonged vasodilator action in the prophylactic management of angina pectoris. A 2% lanolin-based ointment is sometimes applied lightly to a small skin area (one-half to 2 inches) in amounts adjusted to the needs of the individual.

PAPAVERINE HYDROCHLORIDE N.F.

Pharmacology. This opium alkaloid of a different chemical class from morphine and codeine is neither a narcotic analgesic nor an addiction liability. It relieves the pain of biliary and ureteral colic by its smooth muscle antispasmodic action. Despite its potent vascular relaxant action and the increased coronary blood flow seen in experimental animals, this drug has proved disappointing in the management of angina pectoris.

Papaverine is sometimes administered parenterally in other conditions marked by reflex vascular constriction. It is said to increase the collateral circulation to infarcted areas by relaxing the arterioles adjacent to vessels blocked by blood clots. Consequently, the drug may benefit some patients with pulmonary and cerebrovascular embolism, the peripheral vascular blockade of ergot poisoning, and acute coronary occlusion. In coronary thrombosis the drug's depression of heart muscle conduction may reduce myocardial irritability and thus prevent ventricular arrhythmias. Adequate oral doses commonly cause G.I. upset, dizziness, drowsiness, and flushing.

Dosage and Administration. The usual oral dose of papaverine is 100 mg. administered several times daily. A sustained-action capsule containing 150 mg. of this drug is sometimes administered once every 8 to 12 hours. Injectable solutions contain 30 mg./ml., which is the amount usually injected intramuscularly.

PENTAERYTHRITOL TETRANITRATE (PERITRATE, ETC.)

Pharmacology. This coronary vasodilator is a prototype of the long-acting organic nitrate compounds that are commonly employed in the long-term prophylactic management of angina pectoris, coronary insufficiency, and postcoronary attack convalescence. Like other drugs that are claimed to act by increasing the blood flow and oxygen supply of the heart, its actual utility for this purpose is controversial. However, because its side effects and potential toxicity are not great, this agent—like the others—is commonly employed in the management of these coronary conditions, if only for placebo value.

Because of the slow onset of its vasodilator action, pentaerythritol is not likely to cause the drops in blood pressure or increased heart rate sometimes seen with the faster-acting nitrites. Headaches may occur, but these tend to disappear in a few days—a probable reflection of the development of tolerance to nitrites. Early G.I. irritation and late development of methemoglobinemia are rare. Anemia is not considered a contraindication to the use of this drug, but such a condition is treated and the hemoglobin is checked periodically. Like all nitrites, pentaerythritol is used with caution in active glaucoma.

Dosage and Administration. Tablets of 10 to 20 mg. are taken four times daily, one-half hour before meals or 1 hour after meals and at bedtime on an empty stomach. Sustained-action tablets are administered twice daily—immediately upon arising in the morning and 12 hours later.

THEOPHYLLINE N.F. (THEOCIN, ETC.)

Pharmacology. This xanthine derivative possesses the several pharmacological actions characteristic of drugs of this class: it is a relaxant of bronchial and vascular smooth muscle, a myocardial stimulant, and a diuretic. The drug increases the coronary circulation of experimental animals, and numerous clinical reports claim that its routine use reduces the number of acute attacks suffered by some anginal patients. However, some doctors deny that the long-term use of theophylline benefits most patients with angina pectoris, and they warn that the drug's cardiac stimulant effect may increase the work load of the heart undesirably. Theophylline is now used mainly in the management of bronchial asthma.

Theophylline irritates the gastric mucosa somewhat and may be contraindicated in peptic ulcer. Its solubility and degree of absorption increase if it is dissolved in hydroalcoholic solutions or administered in the form of readily soluble double salts, such as theophylline sodium acetate, theophylline sodium glycinate, and theophylline ethylenediamine (Aminophylline; see Drug Digest).

Dosage and Administration. Theophylline itself is administered orally in a usual dose of about 200 mg. It is available as 100 and 200-mg. tablets and as a hydroalcoholic elixir containing 80 mg. of theophylline base in each half ounce (15 cc.)

CHAPTER 23

DRUGS USED IN HYPERTENSION

CHLORISONDAMINE CHLORIDE (ECOLID)

Pharmacology. This quaternary ammonium compound is rapidly but somewhat erratically absorbed. If taken when the stomach is empty, it quickly causes sympathetic ganglion blockade and a fall in the blood pressure in patients with moderate to severe hypertension. The fall in blood pressure is more gradual and less predictable when this drug is given on a full stomach. If the patient is constipated, more of the drug is absorbed than normally, with a consequent exaggeration of postural hypotensive effects. Thus, concurrent administration of laxatives is desirable.

Dosage and Administration. Like other ganglionic blockers, chlorisondamine is used only in cases carefully selected to exclude patients with mild, labile hypertension and those who have severe cardiac, renal, or cerebral disease.

Hospitalized patients, who are observed carefully for signs of toxicity during the period of dosage adjustment, receive more intensive therapy. Treatment is started at 50 mg. twice daily, and dosage is increased by 50 mg. daily until an optimal response is reached.

Ambulatory patients receive only one half tablet (12.5 mg.) to begin with, but this is gradually raised over a period of several days to 50 or 75 mg., and the final daily maintenance dosage reached after several weeks may be as much as 200 mg. daily. Patients with less severe cases and those receiving *Rauwolfia* alkaloids and sulfonamide diuretics concurrently may require less of the drug than do patients with malignant hypertension who are sometimes highly resistant. The drug is usually given only twice daily, in the morning and evening, because of its long duration of action (8 to 12 hours).

GUANETHIDINE SULFATE U.S.P. (ISMELIN)

Pharmacology. This potent antihypertensive agent, which is used in the management of moderate to severe hypertension, does *not* cause parasympathetic blockade-type side effects as do the ganglionic blocking agents. This is related to the drug's site and manner of action: it acts only at sympathetic nerve endings in the arterioles to alter the rate of norepinephrine release and thus reduces transmission of tonic vasomotor impulses.

Side effects of such sympathetic blockade include postural hypotension, nasal congestion, inhibition of male sexual function, slowing of the heart, and diarrhea. The later, which is the result of the relative increase in parasympathetic stimulation of G.I. motor activity, may be reduced by administration of atropine.

The drug is used with caution in patients who have a history of peptic ulcer, and it is contraindicated in patients with pheochromocytoma, in whom it may cause the discharge of norepinephrine from tumor tissue, thus sharply raising blood pressure. It should not be used together with drugs that inhibit monoamine oxidase. Its combined cardiac-slowing and peripheral resistance-reducing effects may tend to precipitate congestive heart failure. This tendency may be counteracted by concurrent administration of a thiazide diuretic drug. Guanethidine should be discontinued two weeks prior to elective surgery, because its catecholamine-depleting action increases the danger of cardiac arrest during anesthesia.

Dosage and Administration. Guanethidine dosage is carefully regulated for each patient by taking the blood pressure in both the standing and supine positions during the period of dosage adjustment. Patients start at doses as low as 25 and 50 mg. Lower doses may be effective and side effects fewer when sulfonamide-type diuretics are administered simultaneously.

HYDRALAZINE HYDROCHLORIDE N.F. (APRESOLINE)

Pharmacology. Hydralazine is a potent antihypertensive drug that differs from most other hypotensive drugs in that it does not cause reduced blood flow to the kidneys. However, its usefulness is limited by many side effects, including general malaise, loss of appetite, headache, flushing, and fever.

Although this drug differs from other blood pressure reducers in that it increases cardiac output and renal blood flow, its tendency to stimulate the heart makes it undesirable in coronary insufficiency and heart failure. An unusual toxic effect of prolonged administration is the development of a syndrome resembling the collagen disease lupus erythematosus, the symptoms of which (e.g., fever and joint pain) disappear when the drug is withdrawn. Numbness and tingling thought to indicate a drug-induced peripheral neuritis may be relieved by adding pyridoxine to the patient's regimen.

Dosage and Administration. Hydralazine is rarely administered alone because of the side effects of full doses. It is prescribed in combination with diuretics such as hydrochlorothiazide and with the bradycrotic *Rauwolfia* and *Veratrum* alkaloids, which may counteract hydralazine-induced heart stimulation. Dosage is low at first—10 mg. four times daily—and is gradually raised to as much as 400 mg. daily, depending on the tolerance of the patient. The drug is administered parenterally in doses of 20 to 40 mg., which are repeated as necessary to reduce high blood pressure rapidly in hypertensive emergencies, including incipient and acute toxemia of pregnancy.

HYDROCHLOROTHIAZIDE U.S.P. (ESIDRIX; HYDRODIURIL; ORETIC)

Pharmacology. This thiazide-type sulfonamide diuretic is used widely either alone, in mild cases of hypertension, or combined with various other antihypertensive agents, for treating more severe hypertension. The drug's usefulness for reducing high blood pressure does not depend on its ability to relieve edema. However, its saluretic action and the resulting reduction in sodium is believed to play a part in the drug's pressure-lowering properties.

As with other sulfonamide diuretics, patients are watched for signs of fluid and electrolyte imbalance, including thirst, weakness, fatigue, and sleepiness. The drug is used with caution in diabetes, gout, and severe liver or kidney disease.

Dosage and Administration. For treating hypertension, hydrochlorothiazide is usually administered by mouth in doses of 75 mg. daily at first. Dosage is then usually adjusted downward to about 25 mg. taken once or twice daily, although it is occasionally raised to 100 to 150 mg. in resistant patients.

Hydrochlorothiazide is commonly combined with *Rauwolfia* alkaloids and is also used to supplement the ganglionic blocking agents, as well as *methyldopa (Aldomet), hydralazine (Apresoline), guanethidine,* and *Veratrum alkaloids.* It is often itself supplemented by potassium chloride or administered together with citrus fruit juices or other sources of dietary potassium to prevent hypokalemia from excessive potassium ion depletion.

MECAMYLAMINE HYDROCHLORIDE U.S.P. (INVERSINE)

Pharmacology. This potent ganglionic blocking agent differs chemically from most other drugs of this class. Because it is a secondary rather than a quaternary amine, it is more readily absorbed through the membranes of the G.I. tract. Thus, it is claimed to lower the blood pressure more smoothly and predictably in moderate to severe hypertension.

The chemical structure of mecamylamine may also account for the C.N.S. side effects sometimes produced by high doses. That is, the toxic psychoses—marked by mental aberrations such as delirium, delusions, and hallucinations—that are sometimes seen with this drug may result because it can penetrate the blood-brain barrier and reach the C.N.S. On the other hand, since these reactions occur mainly in cerebral arteriosclerosis, they could result from reduced local blood flow through the brain—an effect also caused by other ganglionic blockers. Like the others, this drug is used with caution in hypertensive patients with cerebral atherosclerosis, and especially after a recent cerebrovascular accident.

Dosage and Administration. Since mecamylamine may cause all the side effects of the other ganglionic blockers, resulting from excessive inhibition of both sympathetic and parasympathetic ganglionic activity, its dosage is carefully determined and adjusted as necessary. Initial dosage is low—a 2.5-mg. tablet twice daily. Later, as the dose is gradually raised (e.g., 25 mg. daily in three divided doses), the 10-mg. tablet may be employed. Since the latter tablet can be conveniently broken into halves and quarters, the fine adjustment of dosage that is often needed for optimal effectiveness is attained readily.

METHYLDOPA (ALDOMET)

Pharmacology. Methyldopa is said to differ from other potent drugs used to treat moderate to severe hypertension in that it reduces blood pressure while patients are recumbent as well as standing. Although somewhat less potent than some other drugs, it is less likely to cause orthostatic hypertension.

Some patients do not respond at all to this drug; others react only to high doses given in conjunction with sulfonamide diuretics. Side effects seem relatively mild; drowsiness is common in the early days of treatment, as are dryness of the mouth, nasal stuffiness, and G.I. symptoms such as abdominal distention, flatus, and diarrhea. The drug may have to be discontinued if fever and general malaise develop. Blood and liver function tests are made frequently during therapy.

Dosage and Administration. Methyldopa is best given by mouth combined with a sulfonamide diuretic. Initial dosage is about 250 mg. administered two or three times a day; later the dosage is built up or decreased according to the response. A parenteral form, methyldopate HCl (*Aldomet Ester*) is injected intravenously in doses of 250 to 500 mg. every 6 hours to control acute hypertensive crises.

PARGYLINE HYDROCHLORIDE (EUTONYL)

Pharmacology. This drug, like certain agents used in treating mental depression, inhibits the enzyme monoamine oxidase. This may account for its ability to reduce peripheral resistance and arterial blood pressure, but the exact mechanism is obscure. The fall in pressure is mainly of the orthostatic type; thus, patients who become weak and dizzy are warned against getting up too suddenly.

Pargyline is indicated only in selected cases of moderate to severe hypertension. It is not used for either mild or malignant cases, or in treatment of high blood pressure caused by pheochromocytoma. The drug is undesirable for patients with kidney difficulties, which might interfere with its excretion. It is contraindicated in patients with hyperthyroidism, who may be made more nervous and tremorous by the drug's stimulating effects, and in patients with paranoid schizophrenia.

Dosage and Administration. A daily dose of 50 to 75 mg. is the usual amount needed for maintenance after initiating therapy with 25 to 50 mg. and raising the dose after 1 week. Patients who are also taking a sulfonamide diuretic are given only 25 mg. to begin with and may be maintained on lower doses of pargyline than those taking this hypotensive agent alone.

As with other monoamine oxidase inhibitors, other drugs that depress or stimulate the C.N.S are avoided, lest their effects be potentiated. Warn patients, for example, not to use nasal decongestants, weight-reducing medication, antihistamines, sedatives and tranquilizers, hypnotics, and narcotic analgesics or alcohol without the consent of their doctor. Pargyline is not given with guanethidine or reserpine, for a *rise* in blood pressure may result.

PENTOLINIUM TARTRATE (ANSOLYSEN)

Pharmacology. This typical ganglionic blocking agent resembles the prototypes of this class, *tetraethylammonium chloride* and *hexamethonium bromide* in its actions and uses but produces a longer lasting vasodilator and hypotensive effect. This makes it more useful for treating selected cases of moderate to severe hypertension and in the diagnosis and treatment of various peripheral vascular diseases.

Pentolinium produces the side effects that are predictable with all ganglionic blocking agents. Blockade of parasympathetic ganglia, for example, leads to atropine-like reactions such as blurring of vision, mouth dryness, constipation, and urinary retention. Thus, like atropine itself, this drug and other ganglionic blockers are contraindicated in patients with glaucoma

and in elderly male patients with probable enlargement of the prostate gland.

Excessive blockade of sympathetic ganglia causes postural hypotension with faintness, dizziness, and the danger of falls in which the patient may hurt himself. The reduced circulation to the head, heart, and kidneys in such circumstances can be especially dangerous for patients with a history of a recent heart attack or a cerebrovascular accident. The drug is also contraindicated in patients with renal insufficiency, for failure to excrete the drug by way of the kidneys may lead to overdosage.

Dosage and Administration. It is customary to start treatment of hospitalized patients with a single parenteral injection of 2 to 3 mg. and to raise the dose gradually every 4 to 6 hours. The initial oral dose is 20 mg. every 8 hours, and this too is raised gradually until amounts of 60 to 600 mg. daily are taken by mouth.

PROTOVERATRINES A AND B (VERALBA)

Pharmacology. This mixture of two alkaloids from the white hellebore plant *Veratrum album*, has actions and uses typical of all the veratrum products. The alkaloids slow the heart and dilate blood vessels, thus bringing about a drop in blood pressure. The same reflexes responsible for this desirable action indirectly stimulate the vomiting center. The margin between the amount needed for hypotensive effects and that which produces vomiting is often narrow.

Dosage and Administration. These alkaloids are administered orally, alone or combined with other antihypertensive agents in moderate cases of hypertension. Initial dosage for this purpose is 0.5 mg. after each meal and at bedtime; amounts are then adjusted to obtain maximal hypotensive effects with minimal nausea, vomiting, flushing, and other side effects.

These alkaloids are administered parenterally in the management of hypertensive crises. A small amount (0.06 to 0.1 mg.) is injected slowly by vein, and additional doses are repeated at 4-hour intervals. This purified alkaloidal mixture may be infused periodically in the form of a more dilute solution in dextrose. The initial drop in pressure may be maintained, once it has stabilized, by continued slow intravenous infusion or by intramuscular injections of 0.12 to 0.4 mg. every 4 to 8 hours.

RESERPINE U.S.P.
(SERPASIL; SANDRIL; ETC.)

Pharmacology. This most widely employed rauwolfia alkaloid is mainly combined with sulfonamide diuretics (e.g., hydrochlorothiazide) for treating mild degrees of hypertension. However, it is sometimes combined with hydralazine, ganglionic blocking agents, and other potent antihypertensives in the management of moderate to severe hypertension, and it may even be administered parenterally in high doses in the malignant form of the disease and in hypertensive emergencies and toxemias of pregnancy. High doses are occasionally employed to calm severely agitated patients in psychiatric emergencies.

Side effects include nasal congestion, tiredness, drowsiness, headache, dizziness, nausea, frequent loose stools and, rarely, bizarre dreams.

Dosage and Administration. Reserpine is best administered at first in doses of 0.1 to 1.0 mg. daily and later, after stabilization, in a dose of 0.25 mg. The drug is given by mouth after meals to lessen gastric discomfort. Reserpine is sometimes given intramuscularly in doses as high as 5 mg. for treating hypertensive and psychiatric emergencies.

Patients receiving more than 1 mg. daily are watched for signs of mental depression, and those with a history of this condition receive no more than 0.25 mg. daily. Electroshock therapy is delayed for at least a week after the drug is withdrawn because of the danger of severe convulsions and prolonged apnea. Similarly, if possible, the drug is withdrawn at least 2 weeks prior to surgery, because patients taking reserpine have reportedly suffered sharp falls in blood pressure, and marked slowing of the heart, or even cardiac arrest, during anesthesia.

SYROSINGOPINE N.F. (SINGOSERP)

Pharmacology. This semi-synthetic analogue of reserpine is said to act mainly peripherally rather than centrally. Thus, it is claimed to be less sedating than the natural *Rauwolfia* alkaloid and less likely to cause emotional depression. The drug seems weaker than reserpine, however, in its antihypertensive action as well as in tranquilizing effects.

The generally weaker sympatholytic actions of syrosingopine may also account for claims that it causes only mild nasal congestion and little gastric irritation. Caution is required in patients with a history of peptic ulcer.

Dosage and Administration. Patients are started on 1 or 2 mg. daily for at least 2 weeks. The dose is later stabilized at 0.5 to 3 mg., depending on the response. Syrosingopine is also administered combined with the sulfonamide diuretic hydrochlorothiazide, which tends to potentiate its hypotensive actions.

TRIMETHAPHAN CAMSYLATE (ARFONAD)

Pharmacology. This drug lowers blood pressure both by blockade of sympathetic ganglia and by directly depressing the smooth muscle walls of blood vessels. Its vasodilator effects come on almost immediately, but because they last only a few minutes, this drug is not useful for long-term treatment of hypertension. It is used, instead, as a temporary measure in the control of hypertensive crises. By lowering blood pressure rapidly in toxemia of pregnancy and in other acute hypertensive conditions, the drug may prevent encephalopathy and pulmonary edema. It may also act as a hemostatic against severe epistaxis (nosebleed) in patients with acute hypertension.

A unique use of the hemostatic effect of this short-acting ganglionic blocking agent is in the procedure called *controlled hypotension,* which is sometimes employed in certain types of neurosurgery and vascular surgery. By reducing blood pressure to low levels for brief periods, the anesthetist stops excessive bleeding locally in the surgical field, so that the surgeon can better see the operative area. Procedures such as craniotomies and intracranial surgery on aneurysms and vascular tumors can be performed more readily.

Reducing the blood pressure with this drug helps control subdural and subarachnoid hemorrhage in patients with head injuries.

Dosage and Administration. Trimethaphan is infused by vein as a 0.1% solution in dextrose or saline. One to 4 ml./minute (1 to 4 mg.) is the usual rate of infusion when excessive bleeding makes it difficult for the surgeon to see and expose the operative site. The dosage is adjusted to what is required for satisfactory surgery while the blood pressure is maintained to safe levels. (Systolic pressure is never allowed to drop below 60 mm. Hg.) The intravenous drip is gradually discontinued, when the drug's hypotensive and hemostatic actions are no longer needed.

CHAPTER 24

DRUGS AFFECTING BLOOD COAGULATION

ABSORBABLE GELATIN SPONGE U.S.P. (GELFOAM; GELFILM)

Pharmacology. This specially treated sponge of porous gelatin can be left in place when a wound is closed. It is used alone or after being moistened with thrombin solution as a local hemostatic in many situations marked by surface oozing of blood. In brain, chest, and bone surgery it controls bleeding instantly. When left implanted in these areas or in the nose, genitourinary areas, and elsewhere, it is completely absorbed within a few weeks without causing tissue reactions or excessive scar formation.

Dosage and Administration. This material is available in several forms, including sterile and *non*sterile powders and as a pliable film as well as a sponge.

The nonsterile powder, which is used in early attempts to control massive G.I. bleeding, is given every 2 hours in doses of 2 to 4 tablespoonfuls; each is followed by a solution of thrombin. Prior administration of an antacid is also desirable to keep the thrombin from being inactivated and to prevent digestion of the clots that form. The *sterile* powder is used with or without antibiotics for packing bed sores and other slow-healing skin ulcers and wounds.

The gelatin sponge is simply cut to the desired size, held on the wound for 10 to 15 seconds with moderate pressure and left in place after bleeding is controlled. The gelatin film is made rubbery by moistening with saline before being cut into irregular shapes as required to fill in the defects of the dural membrane that are caused by depressed skull fractures or left after removal of large tumors.

ANISINDIONE (MIRADON)

Pharmacology. This is a hypoprothrombinemic anticoagulant of the indanedione class. Unlike some other related compounds of this class, it has *not* caused hypersensitivity reactions such as leukopenia and agranulocytosis, or skin rashes, G.I. upset, and hepatitis. It has, however, a tendency to cause chromaturia, a reddening of the urine. Such a color is due to the presence of a drug metabolite and should not be mistaken for hematuria. This drug, like the other indanediones, has essentially the same actions, indications, and contraindications as the coumarin derivatives.

Dosage and Administration. Anisindione is administered orally in doses similar to those of bishydroxycoumarin. A loading, or priming, dose of 300 mg. is given on the first day; a dose of 200 mg. is given on the second day; 100 mg., on the third day; and thereafter a maintenance dose of 75 to 100 mg. daily.

BISHYDROXYCOUMARIN U.S.P. (DICUMAROL)

Pharmacology. This is the prototype of the coumarin-type anticoagulants, which act by blocking the synthesis of prothrombin and related clotting factors by the liver. Because this hypoprothrombinemic effect is relatively slow in onset, this drug is usually supplemented by heparin for the first few days in acute occlusive conditions involving the peripheral, pulmonary, and coronary arteries. This drug is well-suited for long-term prophylactic maintenance therapy, because its relatively prolonged duration of action facilitates stabilization of the prothrombin time. It helps to prevent extension of the clot in acute coronary thrombosis and to reduce the danger of embolism in thrombophlebitis and other conditions characterized by blood flow stagnation, vascular injury, or abnormal clotting time.

Hemorrhage is the main danger of overdosage, especially in patients with bleeding tendencies. This drug is contraindicated in patients with liver disease, vitamin K deficiency, purpura, and other blood dyscrasias, and acute bacterial endocarditis. Use of bishydroxycoumarin is undesirable during pregnancy and especially in threatened abortion; after recent neurosurgical procedures; and in patients with peptic ulcer, diverticulitis, and colitis and if drainage tubes are in the stomach or small intestine. Caution is required in patients with fever or abnormal menstrual bleeding, or if large doses of salicylates are being taken.

Dosage and Administration. Dosage is individualized according to prothrombin activity as determined by prothrombin time tests. The average adult priming dose is 200 to 300 mg. by mouth, but doses thereafter are 25 to 200 mg. daily, depending on how close prothrombin activity is to the goal of 25 per cent of normal. The drug is withheld when prothrombin activity falls below 25 per cent, and phytonadione (vitamin K_1) is administered whenever activity drops to less than 15 per cent.

FIBRINOLYSIN, HUMAN
(ACTASE; THROMBOLYSIN)

Pharmacology. This clot-dissolving factor is prepared by treating human blood plasma with the enzyme streptokinase. It contains both fibrinolysin (plasmin) and residual activator, which can convert part of the patient's own plasminogen to active plasmin. Administered together with anticoagulants, this preparation destroys recently formed clots and thus speeds the recovery of some patients with thrombophlebitis, phlebothrombosis, pulmonary embolism, and peripheral arterial thrombosis. It is not recommended, however, for treating coronary and cerebrovascular thrombosis.

Febrile reactions marked by chills and about 2° F. rise in temperature are frequent. Headache, backache, muscle pain, nausea, vomiting, and dizziness may also occur but can be counteracted by aspirin, antihistamines, and barbiturates. The possibility of increased bleeding makes the use of fibrinolysin undesirable in some types of patients. However, hemorrhaging may be counteracted by administration of aminocaproic acid, an antidote that reduces the rate of plasmin formation by the activator enzyme.

Dosage and Administration. This product is standardized in arbitrary units set by each manufacturer. The total dose administered varies with the nature and location of the clot. Sometimes, acute thrombophlebitis responds to a single relatively low intravenous dose. Extensive venous thrombi may require many infusions over a period of 5 days or longer. Much larger doses are infused directly into thrombosed arteries. Anticoagulant therapy and other measures for managing thromboembolic episodes must not be neglected.

HEPARIN SODIUM U.S.P.
(LIQUAMIN; PANHEPRIN; ETC.)

Pharmacology. This anticoagulant is effective almost immediately upon injection, and it is thus preferred in thromboembolic emergencies, including pulmonary embolism, and to prevent clotting during cardiovascular surgery and blood transfusions. It reduces the danger of clot formation following vascular, pelvic, and other types of surgery, and, sometimes, in the postpartum period.

Patients receiving heparin for any of these conditions are carefully observed for signs of bleeding from surgical wounds or from mucous membranes. The urine and stool are examined for blood, and its presence is reported to the doctor. The drug is contraindicated in any case in which there is active bleeding. It is not administered following neurosurgical operations or during childbirth. Other contraindications to the use of heparin include pregnancy, active peptic ulcer, and other conditions characterized by bleeding as a result of increased vascular fragility or blood dyscrasias.

Dosage and Administration. Heparin is available in an aqueous solution containing 10 mg. (1,000 units)/cc. This is usually diluted with isotonic salt solution and administered by intravenous drip. An amount of the diluted solution containing 50 mg. of heparin given over a period of one-half hour lengthens the clotting time of blood to about three times normal for about 2 hours, after which the clotting time returns to normal during the next hour, unless further amounts of the solution are injected. Suspensions of heparin in gelatin-dextrose vehicles are also available for deep subcutaneous or intramuscular injection. Dosage and frequency of administration of such depot preparations is regulated to keep the coagulation time of the blood at a level two or three times the patient's normal coagulation time.

MENADIOL SODIUM DIPHOSPHATE U.S.P.
(SYNKAYVITE; KAPPADIONE)

Pharmacology. This synthetic, water-soluble substance with vitamin-K activity (vitamin K_3) does not require bile in order to be absorbed from the intestinal tract as does the lipid-soluble natural vitamin K. Thus it may be preferred for oral administration to patients with obstructive jaundice and biliary fistulas. On the other hand, this synthetic form is less effective than natural vitamin K for counteracting hypoprothrombinemia induced by overdosage of anticoagulant drugs, nor is it as safe as the natural vitamin for treating infants with hypoprothrombinemic hemorrhagic disorders.

Overdosage does *not* cause blood clotting. However, administration of excessive amounts to a patient who had required anticoagulant therapy may make him subject once more to thromboembolic phenomena and render him temporarily resistant to coumarin-type anticoagulants. Adverse reactions are mainly of the allergic type (e.g., skin rashes). However, excessively large doses have caused hemolytic anemia in newborn infants and led to hyperbilirubinemia and kernicterus in premature infants.

Dosage and Administration. This form of vitamin K is administered orally or parenterally in a 5 mg. daily dose. A higher dose—10 to 15 mg.—is sometimes given to prevent bleeding during administration of certain drugs (e.g., salicylates) which reduce plasma prothrombin levels and to prevent hemorrhage following tonsillectomy. The mother may receive 5 mg. parenterally prior to delivery to prevent neonatal hemorrhage.

OXIDIZED CELLULOSE U.S P.
(HEMO-PAK; OXYCEL)

Pharmacology. This local hemostatic substance consists of a specially treated surgical cotton that can be left as a packing in some areas even after the wound is closed. Such implants—in brain surgery, for example—are usually absorbed within a few days. On the other hand, permanent packing is undesirable in some areas. For example, this gauze is not implanted in fractures, where it may interfere with bone regeneration and cause formation of cysts; nor is it left as a surface dressing, where it may prevent epithelization.

Oxidized cellulose is used mainly in neurological, otolaryngolical (adenoidectomy; tonsillectomy), and dental procedures and in other situations in which bleeding from capillaries and small veins or arteries is difficult to control with sutures or ligatures. These include hemorrhages during resections of the bowel, breast, prostate, and thyroid, and following operations on or injuries to the kidneys, spleen, pancreas, biliary tract, and liver. This material does not combine with natural clotting factors in blood; instead it forms an *artificial* clot, because its cellulosic acid component combines with hemoglobin in blood.

Dosage and Administration. Only the least amount needed to control bleeding is used. The gauze strips or pads employed for various procedures are not moistened with thrombin, which is destroyed by oxidized cellulose. In fact, this material is not moistened at all, for it has a greater hemostatic effect when dry.

PHYTONADIONE U.S.P.
(VITAMIN K_1, KONAKION; MEPHYTON)

Pharmacology. This is the naturally occurring form of vitamin K, a substance that is necessary for the biosynthesis of prothrombin and other factors needed in blood clotting. It is employed clinically in the prevention and treatment of hypoprothrombinemia, which occurs as a result of various conditions including overdosage of coumarin and indanedione-type anticoagulant agents.

This vitamin is the form preferred in hemorrhagic disease of newborn infants. It may be administered prophylactically to all mothers or infants or to control hemorrhage in bleeding infants. When given orally to patients with biliary obstruction or other conditions in which this fat-soluble form of the vitamin is poorly absorbed, bile salts must be given simultaneously. However, parenteral forms are used in disorders that interfere with vitamin K absorption, including sprue, celiac disease, and ulcerative colitis.

Dosage and Administration. Oral doses of 2.5 to 25 mg. or more are administered in various medical conditions marked by limited absorption or production of vitamin K. The vitamin is administered orally at least 24 hours prior to surgery in patients who have been taking anticoagulant drugs and to other presurgical patients with prothrombin deficiencies.

An aqueous colloidal solution is available for use by the intramuscular, subcutaneous, and intravenous routes when more rapid onset of action is desired; an aqueous injectable dispersion for intramuscular administration only is used in similar circumstances.

THROMBIN N.F.

Pharmacology. This is an essential blood clotting factor prepared from cow plasma through the same interaction that occurs naturally in the body—that is, by the activation of (bovine) prothrombin with thrombokinase in the presence of calcium ions. When it is applied to a bleeding surface, the thrombin then converts the blood's fibrinogen to fibrin filaments which trap the formed elements of the blood to form a natural clot.

Thrombin controls capillary bleeding and makes wound edges adhere during skin grafting in plastic surgery. Among the conditions in which it is applied topically as a local hemostatic are hemophilia; gastroduodenal hemorrhage; bleeding from bone, tooth sockets, nose and throat, mastoidectomy cavities, and gallbladder beds following cholecystectomy.

Dosage and Administration. Thrombin is usually applied as a sterile powder, or a relatively freshly prepared solution is sprayed over the bleeding area. It may also be given orally, alone or following absorbable gelatin powder. In such cases, it is desirable first to administer milk or a phosphate buffer or other antacid to neutralize gastric acidity. For this purpose 10,000 to 20,000 units is given several times a day.

Thrombin is never injected, for it can cause clotting throughout the vascular system and result in fatal intravascular thromboses.

WARFARIN SODIUM U.S.P.
(COUMADIN; PANWARFIN)

Pharmacology. This coumarin-type compound is both relatively rapid in onset (18 to 36 hours) and prolonged in duration (up to 5 days). Therapeutic levels of hypoprothrombinemia are usually reached within 24 hours and sustained by low daily doses for long-term prophylactic maintenance therapy. The drug is indicated for the same conditions as bishydroxycoumarin and other drugs of this class, and is contraindicated in patients who are susceptible to spontaneous bleeding episodes. Watch patients for the appearance of petechiae, prolonged oozing from small cuts, and microscopic hematuria, because such bleeding may be an early sign of overdosage.

Dosage and Administration. Warfarin is available in both oral and parenteral forms. The average adult dose for initiating therapy is 40 to 60 mg.; only half these amounts are used for aged or weakened patients. The usual maintenance dosage is 2 to 10 mg., and several sizes of tablets are available for flexibility in achieving precise prothrombin levels. Vials for preparation of sterile injection solutions contain 25 mg./ml. for intramuscular or intravenous use in acute thromboembolic conditions.

CHAPTER 25

ANTIANEMIC DRUGS

CYANOCOBALAMIN U.S.P. (VITAMIN B₁₂)

Pharmacology. This substance counteracts the symptoms of vitamin B₁₂ deficiency that develop in patients with pernicious anemia and in others who cannot absorb adequate amounts of the vitamin from food sources. In pernicious anemia, cyanocobalamin quickly brings about remission of the megaloblastic anemia, relieves G.I. disturbances, and stops the progress of nervous system damage. Its value against neuropathies and various other disorders that are not caused by vitamin B₁₂ deficiency is not established.

Dosage and Administration. The parenteral route of administration is more dependable than the oral route for pernicious anemia patients. Cyanocobalamin Injection U.S.P. is given intramuscularly or deep into the subcutaneous tissues in doses of 1 to 100 mcg. Treatment is often initiated with high daily priming doses that are intended to replenish the depleted stores of the vitamin. Later, these doses (e.g., 30 to 100 mcg.) are given at longer intervals—once weekly, and, finally, once a month. Maintenance therapy in pernicious anemia is continued for life.

Vitamin B₁₂ is available both alone and combined with intrinsic factor concentrate for oral use. When used alone, a high daily dose (100 to 1,000 mcg.) is employed. The addition of intrinsic factor aids the absorption of vitamin B₁₂ in pernicious anemia when the stomach does not secrete this substance. The use of oral preparations is largely limited to those patients who refuse parenteral therapy.

FERROCHOLINATE (CHEL-IRON; FERROLIP)

Pharmacology. This iron compound is typical of the newer complexes that are claimed to be less toxic than the single ferrous iron salts. This iron chelate contains the element in a bound form from which it is released only slowly. This is said to account for its low toxicity in animal experiments, a property that should make it less dangerous than ordinary iron salts in case a large quantity were accidentally ingested.

It is doubtful, however, that the frequncy of G.I. upset produced by this compound is less than that caused by simple ferrous salts when both are given in doses that bring about equal hematological responses in anemic patients. A day's treatment costs about four times as much as that of an equally effective dose of ferrous sulfate.

Dosage and Administration. This hematinic compound is administered orally as tablets or in the form of a solution or syrup. The daily dosage recommended for those over 6 years of age is about 1 to 2 Gm., divided into three parts, which it is claimed can be administered on an empty stomach with little G.I. distress. For infants and children under 6, pediatric drops are administered in doses determined by the doctor in accordance with the severity of the anemia.

FERROUS SULFATE U.S.P.

Pharmacology. This relatively inexpensive single iron salt produces rapid hematological responses in hypochromic microcytic anemias. Effective doses cause G.I. upset in some patients, but the incidence of such side effects is said to be no greater than that of other iron compounds that release the same toal amount of free elemental metal more slowly.

This drug is kept out of the reach of children, because overdosage has caused local corrosion of the G.I. tract. Systemic absorption of large amounts of iron through the damaged mucosa has then sometimes led to circulatory collapse and other potentially fatal complications.

Dosage and Administration. The total daily dose of the hydrated salt is about 1 Gm.; the dose of the dried salt is about a third less. (For example, a single ferrous sulfate tablet commonly contains 300 mg., whereas a tablet of the dried salt with equal activity contains only 200 mg.; both are given three or four times daily, preferably after meals). Liquid forms—drops, syrups, and an elixir—are available for treating both children and adults. These are often administered diluted with fruit or vegetable juices. Slow-release capsules of ferrous sulfate are claimed less likely to cause G.I. distress when given twice daily, on account of the wide dispersal and slow absorption of the iron-releasing pellets.

FOLIC ACID U.S.P.
(PTEROYLGLUTAMIC ACID)

Pharmacology. This essential nutrient is found in many foods including fresh, green leafy vegetables, liver, and yeast. It is administered to patients with megaloblastic anemias and symptoms resulting from dietary deficiency of folic acid or failure to absorb enough of it from the G.I. tract. In these conditions, including sprue, celiac disease, and the megaloblastic anemias of pregnancy and infancy, administration of the vitamin promptly corrects the hematological abnormality.

Although it also returns the blood picture of pernicious anemia patients to normal, it is *never* used in place of vitamin B$_{12}$ in that condition. Folic acid cannot counteract the neurological lesions of that disorder, which progress despite the hematological remission brought about by its administration.

Dosage and Administration. Although the daily requirement of folic acid is estimated as only 0.1 mg. daily, it is usually given in oral doses of 10 to 30 mg. daily to correct a diagnosed deficiency. A parenteral preparation containing 15 mg./ml. is injected intramuscularly or deep subcutaneously in G.I. tract malabsorptive disorders. Folic acid is often included in nonprescription panhematinic multivitamin and mineral products in amounts of 0.1 mg. or less. Larger daily doses are considered undesirable, because most anemic patients do not require it and it may obscure the diagnosis of pernicious anemia.

IRON DEXTRAN INJECTION U.S.P.
(IMFERON)

Pharmacology. This parenteral iron preparation is recommended only for treating definitely diagnosed cases of iron-deficiency anemia, in which oral administration of iron has not proved practicable or effective, or in patients for whom oral iron is contraindicated because of severe G.I. tract ulcerations or diarrhea.

When administered intramuscularly, this compound produces few ill effects except occasional local pain. Sometimes, however, systemic allergic reactions are reported in sensitized individuals, including headache, fever, and joint pains. This drug is also sometimes given by vein. However, this may result in the same sort of acute hypotensive reactions that sometimes occur with other intravenously administered iron preparations. Although this compound was once withdrawn from the market because it had reportedly caused sarcomas in animals, there is little reason to believe that injections produce similar malignant tumors in humans.

Dosage and Administration. Iron dextran is usually injected intramuscularly in doses determined by calculation from a formula that takes into consideration the hemoglobin level. A usual initial dose is 1 ml. (equal to 50 mg. of elemental iron); this can then be raised gradually to 5 ml. daily. To avoid staining the skin red at the injection site, it is suggested that a long needle be used for buttocks injections and that the skin and subcutaneous tissues be pushed aside before inserting the needle.

CHAPTER 26

DRUGS USED IN PERIPHERAL VASCULAR DISEASE

AZAPETINE PHOSPHATE (ILIDAR)

Pharmacology. This drug is similar to tolazoline in its combination of adrenergic blocking and direct relaxant effects on vascular smooth muscle in spasm. However, it is claimed less likely to cause adverse G.I. side effects. Nasal congestion, head-

ache, and mouth dryness are among the more common minor side effects. Less common but potentially more serious are cardiac palpitations, tachycardia, and postural hypotension. Thus, this drug is not given to patients with severe coronary artery disease, or any condition in which a sudden fall in blood pressure may be dangerous.

Dosage and Administration. Azapetine is administered orally, starting with doses of 25 mg. three times daily. If patients with Raynaud's syndrome, acrocyanosis, causalgia, and other vasospastic conditions tolerate this dose for one week, it may be raised to 50 or even 75 mg. three times a day in order to attain maximum effects and overcome ulcerations resulting from frostbite or from chronic peripheral vasospasm.

CYCLANDELATE (CYCLOSPASMOL)

Pharmacology. This antispasmodic drug acts directly on the smooth muscle of constricted arterioles to relax them. This is said to increase blood flow to both skeletal muscles and skin. Some physicians have reported that it speeds the healing of refractory skin ulcers and relieves painful intermittent claudication. The drug reportedly counteracts vascular spasm in ergot toxicity as well as in various cases of local frostbite and other vasospastic and occlusive peripheral vascular diseases. It does not ordinarily cause tachycardia or postural hypotension. However, higher doses often cause G.I. upset and flushing, tingling of the skin, and sweating.

Dosage and Administration. Cyclandelate is administered orally in doses of 100 to 400 mg. four times daily, before each meal and at bedtime. If the higher doses are required for full effectiveness, some side effects can be expected. However, most patients are maintained on 200 mg. or less four times a day—a regimen that is claimed to cause few adverse reactions.

NYLIDRIN HYDROCHLORIDE N.F. (ARLIDIN)

Pharmacology. This sympathomimetic drug specifically stimulates adrenergic receptors of the *beta* type in blood vessels of the skeletal muscles. Such stimulation leads to relaxation of the smooth muscle walls of these arterioles and an increase in blood flow to the muscles of the limbs. The drug is used to treat intermittent claudication in cases of arteriosclerosis obliterans, Buerger's disease (thromboangiitis obliterans), diabetic vascular disease, and night leg cramps.

Because the drug is a sympathomimetic agent, it is used with caution in cases of angina pectoris, paroxysmal tachycardia, and hyperthyroidism, and is not employed at all in patients who have suffered an acute myocardial infarction. The drug sometimes causes nervousness and heart palpitations, but it has not had adverse effects on blood pressure.

Dosage and Administration. Nylidrin is ordinarily given by mouth in doses of 6 mg. three to six times daily, depending on the response. Doses of 2.5 to 5 mg. may be injected subcutaneously or intramuscularly one or more times daily.

PHENOXYBENZAMINE HYDROCHLORIDE (DIBENZYLINE)

Pharmacology. This is a relatively long-acting adrenergic blocking agent. This action results in increased cutaneous blood flow and a rise in skin temperature. Relief of excessive vasospasm and ischemia is considered desirable in Raynaud's disease, acrocyanosis, and other peripheral vascular disorders. Besides tending to overcome cyanosis and bring warmth to the cold extremities, the drug's vasodilator action sometimes helps to heal vasospastic ulcers of the extremities and the after effects of frostbite. The pain of causalgia may be lessened.

Like other drugs of this class, it is less useful in vascular diseases marked by arteriosclerosis and thrombotic obstruction. However, in acute arterial occlusion and reflex spasms of collateral vessels, phenoxybenzamine may help to increase blood flow in the unobstructed arterioles. Excessive local vasodilation may be manifested by nasal congestion. More serious is systemic vasodilation resulting in postural hypotension and tachycardia. In most patients this merely causes feelings of dizziness and faintness. However, an excessive drug-induced fall in blood pressure is especially undesirable in cerebral or coronary arteriosclerosis.

Dosage and Administration. It is customary to start treatment with low doses, such as 10 mg. daily. After at least four days this may be increased gradually by another 10 mg. In time, the dosage may be increased to 20 to 60 mg. daily for full benefits, but slow individual adjustments minimize troublesome side effects.

TOLAZOLINE HYDROCHLORIDE (PRISCOLINE)

Pharmacology. This drug produces dilation of blood vessels in various disorders marked by peripheral vasospasm, including Raynaud's disease, scleroderma, and acrocyanosis. It acts by abolishing the tone of vascular smooth muscle, and is, for this reason, used for diagnostic purposes to determine whether surgical sympathectomy might benefit a particular patient. However, this drug's action is not due entirely to sympathetic blockade, for it also has a direct histamine-like effect that helps to relax vascular smooth muscle.

The histamine-like action may also account for the nausea, vomiting, and epigastric distress sometimes caused by this drug. These side effects may be controlled by administering tolazoline together with antacid medications or after meals. However, the drug is undesirable for patients with a history of peptic ulcer or gastritis. It is also contraindicated for patients with coronary artery disease, for it sometimes causes severe tachycardia. Such early skin side effects as flushing, tingling, gooseflesh, and sensations of warmth or chilliness tend to subside during treatment.

Dosage and Administration. Tolazoline may be given orally in doses gradually built up to 25 to 50 mg. four to six times daily. A sustained-release tablet containing 65 mg. given only twice daily produces the same effects. This drug is also administered by various parenteral routes, including intra-arterially. Injection directly into a major artery is usually reserved for conditions marked by sudden arterial occlusion.

CHAPTER 27

PITUITARY GLAND HORMONES

CORTICOTROPIN INJECTION U.S.P. (ACTH, ETC.)

Pharmacology. This purified principle of the anterior pituitary gland stimulates the adrenal cortex to secrete several types of steroids. Thus, it is used to treat all disease that respond to the chief natural adrenal steroid hydrocortisone, with the exception of Addison's disease. In general, the synthetic corticosteroids are preferred in these conditions because they can be given in convenient oral doses which also produce a more predictable response than this injectable product.

Actually, the effects of corticotropin differ from those of the synthetic glucocorticoids in certain significant ways. For example, corticotropin can cause the adrenal glands to secrete steroids with *anabolic* (protein-building) and *mineralocorticoid* (sodium and water retaining) activity. This means that: (1) this hormone may be preferable in multiple sclerosis and other neuromuscular conditions in which the protein wasting effects of corticosteroids are especially undesirable, and (2) the danger of fluid retention and potassium loss in cardiovascular diseases is greater than with

the synthetic corticosteroids. Corticotropin is used mainly as a diagnostic agent and for stimulating the adrenal glands to resume secretion of endogenous steroids during withdrawal of corticosteroid medications.

Dosage and Administration. This preparation is infused intravenously over an 8-hour period in doses of 5 to 50 units. Although it may be injected intramuscularly four times daily in a total dose of 40 to 50 units, the official Repository Corticotropin Injection and the Corticotropin Zinc Hydroxide Suspension are preferred for administration by this route, because a 40 unit intramuscular injection of one of these slowly absorbed dosage forms need be given only once daily.

VASOPRESSIN INJECTION U.S.P. (PITRESSIN)

Pharmacology. This purified extract of the posterior pituitary gland is used mainly to control the polyuria and polydipsia of diabetes insipidus. However, for this purpose the long-continued antidiuretic action of a suspension of vasopressin tannate in peanut oil is often preferred to this aqueous solution.

Much higher doses of this substance may be used to raise the systemic blood pressure. However, since this pressor action, which is brought about by arteriolar vasconstriction, is sometimes accompanied by coronary vascular constriction, vasopressin is not administered to patients with angina pectoris or a history of coronary thrombosis.

Vasopressin, like posterior pituitary extracts containing it, is sometimes given to cause contractions of G.I. tract smooth muscles. This action helps to prevent and control postoperative abdominal distention, and to remove gas from the bowel prior to taking abdominal x-rays.

Dosage and Administration. In diabetes insipidus, the dosage and the intervals of administration are determined for each patient. An average dose is 1 ml. intramuscularly, but the drug may also be given intranasally by dropper, spray, or on cotton pledgets two or three times daily. To produce increased G.I. motility, 5 to 10 units (0.25 to 0.5 ml.) is administered intramuscularly at intervals of 3 or 4 hours for abdominal distention, or 2 hours and one-half hour before roentgenography.

CHAPTER 28

THE ADRENOCORTICOSTEROID DRUGS

DEXAMETHASONE N.F. (DECADRON; DERONIL; DEXAMETH; ETC.)

Pharmacology. This synthetic fluorinated corticosteroid is one of the most potent agents of its class, in terms of the relatively low dosage (fractions of a milligram) that elicits clinically useful anti-inflammatory activity. However, since its margin of safety is no greater than that of other synthetic steroids, patients are watched closely for signs of side effects and typical toxic reactions (see Summary, Chap. 28). Like most other synthetic steroids, dexamethasone has an advantage over the natural glucocorticoids hydrocortisone and cortisone: it is less likely to cause sodium and water retention or loss of potassium even when administered in high daily doses for long periods.

In addition to this base, which is marketed mainly in tablet form for oral administration in treatment of conditions that respond to corticosteroid therapy, a soluble salt, *dexamethasone sodium phosphate* N.F., is available for injection, inhalation, and topical application to the skin and eye. An advantage of such topical therapy is the relatively localized action of the steroid and the lessened likelihood of systemic side effects. However, some is absorbed into the bloodstream during inhalation therapy, so that excessive use can cause side effects. Similarly, when dexamethasone sodium phosphate creams and ointments are applied to the skin under an occlusive dressing during the long-term treatment of psoriasis and other dermatoses, enough absorption may occur through the skin to produce unexpected adverse effects.

Dosage and Administration. A dose of 0.75 mg. of dexamethasone is equivalent to 20 mg. of hydrocortisone in pharmacological activity. The amount administered may be as much as 20 mg. of the salt injected intravenously to help a patient meet an extremely stressful emergency, to as little as 0.5 mg. as oral maintenance therapy in chronic conditions.

The number of inhalations of the spray is limited (e.g., no more than 8 inhalations a day for children at first, with gradual reduction later). Ophthalmic solutions are dropped into the eye frequently during the day (e.g., every hour or two), ointments are preferred for application at night, and both are gradually discontinued after the eye disorder responds to treatment. Dermatologic creams and ointments are applied two or three times daily or covered with an occlusive dressing for longer periods after one application.

HYDROCORTISONE U.S.P. (CORTEF; CORTRIL; HYDROCORTONE; ETC.)

Pharmacology. This is the main natural glucocorticoid secreted by the cortex of the adrenal glands. It is somewhat more potent on a weight basis than the other important adrenal cortex hormone cortisone, but much less potent than most synthetic adrenocorticosteroids. The higher dose of hydrocortisone that is required for clinical anti-inflammatory activity is no drawback, and in its various forms it is widely used in treating steroid-responsive disorders and adrenal insufficiency. Also it is widely employed for topical application in skin conditions.

The chief drawback of this natural steroid compared to the synthetic steroids is its relatively high mineralocorticoid activity. Because of this, salt and water retention with weight gain and edema occur more commonly; thus, synthetic steroids are preferred for patients with cardiovascular disorders. Diuretics are occasionally used to remove edema that develops suddenly if congestive heart failure threatens a patient with diminished cardiac reserve. However, the continued use of diuretics for maintaining such steroid therapy is considered undesirable, because it may have an additive action with hydrocortisone in removing excessive amounts of potassium and, thus, producing hypokalemia. Such potassium loss may be detected when the patient is watched carefully and occasional electrocardiograms are made; and hypokalemia may be avoided by putting the patient on a diet low in sodium and high in potassium with possible additional supplements of that electrolyte.

Dosage and Administration. The basic alcohol hydrocortisone is available in several dosage forms for oral, topical, and parenteral administration. Dosage is individually determined and adjusted after administration of amounts ranging initially from 20 mg. daily in chronic conditions to 240 mg. in acute, life-threatening diseases. Hydrocortisone acetate U.S.P. is a slowly absorbed ester commonly applied topically and injected intrasynovially; hydrocortisone sodium succinate U.S.P. is a highly soluble form that is rapidly absorbed when injected in the treatment of adrenal insufficiency and other acute conditions. Other nonofficial hydrocortisone derivatives are available.

DESOXYCORTICOSTERONE ACETATE U.S.P. (CORTATE; DOCA; PERCORTEN; ETC.)

Pharmacology. This ester of one of the most potent natural mineralocorticoids is used in the management of acute and chronic adrenal insufficiency. It produces prompt retention of sodium and water by the renal tubules of patients with Addison's disease, Simmond's disease, and the Waterhouse-Friderichsen syndrome, as well as in patients who have undergone surgery involving the adrenal gland. The salt-retaining action of this hormone leads to a return of blood pressure to normal levels and an improvement in appetite, weight, strength, and sense of well-being.

Dosage and Administration. Patients usually first receive 5 to 10 mg. daily in an oil solution injected intramuscularly. Later, the daily dose is often lowered to 1 to 5 mg., which may be administered as buccal tablets. Pellets are sometimes implanted to extend the duration of action. However, the longer-acting trimethyl acetate derivative is considered more desirable for this purpose. One depot injection of the latter often keeps a patient in remission for one month. The average dose of this intramuscular depot preparation is 50 to 100 mg. every 4 weeks. Dosage is adjusted to amounts that prevent weight loss and yet do not cause excessive retention of sodium and water or too much potassium loss, with consequent edema, hypotension, hypokalemia, and cardiac failure.

METHYLPREDNISOLONE N.F. (MEDROL)

Pharmacology. This synthetic steroid is a methyl derivative of prednisolone (see Drug Digest), which has slightly greater potency on a weight basis than the latter. Like the parent compound and other synthetic corticosteroids, it lacks the mineralocorticoid activity of the natural adrenal hormones. This is desirable when patients with cardiovascular disease require steroid therapy, but these drugs are not useful as replacement therapy in adrenal insufficiency.

Besides the base, which is taken orally in tablets and sustained-action capsules, this steroid is available as *methylprednisolone sodium succinate* N.F., a highly soluble form suitable for emergency injections, and as the poorly soluble *acetate* N.F., which is applied topically in steroid-responsive skin conditions. A suspension of the latter is injected intramuscularly or directly into inflamed joints, tendons, and bursae. Its local and systemic actions, when administered in this way, are prolonged.

Dosage and Administration. In order to produce the inflammatory action that is desired in treating many disorders while minimizing the likelihood of adverse effects (see Summary, Chap. 28), dosage of this steroid is adjusted to each patient's needs and responses. Treatment is initiated with as little as 4 mg. or as much as 40 mg. daily, depending on whether the condition is chronic or an acute emergency. (Four mg. is equal to 20 mg. of hydrocortisone in anti-inflammatory activity.)

CHAPTER 29

FEMALE SEX HORMONES

DIETHYLSTILBESTROL U.S.P. (STILBESTROL; STILBETIN)

Pharmacology. This nonsteroidal synthetic substance duplicates most of the effects of natural estrogenic hormones on the tissues of the female genital tract. It controls menopausal symptoms occurring naturally or as a result of ovarian surgery. Administered orally or in suppository form, it relieves symptoms of senile vaginitis and pruritus vulvae. It is believed to suppress lactation and ovulation by inhibiting pituitary gland gonadotropin secretion. Diethylstilbestrol is employed in the palliative treatment of male patients with carcinoma of the prostate and in women with breast cancer who are at least 5 years beyond the menopause and whose condition is no longer treatable by surgery or irradiation.

Dosage and Administration. Diethylstilbestrol is available as tablets and suppositories and as an injection. (Various long-acting esters, such as the dipropionate, dipalmitate, and diphosphate, may also be injected intramuscularly.) The average daily oral dose for patients with menopausal symptoms is 0.5 to 1 mg., but treatment begun with lower doses minimizes nausea, vomiting, dizziness, and headache. In prostatic carcinomas, 3 mg. may be given daily; and for mammary cancer, 15 to 25 mg. is the recommended daily dose.

ESTRADIOL VALERATE U.S.P. (DELESTROGEN)

Pharmacology. A single injection of this long-acting ester into an intramuscular depot results in estrogenic actions lasting 2 to 3 weeks. Such prolonged effects are considered especially desirable in the management of patients with carcinoma of the prostate, in which estrogens often induce symptomatic relief and regression of metastatic growths. Elderly women with advanced mammary carcinoma often respond with subjective and objective relief when given high doses biweekly. Injections made at the end of the first stage of labor inhibit lactation and postpartum engorgement of the breasts. This product is employed cyclically with a long-acting progestational preparation in the treatment of various menstrual cycle disorders and ovarian deficiency syndromes.

Dosage and Administration. This preparation is injected deep into the gluteal muscle in doses of 10 to 40 mg., depending on the condition being treated. For example, a 10 mg. injection usually suppresses lactation, whereas repeated weekly doses of 30 to 50 mg. may be required for relief of prostatic carcinoma. Prolonged treatment in women is interrupted every few months to permit the endometrium to regress. A dry, small gauge needle and dry syringe are used.

ESTROGENIC SUBSTANCES CONJUGATED (PREMARIN, ETC.)

Pharmacology. This mixture of water-soluble estrogens excreted by mares after conjugation in the liver, contains sodium estrone sulfate among other active estrogens. It is available in several different dosage forms and is advocated for the management of many conditions besides the relief of menopausal symptoms and the prevention of postmenopausal degenerative disorders.

For example, it is employed in attempts to prolong the lives of poor-risk male cardiac patients with high blood cholesterol, because it is claimed to "protect" against myocardial infarctions. It is said to help counteract incapacitating disorders such as osteoporosis. A vaginal cream is employed for treating senile vaginitis, kraurosis vulvae, and pruritic vulvovaginitis. An intravenous form is used as a hemostatic, not only to overcome dysfunctional uterine bleeding, but also to control capillary bleeding in males and children of both sexes during surgical procedures.

Dosage and Administration. The usual oral dosage for menopausal symptoms is 1.25 mg. daily, and the drug is withdrawn every 3 weeks for a 1-week rest period. Women with atrophic lesions of the vagina and vulva may require much higher oral doses as well as topical therapy. For hemostatic action, 20 mg. may be injected intravenously preoperatively and repeated during or after surgery.

ETHINYL ESTRADIOL U.S.P. (ESTINYL; ETICYLOL; ETC.)

Pharmacology. This semi-synthetic derivative of estradiol is one of the most potent estrogens. Because the ethinyl radical protects the estrogen from decomposition, a low, daily oral dose keeps patients symptom free. This compound, like other estrogens, is employed in menopausal disorders, female hypogonadism, functional uterine bleeding, postpartum breast engorgement, carcinoma of the prostate, and inoperable carcinoma of the breast *post*menopausally. It is *not* given to *præ*menopausal women with cancerous or precancerous lesions; and caution is required in women with a family history of carcinoma.

Dosage and Administration. Dosage of the tablets varies from 0.02 to 3 mg. daily, depending on the condition being treated and the response of the patient. An attempt is made to determine the minimal effective maintenance dose for each patient in order to minimize side effects. Occasional reactions such as headache, vertigo, nausea, and vomiting are said to be reduced when the total daily dose is taken at bedtime.

HYDROXYPROGESTERONE CAPROATE (DELALUTIN)

Pharmacology. This ester derivative of progesterone is long-acting, producing progestational effects for 7 to 14 days on an estrogen-primed endometrium. This, and its lack of virilizing activity, makes it useful for maintaining pregnancy in cases of recurrent and threatened abortion. However, as with other progestins, its true value for this purpose is not established.

This progestogen is employed alone or combined with the potent long-acting estrogen estradiol valerate, in the management of endometriosis, dysfunctional uterine bleeding, and primary or secondary amenorrhea. It is also often administered after ovulation to prevent premenstrual tension, to counteract dysmenorrhea, and to combat chronic cystic mastitis. When the drug's action wears off, the secretory endometrium formed under its influence desquamates, provided that the patient has a source of endogenous or exogenous estrogen. Failure to bleed indicates that endogenous progesterone is being produced—a positive test for pregnancy.

Dosage and Administration. This product is injected deeply into the gluteal muscle in a dose of 250 mg. once every week, or—in cyclic therapy—every 4 weeks. A single dose is given as a therapeutic test for endogenous estrogen production or of pregnancy, or upon completion of delivery to prevent postpartum pains.

MEDROXYPROGESTERONE ACETATE U.S.P. (PROVERA)

Pharmacology. This progesterone derivative is much more active than the parent hormone when taken by mouth and more long-lasting when injected. It is employed in the management of infertility, habitual and threatened abortion, endometriosis, secondary amenorrhea and functional uterine bleeding. Best results are obtained when estrogens are administered simultaneously to develop a proliferative endometrium that can be converted to the secretory type by this progestin. Withdrawal of the drugs then produces menstrual bleeding followed by the start of a new cycle. The treatment is then repeated through three consecutive cycles.

Bleeding usually follows withdrawal of this drug so regularly within 2 to 7 days that failure to menstruate may be considered a positive test for pregnancy. This steroid is combined with the potent estrogen ethinyl estradiol as an oral contraceptive.

Few side effects seem to occur when this progestin is employed alone, but drowsiness and hirsutism are reported occasionally. Patients on prolonged treatment are watched for possible development of adrenocorticoid effects. This steroid and its combinations with estrogens are not used in patients with abnormal uterine bleeding until the presence of genital malignancy has been ruled out.

Dosage and Administration. Dosage schedules vary with the condition being treated and the form of the drug employed. In cyclic therapy, 2.5 to 10 mg. is administered daily for 5 to 10 days beginning on the 16th to 21st day of the menstrual cycle. As a pregnancy test, 10 mg. is given daily for 5 days and then withdrawn. For continuous therapy in habitual abortion, etc., 10 to 40 mg. may be given daily by mouth, or 50 to 100 mg. may be injected intramuscularly daily, weekly, or every 2 weeks, depending on whether symptoms are present and upon the trimester of pregnancy.

CHAPTER 30

THE MALE SEX HORMONES AND ANABOLIC AGENTS

NORETHINDRONE (NORLUTIN)

Pharmacology. This synthetic progestin produces progestational effects upon the endometrium and suppresses ovulation by its action on hypothalamohypophyseal function. These actions account for its usefulness for regularizing menstruation, controlling excessive uterine bleeding, and delaying menstruation in endometriosis and for other medical and social reasons.

This progestin may be useful for treating infertility in women with a demonstrated luteal phase deficiency or in some who have anovulatory cycles, in which case discontinuance of treatment sometimes leads to spontaneous "rebound" ovulation. However, because this progestin also possesses some androgenic activity, it is not continued once pregnancy is established, lest it masculinize the female fetus.

Mild nausea, transient tiredness, and other minor side effects have been reported. The drug, which has occasionally caused jaundice, should not be used in patients with liver dysfunction. Deepening of the voice, hirsutism, and acne are rare manifestations of this steroid's slight virilizing activity.

Dosage and Administration. Norethindrone is administered orally in doses of 5 to 20 mg. daily during cyclic therapy, starting on the 5th day and ending on the 23rd day of the cycle. Withdrawal bleeding then occurs within 5 days. In endometriosis, an initial daily dose of 10 mg. is increased to 20 or 30 mg. daily during a 6 to 9-month course of treatment. Other schedules may be employed in the management of premenstrual tension and dysmenorrhea.

NORETHYNODREL WITH MESTRANOL (ENOVID; ENOVID E)

Pharmacology. This progestin-estrogen combination is employed in the treatment of many gynecological conditions (see text) on account of its varied actions, which are said to imitate the physiological effects of a functioning corpus luteum. These include suppression of pituitary gonadotropin secretion and rapid production of a secretory endometrium followed by the premature atrophy of its glands and its deciduation with menstrual bleeding within 5 or so days of withdrawal.

Conception is prevented in virtually 100 per cent of patients who employ this steroid combination properly. Side effects that resemble the discomforts of early pregnancy occur in a substantial number of women, but tend to lessen or disappear after several cycles. These include nausea and vomiting, weight gain, breast discomfort, and headache. Breakthrough bleeding, or, on the other hand, amenorrhea upon withdrawal occurs sometimes.

The use of this and similar products in patients with uterine fibroids and in those with a history of genital or mammary cancer is considered undesirable. Similarly, although there is no proof that these steroids cause thrombophlebitis, their use in patients with a history of thromboembolic disease is contraindicated. Preexisting liver disease is another contraindication.

Dosage and Administration For contraceptive purposes, a tablet containing 2.5 mg. of norethynodrel with 0.1 mg. of mestranol (Enovid-E) is taken daily from the 5th through the 24th day of the menstrual cycle. In the treatment of menstrual dysfunctions, tablets containing different amounts and ratios of the two steroids (Enovid) are administered in various dosage regimens, up to 20 to 30 mg. daily.

TESTOSTERONE CYPIONATE U.S.P. (DEPO-TESTOSTERONE CYPIONATE)

Pharmacology. This long-acting ester form of the male hormone exerts its masculinizing (androgenic) and anabolic effects over periods of 1 to 4 weeks while being slowly absorbed from the injection site. In the management of hypogonadal male patients with eunuchism and eunuchoidism, it brings about development of secondary sex characteristics. It has been tried for treating the male climacteric, impotence, oligospermia, and cryptorchism in carefully selected patients.

Testosterone cypionate is effective in the management of menstrual disorders such as dysmenorrhea, menorrhagia, metrorrhagia and premenstrual tension. It suppresses lactation and symptoms of metastatic mammary carcinoma, conditions in which, however, shorter-acting forms of the hormone are often preferred. It may be useful in the management of osteoporosis in both men and women.

Caution is required in the use of testosterone cypionate in young hypogonadal boys to prevent precocious sexual development and premature closure of the epiphyses with resulting failure to reach full height. Women are watched for signs of masculinization, including hirsutism, acne, hoarseness or deepening of the voice, clitoral enlargement, and increased libido. In breast cancer, women are carefully observed for signs of hypercalcemia and fluid retention. Edema from salt and water retention is also undesirable in elderly patients.

Dosage and Administration. Doses of 100 to 400 mg. are administered intramuscularly at intervals of 1 to 4 weeks, depending on the condition that is being treated. Typically, hypogonadal males are maintained on doses of 200 to 400 mg. every 3 or 4 weeks, as are patients for whom only anabolic effects are sought.

TESTOSTERONE PROPIONATE U.S.P. (NEO-HOMBREOL; ORETON; PERANDREN, ETC.)

Pharmacology. This testosterone ester of moderate duration offers greater flexibility of dosage in obtaining the androgenic, anabolic, and other desired effects of the male hormone. This is especially desirable in women with advanced breast cancer who could be endangered by the continuing effects of longer-lasting esters in the event that undesirable reactions developed. On the other hand, the necessary frequency of injections of this ester may make it less convenient than the long-acting esters for use in the management of other patients.

Testosterone propionate is used in the treatment of male hypogonadism and in eunuchoidism, and it has been suggested for use in properly diagnosed cases of functional hypogonadism in middle aged men. Also, it halts functional uterine bleeding, relieves symptoms of dysmenorrhea and premenstrual tension, and suppresses lactation, thus preventing painful breast engorgement. As indicated above, this ester has desirable palliative effects in some cases of metastatic mammary carcinoma. It is contraindicated in prostatic carcinoma.

Dosage and Administration. The usual dose of this ester for hypogonadal males is 25 mg. injected intramuscularly three times weekly. However, it may be given daily or as frequently as two or three times daily for up to a week in some cases (e.g., in female disorders) or in doses as high as 100 mg. (e.g., in mammary carcinoma).

CHAPTER 31

THE THYROID HORMONES AND ANTITHYROID DRUGS

METHIMAZOLE U.S.P. (TAPAZOLE)

Pharmacology. This agent has the highest potency among the available antithyroid drugs. Administered in relatively low doses, it rapidly reduces the thyroid gland's ability to biosynthesize the hormones that hyperthyroid patients produce and excrete in excessive quantities.

The drug reduces the symptoms of thyrotoxicosis prior to subtotal thyroidectomy. Many patients who receive methimazole as medical treatment of hyperthyroidism for long periods go into permanent remission and do not require surgery or radiation therapy.

A small proportion may suffer drug reactions, including skin rash, fever, and marked reduction in white blood cells. Patients are warned to report to the physician immediately signs of possible agranulocytosis, such as severe sore throat, so that the drug can be discontinued promptly. Jaundice is watched for, because hepatitis has been reported occasionally. Overdosage can cause hypothyroidism, but this drug does not cause permanent thyroid gland damage, and so the condition can be reversed upon withdrawal of the drug.

Dosage and Administration. The total daily dose of methimazole is 15 to 60 mg. or more, depending on the severity of the condition. The drug is divided into three doses, each taken at 8-hour intervals. Patients are taught to take the drug precisely as ordered.

SODIUM IODIDE I 131 U.S.P. (IODOTOPE; RADIOCAPS; ETC.)

Pharmacology. This isotope of iodine is taken up by the thyroid gland and concentrated there in the same way as other iodides. However, the radiation that is given off makes this radioactive form of the element particularly useful for both the study of thyroid function and the treatment of hyperthyroidism.

The amount of radioactive iodine taken up by the thyroid gland is low in hypothyroidism and abnormally high in hyperthyroidism. Thus, the state of thyroid function is determined by scanning the thyroid gland and measuring the amount of gamma radiation given off some time after administration of the drug in tracer doses. The amount of radioactivity in the urine may also be measured, as an indication of the thyroid's ability to concentrate iodides.

When much larger amounts are administered, the beta rays given off by the radioactive iodine concentrated in the thyroid destroy much of the gland, thus reducing its excessive secretory capacity. This type of therapy for hyperthyroidism is preferred for patients with heart disorders or other conditions which make them relatively poor risks for surgery. It is given only with caution to children and young adults, because the question of whether this compound can cause thyroid cancer or genetic damage in such patients is not yet considered resolved.

Dosage and Administration. This substance is given in the form of a solution that may be administered orally or intravenously in doses that vary with the purpose and the individual's glandular mass. Tracer doses for diagnosis are 1 to 100 *micro*curies. Doses for treating hyperthyroidism are usually about 1,000 times as high—that is, 1 to 100 *milli*curies.

SODIUM LIOTHYRONINE U.S.P. (CYTOMEL; L-TRIIODOTHYRONINE)

Pharmacology. This salt of the most potent of the thyroid gland hormones is more rapid in its onset of action and shorter in duration than other thyroid preparations and derivatives. The greater milligram potency of this preparation does not give it any significant advantage over other forms of thyroid in the treatment of hypothyroidism. However, the faster metabolic response may make this hormone more desirable in certain therapeutic and diagnostic situations.

Patients in myxedema coma and myxedematous patients who require emergency surgery may, for example, profit from the onset of this drug's desirable effects within a few hours. Similarly, because it rapidly suppresses pituitary production of thyrotropin, it may be more useful than slower-acting thyroid preparations in one modification of the radioactive iodine uptake test for hyperthyroidism or thyrotoxicosis.

Sodium liothyronine produces the typical adverse effects of thyroid overdosage, including tachycardia, excessive sweating, nervous irritability, and headache. However, the effects of overdosage may be more readily controlled with this preparation, because of the relative rapidity with which its effects are dissipated when the drug is withdrawn. Although most symptoms of overdosage disappear within a few days after dosage is reduced, caution is required with this drug as with other thyroid preparations in the treatment of patients with a history of angina pectoris and other cardiovascular diseases.

Dosage and Administration. Initial doses as low as 5 mcg. may be raised in gradual increments to maintenance levels of 100 mcg. daily or higher. Usual maintenance dosage for myxedema is 50 to 100 mcg.; in simple goiter 25 to 75 mcg. usually maintains suppression of pituitary thyrotropin secretion.

THYROID U.S.P.

Pharmacology. This is a powder prepared from the dried, defatted whole thyroid glands of domesticated animals that are used as food sources for humans; tablets of various sizes usually contain 15, 30, 60, or 120 mg. of the powder. Administered as replacement therapy in hypothyroidism, it has a slowly cumulative effect. Although appearance and behavior improve within a few days, weeks of treatment are often necessary to bring the metabolic rate back to normal in many cases of myxedema and cretinism.

Overdosage causes nervousness, insomnia, tremors, headache, diarrhea and heart palpitations. Possible thyroid-induced tachycardia makes the use of this hormone undesirable for most patients with angina pectoris and other cardiovascular disorders. Thyroid is also contraindicated for patients with adrenal insufficiency unless this is first corrected, because administration of thyroid may precipitate acute adrenal crisis.

Dosage and Administration. The official usual dose of thyroid is 100 mg., but treatment regimens vary widely depending on the age, condition, and response of the individual patient. Some doctors initiate therapy in full doses of 120 to 180 mg. daily in patients with no history of heart disease; others begin with as little as 30 mg. a day when they feel the need for caution to avoid overdosage. A standard starting dose for cretinous infants is 15 mg.

The daily dose of thyroid is increased at only relatively long intervals—2 to 4 weeks—because of its slowly cumulative effects. For the same reason, the total daily dose is administered all at once rather than divided into several portions. Thus, a patient often receives 30 mg. daily at any time of day for the first 2 weeks; then the dose is doubled, and he receives 60 mg. for another 2-week period. If signs of improvement are far from maximal, the dose is raised to 90 or 120 mg. daily. From the latter point, the dosage is then usually increased more cautiously to the point of optimal effectiveness, which may be 200 mg. but rarely over 300 mg. daily, for toxic effects tend to develop in this dose range with continued treatment.

CHAPTER 32

DRUGS USED IN DIABETES

CHLORPROPAMIDE U.S.P. (DIABINESE)

Pharmacology. This sulfonylurea compound is similar to tolbutamide and the others in its indications. It is sometimes effective in uncomplicated cases of maturity-onset diabetes, which did not respond to treatment with other agents, or in which relapse (secondary failure) developed after initial success. Like the other oral hypoglycemic agents of this class, it should not be used in diabetic patients whose condition is complicated by fever, injury, gangrene, ketoacidosis, or coma.

Chlorpropamide differs from the others in its longer duration of action, because it is bound to the blood plasma and only slowly excreted. Although this prolonged action may increase the convenience of administration, it also adds to the dangers of overdosage. Hypoglycemic reactions, for example, may require close supervision of the patient for several days to a week after this drug is discontinued. This agent is contraindicated in patients with renal impairment which might interfere with its excretion. Liver function is tested before beginning treatment and frequently thereafter, and the drug is discontinued if jaundice develops. Blood dyscrasias have been reported occasionally.

Dosage and Administration. Chlorpropamide is usually administered in a single daily oral dose either with or before breakfast or the evening meal. Most patients require 250 mg. daily, but older patients may need only 125 mg. daily, whereas more severe diabetics may be given up to 500 mg. daily. The drug is sometimes combined with phenformin, when a daily maintenance dose of 500 mg. fails to control severe diabetes.

GLUCAGON U.S.P.

Pharmacology. This purified pancreatic extract is sometimes used to raise the blood sugar of patients who are having hypoglycemic reactions from overdoses of insulin. This *hyper*glycemic substance produces its effects by converting liver glycogen into glucose. The gradual build-up of blood sugar which then follows helps to arouse patients from hypoglycemic coma in 5 to 20 minutes usually.

Glucagon administration may be repeated once or twice if the patient fails to waken. However, the intravenous injection of dextrose is finally required in some cases; and even when the patient does respond to glucagon he should then be given glucose by mouth to keep his blood sugar from dropping once more, when this short-acting substance wears off.

Glucagon causes few side effects; even the nausea and vomiting sometimes reported may actually be the result of the preceding hypoglycemic reaction. However, because it is a polypeptide of animal origin, this substance may cause sensitization-type reactions. Generally, the use of dextrose is preferred whenever possible; the only advantage of glucagon is that it can be given by routes of administration that are more convenient than the intravenous route required with dextrose. This may make it easier to teach members of the family to manage the patient who tends to suffer hypoglycemic reaction. Physicians may also sometimes find it more convenient to bring a psychiatric patient back to consciousness after he has insulin shock therapy, when his restlessness makes an I.V. injection difficult.

Dosage and Administration. A dose of 0.5 to 1 mg. is injected subcutaneously, intramuscularly, or intravenously in the form of a solution made by dissolving the lyophilized powder in the solvent that comes with it. This dose may be repeated at 20-minute intervals. When the patient regains consciousness after use of glucagon, he is given carbohydrates by mouth. The patient or family should always notify the physician of the occurrence of any hypoglycemic reaction, even when the patient recovered without medical aid.

INSULIN INJECTION U.S.P.
(REGULAR INSULIN; REGULAR ILETIN)

Pharmacology. This watery solution of the active antidiabetic principle of beef or pork pancreas is the most prompt acting of the available insulin preparations. It is suitable for use, alone or combined with modified insulins—with which it should never be confused—for initial control of all types of diabetes. Administered in individualized doses, this hormone helps the diabetic patient to utilize dietary carbohydrate and fat in a way that keeps his blood glucose concentration within normal limits and renders his urine free of sugar and of ketone bodies.

This form of insulin is often preferred for stabilizing newly diagnosed diabetes patients. Later, depending on the patient's response, one of the longer-acting modified insulin preparations may be substituted for the many frequent injections of regular insulin that may otherwise be required to achieve and maintain control; this rapid-acting form may then be reserved for only occasional use as a supplement when intermediate and long-acting insulin preparations do not give complete control.

Regular insulin is the preferred form for administration to patients with diabetic ketoacidosis including those in diabetic coma, because of the rapidity of its onset. In such cases, injections are made repeatedly in amounts adjusted in accordance with changes in the patient's blood sugar level in response to each previous dose. Frequent determinations of venous blood sugar avoids the danger of precipitating hypoglycemic reactions; it also aids in the early detection of patients who are relatively resistant to insulin.

Dosage and Administration. Dosage varies widely in amount and frequency of administration, depending on the patient's condition. The official usual dosage range is 5 to 100 U.S.P. units. This is ordinarily administered subcutaneously 15 to 30 minutes before meals. However, some patients in diabetic coma with circulatory collapse may have to receive regular insulin by the intravenous route to assure its absorption.

INSULIN ZINC SUSPENSION U.S.P.
(LENTE INSULIN; LENTE ILETIN)

Pharmacology. This suspension of tiny particles of zinc insulin has a length of antidiabetic action midway between that of regular insulin and protamine zinc insulin. (Its duration of action is almost identical with that of isophane insulin suspension, with which it usually can be used interchangeably). However, this form of insulin is not substituted for any other insulin preparation unless specified by the physician. This suspension is never given by vein.

Dosage and Administration. This form of insulin is usually given before breakfast, in which case it acts quickly enough to counteract the expected rise in blood sugar after that meal. The dosage, which in an average case is about 10 units to begin with, may be raised gradually in increments of 3 to 5 units, until one dose (up to 80 units) can control blood and urine sugar levels for a 24-hour period. While this is usually possible in most patients with maturity-onset diabetes—especially if the diet is adjusted as required—this single dose regimen may have to be supplemented with regular insulin or with the *prompt* insulin zinc suspension; others may require that a long-acting insulin be added to this intermediate-acting one to overcome a tendency toward rises in sugar levels during the night.

This preparation is stored in the refrigerator, but not in the freezer. It should not be shaken vigorously, but the colorless fluid and milky-white suspension should be mixed thoroughly by rotating the vial and inverting it several times from end to end to assure withdrawal of a uniform suspension of particles each time, thus avoiding irregularity in the effects of successive doses.

PHENFORMIN HYDROCHLORIDE (DBI)

Pharmacology. This oral hypoglycemic agent of the biguanide class differs chemically and in its manner of action from the sulfonylurea compounds. It does *not* stimulate pancreatic secretion of insulin but is thought to act on other tissues to step up their rate of glucose utilization. It has been suggested that it does so by increasing the anaerobic breakdown of glucose in a way that avoids fat synthesis. If proved true, this would make phenformin more preferable for treating *obese* diabetics than the sulfonylurea drugs, which, like insulin itself, tend to convert glucose into fat.

Phenformin is sometimes combined with one of the sulfonylurea compounds to control diabetes of the maturity-onset type, in patients who are not adequately managed with the latter drugs alone. It is occasionally used in *combination with insulin* to stabilize brittle *juvenile-onset* and other ketosis and hypoglycemia-prone labile patients. Although this sometimes permits some reduction in insulin dosage, phenformin never entirely does away with the need for insulin in such cases; and it is never used alone in the presence of diabetic complications.

Phenformin has not caused some of the sensitization type reactions seen with the sulfonylurea type hypoglycemic agents. However, G.I. side effects, including anorexia, nausea, an unpleasant bitter metallic taste, and occasional vomiting often occur and indicate that dosage should be reduced.

Dosage and Administration. A 25-mg. tablet is administered with meals from one to four times daily as needed, with a gradual increase in dosage in increments of 25 mg. if needed. A timed-disintegration 50-mg. capsule is also available, which need be given only once or twice daily with breakfast and with the evening meal for relatively prolonged action.

PROTAMINE ZINC INSULIN SUSPENSION U.S.P. (PROTAMINE, ZINC, AND ILETIN)

Pharmacology. This combination of insulin with zinc and with the protein protamine has a prolonged duration of action. Its effects come on only after many hours and may last for several days, in some cases, as the hormone continues to dissolve slowly and to enter the blood stream at a slight, steady rate from the deep subcutaneous or intramuscular depot site of administration.

This preparation is not used in diabetic emergencies, nor is it ever substituted for other insulin preparations except under the doctor's orders. This form of insulin is best for patients whose blood sugar begins to rise at night and stays high during sleep after having been kept at normal levels during the day by other shorter-acting preparations. However, it may have to be supplemented by injections of regular insulin for more rapid onset of antidiabetic activity. Sometimes an extemporaneously prepared mixture is prescribed in a ratio of about 1 unit of this preparation to 2 or 3 units of regular insulin. If hypoglycemia develops, it may be counteracted by administering a combination of a soluble, rapidly utilized source and a slowly digestible source of carbohydrate; treatment may have to be continued at intervals of an hour or two for quite some time.

Dosage and Administration. Ten to 80 units is usually injected before breakfast into the loose tissue beneath the skin of an arm, leg, or the abdomen. (It is injected intramuscularly only when directed by the doctor, and is not injected by vein). The doctor regulates the diet carefully, attempting to balance the intake of food in terms of the prolonged effect of this insulin preparation.

TOLBUTAMIDE U.S.P. (ORINASE)

Pharmacology. This sulfonylurea compound is the oral hypoglycemic agent concerning which the largest amount of clinical experience has accumulated. It is most useful in mild, stable diabetes of the maturity-onset type; and it is contraindicated in the growth-onset type of diabetes or in any case that is complicated by ketoacidosis or coma. Tolbutamide controls glycosuria and prevents polyuria by stimulating the beta cells of the pancreas to release increased amounts of endogenous insulin. If this source of the hormone is missing, as is the case in the juvenile type of diabetes, this drug is ineffective.

Hypoglycemia rarely occurs with tolbutamide, but patients with hepatic and renal disorders are sometimes prone to suffer hypoglycemic reactions; so this drug should probably not be used in patients with a history of liver disease and severe renal insufficiency. Liver function is tested at the beginning of treatment and at intervals during drug therapy.

Toxicity is rare with tolbutamide despite its chemical relationship to sulfonamides known to cause blood dyscrasias and jaundice. G.I. disturbances, headache, and allergic skin reactions, usually of a transient nature, occur in a small percentage of cases and are rarely severe or persistent enough to warrant withdrawal of the drug.

Dosage and Administration. The usual dosage range is 500 mg. to 2 Gm. daily. However, dosage is determined individually for each patient, until the lowest amount that maintains control is established.

Tolbutamide is ordinarily administered alone and *not* together with insulin, for the drug's main advantage is that it does away with the need for daily insulin injections in properly selected patients. (Rarely, patients who are highly resistant to insulin receive tolbutamide in an attempt to lessen their unusual insulin requirements.) Tolbutamide is not uncommonly combined with phenformin to bring about better control than with either drug alone in selected patients.

The sodium salt of tolbutamide is given by vein in a dose of 1 Gm. for diagnostic purposes.

CHAPTER 34

ANTIBIOTIC DRUGS

AMPHOTERICIN B, U.S.P. (FUNGIZONE)

Pharmacology. This antibiotic is often applied topically or administered orally in the treatment and prevention of moniliasis, in the manner described for nystatin. Its use by intravenous injection against various *systemic* fungal infections is of greater significance, however, for it is one of the few agents that are effective for treating such potentially fatal infections. Among the disseminated mycotic infections in which it is employed are: blastomycosis, coccidiomycosis, cryptococcosis, histoplasmosis, leishmaniasis, and candidiasis.

Adverse effects are common, and patients are observed closely to prevent severe toxicity. Anorexia, nausea, vomiting, headache, chills, and fever are frequent early in treatment, but may be minimized by prior administration of aspirin, antihistamines, and antiemetics. Check patients carefully for rises in blood urea nitrogen (BUN) and nonprotein nitrogen (NPN), which indicate the need to interrupt therapy. Kidney, liver, and bone marrow studies are done during long-term therapy, for renal and hepatic failure and anemia have occurred in some cases.

Dosage and Administration. A solution prepared by dissolving a sterile powder in Sterile Water for Injection U.S.P., and dilution with 5% Dextrose Injection U.S.P., is infused slowly by vein over a 6-hour period. The initial daily dose of 0.25 mg./Kg. may be raised gradually to higher levels, provided no toxic effects occur. A total daily dose of 1.0 mg./Kg. is the usual maintenance dose; and while this may be exceeded in severely ill patients, no more than 1.5 mg./Kg. daily is ever employed. Solutions are prepared freshly, protected from light during the infusion, and discarded if a precipitate appears.

BACITRACIN U.S.P. (BACIGUENT, ETC.)

Pharmacology. This antibiotic and zinc bacitracin are commonly employed in ointments for topical application in infections by staphylococci and other gram-positive organisms. Its main advantage over other antibiotics is the rarity with which its use is followed by sensitization and allergic skin rashes. Applied alone or combined with neomycin, polymyxin, tyrothricin, or other agents, it is used in the local treatment of skin ulcers, wounds, impetigo, infected eczema, boils, and pyoderma.

Bacitracin is rarely administered for treating systemic infections because of the availability of safer antibiotics. If it must be used to treat an infection by an organism that is susceptible to it but resistant to other agents, the patient's kidney function is tested often. While proteinuria and hematuria are almost inevitable with its continued administration, the drug need be withdrawn only if signs of renal insufficiency appear.

Dosage and Administration. For topical application to the skin and eye, ointments are available; a powder is used for preparing solutions for injection and for instillation after surgery in osteomyelitis. Bacitracin has long been a common ingredient of troches for use as sore throat remedies. The daily dose by the intramuscular route is 30,000 to 100,000 units daily.

BENZATHINE PENICILLIN G, U.S.P. (BICILLIN)

Pharmacology. This penicillin salt is poorly soluble in water and only slowly absorbable from intramuscular injection sites. This accounts for the long duration of its action (1 to 4 weeks) and the relatively low blood and tissue levels attained when it is administered by this route. Orally administered in adequate amounts, therapeutically effective levels are attained and maintained for up to 8 hours.

This is a preferred form of penicillin for prophylaxis against infection by susceptible organisms in patients with a history of rheumatic fever, especially prior to tonsillectomy and tooth extractions. It is effective against infections by hemolytic streptococci, gonococci, the spirochete of syphilis, etc.

Dosage and Administration. Dosage and frequency of administration vary widely depending on the nature of the clinical situation. A single injection of 600,000 to 1.2 million units may be administered intramuscularly every 2 to 4 weeks to prevent rheumatic fever recurrences. In severe infections, a similar parenteral dose may be administered every other day, or initial injections of 600,000 units may be supplemented by 200,000 unit oral doses every 8 hours.

CHLORAMPHENICOL U.S.P. (CHLOROMYCETIN)

Pharmacology. This broad-spectrum antibiotic is effective against a greater variety of organisms than any other agent, except the tetracyclines. Unfortunately, its clinical utility for treating infection is limited by its potential lethal toxicity in a small but significant number of patients. Because of the possibility of blood dyscrasias following its use, chloramphenicol is reserved for treating certain serious infections by organisms that are resistant to less dangerous drugs, or in individuals who are allergic to other effective drugs.

Among the infections for which chloramphenicol is indicated are typhoid fever, the various types of typhus fevers and other rickettsial diseases, and such illnesses as staphylococcal pneumonia, *Haemophilus influenzae* meningitis, and other miscellaneous infections in which the strain of organisms has been shown by prior testing to be highly susceptible to chloramphenicol. Frequent blood studies are made to detect any changes in cell counts and hemoglobin. The drug is discontinued at the first sign of adverse hematological reactions.

Dosage and Administration. A total daily dosage of 50 mg./Kg. body weight produces blood levels of chloramphenicol that are adequate for treating most infections in adult patients. More severe infections may require 100 mg./Kg. a day for a time. For premature and newborn infants, treatment is initiated with only 25 mg./Kg. and is raised to as much as 50 mg. only after the first 2 weeks of life. The total daily dosage is divided into four equal amounts administered every 6 hours.

For parenteral administration to pediatric patients, chloramphenicol sodium succinate is the preferred form. Chloramphenicol palmitate, a tasteless preparation, is employed in the form of a suspension administered by mouth to children and others. Ophthalmic ointments and suspensions are available for topical treatment of ocular infections.

ERYTHROMYCIN AND ITS ESTERS U.S.P. (ERYTHROCIN; ILOTYCIN)

Pharmacology. This antibiotic has a bacterial spectrum similar to that of penicillin. It is used mainly in patients allergic to penicillin who require treatment for infections such as streptococcal pharyngitis, pneumococcal pneumonia or meningitis, gonorrhea, and syphilis. Although it is sometimes effective against some strains of staphylococci resistant to penicillin G, it is rarely used any longer for treating such infections. This is because doctors generally prefer one of the semi-synthetic penicillinase-resistant penicillins to this antibiotic, against which many strains of hospital staph have acquired resistance.

Except for local irritation in the G.I. tract and at intramuscular injection sites, erythromycin base causes few adverse effects. However, hepatic hypersensitivity reactions have been reported following the use of erythromycin *estolate*. Patients who take this form of the drug for 10 days or more are observed for abdominal complaints, fever, and, finally, jaundice. This derivative should not be used in patients with a history of liver disorders, for it, itself, can cause cholestatic hepatitis.

Dosage and Administration. Adult dosage ranges from 1 Gm. daily to as much as 4 Gm. in severe infections, administered orally or parenterally in several divided doses. Several salts and esters are available for various purposes, including increased palatability when used in lower dosage in drops, etc., for children, and for greater ease in injecting. Erythromycin gluceptate and lactobionate are administered intravenously. The latter drug and the ethylsuccinate derivative may also be administered intramuscularly. However, the ethylsuccinate, like the ethylcarbonate, stearate, and estolate derivatives, is administered mainly by mouth. Attempts are made to protect the base from breakdown by stomach acids. Erythromycin estolate seems least likely to be destroyed in this way, and it is well absorbed, even in the presence of food.

GRISEOFULVIN U.S.P. (FULVICIN U/F; GRIFULVIN V; GRISACTIN)

Pharmacology. This antibiotic, taken internally, reaches skin keratin by way of the bloodstream to exert an antifungal effect against species responsible for superficial infections of the scalp, feet, fingernails, hands, beard, etc. In some cases of ringworm and athlete's foot, inflammation and itching are relieved in a few days. Other conditions, including those involving the nails, may require many months of treatment.

Side effects include epigastric discomfort, heartburn, diarrhea, and headache early in the course of treatment. More serious adverse effects such as symptoms of skin allergy are relatively rare. However, patients who take griseofulvin for long periods are closely observed for signs of chronic toxicity, including impairment of motor coordination and leukopenia. Although the reduced numbers of white blood cells ordinarily return to normal, complete periodic blood counts are recommended, and patients are watched also for clinical signs indicative of blood dyscrasia (e.g., sore throat and fever).

Dosage and Administration. Griseofulvin is taken in tablet form or as a suspension in daily doses of 0.5 to 1 Gm. for several weeks. The microsized particle powder now available, which is more readily absorbed from the intestinal tract, often permits control of fungal infections with doses at the lower end of this range. However, higher doses may be required for more severe infections, just as the duration of treatment may be much longer —many months to a year or more—for infections in locations such as the toenails. Doses are adjusted downward for children.

NEOMYCIN SULFATE U.S.P. (MYCIFRADIN, ETC.)

Pharmacology. This antibiotic is active against a wide variety of gram-positive and gram-negative bacteria. Unfortunately, its toxicity upon systemic administration is so high that it is administered by injection only in severe infections that are not susceptible to treatment with other anti-infective agents.

When taken by mouth, its poor absorption prevents neomycin from attaining blood levels that are either toxic or effective against systemic infections. Instead, when administered orally, the drug attains high local concentrations in the gut. This alters bowel flora, which is considered desirable in the management of hepatic coma and for sterilization of the G.I. tract prior to bowel surgery.

Neomycin is probably most widely used in a great variety of topical preparations for treating infections of the skin, eye, and ear. Used in this manner, it rarely causes sensitization or allergic skin rashes.

Neomycin, which is nephrotoxic, is especially dangerous in patients with renal insufficiency. In such cases, the antibiotic is not excreted and accumulates to levels that damage the auditory nerve and cause deafness. Thus, patients who receive neomycin by injection are hospitalized and are closely followed by audiometry and by tests of renal function.

Dosage and Administration. Neomycin is most commonly applied topically in ointment form for treating bacterial infection in skin wounds, ulcers and burns, and in the eye. The daily oral dose for local action in the gut is 4 to 8 Gm. It is injected intramuscularly for severe infections by susceptible organisms in doses of 0.25 Gm. every 6 hours, or a total of no more than 1 Gm. daily in most cases.

NYSTATIN U.S.P. (MYCOSTATIN)

Pharmacology. This antifungal antibiotic is used to treat and prevent moniliasis of the skin and the mucous membranes of the mouth, vagina, and G.I. tract. Applied topically, nystatin specifically eradicates yeasts and fungi, including *Candida albicans,* without affecting other organisms of the microbial flora. Thus, superinfection is not a problem, and the only side effects are occasional mild symptoms of G.I. upset when the drug is taken orally in large doses.

Dosage and Administration. Nystatin is taken orally in doses of 500,000 units three times a day for the treatment of intestinal moniliasis. It is combined with broad-spectrum tetracyclines in an effort to *prevent* monilial superinfections by overgrowths of *Candida* in case of alteration of the intestinal flora by the antibacterial antibiotic. This prophylactic effort against fungal overgrowths may be particularly desirable in patients with diabetes, lymphoma, or leukemia, or in those being treated with corticosteroids for systemic lupus, since the defenses of such patients against fungal invaders are lowered.

Since nystatin is not absorbed when taken by mouth, it is applied locally to attain adequate concentrations in areas other than the G.I. tract. Thus, for vaginal moniliasis, tablets containing 100,000 or 200,000 units are inserted intravaginally twice daily. For treating monilial stomatitis, or thrush, 1 cc. of a suspension (100,000 units) is dropped into the mouth four times daily. A powder is applied directly to *Candida* skin lesions of the feet; a cream is applies to intertriginous areas; and an ointment containing nystatin is used on rashes of the vulvar and anal regions.

POLYMYXIN B SULFATE U.S.P. (AEROSPORIN)

Pharmacology. This is the least toxic of a group of related polypeptide antibiotics obtained from a soil bacillus, *B. polymyxa.* Although its spectrum is relatively narrow, only gram-negative organisms being affected, polymyxin is valued as one of a very few antibiotics that can inhibit *Pseudomonas aeruginosa* strains.

This antibiotic is used mainly in ointment form, alone or combined with bacitracin and neomycin for a broadened antibacterial spectrum, in the treatment of skin, ear, and eye infections. It is only occasionally administered orally for treating G.I. infections by susceptible organisms. Administered intramuscularly, polymyxin is often valuable in urinary tract, pulmonary, and bloodstream infections causes by *Pseudomonas* and other gram-negative bacteria that are resistant to the tetracyclines and other safer antibiotics.

Injections are frequently followed by persistent local pain. Relatively low blood levels are accompanied by varied systemic side effects and by signs of nephrotoxicity. Patients with renal insufficiency require only low doses; ordinary doses are likely to accumulate in the tissues to cause neurotoxicity.

Dosage and Administration. Polymyxin B sulfate is administered intramuscularly in amounts not exceeding 200 mg. daily; ordinarily, a total dose of 1.5 to 2.5 mg./Kg. is injected in three divided doses, equally spaced over a 24-hour period. In meningitis caused by susceptible organisms, 5 mg., intrathecally, is the average adult total dose. The oral dose is 300 to 400 mg. daily, divided into four equal parts. Topical administration in ointment form is most common, but solutions are sometimes prepared for use as sprays, wet packs, and irrigation.

POTASSIUM PENICILLIN G, U.S.P. (PENTIDS; DRAMCILLIN; ETC.)

Pharmacology. This least expensive form of the antibiotic is considered suitable for the prophylaxis and treatment of infections caused by most penicillin-susceptible organisms. These include gram-positive organisms such as the hemolytic streptococcal strains responsible for most bacterial infections of the upper respiratory tract, pneumococci, and certain *non*-penicillinase-producing strains of staphylococci. Although most gram-negative organisms are affected only by high doses, if at all, penicillin is clinically effective against most infections caused by meningococci and gonococci. The spirochete of syphilis is also readily susceptible to treatment with adequate doses of parenteral penicillin.

Although penicillin G is a drug of very low direct tissue toxicity, sensitivity reactions of varying degrees of severity commonly occur with its use, especially by parenteral administration. Since such allergic reactions are more likely to occur in patients with a history of allergy, patients should be questioned regarding their susceptibility, and the drug withheld from those with previous hypersensitivity reactions to penicillin. The drug is ordinarily discontinued if reactions develop during treatment.

Dosage and Administration. Dosage varies widely, depending on the type and severity of infection. The official oral or intramuscular dose is 400,000 units (250 mg.) every 6 hours, but dosage is best adjusted to individual needs and may vary from as little as 200,000 units (125 mg.) daily by mouth for preventing streptococcal infections in children with a history of rheumatic fever, to as much as 80 million units a day intravenously in patients with severe infections. (The parenteral route is always employed in treating meningitis, syphilis, subacute bacterial endocarditis, etc.; and administration is continued until the acute condition is controlled and blood cultures become negative.)

SODIUM METHICILLIN U.S.P.
(DIMOCILLIN-RT; STAPHCILLIN)

Pharmacology. This semisynthetic penicillin is highly effective against strains of staphylococci that produce penicillinase, an enzyme that inactivates natural penicillins G and V. It is less effective than the latter penicillins in infections caused by other organisms, including streptococci, pneumococci and *non*-penicillinase-producing staphylococci, and, consequently, should not be used in such cases. Among the resistant staph infections that often do respond to this antibiotic are lobar or bronchial pneumonia and lung abscesses, septicemia, endocarditis, osteomyelitis, and infections of the skin and soft tissues.

Dosage and Administration. Methicillin is instable in stomach acids and poorly absorbed from the intestine, so it is administered parenterally. It is injected intramuscularly every 4 to 6 hours in relatively high doses (1 to 1.5 Gm.). Because intramuscular injections are somewhat painful, the I.V. route is often preferred, in which case, 1 Gm. is injected slowly in the form of a freshly prepared dilute solution (50 ml. in 5 minutes) every 6 hours.

SODIUM OXACILLIN U.S.P.
(PROSTAPHLIN; RESISTOPEN)

Pharmacology. This semisynthetic penicillin is useful against infections by staphylococcal strains resistant to penicillin G or V. Its molecule resists destruction, not only by bacterial penicillinase, but also by stomach acids. Thus, it is effective orally as well as parenterally. It may be used to begin treatment in various skin, soft tissue, and respiratory infections believed to be caused by resistant staph organisms, but should be discontinued in favor of penicillin G if sensitivity tests prove the organism to be susceptible to treatment with that natural penicillin.

Allergic reactions typical of other penicillin products have occurred with sodium oxacillin, especially in patients with a history of previous hypersensitivity to penicillin. The drug should be discontinued if such reactions or superinfections by *non*-susceptible microorganisms are seen to develop.

Dosage and Administration. The oral form should be taken on an empty stomach, 1 or 2 hours before meals, for maximal absorption. Oral dosage of 500 mg. every 4 to 6 hours is recommended for mild staph infections, and 1 Gm. for more severe infections. For staphylococcal septicemia or other deep-seated infections, doses of 500 to 1,000 mg. may be administered by intramuscular or slow intravenous injection, although initial therapy with sodium methicillin is usually preferred for such cases.

TETRACYCLINE HYDROCHLORIDE U.S.P.
(ACHROMYCIN V; PANMYCIN;
POLYCYCLINE; STECLIN; TETRACYN)

Pharmacology. This broad-spectrum antibiotic exerts its bacteriostatic action on a wide variety of microorganisms, including not only the common gram-positive and gram-negative bacteria, but also rickettsiae and certain so-called large viruses. It does not affect the small, or true, viruses, nor the pathogenic fungi. Superinfections may occur as the result of overgrowth of *non*-susceptible organisms such as species of *Candida*, *Proteus*, *Pseudomonas*, and resistant staphylococci.

Tetracycline is not ordinarily used for treating infections caused by organisms that are also sensitive to penicillin. However, when administered as a second choice for patients who are allergic to penicillin, it is active against the gram-positive bacteria responsible for common respiratory tract infections, and it is effective against gonorrhea and syphilis. Tetracycline is probably most useful in infections by organisms that are either not susceptible to other available anti-infective agents or are controllable only by more or less toxic doses of other drugs.

Tetracycline is, itself, a relatively safe antibiotic when used in ordinary doses; and most side effects can be minimized by reducing the dose. However, hypersensitivity reactions (e.g., photodermatitis), signs and symptoms of superinfection (e.g., glossitis, stomatitis, proctitis, vaginitis), and, occasionally, true toxicity (e.g., liver damage), do occur, making it necessary to discontinue the drug.

Dosage and Administration. Tetracycline is available in many dosage forms. One gram a day, divided into four 250 mg. doses, is the average amount for most infections in adults. This may have to be doubled in acute illnesses, in which case tetracycline is sometimes administered parenterally. In such cases, blood levels are determined, because the accumulation of excessively large amounts—in the presence of renal dysfunction, for example—may lead to liver failure.

VANCOMYCIN HYDROCHLORIDE U.S.P.
(VANCOCIN)

Pharmacology. This bactericidal antibiotic is effective against the same kinds of gram-positive cocci that ordinarily respond to penicillin, and against some strains of these bacteria that resist penicillin. It is reserved for patients with severe penicillin-resistant staph or nonhemolytic (Group D, etc.) streptococcal infections. However, cephalothin is often preferred for such cases, because it is less toxic than vancomycin. Similarly, in less severe infections of patients allergic to penicillin, the less toxic antibiotics erythromycin, oleandomycin, and lincomycin are ordinarily considered more desirable than this one.

Vancomycin is used cautiously in patients with any kidney complications that might interfere with its renal excretion. If it piles up in the blood and tissues, it may damage the auditory nerve enough to cause deafness. Thus, kidney function and hearing are checked often during long-term treatment. Skin rashes and anaphylactoid reactions are reported occasionally.

Dosage and Administration. A dilute solution of vancomycin is injected intravenously in doses of 1 Gm. every 8 to 12 hours, or 500 mg. every 6 hours. Slow infusion for 20 to 30 minutes is preferred, for it is less likely to cause pain and thrombophlebitis than the more rapid injection of more concentrated solutions. Vancomycin, which is poorly absorbed from the G.I. tract, has recently been given by the oral route in doses of 0.5 to 1 Gm. every 6 hours for its local action in treating staphylococcal enterocolitis.

CHAPTER 35

THE SULFONAMIDES AND OTHER CHEMOTHERAPEUTIC AGENTS

AMINOSALICYLIC ACID U.S.P.
(PARA-AMINOSALICYLIC ACID; PAS)

Pharmacology. This substance, and its salts and derivatives, are of value in tuberculosis when combined with isoniazid, streptomycin, or other tuberculostatic drugs. Although it is itself a relatively weak bacteriostatic agent, combined with other agents it produces added activity against the organism and slows the rate at which resistant strains tend to emerge.

The main side effects are the result of irritation of the G.I. tract and include a feeling of fullness, pressure, or pain in the upper abdomen, anorexia, nausea, vomiting, cramps, and diarrhea. These may be reduced somewhat by administering divided doses of the drug after meals or with antacid-adsorbent drugs. Its use in patients with peptic ulcer is contraindicated, and it is withdrawn if gastric bleeding or other indications of developing ulceration occur.

Other types of toxicity may result from hypersensitivity or as a result of a direct action on the liver or thyroid gland. Goiter may develop during prolonged use as a result of damage to the thyroid; thyroxine may then be required to counteract myxedema. The main types of sensitivity reaction reported may involve the skin, blood-forming organs, and nervous system. High fever and skin eruptions may require withdrawal of the drug to prevent more serious reactions, including fatal blood dyscrasias and liver damage.

Dosage and Administration. A daily dose of 12 Gm. is usually administered in four equally divided doses after meals. Sodium, potassium, and calcium salts as well as the phenyl ester and an amide derivative are available for oral administration. All are claimed to cause less local (G.I.) irritation.

DAPSONE U.S.P. (AVLOSULFON; DDS)

Pharmacology. This sulfone derivative has bacteriostatic and antiprotozoal properties that have led to its experimental use for suppressing tuberculosis and malaria infections, among others. Most important, it is a leprostatic agent in the control of leprosy, or Hansen's disease. Administered over long periods, dapsone gradually brings about variable degrees of improvement in most leprous patients. New lesions do not develop during treatment, and healing of skin nodules is adequate enough to make possible the return of some patients to their communities.

Toxicity is related to dosage and the subsequent blood levels of dapsone. Side effects of low doses affect mainly the G.I. tract (anorexia, nausea, and vomiting) and the central nervous system (headache, nervousness, sleeplessness). More serious are effects on the circulating red blood cells, resulting in methemoglobinemia and hemolytic anemia. These untoward effects are less likely to occur if dosage is built up gradually, and blood levels of the drug are checked periodically to avoid cumulation of the slowly excreted drug to toxic levels.

Dosage and Administration. Initially, dapsone is administered in oral doses of 25 to 50 mg. twice a week for 4 or 5 weeks. It is then increased by 100 mg. at monthly intervals until a maximum dose of 400 mg. two times a week is reached. Doses of 100 to 200 mg. daily are occasionally employed to suppress acute flare-ups of dermatitis herpetiformis.

ISONIAZID U.S.P. (ISONICOTINIC ACID HYDRAZIDE; INH, ETC.)

Pharmacology. This is the most valuable chemotherapeutic agent against tuberculosis. Yet, it is rarely used alone, but is, instead, ordinarily combined with para-aminosalicylic acid (PAS) or streptomycin. These drugs delay the emergence of strains insensitive to INH, and streptomycin synergizes its tuberculostatic activity. The addition of PAS does not significantly add to the suppressive effect of INH, but besides delaying the rate of development of INH-resistant strains, it slows the rate of metabolic conversion of INH to inactive metabolites. This allows higher concentrations of free, active INH to remain in the tissues for longer periods.

Isoniazid causes a variety of autonomic blockade-type side effects, including mouth dryness, constipation, and urinary retention, especially when its dose is raised to maintain tuberculostatic activity against increasingly resistant organisms or in severe infections. Potentially most serious is toxicity to peripheral nerves and the C.N.S. Neurotoxicity may be manifested by paresthesias and pain; optic neuritis with visual disturbances; headache, ataxia, drowsiness and dizziness; muscular twitching,

hyperreflexia, and convulsions. These may be minimized by daily administration of pyridoxine (Vitamin B6). However, special caution is required in patients with a history of epilepsies to avoid increasing the frequency of seizures. Caution is required in patients with a history of psychosis, as the drug sometimes produces mental symptoms.

Dosage and Administration. The usual daily dose is 150 mg. administered orally twice daily. However, dosage may range from 5 to 15 mg./Kg. body weight daily, depending on the type and severity of the tuberculous infection. Isoniazid may be administered parenterally in dosages usually of 300 to 1000 mg. daily.

METHENAMINE MANDELATE U.S.P. (MANDELAMINE)

Pharmacology. This salt of the urinary antiseptics methenamine and mandelic acid breaks down to these compounds in the urinary tract. The methenamine component is converted to formaldehyde in the urine acidified by the mandelic acid. This results in continuous lavage of the urinary tract surfaces by a bactericidal solution that is often effective against organisms resistant to sulfonamides. Unlike sulfonamides, methenamine mandelate rarely causes allergic sensitization. Thus, it is advocated for use in chronic urinary tract infections that require long-term therapy. Side effects are largely limited to occasional G.I. upset, but the drug is contraindicated in moderately severe renal insufficiency.

Dosage and Administration. The average adult dose is 1 Gm. four times daily, alone or combined with antibiotics or with sulfonamides which do not require an alkaline urine. For example, this drug has been combined with sulfamethizole which acts within the urinary tract tissues that cannot be penetrated by this drug.

NITROFURANTOIN U.S.P. (FURADANTIN)

Pharmacology. This furan derivative is used in the treatment of urinary tract infections by a wide range of organisms, including certain strains of gram-negative bacteria resistant to sulfonamides. Bacterial resistance develops only slowly to this bactericidal drug, and crystalluria is unlikely because of its high solubility in urine.

Side effects are ordinarily limited to nausea and vomiting in a few patients and to allergic reactions which usually take the form of skin rashes. A few cases of hemolytic anemia have been reported in patients whose red cells are hypersusceptible to various drugs including the sulfonamides as well as the furans. The drug is administered only with caution to patients with renal insufficiency, for failure to excrete it may result in its accumulation to toxic levels. Peripheral neuritis has been reported in some patients following continued administration of nitrofurantoin in such circumstances.

Dosage and Administration. The oral dosage for most cases of pyelonephritis, pyelitis, cystitis, and prostatitis is 100 mg. four times daily, taken with meals or with milk or food at bedtime. Administration is continued for at least 3 days after the urine becomes sterile. Ordinarily, the drug is given in courses of 10 to 14 days followed by a rest period, but treatment is sometimes continued for longer periods with fractions of the full dose. A soluble sodium salt of nitrofurantoin may be administered intravenously when administration of the oral tablets or suspension is not feasible. For most patients the recommended dose of 180 mg. is infused twice daily by I.V. drip of 500 ml. of solution at a rate of 60 drops/minute.

STREPTOMYCIN SULFATE U.S.P.

Pharmacology. This antibiotic is employed in combination with other antibiotic and chemotherapeutic agents in order to

reduce the rate at which resistant strains of previously susceptible tubercle and gram-negative bacilli emerge when this drug is
given alone. In tuberculosis, streptomycin is commonly combined with isoniazid or with para-aminosalicylic acid; in urinary
tract infections, it may be combined with chloramphenicol,
tetracycline, or a sulfonamide. A streptomycin-sulfonamide
combination may be best for meningitis caused by certain gram-
negative bacteria; and combinations with penicillin are
employed in mixed infections of the respiratory tract.

The most common adverse effect of streptomycin in patients
who receive large doses for long periods is damage to the eighth
cranial nerve. Most commonly, vertigo occurs as a result of
vestibular dysfunction; hearing difficulties leading to deafness
may also develop. Allergic reactions of various kinds sometimes
occur, both in patients and medical personnel frequently
exposed to this drug. Injections are painful, and inflammatory
reactions common.

Dosage and Administration. Streptomycin is most commonly
administered by deep intramuscular injection. For acute infections, 1 Gm. may be injected every 12 hours for about 1 week to
control the condition rapidly, before resistance develops. Dosage schedules for tuberculosis vary. Some specialists employ 1
Gm. once a day; others advocate use of that amount only twice a
week. Sometimes the drug is given at the more frequent rate
early in treatment and, later, less frequently. Dosage varies also
depending on the location of the tuberculous process.

SUCCINYLSULFATHIAZOLE U.S.P.
(SULFASUXIDINE)

Pharmacology. This poorly absorbable sulfonamide concentrates in the intestinal tract, where it inhibits the growth of
coliform bacteria. It is used before bowel surgery to reduce the
danger of secondary infections, such as peritonitis, that might
occur as a result of contamination. It has been employed for
prophylaxis and treatment of bacillary dysentery. However, an
increasing number of *Shigella* strains are proving resistant to
sulfonamides, and, in any case, soluble sulfonamides, such as
sulfadiazine, which are excreted through the bowel wall, are
preferred for treating actual infections. This drug is sometimes
used in the management of nonspecific ulcerative colitis as an
adjunct to dietary and supportive measures, but its benefits are
usually transient.

Systemic toxicity is uncommon, because the small amounts of
sulfathiazole that are absorbed are readily excreted. However,
caution is required in patients with liver or kidney damage or
urinary tract obstruction, and use of the drug is contraindicated
in patients with abdominal obstruction. Typical sulfonamide
hypersensitivity reactions, including various blood dyscrasias,
have occurred with the use of these drugs. Patients require blood
counts as well as kidney and liver function tests periodically.

Dosage and Administration. The average adult dose is 1 Gm.
every 4 hours. A dosage based on body weight is also recommended: 0.25 Gm./Kg. followed by the same amount divided
into six daily doses during maintenance therapy. Antibiotics
such as neomycin are sometimes administered simultaneously in
conjunction with a low residue diet.

SULFADIAZINE U.S.P.

Pharmacology. This sulfonamide is used alone and combined
with sulfamerazine and sulfamethazine, or with such antibiotics
as the penicillins, erythromycin, streptomycin, and chloromycetin in the treatment of infections caused by susceptible bacteria.
These include urinary tract infections by *E. Coli;* meningitis
caused by the meningococcus or by *Hemophilus influenzae;* and
bacillary dysentery by sensitive strains of *Shigella.* The drug is
also used for *prevention* of G.I. infections; for prophylaxis
against meningococcal meningitis in contacts; and for prevention
of streptococcal infections in patients sensitive to penicillin.

Sulfadiazine is readily absorbed from the G.I. tract and distributed into all tissues, including the cerebrospinal fluid. It
becomes highly concentrated in the urine in a short time. These
levels of sulfadiazine in the urine can kill sulfonamide-suscepti-
ble organisms. However, it is important to force fluids in order to
dilute the urinary concentration of the drug and of its acetyl
derivative, both of which are poorly soluble in acid urine. Alkali
may be administered with each dose to alkalinize the urine and
thus increase the solubility of the drug and its metabolite, in
order to avoid crystalluria. Fractional doses of sulfadiazine and of
the other sulfapyrimidines, sulfamerazine and sulfamethazine,
produce a full antibacterial effect with lessened likelihood of
precipitation in the urinary tract.

Sulfadiazine may cause all the types of toxicity known to occur
with sulfonamide therapy; so all the usual precautions with
sulfonamide therapy are taken.

Dosage and Administration. Administered alone, an initial oral
dose of 4 Gm. is followed by 1 Gm. every 4 hours. When
combined with the other sulfapyrimidines, only one third this
amount of sulfadiazine is administered, but the total dose of the
trisulfapyrimidines is the same—a 4-Gm. priming dose followed
by a 1-Gm. maintenance dose.

SULFAMETHOXYPYRIDAZINE
(KYNEX; MIDICEL)

Pharmacology. This unusually long-acting sulfonamide seems
especially suited for treatment of conditions that require
prolonged sulfonamide therapy and for long-term prophylaxis
against streptococcal infections in patients with a history of
rheumatic fever. Among the disorders in which the long-range
suppressive effects of this slowly excreted sulfonamide are sometimes considered especially desirable are the eye infection
trachoma; dermatologic disorders including acne and dermatitis
herpetiformis; and chronic urinary tract infections. The drug is
said to benefit some patients with leprosy.

Although this drug's slow rate of excretion makes crystalluria
unlikely, the difficulty in clearing it from the body if a sulfonamide reaction develops is a disadvantage. Thus, the severity of
the Stevens-Johnson syndrome and other adverse reactions in
hypersensitive individuals may become irreversible even after
the drug is discontinued. In any case, the drug is withdrawn
immediately if a skin eruption develops.

Dosage and Administration. One gram is administered to
adults to initiate therapy, and is followed by 0.5 Gm. once daily
thereafter. Fluid intake is maintained at adequate levels during
treatment and for at least 24 to 48 hours after the drug is discontinued. If larger doses—for example, 2 Gm., then 1 Gm.
daily—are required for severe infections, blood levels of sulfonamide are checked after 3 days of treatment to avoid toxicity.

SULFISOXAZOLE U.S.P. (GANTRISIN)

Pharmacology. This sulfonamide is highly soluble in body
fluids, including urine of normal acidity. Thus, it is less likely
than sulfadiazine to cause crystalluria and such complications as
hematuria and anuria. However, patients should drink enough
water to assure formation of a large volume of urine, in which the
high concentrations of sulfisoxazole excreted by the kidneys
remain dissolved.

Sulfisoxazole is advocated not only for urinary tract infections
such as cystitis, urethritis, prostatitis, and pyelonephritis, but
also for respiratory infections such as pharyngitis, tonsillitis,
otitis, and pneumonia, caused by susceptible organisms including Group A beta hemolytic streptococci, and for wound infections and meningitis. All the usual precautions required in
sulfonamide therapy are observed. This drug is contraindicated
in patients known to be sensitive to other sulfonamides.

Dosage and Administration. Sulfisoxazole is administered
orally in a loading dose of 4 Gm. that is followed every 4 hours by

a maintenance dose of 1 Gm. Acetyl sulfisoxazole is a tasteless form of the drug suitable for use in flavored suspensions and syrups for pediatric patients; it is available in a long-acting homogenized vegetable oil mixture. The diethanolamine salt of sulfisoxazole is a 40% solution for parenteral administration in the usual therapeutic doses. A 10% sulfisoxazole cream is used intravaginally to control bacterial infections and for prophylaxis in postoperative and postpartum patients.

CHAPTER 36

THE CHEMOTHERAPY OF MALARIA AND OTHER PARASITIC INFECTIONS

CHLOROQUINE PHOSPHATE U.S.P. (ARALEN)

Pharmacology. This chemical of the 4-aminoquinoline class of synthetic successors to quinine is the drug most widely used for *suppressive treatment* of malaria and for effecting the *clinical cure* of an acute attack. It acts as a schizonticide in the blood against the erythrocytic forms of the asexual stages in the life cycle of *Plasmodium vivax* and *P. falciparum*. Infections by susceptible strains of *P. falciparum* are usually cured. However, chloroquine does not keep patients with *P. vivax* and similar malarias from relapsing later, as it does not act against the secondary tissue forms of these plasmodia.

Side effects rarely occur with the low dose of chloroquine that is needed for suppressive effects. With the large loading dose given to initiate treatment of an acute ·attack, epigastric discomfort and headache may occur, and as additional doses are administered for aborting the attack, the patient may also complain of pruritus, blurring of vision as a result of disturbances of accommodation, and diarrhea. These adverse effects pass quickly, once the treatment of the malarial attack is completed.

Much more serious toxicity may occur in the prolonged employment of chloroquine for treating chronic diseases such as rheumatoid arthritis and discoid lupus erythematosus. These include possible blindness as a result of irreversible retinal damage, blood dyscrasias, and lichenoid skin eruptions. The drug is contraindicated in patients with psoriasis, as it may set off the acute, progressive phase of that disease. Accidental overdosage in children and massive ingestion by suicidal patients has resulted in cardiac arrest, circulatory collapse, convulsions, and death. Thus, chloroquine should be stored where it cannot be reached by children or depressed patients.

Dosage and Administration. A once-weekly oral dose of 500 mg. is adequate for *suppressive therapy*. It is administered as long as the person remains in the malarious region and for 4 weeks after he leaves the area in which the disease is endemic.

For *clinical cure* of an acute malarial attack, an initial dose of 1 Gm. is followed by 500 mg. in 6 hours and by additional doses of 500 mg. on the second and third treatment days. These may be given with meals to allay gastric distress.

In *extraintestinal amebiasis* with liver abscess 1 Gm. is given daily for 2 days and then 250 mg. is administered twice a day for 2 weeks, or up to a total dose of 11 Gm.

In *discoid lupus erythematosus*, 250 mg. is taken twice daily for 2 weeks and then followed by 250 mg. once a day.

Rheumatoid arthritis requires prolonged daily administration of 250 mg.

PRIMAQUINE PHOSPHATE U.S.P.

Pharmacology. This chemical of the 8-aminoquinoline class has largely replaced all other drugs for producing *radical cure* and thus preventing relapses in malaria caused by *Plasmodium vivax* and other organisms that possess secondary tissue forms. The drug, which does *not* act against erythrocytic schizonts and is thus *not* useful by itself against an acute attack, does eradicate the secondary *exo*-erythrocytic forms of these malarial parasites. It is always administered together with a blood schizonticide, such as chloroquine.

Ordinary doses of primaquine cause few side effects in most persons. Complaints are limited to occasional abdominal distress, headache, itching, and blurred vision. Much more serious is the possibility of a hemolytic reaction in a hypersensitive individual. Negroes and other darkly pigmented people are much more likely than most Caucasians to suffer from sensitivity to primaquine and the many other drugs known to cause hemolysis of red blood cells. Examine the urine of persons taking primaquine for signs of significant darkening. If this should occur, or if the blood shows a sudden drop in hemoglobin or a marked lessening of the leukocyte count, the drug should be discontinued immediately.

Dosage and Administration. A tablet containing 26.3 mg. of this phosphate salt—the equivalent of 15 mg. of primaquine base—is taken by mouth once daily for 14 days together with a drug of the chloroquine-type during the latent period or in an acute attack, in order to achieve a radical cure. Larger daily or weekly doses may be required for radical cure of some malarial strain infections.

PYRIMETHAMINE U.S.P. (DARAPRIM)

Pharmacology. This folic acid antagonist is active against several stages of the plasmodia including primary *exo*-erythrocytic (tissue) forms, erythrocytic forms, and gametocytes. However, in practice, it is recommended for use mainly in suppressive therapy of persons entering endemic areas. The drug is too slow in its action on blood schizonts to be used by itself in an acute attack. When added to the regimen of a person receiving a more rapid-acting schizonticide for clinical cure, it is said to lessen the likelihood of later relapses.

Pyrimethamine has some activity as a causal prophylactic, and it also interferes with transmission of malaria by preventing the fertilized female gamete from going through the steps of sporogony in the mosquito that lead to production of sporozoites. However, it is not used widely in programs of mass prophylaxis and malaria eradication because of concern that this would lead to emergence of plasmodial strains resistant to it.

Pyrimethamine does not produce side effects when administered in the small amounts needed as suppressive therapy. However, the larger doses sometimes used in the management of toxoplasmosis may cause a folic acid deficiency. This may result in vomiting and, more seriously, in bone marrow depression leading to megaloblastic anemia. Pyrimethamine should not be used during the first trimester of pregnancy.

Dosage and Administration. The dose for suppressive therapy is only one 25-mg. tablet weekly. When used in conjunction with other drugs for clinical cure of an acute attack, 25 mg. is administered for 2 days. In toxoplasmosis, treatment is started with 50 to 75 mg. daily (together with sulfadiazine) and continued for 1 to 3 weeks. Treatment with half the initial dose may then be continued for another 4 or 5 weeks.

QUININE SULFATE N.F.

Pharmacology. This is a salt of the main alkaloid of cinchona bark which has been largely replaced by chloroquine and other synthetic chemicals that are less toxic and more effective as suppressive therapy and for producing clinical cures of malaria. It is mainly used for a variety of other medical conditions. However, quinine may be lifesaving in some *Plasmodium falciparum* infections caused by strains of this species that are resistant to treatment with chloroquine and related blood schizonticides.

Quinine possesses analgesic-antipyretic effects similar to those of the salicylates. Like the latter, it relieves headache, fever, and general malaise, but because of its greater toxicity, quinine is not a desirable substitute for the salicylates. Quinine is often useful for relief of skeletal muscle cramps that develop during the night in some patients. It relieves the muscle spasms of the rare condition myotonia congenita.

Overdosage is marked by cinchonism, a syndrome similar to that seen when salicylate dosage is pushed to high levels. Ringing in the ears, blurring of vision, nausea, and headache may be followed by further digestive disturbances, impairment of hearing and sight, and confusion and delirium. Death may follow cardiac arrhythmias, collapse, convulsions, and coma, when massive amounts are taken in misguided attempts to produce an abortion.

Dosage and Administration. For treating an acute malarial attack, 1 Gm. is administered daily for 2 days and followed by 600 mg. daily for the following 5 days. Although the oral route is preferred, the dihydrochloride salt may be given by I.V. drip to patients who are severely ill with *P. falciparum* malaria affecting the brain.

DIETHYLCARBAMAZINE CITRATE U.S.P. (HETRAZAN)

Pharmacology. This nonmetallic filaricide is more effective and less toxic than the antimony compounds formerly employed against filariasis caused by *Wuchereria bancrofti, W. malayi, Onchocerca volvulus,* and *Loa loa.* Taken by mouth, the drug quickly causes the threadlike microfilariae to vanish from the blood of the infected person. Apparently, the drug damages the elongated embryonic organisms so that they are destroyed more easily by body defense mechanisms. The adult worms of most species are killed.

Side effects include transient anorexia, nausea, vomiting, headache, weakness, and muscular or joint discomfort. In onchocerciasis, a condition marked by ocular involvement, rapid destruction of the microfilariae may lead to allergic inflammatory eye reactions. Thus the administration of antihistaminic and corticosteroid drugs along with diethylcarbamazine is advocated.

Dosage and Administration. A dose of 2 mg./Kg. body weight is administered three times daily for 1 to 3 weeks. Available for this purpose are 50-mg. scored tablets and a cherry flavored syrup containing 120 mg./5 ml.

HYDROXYSTILBAMIDINE ISETHIONATE U.S.P.

Pharmacology. This diamidine derivative is active against the invasive fungi that cause blastomycosis and against the protozoal organisms responsible for African trypanosomiasis and leishmaniasis. In each condition it is reserved for cases that do not respond to preferred drugs—amphotericin B in blastomycosis; the organic arsenicals and pentamidine in trypanosomiasis, and the pentavalent antimonials in kala azar. It does not cause trigeminal neuropathy, which occurred with its predecessor, stilbamidine.

During long-term therapy—in blastomycosis, for example—kidney and liver function are observed because of renal and hepatic reactions reported with previous drugs of this class. It has been suggested that light causes breakdown of solutions of these chemicals to hepatotoxic substances. Thus, the solution must not be exposed to sunlight during its preparation and infusion. The solution is injected over periods of 1 or 2 hours, as too rapid administration may result in release of tissue histamine which causes reactions including flushing, fainting, falls in blood

pressure, reflex tachycardia, and other discomforting or disabling symptoms.

Dosage and Administration. Freshly prepared solutions containing 150 to 225 mg. of the drug are infused over a period of 1 or 2 hours. These are repeated every day or two for a total of 10 doses.

LUCANTHONE HYDROCHLORIDE U.S.P. (MIRACIL D; NILODIN)

Pharmacology. This nonmetallic schistosomicide is often effective in treating infections by *Schistosoma haematobium.* Larger doses are required against *S. mansoni,* and it seems to be ineffective in *S. japonicum* infections. Its main advantages are its activity when given by mouth and the likelihood that it will not cause as severe toxicity as stibophen injections.

G.I. upset occurs frequently and C.N.S. and circulatory side effects occasionally. Thus, although this inexpensive oral drug might profitably be taken prophylactically by the population of areas in which schistosomiasis is widespread, the common occurrence of anorexia, nausea, epigastric distress, and vomiting limits this agent's usefulness for that purpose. Adults seem to be more susceptible than children to C.N.S. effects such as headache, dizziness, restlessness, and sleeplessness, and the occasional development of convulsive or psychotic reactions.

Dosage and Administration. A dose of a 5 mg./Kg. body weight is taken three times daily for 1 week, but longer courses with higher doses are employed if required and tolerated.

SODIUM SURAMIN U.S.P. (ANTRYPOL; GERMANIN; BAYER 205)

Pharmacology. This complex urea derivative has both filaricidal and trypanocidal properties. In filariasis caused by *Onchocerca,* this drug is given to kill the adult worms after treatment with the less toxic diethylcarbamazine has caused disappearance of the microfilariae. In the early stages of infection by *Trypanosoma gambiense* and *T. rhodesiense,* suramin may eliminate the protozoal parasite. Similarly, its prolonged presence in the blood after one dose often protects against infection for 2 or 3 months. However, in cases in which the nervous system has already been affected, treatment with this drug alone is inadequate and it is followed by a more potent organic arsenical that can penetrate the blood-brain barrier.

The most common of the varied early reactions to suramin include acute urticaria and other pruritic dermatoses, nausea and abdominal pain, and fever. Rarely, circulatory collapse and coma develop shortly after intravenous injection in highly sensitive individuals. Later reactions include lacrimation and edematous swelling of periocular tissues, skin rashes, and paresthesia or hyperesthesia. Suramin is contraindicated in patients with renal disorders, and the urine of all patients is examined for the presence of blood, protein, and casts.

Dosage and Administration. One Gm. is administered once weekly for 5 to 10 weeks by slow intravenous injection for treatment of trypanosomiasis; prophylaxis is achieved with a 1 Gm. dose. A trial dose of 200 mg. is administered as a test of sensitivity.

STIBOPHEN U.S.P. (FUADIN)

Pharmacology. This trivalent organic antimony compound is a drug of choice for treating schistosomiasis. It readily kills the adult worms of *Schistosoma mansoni,* the main cause of intestinal schistosomiasis; *S. haematobium,* the most common cause of urinary bladder (vesicle) invasion; and *S. japonicum,* an especially dangerous organism found in Japan, the Philippines, and South China.

Watch patients closely for signs of heavy metal toxicity, including blood dyscrasias, and renal or liver damage. Administration of a test dose to determine the patient's sensitivity is desirable before embarking on a course of intensive stibophen therapy. Patients who react with fever, joint pains, and persistent proteinuria should be taken off the drug and treated with the less toxic, nonmetallic compound lucanthone. Stibophen has been employed in leishmaniasis, granuloma inguinale, and lymphogranuloma venereum, but less toxic drugs are generally preferred in these conditions.

Dosage and Administration. The official dose is 95 mg. administered intramuscularly on the first day, followed by 315 mg. on alternate days for 5 weeks up to a total dose of 6.3 Gm. Dosage schedules vary in accordance with what local experience has indicated is generally required. For example, in infections by *S. japonicum* a much larger total dose is administered than when the disease is caused by other species of schistosomes.

TRYPARSAMIDE U.S.P.

Pharmacology. This organic arsenical penetrates into the C.N.S. and destroys the protozoal parasite *Trypanosoma gambiense* or the spirochete *Treponema pallidum*. Thus it has long been employed for treating African sleeping sickness with C.N.S. involvement and in cases of neurosyphilis that are resistant to other treatments. However, it is being replaced by less toxic drugs such as melarsoprol, which is active against *Trypanosoma rhodesiense* as well as *T. gambiense*, and by procaine penicillin G in C.N.S. syphilis.

Typical organic arsenical toxicity occurs fairly frequently. Such reactions affect mainly the skin (dermatoses and angioneurotic reactions) and the G.I. tract (nausea, vomiting, abdominal pain, diarrhea, and possible liver damage). Most serious is the danger of optic nerve damage which can result in blindness. Vision is examined before, after, and during treatment. If signs of visual impairment are noted, or if the patient complains of persistent subjective visual symptoms, the drug is promptly discontinued.

Dosage and Administration. A dose of 1 to 3 Gm. is administered by vein about once weekly up to a total dose of 20 to 45 Gm. in an 8 to 16 week period. A rest period of 6 weeks or more is necessary between courses.

CHAPTER 37

ANTHELMINTIC AND ANTIAMEBIC AGENTS

Antiamebic Agents

CARBARSONE U.S.P.

Pharmacology. This organic arsenical agent is effective against the trophozoite form of *Entamoeba histolytica* in the intestine but does not attain amebicidal concentrations in extra-intestinal tissues such as the liver. Thus, it is used mainly to control acute amebic dysentery in patients who are not as critically ill as those who require emetine therapy. It is employed in chronic intestinal amebiasis, often in alternation with courses of one of the iodoquinoline drugs, such as diiodohydroxyquin.

Although carbarsone is a relatively harmless arsenical, patients are closely observed for skin eruptions and visual changes that may indicate sensitivity to arsenic. A few cases of arsenic-induced exfoliative dermatitis and liver or brain damage have occurred in such patients. Carbarsone is contraindicated in patients with renal damage, which might interfere with its excretion. Its use in patients with hepatic amebiasis, who are being treated with other amebicides, is also undesirable, for the drug,

which is contraindicated in severe hepatitis, may cause further liver damage in such cases. The most common side effects are of the G.I. type—abdominal pain, nausea and vomiting, and an increase in severity of diarrhea.

Dosage and Administration. Carbarsone is administered in 10-day courses with intervening rest periods to avoid cumulation of slowly excreted arsenic. Doses of 250 mg. are taken two or three times daily by adults. Children may receive daily oral doses of 10 mg./Kg. body weight. Rectal retention enemas are employed occasionally.

EMETINE HYDROCHLORIDE U.S.P.

Pharmacology. This amebicidal agent kills the trophozoites, or motile forms, of *Entamoeba histolytica*, in both the intestinal and extra-intestinal tissues. Although the cystic form of the ameba disappears from the intestine during treatment with emetine, the cysts are not eliminated by safe doses of this drug.

These actions of emetine on the parasite, together with its high potential toxicity to the tissues of the host, determine its utility and limitations. It is most valuable for treating amebic hepatitis and amebic abscesses, because of the high amebicidal concentrations reached in the liver. Emetine controls severe diarrhea in acute amebic dysentery and in acute exacerbations of chronic intestinal amebiasis. However, its routine use in mild cases of amebic dysentery is undesirable and its employment in asymptomatic carriers of amebic cysts is contraindicated on account of its high potential cumulative toxicity and low level of effectiveness here.

The toxic effects of emetine vary from relatively mild and transient—for example, increased diarrhea, nausea, and vomiting—to extremely severe and even fatal reactions. The most serious toxicity is the result of emetine's depressant effects on the myocardium. This may be marked by chest pains, tachycardia, and electroencephalographic (ECG) changes, as well as by hypotension and dyspnea in some cases. Emetine is administered to patients with pre-existing heart disease only when the risk from extra-intestinal amebiasis unresponsive to any other therapy seems greater than the danger of drug-induced cardiac damage. It is contraindicated in children under most circumstances and in patients with kidney damage.

Dosage and Administration. Emetine is administered in doses of 1 mg./Kg. body weight, but in a total dose not exceeding 60 mg. daily during a course of 5 to 10 days. The deep subcutaneous or intramuscular injections are made at different sites, and a record is kept so that these can be rotated in order to minimize the degree of local irritation, edema, and necrosis. The injection sites are carefully observed for signs of induration or swelling. Special care is taken to aspirate before injecting in order to be certain that this potent drug is not introduced directly into a blood vessel.

Patients who take emetine are kept at rest in bed throughout the entire treatment period and are warned to avoid strenuous activity for some time after the course of therapy is completed. Rest periods of at least 6 weeks are required before further courses of emetine may be employed safely.

IODOCHLORHYDROXYQUIN U.S.P. (VIOFORM; ENTERO-VIOFORM)

Pharmacology. This iodoquinoline-class compound has antiprotozoal, antibacterial, and antifungal activity. It is used in the management of mild cases of intestinal amebiasis and for patients who show no symptoms but pass cysts in their stool. The drug is also effective in vaginitis caused by the protozoal parasite *Trichomonas vaginalis* or by the yeastlike fungal organism *Candida albicans*. It is employed for its antibacterial effects in secondary skin infections complicating atopic dermatitis, acute psoriasis and eczema and in impetigo. The drug is often taken prophylactically by people traveling in areas where infection by amebae and by bacillae such as *Shigella* strains are endemic.

Side effects are relatively few and mild. Salivation, nausea, abdominal pain, diarrhea, and anal pruritus are sometimes reported, as are headache and skin eruptions. The latter are more likely in patients who are sensitive to iodine. Although frequent or continued use of this drug raises the level of protein-bound iodine of the plasma, this does not indicate altered thyroid gland function.

Dosage and Administration. The adult antiamebic dose is 250 mg. three times daily for 10 days, taken in the form of enteric-coated tablets (N.F.). This course can be repeated after an 8-day rest period, during which an arsenical such as carbarsone is administered. Vaginitis is treated with a 250-mg. suppository or by insufflation of a powder containing this drug in combination with boric acid, lactic acid, zinc stearate, and lactose. Ointments, creams, and a dusting powder are employed in the treatment of skin infections, and for prophylaxis on burns, ulcers, and wounds.

PAROMOMYCIN (HUMATIN)

Pharmacology. This antibiotic, which has a broad spectrum of antimicrobial activity, is used to treat and prevent G.I. infections by pathogenic bacteria and amebae. In amebiasis, it is used mainly in mild to moderately severe chronic cases with subacute or acute excerbations, rather than for patients who are critically ill with acute amebic dysentery. It is not effective for treating extra-intestinal amebiasis.

Paromomycin helps to control the secondary infections by bacteria that sometimes complicate intestinal amebiasis. Similarly, it controls gastroenteritis in shigellosis, salmonellosis and other intestinal infections caused by pathogenic bacteria. It is not effective against the septicemic complications caused by salmonellae and other gram-negative organisms, which are best treated with parenterally administered ampicillin, chloramphenicol or tetracycline.

Paromomycin is sometimes used, like neomycin, to suppress the bacterial flora in hepatic coma and prior to bowel surgery. In such cases, the possibility of overgrowths by candidal organisms and resistant staphylococci exists, as does potential nephrotoxicity in the event of systemic absorption. More common is the occurrence of loose stools or even moderately severe diarrhea.

Dosage and Administration. For amebiasis a minimal daily dose of 25 mg./Kg. daily for at least 5 days is recommended. In bacillary dysentery 35 to 60 mg./Kg. is employed for 6 days or longer. Doses of 35 mg./Kg. are given for 4 consecutive days prior to bowel surgery. Hepatic coma patients may require as much as 75 mg./Kg./day.

Anthelmintics

DITHIAZANINE IODIDE U.S.P. (DELVEX)

Pharmacology. This blue dye is an anthelmintic active against a variety of intestinal worms. It is most effective and least likely to cause adverse effects when used in the treatment of whipworm and *Strongyloides* infections, for which conditions it has proved more effective than any previously available anthelmintic agents. Although it is also active against pinworms and round-worms, its potential toxicity compared with piperazine and other safer drugs precludes its ordinary use in infections by these organisms.

Dithiazanine often causes local irritation of the G.I. tract that results in nausea, vomiting, cramps, and diarrhea. If these symptoms persist, treatment is discontinued. Although this drug is not ordinarily absorbed into the systemic circulation, a number of deaths have been reported, in which hypotension, acidosis, and coma have occurred and postmortem examination revealed blue staining of the skin, sclera, and viscera. Thus, treatment is

discontinued if the urine becomes bluish-green—an indication of systemic absorption. Dithiazanine is contraindicated in patients with G.I. inflammatory disorders or other conditions that may lead to its absorption. It is not given to patients with renal impairment.

Dosage and Administration. Dithiazanine is given after meals to minimize G.I. irritation. Initially, in the treatment of trichuriasis (whipworms), a dose of 100 mg. is administered after each of three meals on the first day. The dose may then be raised to 200 mg. three times daily for the following 4 days. In strongyloides infections, the lower dose—100 mg. t.i.d.—is employed for 14 to 21 days. If infection persists, the dose may be raised to 200 mg. for an additional 10 to 14 days after a 2-week rest period.

HEXYLRESORCINOL N.F. (CRYSTOIDS)

Pharmacology. This anthelmintic of relatively wide spectrum and low toxicity is active against roundworms, pinworms, whipworms, hookworms, and dwarf tapeworms. In practice, however, it is used mainly in special circumstances that do not permit the use of various anthelmintics that are more specifically effective against each particular type of intestinal worm.

In roundworm infections, for example, hexylresorcinol is used mainly when patients cannot tolerate or do not respond to piperazine. Hexylresorcinol may be especially useful for treating mixed infections, such as roundworms with hookworms. Because of its low toxicity, this drug can be given in the repeated courses that are often necessary in such cases.

Dosage and Administration. This drug is available in gelatin-coated pills that are taken by mouth in the morning on an empty stomach. These pills should be swallowed whole and not chewed, for the concentrated hexylresorcinol irritates the mucosa of the mouth and may even cause ulcerations. Such local irritation may also prove harmful to patients with peptic ulcer or other G.I. tract disorders.

Two to 4 hours after taking the average adult dose of 1 Gm., the patient receives a saline cathartic to help remove the round-worms. He may finally eat food about 5 hours after the drug was ingested. Treatment is repeated at intervals of 3 days if required.

PIPERAZINE CITRATE U.S.P. (ANTEPAR; MULTIFUGE; ETC.)

Pharmacology. This is an anthelmintic drug of relatively low toxicity and high effectiveness for treating pinworm and round-worm infestations of the intestinal tract. It is easy to administer to children in the form of flavored tablets and syrups and requires no prior fasting period or post-treatment catharsis or enemas.

Side effects are rare from average doses: only occasional urticaria and diarrhea are reported. Massive overdosage such as may result from a child's drinking an entire bottle of syrup can cause muscular incoordination and weakness, with blurring of vision and possible breathing difficulties.

Dosage and Administration. The official usual dose in pin-worm treatment is 50 mg./Kg. body weight daily for 7 days or a dose of up to 3.5 Gm. daily. In practice, one-half tablet or teaspoon, 250 mg., is given to infants weighing up to 15 lbs.; twice this dose—500 mg.—to children of 15 to 30 lbs.; 1 Gm. to those of 30 to 60 lbs.; and 2 Gm. daily to those over 60 lbs.

The official dose against roundworms is 75 mg./Kg. for 2 days or up to 5 Gm. in infants up to 30 lbs.; 2 Gm. for those from 30 to 50 lbs.; 3 Gm.—50 to 100 lbs.; over 100 lbs., 3.5 Gm.

PYRVINIUM PAMOATE U.S.P. (POVAN; VANQUIN)

Pharmacology. This salt of a cyanine dye has anthelmintic activity against a variety of worms but is recommended specifically for the eradication of pinworms. It is so effective against such organisms that one dose often cures the condition. The usual hygienic precautions are required to prevent early reinfection.

Side effects, which are rare with the currently recommended dose of this insoluble salt, are nausea, vomiting and cramps. Like gentian violet, which it has helped to displace in oxyuriasis treatment, this dye can stain most materials. Thus patients are cautioned to protect underclothing and warned that their stools can be colored bright red by this drug.

Dosage and Administration. An oral dose of 5 mg./Kg. body weight of pyrivinium base (7.5 mg./Kg. of this salt) is taken in the form of a suspension containing 10 mg./ml. or a tablet containing the equivalent of 50 mg. of the base. The tablets should not be chewed but swallowed whole, because they may stain the teeth.

QUINACRINE HYDROCHLORIDE U.S.P. (ATABRINE)

Pharmacology. This substance, once a widely used suppressive agent in malaria, is mainly used in the treatment of tapeworm infestations. It is effective against beef, pork, and fish tapeworms but does not seem useful against the dwarf tapeworm. The drug is not ordinarily toxic to most individuals, but the high doses used in treating tapeworms often cause nausea and vomiting. Some individuals have suffered psychotic reactions following administration of quinacrine. Thus its use is contraindicated in individuals with a history of psychosis.

Dosage and Administration. Careful pretreatment of the tapeworm-infested patient assures maximal contact of quinacrine with the head of the parasite. The intestine is emptied by having the patient eat only a light, fat-free lunch on the evening before treatment, following which a saline cathartic is administered. The next morning, a total of 800 mg. of quinacrine is given in four divided doses over a half-hour period. Each dose is followed by 600 mg. of sodium bicarbonate to reduce nausea and vomiting. About 2 hours following the final dose, a saline purgative is administered. Often, the tapeworm, its head colored yellow, is recovered in the stool in a few hours.

Quinacrine may be administered by duodenal tube in order to reduce gastric irritation. A gram of the drug suspended in 20 ml. of water is introduced into the tube and washed down with a small further quantity of water.

TETRACHLOROETHYLENE U.S.P.

Pharmacology. This chemical safely and effectively removes hookworms from the intestinal tract. Although it is a halogenated hydrocarbon, effective anthelmintic doses administered with proper precautions do not cause toxic reactions of the kind brought about by related agents such as chloroform and carbon tetrachloride. This is because the drug is not absorbed into the systemic circulation to any great extent in ordinary circumstances.

If tetrachloroethylene is absorbed—as it may be in the presence of fat or alcohol in the G.I. tract—the patient may show some signs of C.N.S. depression including giddiness, vertigo, drowsiness, and headache. More commonly, patients may complain of the effects of local irritation, including epigastric distress, nausea, vomiting, and abdominal cramps.

Dosage and Administration. A dose of 0.12 ml./Kg. body weight, but no more than 5 ml., is taken in capsule form on an empty stomach in the morning, after a period of a day or more in which no alcohol or fatty foods have been taken. It is not only not necessary but undesirable to administer a cathartic, according to some authorities who claim that purgation reduces the drug's effectiveness and tends to dehydrate the patient.

The patient rests for at least 4 hours after the drug is taken, and food is withheld for 4 to 6 hours. The treatment may be repeated in about 1 week if stool examination indicates the continued presence of hookworms.

THIABENDAZOLE N.F. (MINTEZOL)

Pharmacology. This broad-spectrum anthelmintic, which was formerly official for veterinary use only, has been introduced recently after extensive clinical trials in the treatment of human helminthiasis. It is claimed to be more than 95 per cent effective against enterobiasis (pinworm disease) and strongyloidiasis (threadworm disease). The drug has been employed in trichuriasis (whipworm disease), ascariasis (large roundworm disease), and uncinariasis (hookworm disease caused by both major infesting organisms). It is claimed to relieve fever, reduce eosinophilia, and produce other benefits in some patients with trichinosis; and it is said to provide the first successful systemic treatment for cutaneous larva migrans (creeping eruption).

Side effects involving the G.I. tract and C.N.S. vary in frequency. Anorexia, nausea, and vomiting occur frequently and epigastric distress and diarrhea less often. Drowsiness, giddiness, and headache sometimes develop, and patients should be warned against driving a car or undertaking other potentially dangerous activities that require alertness. The significance of more serious reactions such as leukopenia, skin rash, and crystalluria, which have been reported occasionally, has not been evaluated fully.

Dosage and Administration. Thiabendazole is available as a pleasant-tasting suspension that is administered after meals in a dose of 10 mg./lb. twice a day. The length of treatment varies in different conditions. In pinworm disease, for example, the drug is usually given for 1 day and repeated 7 days later. It may be given in this condition and in other intestinal parasitoses, cutaneous larva migrans and trichinosis for 2 successive days. In trichinosis, treatment may be continued for 4 successive days. The recommended maximal daily dosage is 3 Gm.

CHAPTER 38

DRUGS ACTING ON THE GASTROINTESTINAL TRACT

ALUMINUM HYDROXIDE GEL U.S.P. (AMPHOGEL; CREAMALIN; ETC.)

Pharmacology. This antacid is widely used in the treatment of peptic ulcer. It acts mainly by neutralizing hydrochloric acid in the stomach with formation of aluminum chloride. Later, aluminum hydroxide is precipitated out once more in the intestine and passes out without being absorbed systemically. This nonsystemic buffering agent is also said to possess adsorbent, demulcent, and astringent properties. Thus, it may form a protective coating over the ulcer crater which slows down the digestive action of pepsin and acid.

The most common side effect of aluminum hydroxide therapy is constipation. This may be counteracted by combining aluminum hydroxide with a mildly laxative antacid, such as magnesium hydroxide, or by administering a bedtime dose of that laxative or of liquid petrolatum. Although high daily doses may, in theory, create a phosphate deficiency, the likelihood that this or other types of systemic toxicity actually occur is slight.

Dosage and Administration. Aluminum hydroxide gel is available as a watery suspension and as tablets of dried material. Large doses of the liquid (e.g., 30 ml. diluted with water) may be given as often as every hour in treating an acute ulcer. Later, the dose is reduced considerably (e.g., 4 to 8 ml. every 2 to 4 hours with water or milk). The dried tablets, which react with acid much more slowly, are chewed and swallowed several times daily in doses of about 600 mg. to relieve acidity.

MILK OF MAGNESIA U.S.P.
(MAGNESIA MAGMA)

Pharmacology. This suspension of magnesium hydroxide is widely used by the public as an antacid and laxative. Part of the suspended powder reacts readily with acid to neutralize it in large amounts. A residue of unreacted material is said to remain in the stomach to combine with new increments of acid secreted later. Thus, the action of this nonsystemic antacid is relatively prompt, prolonged, and complete.

The doses of milk of magnesia required for treating acute ulcers are often in the cathartic range. Consequently, diarrhea may occur unless efforts are made to counteract the drug's laxative action by administering it in combination with constipating aluminum compounds or alternating it with basic calcium salts, such as calcium carbonate.

Dosage and Administration. Milk of magnesia is administered in doses as low as 4 ml. as an antacid and as high as 30 ml. for laxative purposes. However, the larger doses may also be necessary to maintain neutralization of acid in acute peptic ulcer.

OXYPHENCYCLIMINE HYDROCHLORIDE
(DARICON, ETC.)

Pharmacology. This synthetic anticholinergic drug, which is a tertiary rather than a quaternary amine, produces atropinelike effects and is used clinically in the same conditions as the natural belladonna alkaloids. Like other new synthetics, such as glycopyrrolate and isopropamide, it is said to exert a relatively long antisecretory action — up to 12 hours. Thus, it is used as an adjunct to diet, antacids, and rest to relieve pain and promote the healing of duodenal and gastric ulcers. Oxyphencyclimine also reduces G.I. hypermotility and spasm in patients with functional bowel distress. The side effects and contraindications of oxyphencyclamine are like those of other atropinelike drugs (see Summary, p. 267).

Dosage and Administration. Oxyphencyclamine is usually administered in tablet form in a dose of 10 mg. twice daily. However, the dosage may range from 5 mg. to as high as 50 mg. daily, divided into four doses. It is also available with phenobarbital and the minor tranquilizer hydroxyzine which supply a sedative effect.

SODIUM BICARBONATE U.S.P.
(BAKING SODA)

Pharmacology. This soluble, absorbable alkalizer is widely used by the public for relief of hyperacidity symptoms. It is much more rarely employed by physicians for treating peptic ulcer, for although it neutralizes acidity rapidly, this salt has several drawbacks.

Sodium bicarbonate is swept from the stomach rapidly, because it increases the rate of gastric emptying. This, in turn, tends to set off increased acid secretion in the stomach — so-called "acid rebound." The carbon dioxide gas evolved from the action of acid on bicarbonate distends the stomach until relieved by an eructation. The pressure of the gas could be dangerous in a patient with an ulcer that is close to perforation.

Because this salt is a systemic alkalinizer, it is sometimes used to counteract acidosis — for example, in some cases of salicylate and methyl alcohol toxicity — and for alkalinizing the urine in various other conditions. However, this effect is considered undesirable and potentially dangerous, especially in patients with poor kidney function. Metabolic alkalosis, difficult to detect and potentially fatal, may occur in such patients who take large amounts of bicarbonate for ulcer treatment.

Dosage and Administration. Sodium bicarbonate is commonly taken in small amounts (e.g., 200 mg.) in the form of flavored tablets for self-medication of a variety of stomach symptoms. Much larger doses (e.g., 2 Gm. every hour) are occasionally administered in treating acute peptic ulcer. Later, smaller amounts are given at less frequent intervals.

CASCARA SAGRADA U.S.P.

Pharmacology. This is probably the mildest of the anthraquinone class of irritant cathartics. It acts in the large intestine where its active anthracene constituents are liberated. This produces a single soft stool in about 8 hours after it is taken orally. It is preferred for patients who do not require rapid, complete purgation. These include bedridden patients who should not strain at stool because of possible complications. Cascara should be supplemented by other measures for aiding bowel movement, and should be discontinued as soon as normal intestinal activity resumes.

Dosage and Administration. This plant product is available as an aromatic fluidextract (U.S.P.) taken in doses of 5 to 15 ml., as tablets and as an extract and fluidextract, all official in the National Formulary. The solid dosage forms are given in amounts of about 300 mg. and the liquid in a dose of 1 ml. Given at bedtime, all produce a formed movement in the morning.

CASTOR OIL U.S.P.

Pharmacology. This cathartic stimulates peristaltic activity through irritation of the small and large intestine by liberated ricinoleic acid. Its action results in production of a semifluid stool within a few hours. Because of its relatively prompt and complete action, castor oil clears the whole bowel quickly in various situations, including drug poisonings and diarrhea resulting from eating food contaminated by bacteria that cause enteric infections. It is sometimes employed as a purge in hospitals on the day prior to roentgenographic examination of abdominal viscera.

Dosage and Administration. The dose of castor oil for adults is 15 to 60 ml. If given on an empty stomach, it does not slow gastric emptying time. The taste and texture of the oil may be masked in various ways to avoid nausea in patients who find them distasteful. An aromatic castor oil and pharmaceutical emulsions are available, but the taste may also be disguised by making extemporaneous mixtures with fruit syrups and iced carbonated beverages. Castor oil should not be given at bedtime; it is commonly given in the afternoon.

DIPHENOXYLATE HYDROCHLORIDE
(LOMOTIL)

Pharmacology. This drug, which reduces intestinal motility and causes an increase in smooth muscle tone, relieves acute and chronic diarrhea. These G.I. actions are similar to those of the opiate alkaloids, but this drug — although it is a derivative of the opioid meperidine — has a low addiction liability. Because it may be abused, however, it is combined with small amounts of atropine, a drug that would cause discomforting side effects in individuals who might try to take large doses of the diphenoxylate product to attain euphoric effects.

Diphenoxylate has been used in place of paregoric to control diarrhea in gastroenteritis and the irritable bowel syndrome. It is less effective in the chronic diarrhea of ulcerative colitis, regional enteritis, and diverticulitis, although it has been tried in these conditions and in patients who suffer from diarrhea following surgical operations such as gastrectomy, ileostomy, and colostomy.

Side effects include dizziness, depression, and drowsiness; because of possible potentiation, this drug is not administered with barbiturates. The drug, which sometimes causes nausea and abdominal distention, is not administered to patients with impaired liver function. Continued administration can lead to an abstinence syndrome upon withdrawal, but the drug is classed as an exempt narcotic.

Dosage and Administration. Diphenoxylate is available as tablets of 2.5 mg. and as a liquid containing the same amount in 5 ml. A small amount of atropine sulfate (0.025 mg.) is added to each dosage form. The usual daily dose for adults is 15 to 20 mg., administered in divided doses. This is reduced once the acute phase of the diarrhea is controlled.

DIMENHYDRINATE U.S.P. (DRAMAMINE)

Pharmacology. This antiemetic agent is one of the most well-established of the *non*-phenothiazine group. It was tested originally as an antihistaminic agent for allergy but is employed mainly for its C.N.S. action against motion sickness symptoms. In addition to preventing and relieving seasickness, airsickness, etc., this drug is used in various medical and surgical conditions marked by vestibular dysfunction. Such conditions include Meniere's syndrome, labyrinthitis, and streptomycin toxicity. The drug is claimed to control nausea and vomiting occurring in pregnancy and hypertension or following electroshock therapy, anesthesia, and narcotization.

Side effects are few except for drowsiness in some patients. Dimenhydrinate is sometimes combined with low doses of dextroamphetamine to counteract sedation. People who intend to operate vehicles or other motorized machinery are warned that their efficiency may be impaired. Use of this drug together with streptomycin may mask advancing eighth cranial nerve toxicity caused by the antibiotic.

Dosage and Administration. Adults may take 50 mg. every 4 to 6 hours orally. If tablet or liquid forms cannot be retained, the drug may be administered rectally as a suppository, or parenterally, especially when prompt action is desired. Children may receive from one-quarter the adult dose to the full amount in some cases.

PROCHLORPERAZINE MALEATE U.S.P. (COMPAZINE)

Pharmacology. This potent phenothiazine tranquilizer is used not only in psychiatry, but also as an antiemetic in medicine, surgery, and obstetrics to control nausea, retching, and vomiting. Like other phenothiazine-type antiemetics, it is believed to act by blocking the effects of circulating emetic chemicals upon the chemoreceptor trigger zone (CTZ). Thus, it is probably more effective than the *non*-phenothiazine antiemetics against vomiting due to radiation and nitrogen mustard therapy of cancer, uremia, hepatitis, infections, and drugs such as anesthetics and narcotics.

The drugs of this class are used with caution in children and pregnant women. Because the incidence and severity of side effects (e.g., extrapyramidal motor system stimulation) is greater than with the *non*-phenothiazine emetics, prochlorperazine and other drugs of its class are reserved for cautious use in cases of hyperemesis gravidarum not readily controlled by other measures. It is used during labor and postpartum but is not given in eclampsia. Children receive the lowest effective dosage, and parents are cautioned not to exceed the prescribed dosage.

Dosage and Administration. Treatment is begun with the lowest dose of this drug and adjusted in accordance with the patient's response. Dosage for antiemesis is much smaller than the amounts often required by psychotic patients. The drug is administered orally, rectally, and parenterally in single doses of 5 to 10 mg. and in a total daily dosage rarely exceeding 30 mg. Children's dosage is calculated on the basis of body weight, expecially when the drug is to be administered parenterally (e.g., 0.06 mg./lb. body weight by deep intramuscular injection).

TRIMETHOBENZAMIDE HYDROCHLORIDE N.F. (TIGAN)

Pharmacology. This antiemetic drug is used to prevent and treat nausea and vomiting in many conditions, including motion sickness, labyrinthitis, and Meniere's syndrome. It is said to control vomiting caused by circulating chemical substances such as drugs; the toxic metabolites of diseases such as uremia, hepatitis, and malignancies; and the hormones that are present in high amounts in early pregnancy. It is believed to act mainly by blocking the chemoreceptor trigger zone (CTZ), the chemically-sensitive area in the medulla that transmits emetic impulses to the vomiting center.

Side effects, other than occasional drowsiness and allergic reactions, are said to be rare. The possibility of drowsiness makes it desirable that patients not drive until their tolerance of this effect is proved by experience. Patients who show skin reactions or other signs of sensitization should not continue to receive this drug.

Dosage and Administration. This drug is available in the form of capsules, suppositories, and an injectable solution. Adults receive one 250-mg. oral capsule and children one or two 100-mg. capsules—both three or four times daily. A 200-mg. suppository may be administered rectally on a similar dosage schedule; children under 30 lbs. receive only one-half suppository; those weighing over 30 but less than 90 lbs. receive one half to one suppository. An injection is administered intramuscularly (never I.V.) in a dose of 200 mg., and may be repeated after a few hours. To avoid pain, redness, and swelling at the injection site, the needle is inserted deep into the gluteal muscle and leakage of solution is avoided en route.

CHAPTER 39

DRUGS ACTING ON THE MUSCLES OF THE UTERUS

ERGONOVINE MALEATE U.S.P. (ERGOTRATE)

Pharmacology. This is a salt of the ergot alkaloid that is most active in stimulating uterine motility. Taken orally in small doses during the puerperium when the uterus is especially sensitive to its oxytocic action, this drug produces a rapid and relatively prolonged contraction of the myometrium. This prevents puerperal complications, including bleeding and infection, and hastens involution of the uterus when a spontaneous return to normal uterine tone is abnormally delayed. Ergonovine prevents postpartum hemorrhage and checks postabortal bleeding.

This is a relatively safe ergot product, because its effects are largely limited to the uterus when it is administered in moderate doses. However, it is not used for prolonged periods because of the possibility of ergotism. In some patients, rises in blood pressure to abnormal levels are occasionally encountered. The semisynthetic derivative, methylergonovine, is said to be free of this hypertensive side effect.

Dosage and Administration. Ergonovine is administered intramuscularly in a dose of 0.2 mg. (200 mcg.) immediately after delivery of the anterior shoulder of the infant, or, in some cases, after delivery of the placenta, in order to check postpartum hemorrhage. It may be given by vein for this purpose in an emergency and repeated as necessary to control severe bleeding. Ergonovine may be given orally, three or four times daily in a dose of 0.2 to 0.4 mg. during the puerperium to speed involution of the uterus and to prevent late bleeding. It is occasionally given in doses of 0.4 mg. repeated hourly for aborting migraine headaches in patients who cannot tolerate ergotamine.

OXYTOCIN INJECTION SYNTHETIC U.S.P. (PITOCIN; SYNTOCINON; UTERACON)

Pharmacology. This is the oxytocic hormone which was formerly extracted from the posterior pituitary glands of animals and is now prepared synthetically. It is used in obstetrics for prevention and treatment of postpartum atony and hemorrhage and for the induction, stimulation, and management of labor. It is used to induce labor only when certain criteria for determining its safety are met—for example, no cephalopelvic disproportion, normal presentation of the fetus, and a lack of factors that indicate a predisposition to uterine rupture, such as the presence of scars from previous cesarian section or other surgery of the cervix or uterus.

Dosage and Administration. For management of labor and control of postpartum hemorrhage, 3 to 10 units are administered intramuscularly or 1 to 2 units intravenously when the anterior shoulder appears and is delivered. For the induction of labor, 1 ml. (10 units) is added to 1,000 ml. of a 5% dextrose solution and administered by slow intravenous infusion. The rate of drip is adjusted in accordance with uterine response and fetal condition from an initial rate of 10 to 15 drops per minute up to a maximum of 40 drops (2 ml.), if necessary. The patient is kept under constant supervision, and the infusion is discontinued if sustained contractions occur or if changes in the fetal heart rhythm indicate fetal distress.

Other forms of oxytocin include oxytocin citrate for buccal administration. For induction of labor, these tablets are placed in the parabuccal space next to the upper molars. A nasal spray is employed mainly to relieve breast engorgement during lactation. The material is sprayed or instilled into each nostril 2 or 3 minutes before the breasts are pumped or nursing is begun.

CHAPTER 40

DRUGS USED IN ALLERGY, COUGH, AND ASTHMA

Allergy, Hypersensitivity, and Anaphylaxis

BETAZOLE HYDROCHLORIDE U.S.P. (HISTALOG)

Pharmacology. This analogue of histamine is said to stimulate acid gastric secretion when administered in doses less likely to cause typical side effects on the cardiovascular system. Thus, it is used only for testing the ability of the stomach to secrete acid. Failure to evoke a gastric secretory response is one indication of the presence of pernicious anemia (Chap. 25).

Side effects occur less often than with histamine but are essentially similar. Flushing of the face with sweating and a feeling of warmth are most common. Headaches occur much less frequently, and faintness or syncope are rare. Caution is required in patients with bronchial asthma or other severe allergic conditions.

Dosage and Administration. A dose of 0.5 mg./Kg., or often a total dose of 50 mg., is administered subcutaneously or intramuscularly. As with histamine itself, observe patients for flushing, fall in blood pressure, and a reflex increase in the pulse rate. If the reaction seems severe, promptly notify the doctor. Epinephrine (Adrenalin) should be available when histamine or its analogue is to be administered.

CHLORPHENIRAMINE MALEATE U.S.P. (CHLOR-TRIMETON)

Pharmacology. This antihistaminic agent of the alkylamine chemical class counteracts the characteristic effects of histamine when administered in low oral doses that ordinarily cause few side effects. However, because some patients may become drowsy or dizzy, they are cautioned against driving a car at the beginning of treatment or engaging in mechanical activities that require alertness. Injections are sometimes followed by a fall in blood pressure marked by dizziness, weakness, sweating, pallor, and rapid, weak pulse.

The oral forms of the drug, administered alone or combined with aspirin and other analgesic-antipyretics, are employed for symptomatic relief of allergic rhinitis, conjunctivitis, urticaria, angioedema, eczema, drug and serum sickness reactions, atopic and contact dermatoses, insect bites, and generalized pruritus. Parenteral therapy is indicated in the prevention and treatment of penicillin reactions and other severe allergic conditions that require rapid response, or when oral medication has failed to produce the desired response or is contraindicated. It is, however, no substitute for epinephrine in acute auaphylactoid reactions.

Dosage and Administration. The usual oral adult dose is 4 mg. up to four times a day. Prolonged action tablets containing 8 and 12 mg. need be given only once every 8 or 12 hours. An intramuscular dose of 10 mg. may be used prophylactically in attempts to avoid penicillin reactions, and up to 20 mg. may be administered intravenously in the treatment of actual anaphylactic reactions. This may be followed by an additional 10 mg. subcutaneously or intramuscularly to prevent recurrence of symptoms.

DIPHENHYDRAMINE HYDROCHLORIDE U.S.P. (BENADRYL)

Pharmacology. This prototype antihistamine drug of the ethanolamine chemical class has moderately high central sedative and peripheral anticholinergic properties. Thus drowsiness and dryness of the mouth are not uncommon side effects, and people prone to become lethargic or less alert than normal should not drive a car or undertake other activities of a potentially dangerous nature. The drug may add to the depressant effects of barbiturates or other sedatives, tranquilizers, or hypnotics.

Diphenhydramine has proved effective in allergic disorders such as hay fever, vasomotor rhinitis, atopic and contact dermatitis, acute and chronic urticaria, angioedema, drug reactions, serum sickness, transfusion reactions, and G.I. allergy. It has been employed for its C.N.S. effects in parkinsonism, and for control of dystonic reactions to the phenothiazine tranquilizer drugs, as well as for motion sickness and other conditions in which nausea, vomiting, and vertigo occur.

Dosage and Administration. Diphenhydramine is administered orally to adults in doses of 25 to 50 mg. three or four times daily. Doses as high as 300 to 400 mg. daily may be required and tolerated. Doses of 10 to 50 mg. may be injected parenterally. The drug is available in a cream for topical application.

HISTAMINE PHOSPHATE U.S.P.

Pharmacology. Histamine has a number of diagnostic and therapeutic uses, but its clinical value is limited by the widespread undesired effects that are often elicited simultaneously.

The most important use of histamine is as a diagnostic aid in determining the stomach's capacity to secrete acid. Although histamine can cause functioning gastric glands to increase their production of acid secretions when administered in relatively low doses, its use is often accompanied by side effects such as flushing, fall in blood pressure, tachycardia, vertigo, nausea, and abdominal cramps. It is contraindicated in patients with peptic ulcer, bronchial asthma, and other allergies, and the less toxic analogue *betazole* (see Drug Digest), is preferred in patients who are particularly sensitive to histamine.

Histamine is used occasionally in one of a battery of tests employed to detect pheochromocytoma (Chap. 17), and in the desensitization treatment of various vascular headaches believed to be of allergic origin. It is employed to relieve vertigo in Meniere's disease. Here, too, a related compound of lesser toxicity, *betahistine hydrochloride* (Serc), is claimed less likely to cause undesired side effects.

Dosage and Administration. For testing gastric acidity, the usual dose for subcutaneous injection is 800 mcg., which is the equivalent of 300 mcg. of histamine base. Doses up to 2,000 mcg. are sometimes administered after first protecting the patient by prior administration of an antihistaminic agent. The patient is first tested for histamine hypersensitivity with a small test dose.

TRIPELENNAMINE HYDROCHLORIDE U.S.P. (PYRIBENZAMINE)

Pharmacology. This antihistamine drug of the ethylenediamine chemical class is available alone or combined with various drugs to relieve the symptoms of hay fever and other upper respiratory tract allergies; urticarial and other skin reactions marked by pruritus, redness, and edema; contact dermatitis caused by poison ivy, poison oak, poison sumac, and other skin-sensitizing allergens; reactions to drugs including penicillin; pyrogenic transfusion reactions; and for asthmatic cough and bronchoconstriction.

Drowsiness, the most common side effect, is counteracted by combining tripelennamine with methylphenidate, or by drinking coffee containing caffeine. Mouth dryness, epigastric distress, nausea, vertigo, and occasional dysuria are sometimes felt but are rarely severe enough to require discontinuing the drug. It is administered with caution to patients taking sedative, hypnotic, or tranquilizer drugs.

Dosage and Administration. The usual oral adult dose is 50 mg. taken once or twice daily, but dosage may be 25 to 600 mg. or more daily, depending on individual need and tolerance. The drug may be administered intramuscularly or by slow intravenous injection of 25 mg. for rapid control of severe drug and transfusion reactions. It is available in the form of an ointment or cream for topical application in pruritic dermatoses and as a nasal spray combined with an adrenergic decongestant, naphazoline HCl.

Management of Cough

CODEINE PHOSPHATE U.S.P.

Pharmacology. This salt of an alkaloid of opium is used both for the relief of pain of mild to moderate intensity and as a centrally acting antitussive. In the latter case, adequate doses of codeine tend to reduce the frequency of cough volleys caused by inflammatory irritation of the respiratory tract mucosa. Since codeine is less likely than morphine to produce dependence or cause respiratory depression, it is preferred to the more potent opiates and opioids in most clinical situations that require cough control.

Although C.N.S. and peripheral side effects occur less frequently with codeine than with morphine, some patients seem to be sensitive to this alkaloid. This may be manifested by anorexia, nausea, vomiting, or constipation, and by dizziness, drowsiness, and headache.

Dosage and Administration. Many cough mixtures contain 8 mg./teaspoonful dose. A more adequate dose is 15 mg. This may be repeated every 4 hours. Doses as high as 60 mg. are sometimes administered orally or subcutaneously for analgesic action. The traditional preparation Terpin Hydrate and Codeine Elixir N.F. which contains only 8 mg. of codeine per teaspoonful together with a therapeutically inadequate dose of the expectorant terpin hydrate, is not very effective for cough relief. Equally weak is the commonly sold Compound Syrup of White Pine with Codeine.

DEXTROMETHORPHAN HYDROBROMIDE N.F. (ROMILAR, ETC.)

Pharmacology. This synthetic morphinan derivative is, unlike the levo isomer of the same compound, devoid of analgesic and addictive properties. It is the most thoroughly investigated of the centrally acting non-narcotic depressants of the cough reflex, and apparently effectively controls most minor coughs, such as those caused by the common cold. Although about as effective an antitussive as codeine in such cases, it seems less likely than that opium alkaloid to cause G.I. and C.N.S. side effects, such as constipation and drowsiness.

Dosage and Administration. The official usual dose is 10 to 20 mg. one to four times daily. It is most commonly available in syrups containing 15 mg./teaspoonful (5 ml.) dose.

Management of Asthma

AMINOPHYLLINE U.S.P. (THEOPHYLLINE ETHYLENEDIAMINE)

Pharmacology. This solubilized form of theophylline is the most commonly employed derivative. Its several pharmacological effects are shared to various degrees by all drugs of the xanthine class, including caffeine and theobromine: smooth muscle relaxation, myocardial and C.N.S. stimulation, and diuresis.

Aminophylline has a direct spasmolytic action on bronchial smooth muscle, which makes it especially useful for relief of dyspnea in patients with status asthmaticus who fail to respond to epinephrine. For this purpose, a dilute solution is administered by slow intravenous injection in order to avoid adverse cardiovascular effects. Smaller oral doses of aminophylline, administered alone or combined with ephedrine and barbiturates, are employed in the long-term treatment of chronic bronchial asthma cases. The barbiturate tends to counteract restlessness and insomnia induced by the C.N.S. stimulating actions of the combination of xanthine and adrenergic drugs.

Aminophylline often relieves pulmonary edema and dyspnea following acute left ventricular failure. In such cases, its effects are mainly the result of its direct myocardial stimulating and diuretic effects. That is, it acts like the digitalis glycosides (but more rapidly than most of the latter) to increase cardiac output, reduce venous pressure, and speed removal of edema fluid by the kidneys.

Dosage and Administration. Aminophylline is administered orally, rectally, and by injection. Oral dosage is 100 to 200 mg. three times daily. Rectal dosage by suppository or retention enema is 250 to 500 mg. once a day, or twice daily, in the morning and evening. Intravenously, dilute solutions containing 250 to 500 mg. are injected slowly up to three times a day. The drug is occasionally injected intramuscularly but may cause prolonged pain as a result of tissue irritation. Local irritation may also be manifested in the anorectal area with the continued use of suppositories; and nausea, vomiting, and epigastric distress are common side effects resulting from irritation of the upper G.I. tract by orally administered tablets.

HYDROCORTISONE SODIUM SUCCINATE U.S.P. (SOLU-CORTEF)

Pharmacology. This highly soluble ester-salt of the adrenal hormone hydrocortisone is especially useful for parenteral administration in status asthmaticus and other emergencies that respond to intensive treatment with corticosteroids. These conditions include acute allergic reactions, severe fulminating infections, acute adrenal insufficiency, and acute exacerbations of potentially fatal diseases such as lupus erythematosus. Although this form of hydrocortisone shares the hazards of the parent compound, its use for short-term therapy in emergencies is unlikely to cause cushingoid signs and symptoms.

Dosage and Administration. This preparation is administered intravenously or intramuscularly in doses of 50 to 300 mg. daily. An initial dose of 100 mg. is administered intravenously dissolved in 2 ml. of water or isotonic salt solution and followed by repeated I.V. or intramuscular 50-mg. doses as needed during continued emergency treatment. The drug may be administered by intravenous drip dissolved in a saline-dextrose solution. Oral therapy is substituted for parenteral steroids as soon as practicable.

POTASSIUM IODIDE U.S.P.

Pharmacology. This inorganic iodine salt is used mainly as a mucolytic expectorant for liquefying tenacious sputum in the treatment of bronchial asthma, bronchiectasis, and the later stages of bronchitis. It stimulates secretion by the bronchial glands mainly as a result of reflex actions induced by gastric irritation. Thus moderate doses may cause epigastric distress, nausea, and diarrhea in some patients.

Sensitivity to iodides may be manifested by painful swelling of the parotid glands within a day or two of the start of treatment or by acneform skin lesions after 4 to 7 days. Such parotitis and ioderma require the prompt withdrawal of iodides. Other patients on long-term therapy may develop iodism, or chronic iodide poisoning. This may begin with soreness of the mouth and a brassy, burning taste, followed by sore throat, sinus headache, and symptoms of a heavy head cold such as excessive secretion of the nasal and lacrimal glands and chest congestion.

The doctor is careful not to confuse these signs and the accompanying pharyngitis, laryngitis, and tonsillitis with those of a secondary respiratory infection, for their occurrence requires withdrawal of iodides rather than administration of anti-infective therapy. Removal of excess iodides from the body is sometimes speeded by administration of saline solutions or osmotic diuretics. The use of iodides is considered undesirable in patients with thyroid disease or tuberculosis.

Dosage and Administration. Potassium iodide may be administered in the form of a saturated solution containing 1 Gm./ml. or as tablets or capsules, or dissolved in a syrup. The usual dose is 300 mg. up to four times daily, but up to 2 Gm. a day is sometimes ordered. Give each dose with a glass of water or milk to hydrate the patient and to reduce gastric irritation.

CHAPTER 41

DRUGS USED IN THE MANAGEMENT OF RHEUMATIC DISORDERS AND HEADACHE

Headache

ERGOTAMINE TARTRATE U.S.P. (GYNERGEN, ETC.)

Pharmacology. This ergot alkaloid is relatively specific for aborting acute attacks of migraine. Administered early in an attack in adequate dosage, ergotamine often brings about dramatic relief. The drug is believed to act by constricting dilated cranial arteries and thus reducing their painful pulsations. This action is said to be potentiated by the addition of caffeine, a much weaker constrictor of cerebral blood vessels.

Employed in ordinary dosage, ergotamine rarely constricts peripheral vessels. However, patients who take this drug more frequently than once weekly are watched closely for numbness and tingling of toes and fingers and other signs of ergotism. Like other ergot alkaloids, this one is not used in patients who show signs of peripheral vascular disease, coronary artery insufficiency, or other conditions marked by arteriosclerosis.

Dosage and Administration. Ergotamine is most promptly effective when injected intramuscularly in a dose of 0.25 to 0.5 mg. during the period before the attack becomes severe. This dose may be repeated twice at half-hour intervals if necessary, but no more than 1 mg. is given this way in 1 day. (The total I.V. dose permissible in a 24-hour period is only 0.5 mg.)

The drug is available for oral, sublingual, and rectal use in the form of tablets, suppositories, and retention enemas and even as an aerosol for oral inhalation. Administered orally in combination with caffeine, 2 tablets (2 mg.) followed every half hour by a 1-mg. tablet often controls mild migraine symptoms within a few hours, especially when taken at the first sign of an approaching attack. The maximum amount recommended for oral use is 6 mg. Some patients may take this all at once, if they know that this is the minimal amount that will prove effective.

METHYSERGIDE MALEATE (SANSERT)

Pharmacology. This drug has proved to be an effective *prophylactic* against vascular headaches, including migraine and cluster headaches, but it is of no value for the management of acute attacks. Its exact mechanism is uncertain, but its preventive effect may stem from an ability to antagonize serotonin, histamine, and neurokinin—chemicals believed to be responsible, in part, for cranial vasodilation and local edema and tenderness during attacks of head pain.

Side effects similar to those sometimes seen with related ergot derivatives may occur. Most common early in treatment are epigastric distress, nausea, and vomiting. More serious is possible vasospasm, manifested by painful muscle spasms of the legs, numbness and cold in the hands, and chest pain—symptoms which patients should be warned to report immediately. These symptoms usually disappear when dosage is reduced. Symptoms of abdominal distress resulting from mesenteric arteriolar constriction and retroperitoneal fibrosis are reported occasionally. The latter condition, which is marked by pelvic area growths of fibrous tissue that may cause urinary obstruction, requires withdrawal of the drug. A related condition, pleuropulmonary fibrosis, has recently been recognized. Such symptoms as shortness of breath and chest pains are said to be relieved soon after this medication is stopped.

Like other ergot derivatives, methysergide is contraindicated in the presence of peripheral vascular and coronary artery disease. It is not given to pregnant migrainous patients nor to those with liver or kidney disease or sepsis.

Dosage and Administration. Patients are often started on a single 2-mg. tablet taken at bedtime with food and liquid. Later, equal doses are also administered with each meal, until the patient is taking a total dose of 8 mg. daily. This may be increased to 12 mg. or more daily or reduced temporarily if necessary. A drug-free interval of several weeks is recommended after 6 months of therapy. The drug should be discontinued slowly to avoid rebound headaches.

Rheumatic Disorders

GOLD SODIUM THIOMALATE U.S.P. (MYOCHRYSINE)

Pharmacology. This gold salt is used for managing cases of active rheumatoid arthritis that are not adequately controlled by salicylates and corticosteroids alone. Although the drug often produces rapid partial or complete remissions, the incidence of side effects is relatively high, and patients must be closely observed in order to detect early signs of potentially severe toxicity.

Among the abnormalities that may require discontinuance of the drug are skin reactions (itching, redness); albuminuria; G.I. inflammation including stomatitis, glossitis, gingivitis, and colitis; and blood cell count alterations. Thus, patients are questioned concerning their condition and examined for signs of reactions. Urinalyses and differential blood counts are carried out routinely at frequent intervals.

Gold salts are used with extreme caution, if at all, in the presence of kidney, liver, or cardiac diseases and in patients with chronic skin, blood, and G.I. disorders, such as lupus, anemia, or colitis. Severe toxic reactions are counteracted to some extent by treatment with dimercaprol (BAL).

Dosage and Administration. This drug is administered intramuscularly in doses that are individualized. A typical schedule of 24 weekly injections may be initiated with 10-mg. doses, which are gradually raised to 25 mg. and then 50 mg. Maintenance schedules usually call for less frequent administration of larger amounts—for example, 35 mg. every 2 weeks, or 45 mg. every 3 weeks.

HYDROXYCHLOROQUINE SULFATE U.S.P. (PLAQUENIL)

Pharmacology. This agent, introduced originally as an antiparasitic in malaria and giardiasis, is also employed in the collagen diseases, rheumatoid arthritis, and chronic discoid lupus erythematosus, as well as for control of polymorphic light eruptions.

Side effects that are frequent but are usually controlled by reducing the dosage, include G.I. upset, headache, dizziness, and skin eruptions. More serious are various visual defects that may develop. The eyes are examined periodically to detect corneal changes or early evidence of retinopathy, while it is reversible. The drug is discontinued immediately if retinal changes or visual field restrictions are noted. Complete blood cell counts are made at frequent intervals during long-term therapy.

Dosage and Administration. Hydroxychloroquine is taken in daily doses of 400 to 600 mg. during the first 4 to 12 weeks of rheumatoid arthritis treatment, and dosage is later reduced to a maintenance level of 200 to 400 mg. daily. Maintenance dosage in cases of lupus and light eruptions are similar, after initiating therapy with doses as high as 800 mg. daily.

PHENYLBUTAZONE N.F. (BUTAZOLIDIN)

Pharmacology. This chemical relative of the pyrazolon-type analgesic aminopyrine (Chap. 10), shares the analgesic-antipyretic, and anti-inflammatory actions of that drug. Like the latter, it can cause agranulocytosis and other toxic reactions. These limit its usefulness for most patients with rheumatoid arthritis, whose condition can usually be just as adequately and much more safely controlled with salicylates.

However, the potent anti-inflammatory activity of this agent is sometimes especially useful in ankylosing spondylitis not responsive to salicylates; in acute gout attacks not controlled by colchicine; and in some cases of acute thrombophlebitis.

Side effects have been reported in as many as 40 per cent of patients who take phenylbutazone. These include G.I. upset, which may be partially counteracted by administration of phenylbutazone in combination with antacids such as aluminum hydroxide gel and magnesium trisilicate. The drug is contraindicated in patients with peptic ulcer to avoid reactivating this condition. Its use is considered dangerous for patients with cardiac decompensation, in whom its tendency to cause fluid retention and edema may precipitate congestive failure. Caution is also required in patients with a history of drug-induced dermatitis or hematological disorders, because of their possible

sensitivity to this drug, which is known to cause skin rashes and blood dyscrasias occasionally.

Dosage and Administration. Treatment of most rheumatoid conditions is begun with about 100 mg. three or four times daily. In acute gouty arthritis, an initial dose of 400 mg. is followed by doses of 100 mg. every 4 hours until the attack subsides. The drug is usually taken with food or a full glass of milk to minimize gastric upset.

PREDNISOLONE BUTYLACETATE (HYDELTRA-T.B.A.)

Pharmacology. This is an only slightly soluble ester of the synthetic corticosteroid prednisolone. When injected locally into a joint, bursa, or soft tissue sites, its anti-inflammatory activity often provides prolonged relief in rheumatoid arthritis, osteoarthritis, acute gouty arthritis, bursitis, and tendinitis. Relief begins in a day or two and lasts from a few days to a few weeks.

Patients are told that their discomfort may actually become worse for a while before improvement becomes apparent. They are also warned to avoid excessive use of the joint, for this may lead to its deterioration despite the symptomatic relief. A continued increase in local pain and swelling accompanied by fever and general malaise may indicate the development of a joint infection requiring immediate and prolonged antibiotic therapy.

Dosage and Administration. The dosage of this drug depends mainly on the size of the joint involved. Thus finger or toe joints may require 8 to 10 mg., whereas knee joints may need 20 to 30 mg. for full relief. If the response is too weak or transient, the amount of suspension deposited in the joint may be raised. Injections are repeated at appropriate intervals ranging from 1 week to as much as 1 month.

COLCHICINE U.S.P.

Pharmacology. This alkaloid is specific for aborting or relieving acute attacks of gout, and aids in reducing the frequency and severity of such attacks when taken prophylactically in low doses during the intercritical period. It is neither an analgesic nor an antirheumatic but somehow suppresses the inflammatory response to uric acid crystals that are being deposited in gouty joints during an attack.

Overdosage of colchicine results in nausea, vomiting, and diarrhea. Since such symptoms are likely to occur during treatment of an acute attack, especially when the patient is still uncertain of the required dosage, patients should have available paregoric and other antidiarrheal medications for counteracting this side effect.

Dosage and Administration. For aborting an acute attack, colchicine is taken in doses of about 1 mg. every 2 hours until pain diminishes markedly or side effects develop. This usually requires 4 to 8 mg. total dosage. During the intervals between attacks, patients take about 1 mg. daily, usually in divided doses of 0.5 mg. every 12 hours. However, other amounts and schedules may be employed.

PROBENECID U.S.P. (BENEMID)

Pharmacology. This drug's action upon the renal tubules accounts for its therapeutic usefulness in two different conditions: (1) for treatment of gout and gouty arthritis and (2) as an adjuvant to certain anti-infective agents in the management of infections (see Chaps. 34 and 41).

When used in the interval treatment of gout, probenecid promotes the excretion of uric acid by interfering with reabsorption of filtered urates by the renal tubules. As a result, plasma levels of uric acid are reduced. Although this lessens the likelihood of acute attacks, too high initial dosage actually sets off such an attack occasionally. If this occurs, this drug is *not* discontinued, but colchicine is administered to control the acute gout attack.

Probenecid's action in keeping urates from being reabsorbed may so raise the concentration of that metabolite in the urine that uric acid stones may form. To prevent this, the urine may be alkalinized by administering a teaspoonful of sodium bicarbonate with each dose of this drug. Probenecid is not recommended for use in patients who already have uric acid kidney stones.

Other side effects are few except for occasional headache, anorexia, nausea, and sensitivity reactions such as skin rash.

Dosage and Administration. During the first week, patients take only 250 mg. twice daily. This is then raised to 500 mg. twice a day, or occasionally to as much as 2 Gm. administered in four divided doses. Salicylates are *not* given for pain relief together with probenecid, for although salicylates are themselves uricosuric (Chap. 10), they tend to interfere with the uricosuric activity of probenecid.

CHAPTER 42

DRUGS USED IN THE TREATMENT AND DIAGNOSIS OF EYE DISORDERS

CARBACHOL U.S.P. (CARBAMYLCHOLINE; CARCHOLIN; DORYL)

Pharmacology. This potent synthetic choline ester is used mainly for its ophthalmic effects in open-angle glaucoma. It produces a drop in intraocular pressure as a result of its ability to cause miosis and spasm of accommodation by its direct action on cholinergic neuroeffectors in the sphincter muscles of the iris and ciliary body. The contraction of these muscles results in improved fluid outflow from the eye.

Systemic absorption may lead to such parasympathomimetic side effects as G.I. cramps and diarrhea. It may set off asthmatic attacks or cardiac arrhythmias in susceptible patients. The drug is no longer given by injection because its widespread cholinergic effects are difficult to control. It is undesirable in narrow-angle glaucoma because of its local vasodilating action in the eye.

Dosage and Administration. An ophthalmic solution (0.1 ml.) is instilled into the conjunctival sac one to six times daily. Solutions of 0.75, 1.5, and 3% strengths are available.

CYCLOPENTOLATE HYDROCHLORIDE U.S.P. (CYCLOGYL)

Pharmacology. Applied topically to the eye, this anticholinergic agent rapidly penetrates the mucosa to produce complete mydriasis and cycloplegia of comparatively short duration. It is used in ophthalmology for refraction and in the treatment of iritis, iridocyclitis, choroiditis, and keratitis.

Normal vision is usually recovered within one day compared to as much as a week or more with atropine. Recovery time can be further reduced—to about 6 hours—by dropping a pilocarpine solution into the eye. Also, pilocarpine antagonizes any peripheral atropinelike effects that may occur as a result of systemic absorption in young children who are especially sensitive to atropine-type drugs.

Dosage and Administration. Ophthalmic solutions of 0.5, 1, and 2% strengths are available. One or 2 drops of the less concentrated solutions are usually effective for children and adult Caucasians; the stronger drops are employed for adult Negroes and others with darkly pigmented irises, which are relatively resistant to the action of anticholinergic mydriatic drugs. However, the 2% solution may be required for children

and adult whites when instillations of 1 or 2 drops of a weaker solution have proved ineffective.

DEMECARIUM BROMIDE U.S.P. (HUMORSOL)

Pharmacology. This potent cholinesterase-inhibiting agent is used mainly as a long-acting miotic in the management of chronic, simple glaucoma. It may be useful in glaucoma secondary to removal of the lens (aphakia) and in children with accommodative convergent strabismus. However, the drug is contraindicated in narrow-angle glaucoma and in glaucoma secondary to iritis, because it may, in such cases, cause a rise in intraocular pressure instead of the long-lasting reduction in tension that ordinarily occurs.

Local side effects include browache, headache, and blurring of vision as a result of ciliary muscle spasm; photophobia, myopia, and twitching of the eyelids may occur; the conjunctiva may redden as a result of vasodilation; and nodules may develop on the iris margins. Systemic absorption from the conjunctiva may cause cholinergic effects including bronchial constriction, abdominal pain, and diarrhea. Severe poisoning may be marked by convulsions and respiratory failure.

Dosage and Administration. Systemic absorption of solutions being instilled into the eye may be minimized by holding the lids open for several seconds and by pressing upon the nasolacrimal ducts for a minute or two. Optimal dosage, which is determined by tonometric measurements, is 1 or 2 drops of a 0.25% solution twice daily to twice weekly. Paradoxical rises in intraocular tension should be counteracted by appropriate measures, including the use of vasoconstrictors locally and carbonic anhydrase inhibitors.

DICHLORPHENAMIDE U.S.P. (DARANIDE; ORATROL)

Pharmacology. This carbonic anhydrase inhibitor is used mainly to reduce intraocular pressure in glaucoma rather than as a diuretic for treating edematous disorders. Administered alone, or together with topically applied miotics, it often produces a prompt fall in intraocular pressure. This is thought to be brought about by a reduction in the rate at which fluid is secreted into the chambers of the eye.

Side effects involve mainly the G.I. tract and nervous system. Loss of appetite, nausea and vomiting, dizziness, headache, mental confusion, and fatigue are sometimes seen. Paresthesias—numbness and tingling of fingers and toes, lips, and anus—are reported occasionally. Watch patients for signs of hypersensitivity including red, itchy skin rash or hives. Agranulocytosis and thrombocytopenia have been reported. Potassium salts may be administered to counteract any indications of hypokalemia. The drug should not be used in patients with acid-base imbalance or renal or hepatic insufficiency.

Dosage and Administration. Patients with open-angle glaucoma are often maintained on doses of 25 to 50 mg., one to three times daily. Larger doses—100 to 200 mg.—may be needed in initiating therapy and especially during an acute attack.

ECHOTHIOPHATE IODIDE U.S.P. (PHOSPHOLINE)

Pharmacology. This long-acting anticholinesterase drug controls intraocular pressure in selected cases of chronic, simple (wide-angle) glaucoma. It acts like other cholinergic miotics to increase the flow of fluid out of the anterior chamber of the eye. Its longer duration of action permits less frequent administration than is required with pilocarpine and other direct-acting drugs.

However, because echothiophate is more irritating than pilocarpine and physostigmine, it is usually reserved for patients whose intraocular tension is not adequately controlled by these less potent miotics. This drug is contraindicated in narrow-angle glaucoma because its potent action may cause congestion and a paradoxical rise in intraocular pressure.

Other local ocular effects include aching of the eye and blurring of vision as a result of spasm of the ciliary muscle. Cysts may develop in the pupillary margin of the iris, especially in children. Systemic absorption may occasionally cause cramps, diarrhea, salivation, nausea, and vomiting.

Dosage and Administration. One drop of a solution of echothiophate is instilled into the conjunctival sac usually once daily at bedtime. Occasionally, administration on alternate days is adequate; sometimes two daily instillations are required, but never more. Solutions of 0.06, 0.125, and 0.25% are employed in accordance with individual requirements.

EPINEPHRINE BITARTRATE U.S.P. (EPITRATE, ETC.)

Pharmacology. This salt of epinephrine is used in 1 and 2% ophthalmic solutions which are applied topically to constrict the vessels of the eye and, thus, reduce the rate of aqueous secretion in chronic, simple (wide-angle) glaucoma. Its use in narrow-angle glaucoma is contraindicated because mydriasis may precipitate an acute congestive attack.

Instillation is often followed by stinging and ocular discomfort or pain. However, this is transitory and tends to lessen with continued treatment. A secondary redness commonly occurs, and this reactive hyperemia may cause a chronically boggy and discolored conjunctiva.

The drug's initial vasoconstrictor action tends to prevent its systemic absorption. However, it is used with caution in elderly patients and others who may be especially sensitive to adrenergic stimulation, including those with hypertension, heart disease, hyperthyroidism, and diabetes.

Dosage and Administration. Dosage varies with the requirements of different patients. Some require 1 drop every 2 or 3 days; others need 2 drops, twice daily. Initial dosage is determined on the basis of careful studies of the pressure changes and the width of the angle. When used in combination with miotics, such as pilocarpine, the latter is instilled first, a few minutes before epinephrine.

EUCATROPINE HYDROCHLORIDE U.S.P. (EUPHTHALMINE)

Pharmacology. This anticholinergic agent produces rapid mydriasis without cycloplegia when applied topically to the eye. The drug is used alone or combined with an adrenergic mydriatic, such as phenylephrine or ephedrine, for aiding the ophthalmoscopic examination of the retina and optic disk.

Maximal dilation occurs within 1 hour, and the iris returns to normal in a few hours. Blurring of vision does not occur because there is little or no interference with accommodation. Although the drug's mydriatic action causes no increase in the intraocular pressure of normal eyes, it is, of course, contraindicated for patients with glaucoma.

Dosage and Administration. One or 2 drops of a 2 or 5% solution are applied topically to the conjunctiva for rapid mydriatic action.

HOMATROPINE HYDROBROMIDE U.S.P.

Pharmacology. This anticholinergic agent is employed to dilate the pupil prior to retinoscopy and to paralyze accommodation temporarily prior to refraction and in the treatment of keratitis and uveitis. Although relatively weak compared to atropine, it has the advantage of wearing off rapidly, so that recovery is usually complete within 1 day. The solution is used with caution in patients over the age of 40, for they are more subject to precipitation of glaucoma attacks by atropinic agents.

Dosage and Administration. A 1% solution is employed to produce mydriasis. Repeated instillations (up to 6 times daily) of a 2% solution may be required to produce and maintain cycloplegia.

IDOXURIDINE (HERPLEX; STOXIL; IDU)

Pharmacology. This is an antiviral chemotherapeutic agent specifically indicated in the treatment of herpes simplex keratitis. Topical application in infections that are limited to the corneal epithelium often checks such infections. Responses are less favorable in more deeply localized infections.

Idoxuridine may be combined with antibiotics to control secondary infections by bacteria. Its use in combination with corticosteroids is ordinarily contraindicated in *superficial* keratitis, for such steroids may accelerate the spread of the herpes simplex virus to deeper structures. However, some ophthalmologists employ such combinations of topical idoxuridine and systemic steroids cautiously for treating deep-seated virus infections of the eye.

Some local irritation and edema of the eyes and lids has been reported after instillation of solutions of idoxuridine, but these may be manifestations of the condition being treated rather than side effects of the drug. The simultaneous use of boric acid solutions is undesirable for it can cause irritation in the presence of idoxuridine.

Dosage and Administration. Idoxuridine is available in ophthalmic solutions and ointments. One drop of the solution is placed in each infected eye every hour during the day and every 2 hours at night, until definite improvement occurs. The ointment need be instilled only about every 4 hours. Treatment with these ophthalmic products is continued at reduced dosage for several days after the corneal lesions seem healed.

PHYSOSTIGMINE SALTS U.S.P. (ESERINE)

Pharmacology. The salicylate and sulfate salts of this alkaloid are applied topically to the eye to produce miosis and spasm of accommodation. These actions are the result of increased cholinergic activity that stems indirectly from the drug's ability to inhibit activity of the enzyme cholinesterase.

Contraction of the sphincter muscles of the iris and ciliary body often quickly brings about increased outflow of fluid from the anterior chamber and a resulting reduction of intraocular pressure in glaucoma of the open-angle type. This drug is ordinarily avoided in narrow-angle glaucoma, except in acute attacks when it may be instilled alternately with pilocarpine as part of emergency medical measures to reduce pressure prior to surgery. The drug is occasionally employed to counteract drug-induced mydriasis.

Local side effects include conjunctivitis and ciliary muscle spasm leading to blurred distant vision and headache. Systemic absorption may cause increased G.I. motility symptoms and other signs of parasympathomimetic activity. The drug has anticurare and antimyasthenic actions on skeletal muscle fibers, which is occasionally manifested in twitching of the eyelids.

Dosage and Administration. Ophthalmic solutions (0.1 ml.) of 0.25 to 0.5% strength are ordinarily instilled. Stronger solutions (1 to 2%) may be required in glaucomatous eyes that have become resistant to miotics. An ophthalmic ointment of 0.25% strength is sometimes preferred for use at bedtime.

PREDNISOLONE SODIUM PHOSPHATE OPHTHALMIC SOLUTION U.S.P.

Pharmacology. This salt and the acetate ester of the same synthetic corticosteroid are commonly applied topically as ophthalmic preparations because of their superior ability to penetrate into the anterior segment of the globe by way of the cornea. They are combined with anti-infective agents such as sulfacetamide or neomycin or with antihistaminics such as chlorpheniramine in the management of certain inflammatory disorders of external eye structures.

Among the infectious, allergic, and traumatic inflammatory conditions in which such solutions or suspensions are employed are the following: blepharitis, conjunctivitis, keratitis, iritis, and iridocyclitis. Their use is supplemented with systemic corticosteroids in severe forms of these conditions. Both local and systemic steroids are contraindicated in the early stages of acute viral diseases of the cornea, including herpes simplex infections. They are not used in the presence of active tuberculosis of the front of the eye or in fungal disease of the conjunctiva and lids.

Dosage and Administration. Acute inflammatory disorders are treated by frequent instillation of 2 or 3 drops into the conjunctival sac—every hour or two during the day and somewhat less often at night. (Ophthalmic ointments applied at bedtime provide relatively prolonged anti-inflammatory action.) If the response is favorable, dosage may be reduced gradually but is not discontinued prematurely.

SULFACETAMIDE SODIUM U.S.P. (SULAMYD)

Pharmacology. This sulfonamide is available in an official (U.S.P.) ophthalmic ointment and solution for use in the prophylaxis and treatment of external eye infections, including blepharitis, conjunctivitis, and keratitis. It penetrates readily into ocular tissues without ordinarily causing irritation or allergic sensitization. However, the use of sulfacetamide in patients already sensitive to sulfonamides is not desirable; and if employed cautiously in such cases, this drug should be discontinued at the earliest sign of an allergic reaction.

Dosage and Administration. The 10% ointment is used mainly for styes or as an adjunct to the more frequent instillation of the solutions. The 30% solution is instilled (0.1 ml.) into the conjunctival sac every 2 to 4 hours. Simultaneous systemic therapy with this drug or other sulfonamides is recommended in the treatment of trachoma.

CHAPTER 43

DRUGS USED IN DERMATOLOGY

ALUMINUM ACETATE SOLUTION U.S.P. (BUROW'S SOLUTION)

Pharmacology. This solution is used as a soak and for making wet dressings that are employed in the treatment of acute inflammatory reactions of the skin and mucosa. Its main action is as a mild astringent to exert a slight coagulant effect upon tissue protein. Applied to oozing, or weeping, lesions in acute contact dermatoses (e.g., poison ivy), acute fungal infections of the skin, and bacterial infections, especially in intertriginous areas, this solution gives some relief of itching and pain. Its cleansing and antiseptic actions exert a favorable effect upon the local environment that helps healing after opening of vesicles. The solution is said to be nonirritating and nonsensitizing.

Administration. The official 5% solution is diluted with 10 to 40 parts of water for use as a wet dressing that may be applied cold, tepid, or warm. Depending on the part of the body involved, the solution is used as a simple soak, Sitz bath, douche, or gargle. Powders in packets and tablets are also available, from which solutions of the proper strength may be prepared conveniently.

AMMONIATED MERCURY U.S.P.

Pharmacology. This insoluble compound releases the free mercury ion slowly in small amounts that have an antiseptic action on the skin without being excessively irritating. It is used in ointment form in impetigo and fungal infection of the skin, and as an ophthalmic preparation for application to the conjunctiva. The official ointment is one of the mildest medications for accelerating the scaling and healing of dry lesions in chronic psoriasis. It may be useful in pediculosis, pinworms, and pruritus ani. However, the continued use of ammoniated mercury in infants and young children with these conditions is contraindicated.

Administration. A 5% ointment is available for topical application to the skin, and a 3% ophthalmic ointment is used topically on the conjunctiva.

BENZALKONIUM CHLORIDE U.S.P. (ZEPHIRAN)

Pharmacology. This cationic-type detergent and antiseptic is used in nonirritating low concentrations to prevent and treat infections of the skin and mucous membranes. Higher concentrations are employed for sterilizing surgical instruments and other operating room materials that are to be stored in a sterile state.

Certain precautions are required in both the above uses. When they are to be applied to the skin preoperatively, benzalkonium solutions are used only after all soap has been rinsed from the skin site and it has been swabbed with alcohol. This keeps the cationic detergent from being inactivated through the antagonistic anionic action of ordinary soaps. Similarly, in storing cotton sponges, rubber gloves, and other materials, loss of activity is avoided by using fresh solutions, since these materials tend to absorb the antiseptic. Thus repeated use of the same solution reduces its concentration below effective germicidal levels.

Administration. An alcohol-water solution, or tincture, applied preoperatively in a 1:1,000 dilution disinfects the patient's skin and the surgeon's hands. Although this preparation may be used in minor wounds, more dilute aqueous solutions are ordinarily preferred for irrigating deep wounds, widely denuded skin areas, and mucous membranes of the eye and the genitourinary tract (e.g., 1:2,000 to 1:5,000 as a vaginal douche; 1:3,000 to 1:10,000 for eye irrigation; 1:5,000 to 1:20,000 for urethral irrigation; and 1:20,000 to 1:40,000 for retention lavage of the urinary bladder).

BENZYL BENZOATE U.S.P. (ALBACIDE: BENYLATE)

Pharmacology. This safe and effective scabicide kills lice as well as mites. It should be kept from coming in contact with the eyes and thus is best not applied to the face at all. Persons with especially sensitive skin may feel a burning sensation and even suffer from severe skin irritation as a result of treatment.

Administration. The official lotion contains 25% of this chemical. It is applied over the entire body except the face while the skin is still wet after a bath in warm, soapy water. A second application is made on the obviously involved areas after the first has dried. The following day another warm bath is taken, and after such a soaking, clean clothing is put on. Further treatments are administered if the parasite infestation persists.

BORIC ACID U.S.P.

Pharmacology. This substance, which is widely used by the public as a household remedy, has an unwarranted reputation as an antiseptic and astringent healing agent. It is an ingredient of numerous preparations employed in the treatment of bacterial and fungal skin infections, burns, bedsores, and diaper rash.

In the concentrations ordinarily employed topically, boric acid is harmless. However, systemic absorption of undiluted boric acid powder through skin abrasions or after accidental ingestion has resulted in severe toxicity. Some authorities have suggested that this substance be colored blue as a warning against accidental misuse; others feel that its virtues are so limited that boric acid might well be dropped from medical use.

Administration. Boric acid is available as a saturated solution of about 5% and in dusting powders and ointments containing about 4 to 10% of this ingredient combined with other protectives and emollients. The solution is used undiluted or in various lower concentrations for making wet dressings for the skin or for irrigating the mucous membranes of the mouth, eye, or genitourinary tract.

CARBOL-FUCHSIN SOLUTION N.F. (CASTELLANI'S PAINT)

Pharmacology. This alcohol-acetone solution of the antiseptic dye fuchsin and other antifungal agents such as benzoic and boric acids and phenol is often effective against ringworm in interdigital areas and intertriginous sites. Painted between the toes, on the axillae, or in the anogenital region, the medication tends to dry the moist tissues and relieve itching. It is rarely irritating or sensitizing but may cause excessive drying and thus add to the chronic fissuring if applied too frequently.

Administration. The solution is applied with an applicator no more than once daily. It is kept tightly closed to avoid evaporation and concentration of the solution. Take care to avoid staining clothing. A fresh solution should be used, for it deteriorates in a few weeks.

CYPROHEPTADINE (PERIACTIN)

Pharmacology. This antihistamine drug is recommended for relief of itching in various dermatologic disorders, including acute and chronic urticaria and angioneurotic edema; atopic dermatitis (disseminated neurodermatitis) and localized neurodermatitis, pruritus ani and vulvae. It may be useful in respiratory allergy, including perennial rhinitis and hay fever.

In addition to its antihistaminic, antiserotonin, and anticholinergic actions, cyproheptadine is a C.N.S. depressant. This may be the main source of its antipruritic activity. It is certainly the cause of the drug's most common side effect—drowsiness. While such sedation is often desirable for reducing perception of itch stimuli and decreasing emotional tension in pruritus, the resulting loss of alertness is dangerous in some circumstances. Warn patients against driving a car if they are made drowsy by cyproheptadine; and caution them against drinking alcoholic beverages while taking this medication.

Dosage and Administration. Dosage is individualized in accordance with the severity of the symptoms and the age and tolerance of the patient. Adult dosage ranges from 4 mg. three times daily to no more than a total of 32 mg. given in four divided doses. Children receive reduced dosage in accordance with their age, size, and response. The usual dose for children aged 2 to 6 is 2 mg. t.i.d.; for those 6 to 14 it is 4 mg. t.i.d. This drug is available in combination with the corticosteroid dexamethasone.

GAMMA BENZENE HEXACHLORIDE U.S.P. (GEXANE; KWELL)

Pharmacology. This insecticide has helped to make the control of pediculosis and scabies relatively simple, once these conditions are recognized. Although it is theoretically toxic when absorbed through the skin or ingested, side effects do not occur when the products are employed properly. Avoid contact with the eyes and mucous membranes.

Administration. Creams, lotions, and shampoos containing 1% of this chemical are applied topically directly to the skin and hair, after first thoroughly cleaning the involved skin areas, or cutting the hair if it is lengthy. Instruct patients not to bathe or wash for 24 hours after treatment. Application may be repeated once more in the same week if necessary. Other family members should also be treated, and contaminated clothing should be cleaned, sterilized, or fumigated to avoid reinfection.

HEXACHLOROPHENE U.S.P. (GAMOPHENE; pHisoHex; SURGICEN; SUROFENE, ETC.)

Pharmacology. This chlorinated diphenol antiseptic is commonly incorporated into bar soaps for home use and into detergent solutions such as Hexachlorophene Liquid Soap U.S.P. for professional use. A single washing with such soaps does not seem superior to that with nonmedicated soap as a means of affecting the bacterial flora of the skin. However, the frequent use of hexachlorophene-containing soaps for detergent solutions is said to exert a cumulative antibacterial effect which is attributed to the deposit of a film of the antiseptic upon the skin surface. The repeated routine use of this compound in this manner does not irritate the skin, and bacterial resistance to it does not develop.

Soaps containing hexachlorophene are sometimes used in part of the preoperative scrub procedure for the hands of surgeons and other O.R. personnel. Patients may use such soaps on their skin at home for several days prior to surgery. Although this may reduce the bacterial skin count, it does not, of course, obviate the need for the usual preparation of the skin with strong antiseptic solutions in the final preoperative prepping of the site of the surgical incision. Patients with various skin disorders, and especially with staphylococcal infections, are often advised to cleanse their skin surfaces routinely with hexachlorophene products. Thus, such soaps and solutions are used as adjuncts in the treatment of acne, impetigo, furuncles, carbuncles, and allergic dermatoses.

Administration. Solutions or soaps containing hexachlorophene are applied topically to the previously wetted skin and worked into a lather which is spread over the entire area that is to be cleansed. Techniques for prepping the skin vary widely. However, it is claimed that in all techniques, the time spent in preparation can be shortened by the use of a hexachlorophene soap solution routinely in place of ordinary proprietary soaps.

IODINE U.S.P.

Pharmacology. This element is a highly active antiseptic against a wide variety of microorganisms, when applied to tissues in solutions of relatively low toxicity. Such solutions are employed preoperatively to disinfect the skin, are applied to skin wounds and infections, and are used to disinfect drinking water.

Although weak dilutions can be taken internally without harm—for example, as a gavage fluid for counteracting alkaloidal poisons chemically in the stomach—concentrated solutions may be corrosive to the mucosa of the G.I. tract. Deaths have sometimes resulted from circulatory collapse following ingestion of strong solutions for suicidal purposes. Starch solution lavages are used to precipitate and remove iodine in such cases.

Administration. Tincture of iodine U.S.P., a 2% solution in dilute alcohol, is the preferred form for preoperative skin preparation. Aqueous solutions, such as Iodine Solution N.F. and Strong Iodine Solution U.S.P., may be diluted to 0.5 to 1.0% concentrations for application to skin and mucous membrane wounds, abrasions, and infections. As little as 3 drops of the tincture added to a quart of water kills bacteria and amebae and yet leaves the water palatable enough for drinking.

PHENOLATED CALAMINE LOTION U.S.P.

Pharmacology. This lotion offers the protective action of calamine and zinc oxide and the mild antipruritic action of a low dilution of phenol. It is often applied to the oozing lesions of poison ivy and other contact dermatoses, or acute skin infections following application of compresses or soaks containing astringent solutions.

Other substances may be added to the basic lotion, including 1% camphor or menthol, which possess cooling and antipruritic actions that also relieve the discomfort of itchy, oozing eruptions. This lotion may be made more drying by the addition of alcohol, or it may be made more soothing by the addition of emollients such as glycerine and lanolin.

Administration. After *shaking* the lotion, apply it in small amounts to the affected areas. Application with cotton pledgets or a brush at frequent intervals is preferred to the occasional use of large amounts, as the formation of a hard residue of dried material is undesirable. A firm touch is used, as light dabbing may increase itching sensations.

The use of this lotion in the presence of infection is not desirable, and its accumulation in excessive quantities in hairy areas may cause discomfort and irritation. In the later stages, when the skin is scabby, or dry, cracked, and fissured, Calamine Ointment N.F., containing skin-softening lanolin and petrolatum, may be preferred, as may be the use of the oilier Calamine Liniment.

POTASSIUM PERMANGANATE U.S.P.

Pharmacology. This oxidizing type of antiseptic and deodorant is sometimes applied in dilute solution to weeping skin lesions or to the vaginal mucosa as a douche. The solutions have a mild astringent action that aids drying of oozing areas in the acute stages of contact dermatitis and fungal or bacterial infections. Strong solutions are sometimes used to disinfect organic matter, and much weaker solutions are sometimes used internally as gavage fluids for oxidizing certain ingested poisons (e.g., strychnine).

Administration. Complete solution of the purple crystals in adequate amounts of water to avoid irritant and caustic actions is essential. Fresh solutions of 1 part per 4,000 parts to 10,000 parts of water are effective, nonirritating, and nonsensitizing, even when used on delicate vaginal tissues. On the other hand, severe local trauma has occurred when the tablets intended for dilution have been deliberately inserted into the vaginal vault in misguided, futile, and dangerous attempts to produce an illegal abortion.

POVIDONE-IODINE N.F.
(BETADINE; ISODINE)

Pharmacology. This chemical contains iodine in a complex with polyvinylpyrrolidone, from which it is released when it comes in contact with the skin or mucous membranes to which the solution is applied. The iodine let loose in this way is less irritating to tissues than iodine applied in form of the tincture. Thus, it is often preferred for application to abraded skin and intravaginally. However, it is doubtful that this complex is as effective as iodine tincture for preoperative preparation of the skin. Patients who are sensitive to other iodine products are likely to prove allergic to this compound also.

Administration. Among the products available are: an antiseptic solution for painting on the proposed surgical site preoperatively; an aerosol for spraying on burns, wounds, and ulcers; an ointment for application to bacterial and fungal infections, lacerations, and abrasions; a gargle for use following oral surgery and in stomatitis and Vincent's infection; and a douche for cleansing the vaginal tract in the management of moniliasis, trichomoniasis, and nonspecific bacterial infections.

RESORCINOL U.S.P.

Pharmacology. Since this phenolic substance has a variety of actions on the skin, it is included in numerous dermatologic preparations employed for treating many conditions. As a mild irritant, resorcinol helps to speed the loosening and removal of the outer layer of dead skin cells or scales. This keratolytic action is useful in the management of eczema, psoriasis, and seborrheic dermatitis. In fungal infections such as ringworm and athlete's foot, this chemical has a desirable fungicidal as well as desquamating action. Its antibacterial and mild drying and peeling actions are thought to be useful in the management of acne and in various pyodermas.

Administration. Resorcinol is applied topically in ointments, pastes, and lotions varying in concentration from 2 to 20%. It is frequently combined with sulfur and with salicylic acid in lotions and soaps. Resorcinol monoacetate N.F. releases resorcin at a slow rate and is thus said to be longer-acting.

SELENIUM SULFIDE U.S.P. (SELSUN)

Pharmacology. This antiseborrheic agent, available in the form of Selenium Sulfide Detergent Suspension U.S.P., a 2.5% suspension, is effective in the control of seborrheic dermatitis of the scalp. It is most successful against the dry form of seborrhea—that is, dandruff marked by profuse, dry, powdery scales, and prevents spread of the condition to facial areas. The oily type of seborrhea with heavy, greasy, crusting patches is treated with more potent antiseborrheics, such as sulfur, salicylic acid, and, sometimes, tars, applied in ointment form and then shampooed out in the morning.

The suspension is kept from coming in contact with the eyes, for it may cause irritation, stinging, and conjunctivitis or keratitis. Although selenium is a toxic substance, systemic absorption from the scalp is unlikely, except in extensive acute inflammation. Taken orally, however, salts of this element can cause kidney and liver damage. Thus, patients are warned to keep the suspension out of the reach of children, and to wash their own hands and fingernails thoroughly after working this material into the scalp.

Administration. The hair and scalp are first washed with soapy water and rinsed. Then 1 or 2 teaspoonfuls of the suspension are massaged in and allowed to remain on the scalp for 2 or 3 minutes before rinsing thoroughly. The application is then repeated. This procedure is followed only once or twice weekly at first and less frequently later to avoid excessive oiliness or sensitization. An ointment containing selenium sulfide combined with hydrocortisone is employed on the eyelids, external ear canal, and other areas with seborrheic involvement.

SILVER NITRATE U.S.P.

Pharmacology. This silver salt is bactericidal in low concentrations. Higher concentrations have astringent and caustic actions. A 1% ophthalmic solution is employed routinely to prevent gonorrheal eye infections in newborn babies. This use in the prophylaxis of ophthalmia neonatorum is required by law to prevent blindness that might result from this eye disease. Yet silver nitrate solutions themselves frequently cause a chemical conjunctivitis, and accidents in their use has resulted in cauterization of delicate eye tissues with subsequent blindness.

A high local concentration of silver nitrate is sometimes attained deliberately by moistening a solid stick of the salt and applying it to tissues for caustic effect. This is sometimes used to remove warts and granulomatous tissues and to cauterize wounds.

Administration. The official 1% ophthalmic solution is available in collapsible capsules containing 5 drops for topical application to the conjunctival sacs of the eyes of infants. Toughened Silver Nitrate U.S.P., or Lunar Caustic, comes in pencils, the ends of which are moistened just prior to topical application of the area to be treated. Solutions ranging from 1:10 to 1:10,000 concentration are sometimes ordered. Care is required to see that solutions of the proper strength are employed for the intended purposes.

TRIAMCINOLONE ACETONIDE (ARISTOCORT; KENALOG)

Pharmacology. This synthetic corticosteroid is applied topically or sometimes injected intradermally in the management of certain skin disorders. Topical application often provides prompt and prolonged relief of pruritus in conditions marked by itching, burning, and inflammation. Among the specific indications for this and other topical steroids are eczematous dermatoses such as atopic dermatitis, contact dermatitis, seborrheic dermatitis, neurodermatitis, pruritus ani, pruritus vulvae, and—when combined with systemic measures—exfoliative dermatitis and psoriasis. In the latter condition, stubborn localized lesions are sometimes infiltrated with an aqueous suspension of this steroid.

When applied under occlusive dressings in the treatment of resistant dermatoses, deeper penetration is obtained, but at the risk of possible systemic absorption. Although hypercorticism has not occurred often as a result of this, the patient's own adrenocortical function may be somewhat suppressed, as indicated by a decrease in adrenal hormone metabolites in the urine. To avoid this, intermittent therapy with low concentrations applied topically to varied sites is recommended.

Dosage and Administration. This steroid is available in the form of cream, lotion, ointment, foam, and spray, and as aqueous injectable suspension. Concentrations of most preparations are 0.01% to 0.1%, the stronger forms being used to control dermatoses, whereas the less concentrated forms (e.g., 0.025%) are preferred for maintenance therapy. Creams and lotions are considered best for moist, weeping areas, and ointments for dry, scaly lesions. The very dilute spray (0.007%) is for coverage of extensive and hard-to-reach areas.

TRIOXSALEN (TRISORALEN)

Pharmacology. This drug produces repigmentation in vitiligo and increases tolerance to sunlight of some fair-skinned persons who fail to tan. Taken by mouth, trioxsalen is thought to concentrate in melanocytes in the basal layers of the epidermic. There it stimulates production of melanin by the melanocytes when activated by ultraviolet light.

The photosensitizing action of trioxsalen during the first days of administration makes the skin more subject to sunburn than usual. Thus, exposure to sunlight is carefully controlled in order to prevent severe reactions that may result in skin damage. After the drug has been taken for a week or two with gradually increased exposure to sunlight, the skin seems to be protected from amounts of ultraviolet light that ordinarily cause burning or peeling in some light-skinned persons. This late photoprotective effect is the result of retention of stimulated melanin pigment in epidermal strata of increased thickness—a speeding up of the tanning processes that ordinarily occurs in normal skin.

Dosage and Administration. A dose of 5 to 10 mg. is taken by mouth, preferably with milk or a meal to avoid abdominal discomfort. The patient then waits 2 to 4 hours before exposing himself to a source of ultraviolet light for brief periods, which may be lengthened gradually as tolerance to light increases. The dose of trioxsalen and exposure time to light are carefully controlled in order to avoid severe burning and injury to the skin.

CHAPTER 44

DRUG TREATMENT OF NEOPLASTIC DISEASES

BUSULFAN U.S.P. (MYLERAN)

Pharmacology. This alkylating agent is more selective for the myeloid cells of the bone marrow than nitrogen mustard or other neoplastic drugs. It is thus especially effective for bringing about remissions in many patients with chronic granulocytic leukemia. Patients feel better and have a better appetite soon after beginning treatment. Later, there is a lessening of immature white cells in the blood and a reduction in the size of the enlarged spleen.

Overdosage may depress platelet and red blood cell formation. Thus, complete blood cell counts are made regularly, and busulfan is discontinued in the event of any sudden drop in leukocyte count. Such careful hematological control avoids pancytopenia and the danger of irreversible bone marrow depression. Although busulfan has relatively little effect on the G.I. mucosal epithelium, nausea, vomiting, and diarrhea occur in some cases.

Dosage and Administration. The usual dosage is 1 to 6 mg. orally. Treatment is usually initiated with 4 mg. daily and continued until clinical and hematological improvement are maximal. The dosage may then be reduced to a suitable maintenance level—usually 1 to 3 mg. daily.

CHLORAMBUCIL U.S.P. (LEUKERAN)

Pharmacology. This nitrogen mustard derivative acts primarily on lymphoid tissue and only to a lesser extent on other hematopoietic tissues or on the G.I. mucosal epithelium. Thus, it often brings about remissions in patients with chronic lymphocytic leukemia, Hodgkin's disease, and lymphosarcoma, while producing relatively little G.I. discomfort or toxicity stemming from bone marrow depression.

However, dosage must be carefully regulated in accordance with the results of frequent differential leukocyte counts. If the count drops to half of the pretreatment level, chlorambucil must be withdrawn to avoid the danger of irreversible bone marrow injury. The depressed white cell count then usually returns to normal rapidly. Because the myelosuppressive effects of this drug come on relatively slowly and are readily reversible, chlorambucil is considered one of the safest drugs of its class.

Among other conditions occasionally treated with chlorambucil are chronic granulocytic leukemia and advanced carcinomas of the ovaries and testes. Although the drug often produces prolonged palliation and can be given in repeated courses with relatively little danger of serious side effects, it tends, as do other antineoplastic agents, to become progressively less effective with continued use.

Dosage and Administration. The usual dosage range is 2 to 12 mg. daily. Because chlorambucil is readily absorbed upon oral administration with few G.I. side effects, it is given 1 hour before breakfast or 2 hours after the evening meal. It is administered in several successive short courses rather than as continuous maintenance therapy.

CYCLOPHOSPHAMIDE N.F. (CYTOXAN)

Pharmacology. This derivative of mechlorethamine is metabolized to the nitrogen mustard in the plasma, liver, and neoplastic tissues. Since it is inert until broken down within the body, this drug does not exert the local irritant-type toxicity of the parent compound. Thus it is administered safely by several parenteral routes besides intravenously, as well as by mouth.

Another advantage of cyclophosphamide is its relatively greater toxicity for lymphatic and neoplastic tissues compared to platelets and megakaryocytes. Thus, when administered in doses effective in Hodgkin's disease, lymphosarcoma, multiple myeloma, leukemias, and certain solid tumors, this drug rarely causes severe thrombocytopenic bleeding. G.I. upset is less common than with nitrogen mustard, but nausea and vomiting occur often enough to warrant pretreatment with antiemetics and sedatives.

The most common adverse effect of cyclophosphamide is the loss of hair that frequently occurs. Warn patients of the possibility of alopecia and assure them that their hair will grow back after the course of drug therapy is discontinued. White blood cell and thrombocyte counts are made often early in treatment and periodically during maintenance therapy with the safe dose arrived at with the aid of such blood tests.

Dosage and Administration. Cyclophosphamide can be given orally, preferably on an empty stomach but with meals in the event of local G.I. distress. The loading dose of about 40 mg./Kg. is given in divided doses of 10 to 20 mg./Kg. each day for 2 to 4 days to reduce G.I. upset. A single intravenous total dose is sometimes administered instead. In either case, treatment is continued only after the leukocyte count has recovered and an individualized maintenance dose has been determined.

MECHLORETHAMINE HYDROCHLORIDE U.S.P. (MUSTARGEN)

Pharmacology. This first of the nitrogen mustards is considered the most effective of the alkylating agents for bringing about rapid and prolonged remissions in advanced stages of Hodgkin's disease; months of symptomatic relief are often gained from a single course of treatment. The drug produces desirable but less readily predictable palliative effects in other lymphomas, such as lymphocytic lymphosarcoma, and in some solid tumors, including carcinomas of the breast, bronchi, testes, and ovaries. However, certain of its less reactive derivatives are preferred for treating lymphocytic leukemias and most other neoplasms.

Mechlorethamine has certain drawbacks in addition to the danger of producing bone marrow depression that limits the utility of all antineoplastic agents. For example, it can cause local tissue damage and must be administered with special care to avoid leakage which can lead to severe pain and even to sloughing of the involved tissues. Anorexia, nausea, and vomiting occur commonly, but may be minimized by the adjunctive use of a phenothiazine-type antiemetic combined with short-acting barbiturates.

Dosage and Administration. Mechlorethamine is administered by vein in doses of 200 to 600 mcg./Kg. body weight per course of treatment, which may be spread over several days or given all at once. The solution is prepared freshly just prior to injection. Care is required to avoid contaminating one's eyes when handling the concentrated solution which can have severe local vesicant effects. The injection is made directly into the tubing of a fast-flowing intravenous infusion, in order to dilute the vesicant and thus avoid damage to the lining of the vein which can result in thrombophlebitis.

MERCAPTOPURINE U.S.P. (PURINETHOL)

Pharmacology. This analogue of certain purine metabolites is believed to interfere with the biosynthesis of nucleic acid through its action as a metabolic antagonist. It most readily damages rapidly growing cells such as those of bone marrow neoplasms. Thus mercaptopurine often brings about bone marrow remissions in acute leukemia of children and occasionally of adults. Chronic myelocytic leukemia is sometimes responsive, but the drug is ineffective in chronic lymphocytic leukemia, Hodgkin's disease, and other lymphomas or solid tumors.

Patients are carefully managed on an individual basis to obtain optimum therapeutic response with minimal bone marrow depression. Complete blood counts are made at frequent intervals so that mercaptopurine can be discontinued temporarily if leukopenia or thrombocytopenia appear suddenly as a result of excessive suppression of normal bone marrow elements. These effects and G.I. complications are less likely to occur with this drug than with antifolic agents such as methotrexate. However, nausea, vomiting, diarrhea, and ulcerative stomatitis develop occasionally in adults and less often in children. Skin rash and jaundice are sometimes seen but often disappear if the drug is withheld for a while. Hyperuricemia, which sometimes results from purines released from the destroyed cells, may be controlled by the use of allopurinol.

Dosage and Administration. The usual oral dose is 2.5 mg./Kg. body weight daily. If remission occurs within a few weeks,

dosage is adjusted downward during maintenance of improvement. If no significant change occurs in about 1 month after initiating treatment, dosage may be raised to 5 mg./Kg. daily.

METHOTREXATE U.S.P.(AMETHOPTERIN)

Pharmacology. This antimetabolite disrupts the reproductive processes of neoplastic cells by preventing synthesis of nucleic acid. It does so because it is chemically analagous to folic acid, an essential growth factor with which its molecule competes for a place in an enzyme system. When deprived of the coenzyme that would ordinarily be formed by the folic acid-enzyme reaction, the rapidly growing cells fail to reproduce. This often leads to remission of various neoplastic diseases.

Among the conditions that respond to methotrexate treatment are: acute leukemias, uterine choriocarcinoma and hydatidiform mole, lymphosarcoma, mycosis fungoides, and tumors of the breast, head, neck, and pelvis. It has been employed to control acute psoriasis, a *non*-neoplastic skin disorder.

Patients are observed closely for signs of hematopoietic system and G.I. system toxicity. These include stomatitis, gingivitis, and gastroenteritis with nausea, vomiting, and bloody diarrhea. Itching skin eruptions, alopecia, chills, and fever also occur. Caution is required in patients with infections, kidney function impairment, or liver or bone marrow damage. Use of the drug is contraindicated during pregnancy, for it may damage the fetus.

Dosage and Administration. The average oral dose in children with acute leukemia is 2.5 to 5.0 mg. three to six times weekly, and 5 to 10 mg. for adults with this disease. However, dosage is adjusted according to the individual's response to therapy and his tolerance of the drug's adverse effects. Dosage for women with choriocarcinoma is 10 to 30 mg. orally or intramuscularly daily for each 5-day course given at intervals of 7 to 10 days. Methotrexate is sometimes administered intravenously, intra-arterially, and intrathecally.

SODIUM PHOSPHATE P 32 SOLUTION U.S.P.

Pharmacology. Phosphate is taken up by all body tissues but concentrates especially in cells that have a high reproductive rate, including the bone marrow, lymph nodes, and spleen. The disintegrating atomic nuclei of P 32 give off beta particles which damage the cells that they penetrate. Although the range of penetration is only 2 to 8 mm., this causes a significant drop in the number of cells being produced by the bone marrow and appearing in the peripheral blood.

Such ionizing radiations from radiophosphorus are utilized particularly in the treatment of polycythemia vera and to a lesser extent in chronic granulocytic leukemia. In these conditions the excessive numbers of cells produced by the erythroid and myeloid bone marrow elements are reduced, with clinical remissions following normalization of the blood picture.

The blood is examined between courses of radioactive phosphorus in order to avoid administering too much too frequently, for this can depress the bone marrow excessively and cause leukopenia, thrombocytopenia, and anemia.

Dosage and Administration. A dose of about 3 millicuries is given intravenously usually, or occasionally by mouth, for treating polycythemia vera. Later doses and the intervals at which they are given are determined by the results of blood tests. In chronic myelogenous leukemia, lower doses (1 or 2 millicuries) are administered more often (once weekly for several weeks), with frequent checks of peripheral blood.

THIOTEPA U.S.P. (THIO-TEPA; TESPA; TSPA)

Pharmacology. This alkylating agent produces cytotoxic effects similar to those caused by nitrogen mustard, to which it is chemically related. However, it is slower in onset of action and does not irritate local tissues. Thus, although its generalized systemic effects are no greater than those of the nitrogen mustards, thiotepa has advantages when applied locally in the vicinity of various neoplastic lesions.

For example, thiotepa controls the effusion of fluid into various body cavities containing breast cancer metastases. For this purpose, it is instilled directly into the pulmonary, pleural, or peritoneal cavities immediately after aspiration of the serous effusion. This often relieves symptoms such as cough and dyspnea caused by pressure of fluid effusions from the growth.

Thiotepa is used as an adjunct to surgery in order to reduce seeding and to support the palliative effect of the operation.

When administered in this way as an adjunct to radical mastectomy in patients whose breast cancer does not yet appear to have metastasized, thiotepa is thought to reduce the rate of recurrences of breast cancer at other sites in the body.

Dosage and Administration. Dosage is carefully individualized in accordance with the guidance offered by frequent checks of the white blood cell counts. The usual intravenous dosage range runs up to 200 mcg./week, if indicated. Thiotepa may be mixed with procaine HCl 2% and epinephrine 1:1,000 for local infiltration of tumors. It is also injected intrapleurally, intraperitoneally and elsewhere, including the sites of surgical operations.

Drug Digest Index

General Index

Page numbers in *italics* refer to tabular material.

DD, Drug Digest.

716